Improve International Manual of Feline Practice

Improve International Manual of Feline Practice

Improve
Veterinary Education

First published 2023

Published by
Improve International Ltd.
Alexandra House, Whittingham Drive
Wroughton, Swindon,
Wiltshire SN4 0QJ
United Kingdom

Tel: +44 (0) 1 793 759 159
https://improveinternational.com/uk/

Important note
Medicine is an ever-changing science, so the contents of this publication, especially recommendations concerning diagnostic and therapeutic procedures, can only give an account of the knowledge at the time of publication. While utmost care has been taken to ensure that all specifications regarding drug selection and dosage and treatment options are accurate, readers are urged to review the product information sheet and any relevant material supplied by the manufacturer, and, in case of doubt, to consult a specialist. From both an editorial and public interest perspective, the publisher welcomes notification of possible inconsistencies. The ultimate responsibility for any diagnostic or therapeutic application lies with the reader.

A Catalogue record for this book is available from the British Library.

ISBN: 9781913352165

Copywriter: Dr Pippa Elliott.
Illustrator: Elaine Leggett.
Book layout by Cheshire Typesetting Limited, Cuddington, Cheshire
Photos by the authors unless otherwise indicated.

Contents

Authors

Valentina Aybar Rodríguez

DVM, GPCert (Feline Medicine)

Originally from Chile, Valentina graduated in Veterinary Medicine from the Complutense University of Madrid in 1996. She is AVEPA accredited in Feline Medicine as well as being certified as a specialist in Feline Medicine by the European School of Veterinary Postgraduate Studies (ESVPS) with the General Practitioner Certificate in Feline Medicine GPCert (Feline Medicine). During 2017 she completed a Postgraduate Specialty in Feline Medicine at the University of Sydney.

She is a founding partner of the Hospital Felino Ventas, where she has specialized in feline medicine since the beginning of her career, with a special interest in internal medicine, infectious diseases, diagnostic imaging, and anaesthesia.

Currently, she is founding partner of the Hospital Felino Madrid, member of the Scientific Committee of AVEPA (Association of Spanish Small Animal Veterinarians), president and member of the Scientific Committee of GEMFE (Group of Feline Medicine Specialists) and member of FAB (Feline Advisory Bureau) and ISFM (International Society of Feline Medicine).

Domingo Casamián Sorrosal

DVM, Cert. SAM, DVC, Dipl. ECVIM-CA, MRCVS

Domingo is a dual diplomate in both Veterinary Cardiology and Internal Medicine of small animals and currently works as Head of the Cardiology and Cardiopulmonary Service of the referral practice Southfields Veterinary Specialists (United Kingdom) and as a lecturer and clinician in cardiology and respiratory medicine at the Referral Hospital and the Veterinary Faculty of the Catholic University of Valencia.

He graduated from the University of Zaragoza and completed an internship at Manchester's Animal Medical Centre in 2000. From 2001 to 2005 he worked at two hospitals in the United Kingdom, which he combined with long stays at the Cardiorespiratory Centre in Kenilworth. During this time, he obtained British certificates in Cardiology and Internal Medicine. In 2006 he entered the University of Bristol as a resident and completed his training as a specialist in Internal Medicine (three years) and then in Veterinary Cardiology (four years) becoming a clinician and then Head of service at the university hospital until 2016. Domingo is a diplomate and specialist of the British College of Veterinary Cardiology and the European College of Small Animal Internal Medicine. He has published numerous articles in scientific journals and is a regular reviewer in journals such as JVIM, JFMS and JSAP. He has been a speaker at numerous national and international congresses. His main areas of interest include arrhythmias, pacemaker therapy, and interventional cardiology.

José Joaquín Cerón Madrigal

DVM, PhD, Dipl. ECVCP

José Cerón is the head of the Clinical Pathology laboratory of the Faculty of Veterinary Medicine of Murcia, a laboratory accredited by the Laboratory Standardization Committee of the European College of Clinical Pathology (ECVCP) that performs and provides clinical interpretation of haematological, biochemical, and cytological analyses.

He is a ECVCP diplomate, has obtained the Heiner Sommer Prize for his scientific career and has been a speaker at various congresses organized by the ESVIM, ESCCP or ESVCP.

María Chie Niimura

DVM, DVMS, Dipl. ECVAA, GP(EqCert), MRCVS

Dr María Chie Niimura del Barrio graduated from Universidad Complutense in Madrid (Spain) in 2008 and for three years she was an equine vet in Spain. In 2012 she joined the University College Dublin (UCD) Veterinary School

(Dublin, Ireland) to complete her European Residency in Veterinary Anaesthesia and Analgesia and her Doctorate of Veterinary Medical Specialization. In 2017 she achieved the Diplomate status in Veterinary Anaesthesia and Analgesia and in 2018 the Doctor status. For almost three years she worked as an Assistant Professor in Veterinary Anaesthesia and Analgesia in UCD. In February 2019, Maria Chie joined Lumbry Park Veterinary Specialists as a veterinary specialist in Anaesthesia and Analgesia.

Francisco Clemente Vicario
DVM, MS, Dipl. ACVIM (Oncology)
Francisco graduated in Veterinary Medicine from the University of Extremadura in 1993 and he has since dedicated his career to small animal medicine, with a special interest in Oncology. From 2003 to 2012 he combined clinical work with teaching as an associate professor at the Cardenal Herrera CEU University of Valencia, where he was responsible for the Oncology service of the University Hospital.

Between 2012 and 2015 he completed a residency in Medical Oncology at the American College of Veterinary Internal Medicine, Ohio State University, where he also completed a master's degree in Comparative and Veterinary Medicine.

Since August 2015 he has been working at La Merced OncoVet, a clinic specialized in veterinary oncology in Calpe (Alicante) and collaborating with other veterinary centres.

Patricia Darder Solé
DVM, MSc, Res ECAWBM, AVEPA Behavioural Medicine Accredited
Patricia gained her Master of Science degree from the Autonomous University of Barcelona. She is Accredited in Behavioural Medicine by AVEPA, and since 2019 she has been implementing the residency program for the European College of Animal Welfare and Behavioural Medicine Diploma.

She is a member of Ethogroup-Medicina del Comportamiento, a behavioural medicine referral service based in Barcelona and has been collaborating on research as the Chair of Affinity Foundation Animals and Health since 2014. In addition, she is a member of the small animal welfare commission at the Veterinary College of Tarragona from 2004 and has been a member of Scientific Committee at GEMCA-AVEPA from 2017. She attends and actively participates in both national and international conferences and meetings (ECAWBM annual meeting, Canine Science Forum, ESVCE congress, SEVC-AVEPA, GTA-AVEPA) with oral communications and posters.

Her main research areas of interest are the analysis of owner-related factors in the expression of behaviour problems and the impact that behaviour problems have on the wellbeing of the family and the veterinary team.

Jaume Fatjó
DVM, PhD, Dipl. ECAWBM(BM)
Jaume gained his degree in Veterinary Medicine and a PhD from the Autonomous University of Barcelona. He is a Diplomate of the European College of Animal Welfare and Behavioural Medicine. Since 2010 he has been an assistant professor at the Department of Psychiatry and Forensic Medicine at the Autonomous University of Barcelona. In 2012, he became the Director of the Affinity Foundation for Animals and Health at the Department of Psychiatry and Forensic Medicine (Autonomous University of Barcelona) and PSMAR. He is the co-founder of Ethometrix Ltd. He is the director of Ethogroup, a behavioural medicine referral service based in Barcelona. Since 2023 he has been Head of Behavioural Medicine and Animal Welfare at VetPartners Spain. His research interests are focused on understanding the relationships between people and animals, the development of tools to assess canine and feline behaviour, as well as the comparative study of human psychiatric disorders and animal behavioural problems.

Nicola Grint
BVSc, PhD, CertVA, DVA, Dipl. ECVAA, MRCVS
Nicki graduated from Bristol Vet School in 2000 and stayed on to undertake an internship and then residency in veterinary anaesthesia. In 2005, she moved to Liverpool Vet School to undertake a three-year lectureship post, becoming Head of Division in 2007.

After leaving Liverpool, Nicki worked as a locum at the Animal Health Trust, the Royal Veterinary College, and Ross University School of Veterinary Medicine. She completed her PhD in Analgesia at Bristol University and holds the RCVS Certificate and Diploma in Veterinary Anaesthesia and is also a European Diplomate in Veterinary

Anaesthesia and Analgesia. She ran the anaesthesia service at Cave Veterinary Specialists for eight years and is now an independent anaesthesia consultant.

María Ángeles Jiménez Lozano
DVM, CertVA, MRCVS, Dipl. ECVAA
Angie got her degree in Veterinary Medicine from the Autonomous University of Barcelona (UAB) in 1999. Shortly after in 2000 she moved to UK to specialise and progress in her veterinary career. Between 2003 and 2007 she completed an anaesthesia internship and a residency in the Royal Veterinary College (RVC). She obtained her RCVS certificate in Veterinary Anaesthesia during her residency. Shortly after finishing her training, she started a job as clinical instructor in anaesthesia working alone students, nurses, and residents in the Queen Mother Hospital in the RVC. She obtained her European diploma in 2010 so she has been a European specialist in Veterinary Anaesthesia and Analgesia since. In 2011 she moved to the United States to work for two years as an assistant professor in Veterinary Anaesthesiology in the University of Minnesota. After that she moved back to UK to work as an anaesthetist in the Animal Health Trust (AHT) for almost a year until her current job came along. She got her current position as senior clinician in anaesthesia in North Down Specialists Referrals at the beginning of 2015 and she has been happily working there up to this date.

Alejandro Luján Feliu-Pascual
DVM, MRCVS, Dipl. ECVN
Alejandro gained his degree in Veterinary Medicine from the University of Murcia (1994). He completed a rotating internship at Davies Veterinary Specialists (2000–2001) and went on to complete a residency in Neurology and Neurosurgery approved by the European College of Veterinary Neurology (ECVN) at the Faculty of Veterinary Medicine in Glasgow (2001–2004). He then became registrar in Veterinary Neurology at the Faculty of Veterinary Medicine, University of Glasgow (2004–2005). He became a Diplomate of the European College of Veterinary Neurology (ECVN) in 2006. He has been a registered European EBVS and Royal College of Veterinary Surgeons (RCVS) London specialist in Veterinary Neurology since 2006. After this he became Senior Clinical Neurologist at the Animal Health Trust (2005–2008) and Senior Clinical Neurologist at Ars Veterinaria Barcelona (2008–2015). He is founding partner and head of the Neurology/Neurosurgery Service of the referral hospital Aúna Especialidades Veterinarias of which he is currently Clinical Co-Director. He was Chairman of the Education Committee of the ECVN from 2009–2012. He is a scientific reviewer of the journals JSAP, Veterinary Surgery, JFMS, JVIM and Veterinary Clinics for AVEPA as well as being a regular speaker at training courses throughout Spain.

Alejandro was President of the Association of Veterinary Specialists Diplomates of Spain AVEDE from 2013–2022 and Vice-president of the ECVN from 2019–2022. He was also President of the Neurology / Neurosurgery Group of AVEPA 2012–2014.

His main areas of interest include medical and surgical treatment of brain tumours, congenital vertebral and cerebral malformations, and neuromuscular diseases.

Albert Lloret Roca
DVM, MANZCVS Feline
Albert graduated in Veterinary Medicine from the Autonomous University of Barcelona (UAB) in 1990. After seven years in practice, he began working at the Internal Medicine Service of the Hospital Clínic Veterinari Foundation of the UAB as a clinician and teaching collaborator in internal medicine. He was also a visiting veterinarian at Colorado State University (Internal Medicine and Oncology Services) in 1999 and 2002.

Accredited in Feline Medicine by AVEPA and accredited in Feline Medicine by examination by the College of Scientific Veterinarians of Australia and New Zealand (MANZCVS Feline Medicine). Member of the scientific committee of GEMFE and of the veterinary subcommittee of the ISFM. Member of the European group ABCD (Advisory Board on Cat Diseases). Associate editor of the official magazine of AVEPA. Author or co-author of various international publications and speaker on feline internal medicine in numerous national and international courses and congresses.

Rosa Novellas Torroja
DVM, PhD, Dipl. ECVDI
Rosa graduated in Veterinary Medicine from the Autonomous University of Barcelona in 2003 and obtained her PhD from the same University in 2007. From 2007 to 2010 she completed a residency in diagnostic imaging at the

Royal (Dick) School of Veterinary Medicine at the University of Edinburgh and Glasgow Veterinary School. In 2010 she became a Diplomate of the European College of Veterinary Diagnostic Imaging.

From 2010 until present she has combined her work at the Diagnostic Imaging service at the Hospital Clínic Veterinari with that of Associate Lecturer at the Veterinary Faculty at the Autonomous University of Barcelona.

Dolores Pérez Alenza
DVM, PhD
Dolores graduated (1989) and gained her Doctor in Veterinary Medicine (1994) from the Complutense University of Madrid (UCM). She completed her training with stays at the University of Utrecht (Holland), California-Davis and Florida (USA).

She is Professor of the Department of Animal Medicine and Surgery of the Faculty of Veterinary Medicine of the UCM, Director of the Complutense Veterinary Clinical Hospital (HCVC) of the UCM and head of the Endocrinology and Mammary Oncology Department, within the Small Animal Service of the HCVC. She has more than 90 publications in scientific journals as well as book chapters. She is AVEPA (Association of Spanish Veterinary Specialists in Small Animals) accredited in the specialties of Internal Medicine and Oncology. She belongs to the EAEVE (European Association of Establishments for Veterinary Education) as an expert in Clinical Sciences.

Dolores María Porteiro Vázquez
DVM, Dipl. ECVIM-CA (Cardiology)
Dolores graduated in 2005 from the Faculty of Veterinary Medicine Lugo, University of Santiago de Compostela. From 2005 to 2011 she worked at different practices in Madrid, mainly in internal medicine and diagnostic imaging. From February 2012 to July 2013, she completed an internship, specialising in Cardiology with Dr Claudio Bussadori and Roberto Santilli in Milan (Italy). In August 2013 she started the European residency programme in Cardiology under the supervision of Dr Santilli (ECVIM-CA Cardiology) and has recently become a diplomate. She is head of the Cardiology Service of the Puchol Veterinary Hospital (Madrid) and collaborates with the ecgontheweb Telemedicine Service (Milan). She is the author of numerous publications in national and international journals, has presented at national and international congresses, has collaborated in the writing of several chapters on veterinary cardiology books and is editor of the book "Clinical Cardiology in Dogs and Cats". Her main areas of interest are the diagnosis and treatment of arrhythmias.

Fernando S. Reina Rodríguez
DVM, MSc, PhD, Dipl. ECVS, MRCVS
Fernando obtained his degree in Veterinary Medicine from the University of Córdoba in 2004. After working as a small animal clinician in Spain and later in the United Kingdom, he carried out a rotating internship at a private referral hospital in the south of England, followed by an internship in surgery at the University of Dublin, Ireland. After the specialty internship, he completed a residency in surgery with the European College of Veterinary Surgeons ending in August 2016. He remained as a senior clinician in this institution whilst finishing the experimental part of his doctoral thesis, which he defended the following year and obtained his PhD.

After a short period working in private referral centres in Spain, he moved to Scotland to work as an Associate lecturer at the University of Edinburgh until obtaining the title of European Specialist in Small Animal Surgery at the beginning of 2019. Subsequently, he has worked in private referral centres in Spain as a senior surgeon. Currently, he undertakes his professional work as a specialist in surgery at the veterinary referral centre Anicura Bahía de Málaga, performing traumatology, orthopedics, neurosurgery, and soft tissue surgery procedures.

He is a regular speaker at national training courses and reviewer of scientific articles for international journals.

Susana da Rocha e Silva
DVM, Cert. SAM, Dipl. ECVIM-CA, MRCVS, European Specialist in Veterinary Small Animal Medicine
Susana graduated from the University of Porto (Portugal) in 2001 and spent four years working in small animal practice. She moved to the UK in 2005, with the aim of completing her training, and obtained the European Diploma in Internal Medicine of Companion Animals. In 2007 she obtained the RCVS Small Animal Medicine Certificate (Cert. SAM) and completed a residency at the University of Bristol in 2009. In 2010 she obtained the European Diploma in Veterinary Small Animal Medicine (Dipl.ECVIM-CA).

After several years working in referral practice, she now works as a consultant in internal medicine at Idexx laboratories and at Virtual Veterinary Specialists in the United Kingdom.

Kerry Rolph

BVM&S, CertVC, PhD, FANZCVS (Feline Chapter), Dipl. ECVIM-Ca, FRCVS, RCVS Specialist in Feline Medicine, European Specialist in Small Animal Medicine

Kerry graduated from the University of Edinburgh in 1998 and worked in small animal practice for two years before returning to Edinburgh to gain her PhD. She gained both her certificate in Veterinary Cardiology and PhD in 2004. In 2010, Kerry passed her Feline Medicine Australian College of Veterinary Scientists Fellowship examinations. Gaining this diploma level qualification made her eligible to apply for Specialist status, and she was made a Specialist of the Royal College of Veterinary Surgeons in Feline Medicine in 2011. In 2014 Kerry became a European diplomate in Companion Animal Medicine and became a European Specialist in Companion Animal Medicine. She then worked at a private referral hospital in Bristol for three years. Before moving to Ross University School of Veterinary Medicine, in St Kitts, where she holds the post of Professor of Small Animal Medicine and is Director of the Centre for Integrative Mammalian Research and Chair of the Educator Development Committee. Throughout her career Kerry has been invited to lecture in over twenty different countries and has delivered over 2000 hours of CE presentations. In addition, she is an associate editor for the Journal of Small Animal Practice, and a member of the Academy of Feline Medicine. In 2020, Kerry was awarded Fellowship of the Royal College of Veterinary Surgeons for meritorious contributions to clinical practice.

Kerry Smith

Kerry Smith graduated from the Royal Veterinary College, London, in 1994. She spent the next nine years in general practice during which she obtained the RCVS Certificate in Veterinary Ophthalmology. In 2003 she commenced a Residency at the Animal Health Trust, obtaining her European Diploma in 2007. She became a member of the BVA/KC/ISDS Eye Panel in 2008. From 2006 she was a Senior Clinical Ophthalmologist at Davies Veterinary Specialists in Hertfordshire, becoming Head of Ophthalmology in 2020. She has lectured for Improve International since 2014 and was External Examiner for the BSAVA postgraduate Certificate in Veterinary Ophthalmology from 2017–2021. She was a member of the ECVO Education and Residency Committee from 2010–2021, the BVA/KC/ISDS Eye Panel Working Party from 2018–2023, and Linnaeus Subject matter Expert in Ophthalmology from 2021–2023. She is currently Clinical Director of the multidisciplinary hospital Southfields Veterinary Specialists in Essex. Her professional interests are corneal surgery, and postgraduate education in Veterinary Ophthalmology.

Fernando Tecles Vicente

DVM, PhD

Fernando obtained both his degree in Veterinary Medicine in 1997 and Doctor of Veterinary Medicine from the University of Murcia in 2001. He is a lecturer in Veterinary Clinical Pathology and Clinical Propedeutics in the Veterinary Medicine Degree at the University of Murcia, and in Clinical Pathology and Oncology which forms part of the Master of Veterinary Medicine. He is Head of the Haematology and Cytology areas of the Interdisciplinary Clinical Analysis Laboratory of the University of Murcia (INTERLAB-UMU).

JuanJo Vega Guerrero

DVM, AVEPA accredited, GPCert (SAS)

JuanJo graduated from the Complutense University of Madrid in 1994, he is accredited by AVEPA in Feline Medicine and is a certified veterinary specialist in small animal surgery GP-Cert (SAS).

He is a member of the FAB (Feline Advisory Bureau) and the ISFM (International Society of Feline Medicine), and has given lectures in multiple congresses, specialising in Feline Medicine. He has presented numerous communications in congresses such as the AVEPA Specialties Congress (GTA), the AMVAC Congress and the ISFM International Feline Medicine Congress. He has been a Founding partner of the Hospital Felino Madrid since its inception in 1996, where he has worked since.

Giordana Zanna

DVM, PhD, Dipl. ECVD

Giordana graduated from the University of Veterinary Medicine of Bari (Italy), 2000. After working in private veterinary practice, she undertook an externship program at the universities of Liverpool and Bristol until starting a residency in Veterinary Dermatology in 2005 at the Autonomous University of Barcelona, obtaining the Diploma of the European College of Veterinary Dermatology (Dipl. ECVD).

She received her doctorate from the UAB with a thesis on the pathogenesis of cutaneous mucinosis-hyaluronosis in Shar Pei dogs.

She is scientific leader and speaker of the didactic itinerary of Dermatology of the Italian School of Continuing Professional Development (SCIVAC) and President of the Italian Society of Dermatology (SIDEV).

She is head of the Dermatology Service of the Veterinary Institute of Novara (Italy), her areas of interest are genetic diseases, veterinary applications for dermoscopy and veterinary training. She is the author of scientific articles in national and international journals and co-author of several books.

Laboratory diagnostics and clinical pathology

1

Fernando Tecles and *José Joaquín Cerón*

Contents

Red blood cells: basic interpretation

Haematocrit

The **haematocrit represents the volume of red blood cells as a ratio of the total volume of a blood sample**, and is usually expressed as a **percentage**.

Haematocrit is measured manually (the micro-haematocrit technique, using a capillary tube and a centrifuge) or by **automated analyser** methods (Meyer DJ and Harvey JW, 1998). The advantage of the **manual microhaematocrit technique is it provides additional information** of clinical importance, whilst acting as quality control for the automated analysis.

Interpretation of haematocrit values should always be **done in conjunction with the total protein levels.**

Raised or elevated haematocrit

An **elevated haematocrit** value can be accompanied by (Meyer DJ and Harvey JW, 1998):

- **Normal or low total proteins** (the latter is less common) and indicates **polycythaemia** (a raised concentration of red blood cells).
- **Increased total proteins and symptoms of dehydration** would indicate a relative polycythaemia caused by dehydration, where there is no true increase in erythrocyte numbers. In this situation the increase in haematocrit value is due to **loss of the plasma component.**
- With **dehydration there is a false increase in the haematocrit value** which can mask mild anaemia.

Decreased or low haematocrit

- A **low haematocrit value always indicates anaemia.** Total proteins can provide information as to the aetiology of anaemia:
  - With the exception of haemorrhagic anaemia, **all anaemias** (including chronic anaemia) **are accompanied** by **normal or increased total proteins**, for example in cases of immune-mediated haemolytic anaemia.
  - **Anaemia due to acute haemorrhage** is associated with **decreased levels of total proteins.**

Advantages of the microhaematocrit

Once the haematocrit value and total proteins have been measured and interpreted, the micro-haematocrit can provide further information.

- The depth of the **platelet and leukocyte layer (grey layer or buffy coat)** increases with **increased leukocyte numbers.**
- **Variations in plasma colour** may be observed. **Plasma is usually clear** and does not have a defined colour in small animals. The most frequent variations in colour are:
  - **Yellow** (**icteric**) in cases of **mild haemolysis or liver problems.**
  - **Red or pink** in cases of more **severe haemolysis.**
  - **Turbid** in cases of **lipaemia.**

Reticulocyte numbers

Reticulocyte (immature red blood cells) numbers give a useful indication of the body's ability to replace lost erythrocytes, and whether or not **anaemia is regenerative.**

Reticulocyte numbers are obtained automatically via laser counters or by counting slides stained with new methylene blue (the number of reticulocytes per 100 or 1,000 erythrocytes is counted and multiplied by the total number of erythrocytes). Values greater than 50–60,000 reticulocytes/mm^3 indicate a regenerative anaemia. In the case of the cat, determining if reticulocytes are aggregate or punctate is important, which is discussed later.

Erythrocyte parameters or indices

Erythrocyte parameters are calculated using **the total erythrocyte count and haemoglobin concentration.** These values are most commonly obtained via automatic analysers. The most important indices include (Thrall MA, 2004).

Mean corpuscular (cell) volume (MCV)

The MCV represents the average volume of each erythrocyte. An increase in MCV indicates **erythrocytes of larger than normal size** such as occurs in a **regenerative response to anaemia** with the presence of a large number of **reticulocytes** (macrocytic anaemias) or in cases of agglutination.

A **decreased MCV** indicates **smaller than normal erythrocytes** and usually occurs in **iron deficiency anaemias.** They have also been described in cases of **portosystemic shunts.**

Mean cell haemoglobin concentration (MCHC) and mean cell haemoglobin (MCH)

MCHC and MCH are two parameters relating to **erythrocyte haemoglobin content.** Both parameters provide similar information, with **MCHC preferred** as it is more precise.

Decreases in MCHC or MCH occur secondary to **iron deficiency** or **the presence of reticulocytes** (the latter contain less haemoglobin than mature red blood cells).

Erythrocyte distribution range (RDW, Red Cell Distribution Width)

The RDW is a coefficient of variation of the MCV, and **provides information about the degree of anisocytosis** (variation in red blood cell size) **amongst erythrocytes.** An increase in RDW is associated with **regenerative anaemias.**

Erythrocyte indices allow classification of anaemias into (Figure 1):

- **Macrocytic and hypochromic**: correspond with regenerative anaemias.
- **Macrocytic and hyperchromic**: hyperchromia is considered an artefact caused by haemolysis or lipaemia, therefore, in the case of a macrocytic anaemia that occurs with an increase in MCHC and MCH, the hypothesis that these anaemias are of a haemolytic nature is highly likely.

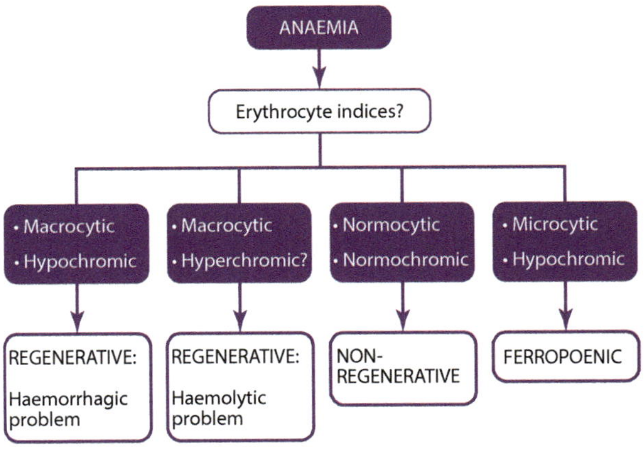

Figure 1. Flow chart for the interpretation of anaemia using erythrocyte indices.

- **Microcytic and hypochromic**: commonly found in iron deficiency anaemias.
- **Normocytic and normochromic**: typically associated with non-regenerative anaemias.

Blood smears

In addition to a differential count, blood smears serve to provide quality control for automatic blood analysis equipment. They also provide important clinical data such as:

- An appreciation of any **erythrocyte abnormalities in colour, size, distribution**, and **shape**, plus the presence of parasites or inclusion bodies.
- An estimate of the number of **morphological abnormalities in leukocytes**.
- An estimate of the number of **morphological abnormalities in platelets**.

The **basis of a blood smear is to achieve a thin film or layer of blood**, so that its different cellular components appear clearly individualized and evenly spread for better evaluation.

In a **well-executed smear, three areas can be distinguished**: the head, the body and the tail. The head is the area near the application of the blood where the drag begins, the body constitutes the greater part of the extension and the tail is very thin with frayed edges (Cerón JJ et al., 2007).

The most important aspect of a smear is to obtain a sufficiently large area of monolayer cells. This **monolayer has two characteristics:**

1. The **cells do not contact each other** and do not show deformities or ruptures due to the extension of the smear.
2. A thin area located in the final part of the body (near the tail) of the smear.

To stain the smears, coloured substances that dye each cell type on the smear differently are used. The most widely used are those from the Romanowsky group of dyes, among which are the May Grünwald-Giemsa, Leishman or Wright stains.

In general, Romanowsky type dyes stain (Cerón JJ, 2014):

- Blue: the acid groups (DNA, RNA).
- Orange: the basic groups (proteins such as erythrocyte haemoglobin or eosinophil granules).

Rapid staining using Diff-Quick is popular in practice. This system is a modification of Romanowsky staining, using three quick stages (fixative, basic dye and acid dye). The advantages include the **speed of staining**, whilst providing **acceptable staining quality**. Its disadvantages include some commercial formats that are not useful for appreciating the polychromasia of immature erythrocytes and, in turn, can **defectively stain basophil and mast cell granules** (Harvey JW, 2001). Therefore, it is sometimes preferable to use other staining systems, even if slide preparation takes longer.

Red cell peculiarities in cats

Sample processing

It is advisable to **prepare smears immediately** after drawing the sample and then keep the blood refrigerated until it is processed.

The **general blood count evaluation system** for red cells should be as follows:

1. Haematocrit value (HV), reticulocytes and total proteins.
2. Erythrocyte indices.
3. Smear.

Normal ranges

It should be noted that the **HV and associated parameters are significantly lower in the cat compared to the dog** (Table 1). This should be taken into account to avoid interpretation errors.

Young animals also have lower erythrocyte values compared to adults. Although there is no consensus between different authors establishing normal values, the idea is that between one and four-months of age cats have red cell values towards the lower end of the confidence interval (Weiss DJ and Wardrop KJ, 2010).

In the **last third of pregnancy**, cats usually have moderate normocytic and normochromic anaemia with approximately an **8% decrease in haematocrit**. Likewise, **anaesthetics that cause splenic sequestration**

Table 1. Comparison of the physiological values as used by INTERLAB-UMU, for the main parameters relating to red cells in adult dogs and cats.

	Cat	Dog
HV (%)	24–45	38–58
Erythrocyte numbers ($\times 10^6$/mm^3)	5.0–10.0	5.69–8.56
Hb (g/dl)	8.0–15.0	13.7–20.6
MCV (fl)	37.0–49.0	61.7–74.1
MCH (pg)	13.0–18.0	21.4–25.5
MCHC (g/dl)	30.0–36.0	33.2–36.8
RDW (%)	14.0–18.0	11.3–15.1

HV: haematocrit value; Hb: haemoglobin; MCV: mean cell volume; MCH: mean corpuscular haemoglobin; MCHC: mean corpuscular haemoglobin concentration; RDW: red cell distribution width.

such as ketamine, acepromazine, barbiturates or halothane, will **lower haematocrit values**.

In **healthy cats, rouleaux can sometimes be seen**, and there are usually between 0–1% of Howell-Jolly bodies and less than 5% of Heinz bodies.

Reticulocytes

In the cat there are **two types of reticulocyte** (Weiss DJ and Wardrop KJ, 2010):

- **Aggregate:** which have relatively large RNA aggregates and constitute the **first phase of reticulocyte maturation**. They transform into punctate reticulocytes in 12–24 hours.
- **Punctate**: have two to six small reticule granules. In normal cats these can form up to **10% of total erythrocytes**.

Laser analysers do not always differentiate cat reticulocyte types and therefore the use of methylene blue is recommended for this purpose (Bauer N et al., 2012). A **regenerative response is indicated by a total reticulocyte count above 50,000/mm³**. If the **aggregate form predominates, they are from a recent response**, while if punctates are the most abundant this indicates a longer lasting process.

The algorithm shown (Figure 2) is helpful for classifying anaemias according to their regenerative nature or not.

Macrocytosis

As seen previously, macrocytosis is usually associated with **circulating reticulocytes due to a regenerative response**. In addition, in cases of **immune-mediated haemolytic anaemia the presence of agglutination** may also lead to an elevation of MCV. In cats, an **increase in MCV associated with non-regenerative anaemia is highly indicative of feline leukaemia** (Thrall MA, 2004). In these cases, there are alterations in the maturation of erythropoietic precursors and there is a non-regenerative response with the presence of larger than normal erythrocytes in circulation (**megaloblastic anaemia**) (Figure 3).

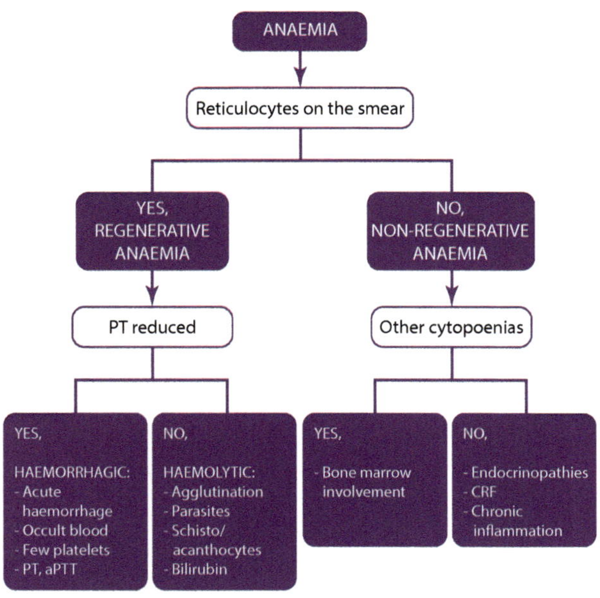

Figure 2. Flow chart for interpretation of anaemias depending on their regenerative nature.

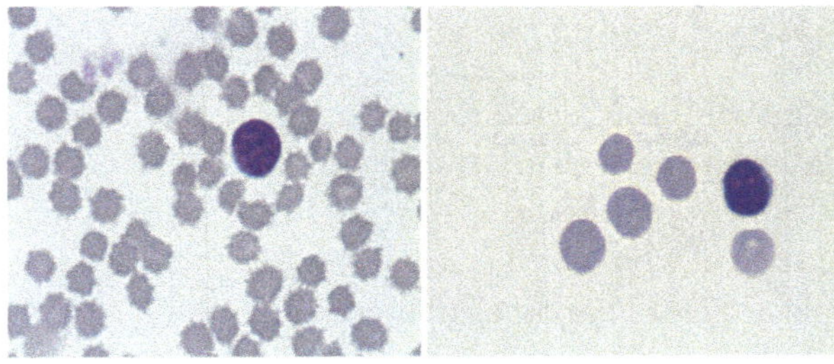

Figure 3. The image on the left is from a blood smear from a cat with normal sized erythrocytes and the one on the right is an example of a megaloblastic anaemia from a cat with feline leukaemia, where giant sized erythrocytes can be seen (macrocytosis). The lymphocyte which is present in both images acts as a reference for evaluation of their size.

Of special note regarding blood smears

When examining a cat blood smear two factors should be kept in mind:

1. Cat erythrocytes are predisposed to **Heinz bodies**. Haemoglobin in cats contains many sulphhydryl groups that are easily oxidised, which together with a non-sinusoidal spleen that is ineffective at eliminating erythrocytes with Heinz bodies, means the possibility of a greater amount of these erythrocytes (less than 5%) (Thrall MA, 2004).
2. **Cats have smaller erythrocytes** (between 5.5 and 5.8 microns compared to 7 microns) than the dog and they have **no central pallor**, so **differentiating normal erythrocytes from spherocytes is very difficult**. Therefore, **immune-mediated haemolytic anaemia is diagnosed due to the presence of agglutination and/or a positive Coombs test** (Weiss DJ et al., 2008; Tasker S et al., 2010).

In order to **detect the presence of spherocytes**, the **osmotic globular fragility test** can be useful. This is because with immune-mediated haemolytic anaemia there is a reduction in erythrocyte surface and therefore the cells are more sensitive to rupture when subjected to hypotonic solutions, leading to a positive result. However, an increase in positive test results has also been found in cases of mycoplasmas, lymphoma, leukaemia and peritonitis.

Interpretation of anaemia

An animal is considered to have a **regenerative anaemia when more than 50–60,000 reticulocytes/mm^3 are present** (unless the anaemia has a duration of less than five days in which case regeneration may not yet be detectable in the circulation).

A **regenerative anaemia** can be (Thrall MA, 2004):

- **Haemorrhagic**: Usually occurs with low total proteins.
- **Haemolytic**: Normal or high total proteins, with signs of erythrocyte rupture (haemoglobinaemia-urea or bilirubinaemia-urea).
- **Immune mediated haemolytic anaemia**: Agglutination (Note: spherocytes are difficult to see in cats).
- Anaemia due to **DIC**: presence of schistocytes.
- Anaemia due to **oxidizing agents**: presence of Heinz bodies.
- Anaemia due to **parasitic agents** (Babesia, Mycoplasma): sometimes these agents are present on the smear.

For some other cases of regenerative anaemia, such as phosphorus deficits or genetic problems, clues to these underlying causes are not identifiable on smears.

Anaemia is considered non-regenerative when the animal **has less than 50–60,000 reticulocytes/mm^3.**

This type of anaemia can be caused by:

- **Kidney disorders:** (elevated urea and creatinine).
- **Bone marrow** disorders (bicytopoenia or pancytopoenia).
- **Chronic inflammation** (signs of inflammation, such as alterations in acute phase proteins).

Common causes of anaemia in cats

Haemolytic anaemia

The following are **causes of haemolytic anaemia**:

- **Infectious agents** (*Mycoplasma, Babesia*). Anaemia caused by *M. haemofelis* has two components (Tasker S and Lappin MR, 2002):
  - The **direct action of the parasite** causing erosions and damage to the red cell membrane in the areas where it is attached.
  - An immune mediated component by **inducing antibodies against erythrocytes**.
- Alterations to vessel walls (disseminated intravascular coagulation, **DIC**) (Estrin MA et al., 2006).
- **Oxidative damage** due to exposure to toxins (onion, paracetamol) (Robertson JE et al., 1998).
- Hypophosphataemia (Brenner K et al., 2011).
- **Hereditary disorders** (pyruvate kinase deficiency).
- Immune-mediated haemolytic anaemia (**IMHA**) (Kohn B et al., 2006):
  - Idiopathic
  - Secondary to:
    - **Infectious diseases** such as leukaemia, feline infectious peritonitis or mycoplasmas due to *M. haemofelis*. This aetiological agent is one of the most frequent causes of IMHA, so some authors recommend if cytology is negative in a cat where suspicions of *M. haemofelis* infection are high (regenerative, haemolytic anaemia with agglutination) the cat should be treated regardless, due to the high incidence of false negatives on cytology (Alleman AR et al., 1999).
    - **Neoplasms**, such as lymphoma.
    - Medications.

Primary immune-mediated haemolytic anaemia (without associated cause) has been described after vaccination, but is not common. For example, it has been seen in just 19 cases in a study over almost 7 years at the University of Berlin (Kohn et al., 2006).

Non-regenerative anaemia

The most common causes of non-regenerative anaemia in the cat are:

- **Renal** problems.
- **Bone marrow abnormalities**: live agents (feline leukaemia), neoplasms or drugs.
- **Chronic inflammation** as in cases of feline infectious peritonitis.

White cells

Basic interpretation and characteristics in cats

Differential count (leukocyte formula)

The differential count or leukocyte formula **represents the percentage of the different white cell types present on a blood smear**. Table 2 shows the morphology of the types of leukocytes found on a smear.

Detection of toxic neutrophils

Toxic neutrophils appear due to deficient bone marrow maturation and the effect of toxins in the circulation, hence why they are **associated with inflammatory conditions**.

Toxic neutrophils typically present with an increase in size, basophilic cytoplasm with vacuolisations, and Döhle bodies (endoplasmic reticulum aggregates), which appear as **small basophilic granules** (Segev G et al., 2006).

Table 2. Microscopic characteristics of each type of leukocyte.

	Characteristics	Image on a smear
Band neutrophil	Narrow nucleus with a smooth outline and parallel sides in a "U" shape with dense chromatin. The cytoplasm is white or slightly blue.	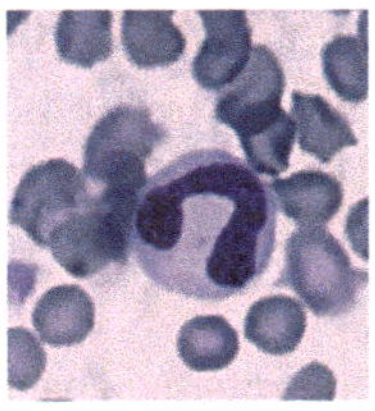
Segmented neutrophil	Nucleus separated into more lobes by constrictions. The cytoplasm is white in colour.	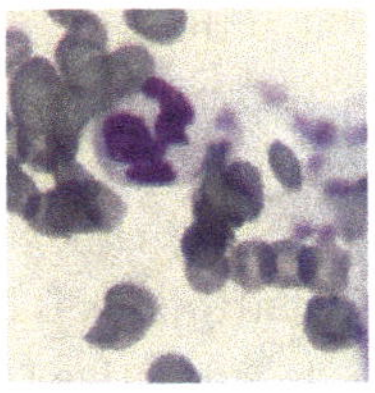
Lymphocyte	Rounded nucleus. Small amount of blue cytoplasm.	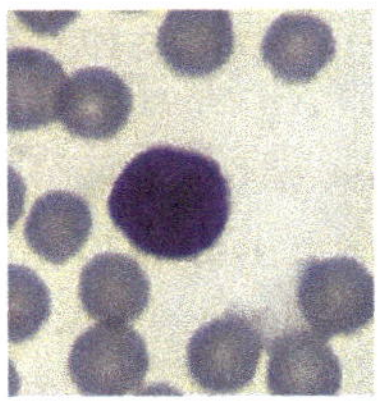
Monocyte	Large cell with bulky nucleus with irregular edges in an ameboid or kidney shape, with intensely stained reticular chromatin. The cytoplasm is blue grey and may contain vacuoles.	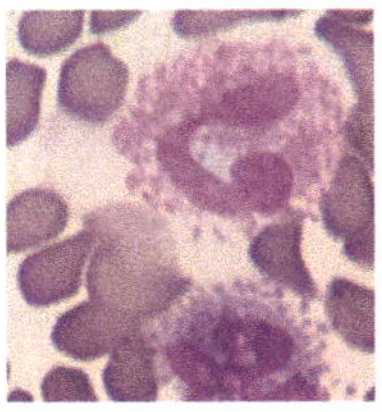
Eosinophil and basophil	The nuclei are less segmented than in the neutophil and they are characterised by their cytoplasmic granules: the granules found in eosinophils are red orange in colour and those in basophils are blue.	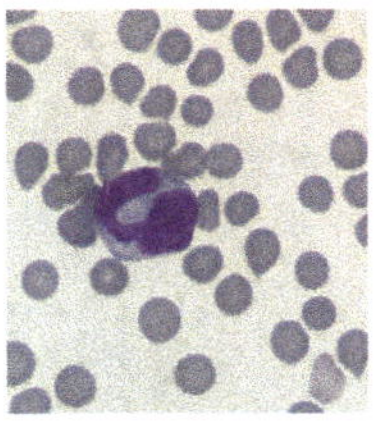

Reactive lymphocytosis

Cats have a high number of lymphocytes in the marginal zone and are **sensitive to stress lymphocytosis** (Thrall MA, 2004). Thus, the number of lymphocytes can sometimes double and even triple. It can be distinguished from lymphoid neoplasms by the animal's clinical history and because the lymphocytes are mature.

Low levels of neutrophils

Cats may have lower levels of neutrophils than dogs. Thus, **in cats the reference values for neutrophils are between 2,500–12,500/mm³**, while in the dog they are 3,000–11,500/mm³ (Thrall MA, 2004).

Some authors point out that values of even 2,000/mm³ may be normal. In these cases, assessing whether there is fever or any symptoms, as well as signs of neutrophil toxicity, a left shift or increase in acute phase proteins is recommended. If there are no abnormalities, it may be normal for the cat.

Possible **differentials for leukopoenia** in cats include **severe inflammation, bone marrow depression** (usually caused by living agents or malignancies) or a combination of both as is in feline panleukopoenia.

Eosinophils as markers of inflammation

Eosinophils are increasingly recognized as important **markers of inflammation in the cat** and some authors suggest that in the cat eosinophils "are like neutrophils in dogs".

Hypereosinophilic syndrome, which causes chronic vomiting, diarrhoea and weight loss, has also been described. These animals show marked leukocytosis and eosinophilia and the bone marrow and other organs are infiltrated by eosinophils. In many cases it is difficult to differentiate from an eosinophilic leukaemia.

In any case, the prognosis is usually poor (Weiss DJ and Wardrop KJ, 2010).

Importance of band neutrophils

Band neutrophils are **markers of acute-active inflammation** and will help establish a diagnosis of inflammation.

- An increase in band neutrophils is called a **left shift (LS)**:
  - If at the same time the number of **mature neutrophils is increased,** it is a **regenerative LS** and indicates an adequate response to inflammation.
  - If at the same time the number of **mature neutrophils is diminished** or normal, it is a **degenerative LS** and indicates an **inappropriate response to inflammation**.

How often should neutrophils be measured?

The **half-life of neutrophils in peripheral blood is 6–12 hours**. A healthy animal replaces all neutrophils once or twice a day.

Therefore, the white blood cell count can vary very rapidly during the course of an illness.

It takes **4–6 days for a neutrophil to develop in the bone marrow to be released** into peripheral blood, which is the time that should be expected for a response to treatment in animals with leukopoenia to be seen.

Platelets and coagulation

Basic interpretation and particularities in cats

Methods of evaluation

The methods used to evaluate platelets and the coagulation system are (Tvedten HW et al., 2013):

- **Automated count** or a smear with **morphological evaluation of platelets**.
- **Estimation of platelet number**. With the oil immersion lens, the average number of platelets per field should be counted (**the normal value is eight to ten platelets**) and multiplied by 15,000. If after examining at least 10 fields the number of platelets per field is seen to be **less than three, a significant decrease in platelets** should be considered. In these cases, before diagnosing the animal with thrombocytopaenia the following is recommended:
  - **Examination of the tail (end part)** of the extension to see if platelet aggregates are present.
  - Check the blood sample for clots that may have consumed platelets. This can occur despite having used anticoagulant, especially if there are difficulties with blood collection.
- **Identification of morphological abnormalities.** Platelets appear in the smear as small (diameter between 2–4 µm), un-nucleated, rounded or oval forms, and with small reddish granules which are often difficult to differentiate. The volume of platelets in the cat is 14–18 femtolitres (fl) (that of the dog is 6–9 fl).
  - An **increased number of large platelets** may indicate **an increase in bone marrow production.** Also, although more difficult to appreciate, parasites such as *Ehrlichia platis* can be observed.
- Measurement of **prothrombin time** (PT, evaluation of the **extrinsic** coagulation system) and activated **partial thromboplastin time** (APTT, evaluation of the **intrinsic** coagulation system).
- Measurement of **D-dimers** to assess the **risk of thrombosis**.
- More specialized tests include the measurement of
  - **Von Willebrand factor**, which evaluates the ability of platelets to adhere to vessels.
  - **Fibrinogen degradation products** (FDPs), which evaluate the action of plasmin on fibrinogen-fibrin complexes (if it increases, it indicates DIC or fibrinolysis).
  - **Antithrombin-III** (AT-III), which assesses the ability of blood to resist coagulation.

Problems with blood analysis machines

Cats can have low platelet counts as a result of two causes (Tvedten HW et al., 2013):

1. The platelets of the cat are very large and may even be larger than erythrocytes. Thus, there are analysers that **count platelets as erythrocytes**, especially impedance analysers.
2. It is frequent, particularly if the samples are not analysed straight away, for **platelet aggregates to form** (Figure 4) which can cause low counts.

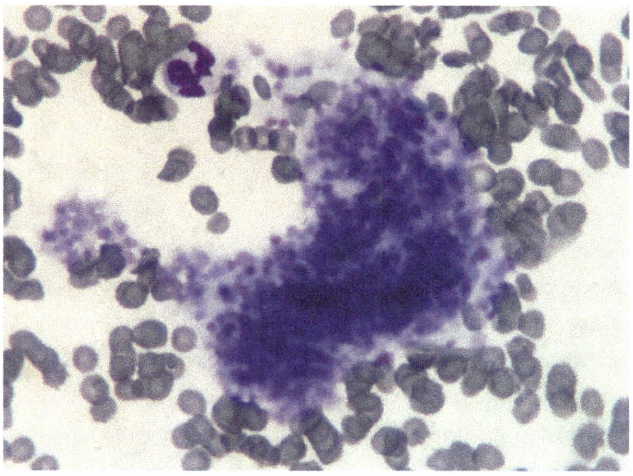

Figure 4. Platelet aggregates on a blood smear from a cat.

As a result, even laser analysers such as CELLDYN and ADVIA, can give up to a 25% error for diagnosis of cases of thrombocytopaenia, especially in samples which are more than 24 hours old. One advantage of ADVIA is that it can detect platelet aggregates and thus alert to this problem (Furlanello T et al., 2006).

In any case, the **estimation of platelets on a smear** is considered gold standard when in doubt.

Platelet abnormalities

There may be variations in the number (thrombocytopaenia or thrombocytosis) or function.

Low blood platelet count

Low platelet numbers should first be **confirmed on a smear**, especially when the same was not analysed promptly. **False thrombocytopaenia** can be caused by the presence of **platelet aggregates.** Values of less than 20,000/mm^3 usually cause obvious petechiae and ecchymosis. If these values are present and the animal shows no clinical signs, the search for platelet aggregates should be continued, especially at the edges and end of the smear.

If platelet aggregates are not found, the **cause of thrombocytopaenia** should be established, and this can be (Weiss DJ and Wardrop KJ, 2010):

- **Decrease in production** (bone marrow abnormality). This can occur for several reasons:
  - **Living agents**. In cats FeLV PCR serology is recommended, although it has also been described secondary to *Ehrlichia spp*.
  - **Neoplasms**.
  - **Immunosuppressive treatments.**
- **Increase in consumption**, as is the case in disseminated intravascular coagulation (DIC). The most common characteristics of this problem are:
  - Clinical signs of a platelet problem (petechiae/ecchymosis), along with **haemorrhage and thrombosis.**
  - Regenerative anaemia with schistocytes.
  - Abnormalities in everything related to coagulation: platelets, times, FDPs.
- **Increase in the rate of destruction** (immune mediated). The most characteristic findings when this is the cause are:
  - **Very, very low platelet numbers** (less than 10,000/mm^3).
  - Regenerative response (variability in size).
  - Responds very well to glucocorticoid treatment.

Vascular and platelet abnormalities are characterized in that the bleeding is almost never severe. In this way, affected animals show bleeding in the form of **petechiae or ecchymosis** on any external or internal body area. They can also **bleed spontaneously** through any mucosal surface (epistaxis, haemoptysis, haematuria and gastrointestinal bleeding).

Increased platelet count

The main causes are:

- Chronic inflammation leading to chronic bleeding (especially in the intestines).
- Increase in levels of glucocorticoids.
- After a splenectomy.
- Tumour problems.

Platelet function abnormalities

Suspicions of platelet function abnormalities should be suspected when petechiae, ecchymosis, epistaxis and sometimes **major bleeding are seen, but platelet numbers are within normal values** and coagulation factor tests (PT, aPTT, FDPs) also are not affected.

Given these findings, the first thing is to think about a functional defect. The main causes include:

- Acquired:
  - NSAID administration.
  - Excess oestrogen.
  - Renal or hepatic failure.
  - DIC.
  - Neoplasia with hyperglobulinaemia (multiple myeloma).
- Hereditary:
  - Von Willebrand disease (although much less common than in dogs, this disease has also been described in the feline species).

Coagulation factor abnormalities

These are characterized clinically by the presence of **prolonged haemorrhages and bruises, caused by wounds, minor trauma or even local venous punctures**. Haemorrhages can also appear in body cavities and joints.

There may be **inherited or acquired** causes (Peterson JL et al., 1995).

Hereditary-haemophilia deficits

These usually **only affect one factor** and cause lower production or absence of synthesis of active factors. Symptoms usually begin at an early age and affected animals usually have a family history of the condition. The main problems being:

- **Factor VIII**: haemophilia A.
- **Factor IX**: haemophilia B.

- **Factor X**: uncommon, it has been described in a cat with seizures and increased bleeding time.
- **Factor XI**: at least one case described, detected after an ovariohysterectomy and onychectomy.
- **Factor XII**: the most frequent in cats but does not give rise to clinical signs in vivo. It has been described in combination with Factor VIII and Factor IX deficiencies.

Acquired deficits

These should be suspected where adult animals bleed without any obvious inciting trauma. The main causes include:

- Vitamin K antagonist poisoning (**rodenticides**): cause very significant increases in PT.
- **DIC**: affects all coagulation tests.
- **Liver disease**: abnormal liver function tests. It usually causes abnormally high clotting times but no clinical symptoms.

Thrombosis

It is seen on tests as an **increase in the D-dimer** and can occur in cases of (Estrin MA et al., 2006; Rogers CL et al., 2008):

- **DIC.**
- **Nephrotic syndrome**: loss of AT-III.
- **Cardiomyopathies**. This is a common cause of **thromboembolism in cats**. Cats with heart disease can develop thromboembolic complications **secondary to blood stasis in the left atrium** and myocardial damage. The thrombus is often located at the bifurcation of the terminal aorta, resulting in clinical signs such as **hindlimb paralysis** with pain (since vasoactive substances are released) and ischaemic myopathy. Therefore, heart disease should be considered as a frequent cause of thromboembolism in this species. Ideally, D-dimers should be measured in these cases, although it seems that in studies carried out so far this test has a low sensitivity in cats.
- **Diabetes mellitus, hyperadrenocorticism:** an increase in procoagulant factors (especially VIII) and a decrease in AT-III have been seen.

Disseminated intravascular coagulation (DIC) in cats

One criterion used to identify DIC in cats is the presence of **three out of five** of these abnormalities (Estrin MA et al., 2006):

1. Increase in PT.
2. Increase in APTT.
3. High levels of FDPs.
4. Low fibrinogen.
5. Thrombocytopaenia.

In a study published where 46 cats were found to comply with these criteria (Estrin et al., 2006), it was observed that specific clinical symptomatology was very scarce, since the majority of cats presented depression, lethargy, anorexia or weakness, and haemorrhage was only seen in 7 of 46 cats (haemothorax, haemoabdomen, rectal blood, epistaxis, haematuria) and petechiae in five. Survival was limited (only three survived).

The main causes of DIC include:

- Lymphoma and other neoplasms.
- Inflammation: pancreatitis, sepsis.
- Infectious diseases.

Care should be taken because cats with liver disease (such as hepatic lipidosis or cholangitis) may show increases in PT and APTT due to **decreased synthesis of clotting factors in the liver**. In addition, fibrinogen concentrations may be low due to a decreased synthesis of this substance. Additionally, FDPs may be high due to decreased hepatic degradation. Therefore, it is difficult to differentiate between cats with liver disease and DIC (Peterson JL et al., 1995; Dirks B et al., 2012).

Biochemical idiosyncrasies of the cat

Liver

Hepatic enzymes

Hepatic enzymes act as markers of primary or reactive liver damage. Serum levels may increase due to primary liver disease or secondary to external causes that produce reactive liver disease: for example pancreatitis, hyperthyroidism, hypoxic-anaemia, or traumatic causes.

Cholestatic problems are more frequent in cats than dogs. These cause an increase in the parenchymatous enzymes alkaline phosphatase (**ALP**) and gamma glutamyl transferase (**GGT**), and increases in alanine aminotransferase (**ALT**) or aspartate aminotransferase (**AST**).

ALP is characterised by the following:

- It has a very short half-life. The **half-life of ALP and AST in the cat is seven hours**, while in the dog it is 72 hours. Thus, even small increases can be significant.
- Glucocorticoids do not cause increases in ALP, as is the case in the dog (Lowe AD et al., 2008).

Table 3. Comparison of average values of T4, ALT, AST, ALP and GGT in cats with and without hyperthyroidism (Berent et al., 2007).

	T4 (mg/dl)	ALT (IU/l)	AST (IU/l)	ALP (IU/l)	GGT (IU/l)
Hyperthyroidism	11.7	239	77	92	5.0
Control	2.15	60	31	40	5.5

- **ALP is mostly found in hepatocytes,** while **GGT** is present in greater quantities in the **bile ducts** (Center SA et al., 1993).
- Between **43–75% of hyperthyroid cats** have increased ALP (usually due to increases in the bone isoenzyme). Cats with hyperthyroidism usually have increased ALT, AST and ALP, but GGT is not usually high.

In an experimental study in 19 cats with hyperthyroidism (Berent et al., 2007), 14 had increased ALT, 14 AST and 8 ALP. At least 15 had abnormalities in one of the three enzymes. Table 3 shows the average values found in this study, compared with those in a group of normal animals.

This same study found the **raised liver enzymes were not associated with abnormalities of the liver parenchyma** or liver function, and levels returned to normal once the hyperthyroidism was controlled. Therefore elevated liver enzymes in hyperthyroid cats are not generally a great cause for concern.

Bilirubin

Anorexic cats can show an increase in bilirubin levels, as is also the case for fasting horses; however, the mechanisms differ between the two species. For the anorexic horse, free fatty acids compete with bilirubin for hepatic metabolism, while in **the cat the rise in levels occurs secondary to hepatic lipidosis** (Meyer DJ and Harvey JW, 1998) (Figure 5).

The **plasma becomes icteric when bilirubin concentrations are greater than 1.5–2 mg/dl.** Mucous membranes are icteric when bilirubin exceeds a concentration of 3–4 mg/dl and, normally **icteric mucous membranes indicate a primary liver problem** (Cerón JJ, 2014).

The most common causes of **primary liver damage** with marked increases in bilirubin are:

- **Hepatic lipidosis.**
- **Cholangiohepatitis** – often associated with pancreatitis and inflammatory bowel disease.
- **Neoplasia**: lymphoma.

Unlike the dog, the cat does not normally have traces of bilirubin in urine, so the presence of **bilirubin in cat urine is significant.**

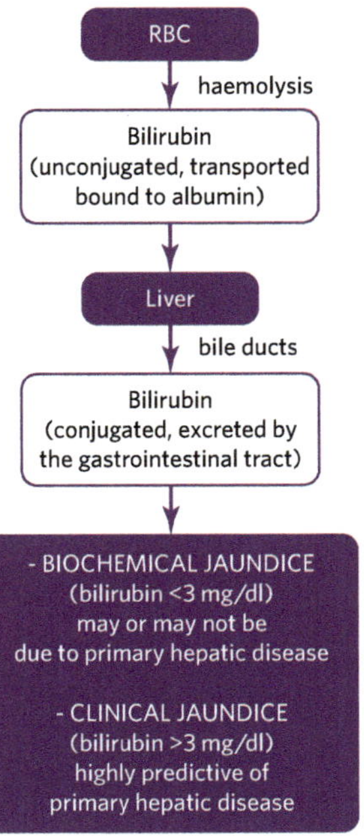

Figure 5. Diagram showing bilirubin metabolism with a description of biochemical and clinical jaundice.

Bile acids

Bile acids are a sensitive marker for assessing liver functionality, although they can also be raised in cases of portocaval shunts and cholestasis. It has been shown that the **sensitivity for diagnosis of liver disease increases from 73% to 100% when it is measured after food intake** (Center SA et al., 1995).

Kidney

Renal parameters (urea, creatinine and urinalysis) are interpreted similarly to the dog. It should be noted that **not all increases in urea and creatinine are caused by primary kidney problems** and **feline urine density values are usually around five units higher than the dog.**

For a cat to be considered as having **renal failure the following findings must be present**:

- **Azotaemia** (increased urea and/or creatinine in plasma), indicates a failure in ability to eliminate metabolic waste from plasma.
- **Isosthenuric urine (1.008–1.020)** indicates a failure of the ability to concentrate urine.

Blood glucose levels

Increases in blood glucose can be associated with diabetes mellitus or stress. These conditions can be **differentiated by measuring serum fructosamine levels**, which is an estimate of the average blood glucose during the previous 2–3 weeks (Link KR and Rand JS, 2008).

In cases of poorly regulated diabetes mellitus, where glucose does not drop despite administering insulin, **measuring IGF-1 levels can help detect acromegaly** as a cause of insulin resistance (Berg RI et al., 2007; Niessen SJ et al., 2007).

Pancreas

There is conflicting data on the trends in amylase and lipase levels in cats suffering from pancreatitis. In cats with spontaneous pancreatitis, amylase may be normal or moderately elevated (three times normal concentrations) and lipase may be normal or elevated (five times). However, in experimental pancreatitis in six cat's **serum amylase did not increase,** although **lipase was raised up to six times from day one** and after one week this increase in lipase was reduced by up to half.

The **feline pancreatic lipase immunoreactivity (fPLI) test** is currently available. This test has a **sensitivity of 100% for detection of acute pancreatitis,** while for **chronic patients the sensitivity is 37–54%.** On the other hand, its specificity is 63–67% since other pathologies (e.g. IBD or diabetes mellitus) can lead to increases in fPLI (Forman MA et al., 2004; Oppliger S et al., 2013). Spectrophotometric tests that have been traditionally used for lipase measurements provide similar sensitivity and specificity than fPLI for the diagnosis of pancreatitis.

It should be noted that the main problem pancreatitis presents in cats is that clinical signs are vague and **nonspecific.** In the acute form the following are seen (Forman MA et al., 2004):

- Lethargy, anorexia, dehydration and hypothermia.
- Only a third of cases suffer from vomiting and abdominal pain.
- Other less common clinical signs are ataxia, dyspnoea, diarrhoea and constipation, fever or jaundice.

It is important to highlight that **pancreatitis in the cat often occurs concurrently** with other conditions such as inflammatory bowel disease, cholangiohepatitis, hepatic lipidosis, interstitial nephritis and diabetes mellitus (Cerón JJ, 2014).

Acute phase proteins

In the cat the principal major **acute phase protein is serum amyloid A** (increases up to 100 times in the presence of an inflammatory condition), while **fibrinogen and haptoglobin are moderate acute phase proteins** (they increase between 2–10 times in the face of inflammation). Recent work indicates the usefulness of **serum amyloid A for the diagnosis and monitoring of feline pancreatitis** (Tamamoto T et al., 2009 and 2013).

Electrolytes

The main causes of the **decrease in the Na/K ratio** in cats are (Bell R et al., 2005):

- **Gastrointestinal disease** (diarrhoea and vomiting) with loss of Na, on the one hand, and also bicarbonate, which causes acidosis and increased K, on the other.
- **Renal disorders**: urethral obstruction and renal failure, which lower tubular flow.
- **Endocrine problems**: diabetes mellitus (Na is lost with glucose via the kidney).
- **Heart problems linked to effusions.**

In cats, **refeeding syndrome,** (which occurs when food is introduced very quickly in animals with hepatic lipidosis) should be monitored. Hypophosphataemia may occur, resulting in haemolytic anaemia (Brenner K et al., 2011).

Folate and cobalamin

The detection of an **increase in folate accompanied by a decrease in vitamin B12** (Figure 6) indicates **intestinal bacterial overgrowth,** but has **low sensitivity and specificity** (Meyer DJ and Harvey JW, 1998; Cerón JJ, 2014):

- If folate concentrations fall, abnormalities in the proximal small intestine can occur.
- If the concentration of vitamin B12 decreases, distal small intestine abnormalities or the absence of pancreatic factors can occur (Simpson KW et al., 2001; Maunder CL et al., 2012).

Infectious diseases and clinical pathology

Feline leukaemia (FeLV) and feline immunodeficiency virus (FIV)

There are some haematological and biochemical differences between leukaemia resulting from FeLV or FIV.

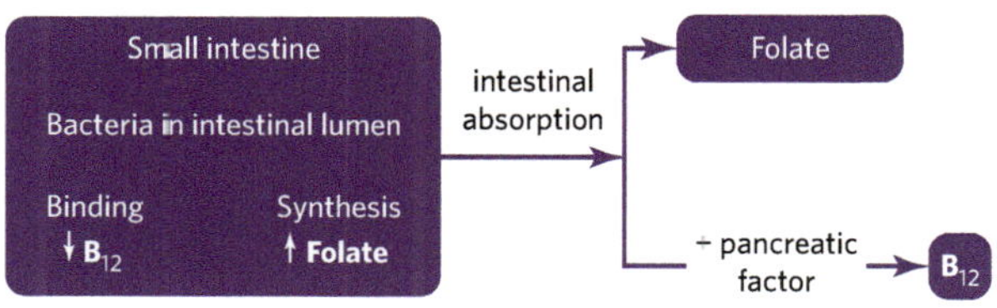

Figure 6. Diagram explaining folate and vitamin B_{12} metabolism in the intestine.

Feline leukaemia

In cats suffering from FeLV related disease, a **non-regenerative anaemia with macrocytosis** usually occurs. The causes of this anaemia are (Thrall MA, 2004):

- The virus inhibits maturation and division of progenitor cells. However, maturation of megaloblastic cells to macrocytes does occur.
- Anaemia as a result of chronic disease related to concurrent infection or neoplasia.

In rare cases **regenerative anaemia** occurs due to **haemolysis or blood loss secondary** to mycoplasma or immune mediated disease.

Neoplasms (lymphomas, lymphocytic leukaemia) occur with high frequency in white cells. In any cat, with leukaemia or lymphoma, an **assessment of feline leukaemia status** should be made. With FeLV related disease there is usually no increase in gamma globulins or total proteins, although if there is secondary infection, the T-helper lymphocyte response is affected.

Feline immunodeficiency virus

Complete blood counts are not usually particularly helpful in FIV cases since:

- **Anaemia is not frequent** and if it occurs is non-regenerative.
- Animals usually have **neutropoenia in the acute phase of infection**, although in the chronic phase it is rarely present (22%) and lymphopoenia occurs more often.

Affected cats usually have **high levels of globulins** (both due to the virus itself and associated infections), and that is **good indicator to look for to diagnose the disease.**

These data were confirmed by Hofman-Lehmann et al., (1997), who indicated that the most common characteristic of **immunodeficiency is the increase in gamma globulins**, while in **feline leukaemia it is the increase in MCV**.

Mycoplasma types and anaemia

Of the three most common haemoplasms: *Mycoplasma haemofelis*, *Candidatus* M. *Haemominutum*, and *Candidatus M. turicensis*, only *M. haemofelis* is capable of causing anaemia. Likewise, anti-erythrocyte antibodies (immune mediated anaemia) are only evident in infections caused by this species. The resulting anaemia is severe and macrocytic (possibly due to being regenerative or immune mediated) (Gentilini F et al., 2009; Tasker S et al., 2009).

Feline panleukopaenia

Feline panleukopaenia virus a **highly resistant parvovirus** which can persist in the environment for several months

Clinical signs include (Truyen U et al., 2009; Kruse BD et al., 2010):

- **Leukopoenia and pancytopoenia**. The lower the white blood cell count, the worse the prognosis.
- **Haemorrhagic diarrhoea**.
- Immunosuppression.
- Intrauterine infections: **cerebellar ataxia in kittens.**
- Effusions due to vasculitis.

Ehrlichiosis

Cats infected with *Ehrlichia spp*. are usually over two years of age.

Clinical signs include:

- anorexia
- fever
- lack of appetite
- lethargy
- weight loss
- hyperaesthesia/joint pain
- pale mucous membranes
- splenomegaly
- lymphadenopathy.

On tests, cases demonstrate **non-regenerative anaemia, leukopoenia** (with lymphocytosis) or **leukocytosis, and intermittent thrombocytopaenia**.

A definitive diagnosis should be based on compatible clinical signs, serology (although positive serologies to *E. canis* and *N. risticii* can be seen in healthy cats), PCR and response to the administration of doxycycline (Ayllón T et al., 2012).

Cytology

Advantages and limitations of cytology

As a diagnostic technique cytology has many advantages, including:

- Rapid results.
- **Inexpensive** (only requires a needle, slides and microscope).
- **Minimally invasive** (no need for anaesthesia on most occasions).

- Safe (the only problems described were in cases of astrocytoma in the thoracic cavity).
- In certain cases facilitates a specific diagnosis.

Cytology enables **detection and differentiation of types of inflammation**. It can also detect and **identify neoplasms,** including the **diagnosis of malignancy** and, in some cases, the type of malignancy. It also detects **metastases in the lymph nodes** and allows differentiation between different types of fluids.

But cytology also has limitations. The most commonly encountered problems include (Cerón JJ, 2014):

- Low quality samples:
  - Insufficient sample size.
  - **Cells are damaged** during aspiration, taking an imprint, or smearing.
  - Overly "thick" smear, with too many cells.
  - **Sample not representative** of the organ or tissue to be analysed.
  - Presence of contaminants, such as glove powder or ultrasound gel.
  - Poor staining technique.
- Possibility of **false negatives**. A false negative means the condition goes undetected and can occur in cases of malignancies due to:
  - A **poorly exfoliative neoplasm,** such as a sarcoma.
  - Lots of inflammation and/or necrosis masking a neoplasm.
  - Neoplasia of well-differentiated cells (e.g. small cell lymphomas).

There can also be **false positives**, where a neoplasm is diagnosed in an animal that does not have one. They occur when **multinucleate cells, fibroblasts or dysplasia associated with chronic inflammation** are present and are interpreted as signs of malignancy associated with neoplasia.

Thus, it should be noted that **chronic inflammation, can lead to cellular changes (dysplasia) which appear neoplastic,** and care should be taken in these cases. In these situations, **treatment of the inflammation followed by repeat cytological samples** is recommended.

Obtaining a cytology sample

There are four steps to obtaining a good quality, diagnostic cytology sample:

1. Sample taking.
2. Performing the smear.
3. Staining.
4. Observation under the microscope.

Sample taking

The following methods can be used to obtain a sample from a mass (Raskin RE and Meyer DJ, 2009):

- **Fine needle aspiration**. A 21–25-gauge needle without suction (a simple technique which produces less cell damage) or a needle attached to a 5 ml or smaller syringe and suction is applied (appropriate when a larger sample volume is required).
- **Mass imprinting**. This is done in many biopsy cases. Removing contaminating blood with blotting paper prior to the imprint is recommended.
- **Scraping**. The tissue or lesion is scraped with a scalpel blade, spatula, or the edge of a slide, and the material collected is spread on a slide.
- **Swab**. Used to collect samples from fistulous lesions or secretions.

In the **case of fluids, an EDTA tube** is recommended, since the high fibrinogen content of some liquids can cause them to coagulate quickly. In this tube, **haematocrit** can be measured (in cases of haemorrhagic fluids), **cell count** (to differentiate exudates from transudates) and **smears** (directly and/or after centrifuging samples).

Performing the smear

To correctly perform a smear, it is essential not to press down with the slide spreading the sample, as this will break cells. This is especially important for samples from lymph nodes and some effusions.

- A slide should be used to extend the sample as if it were a blood smear, in parallel or perpendicular. In any case, the following are very important:
  - smears should be **performed quickly**
  - smears should be **dried quickly**
  - if they cannot be stained straight away, they should **at least be fixed**.

Staining

Rapid staining systems should be used routinely. It is important to **keep the dyes clean** (Note from the author: in our laboratory they are changed every week). It is advisable to have **two sets of stains:** one for clean-haematology stains and the other for dirtier stains such as dermatology samples.

New methylene blue should be used for **reticulocyte count** and also on occasion for staining urine sediments.

To avoid problems associated with staining, the following must be taken into account:

- Use new, clean slides.
- Slides should be **stained immediately** after the sample is air dried or at least fixed with methanol for five minutes.
- Re-stain in case of poor staining.
- As already mentioned, stains should be filtered or renewed frequently.

Examination of the sample

The technique recommended by the author is:

- Put a cover slip on top (or drop of oil and cover slip).
- Observe with the **×10 and ×40 objectives**:
- Check the quality of the staining.
- Check that cells are **mono-layered**, separated and not damaged.
- **Evaluate several fields.**
- Observe with the **×100 lens** for more detail.

Where possible, take photos of the samples. It is highly recommended before sending to an outside laboratory, to check the cytology to ensure they are of good enough quality.

General rules of interpretation for cytology

The following can be used as general rules of interpretation:

1. Do not make a diagnosis from poor quality smears. Particularly when inexperienced, people have a tendency to try to make diagnoses, even if material is not good quality.
2. It is **better to have doubtful false negatives** than false positives. For example, in the case of cancer, a false positive can lead to inappropriate treatment – chemotherapy, surgery – or even euthanasia.
3. In case of doubt:
   - If it is due to the **presence of inflammation, treat with antibiotics for 7–15 days** and re-evaluate.
   - Carry out other diagnostic procedures (histology).
4. To send or save samples:
   - Clean the immersion oil with pure xylene.
   - Use a large coverslip with mounting medium.
   - Send the smear well packaged and away from the formalin container, as the vapours can damage the preparation. Even if you are going to make an imprint and then put in formalin, it is advisable to carry out each step-in different room.

Benign lesions

Inflammation

Inflammation can be of **two types, acute or chronic** (Cerón JJ, 2014).

Acute

More than **85% of nucleated cells that can be observed are granulocytes, usually neutrophils**. The remainder can be mononucleated cells such as monocytes, macrophages, lymphocytes, and plasma cells.

Several types of acute inflammation can be differentiated between:

- **Non-septic or sterile:** Well preserved neutrophils. Occurs in autoimmune conditions, viral infections, neoplasms, trauma, due to irritative agents.
- **Septic:** Neutrophils with signs of toxicity, such as karyolysis or pyknosis, predominate and/or there are bacteria. Sometimes only degenerative changes are seen in neutrophils. **Karyolysis** is defined as rupture of the nuclear membrane and loss of lobulation, while in **pyknosis** the nuclear material "retracts" giving rise to hyperchromatic masses.
- **Eosinophilic:** Eosinophils predominate. It occurs in **allergic inflammations** (e.g. feline asthma), caused by parasites and fungi, eosinophilic granuloma and in some neoplasms.

Chronic

More than **15–30% of the nucleated cells are mononuclear** (monocytes, macrophages, lymphocytes, and plasma cells). Multinucleated cells may be present on many occasions.

This type of inflammation is usually seen in:

- **Chronic injuries** in general/foreign bodies.
- **Protozoal lesions** (Leishmania, although not as common in the cat as the dog).
- **Intracellular fungal-bacterial** lesions (e.g. *Mycobacterium*).

Haematoma

Presents the following characteristics (Raskin RE and Meyer DJ, 2009):

- Contains a blood-like, dark-looking fluid that **does not clot.**
- This fluid shows cell counts and protein levels similar to those in the blood.
- When examining a smear, it should be treated like blood, except for:

- There are **no platelets**.
- Macrophages with erythrophagy and haematoidin are seen if it is of long duration.

Lipoma

Tend to have **low cellularity** and are sometimes accompanied by connective tissue cells.

They are characterized by the **presence of adipocytes**, which are very large cells with an abundant light-coloured cytoplasm and a small nucleus (oval and flat) on one edge of the cell (Cerón et al., 2014).

Neoplasms

Neoplasia nomenclature is based on whether the lesions are **benign or malignant** and is articulated using suffixes:

Epithelial tumours:

- Benign: "-oma".
- Malignant: "-carcinoma."

Mesenchymal tumours:

- Benign: "-oma".
- Malignant: "-sarcoma."

Benign neoplasia

In many cases, **cytology alone does not differentiate a malignant neoplasm from a benign one**. Benign lesions usually have **cells uniform in shape and size, with a similar nucleus/cytoplasm ratio.**

Malignant neoplasms

Cells from healthy tissue with the same function must be similar and well-ordered. In a **malignant neoplasm there is uncontrolled and anarchic growth** and differences appear between cells. Small cell lymphoma is perhaps an exception to this.

The main criteria for malignancy are (Cerón JJ, 2014):

Nuclear criteria:

- **Wide pleomorphism** (variation in shape) and **anisokaryosis** (variation in size).
- Increase of the **nucleus/cytoplasm ratio** or variable ratio.
- **Multi-nucleation**.
- Mitosis.
- Moulding: compression or deformation of the nucleus by other nuclei of the same or adjacent cells.
- More than one visible nucleolus.

Cellular criteria:

- Ample pleomorphism (variation in shape) and anisocytosis (variation in size).
- High and/or variable nucleus/cytoplasm ratio.
- **Foreign cells ("alien")** to the location where they are found.

Cytoplasmic criteria:

- **Basophilia**, vacuoles.
- Apparent phagocytosis of other cells.

Epithelial neoplasms

Characterized by (Figure 7) (Raskin RE and Meyer DJ, 2009):

- **High cellularity.**
- Joined cells (**sheets**/cell clusters).
- **Variable morphology** (polygonal, round, oval cells).

An example of this type would be **squamous cell carcinoma**, which appears mainly on the face (nasal plane, eyelids, lips) and in the ears, and is characterized by isolated or groups of cells with a keratinized cytoplasm and a large, active core.

Mesenchymal neoplasms

Characterized by (Figure 8) (Raskin RE and Meyer DJ, 2009):

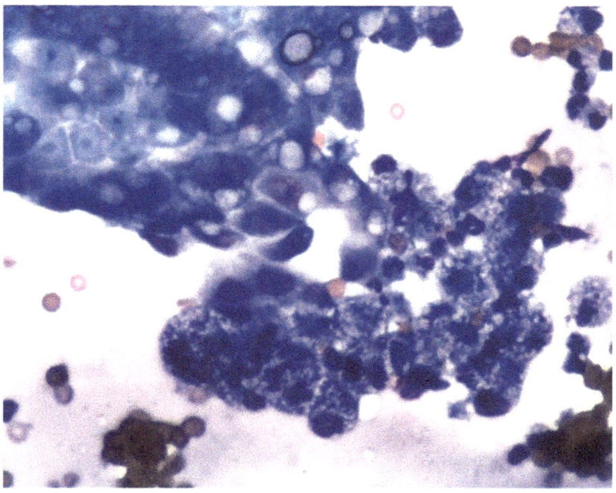

Figure 7. Representative image of an epithelial neoplasm (apocrine gland adenoma in the external auditory duct). Cells are seen to form groups, and an acinar structure can be appreciated in the centre of the image. The highly vacuolated cytoplasm indicates a glandular origin.

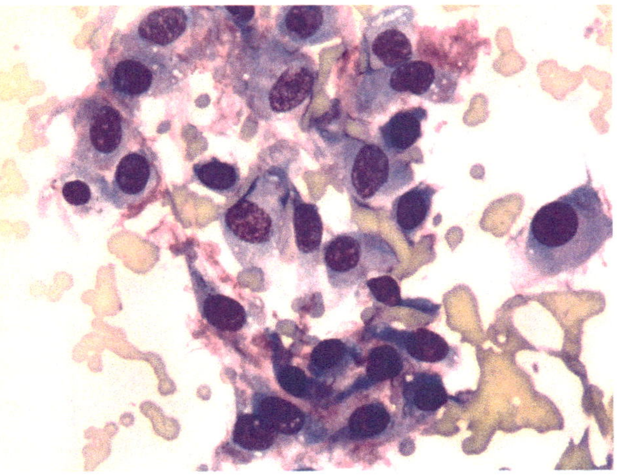

Figure 8. Representative image of a mesenchymatous neoplasia in a cat (an osteosarcoma). Cells of different sizes with a fusiform appearance can be seen in an eosinophilic matrix, with a rounded or oval eccentric nucleus and anisokaryosis.

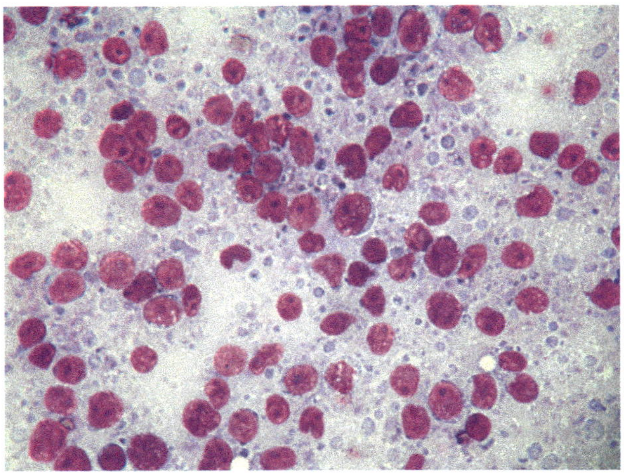

Figure 9. Representative image of a round cell neoplasia, in this case an intestinal lymphoma. Rounded, isolated cells with a high nucleus to cytoplasm ratio stand out with a large quantity of lymphoglandular bodies in the background of the preparation.

- Low cellularity.
- The cells are usually individualized.
  - **Cell morphology is abnormal**, with the presence of elongated/tailed cells.
  - Cellular edges are difficult to identify.

An important example of this type of neoplasm in cats is **fibrosarcoma.** Like all sarcomas, they are characterized by the appearance of very large cells, with a very large and active nucleus and a blue cytoplasm with poorly defined vacuoles, which may present reddish granules. They usually exfoliate a little. It is important to check that there are no neutrophils or signs of inflammation.

Round cell neoplasms

Included in this group are:

- **Lymphoma** (Figure 9). Considered when there are **more than 50% of lymphoblasts** in a tissue. Lymphoblasts are characterized as being **larger than lymphocytes and having more than one nucleolus**. Diagnosis of lymphoma is greatly helped if there are no signs of associated inflammatory activity (no neutrophils or plasma cells are observed).
- **Plasmacytomas**. Have the following main characteristics:
  - Round cells have an **eccentric nucleus** plus a perinuclear halo (sometimes bi or multinucleation can occur). Chromatin may be lumpy.
  - Basophilic and well delimited cytoplasm.
  - Anisocytosis and anisokaryosis.
- **Mastocytoma**. Population of round cells with **metachromatic granules in the cytoplasm**. In the cat, they can be cutaneous or visceral (especially affecting the spleen and gastrointestinal tract). Cutaneous ones can be divided into (Blackwood L et al., 2012):
  - **Mastocytic**. In turn, they can be low-grade (more common, with a more uniform cell population and low mitotic index) or high-grade (less frequent and with a more pleomorphic cell population, as there may be multinucleated cells).
  - **Atypical**. More common in young animals (less than 4 years of age), they affect Siamese cats and can be self-limiting.

Fluids

In fluids, the following parameters are usually evaluated (Cerón JJ et al., 2007; Cerón JJ, 2014):

- **Appearance.**
- **Protein content**, with the refractometer.
- **Cell count** (manual or automated). Care should be taken when centrifuging and concentrating cells as this may give the impression that there are higher numbers than in reality.
- **Smear.** Very important to take into account the **reactive mesothelial cells**. They appear individually or in groups in all body cavity fluids and increase in number and can be dysplastic when there is **irritation, inflammation or chronicity**.

If there is **dysplasia**, they appear:

- Very large.
- With a markedly **basophilic cytoplasm.**
- **Multinucleated or binucleated**, with lumps of chromatin and evident nucleoli.
- In some cases, with a pinkish halo around them.

On some occasion's biochemistry can be used:

- **Amylase and lipase**, when acute pancreatitis is suspected.
- **Bilirubin** if gallbladder or bile duct rupture is suspected.

For this centrifugation of the fluid before analysis is recommended, along with **comparison of values obtained from the fluid with those from serum-plasma**: increases indicate that there is release of these analytes in the abdomen.

Fluids can be **classified into five groups**, according to their characteristics:

1. Transudate.
2. Modified transudate.
3. Exudate.
4. Neoplastic effusion.
5. Other fluids.

Transudate

The main cause is **hypoproteinaemia**, and effusions usually form when a level of **1.4 g/dl of albumin is reached in serum** (although most effusions start at 1 g/dl).

It occurs in:

- **Liver disease**: due to hypo-albuminaemia plus increased portal pressure.
- **Nephrotic syndrome**.
- **Protein losing enteropathy**.
- **Heart failure** with increased blood pressure, at first it is transudative but is then modified.

Transudates have the following characteristics:

- Appearance: clear, water-like (see through).
- **Total proteins: less than 2.0 g/dl.**
- Nucleated cells: less than 1000/mm^3.
- Smear: few cells in general. Few erythrocytes. Few white cells (neutrophils up to 60%).

Modified transudate

The main cause is **increased hydrostatic venous pressure** (heart failure, hepatic fibrosis). It can also be associated with **neoplasms.**

There are two theories which explain how it is produced:

- The increase in hydrostatic pressure causes mild inflammation/activation of mesothelial cells and extravasation.
- Some authors claim that it is a long-lasting transudate.

It presents the following features:

- Appearance: clear/cloudy/sero-sanguinous.
- **Total proteins: between 2 and 3.5 g/dl.**
- Nucleated cells: between 1000 and 5000/mm^3.
- Smear: moderate numbers of cells.

Exudate

The main cause is **inflammation**, although it can also be associated with **neoplasms**.

It presents the following features:

- Appearance: cloudy/sanguinolent/purulent.
- **Total proteins: greater than 3.5 g/dl.**
- Nucleated cells: more than 5000/mm^3.

Smear:

- High numbers of erythrocytes.
- The majority of nucleated cells are **neutrophils.**
- There may be **karyolysis and bacteria.**

Neoplastic effusion

Cells with malignant characteristics may be present.

Other fluids

Haemorrhage

The appearance of a haemorrhage is **blood that does not clot**. Total proteins and the proportion of nucleated cells are similar to those in blood.

Smear:

- Erythrocytes.
- There are **no platelets**.

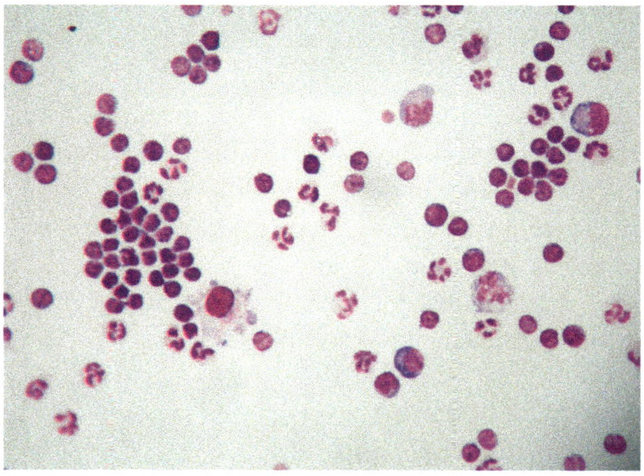

Figure 10. Image showing a chylous effusion, where mature lymphocytes predominate in addition to the presence of neutrophils which indicate an inflammatory component.

- Erythrophagia and possibly haemosiderin and haematoidin crystals.

Chyle

It occurs due to **trauma (rupture) of the thoracic duct.** It can also occur due to an increase in hydrostatic pressure in the lymphatic system, causing chyle output (lymph and lipids), as occurs in **cardiac failure and neoplasia**.

It presents with the following characteristics (Figure 10):

- **Appearance: milky, white or pink.**
- Total proteins-nucleated cells: varies greatly, from 1–3 g/dl and from 5–20×10^3/mm^3 respectively.
- Mature lymphocytes on the smear.

Bibliography

Alleman AR et al. *Western immunoblot analysis of the antigens of Haemobartonella felis with sera from experimentally infected cats.* J Clin Microbiol. 1999, 37:1474–9.

Ayllón T et al. *Vector-borne diseases in client-owned and stray cats from Madrid, Spain.* Vector Borne Zoonotic Dis. 2012, 12:143–50.

Bauer N et al. *Evaluation of the automated hematology analyzer Sysmex XT-2000iV ™ compared to the ADVIA ® 2120 for its use in dogs, cats, and horses.* Part II: Accuracy of leukocyte differential and reticulocyte count, impact of anticoagulant and sample aging. J Vet Diagn Invest. 2012, 24:74–89.

Bell RI et al. Decreased sodium:potasium ratios in cats: 49 cases. Vet Clin Pathol 2005, 34:110–114.

Berent AC et al. *Liver function in cats with hyperthyroidism before and after 131I therapy.* J Vet Intern Med 2007, 21:1217–23.

Berg RI et al. *Serum insulin-like growth factor-I concentration in cats with diabetes mellitus and acromegaly.* J Vet Intern Med. 2007, 21:892–8.

Blackwood L et al. European consensus document on mast cell tumours in dogs and cats. Vet Comp Oncol 2012, 10:e1-e29.

Brenner K et al. Refeeding syndrome in a cat with hepatic lipidosis. J Feline Med Surg 2011, 13:614–7.

Center SA et al. Measurement of serum bile acids concentrations for diagnosis of hepatobiliary disease in cats. J Am Vet Med Assoc 1995, 207:1048–1054.

Center SA et al. *A retrospective study of 77 cats with severe hepatic lipidosis: 1975–1990.* J Vet Intern Med 1993, 7:349–59.

Cerón JJ et al. *Veterinary clinical pathology. An integrated undergraduate course.*

Cerón JJ. *Análisis clínicos en pequeños animales.* Inter-Médica. 2014.

Dircks B et al. *Haemostatic abnormalities in cats with naturally occurring liver diseases.* Vet J. 2012, 193:103–8.

Estrin MA et al. *Disseminated intravascular coagulation in cats.* J Vet Intern Med 2006, 20:1334–9.

Forman MA et al. *Evaluation of serum feline pancreatic lipase immunoreactivity and helical computed tomography versus conventional testing for the diagnosis of feline pancreatitis.* J Vet Intern Med 2004, 18:807–15.

Furlanello T et al. *Artifactual changes in canine blood following storage, detected using the ADVIA 120 hematology analyzer.* Vet Clin Pathol 2006, 35:42–6.

Gentilini F et al. *Use of combined conventional and real-time PCR to determine the epidemiology of feline haemoplasma infections in northern Italy.* J Feline Med Surg 2009, 11:277–85.

Harvey JW. *Atlas of veterinary haematology. Blood and bone marrow of domestic animals.* WB Saunders Company. 2001.

Hoffmann-Lehmann R et al. Parameters of disease progression in long-term experimental feline retrovirus (feline immunodeficiency virus and feline leukemia virus) infections: hematology, clinical chemistry, and lymphocyte subserts. Clin Diagn Lab Immunol 1997, 4:33–42.

Kohn B et al. *Primary immune-mediated hemolytic anemia in 19 cats: diagnosis, therapy, and outcome (1998–2004).* J Vet Intern Med 2006, 20:159–66.

Kruse BD et al. *Prognostic factors in cats with feline panleukopenia.* J Vet Intern Med 2010, 24:1271–6.

Link KR, Rand JS. *Changes in blood glucose concentration are associated with relatively rapid changes in circulating fructosamine concentrations in cats.* J Feline Med Surg 2008, 10:583–92.

Lowe AD et al. *Clinical, clinicopathological and histological changes observed in 14 cats treated with glucocorticoids.* Vet Rec 2008, 162:777–83.

Maunder CL et al. *Serum cobalamin concentrations in cats with gastrointestinal signs: correlation with histopathological findings and duration of clinical signs.* J Feline Med Surg 2012, 14:686–93.

Meyer DJ, Harvey JW. *Veterinary Laboratory Medicine. Interpretation and diagnosis.* WB Saunders Company. 2nd ed. 1998.

Niessen SJ et al. *Feline acromegaly: an underdiagnosed endocrinopathy?* J Vet Intern Med 2007, 21:899–905.

Oppliger S et al. *Agreement of the Serum Spec fPL™ and 1,2-O-Dilauryl-Rac-Glycero-3-Glutaric Acid-(6'-Methylresorufin) Ester Lipase Assay for the Determination of Serum Lipase in Cats with Suspicion of Pancreatitis.* J Vet Intern Med 2013, 27:1077–82.

Peterson JL et al. *Hemostatic disorders in cats: a retrospective study and review of the literature.* J Vet Intern Med 1995, 9:298–303.

Raskin RE, Meyer DJ. *Atlas of canine and feline cytology.* WB Saunders Company. 2001.

Robertson JE et al. *Heinz body formation in cats fed baby food containing onion powder.* J Am Vet Med Assoc 1998, 212:1260–6.

Rogers CL et al. *Portal vein thrombosis in cats: 6 cases (2001–2006).* J Vet Intern Med 2008, 22:282–7.

Segev G et al. *Toxic neutrophils in cats: clinical and clinicopathologic features, and disease prevalence and outcome--a retrospective case control study.* J Vet Intern Med. 2006, 20:20–31.

Simpson KW et al. *Subnormal concentrations of serum cobalamin (vitamin B12) in cats with gastrointestinal disease.* J Vet Intern Med 2001, 15:26–32.

Tamamoto T et al. *Time-course monitoring of serum amyloid A in a cat with pancreatitis.* Vet Clin Pathol 2009, 38:83–6.

Tamamoto T et al. *Serum amyloid A as a prognostic marker in cats with various diseases.* J Vet Diagn Invest. 2013, 25:428–32.

Tasker S, Lappin MR. *Haemobartonella felis: recent developments in diagnosis and treatment.* J Feline Med Surg 2002, 4:3–11.

TASKER S et al. *Description of outcomes of experimental infection with feline haemoplasmas: copy numbers, haematology, Coombs' testing and blood glucose concentrations.* Vet Microbiol 2009, 139:323–32.

TASKER S et al. *Coombs', haemoplasma and retrovirus testing in feline anaemia.* J Small Anim Pract. 2010, 51:192–9.

THRALL MA. *Veterinary hematology and clinical chemistry.* Lippincott Williams & Wilkins. 2004.

TRUYEN U et al. *Feline panleukopenia. ABCD guidelines on prevention and management.* J Feline Med Surg 2009, 11:538–46.

TVEDTEN HW et al. *Enumeration of feline platelets in ethylenediamine tetra-acetic acid anticoagulated blood with the ADVIA 2120 system and two manual methods: Leucoplate and Thrombo-TIC.* J Vet Diagn Invest 2013, 25:493–7.

WEISS DJ. *Bone marrow pathology in dogs and cats with non-regenerative immune-mediated haemolytic anaemia and pure red cell aplasia.* J Comp Pathol 2008, 138:46–53.

WEISS DJ, WARDROP KJ. *Schalm's Veterinary Hematology.* Wiley-Blackwell. 6th ed. 2010.

Test

1. Regarding reticulocytes in cats:
A) Aggregates indicate a recent regenerative response.
B) Spikes only appear after heavy bleeding.
C) Only the spiked ones should be counted.
D) An increase in reticulocytes is compatible with FeLV.

2. An increase in MCV can be caused by:
A) FeLV, only if accompanied by regeneration of red cells.
B) FeLV, even though there is no regeneration of red cells.
C) Liver diseases.
D) Endocrinopathies.

3. In the cat, Heinz bodies are common because:
A) Haemoglobin is easily oxidised.
B) They are prone to liver failure.
C) Anaemias are usually non-regenerative.
D) They eat a lot of onion.

4. Regarding immune-mediated haemolytic anaemias:
A) They are usually idiopathic.
B) Numerous spherocytes can be seen on smears.
C) The haematocrit value is usually close to the lower limit.
D) Secondary types are more common.

5. In the case of feline leukaemia and immunodeficiency:
A) Non-regenerative anaemias are more frequent than regenerative ones.
B) In both conditions, macrocytosis can be seen.
C) In both cases leukocytosis can be seen.
D) There is an increase in punctate reticulocytes.

6. Regarding mycoplasmosis:
A) Observation on a blood smear is the gold standard for diagnosis.
B) *M. haemofelis, Candidatus M. haemominutum* and *Candidatus M. turicensis* are equally pathogenic.
C) They are usually associated with feline leukaemia and immunodeficiency.
D) They cause non-regenerative anaemia by supressing the bone marrow.

7. A cat with a neutrophil count of 2,000/mm^3:
A) This could indicate possible bone marrow disease.
B) It would be useful to perform a differential count to evaluate the presence of toxic neutrophils.
C) It may be compatible with feline leukaemia.
D) This indicates that antibiotic treatment should be implemented.

8. A cat with pneumonia has 24,000 leukocytes/mm^3 (reference 6,000–17,000), of which 22,000 are segmented (reference 3,000–11,500) and 1,500 are banded (reference 300). Here are two possibilities of how this may progress in this animal over a period of 3 days: A) 22,000 total leukocytes, 20,000 segmented, 500 banded B) 5,000 total leukocytes, 2,200 segmented, 2,800 banded.

A) A is a degenerative left shift.
B) B is a regenerative left shift.
C) The prognosis for B is worse than that for A.
D) The prognosis for A is worse than that for B.

9. Regarding disseminated intravascular coagulation (DIC) in cats:

A) Its diagnosis is simple since it causes obvious clinical signs.
B) D-dimer measurement is highly sensitive for the diagnosis of DIC.
C) It should be suspected if the platelet count is low.
D) It is not often diagnosed since haemorrhages are uncommon.

10. In cats the enzyme alkaline phosphatase (ALP):

A) Is more likely to be elevated in cholangiohepatitis than in hepatic lipidosis.
B) If it is found to be high, one of the possible differentials would be hyperthyroidism.
C) If it is found to be high, it could indicate a cortisol excess.
D) It has a longer half-life than in the dog.

11. Regarding bilirubin levels in the cat:

A) Clinical jaundice, where the mucous membranes are yellowish, is highly suggestive of primary liver disease.
B) Any increase in bilirubin, even if it is subclinical (yellowish but not mucous serum), is highly suggestive of primary liver disease.
C) Cholangiohepatitis rarely causes clinical jaundice.
D) There are normally traces of bilirubin in urine.

12. Regarding pancreatitis in cats:

A) The feline pancreatic lipase immunoreactivity (fPLI) test has a high sensitivity for both acute and chronic pancreatitis.
B) The fPLI test has a specificity close to 100% for the diagnosis of pancreatitis.
C) The most suitable tool for diagnosis is measurement of amylase and lipase enzymes in serum.
D) The fPLI test presents greater sensitivity for the diagnosis of acute pancreatitis than for chronic pancreatitis.

13. Regarding feline infectious diseases:

A) An increase in globulins may be the only abnormal parameter in cases of feline immunodeficiency.
B) In feline leukaemia there are usually increases in total proteins and globulins.
C) In feline leukaemia, the most characteristic feature of the blood count is microcytic anaemia, because the bone marrow is affected.
D) Ehrlichiosis has not been described in cats.

14. When eosinophilic inflammation is identified on cytology:

A) It does not indicate anything in particular, since eosinophils usually increase in any type of inflammation.
B) Allergic inflammation, such as asthma or eosinophilic granuloma, should be considered among the differential diagnoses.
C) There must have been contamination of the sample with blood, so sampling should be repeated.
D) The sample should be checked for the presence of bacteria.

15. Regarding fluid analysis:

A) The main cause of a pure transudate would be a possible neoplasm in a body cavity.
B) The presence of different sized mesothelial cells undergoing mitosis are always indicative of the existence of a mesothelioma.
C) A chylous effusion is characterized by the presence of large numbers of mature lymphocytes.
D) In a haemorrhagic effusion a large number of platelets will be seen.

Clinical case

Signalment: 13 year 10-month-old, female, Common European cat, weighing 5 kg with a body condition score of 3 (scale 1–5).

Reason for consultation: weight loss of unknown origin.

Physical examination: no relevant abnormalities.

Complete blood count and biochemistry: the sample is taken and sent to the laboratory and arrives the next day. The results submitted by the laboratory are shown in the attached table.

	Parameter	Result	Reference
Red cells	Haematocrit	47%	24–45
	Erythrocytes	8.46 × $10^6/mm^3$	5.5–10.0
	MCV	55.5 fl	37–49
	Haemoglobin	14.0 g/dl	8–15
	MCHC	29.9 g/dl	30–36
	RDW	15.9%	14–18
	Total protein	7.8 g/dl	5.4–7.8
White cells and platelets	Leukocytes	8.27 × $10^3/mm^3$	5.5–19.5
	Segmented	6.53 × $10^3/mm^3$	2.5–12.5
	Band	0.25 × $10^3/mm^3$	0.0–0.3
	Lymphocytes	0.58 × $10^3/mm^3$	1.4–7.0
	Monocytes	0.25 × $10^3/mm^3$	0.1–0.8
	Eosinophils	0.66 × $10^3/mm^3$	0.1–1.0
	Basophils	0.1 × $10^3/mm^3$	<0
	Platelets (platelet aggregate are seen on smears)	138 × $10^3/mm^3$	175–500
Biochemistry	ALT	55 UI/l	<50
	AST	35 UI/l	<50
	g GT	<1.0 UI/l	1.0–6.5
	ALP	66 UI/l	20–6.3
	CK	821 UI/l	50–450
	Lipase	57 UI/l	5–80
	Amylase	1277 UI/l	250–1300
	Na	149 mEq/l	140–154
	K	3.3 mEq/l	4.1–5.3
	Cl	119 mEq/l	105–116
	Ca	9.84 mg/dl	8.0–11.7
	P	3.4 mg/dl	4.0–8.0
	Albumin	3.1 g/dl	2.3–3.4
	Globulins	4.7 g/dl	2.6–3.8
	Haptoglobulin	3.23 g/l	<3.0
	Serum amyloid A	<1.0 µg/ml	<10.0
	Urea	53.3 mg/dl	20–50
	Creatinine	1.48 mg/dl	0.5–1.5
	Total bilirubin	0.1 mg/dl	<0.4
	Cholesterol	211 mg/dl	100–300
	Triglycerides	29 mg/dl	30–200
	Glucose	110 mg/dl	70–110

1. **What clinical significance does the increase in mean corpuscular volume (MCV) have?**
   A) Microcytosis.
   B) Possible artefact due to sample storage.
   C) Feline immunodeficiency.
   D) An increase in MCV can occur with inflammation.
2. **What does the low platelet count indicate?**
   A) It is due to the existence of an inflammatory condition in the intestines.
   B) It is an artefact.
   C) Platelet count decreases in geriatric animals.
   D) The cat has disseminated intravascular coagulation.
3. **What would be the most likely cause of the azotaemia?**
   A) Chronic renal failure.
   B) Increased protein catabolism.
   C) Prerenal origin because the animal would be dehydrated otherwise.
   D) Intestinal bleeding.
4. **Which of the following differential diagnoses would be the most likely?**
   A) Chronic renal insufficiency.
   B) Intestinal lymphoma.
   C) Hyperthyroidism.
   D) Hyperadrenocorticism.
5. **Total T4 values are 44.8 mg/ml (10–35) and canine TSH values are <0.03 ng/ml (0.03–0.4). What do these values mean?**
   A) They rule out hyperthyroidism.
   B) These results are compatible with a sick euthyroid syndrome due to liver disease.
   C) Hyperthyroidism is confirmed.
   D) The measurement of canine TSH is not useful in the cat.

Answers

Test

1: A	6: C	11: A
2: B	7: B	12: D
3: A	8: C	13: A
4: D	9: D	14: B
5: A	10: B	15: C

Clinical case

1: B
2: B
3: C
4: C
5: C

Diagnostic imaging techniques

2

Rosa Novellas Torroja

Contents

Thoracic radiology

Heart

The heart is located **within the mediastinum**, between approximately the **third and sixth intercostal spaces**. It is important to remember the **cardiac silhouette includes the heart, pericardium, pericardial content** (such as fat and a minimal amount of fluid), plus the origin of the **aorta and pulmonary trunk**.

The internal appearance of the cardiac chambers cannot be visualized on radiography. However, it is possible to **locate the approximate boundaries of the various chambers**, to facilitate assessment of cardiomegaly or enlargement of the great vessels.

To **locate the structures of the heart the clock-face analogy** can be used (Figure 1):

- Lateral projection:
  - 12.00–02.00: left atrium (LA). More cranial position than in dogs and more difficult to visualize.
  - 02.00–05.00: left ventricle (LV).
  - 05.00–09.00: right ventricle (RV).
  - 09.00–10.00: pulmonary trunk and right auricle (RAu).
  - 10.00–11.00: aortic arch.
- Dorsoventral projection (DV):
  - 11.00–01.00: aortic arch.
  - 01.00–02.00 left atrium and auricle. Pulmonary trunk more cranial or not visible.
  - 02.00–05.00: left ventricle (LV).
  - 05.00–09.00: right ventricle (RV).
  - 09.00–11.00: right atrium (RA).

As a guideline the following **radiographic measurements** of the heart are considered normal:

- **Width:** 2 – 2.5 intercostal spaces in the lateral projection. The maximum width in the lateral view should be approximately the same as the distance between the cranial margin of the 5th rib and the caudal margin of the 7th.

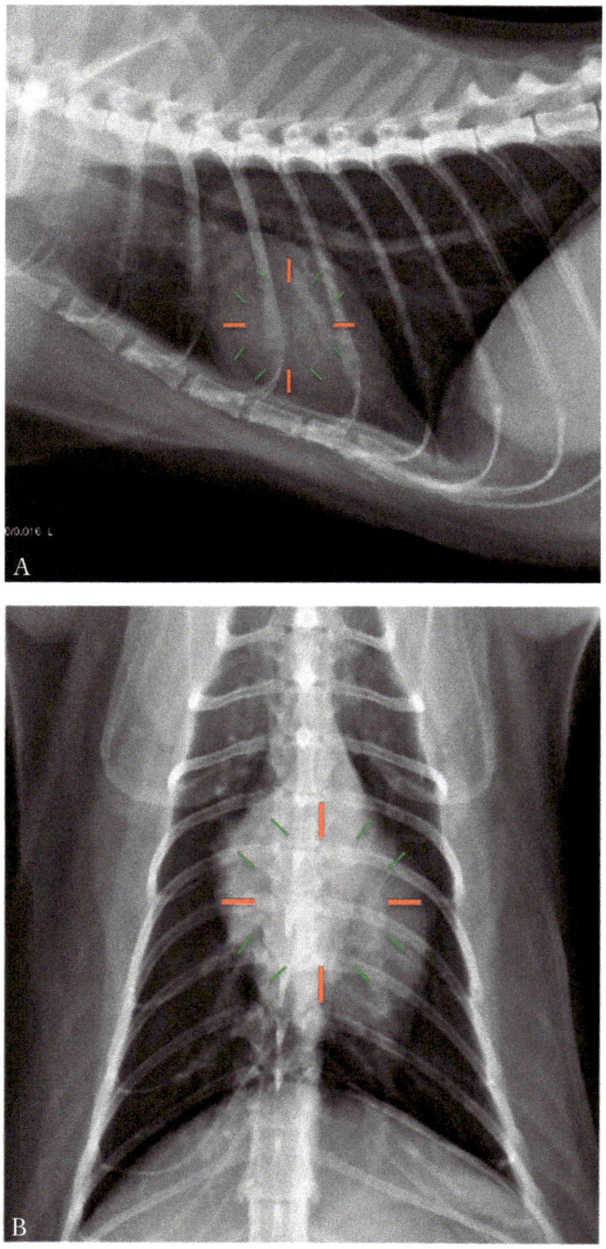

Figure 1. Position of heart structures on a radiograph of a normal heart: clock analogy.

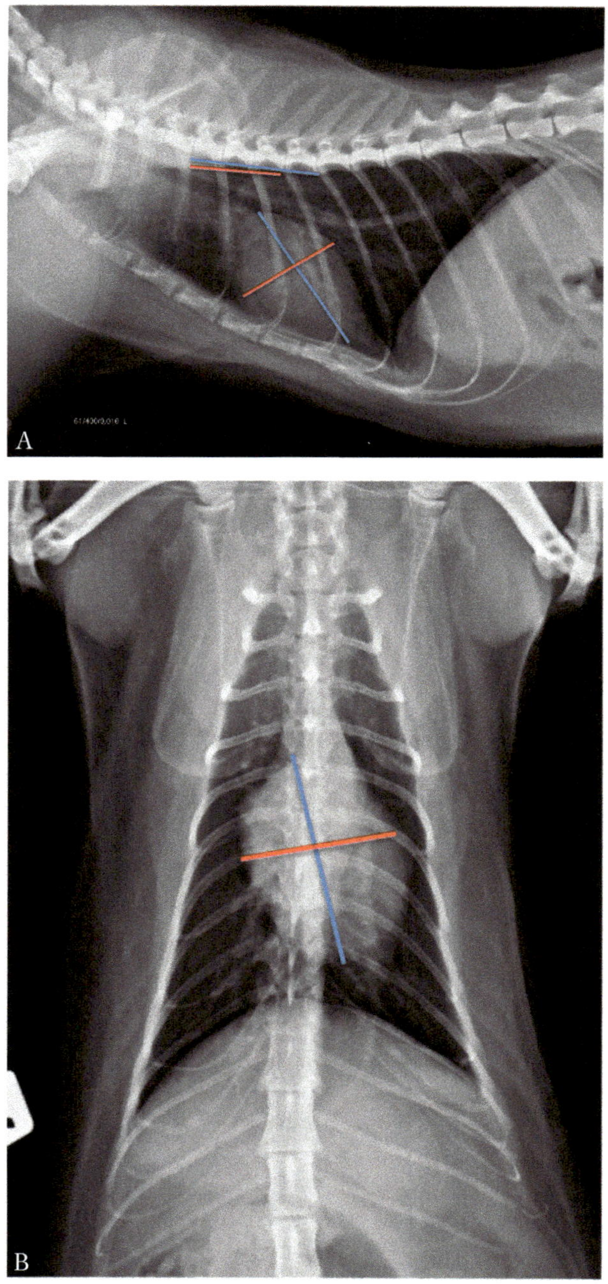

Figure 2. Calculation of the vertebral heart score on a lateral (A) and VD (B) projection.

- **Vertebral heart score (VHS)** (various cat breeds) (Figure 2):
  - 7.5 ± 0.3 vertebrae in lateral projection (normal limit 8.1).
  - 8.1 ± 0.45 vertebrae in DV projection.
  - Width in DV/VD 3.4 ± 0.25 vertebra measured perpendicular to the long axis.

A more recent study suggests slightly lower values for the vertebral heart score: 7.3 ± 0.49 on the right lateral view (RL) and 7.5 ± 0.58 on the DV view.

Factors which can affect the radiographic size of the cardiac silhouette include:

- **Pericardial fat**: it can be found in large quantities and even lead to the erroneous diagnosis of cardiomegaly, especially in DV/VD projections where it can show a **characteristic triangular shape on the right cranial margin** of the cardiac silhouette. Normally fat is less opaque but a clear difference between fat and the heart is not always evident. Occasionally, increasing the mA and reducing the KVp can improve differentiation between the heart and pericardial fat (Figure 3).
- **Age**: Kittens' hearts generally appear larger than adult cats hearts due to lower lung volume, resulting in an increased cardiothoracic ratio. **40% of cats over 10 years of age have a heart with a more cranial inclination, with greater sternal contact.** In 28% of cats over 10 years of age, a redundant or

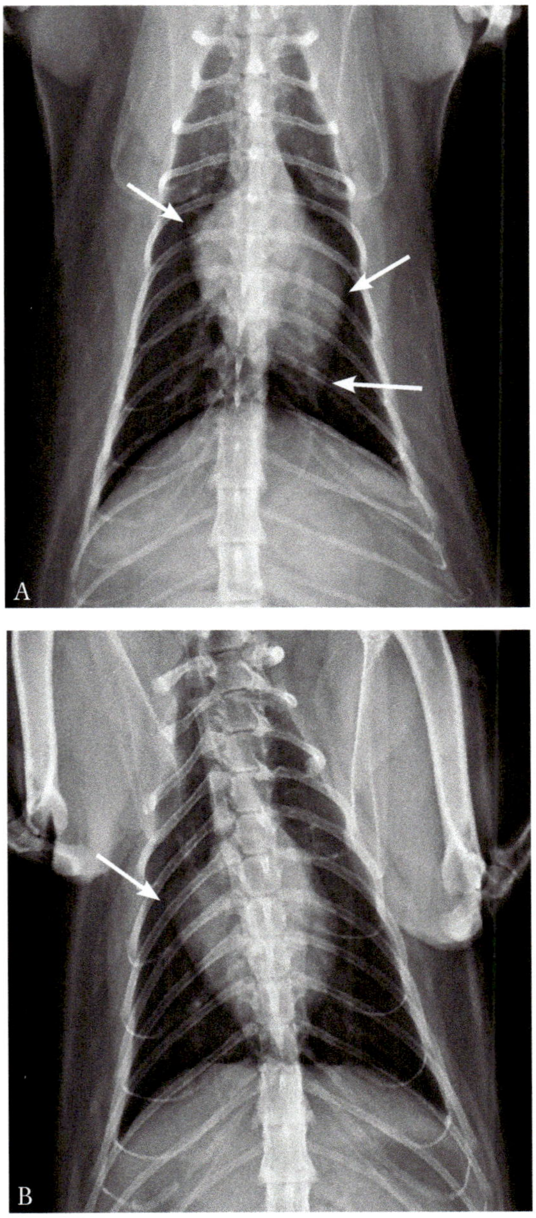

Figure 3. VD projection of two cats with pericardial fat. In the top image (A), the fat can be better differentiated because it has a reduced radiopacity in comparison with the cardiac silhoutte in addition to a more angular shape. In the bottom image (B), at the point indicated by the arrow, the border between the fat and the heart shows poorer definition, but the position and shape are typical, in addition to the presence of fat on the left side which also allows identification of this area as pericardial fat.

tortuous aorta can be observed which is not associated with pathology (Figure 4).

- **Cardiac cycle**: in diastole the heart may be slightly wider than in systole, these differences being more evident in the DV projection.
- **Sedation**: the administration of dexmedetomidine (40 µg/kg IM) has been associated with a slight increase in the radiographic size of the cardiac silhouette (mean VHS in RL projection of 7.8: 7.25–8.25).

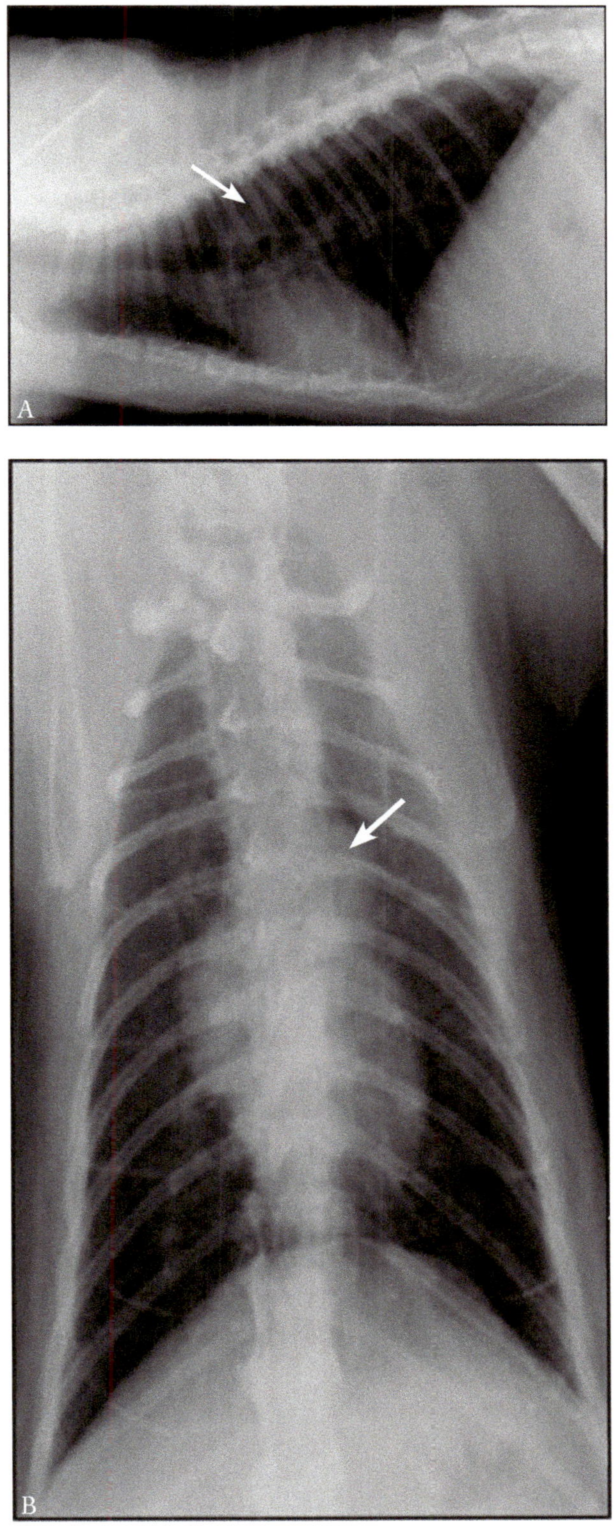

Figure 4. RL and VD projections from a geriatric cat where increased sternal contact of the cardiac silhouette and redundant aorta (arrow) can be seen.

Radiographic diagnosis of cardiac pathologies

Echocardiography is the diagnostic technique of choice for the diagnosis of cardiac pathology. Radiography is helpful for an initial assessment and to detect signs associated with heart failure, as well as ruling out other thoracic pathologies.

Right-sided cardiomegaly

Radiographic signs suggestive of right-sided cardiomegaly include (Figure 5):

- DV/VD and lateral views respectively: increased convexity or **bulging of the right and cranial aspects of the heart**
- DV/VD projection: **displacement of the apex** cranially and to the left
- Lateral view **elevation of the cardiac apex** with respect to the sternum
- Lateral view: Slight elongation of the cardiac silhouette with **elevation of the trachea**

Abnormalities causing right heart disease include:

- tricuspid regurgitation
- pulmonary stenosis
- dirofilariasis
- chronic lung disease with pulmonary hypertension
- atrial septum defect

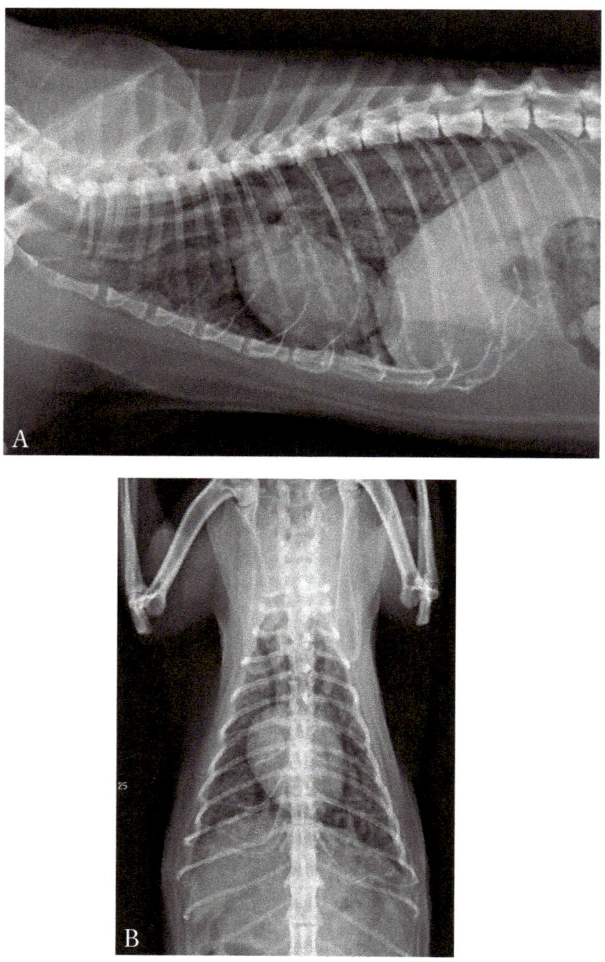

Figure 5. Left lateral (A) and VD (B) projection from a patient with right-sided cardiomegaly where bulging of the right cranial aspect of the heart can be seen in both projections, with elevation of the apex with respect to the sternum and elevation of the trachea in the lateral projection.

- arrhythmogenic cardiomyopathy of the right ventricle.

Left-sided cardiomegaly

Radiographic signs suggestive of left-sided cardiomegaly (Figure 6) include:

- Increased convexity or **bulging of the caudal** (lateral) and **left border** (DV/DV).
- **Rounding** of the cardiac apex.
- **Increased length and width** of the cardiac silhouette and elevation of the trachea in RL projections.

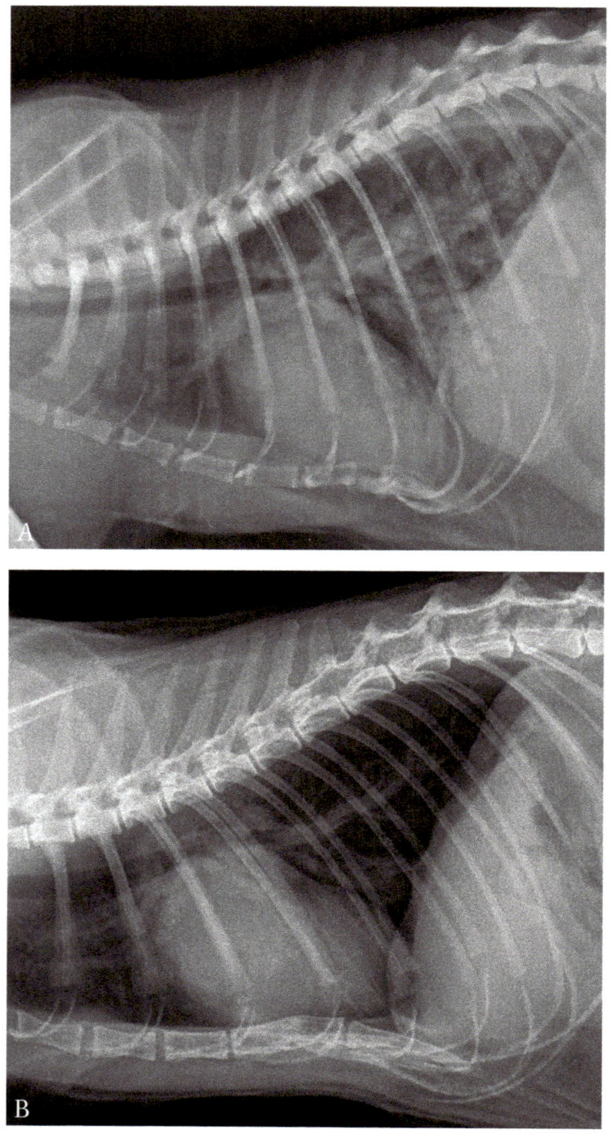

Figure 6. Lateral projections in patients with left-sided (A: HCM) and generalized (B: unclassified) cardiomegaly. Components of left-sided cardiomegaly such as bulging of the caudal border of the heart in both projections, with the presence of a notch in B, an increase in length and width of the cardiac silhouette, with tracheal elevation and slight rounding of the cardiac apex can be seen. In Image A pulmonary oedema can also be seen with an interstitial pattern with a caudo-dorsal distribution and mild pleural effusion.

- **A notch** can also be seen at the caudal edge of the heart.

The most frequent left-sided heart disorders include:

- congenital defects with shunts from left to right (septal defects, PDA)
- mitral valve dysplasia
- primary cardiomyopathies.

Severe enlargement of the left atrium or bi-atrial enlargement is a frequent finding in **advanced cardiomyopathies**. The cardiac silhouette adopts a **Valentine heart shape**, wider cranially and narrower caudally in the DV/VD projection. Although the Valentine's heart shape has been frequently considered a characteristic of hypertrophic cardiomyopathy (HCM), recent studies found this shape is also observed in other primary cardiomyopathies and congenital diseases. This **shape is mainly due to an increase in size of the left atrium** instead of right-sided atrial enlargement or bi-atrial enlargement. This form can be seen occasionally in cats without true cardiomegaly.

Generalised cardiomegaly (Figure 7) can be seen in almost all **cats** with DCM, atrioventricular valve dysplasia, cardiac shunts, peritoneopericardial diaphragmatic hernia, and pericardial effusion, and less frequently in cats with restrictive, unclassified, or hypertrophic cardiomyopathies.

In a lateral view a **VHS above 7.9** was considered to have high diagnostic precision to distinguish normal cats from those with moderate and severe left-sided heart disease and left atrial enlargement. In another study, VHS was found to be useful in distinguishing between cardiac and non-cardiac causes of respiratory distress. **A VHS> 9.3 was very specific for heart disease,** while values between 8–9.3 were equivocal as to the cause of dyspnoea. Values of 8 or less indicate heart disease is highly unlikely to be the cause of dyspnoea. In cats with severe anaemia, volume overload has been observed on the left side of the heart, with increases in VHS in these patients (9.1 vertebrae).

However, it should be remembered that **the absence of signs of an enlarged left atrium on radiography does not completely rule out the presence of heart failure**. In one study, 36% of cats with congestive heart failure had no radiographic evidence of increased left atrial size.

Radiographic signs of congestive heart failure frequently include **pulmonary oedema and/or pleural effusion**. Pulmonary oedema is more common than pleural effusion in cats with HCM-associated congestive heart failure, but pleural effusion occurs more frequently than pulmonary oedema in other cardiac conditions.

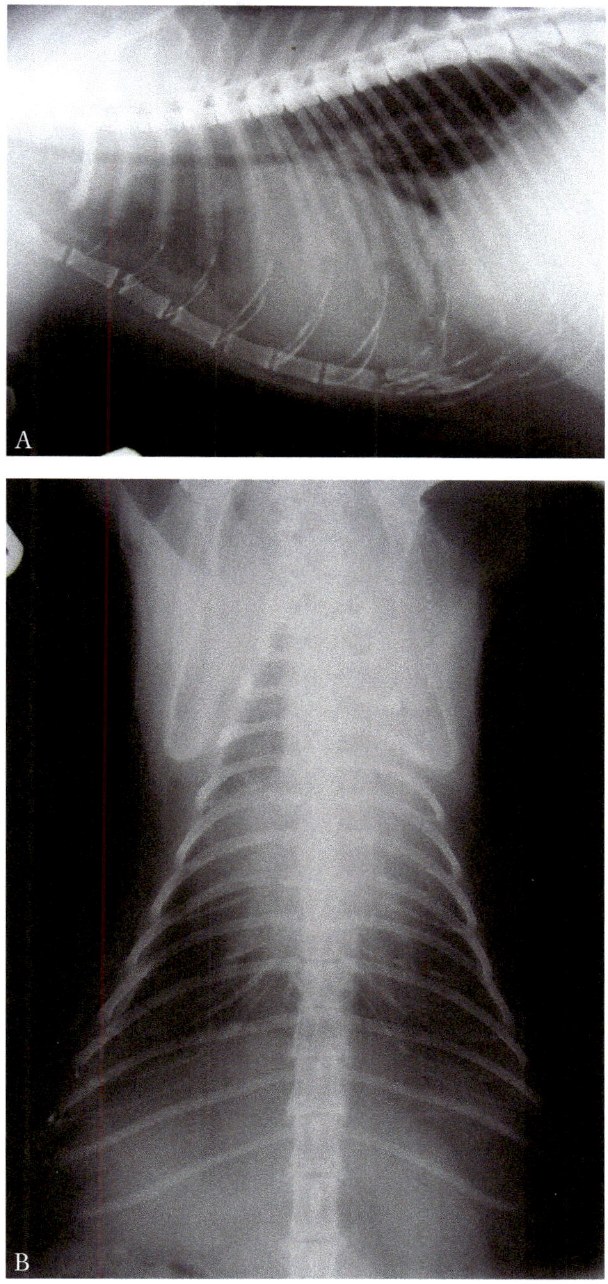

Figure 7. Patient with generalised cardiomegaly due to pericardial effusion. The cardiac silhouette appears globoid like in both projections, in particular in the VD view. In the VD projection the right margin of the cardiac silhouette is well-defined. In the lateral projection the edges of the cardiac silhouette are less well-defined due to the concurrent presence of pleural effusion.

Pulmonary oedema (Figure 8) can present a wide variation of radiographic characteristics, including an **unstructured interstitial pattern** in transition to an **alveolar pattern**, depending on severity and sometimes affecting the **peribronchial interstitium**. The distribution is predominantly **diffuse/non-uniform** (61%), followed by diffuse/uniform (17%), multifocal (17%) and focal (4%). The distribution, according to another classification, is **predominantly regional** (39%)—with a ventral distribution being the most frequent (22%),

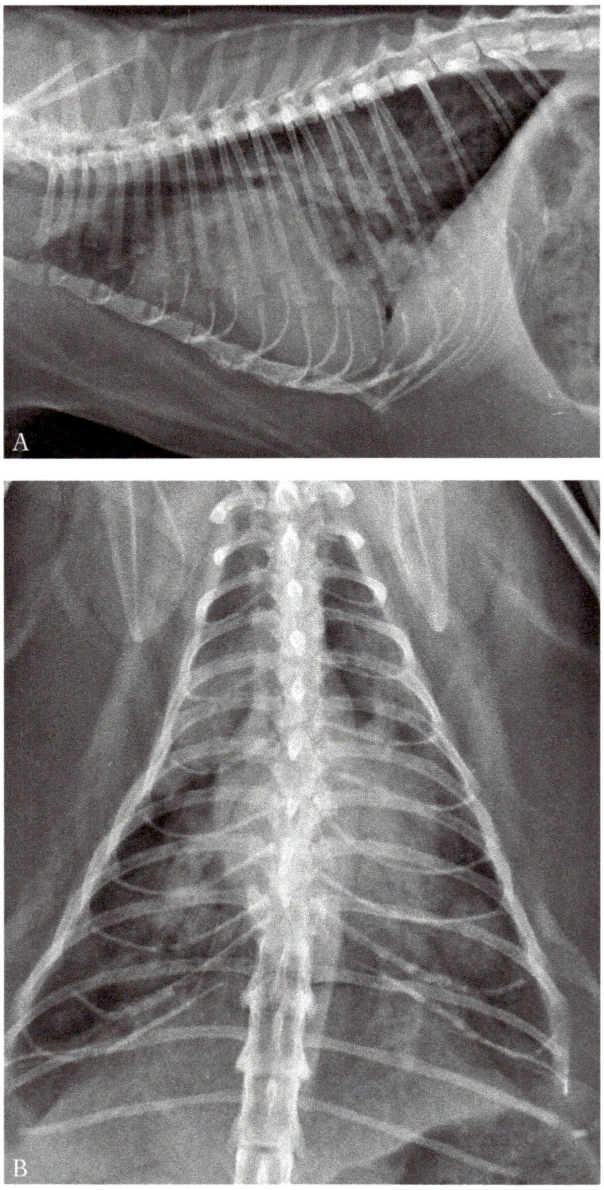

Figure 8. Patient with cardiomegaly and pulmonary oedema. A multifocal interstitial alveolar pattern affecting the ventral areas of the right and left cranial lobes, and diffuse interstitial pattern in the caudal lobes with a nodular focal area in the left caudal lobe can be seen. An increase in the pulmonary veins in the caudal lobes can also be seen. See also figure showing left-sided cardiomegaly (Figure 6A).

followed by caudal (13%) and hilar (4%)—or bilateral and symmetrical (22%).

Differential diagnoses of this pattern include:

- non-cardiogenic pulmonary oedema
- bronchitis
- pneumonia
- bronchopneumonia
- neoplasia
- haemorrhage
- dirofilariasis
- pulmonary fibrosis.

Enlargement of the pulmonary veins and arteries may be found, with variable frequency depending on the study.

In cases of right congestive heart failure, other radiographic changes include enlargement of the caudal vena cava and hepatomegaly.

Thoracic wall and diaphragm

The wall or margins of the thoracic cavity include the thoracic skeleton, the cranial and caudal apertures, the diaphragm, and the overlying soft tissue structures.

- The **cranial thoracic aperture (or thoracic inlet)** corresponds approximately to the region of the first two ribs and consists of the opening through which the trachea, oesophagus, vessels and nerves pass.
- The **thoracic skeleton** consists of 13 ribs, the sternum with 8 sternebrae, and the 13 vertebrae of the thoracic spine. It is important to assess these structures on thoracic radiography including their number, location and symmetry (ribs), as well as the opacity and shape of the bony structures.
- The **diaphragm** covers the caudal thoracic opening. It is made up of two crura and a cupola, and these structures take different positions and shapes depending on the projection, although this is less evident in cats than in dogs.

The diaphragm can be distinguished in animals with abundant falciform fat as a thin curved line with soft tissue opacity in the ventral aspect of the thorax/abdominal cavity, between the lung field and the falciform fat. The **dorsal aspect of the crura inserts at the level of L3 and L4.**

The normal diaphragm has three openings:

1. the **aortic hiatus** (dorsal)
2. the **oesophageal hiatus** (central)
3. the **caval foramen** (ventral and to the right).

The **diaphragm forms four recesses** where it inserts into the chest wall: the dorsal, ventral, right and left costodiaphragmatic recesses.

The soft tissues of the chest wall should be thin and regular.

Wet hair (for example, if the radiograph is taken after an ultrasound), or subcutaneous changes, such as emphysema and oedema, can also create overlapping opacities in the thoracic cavity which can cause confusion. **Nipples or other nodules can create nodular opacities** that should not be confused with lung nodules. The prominent nodules or nipples in the patient should be identified, and when in doubt, the radiograph can be repeated by marking the structure with barium or a radiopaque marker.

Radiographic diagnosis of thoracic wall and diaphragm pathologies

Congenital skeletal malformations

Congenital abnormalities of the thoracic skeleton are relatively rare in cats compared to dogs. Possible abnormalities include findings of no clinical importance, such as **supernumerary or infranumerary ribs** associated with transitional vertebrae. Significant abnormalities of the sternum, such as ***pectus excavatum*** can also be found.

Fractures

They can be **traumatic, pathological or stress fractures** (Figure 9). Traumatic fractures are often multiple, usually transverse or oblique or segmental (more than one fracture in the same rib). They can be associated with **pneumothorax or pulmonary contusion.** If there are three or more ribs with segmental fractures or five or more ribs with single fractures, a **flail chest** can occur, which is observed as a paradoxical movement of the affected segment (inward on inspiration and outward on expiration).

A **flail sternum** occurs when there are **multiple bilateral fractures of the costal cartilage** and a paradoxical movement of the sternum is observed.

Pathological fractures can be caused by diseases that **weaken the bone structure** (chronic feline kidney disease or other causes of hyperparathyroidism, neoplasia) or as a result of **hyperinflation or chronic coughing** (feline asthma).

Fractures due to **metabolic disease or respiratory conditions are usually serial and located dorsally and caudally**. If the fracture margins are not sharp and do not show remodelling, they are suggestive of a pathological fracture due to an osteolytic condition.

Traumatic fractures are normally ipsilateral to trauma.

Neoplasms

Primary rib tumours are very rare in cats (Figure 10), and the most frequent are osteosarcomas and chondrosarcomas. They are usually located in the distal third of the rib, near the costochondral junction.

Metastases with osteolytic lesions and periosteal reaction in the ribs have been described in cats with lung carcinoma.

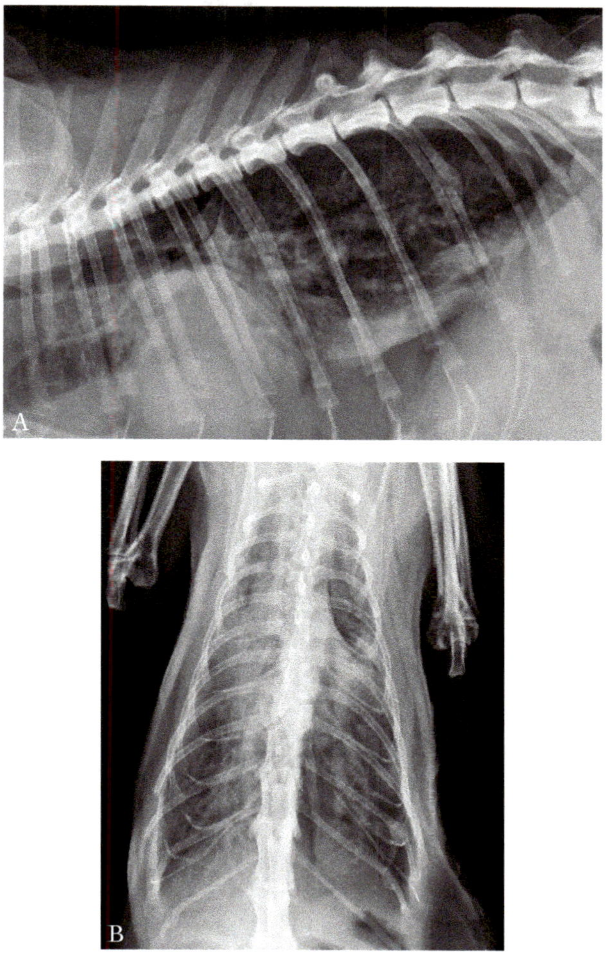

Figure 9. Cat with chronic respiratory problems. Multiple, bilateral rib fractures can be seen on the more caudal vertebrae at different stages of healing.

Diaphragm ruptures of traumatic origin

These are often referred to as acquired diaphragmatic hernias (incorrectly, since the organs are not found within a hernia sac).

Radiographic features include:

- Loss of visualization of the **diaphragmatic contour**.
- Loss of visualization or displacement of the **cardiac silhouette**.
- Increased opacity of the ventral thorax.
- **Mediastinal shift**.
- Presence of tubular structures with **air content** or other digestive content.
- Pleural effusion.
- Collapse of lung lobes.
- **"Empty" abdomen**, with absence of abdominal organs in their normal position (in cats, falciform fat may be the only "herniated" structure) (Figure 11).

Hiatal hernias

A hiatal hernia is the result of **organ herniation through the oesophageal hiatus.** They can be **congenital or**

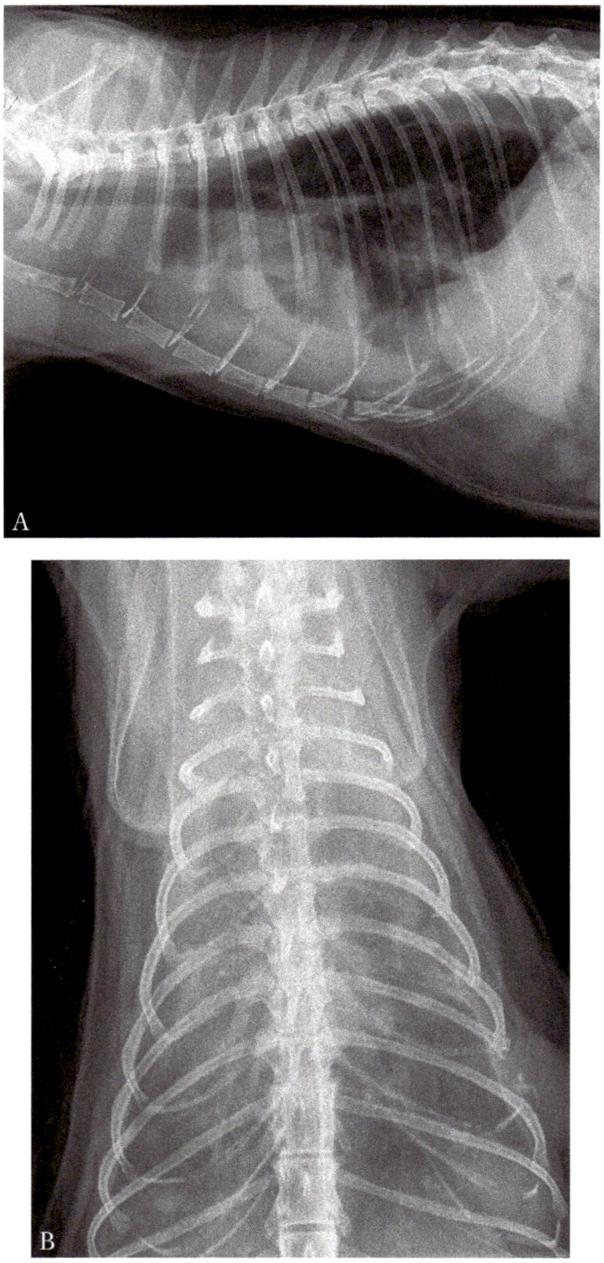

Figure 10. Geriatric patient which presented due to pleural effusion. A soft tissue mass can be seen on the ninth right rib which is causing lysis of the distal half of the body of the rib.

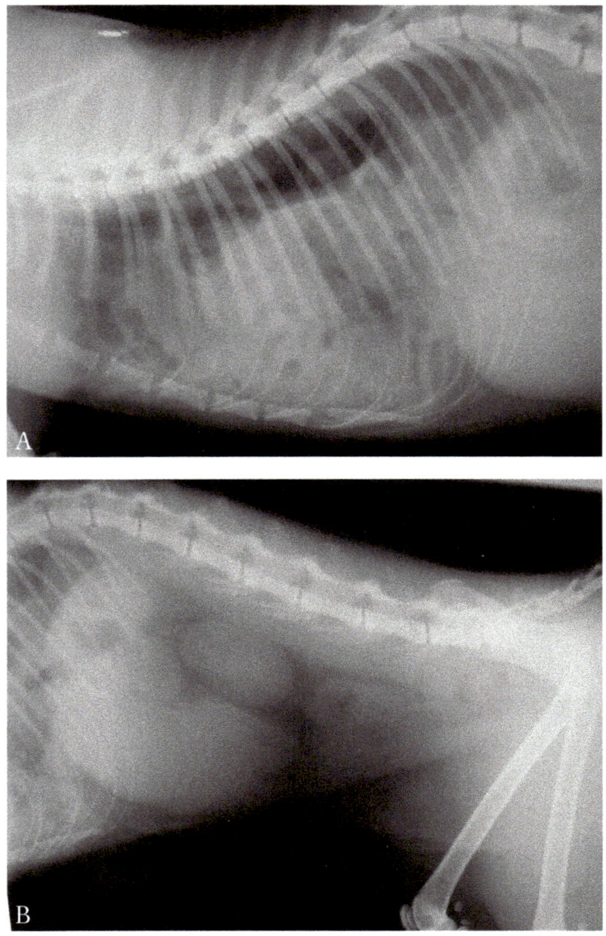

Figure 11. Cat with polytrauma where the presence of structures with gas compatible with the small intestine in the thorax can be seen. The abdomen appears empty of small intestine.

acquired and are often **secondary to upper-airway pathologies**. **Sliding hiatal hernias** are included in this group: the caudal oesophageal sphincter moves back and forth in the caudal mediastinum followed by the stomach. In this type of hernia, oval soft tissue opacity and variable presence of gas between the vena cava and the aorta in the lateral view and widening of the caudal mediastinum in the VD view are observed radiographically.

If the stomach is herniated and contains gas, it is possible to distinguish the gastric folds. Associated aspiration pneumonia may be seen, and radiographic signs may not be observed, especially during expiration. Sometimes contrast studies or fluoroscopy are necessary for diagnosis.

Peritoneopericardial hernias

A peritoneopericardial hernia is **an embryological fusion defect** in the ventral diaphragm that produces a **communication between the pericardial and peritoneal cavities**. This can be associated with sternal and heart defects. In most cases they **do not cause clinical signs**.

Radiographically (Figure 12), a moderate or **marked increase in size of the cardiac silhouette** is observed, which converges with the diaphragm, without signs of cardiac failure. Heterogeneous opacity of the cardiac silhouette (soft tissue, fat, mineral, gas) is also seen if it contains mesenteric fat and the gastrointestinal tract. Radiographs show **cranial displacement of the stomach** or other abdominal organs. Ultrasound confirms the diagnosis and is used to assess which organs are in the pericardial sac.

Pleura and pleural cavity

The pleura is divided into parietal and visceral.

The **parietal pleura lines the interior aspect of the chest wall and diaphragm**, and envelops the heart,

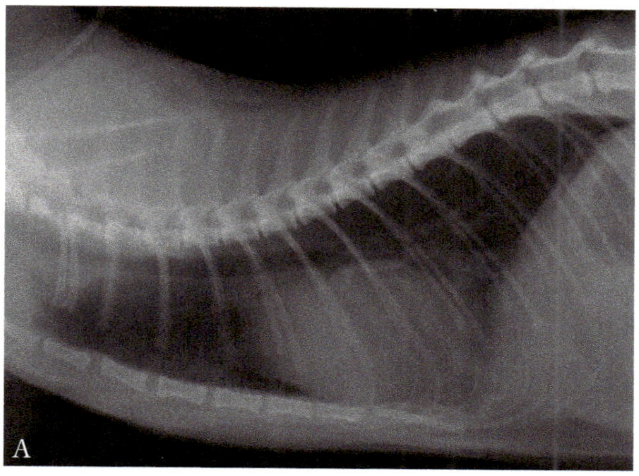

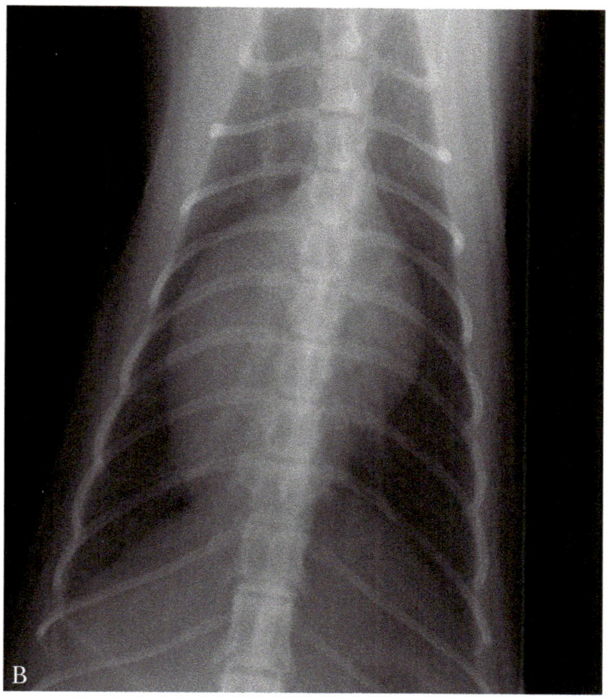

Figure 12. 9-month-old cat, which has fallen from a height. Right lateral and VD projections showing a cardiac silhouette which is markedly increased in size with a silhouette sign between its caudal border and the diaphragm and a hepatic silhouette which is reduced in size, compatible with a peritoneal pericardial diaphragmatic hernia, an incidental finding in this patient.

great vessels, and oesophagus to form the the mediastinum. The visceral pleura lines the lungs and **forms the interlobar fissures**.

The visceral and parietal pleurae are separated by the pleural space, which is a potential space, usually less than 1 mm thick, and contains a small amount of fluid. As a general rule, **the pleura is not visualized radiographically**. It is useful to be aware of the position of the pleural fissures (between the lung lobes), in order to identify them in pathological cases (Figures 26, 27 and 28).

Radiographic diagnosis of pathologies of the pleura and pleural cavity

The **pleural space is radiographically visible when distended with gas, fluid, or fibrin and cellular debris.**

Pleural effusion

Pleural effusion is the accumulation of **any type of fluid in the pleural space** (Figure 13). Radiographic features include:

- **Soft tissue opacity** in the pleural space.
- **Loss of visualization** of the margins of the heart and diaphragm, depending on the amount of fluid.
- Visualization of **pleural fissures.**
- **Retraction of the margins of the lung lobes** away from the sternum, ribs and spine.
- In acute or non-reactive effusions, the lobe margins tend to remain sharp, whereas in chronic or reactive effusions (pyothorax or chylothorax) they tend to become rounded.
- Increased lung opacity due to **collapsed lobes**.
- Normally bilateral, although it can be unilateral especially with very dense effusions that plug the mediastinum.

In the different recumbent positions, the **liquid accumulates towards the dependent part of the thorax.** In a DV projection, the liquid accumulates around the heart, preventing the visualization of its silhouette. To better visualize the heart, a VD view will move the fluid to the dorsal part of the chest, leaving the heart surrounded by the lung, and therefore with more visible margins. However, the animal will probably be less tolerant of this position, and it is safer to repeat the radiographs after draining the thorax.

Repeating post-drainage radiographs is also helpful in identifying chest masses which cannot be seen with effusion.

Pericardial fat can help visualize part of the heart's silhouette and thereby identify any possible associated cardiac pathologies. The fat, which is less opaque than the effusion and the heart, continues to be visualized showing the position and shape of the organ's cranial border (Figure 10).

Pneumothorax

Pneumothorax is the accumulation of air in the pleural space. Pneumothorax can be classified as **traumatic** (open or closed) and **spontaneous**. Spontaneous pneumothorax in cats are **secondary to an underlying pulmonary pathology** such as inflammatory disease of the respiratory tract, neoplasia, dirofilariasis, abscesses or pulmonary verminosis.

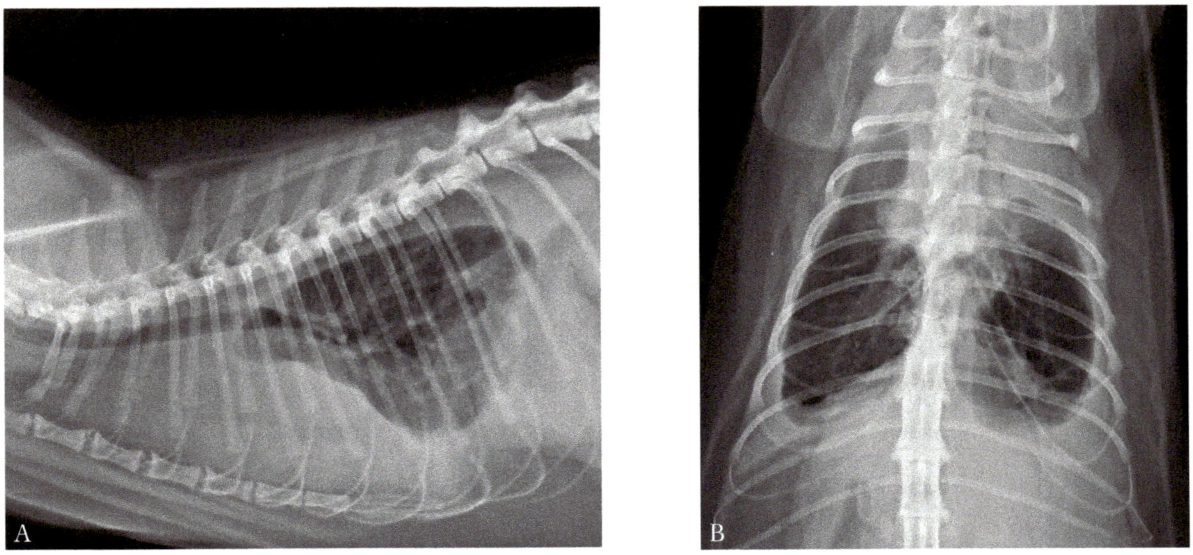

Figure 13. Patient with a chronic chylothorax. Take note of the markedly rounded edges of the pulmonary lobes.

A particular type is **tension pneumothorax**, which occurs when the pressure of the pleural gas is above atmospheric pressure. This occurs when a one-way valve effect occurs between the air source and the pleural space: air enters during inspiration but does not exit during expiration. There is a rapid increase in pressure in the pleural space which is **life-threatening**.

Radiographic features:

- **Pulmonary margins retracted** from the costal wall, spine, and diaphragm.
- **Collapsed lung lobes** (with increased opacity) and well-defined margins.
- Pulmonary pattern not visible on the peripheries of the thorax.
- **Cardiac silhouette elevated** from the sternum due to air opacity.
- Usually bilateral.
- Uneven collapse of the lung lobes may indicate concurrent lung disease.

In cases of **tension pneumothorax,** in addition, the following may be present:

- **Rapid worsening** of radiographic changes.
- Severe lung compression/collapse.
- **Flattened diaphragm.**
- **Thoracic distension,** with widened intercostal spaces.

Hydropneumothorax

Hydropneumothorax refers to the presence of air and liquid in the pleural cavity (Figure 14), therefore radiographic features of both pneumothorax and pleural effusion are present.

Some **special projections, using a horizontal beam** with the animal lying or standing, may be helpful in showing a soft tissue-liquid interface. Causes include trauma, iatrogenic (e.g. after thoracentesis), perforation or inhaled oesophageal foreign body, and malignancy. If the distribution of liquid and air is not homogeneous between the two sides, the appearance of the lateral projection can be very different between right and a left sides.

Pleural masses

The potential causes of the presence of masses in parietal and/or mediastinal pleura, includes **neoplasia** (mesothelioma, metastasis), **haematoma**, and **abscess.** They are often accompanied by **pleural effusion**, which can make diagnosis very difficult.

Radiographically, regions with **soft tissue opacity** are visualized, which are frequently fusiform in shape, displacing the lung from the chest wall or mediastinum (although in the latter case they are more difficult to visualise). The pleural effusion that usually accompanies them makes them difficult to visualize, but they can be suspected if a non-uniform compression or displacement of the lung or a soft tissue opacity is observed that maintains its position and shape despite changes in the position of the patient (Figure 15).

Differential diagnoses include encapsulated fluid.

Mediastinum

The mediastinum is the space between the left and right pleural cavities. Its lateral limits are the mediastinal pleura, which are reflections of the parietal pleura. The mediastinum communicates cranially with the fascial planes of the neck through the thoracic inlet and caudally with the retroperitoneal space through the aortic hiatus.

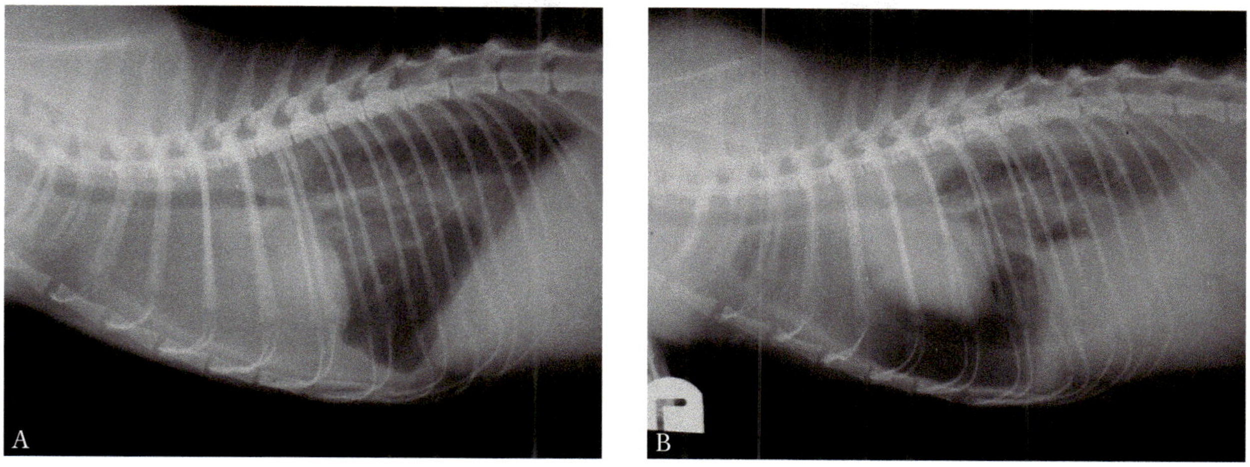

Figure 14. Cat with hydropneumothorax. The different appearance of both lateral projections can be observed. In A (right lateral projection) the pleural effusion impedes visualisation of the cardiac silhouette, while in B (left lateral projection) the cardiac silhouette is seen to be elevated due to the presence of pleural air.

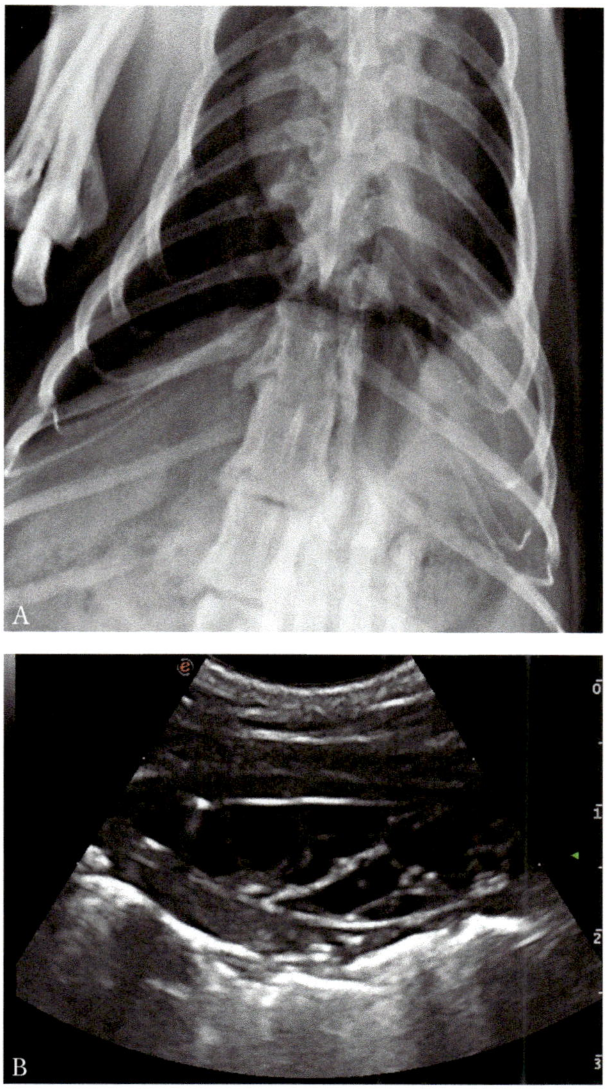

Figure 15. DV projection (A) and ultrasound image (B) from a patient with a history of pyothorax and thoracotomy tube placement, where a mass with soft tissue opacity which displaces the left caudal lung is visible. On ultrasound the mass contains liquid, which on aspiration was compatible with a seroma (at the site of prior thoracotomy tube placement).

It contains the midline thoracic structures, including:

- Heart and large vessels.
- Trachea.
- Oesophagus.
- Thymus in young animals.
- Lymph nodes (not visible radiographically if normal):
  - sternal (Figure 16A), dorsal to the 2nd-3rd sternebra
  - tracheobronchial, at the bifurcation of the trachea
  - cranial mediastinal, ventral to the trachea
- Thoracic duct and nerves.

The mediastinum can be divided into:

- Cranial mediastinum (cranial to heart).
- Middle mediastinum (level with and containing the heart).
- Caudal mediastinum (caudal to the heart).
- Dorsal mediastinum (dorsal to the carina).
- Ventral mediastinum.

In the cat, the width of the cranial mediastinum measured on a DV/VD view should be no greater than the width of the cranial thoracic vertebrae (Figure 16B). However, in patients with a high body condition, the mediastinum may contain a large amount of fat and be wider.

The **thymus is seen in young animals**. In the lateral projection it can be seen as a triangular opacity, which is often not well defined, cranial to the heart, while in the VD projection it is seen as a triangular opacity extending from the midline cranial to the heart (called thymic sail) or as a widening of the mediastinum (Figure 17).

The oesophagus is not usually seen under normal conditions. In some sedated or anaesthetized patients, it can be visualized with gas content at times without being abnormal.

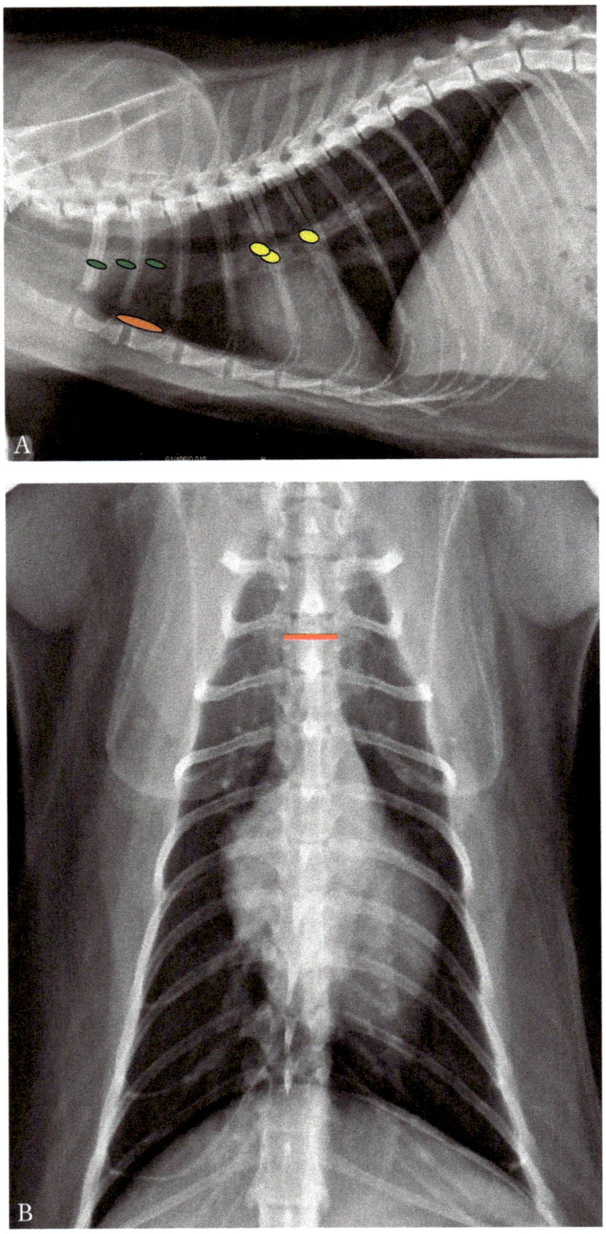

Figure 16. Right lateral projection (A) showing the approximate position of the most common lymph nodes in the mediastinum (sternal in orange, tracheobronchial in yellow and cranial mediastinal in green). VD projection (B) showing the normal size of the cranial mediastinum, not wider than the width of the vertebra.

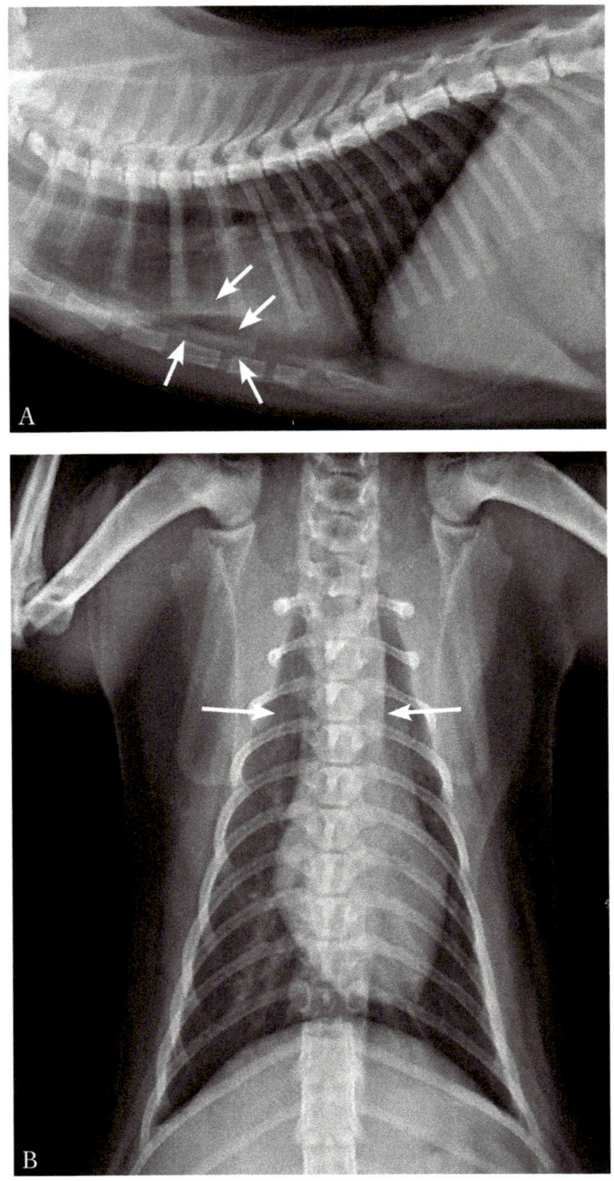

Figure 17. Right lateral (A) and VD (B) projections of a 6 month old cat where the thymus can be visualised as an approximately triangular shaped area with soft tissue opacity, but with poorly defined edges and which is difficult to distinguish from the heart in the RL projection and as a thickening of the mediastinum in the VD projection.

The trachea is best visualised in the lateral view. The normal position of the carina is at the level of the 4th-5th intercostal spaces.

Radiographic diagnosis of pathologies of the mediastinum and its contents

Pneumomediastinum

This is the accumulation of air in the mediastinum. Consequently, the structures that normally form part of the joint soft tissue opacity become individually visible. It is important to remember that the mediastinum communicates both with the fascia of the neck (and therefore with the subcutaneous space) and with the retroperitoneal space, since associated abnormalities can be found in these regions. Pneumomediastinum can lead to a pneumothorax; the reverse is much more unusual.

Radiographic characteristics (Figure 18):

- Decreased radiopacity of the mediastinum.
- Visualization of mediastinal structures previously not visible individually:
  - Ventral serosal surface of the trachea.
  - Individualized cranial mediastinal vessels (left subclavian artery, brachiocephalic trunk, CrVC).
  - Better visualization of the contour of the aorta.

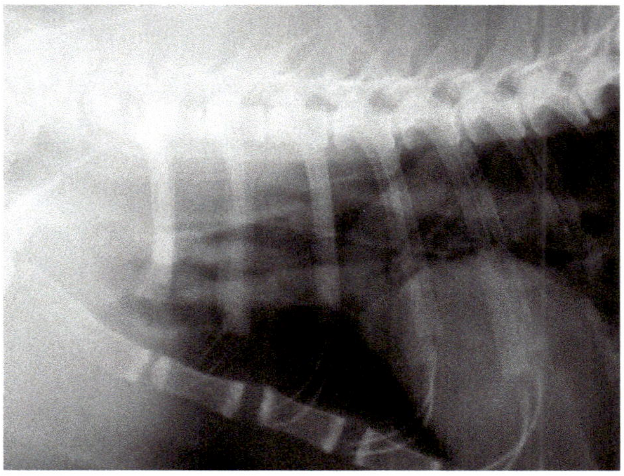

Figure 18. Lateral projection of the cranial thorax in a patient with pneumomediastinum. Vessels in the cranial mediastinum can be seen clearly, as can the ventral serosa of the trachea.

- Visualization of the azygos vein in the dorsal thorax.
- Visualization of the ventral edge of the longissimus colli muscle (inserted on the ventral aspect of T6).
- Possible emphysema of the neck and subcutaneously. Radiographs of the neck can show the cause of pneumomediastinum.
- Possible pneumoretroperitoneum. Usually incidental but must be differentiated from pneumoperitoneum.

The most common causes in cats include positive ventilation with the endotracheal tube, thoracic trauma, tracheal foreign bodies, underlying lung disease, and venepuncture. It can also be caused by extension of injuries from the neck.

Mediastinal masses

These can occur anywhere in the mediastinum, but the **most frequent location is in the cranioventral area.** The clinical and radiographic signs vary depending on the location.

Cranioventral mediastinum

Radiographic characteristics (Figure 19):

- Increased soft tissue opacity in the **cranioventral thorax**.
- Elevation +/– compression of the trachea.
- Cranial mediastinum thickening in VD/DV.
- Caudal displacement of the heart and carina.
- Caudal displacement/compression of the lung lobes.

Differential diagnoses include:

- Lymphoma.
- Thymic lesions (thymoma, thymic lymphoma, cyst).
- Sternal lymph adenomegaly (may represent abdominal pathology).

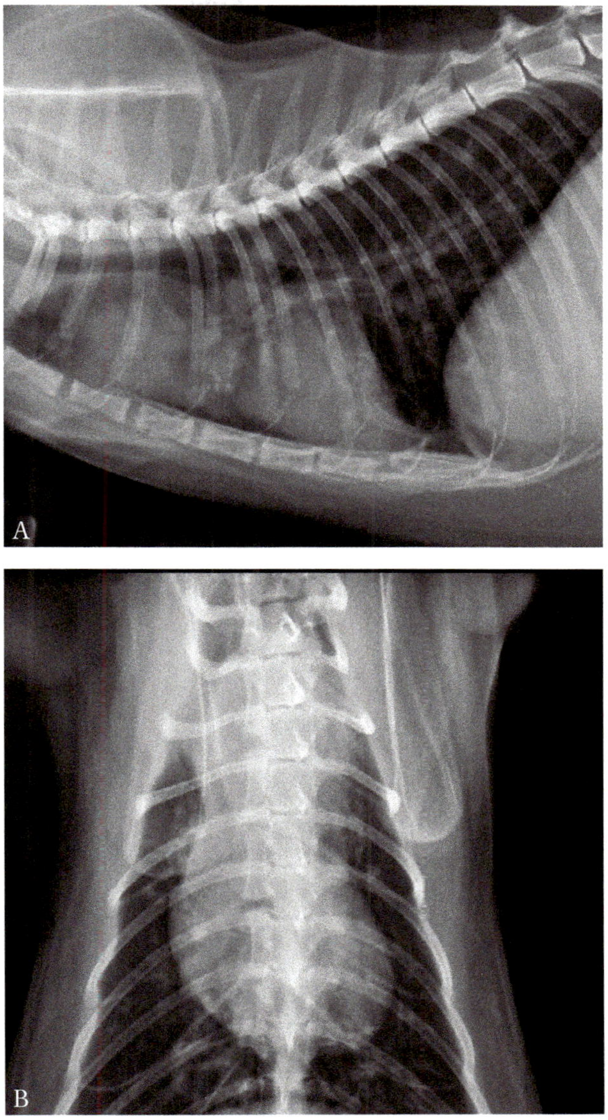

Figure 19. Lateral (A) and VD (B) projections from a patient with a cranial mediastinal mass which is causing dorsal displacement of the trachea in the lateral projection and widening of the mediastinum in the VD projection.

- Ectopic thyroid/parathyroid tumours.
- Mediastinal cyst.
- Haemorrhage.

Perihilar

Radiographic features:

- Increased peri-hilar opacity.
- Ventral displacement of the terminal trachea/carina.
- Possible bronchial obstruction +/– pulmonary collapse.

Differential diagnoses include:

- Tracheobronchial lymphadenopathy (lymphoma, metastasis, tuberculosis, nocardiosis, fungal disease).
- Neoplasm of the heart base.

Caudodorsal mediastinum
Radiographic features:

- Widening of the caudal mediastinum (DV/VD).
- Displacement or compression of the oesophagus.
- Silhouette sign with the diaphragm.

Differential diagnoses include:

- Oesophageal lesions (foreign body, tumour, granuloma).
- Hiatal hernia.
- Diaphragmatic lesions (mass, abscess, haematoma).
- Neural tumours.

Craniodorsal mediastinum
Radiographic features:

- Ventral displacement of the trachea.
- Silhouette sign with aorta.
- Difficult to visualize if the mass is not mineralized.

Differential diagnoses include:

- Oesophageal diseases.
- Neural or neuroendocrine tumours.
- Aortic aneurysm.
- Vertebral/paravertebral tumours.
- Haemorrhage/haematoma.

Oesophageal diseases

Radiographic interpretation of oesophageal disease

Megaoesophagus
Megaoesophagus can be segmental or generalized, **congenital or acquired**, but it is rare in cats. Acquired causes include obstruction of the upper airways, neuromuscular diseases (including dysautonomia), and vascular ring abnormalities.

Radiographic characteristics (Figure 20):

- Generalized or focal **distention of the oesophagus** (gas or food).
- Tracheal stripe sign.
- Right, ventral **tracheal displacement**.
- It can also cause ventral displacement of the base of the heart.
- +/– aspiration pneumonia.

Failure to identify megaoesophagus on plain radiographs does not completely rule out its presence and contrast studies may be necessary. **Barium mixed with food** usually gives better results for visualization

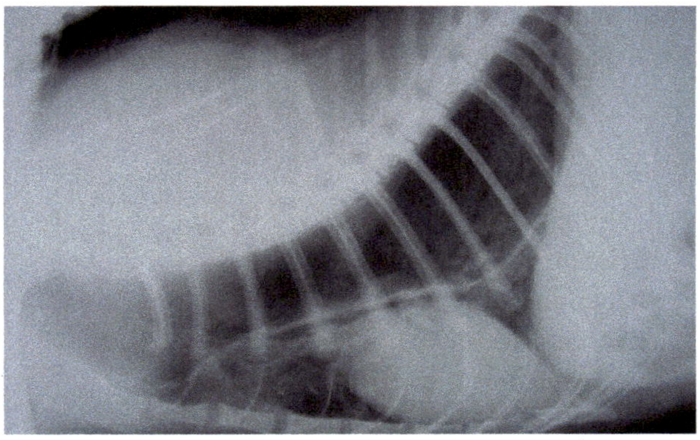

Figure 20. Lateral projection of a cat with dysautonomia. Marked distension of the oesophagus with ventral displacement of the heart and trachea can be seen with an increased opacity in the ventral lung field which may correspond with aspiration pneumonia.

of oesophageal disorders, but the **risk of aspiration** should be considered.

Foreign bodies
Oesophageal foreign bodies are rare in cats, excluding linear foreign bodies that extend from the base of the tongue to the stomach and intestine. V-shaped bird bones can cause obstruction in the pharynx and proximal oesophagus (Figure 21).

Radiographic features:

- Visualization of the foreign body depending on radiopacity.
- +/– oesophageal distention.

Oesophageal strictures
These have been described in cats associated with **administration of doxycycline and clindamycin, as well as secondary to reflux during anaesthesia.** Plain radiographs are usually not diagnostic and **an oesophagogram is required** to visualize the stenosis.

Vascular ring anomalies
Congenital malformations of the aorta and its branches, most often **persistence of the fourth right**

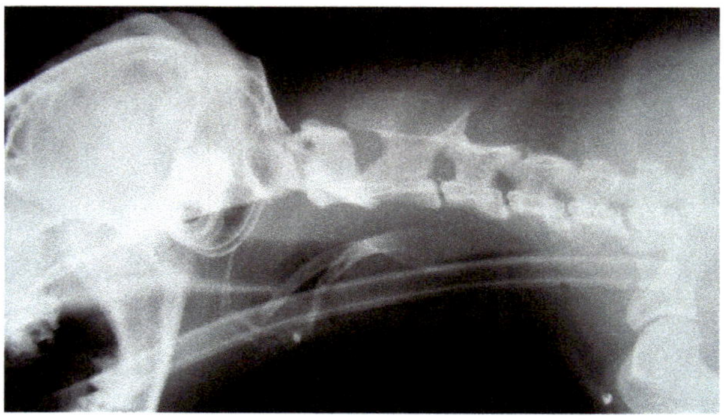

Figure 21. Lateral projection of the neck area. A chicken bone can be seen trapped in the pharynx and oesophagus.

aortic arch, causing obstruction of the oesophagus at the base of the heart, with cranial oesophageal distension.

Radiographic features:

- **Dilation of the oesophagus cranial to the obstruction**, with acute narrowing between the 4th intercostal space and the 6th rib.
- Ventral deviation of the trachea.
- Moderate or marked deviation of the trachea to the left (DV/VD) near the cranial border of the heart.

Neoplasia

Neoplasia is rare. In cats, squamous cell carcinoma is most common.

Radiographic features:

- Oesophageal dilatation.
- Soft tissue mass in the caudodorsal mediastinum.
- Mineralization of the mass is possible.

Tracheal disorders

Tracheal collapse

Primary tracheal collapse is very rare in cats with only a few cases described. It is important to know that **collapse of the cervical trachea can occur as a consequence of laryngeal or nasopharyngeal obstruction** (Figure 22). Therefore, in cases of tracheal collapse always consider obstruction of the upper respiratory tract.

In cats, degeneration of tracheal cartilage has only been described in cases with mucopolysaccharidosis.

Tracheal masses

Tracheal masses are uncommon in the cat.

Radiographic characteristics (Figure 23):

- Lesion with **soft tissue opacity within the tracheal lumen.**
- If masses cause intrathoracic obstruction this can result in air retention and **pulmonary hyperinflation.**
- In cases of cervical obstruction, lung volume may be reduced.

Differential diagnoses include:

- Neoplasia.
- Granuloma.
- Polyps.
- Haematoma.

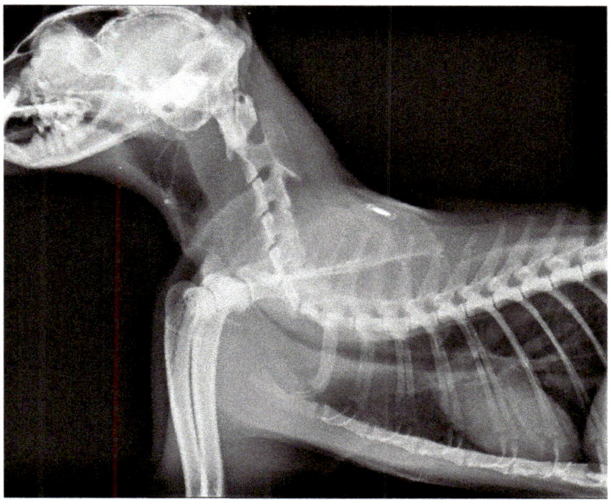

Figure 22. Lateral projection from a patient with a nasopharyngeal mass. Note the tracheal collapse in the neck region as well as the oesophageal distension, which is most marked in the most caudal part of the thorax.

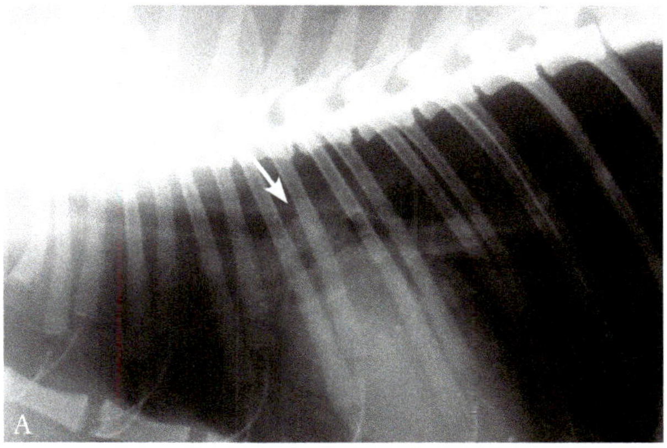

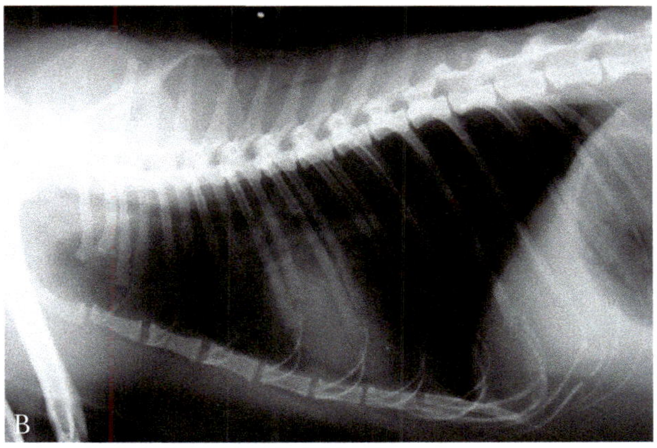

Figure 23. Lateral projection magnified around the carina (A) and the full view (B) of a cat with a mass with soft tissue opacity just cranial to the carina. The lung fields appear hyperinflated.

Foreign bodies

Tracheal foreign bodies are more frequent in **young animals**, and may be visualized on radiographs depending on their size, opacity, and position. In the trachea they cause changes similar to those caused by masses, with variable opacity depending on the

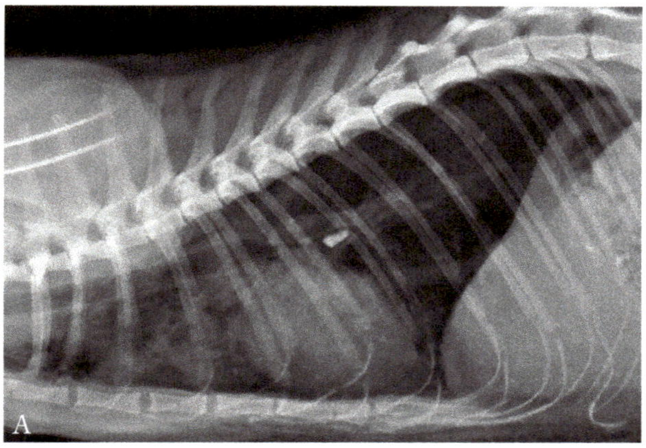

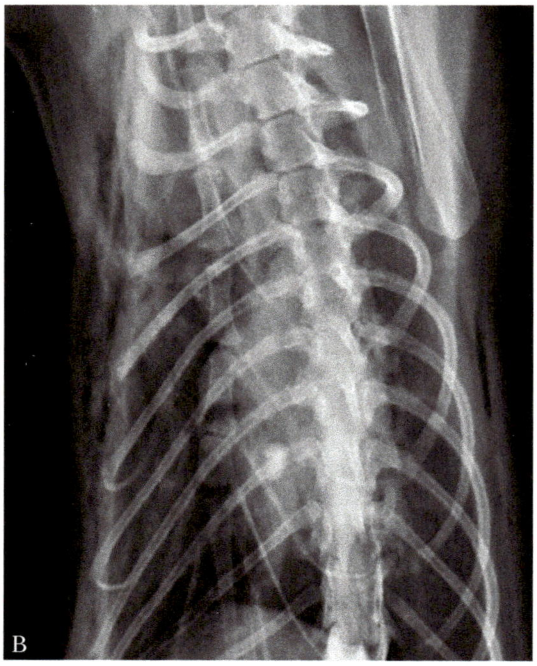

Figure 24. Cat treated after being bitten by a dog. A mineral-opaque structure can be seen in the bronchus of the right caudal lobe (stone). There is also subcutaneous emphysema and mild pneumothorax.

material. **Larger foreign bodies stop at the tracheal** bifurcation and the smallest ones **pass through to the bronchi**, more frequently to those in the **caudal lobes** because they follow a straighter path from the trachea (Figure 24).

Tracheal avulsion

This is a **rare lesion** but has been described in cats (Figure 25). Tracheal avulsion can be caused by **trauma with hyperextension of the neck and head**, which causes an avulsion usually **between 1–4 cm cranial to the bifurcation of the trachea.** Avulsion of the main bronchus can also occur.

After injury, the lumen of the airway is maintained by intact tracheal adventitia and thickening of the mediastinum, creating a **pseudo airway**. Subsequently, narrowing of the avulsed margins can result in stenosis.

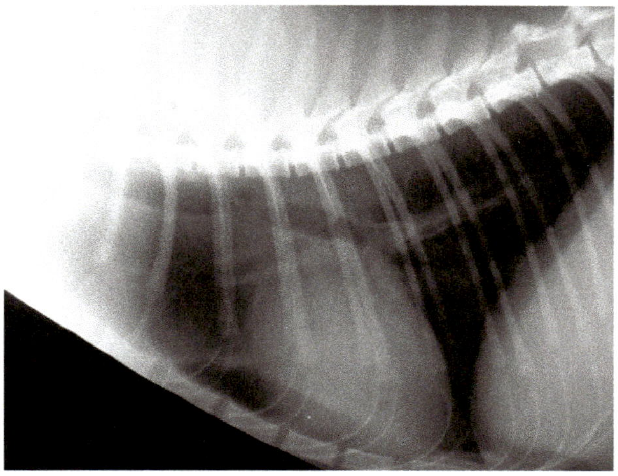

Figure 25. Patient with tracheal avulsion. Localised, focal stenosis can be seen cranial to the carina and dorsal to this an oval gas containing structure can be see, which corresponds with the pseudo trachea.

Lung

Cats have two lungs that divide into several lobes, according to the branching of the bronchi (Figures 26, 27 and 28).

Right lung:

- Cranial lobe.
- Middle lobe.
- Caudal lobe.
- Accessory lobe.

Left lung:

- Cranial lobe.
  - Cranial part.
  - Caudal part.
- Caudal lobe.

The **pulmonary vessels** are seen as soft tissue opacities which **branch from the perihilar region**, decreasing in size towards the periphery. Lateral radiographs show the vessels of the cranial lobes, with the **arteries located more dorsally than the veins**, although both should have a similar diameter.

The vessels of the caudal lobes are seen in the DV projection (preferable to a VD projection) since the **caudal lobes are better ventilated** in this projection and display greater contrast between the aerated lung and the vessels. **On a DV projection the arteries are lateral to the veins.**

The arteries of the **cranial lobes should measure 0.5–1 times the proximal third of the 4th rib** (average ratio between the artery and the rib is 0.7), measured at the 4th rib. The veins of the cranial lobes should

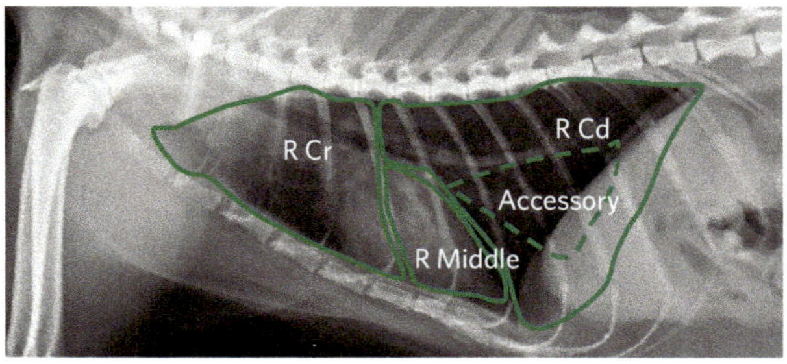

Figure 26. Left lateral projection showing the approximate position of the right lung lobes.

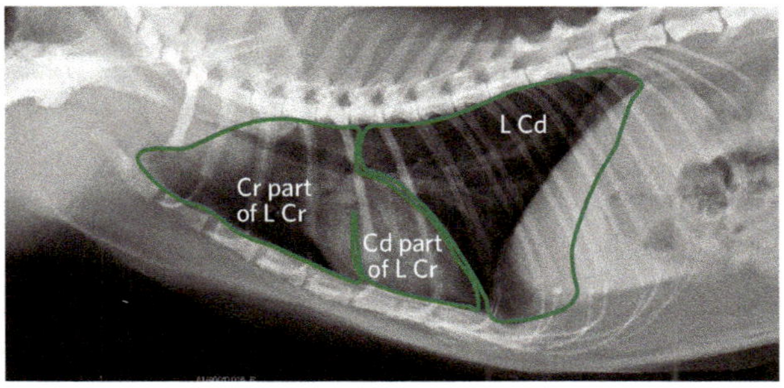

Figure 27. Right lateral projection showing the approximate position of the left lung lobes.

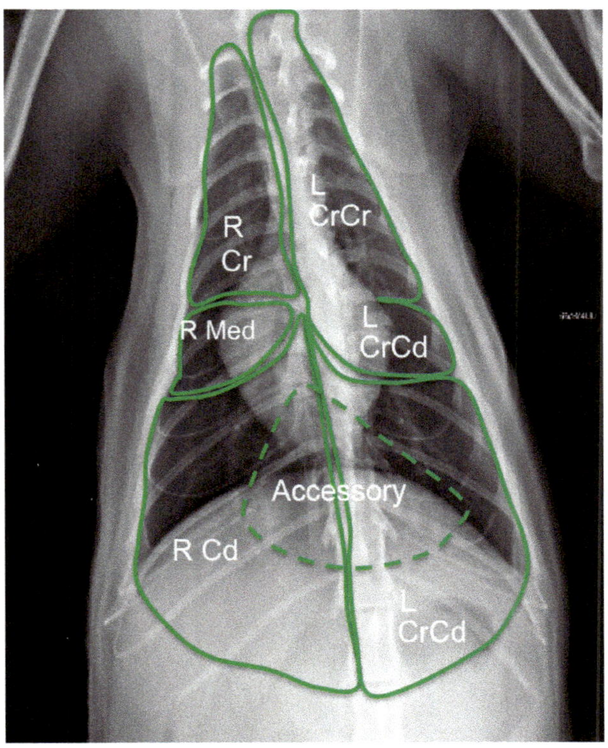

Figure 28. VD projection showing the approximate position of the lung lobes.

measure about 0.2 cm (± 0.03 cm) in diameter in the same place (Figure 29).

In cases of **dirofilariasis, an upper limit for the normal diameter of the arteries to the caudal lobes, 1.6 times the diameter of the 9th rib** has been suggested.

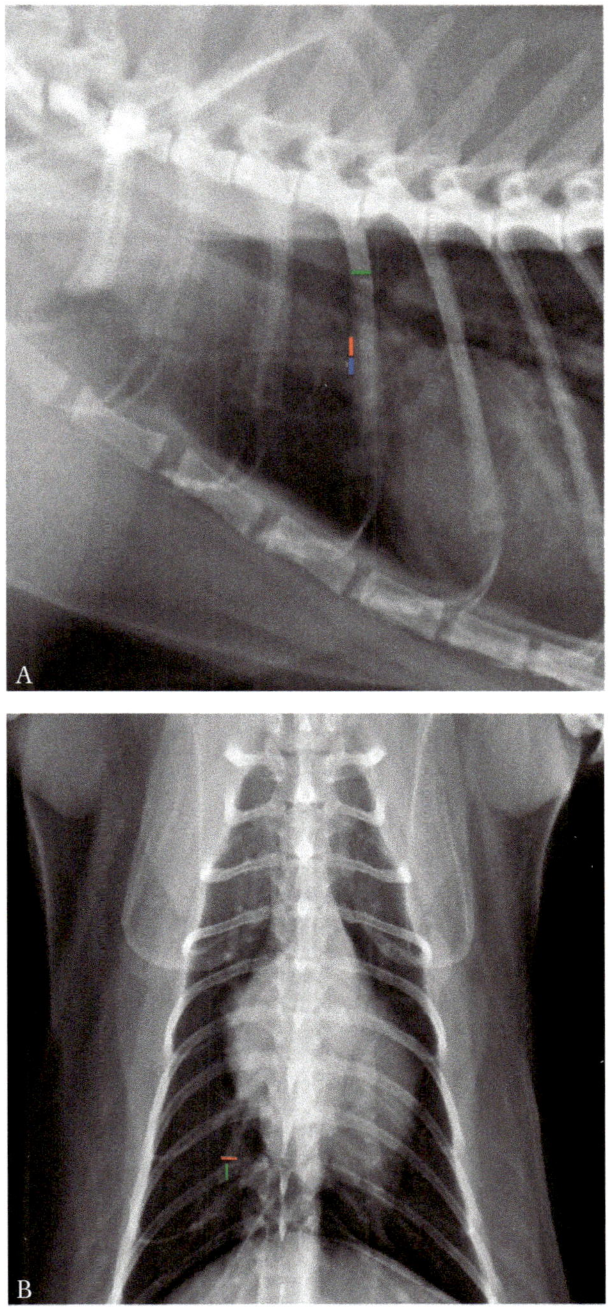

Figure 29. Right lateral and VD projections showing the comparative measurement between the pulmonary artery (red) and vein (blue) diameters with the diameter of the fourth rib (RL) and ninth rib (VD).

Factors influencing the radiographic interpretation of lung pathology

Recumbency effect

The dependent lung lobe is partially compressed and less aerated, so **lesions are better visualized in the non-dependent part of the lung** (for example: a nodule in the right lung is better visualized in a left lateral view – left sided recumbency).

Age

Kittens have more opaque lungs due to a higher water content in the interstitium and presence of the thymus.

Older cats may have a more evident bronchial pattern without this being associated with pathology.

Body condition

In **obese animals**, the overlap of fatty tissue produces an **increase in the opacity of the lung** field, causing worse visualization of the bronchovascular structures. In very thin animals the lungs may appear more radiolucent.

Radiographic diagnosis of lung pathologies

Lung patterns

Lung patterns are a descriptive method that tries to relate the **radiographic characteristics of increased lung opacity to the morphological changes in the lung.**

Bronchial pattern

The **bronchial pattern consists of increased visualization of the walls of the** bronchi due to an increase in their opacity. The increased opacity may be caused by **mineralization** or by **thickening** of the bronchial wall. The increased visualization of the bronchi may also be due to an increase in their diameter and changes in their shape (bronchiectasis).

Radiographic characteristics of the bronchial pattern:

- Circular structures with a radiopaque wall and radiolucent centre ("**donuts**") representing bronchi when viewed transversely (end-on).
- Radiopaque parallel linear structures ("**tram lines**"), representing bronchi when visualized longitudinally.

Normally, if the walls are thin and well defined, this represents mineralization of the bronchi, whereas, if they are thick and less defined this is more indicative of inflammation or infiltration.

Bronchiectasis is seen as distended and irregular bronchi that do not taper towards the periphery of the lung field as would be normal. This is **rare in cats** and is usually a sequel to chronic inflammatory bronchopulmonary disease, especially chronic bronchitis, neoplasia, or bronchopneumonia.

In **older cats, a mild or moderate bronchial pattern** can be observed with **no associated clinical signs.** It is unclear whether this is due to normal degeneration or previous or subclinical disease.

Differential diagnoses:

- Normal in old cats.
- Bacterial, viral or allergic (asthma) bronchitis (Figure 30).
- Neoplasia (Figure 31).
- Lymphoma (along with masses and nodules).

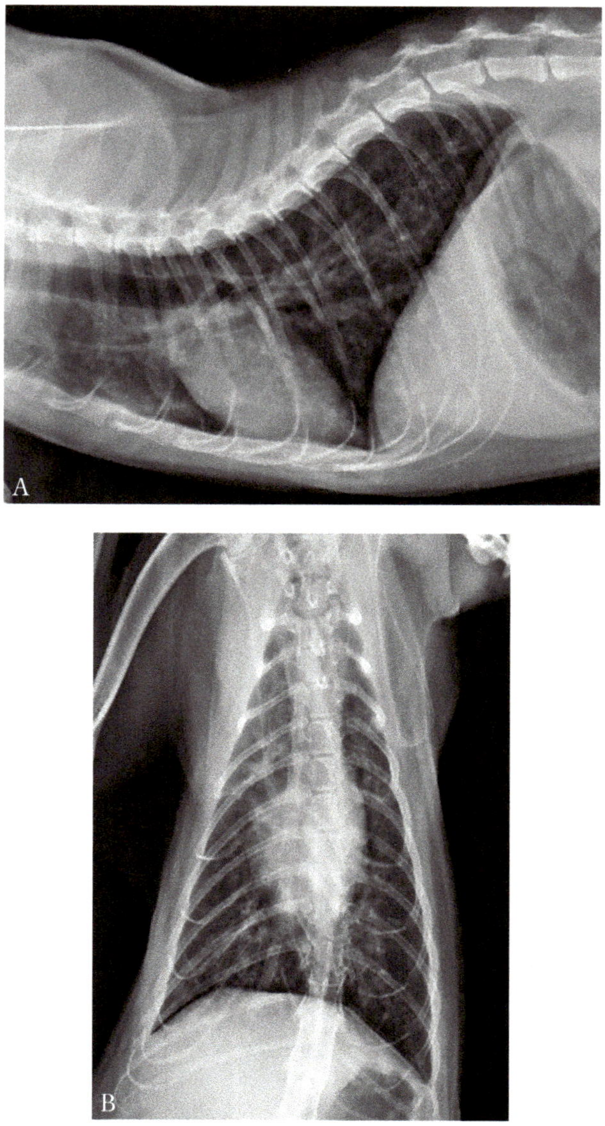

Figure 30. Partial enlargements of lateral (A) and VD (B) projections in a patient with infectious bronchitis where a marked bronchial pattern can be seen.

- Oedema of the bronchial wall. It can be part of alveolar or interstitial oedema.

Alveolar pattern

Seen as **an increase in the opacity of the lung because the alveoli are filled with fluid or soft tissue**, or completely collapsed and without air.

Radiographic features:

- Increased soft tissue opacity in the lung field.
- Presence of **air bronchograms**.
- **Border effacement** (silhouette sign) of adjacent soft tissue or liquid structures.
- Loss of visualization of vessels.

Air bronchograms are a reliable indicator of an alveolar pattern. However, the **absence of bronchograms**

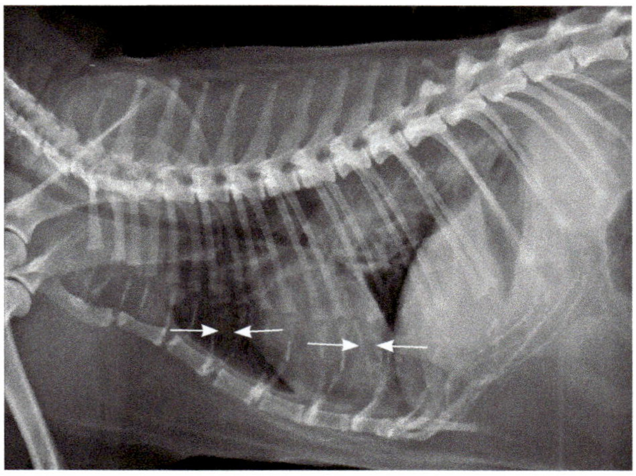

Figure 31. Patient with a pulmonary mass in the left caudal lobe in addition to a diffuse bronchial pattern. Mild distension and decreased tapering of several bronchi (arrows) can be seen, compatible with bronchiectasis.

does not exclude an alveolar pattern, since, if the bronchus fills with tissue or fluid and no longer contains air, the effect of the bronchogram will disappear.

If the area affected with the alveolar pattern is smaller than the lobe, it will have poorly defined margins, showing a **cotton or cloud like appearance**. If an entire lobe is affected, the edges (silhouette sign) with adjacent soft tissue structures (heart, diaphragm) will be effaced and/or a lobar sign will occur with the adjacent aerated lung. The lobar sign occurs when the lobe is fully consolidated or collapsed, so that its edge with the adjacent aerated lung becomes visible.

The causes of an alveolar pattern include any type of **material filling the alveoli** or its collapse/atelectasis (absence of air). The main differential diagnoses can be summarized as:

- Oedema
  - Cardiogenic
  - Non cardiogenic
- Pneumonia (Figure 32)
  - Bronchopneumonia
  - Aspiration pneumonia
  - Foreign body aspiration
  - Bacterial
  - Parasitic
  - Fungal
- Haemorrhagic
  - Trauma
  - Coagulopathy.
- Neoplasia.
- Atelectasis:
  - Due to recumbency.
  - Pleural effusion/pneumothorax.
  - Pleural/costal mass.
  - Small airway obstruction/asthma (right middle and cranial lobes).
  - Bronchial obstruction.
- Lobe torsion.
- Pulmonary thromboembolism.

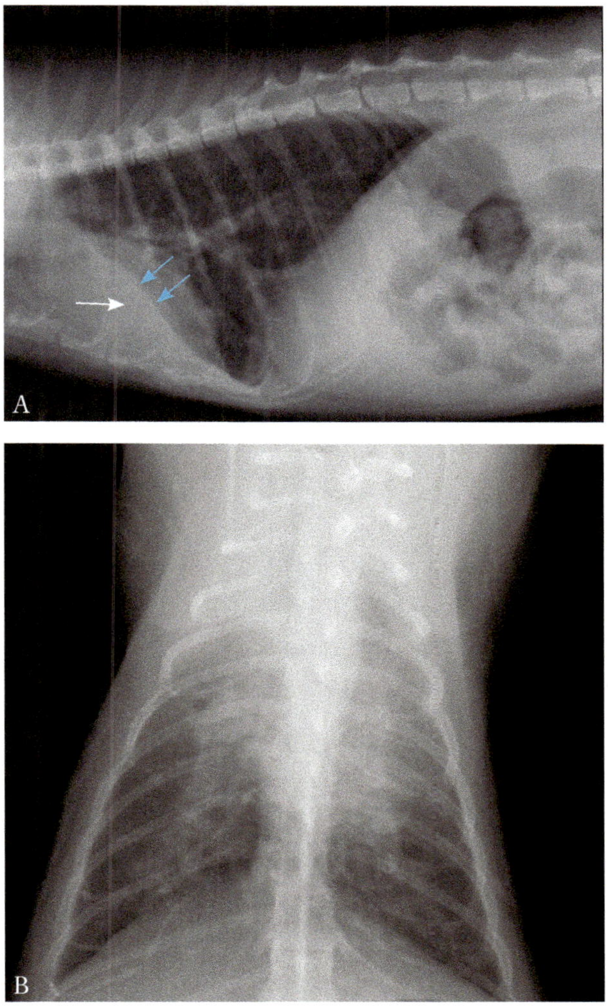

Figure 32. Right lateral (A) and VD (B) projections of a cat with verminous pneumonia (*Aelurostrongylus*). An alveolar pattern can be seen in the cranial lobe with a lobar sign (blue arrows) between this and the right middle lobe and an air bronchogram (white arrow).

Interstitial pattern

The interstitial pattern is divided into:

1. **Nodular**: caused by nodular lesions originating in the interstitium.
2. **Unstructured**: caused by diffuse infiltration of the interstitial space.

Nodular interstitial pattern

Radiographic features:

- Soft tissue opacity nodules (**minimum 3–5 mm to be visible**).
- Its opacity depends on size and number of nodules.

- Lesions less than 3 mm may be visible in case of **multiple overlapping small lesions** – miliary lesions.
- The nodular pattern also includes cavitated nodular lesions, which contain gas.

Differential diagnoses:

- Nipples, cutaneous nodules
- End-on vessels
- Metastasis
- Abscesses
- Granulomas
- Lymphosarcoma
- Haematoma
- Cysts
- Pulmonary fibrosis
- Alveolar nodules due to aspiration of radiopaque material (barium)
- Cavitated nodules:
  - With a thin wall
    - Bulla (+/– pneumothorax)
    - Healed abscesses
  - With thick and irregular wall:
    - Neoplasia
    - Abscesses
    - Granulomas.

Primary lung neoplasms usually appear as lung masses (Figure 33), but can present as disseminated lung lesions without a defined mass. They are most commonly seen in the **caudal lobes** and frequently show gas cavities and mineralization (63% and 56% respectively, in a computed tomography study) (Figure 34). In many cases (53% in the same study) they are accompanied by metastasis. Metastatic lung masses and nodules often have less defined margins than in dogs.

The **digits may be sites of predilection for metastasis** of primary lung neoplasms (adenocarcinoma, squamous cell carcinoma, bronchogenic carcinoma) (Figure 35).

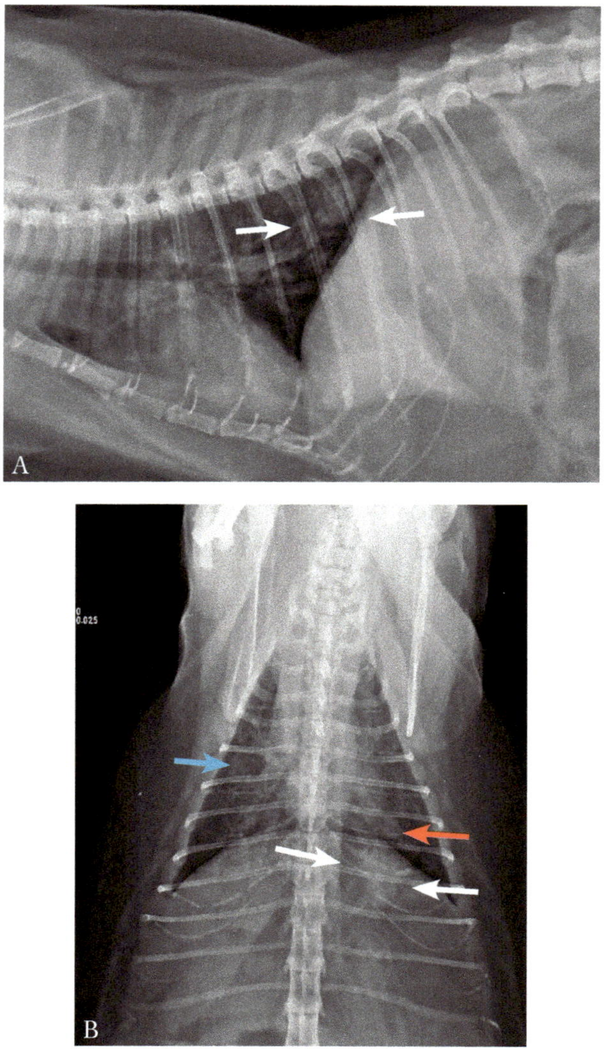

Figure 33. Right lateral (A) and VD (B) projections in a patient with a mass in the left caudal lobe (white arrows), with poorly defined margins, especially in the VD projection (B). Another nodule can also be seen in the VD projection (red arrow), cranial to the mass, but is not seen so clearly in the lateral view. The patient's obesity makes evaluation of the lung field (blue arrow indicating pericardial fat) difficult.

Unstructured interstitial pattern

It is easily **caused by artefacts** and the majority of pathologies in transition (**resolving or initiating**) can present with this pattern.

Radiographic features:

- Mild or moderate increase in lung opacity.
- It can be homogeneous or with **linear, reticular or honeycomb opacities**.
- Compared to an alveolar pattern, the pulmonary vessels are visible, but the margins are not as clear.

Differential diagnoses are the same as for an alveolar pattern. Once possible artefacts (caused by expiration, obesity, movement, etc.) or physiological causes (young or old animals) have been ruled out, the main causes of an unstructured interstitial pattern are:

- Oedema.
- Pneumonia.
- Haemorrhage.
- Neoplasia.
- Allergic disease.
- Pulmonary fibrosis (Figure 36).

Vascular pattern

The vascular pattern may be due to both an **increase in the size of the vessels** (more frequent) and a decrease,

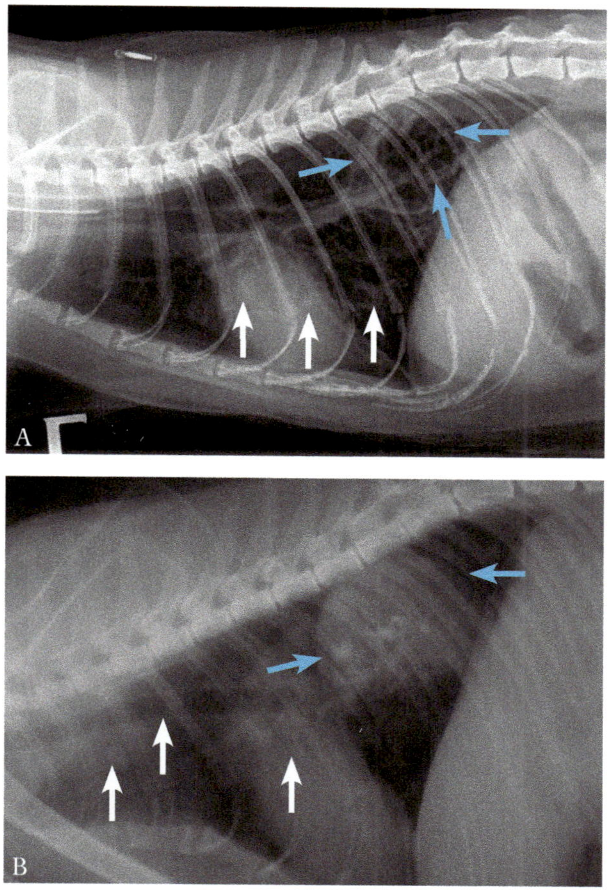

Figure 34. Lateral projections of two cats with pulmonary neoplasia, both with primary masses in the caudal lobes (blue arrows) and other pulmonary nodules (white arrows). Note the cavitation of the mass in image A and mineralisation in image B.

as well as changes in **shape, opacity or number**. In the first case, a difference may be observed between **the size of the veins and the arteries**.

Differential diagnoses for a vascular pattern are:

- Generalized increase in veins and arteries (Figure 37):
    - Passive pulmonary congestion – **left-sided heart failure**.
    - Active pulmonary congestion – **pneumonia**.
    - Left to right shunts:
        - Patent ductus arteriosus.
        - Ventricular septal defect (VSD) and atrial septal defect (ASD).
    - Iatrogenic **overhydration.**
- Veins larger than arteries:
    - Left-sided heart failure.
    - Right to left shunts (relatively smaller arteries).
    - Left to right shunts (in some cases, the veins are more distended than the arteries – septal defects).
- Arteries larger than veins (Figure 38):
    - *Dirofilariasis, Aelurostrongylus*.
    - Large left to right shunts.

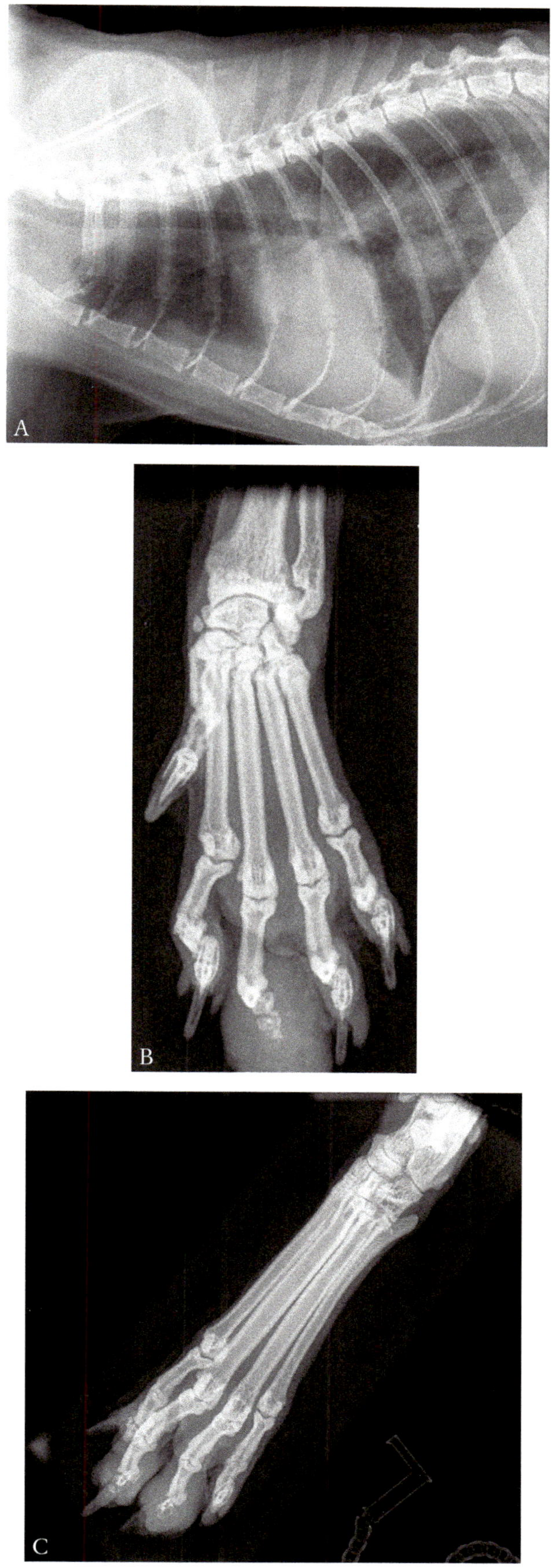

Figure 35. Right lateral projection (A), dorsopalmar projection of the left forelimb (B) and dorsoplantar projection of the left hindlimb (C) in a geriatric patient. In B and C lytic lesions and surrounding soft tissue swelling can be seen in the phalanges due to metastasis of the pulmonary neoplasia visible in image A.

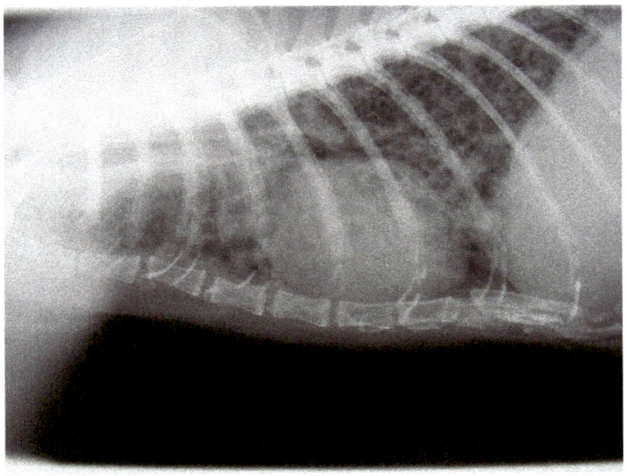

Figure 36. Patient with a history of asthma and pulmonary fibrosis. A mixed pattern can be seen with a diffuse bronchial interstitial pattern and poorly defined alveolar foci cranially on the ventral aspect and superimposed on the cardiac silhouette.

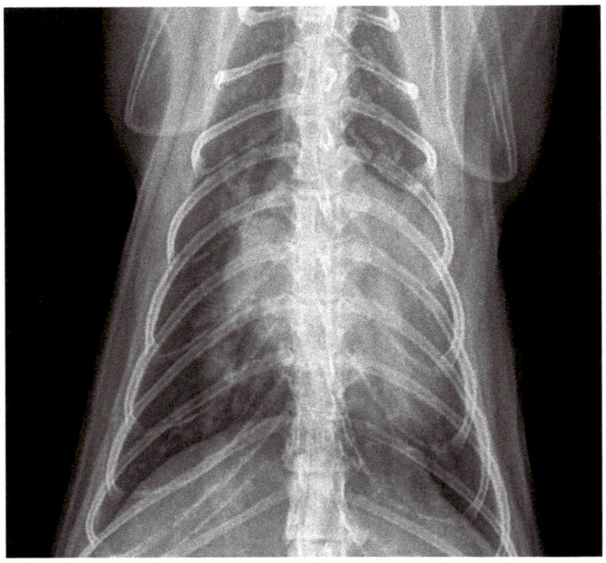

Figure 37. VD projection in a patient with cardiomyopathy. An increase in pulmonary vessels, both veins and arteries, can be seen in the caudal lobes.

- Pulmonary thromboembolism – distended perihilar artery, with abrupt decrease in diameter in the centre or periphery of the lobe, with peripheral hypoperfusion and small or absent return vein.
- Pulmonary hypertension.

Mixed pattern

Many lung pathologies show **more than one pattern**. In these cases, the **predominant pattern should be treated as the most important**. It must also be taken into account that some of the components (for example, bronchial pattern in an old cat) may be incidental.

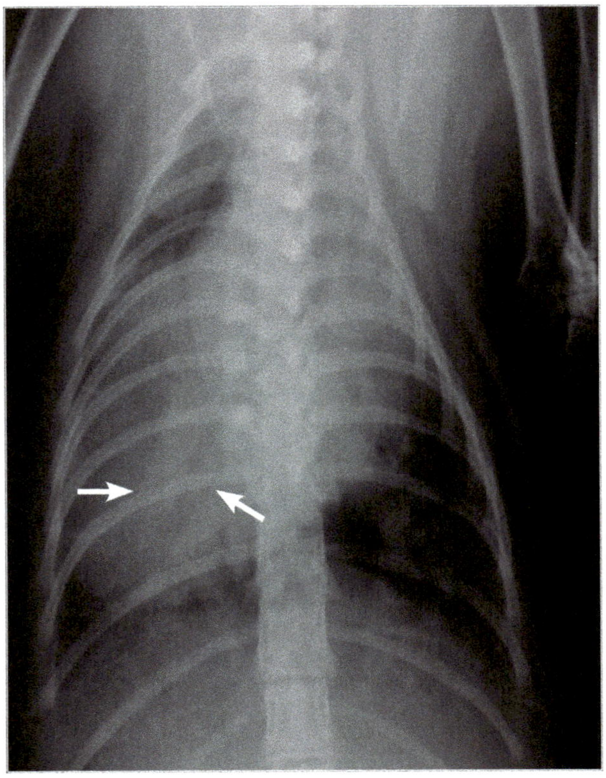

Figure 38. VD projection in a cat with a persistent ductus arteriosus. Note the marked increase in the pulmonary arteries level with the ninth rib.

Decreased lung opacity

Although less frequent, a decrease in normal lung opacity can sometimes be observed. Once the presence of **artefacts** has been ruled out, it may be due to a decrease in one of the components that create soft tissue opacities in the lung field (basically the **blood in the vessels**) or to **an increase in the amount of air.**

Differential diagnoses for a generalized decrease in pulmonary opacity:

- Artefact:
  - Overexposure.
  - Manual forced ventilation/deep inspiration.
  - Emaciation.
- Pulmonary hypoperfusion (hypovascular pattern):
  - Shock.
  - Severe dehydration.
  - Cardiac tamponade.
  - Congenital heart disease with right to left shunt.
  - Severe pulmonary stenosis.
- Air trapping due to expiratory obstruction (+/− increase in the area of the lung field, flattening of the diaphragm):
- Asthma (Figure 39).
- Bronchial or tracheal foreign body.
- Chronic bronchitis.

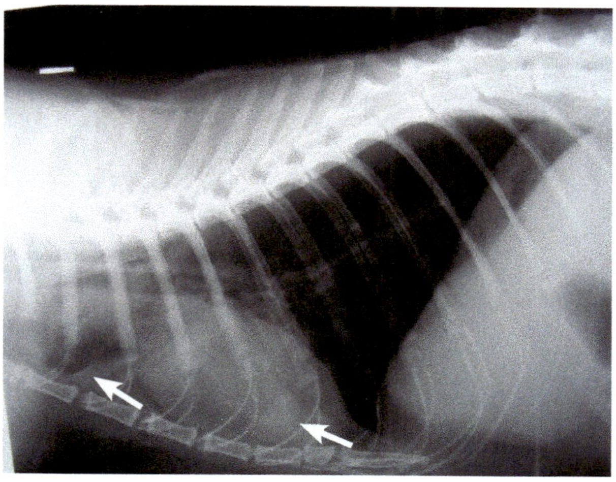

Figure 39. Lateral projection of an asthmatic patient. There is a reduced opacity in the caudodorsal lung lobe. Right cranial lobe collapse and a middle right lobe collapse (on its ventral aspect), can also be seen with the presence of air bronchogram (arrows).

- Obstruction of the upper respiratory tract (nasopharyngeal polyp).
- Pulmonary emphysema.

Abdominal radiology

Peritoneum

Adult cats have a **moderate or marked amount of fat in the peritoneum**, especially in the **falciform ligament.** In **obese cats** (Figure 40), the **small intestine is observed displaced** towards the central aspect of the abdomen and to the right due to the accumulation of peripheral peritoneal fat.

Pneumoperitoneum

Pneumoperitoneum refers to the **accumulation of air in the peritoneum**. The most frequent cause is **iatrogenic**, after a laparotomy, and can persist for up to a month. Pathological causes include **penetrating trauma or perforation of a hollow viscera**, usually the gastrointestinal tract (gastric perforations due to lymphoma and after treatment with anti-inflammatory drugs) and more rarely as a complication of pneumocystography.

Radiographic changes include **increased serosal detail,** due to the presence of gas accumulation, which often appears triangular. The largest volumes accumulate under the ribs, delineating the lobes of the liver, diaphragm, and cranial poles of the kidneys.

Loss of serosal detail

The most frequent causes of a **loss of abdominal detail** include very young patients (due to the presence of brown fat), **emaciation, free fluid, peritonitis** (including steatitis), carcinomatosis, and **large abdominal masses.**

In the presence of abdominal fluid, the displacement of the gastrointestinal tract may indicate a concomitant organomegaly (Figure 41).

In the **wet form of FIP, abdominal effusion** is observed, while in the dry form, with the presence of multiple pyogranulomas, the appearance is similar to a carcinomatosis.

In cats, **steatitis** secondary to vitamin E deficiency, a diet rich in fish or chronic pancreatitis can be seen. Radiographically, it is similar to **focal peritonitis, affecting falciform fat, perirenal fat,** and also large extra-abdominal fat accumulations, such as inguinal fat.

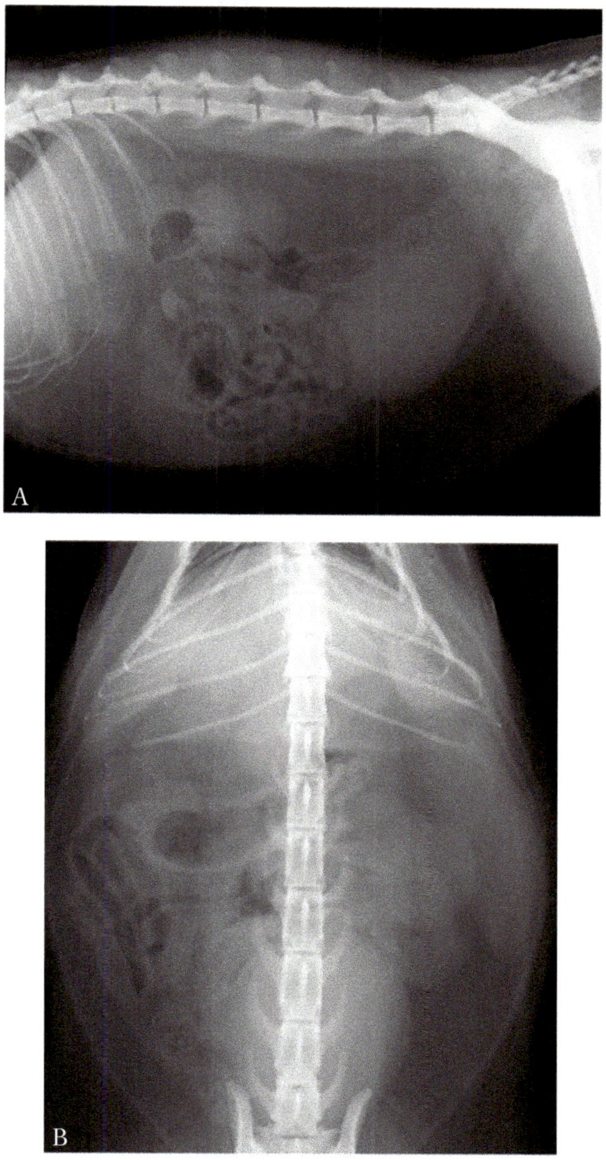

Figure 40. Obese patient with a large amount of peritoneal and retroperitoneal fat. Note the bunched appearance of the small intestine in the central ventral area of the abdomen in the right lateral projection (A) and towards the right in the VD projection (B).

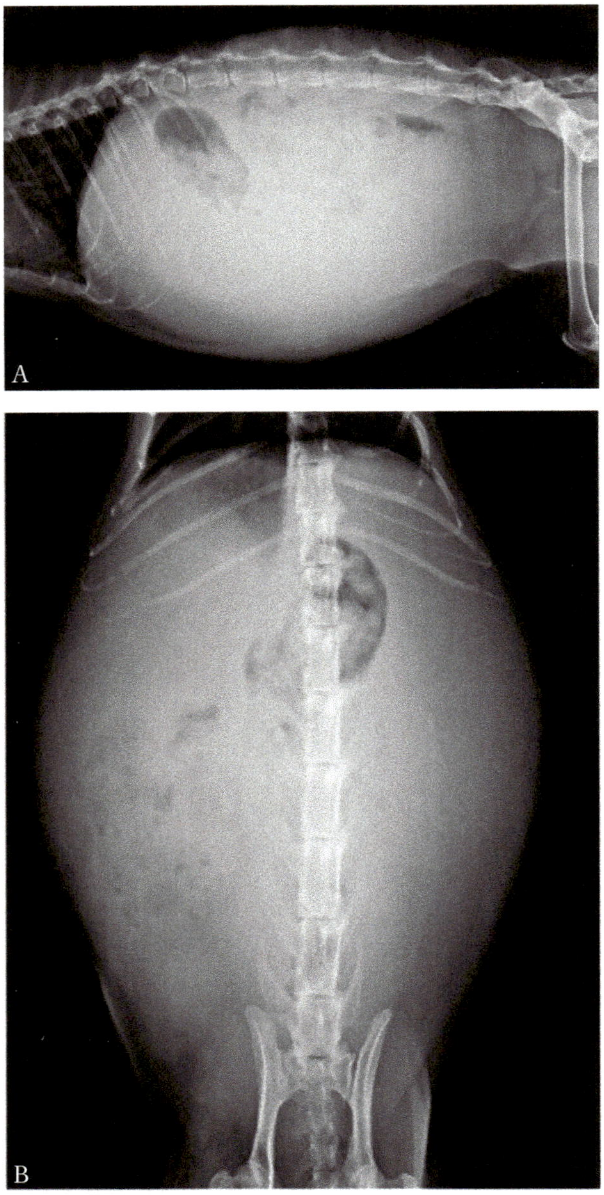

Figure 41. Patient with marked abdominal effusion. The caudal displacement of the stomach with rotation of the gastric axis suggests the presence of concurrent hepatomegaly.

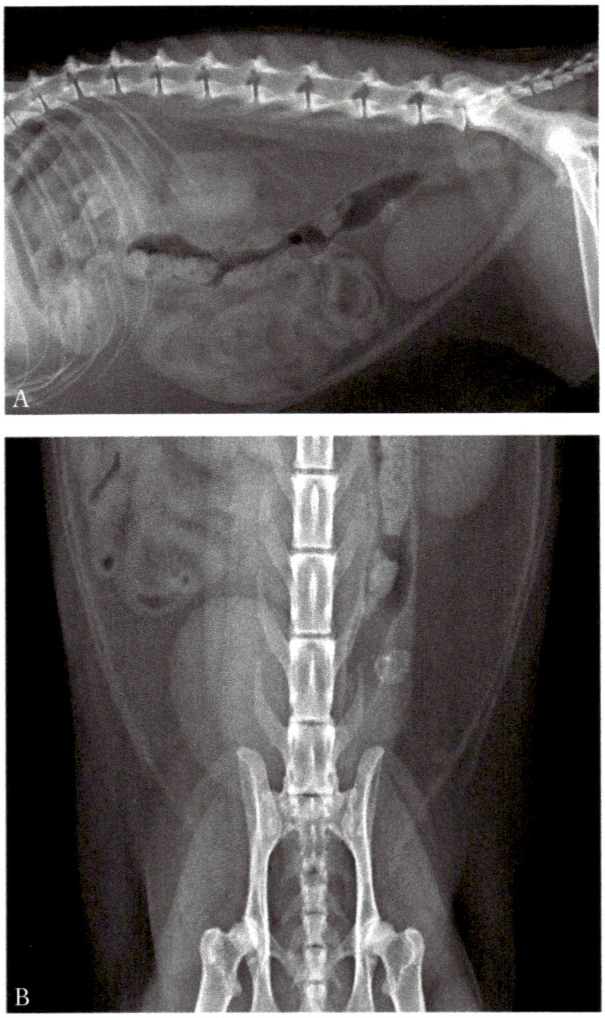

Figure 42. Lateral (A) and cropped VD (B) projections of the abdomen in an obese patient. The presence of an irregular, partially mineralised nodule between the colon and the bladder in the lateral projection and laterally and partially superimposed on the colon in the VD projection can be observed.

Peritoneal masses

Masses of peritoneal origin include **neoplasms, haematomas, abscesses** (perforation, penetrating wounds), or **retention of surgical gauze**. In the case of abscesses, in addition to a mass with soft tissue opacity, a mottled appearance with gas bubbles can be observed.

Occasionally, **nodules of fat necrosis** can be found (Figure 42), which are observed as structures with mineralized edges, with an eggshell appearance. These are not of clinical importance.

Gastrointestinal tract

The stomach in cats (Figure 43) is located towards the **left of the abdomen, and has a J shape**, with the long axis more parallel to the spine than in the dog and with the **pylorus superimposed on the spine. Gastric folds are less prominent** than in dogs. In obese cats, fat opacity in the gastric wall can be seen, which corresponds to fat in the submucosa.

In cats, under normal conditions the **small intestine contains very little gas**. The diameter of a normal small intestinal loop should be similar between loops and should **not exceed 12 mm**.

The **duodenum creates a sharper angle with the pylorus** and, due to the more central position of the stomach, it is also located **closer to the midline** than in dogs. Under normal conditions, symmetric segmental peristaltic waves can be observed that give a pearl necklace appearance (Figure 44).

The caecum is small, non-compartmentalized, and rarely radiographically visible. Both the **caecum and the ascending colon are located medial to the descending duodenum**. The ascending colon continues cranially from the caecum and runs for a

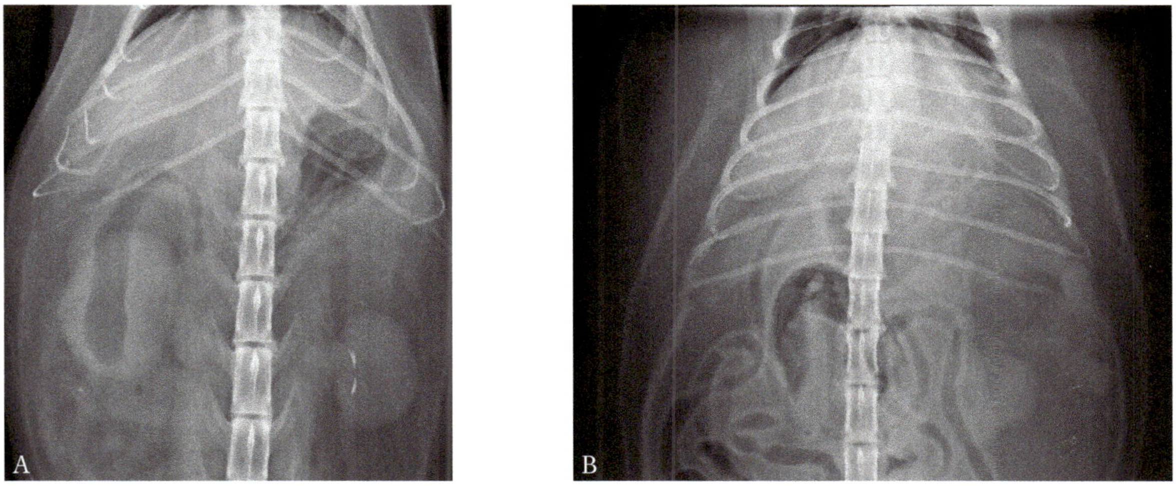

Figure 43. VD projections from two cats with normal stomachs. The cat on the right (B) is obese (note the large amount of subcutaneous fat) and an empty stomach with a fat opacity in the wall, between the mucosa and the most external layer which is of soft tissue opacity can be seen. In image B, the duodenum can also be seen containing gas from the pyloric region.

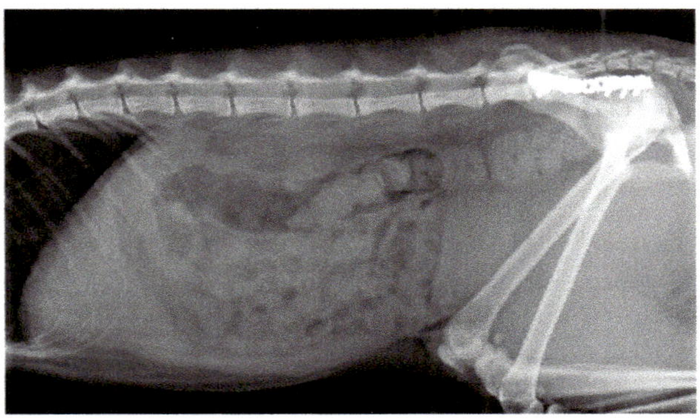

Figure 44. Right lateral projection of a cat with a previous pelvic fracture. The gastrointestinal tract appears within normal limits, with loops of small intestine with small amounts of gas in the lumen and a pearl necklace appearance.

short distance down the right side of the abdomen. Anatomical variations in length and location of the ascending colon can be observed in some animals. When this is the case, it may not be possible to locate the ascending colon, or it may be located further left than normal. The **transverse colon is located caudally to the stomach** and the descending colon along the left side of the abdomen. The **normal diameter of the colon on radiographs should not be more than 1.5 times the length of L5: higher values are indicative of megacolon.**

Foreign bodies

The foreign body's opacity determines whether or not they are directly visible on a radiograph. In cats **linear foreign bodies are common** (Figure 45), and the majority of these are non-radiopaque. The visible changes in these cases include the presence of **bunched together, plicated intestinal loops**, often without a distended appearance. **Teardrop-shaped, triangular, or crescent gas bubbles** are frequently observed.

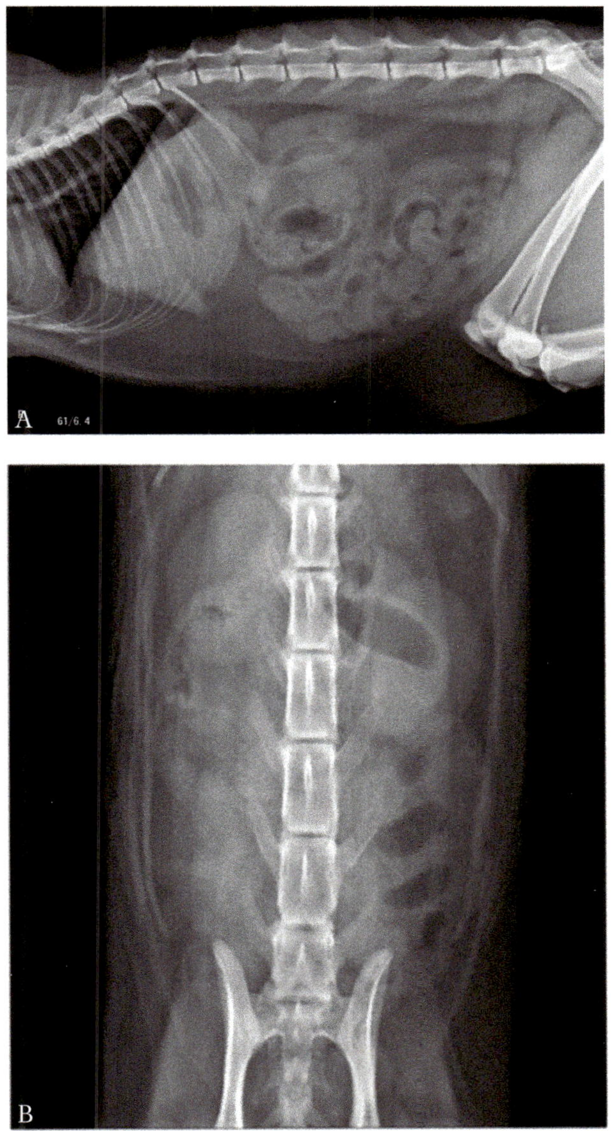

Figure 45. Lateral and VD projections of a patient with a linear foreign body. The loops of the small intestine can be seen bunched together in the caudoventral abdomen, with a plicated appearance and some tear and half-moon shaped gas bubbles.

Non-linear foreign bodies can produce more typical images of obstruction (Figure 46), with **marked distension of intestinal loops**, focally or regionally, with gas and fluid in the lumen.

Neoplasia

The most frequent gastrointestinal neoplasia includes **lymphoma, mastocytoma, or adenocarcinoma**. The first two can occur with diffuse changes that are not detected radiographically. They can also appear as masses (Figure 47), which can be observed radiographically as irregular thickenings of the wall if they are surrounded by gas from the gastrointestinal tract itself. The **lesions tend to be non-obstructive**, so intestinal distention is not frequent.

Invagination

Invaginations can sometimes be detected radiographically, as **elongated tubular structures with soft tissue opacity**. Ileocolic invaginations are located in the middle abdomen, caudal to the stomach. Sometimes gas in the colon can highlight the crescent-shaped edge of the invaginated segment.

Inflammatory lesions

In most cases, radiographic changes in inflammatory lesions are either non-specific or do not even occur.

Liver and gallbladder

The **liver has a constant shape in cats**, it is approximately triangular in lateral projections and does not protrude or only slightly protrudes from the costal arch. In VD projections, the right caudal border is usually more visible and extends more caudally than the left. The **gallbladder** can sometimes be seen as a rounded soft tissue opacity on the ventral aspect of the liver in the lateral view (Figure 48).

Microhepathy

Microhepathy is a reduction in the size of the liver, seen radiographically as a reduction in the anatomical extension of the organ, with **cranial rotation of the gastric axis** (clockwise).

Causes include:

- **Portosystemic shunt** (although microhepathy is less frequent in cats than in dogs with PSS).
- Absence of liver tissue in the abdomen due to **hernias or diaphragmatic ruptures** (Figure 49).

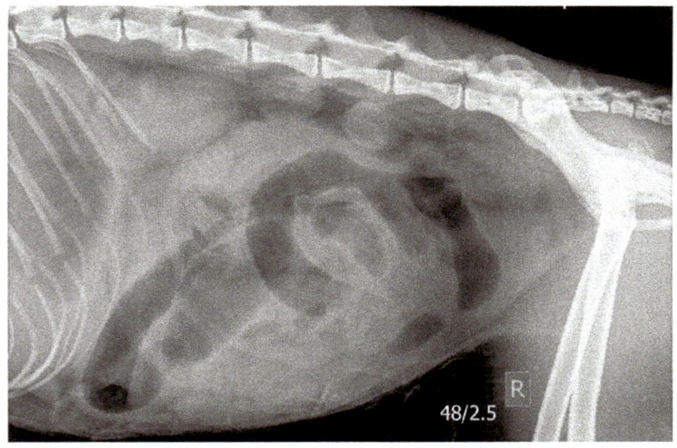

Figure 46. Patient with acute vomiting. Various loops of small intestine can be seen to be markedly distended with gas and liquid while others in the ventral abdomen have a normal diameter. This is suggestive of an obstruction. On abdominal ultrasound a foreign body (button) was seen in the jejunum.

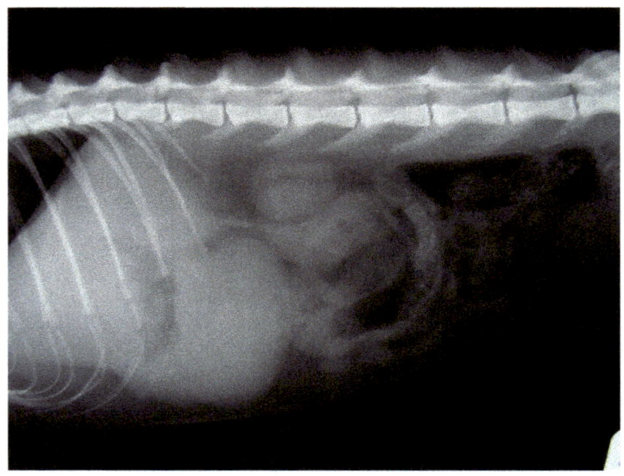

Figure 47. Gastric mass which is growing caudally in a particularly eccentric manner. A small amount of granular mineral material can be seen in the stomach which may be compatible with a mild gravel sign, indicative of a chronic partial obstruction.

Hepatomegaly

An indication of increased liver size (in the lateral view) is the **caudal rotation of the gastric axis (counter clockwise).**

Among the causes of generalized hepatomegaly are the following:

- Passive **congestion** (right heart failure, pericardial tamponade)
- Lipidosis
- Diabetes
- Amyloidosis
- Infiltrative neoplasms (such as lymphoma or other round cell neoplasia).

Local hepatomegaly can be difficult to differentiate from generalized hepatomegaly unless the lesion is in

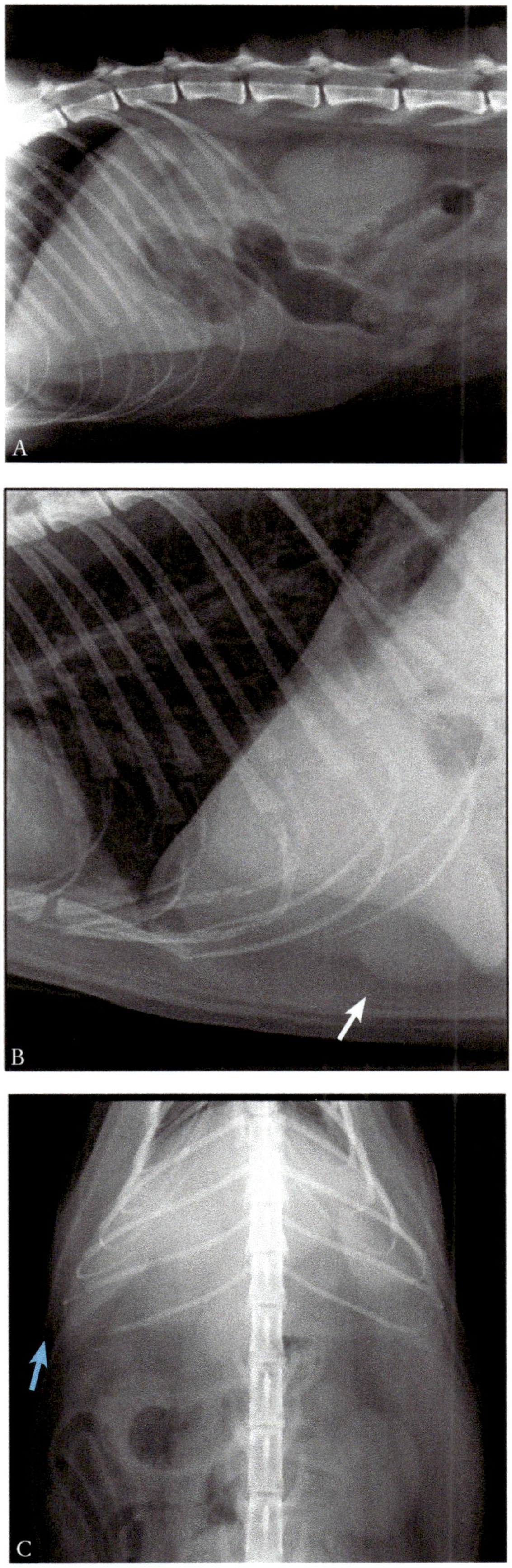

Figure 48. Right lateral (A and B) and VD (C) projections of normal cats. In image A a normal liver can be seen in the lateral projection. In image B the gallbladder can be seen protruding from the ventral border of the liver (white arrow). In image C the right caudal border of the liver is indicated.

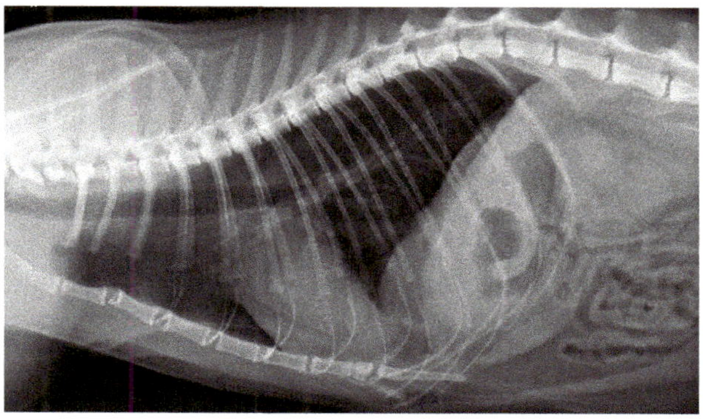

Figure 49. Right lateral projection of a patient involved in a trauma with the presence of soft tissue ventral to the heart. The normal hepatic silhouette cannot be seen in the abdomen and the pyloric antrum is displaced cranially. The patient presented with a diaphragmatic rupture with the left liver lobes in the thorax.

the caudal margin of the liver, allowing differentiation of its edges.

Differential diagnoses of focal hepatomegaly include:

- Primary neoplasms (biliary cystadenoma, hepatocellular or ductal carcinoma)
- Cysts
- Abscess
- Gallbladder distention.

Mineralisation

Mineral opacities can be observed in the gallbladder and bile ducts, which can adopt a branching appearance in the latter. They can be associated with chronic inflammation and obstruction, although they do not always cause clinical signs (Figure 50).

Pancreas

In some obese cats, the left lobe of the pancreas (Figure 51) can be seen on the VD projection as a focal area of soft tissue opacity caudal to the stomach, medial or caudal to the head of the spleen, and cranial to the left kidney.

Pancreatic pathologies

Pancreatic abnormalities are rarely directly visualized radiographically.

Abnormalities associated with pancreatic disease include:

- Loss of peritoneal detail.
- Irregular, ground glass opacity in the pancreatic region.
- Mass effect with lateral displacement of the descending duodenum.

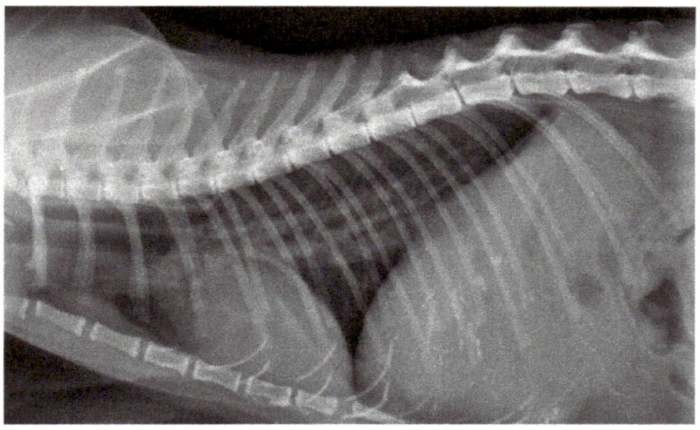

Figure 50. Lateral projection of the thorax in a cat with no hepatobiliary clinical signs at the time she presented. Several mineralizations are seen in the bile ducts and calculi in the gallbladder.

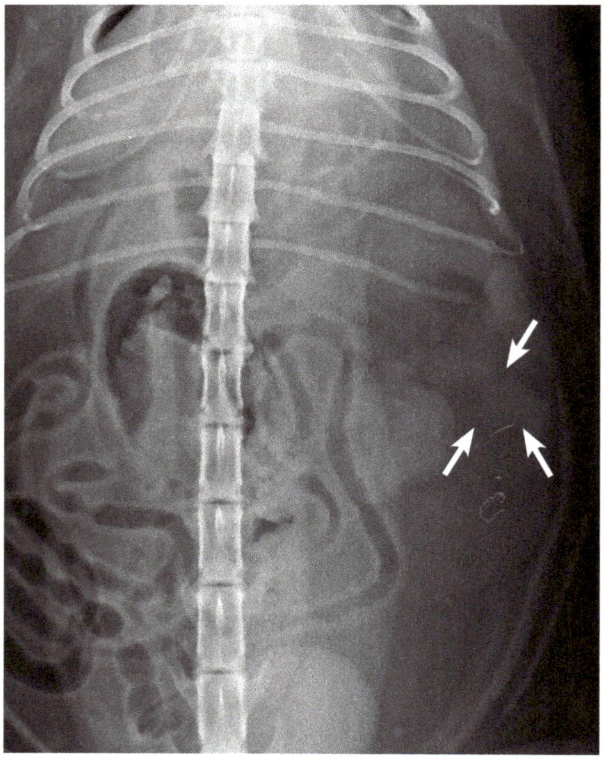

Figure 51. VD projection of an obese patient. The left lobe of the pancreas can be seen (arrows).

- Cranial displacement of the stomach and/or caudal displacement of the transverse colon.
- Gaseous distension of the duodenum.

Spleen

In **lateral views, the head of the spleen is seen as a triangular soft tissue opacity located in the cranio-dorsal abdomen**, between the fundus and the kidneys. The tail of the spleen is not normally seen in the lateral view in the mid-ventral abdomen, although some cats have longer spleens that do reach this region.

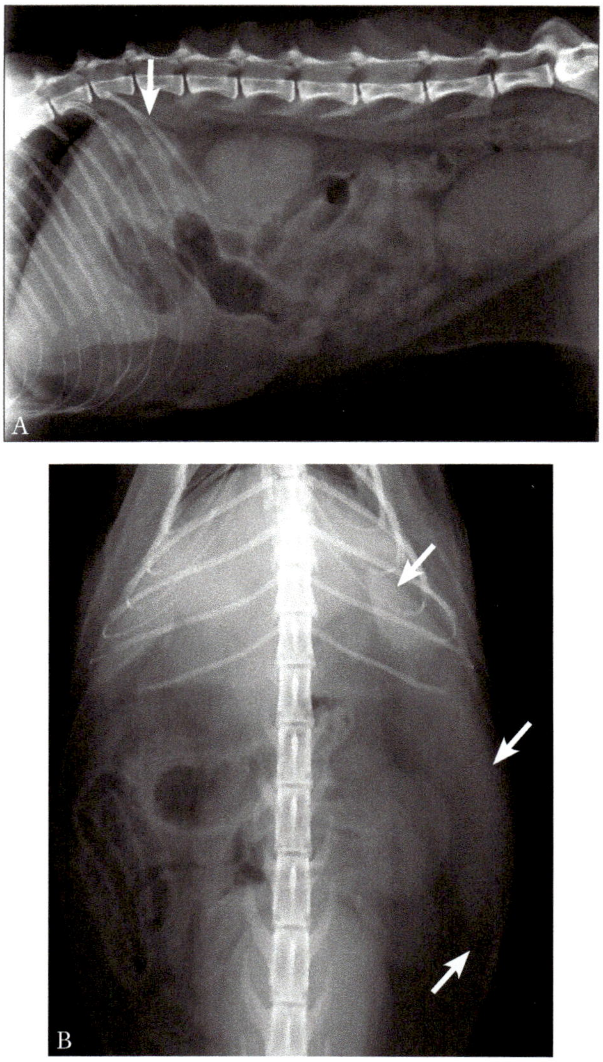

Figure 52. Lateral (A) and VD (B) projections of a cat. In the lateral projection only the head of the spleen can be visualized. In the VD projection the whole length of the spleen can be seen with the head caudal to the liver and body and tail throughout the left lateral abdomen.

In VD projections, the head of the spleen is also visualized in an approximately triangular shape, in the left cranial abdomen, caudal to the liver, and the body and tail are generally visualized caudal to it, in the left lateral abdomen (Figure 52).

Splenomegaly

Splenomegaly is normally suspected when the tail of the spleen is seen in the lateral view in the ventral abdomen. Enlargement of the head of the spleen can also cause caudal displacement of the intestines and left kidney. In cases of diffuse splenomegaly (Figure 53), an enlarged spleen can also be observed, with **rounded margins**.

Focal lesions, such as neoplasms or haematomas, can be visualized if they are large and/or reach the surface of the spleen deforming its normal contour.

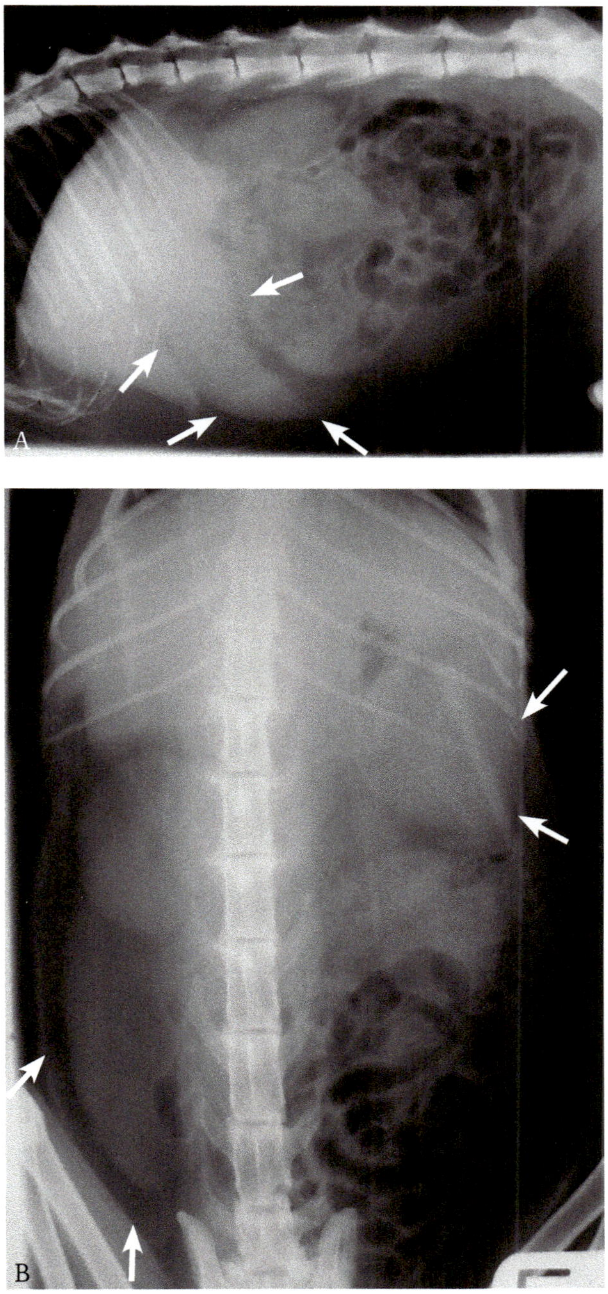

Figure 53. Patient with diffuse splenomegaly due to lymphoma. The large spleen can be seen in both projections, with the body and tail in the cranial and ventral abdomen visible in the lateral projection (A) and the head in the left cranial abdomen with the body extending towards the right lateral ventral abdomen in the VD projection (B).

Adrenal glands

Normal adrenal glands are not usually visualized on radiographs. However, in geriatric cats the adrenal glands can develop **mineralized foci** and be seen radiographically (Figure 54). This is considered a finding with no clinical importance.

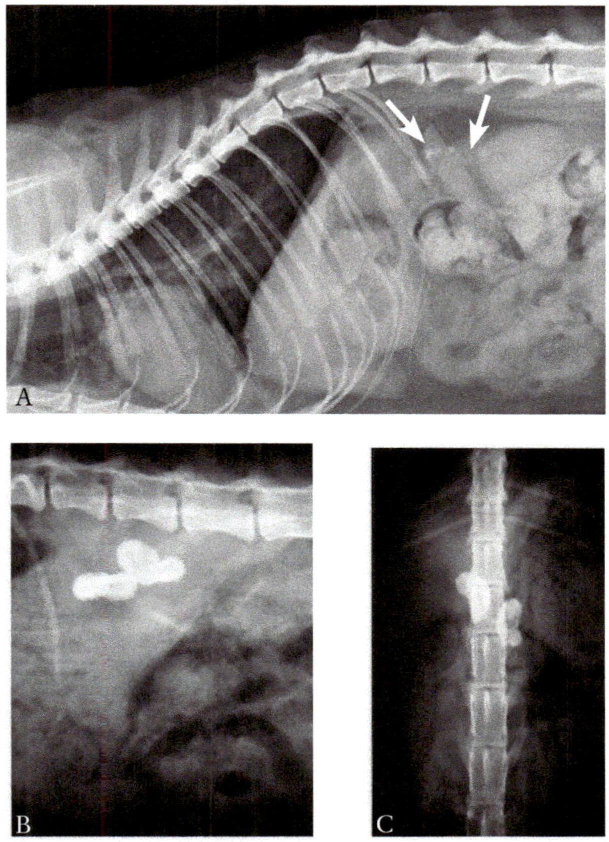

Figure 54. Lateral (A and B) and ventrodorsal (C) projections of the cranial abdomen of two geriatric cats. In image A mineralised foci can be seen in both adrenal glands. Images B and C are from another patient where marked mineralisation can be seen in both adrenal glands, although they maintain their normal shape and size. Mild changes, such as those in image A are seen most commonly.

Adrenal gland abnormalities

Radiographic visualization of adrenal gland abnormalities is rare. Signs of an **adrenal mass can be visualized if they exceed 2 cm in diameter** (Figure 55) or even earlier in cats if they are surrounded by fat.

Kidneys and ureters

Radiographically, in cats normal kidneys (Figure 56) are **between 2.1–3.2 times the length of L2 in unneutered cats** with slightly lower values in neutered cats (1.9–2.6). They present a regular contour with soft tissue opacity, although the renal pelvis can be seen as a more radiolucent region due to the presence of fat. The **right kidney may be more cranial** or at the same level as the left.

The **ureters are not visualized** in most cases, but in patients with a large amount of retroperitoneal fat they may become visible as thin structures with soft tissue opacity in the retroperitoneum.

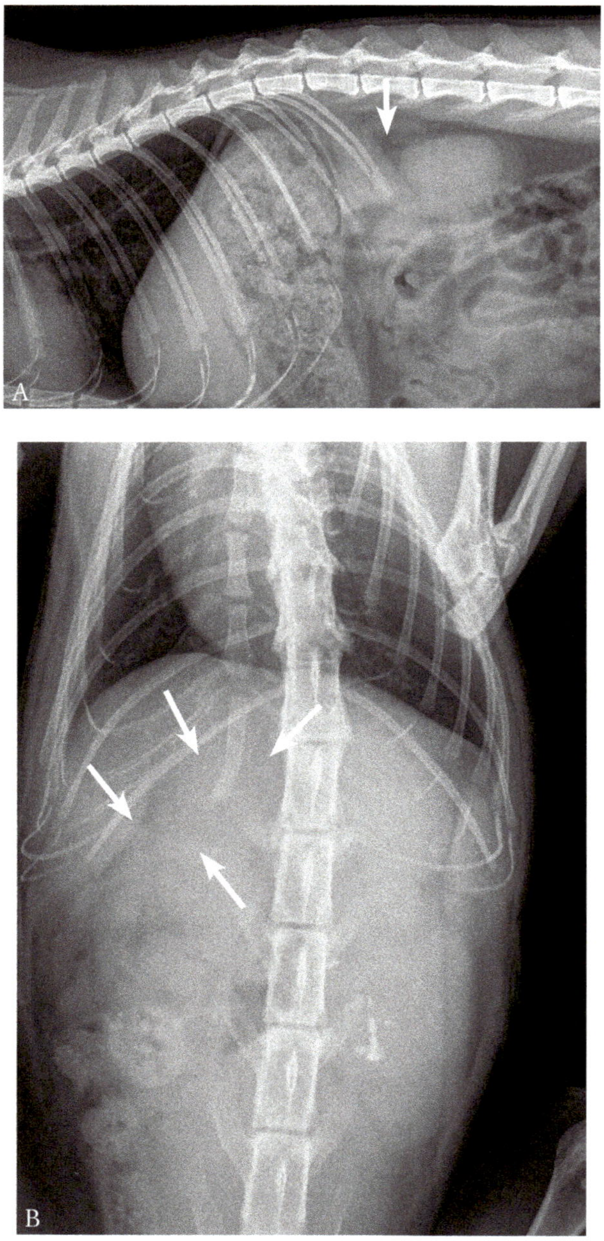

Figure 55. Lateral (A) and VD (B) projections from two different patients, with enlarged adrenal glands. In the lateral projection an oval soft tissue opacity measuring approximately 1 cm in thickness can be seen, positioned dorsal to the cranial pole of the kidneys. In the VD projection a rounded mass can be seen, measuring just over 2 cm in the right cranial abdomen. Both lesions were confirmed ultrasonographically. In the VD projection calculi in the left kidney can also be seen along with an increase in size due to hydronephrosis.

Renomegaly

In **severe cases, a mass effect** can be observed radiographically which displaces the abdominal viscera, either caudally or medially, especially the intestine.

Differential diagnoses for renomegaly with a regular contour (Figure 57) include:

- Compensatory hypertrophy
- Lymphoma

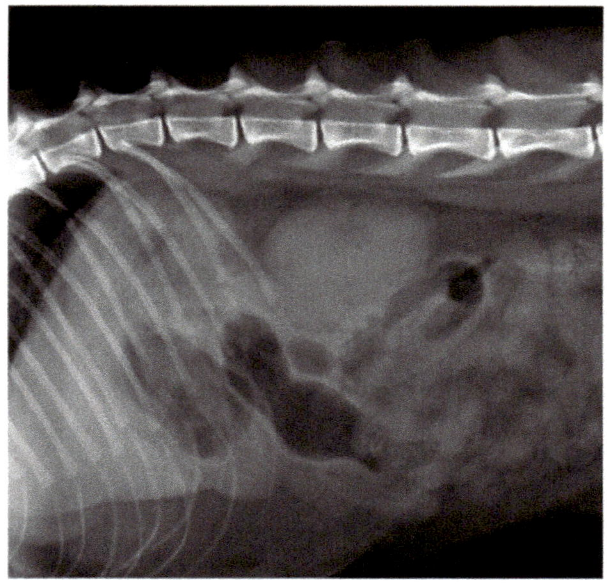

Figure 56. Lateral projection from a patient with normal kidneys, which are both practically at the same level and superimposed. The renal pelvis can be seen in the hilar regions as a more radiolucent area with a fat opacity.

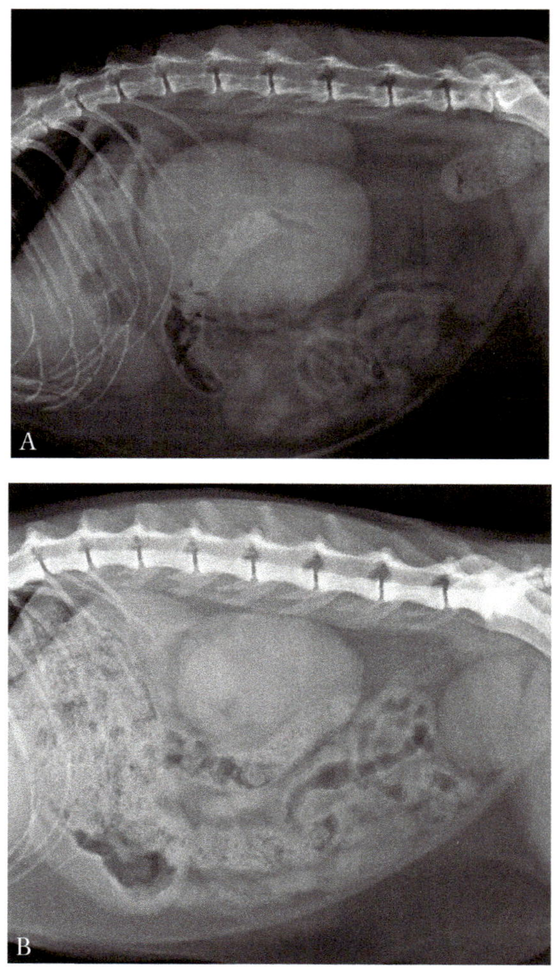

Figure 57. Lateral projections of two patients with renomegaly. The patient in image A presents with renomegaly with smooth, well-defined edges, due to a perinephric pseudocyst. In the patient in image B the edges of the kidneys are more irregular, a consequence of, in this case a renal carcinoma.

- Hydronephrosis
- Perinephric pseudocyst
- Acute nephritis
- Intoxication
- Acute renal failure
- Amyloidosis
- FIP.

In cases of renomegaly with irregular margins, differential diagnoses include:

- Neoplasia
- Renal cysts (including polycystic kidney disease)
- FIP
- Abscess
- Haematoma.

In cases of **acute renal failure, a slight retroperitoneal perirenal effusion** can sometimes be observed, with a reduction in detail in this area and consequent blurring of the margins of the kidneys (Figure 58).

Reduction in renal size

Differential diagnoses for reduced-size kidneys include:

- **Chronic kidney disease** (irregular margins are usually seen in addition) (Figure 59).
- Hypoplasia.
- Amyloidosis.

Calculi

Calculi in cats are frequently composed of **calcium oxalate and therefore radiopaque**.

They can be seen in the pelvis and pelvic diverticula and along the ureters, and in the retroperitoneal space as focal structures with mineral opacity. Calculi in the ureters are usually well visualized in lateral views (Figure 60) but are more difficult to visualize in VD

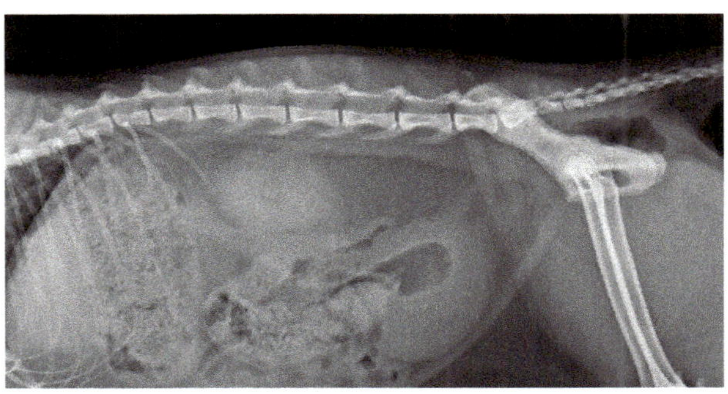

Figure 58. Lateral projection in a patient with a urethral obstruction and acute associated post-renal kidney failure. Slight retroperitoneal effusion can be seen which reduces the visibility of the renal contour, along with loss of detail of the periurethral serosa due to inflammation of the fat and/or a small quantity of liquid in this area.

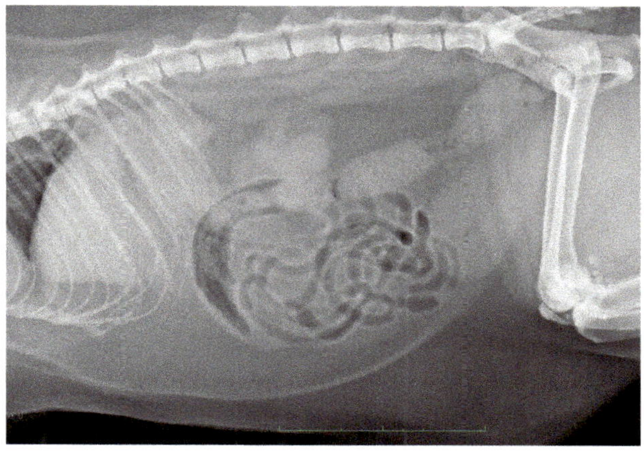

Figure 59. Lateral projection of the abdomen of a cat with chronic renal disease. One kidney (possibly the right) can be seen reduced in size, with an irregular contour.

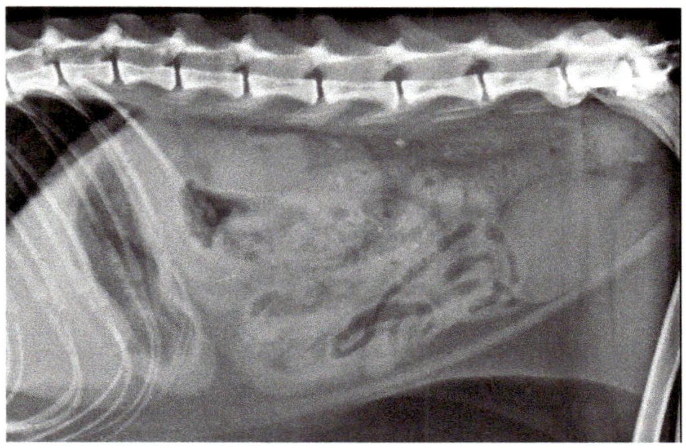

Figure 60. Lateral projection of a cat. Renomegaly of one of the kidneys can be seen and multiple mineral structures in the retroperitoneal space in a linear structure, following the path of the ureters. Just dorsal to the area of the trigone and ventrally and partially superimposed on the colon a group small-sized calculi can be seen.

projections and therefore **lateral views should be used for identification**.

Ectopic ureters

Ectopic ureters are rarely seen in cats. If the ureters are markedly distended, they can be seen as tubular structures in the retroperitoneal space. However, contrast studies are often necessary to visualize the ureters and determine their point of insertion.

Urinary bladder and urethra

In cats the position of the bladder is **intra-abdominal, with the bladder, the trigone and a long part of the urethra in the abdomen**. In animals with good body condition, the urethra is seen as a well-defined tubular structure (Figure 61).

It is important to be aware that male cats may have a **small penile bone** (*os penis*), which should not be confused with a calculus (Figure 62). Radiographically

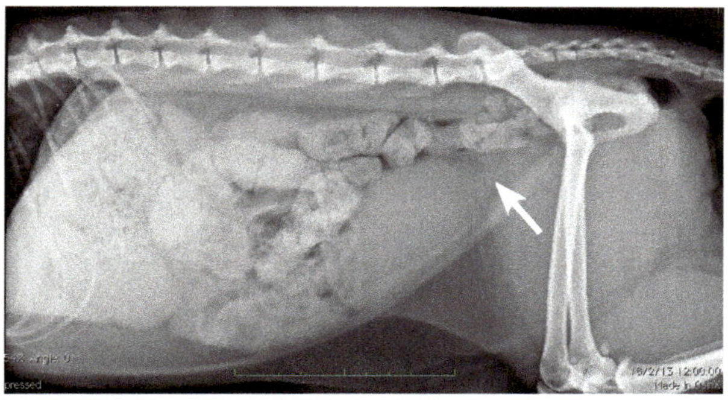

Figure 61. Right lateral projection showing a moderately distended bladder and normal urethra (arrows).

this was detected in approximately 50% of cats, whereas on computed tomography it is visible in 90% of animals.

Bladder rupture

Radiographically a loss of serosal detail can be seen due to the presence of uroabdomen. Viewing the bladder with content inside does not completely rule out bladder rupture, as it may remain partially full. To confirm suspicions, **positive contrast cystography** is necessary.

Bladder diverticula

Diverticula can be seen in some cats in the region of the origin of the urachus at the apex of the bladder. They may be **incidental findings** and, in some cats with a history of urethral obstruction, they seem to resolve after bladder decompression, suggesting that they are not the primary cause.

Wall abnormalities

Thickening of the wall, whether in cases of cystitis or neoplasia, is not visualized on plain radiographs and **contrast radiographs** are necessary to observe its presence (preferably double contrast). However, **ultrasound** has largely replaced radiography when these injuries are suspected.

On plain radiographs, **mineralisation** associated with the lesions can be detected, which can be found both in cases of **chronic cystitis and neoplasms** (Figure 63).

Urethral abnormalities

The most frequent urethral abnormalities in cats include **urethral calculi and plugs**.

Calculi can be visualized more or less easily depending on their location, although they can be difficult to see in the pelvic urethra. Oblique projections can be useful when in doubt (Figure 64).

Urethrography may be required to locate calculi and detect other obstructive causes such as stenosis.

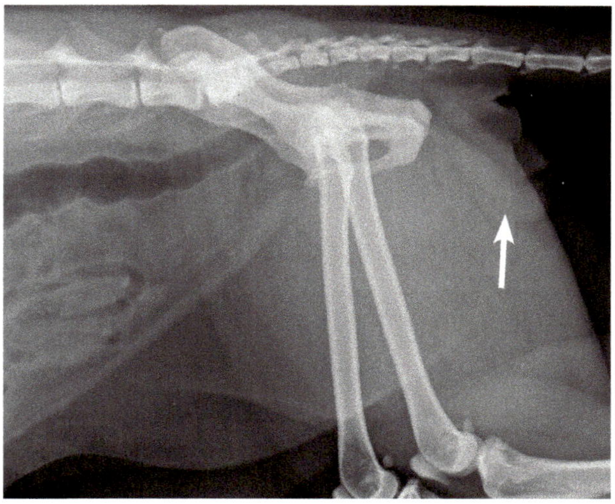

Figure 62. Perineal region of a castrated male cat. A small-sized, elongated structure with a mineral opacity can be seen in the area of the penis, compatible with the penile bone.

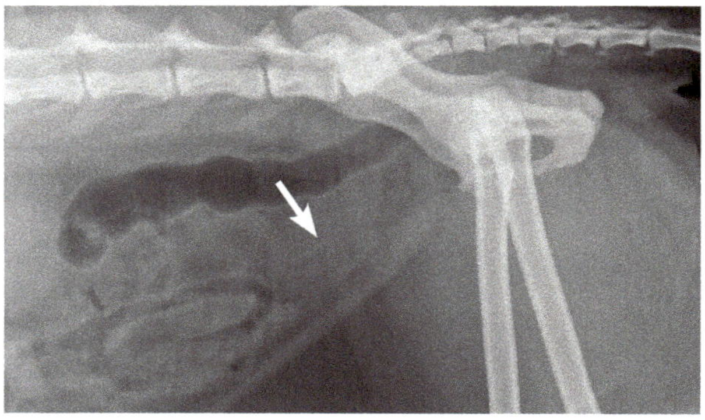

Figure 63. Lateral projection of a patient with chronic cystitis. An irregular, roughly linear mineralization can be seen in the central area of the bladder, which corresponds with mineralisation of the wall.

In cases of **urethral obstruction, a loss of detail of the serosae around the abdominal** urethra can be seen, due to **inflammation of the periurethral fat** and/or the presence of a slight amount of associated free fluid (Figure 65).

Reproductive tract

In healthy unneutered females, the neck of the uterus can sometimes be visualized as a tubular structure with **soft tissue opacity between the colon and the bladder**. Normal ovaries are rarely seen radiographically.

The gravid uterus can start to be visualized enlarged between 25–35 days and **foetal mineralization between 36–45 days.**

In the male's reproductive tract, testicles can be radiographically visualized in uncastrated cats. The prostate cannot be visualized.

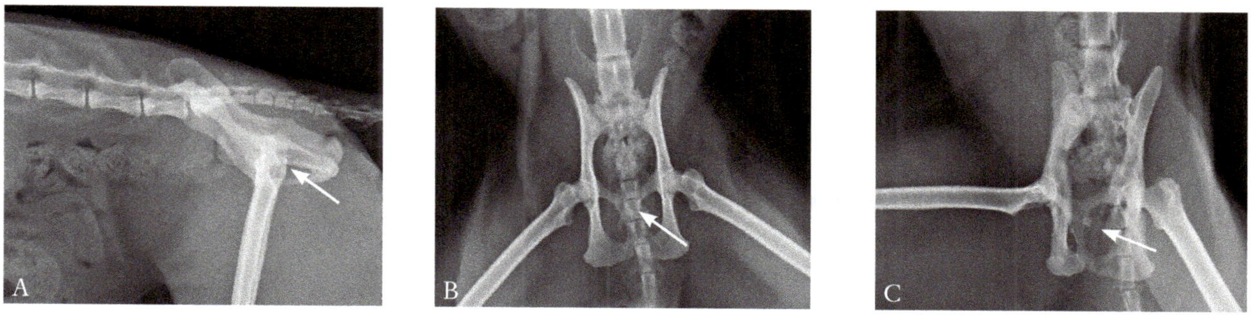

Figure 64. Right lateral (A), VD (B) and oblique (C) projections of a cat with a history of urinary obstruction and suspicions of urethral calculi where difficulty was experienced whilst catheterising. In projections A and B the presence of an intrapelvic calculus superimposed on the pelvis and caudal vertebrae was suspected, which is more evident in the oblique projection.

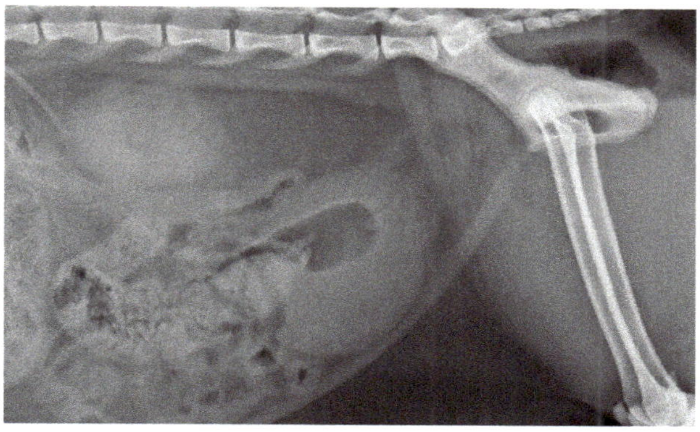

Figure 65. Lateral projection of a patient with urethral obstruction. A loss of serosal detail is seen around the bladder neck and the urethra due to inflammation and/or mild associated periurethral effusion.

Uterine abnormalities

A generalized increase in the size of the uterus is visualized as a tubular structure in the caudoventral abdomen in lateral views and on the lateral sides of the abdomen in VD views. **Pathological thickening (pyometra, mucometra, hydrometra) cannot be distinguished radiographically from a pregnancy before foetal mineralization.**

Occasionally, pyometras may appear as non-uniform focal or multifocal thickenings. Uterine neoplasms, although rare, can also be seen as focal thickenings, although it can be difficult to identify them radiographically as a uterus.

Contrast techniques

Contrast media

There are **two types of radiographic contrasts**, which are described depending on their opacity: **negative (radiolucent)** and **positive (radiopaque)** contrasts.

Negative (radiolucent) contrast

Gases are used to fill hollow organs. The most widely used gas is atmospheric air. CO_2 and N_2O are soluble in plasma and in theory they present a lower risk of gas embolism than atmospheric air.

Positive (radiopaque) contrast

This contains elements with a **high atomic number** (barium, iodine), so **they absorb more X-rays** and present metallic opacity.

Barium

Barium preparations can be found in **different formulations** (powder, liquid, paste, BIPS-Ba impregnated polyethylene spheres) and are used to study the **gastrointestinal tract.** However, their use is **contraindicated if there is suspicion of oesophageal or gastrointestinal perforation**, since they can cause a granulomatous reaction. If the patient is to undergo an endoscopic procedure later, the use of iodinated contrast is preferable.

Iodine-based contrasts

Iodine-based contrasts are marketed in different chemical forms. Iodinated contrasts can be ionic or non-ionic and of high or low osmolality:

- **High osmolar contrast media.** These are ionic compounds, cheaper than those of low osmolarity and can be used for **urinary, gastrointestinal or vascular contrasts** (diatrizoate meglumine/sodium: Gastrografin, Urografin; iotalamic acid: Conray). However, there are **contraindications**, such as their gastrointestinal use in **dehydrated or neonatal patients** since their high osmotic potential attracts water to the gastrointestinal tract, which not only dilutes the contrast but can increase the patient's level of dehydration. In such cases it is preferable to use agents with a low osmolality. These agents are also more irritating to the mucosa and, especially in cats with **cystitis, can irritate the mucosa**. They can also cause **pulmonary oedema** if aspirated, therefore, when there is a possibility of aspiration, agents with a low osmolarity should also be used.

- **Low osmolar contrast media.** These can be ionic or non-ionic (iohexol: Omnipaque; iomeprol: Iomeron; Iopamidol: Scanlux; Ioversol: Optiray, etc.). The use of low osmolar and non-ionic media causes fewer adverse effects (cardiovascular effects, allergic reactions, toxicity). If gastrointestinal or **oesophageal perforation is suspected, or if an endoscopy is to be performed later, low osmolality media should be used.**

Before using these contrast media, it is necessary to **be aware of any renal abnormalities** in the patient and correct alterations of renal parameters, electrolytes and degree of hydration, since a possible complication is acute renal failure, especially in animals with altered renal function or dehydration.

Double contrast

Negative and positive contrast are combined in the same study.

General technical considerations

The study should be properly planned, and the patient prepared. **Plain radiographs should be performed initially**, as some diagnoses may be possible with these radiographs alone, and **contrast may mask injuries** (some foreign bodies for example). Taking plain radiographs before starting the contrast study also ensures that the **exposure factors are correct** and can be used to check whether the patient has been adequately prepared (fasting, enemas).

For **urinary or large intestinal studies**, carrying out **2–3 enemas** the night before +/− in the morning is recommended, **avoiding soapy enemas** since they cause formation of bubbles in the colon. The last enema should be administered about **2–3 hours before the study**.

If urinalysis is necessary, this must be done prior to the contrast study since iodinated contrast will affect the analysis, inhibiting bacterial growth and affecting urine density. Emptying the bladder after urinary contrast techniques is recommended.

If the possibility of performing ultrasound and/or a gastrointestinal barium study is being considered, the **ultrasound must be performed first** since the barium produces a marked acoustic shadow and prevents the evaluation of the gastrointestinal tract with ultrasound. Contrast studies require that the patient be anaesthetized, except for with some gastrointestinal contrasts.

Exposure values should be modified for contrast studies (especially in analogue radiography), reduced slightly (about 5 kVp) for negative contrast studies and increased (between 5–10 kVp) for positive contrasts.

Barium oesophagogram or swallow

Uses

Used for the **diagnosis of oesophageal disorders** (megaoesophagus, oesophageal masses or foreign body, perforation, oesophagitis, diverticulum, motility disorders), differentiation of mediastinal masses, hiatal hernias and vascular ring anomalies.

Fluoroscopy allows better assessment of motility as well as detecting causes of dysphagia in the mouth or oropharynx.

Patient preparation

The patient should be fasted for 24 hours and deprived of water for 12 hours.

Technique

The use of fluoroscopy or **horizontal beam radiography** allows the patient to remain standing and therefore in a normal physiological position during swallowing (Figure 66). This reduces the risk of deviant swallowing, which increases if the patient has to be placed in lateral recumbency.

Preferably barium should be administered (if there is no suspicion or risk of perforation) since it allows better filling of the oesophagus. **Mixing barium with both soft food** (canned/pate) **and dry food** is recommended, since false negatives can be seen if only one of the two is used.

Complications

Inhalation

Barium is usually eliminated by coughing and ciliary movement. Sometimes it is phagocytosed and can remain visible in the lung and/or in the tracheobronchial lymph nodes long after its aspiration. On rare occasions, it can cause pneumonia or a granulomatous reaction.

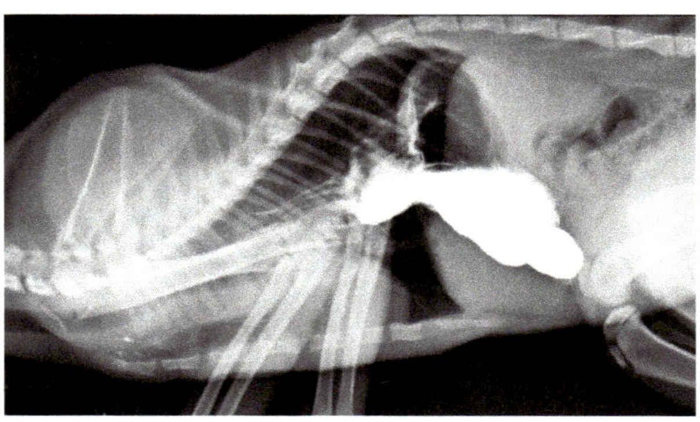

Figure 66. Lateral projection with the patient standing performed with the horizontal beam. Contrast can be seen in the oesophagus and stomach, with the latter partially located in the caudal mediastinum, compatible with a hiatal hernia.

Positive gastrography

This technique is **rarely used** nowadays and has been replaced by ultrasound and gastroscopy.

Uses

Indications include confirming gastric pathologies, **assessing stomach position, size, and shape** when not visible on plain radiographs, and assessing gastric motility.

Patient preparation

The same as for an oesophagogram.

Sedation is not normally required, but if required, **low doses of acepromazine or ketamine** may be used as they do not have a significant effect on gastric motility.

Technique

Administration of **diluted barium sulphate to obtain a suspension with a 30% weight/volume ratio at a dose of 10–15 ml/kg.** Administration via gastric tube.

Right and left lateral projections are performed immediately afterwards and subsequently VD and DV projections should be obtained, which are centred on the stomach and include the caudal oesophagus.

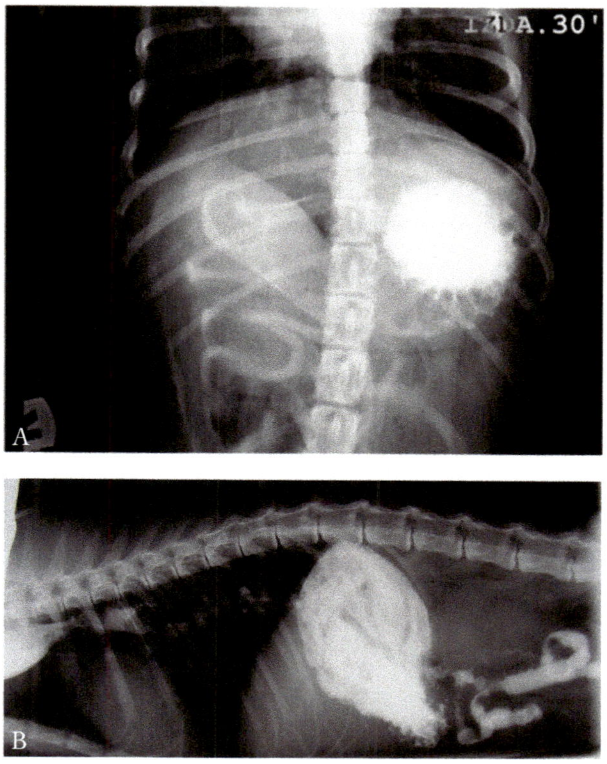

Figure 67. VD (A) and lateral (B) projections in a patient who has been administered contrast due to suspicions of an oesophageal abnormality. The presence of the contrast in the stomach can be seen.

Complications

Introduction of the tube and/or contrast into the trachea.

Contraindications

Suspected **gastrointestinal perforation**. In such cases, non-ionic iodinated contrast should be used to avoid granulomatous barium-induced peritonitis.

Normal appearance

Gastric emptying should begin within one hour after contrast administration and have been **completed in less than five hours in cats**, although gastric emptying and gastrointestinal transit times may vary due to several factors, including patient stress in an unknown environment. Therefore, the usefulness of the technique to assess gastric emptying disorders is limited. As a general rule **the stomach should be empty when the contrast has reached the colon**. The gastric wall and folds should be of uniform thickness and the lumen should be free of filling defects. Distribution of contrast in the stomach should also be uniform, without abnormal displacements (Figure 67).

Pneumogastrography

This is a simple technique, with the same preparation as described previously for an oesophagogram. Approximately **20 ml/kg of air** (or until the distended stomach is palpated) should be administered via a gastric tube. This allows visualization of the interior of this organ and sometimes identification of masses or foreign bodies.

This can also be done when the stomach has been almost completely emptied of barium (double contrast gastrography) to allow for better visualization of the gastric walls.

Upper gastrointestinal series

Uses

Again, the technique has been replaced by **ultrasound**. Its uses include assessment of the stomach and small intestine in cases of vomiting and diarrhoea, especially when a **foreign body or other cause of obstruction is suspected.**

Patient preparation

The same as for the previous techniques, in addition to enemas to eliminate faecal material.

Technique

Administration of barium **13 ml/kg orally or by gastric tube**. Lateral and VD projections should be taken every **10–30 minutes** (depending on the speed of passage observed), until the contrast reaches the colon. If an abnormality is suspected, the projection must be repeated immediately to confirm that it is real, since peristaltic waves can simulate injuries. Real injuries have to be seen in multiple projections and at different times. It is important to note the time elapsed on the radiograph. If a diagnosis has not been reached on the initial radiographs, they must be **repeated after 24 hours**.

Contraindications and complications
The same as for positive gastrography.

Normal appearance
The normal **intestinal mucosa is smooth and uniform.** The distribution of contrast inside must also be uniform, without abnormal displacements. In cats visualisation of **a pearl necklace appearance** due to peristaltic contractions is normal. The typical **small intestine transit time in cats is approximately 1 hour.**

Barium enema, pneumocolonography and double contrast colonography
Uses
Study of **rectal masses, narrowing, and ulcers,** diverticula, hernias, intussusception, location of the colon to differentiate it from the small intestine.

Patient preparation
Fasted for 24 hours. Enemas. It is very important for the colon to be completely empty of stools, as these can create irregularities that simulate injuries.

Technique
- **Barium enema:** the patient must be **anaesthetized.** About **8 ml/kg of barium suspension (one barium part with 2 parts water)** +/– **4 ml/kg** are administered as needed to fully distend the colon. They are administered in the colon, through a **balloon catheter** to prevent leakage. Administration must be slow, and radiographs can be taken to monitor the degree of distension. Lateral and ventrodorsal radiographs should be performed once the colon is distended. Oblique projections may be necessary.
- **Pneumocolonography:** sedation may not be necessary. The catheter (preferably Foley) is placed into the rectum. Administration should be **slow at 8 ml/kg,** avoiding patient discomfort. Lateral, VD and +/– oblique projections are performed immediately, with the catheter still in place to prevent leakage.
- **Double contrast:** after draining the positive contrast from the colon, the same volume of air is injected. This allows evaluation of masses in the colon wall and localization of narrowings or intramural lesions.

Contraindications
Suspected perforation. In these cases, the use of ionic or non-ionic contrast diluted to 20% is recommended.

Complications
Intestinal rupture due to overdistension, especially in cases with obstructive lesions.

Normal appearance
In normal patients (Figure 68), the interface between the barium and the mucosa should be smooth. Peristaltic waves have a corrugated appearance that disappear or differ in subsequent projections. The catheter tip can produce symmetrical narrowing associated with transient local spasticity.

Excretory urography
Uses
Indications for excretory urography include haematuria, incontinence (suspected ectopic ureter), uroabdomen (suspected rupture of the kidney, ureter, or bladder), retroperitoneal effusion, mass in the dorsal abdomen, evaluation of kidney size, shape, or location.

Patient preparation
The patient is preferably **fasted for 24 hours** (12 hours minimum). **Enemas** should be administered the day

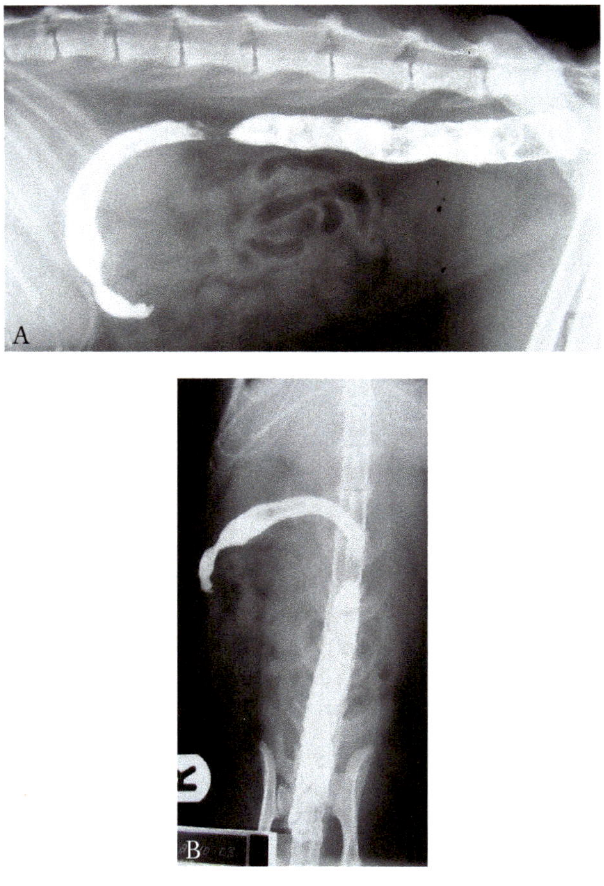

Figure 68. Right lateral (A) and ventrodorsal (B) projections of a patient where contrast was administered orally but has reached the colon. The whole colon and caecum can be seen with contrast and a normal appearance. The filling defect in the descending colon is probably due to peristalsis.

before and two hours before the study. If this is not possible then an enema should be used once the patient is anaesthetized but before the study, to avoid overlapping of faecal material from obscuring the path of the contrast agent.

Technique

Fluid therapy is recommended from the beginning of anaesthesia. An intravenous catheter with as large a gauge as possible should be used. **Warming the contrast agent to body temperature** improves its fluidity and is recommended. In order to achieve adequate opacity the recommended dose is **600–700 mg iodine/kg** (with concentrations of 300–400 mg iodine/ml).

Plain radiographs should be taken first, followed by **penumocystography** to visualize the bladder neck and ureteral insertions.

VD projections should be taken immediately after the contrast is injected, and then at **1, 5, 10 and 20 minute intervals, with lateral +/– oblique projections at 5, 10 and 20 minutes.** Normally this provides good visualization of the ureters and by this time the contrast will have already reached the bladder.

Contraindications

Contraindications for excretory urography include **anuria, dehydration**, and hypersensitivity to iodinated contrast media.

Complications

Complications are less frequent when non-ionic iodine compounds are used. Complicatons include **nausea, vomiting, hypotension, local irritation and acute kidney failure**. In the latter case, persistence of the nephrogram phase or a late pyelographic phase is observed.

Normal appearance

The nephrogram occurs between 5–30 seconds and 5 minutes after injection. Kidneys with increased opacity are seen, where the cortex is more opaque than the medulla in some patients. **The pyelogram** (presence of contrast in pelvic diverticula and the pelvis) occurs between **2–5 minutes after injection.** The normal renal pelvis will be visible as a curvilinear region in the renal hilum.

The ureterogram is first visible 5–10 minutes after administering the contrast medium. The ureters appear as linear structures of regular thickness. Peristalsis of the ureters means they cannot always be followed completely, but "filling defects" appear that change between serial radiographs. For this reason, several radiographs are necessary to visualize the entire ureter. In the trigone region, the ureters are J-shaped or hook-shaped (Figure 69).

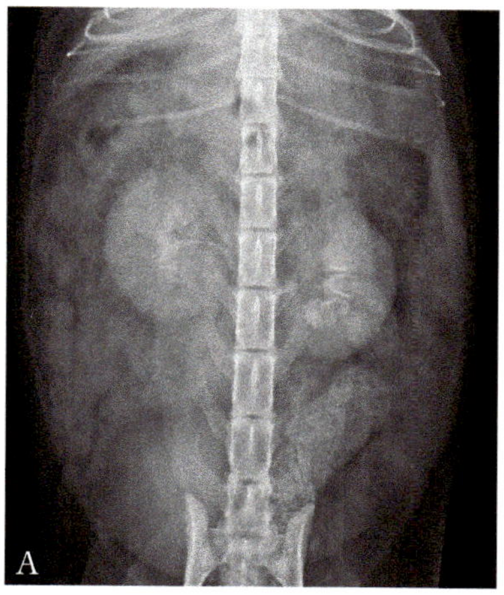

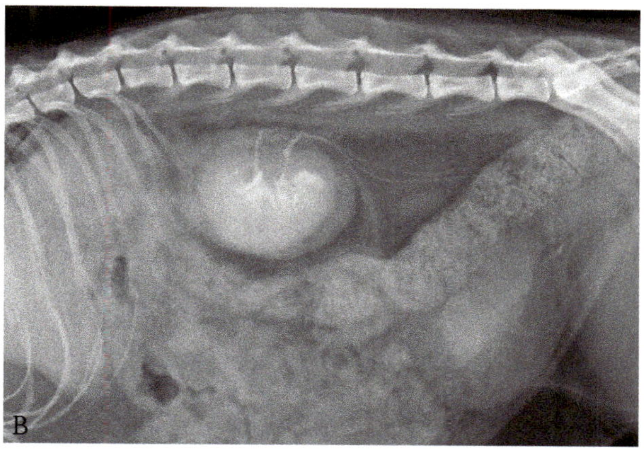

Figure 69. VD (A) and lateral (B) projections showing the pyelogram and ureterogram phase. A reduction in serosal peritoneal detail due to abdominal effusion can also be seen.

Percutaneous positive antegrade pyelography

Uses

This is an alternative method to visualize the kidney and ureter, that is **not limited by poor kidney function** and less likely to cause adverse reactions. It allows **visualisation of the ureter and renal pelvis in a consistent way,** to evaluate the size, shape, diameter and whether the ureter is patent. It is very useful to assess the patency/obstruction of the ureter, especially in cases of hydronephrosis and hydroureter.

Preparation

Preparation is the same as for urography.

Technique

Under ultrasound guidance **iodinated contrast is introduced directly into the renal pelvis**. A needle is inserted into the renal pelvis through a thin area of the renal cortex.

A variable volume of urine is withdrawn and half of that volume of iodinated contrast is injected slowly. Fill can be monitored with fluoroscopy or immediate lateral and VD radiographs.

Complications
Complications include contrast leaking out of the renal pelvis or renal capsule, and renal or subcapsular haemorrhage.

Pneumocystography
Uses
Complementary technique to the majority of urinary contrast studies or, in isolation, above all to locate the bladder with respect to other structures, providing better contrast of the bladder-ureteral junction.

Preparation
The same as for urography.

Technique
The patient should be catheterised with a normal urinary catheter, and the bladder emptied of urine. The catheter must be of a diameter similar to that of the urethra to prevent leakage. Subsequently about **5 ml/kg (up to about 12 ml/kg) of air** should be introduced, monitoring until a firm bladder or pressure in the syringe can be felt.

Contraindications
If severe cystitis is suspected, **gas embolism may occur.** In these cases, plasma soluble gases (CO_2) should be used to avoid possible fatal consequences.

Complications
Complications include **bladder rupture** due to over-distension or previous intervention and intramural air due to traumatic catheterization. **Gas embolism and death** are possible (plasma soluble gases should be used and the patient placed in left lateral recumbency so that the air dissipates on the right side of the heart).

Normal appearance
The **bladder appears uniformly distended with a tear shape**, without filling defects and with a thin wall. Under normal conditions, the ureters and renal pelvis should not be filled.

Positive cystography
Uses
Positive cystography is used to assess suspicions of **bladder or urethral rupture**, although it is not currently widely used (Figure 70).

Preparation
As above for urography, although in many cases it is performed in an emergency situation and there is no time to prepare the patient.

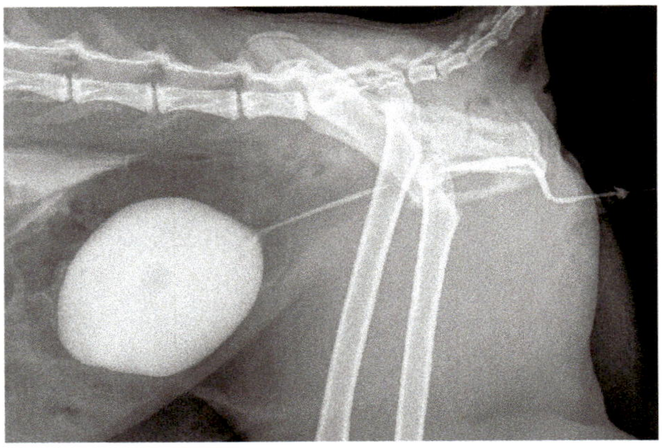

Figure 70. Normal positive urethrocystography in a patient with ureteral rupture (note the presence of retroperitoneal contrast due to the ruptured ureter). An excretory urography had been performed prior to this.

Technique
The patient's urethra is catheterized and contrast introduced. If the urethra needs to be assessed at the same time, the catheter is placed in the penile urethra or in the vaginal vestibule. A volume of 150 mg/kg should be administered (diluting the contrast, using 50% PSS (physiological saline solution), and 50% iodinated contrast at 300 mg/kg).

Contraindications
If very severe cystitis is suspected, it is advisable to use non-ionic iodinated contrast.

Complications
Bladder rupture or wall injury.

Normal appearance
The bladder appears uniformly teardrop-shaped, without filling defects and with a thin wall. Under normal conditions, the ureters and renal pelvis should not be filled. The urethra should be filled evenly and without filling defects.

Double contrast cystography
Uses
This technique is currently **not widely used.** Indications include suspected cystitis, intraluminal and bladder wall lesions.

Preparation
As for urography.

Technique
Pneumocystography is performed in a **lateral projection**. Subsequently, between **1–5 ml of undiluted iodinated contrast medium** is introduced into the bladder and the patient rotated to ensure the distribution of the contrast, although this may produce bubbles. To

avoid this, the alternative is the introduction of the positive contrast into the empty bladder, it should then be massaged to distribute it and subsequently the air introduced.

Lateral +/– VD projections should be performed immediately.

Contraindications
The same as for positive cystography.

Complications
Also, as for positive cystography.

Normal appearance
The bladder appears **uniformly distended with a teardrop shape**, without filling defects and with a **thin wall**. The contrast should be observed accumulating in the centre, surrounded by air and should not adhere to the walls.

Retrograde vaginourethrography
Uses
Urethral diseases (dysuria, stranguria, calculi) or of the **bladder neck**. As a complement to urography to search for ectopic ureters, or even without urography.

Patient preparation
As for urography.

Technique
Pneumocystography facilitates filling and maximum distension of the urethra due to the pressure it exerts contrary to the injection.

A cut tip Foley catheter should be placed in the vaginal vestibule, with the balloon inflated and atraumatic forceps placed on the vulva. As an alternative a normal catheter and clamps covered with cotton or similar material can be used. The catheter is filled with contrast before placing it to avoid the formation of bubbles.

A dose of approximately **1 ml/kg (or 5 ml/cat) of iodinated contrast, diluted to 50% with PSS should be used.** Addition of more contrast may be necessary, to achieve complete filling of the urethra, however, it must be ensured that the absence of filling is not due to obstruction of the urethral papilla due to the balloon, since if contrast continues to be injected in such circumstances, it can cause vaginal rupture. The radiograph should be taken towards the end of the injection.

Contraindications
It is preferable **not to carry out this technique in females in season**, since the vagina is larger and it is harder to fill the urethra in a retrograde manner, as well as due to the possible risk of causing pyometra if the uterine horns are filled.

Complications
Vaginal or urethral rupture.

Normal appearance
The urethra and vagina have **smooth, uniform walls** with no filling defects.

Retrograde urethrography
Indications and patient preparation
As for the retrograde vaginourethrography technique.

Technique
Pneumocystography is performed using an atraumatic catheter (+/– clamps) placed, with the catheter previously filled with iodinated contrast to avoid air bubbles. A **dose of 2–4 ml/cat, diluted 50% with PSS should be used**. The catheter is placed in the penile urethra and the penis and the prepuce are fixed with clamps. The radiograph should be taken at the end of the injection.

Normal appearance
Urethra with smooth, uniform walls. An area of narrowing due to spasm may occur in the area of the ischial arch.

Ultrasound

Liver and gallbladder

The liver is mainly **located cranial to the costal arch**, although on the **right side it may protrude slightly caudal to the costal arch**. The gallbladder is located between the right medial and the quadrate lobes.

The **normal liver parenchyma is hypoechoic with respect to the spleen** and has a more granular texture than the spleen, and is between hypo and hyperechoic with respect to the renal cortex.

For cats in good body condition a variable amount of **falciform fat** can be seen, which is normally **iso or hyperechogenic with respect to the liver** and presents a rougher or striated ultrasonographic appearance. It can also protrude between the left and right sides of the liver. It can sometimes be seen clearly separated from the liver by the liver capsule. In clinically normal obese cats, hyperechogenic liver parenchyma can be observed with respect to falciform fat (Figure 71).

The **gallbladder is seen as an oval or teardrop-shaped structure and anechogenic content**. In cats, it often has a bilobed appearance and some patients

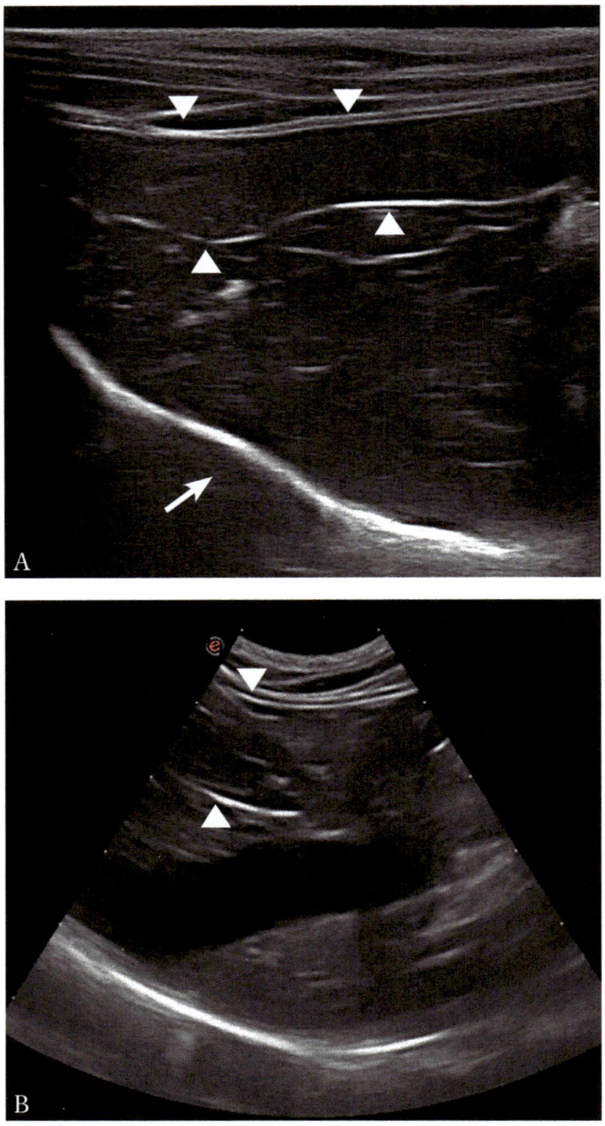

Figure 71. Sagittal sections of the liver in two cats. In image A the tips of the arrows delineate the falciform fat which is hyperechogenic with respect to the liver. In image B with a higher body condition than the cat in image A, the fat is hypoechoic with respect to the liver.

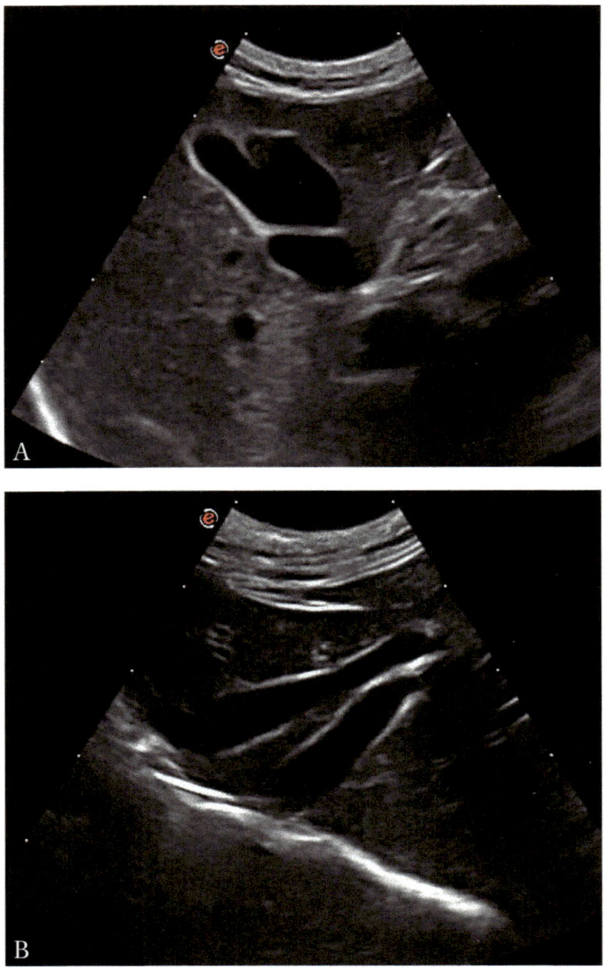

Figure 72. Sagittal sections of the liver and gallbladder in two different patients. A bilobed gallbladder can be seen in the patient image A and a double one in image B.

may have bilobed or double gallbladders, with two separate compartments (Figure 72). **The normal wall of the gallbladder is hyperechogenic and smooth**, measuring less than 1 mm. The size of the gallbladder is variable, and larger in patients which are fasted or anorexic, and cannot be used as a reliable indication of obstruction.

Intrahepatic bile ducts are not visible in normal patients. The cystic duct begins at the neck of the gallbladder and after receiving the last tributary of the hepatic bile duct, forms the common bile duct. In the cat the **common bile duct is more tortuous and can be viewed ultrasonographically ventral to the portal vein near the hepatic hilus** (Figure 73), dorsal to the duodenum, and running parallel to the portal vein for a few centimetres until it reaches the major duodenal papilla. The common bile duct is up to 4 mm in diameter in normal cats. The pancreatic duct joins the common bile duct before the latter enters the sphincter. 20% of cats have an accessory pancreatic duct that drains into the minor duodenal papilla, more distally into the duodenum.

Diffuse liver abnormalities

Changes in the echogenicity of the liver can be assessed by **comparing its echogenicity with that of the spleen at the same depth**, as well as by visualizing the walls of the portal vessels. In a liver with increased echogenicity, visualization of the walls of the portal vessels (which in normal conditions are hyperechoic) is reduced, whereas when the liver is more hypoechogenic, the walls of the portal vessels are more evident.

These changes can also affect the size and contour of the liver.

Lipidosis

Ultrasonographic findings in patients with lipidosis include **diffuse hepatomegaly** and a diffuse **increase**

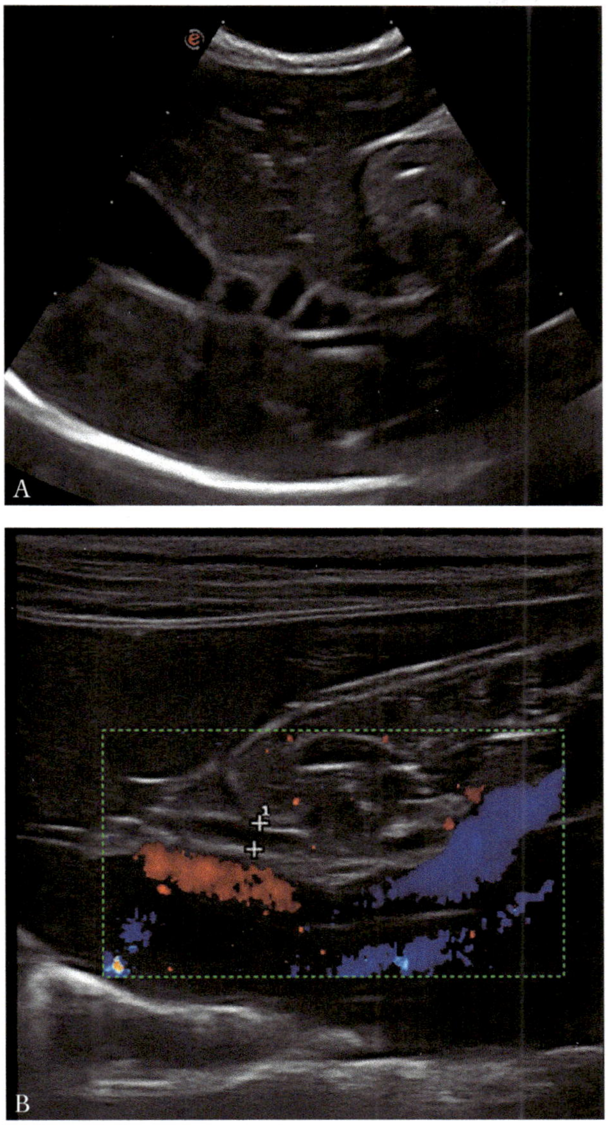

Figure 73. Sagittal sections near the hepatic hilus where the tortuous cystic duct/choledocus can be seen in image A and where the common byle duct is seen ventral to the vena porta, where flow is shown with colour Doppler in image B.

in echogenicity (Figure 74). Lipidosis can also increase the attenuation of the ultrasound waves.

Inflammatory/infectious abnormalities

Cholangitis (Figure 75) is usually seen as a decrease or increase in echogenicity of the liver and associated with changes in the biliary system, such as thickening of the gallbladder wall, biliary sludge, cholelithiasis, and bile duct distension. Concomitant changes in the echogenicity of the pancreas and an increase in its thickness can also be observed.

However, many cats with cholangitis do not show ultrasonographic changes.

Feline infectious peritonitis can cause diffuse changes in the liver, sometimes with hepatomegaly, hypoechogenic parenchyma, or, less frequently, a diffuse hyperechoic appearance, with hypoechogenic focal or multifocal regions and irregular edges. In many cases ultrasonographic changes may not be seen despite the presence of histopathological lesions. The presence of granulomas has also been described, which appear in the form of hyperechogenic nodules.

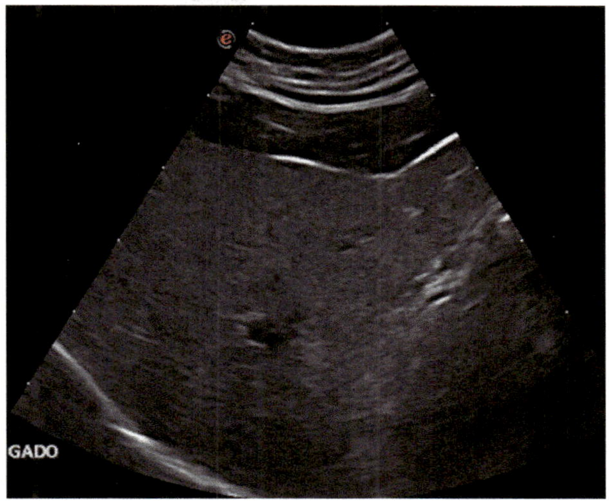

Figure 74. Sagittal section of the liver in a patient with lipidosis. An increase in the echogenicity of the liver with reduced visualisation of the walls of the portal veins is seen.

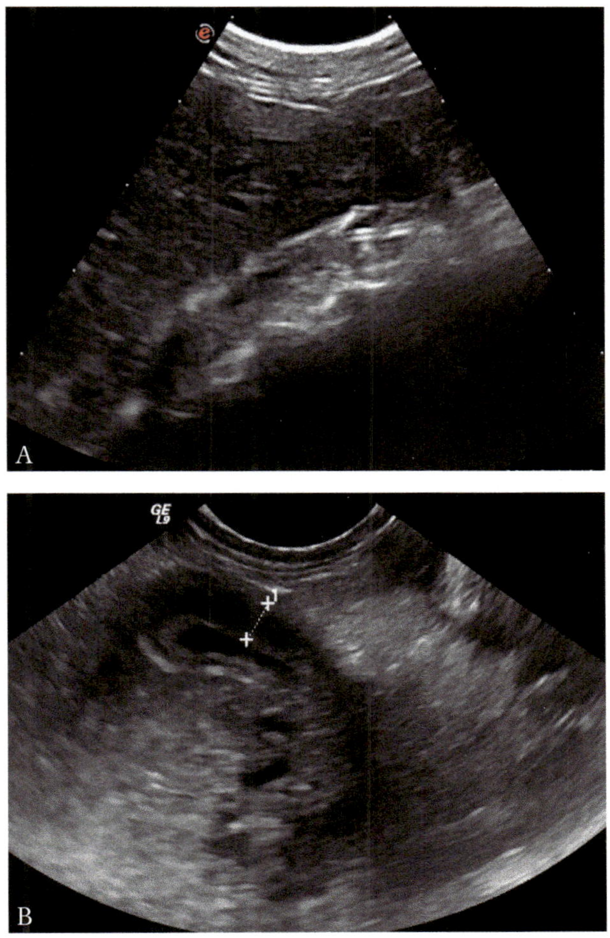

Figure 75. Images of patients with cholangitis. In image A a reduction in echogenicity and hepatomegaly are seen, with rounded hepatic edges. In image B an increase in the echogenicity of the liver and thickening of the wall of the gallbladder are seen.

Neoplasia

Diffuse neoplastic infiltration of the liver is usually due to infiltration of round cell tumours. Normally there is also hepatomegaly, although the degree of this can be variable.

In patients with **lymphoma** (Figure 76), the liver may show no ultrasonographic changes, or may present diffuse changes with hypoechoic, hyperechoic, or mixed echogenicity parenchyma.

With **mastocytomas** the liver may appear diffusely hyperechogenic. Liver carcinomas can also be diffuse or affect multiple lobes and have a variable ultrasonographic appearance.

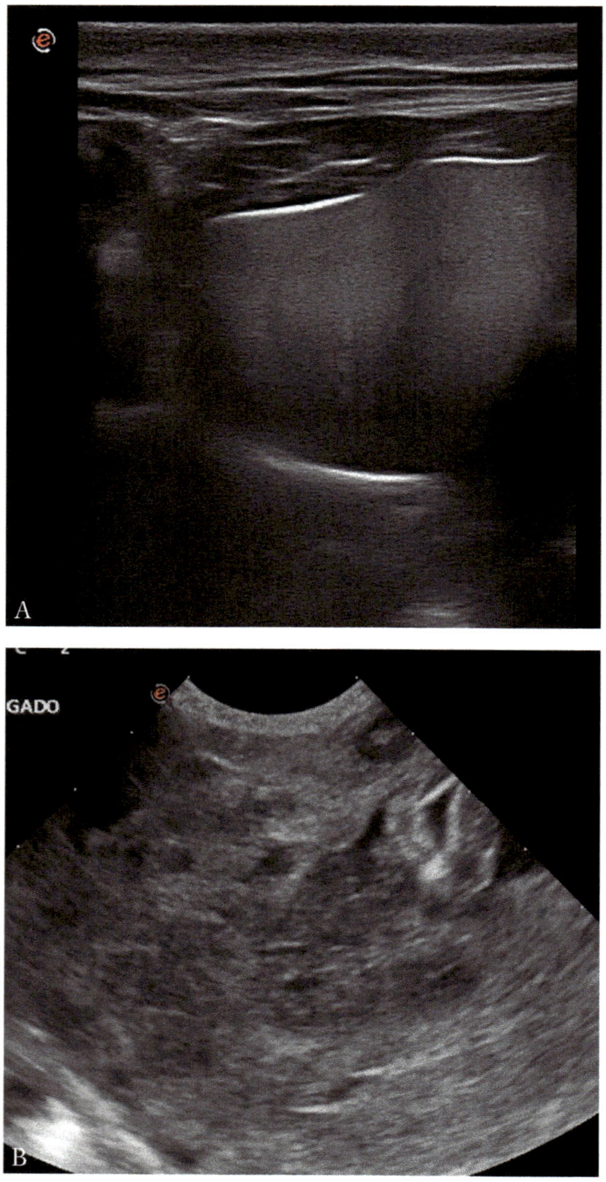

Figure 76. Images of two patients with lymphoma in the liver. The one in image A shows an increase in echogenicity and the one in image B has a heterogeneous parenchyma with hypoechoic nodular regions.

Focal and multifocal liver abnormalities

Neoplasia

Biliary cystadenomas (Figure 77) are benign lesions found in geriatric cats and appear as focal or multifocal cystic lesions. Their ultrasonographic appearance may vary:

- Multilocular masses containing thin-walled cysts.
- Hyperechogenic masses with cystic components.
- Masses of mixed echogenicity with cystic components.

Typically, a variable degree of posterior enhancement is observed in most masses.

Liver carcinomas can appear as focal or multifocal lesions of variable echogenicity. The liver is a frequent location for visceral haemangiosarcoma in cats. The lesions are usually hypoechogenic and heterogeneous and may be accompanied by haemoabdomen.

Metastases may appear with a varied appearance and may be hyperechoic, hypoechoic, or present mixed echogenicity. Target lesions (Figure 77), with a hyperechoic centre and hypoechoic periphery, are frequently associated with malignant lesions, especially metastases, but they have also been described in dogs with nodular hyperplasia.

Cysts

Liver cysts can be **isolated findings without clinical significance** or associated with polycystic kidney disease. They normally appear as spherical, well-defined lesions with a hyperechogenic, thin wall.

Other focal lesions

Other focal lesions include **nodular hyperplasia** (less frequent than in dogs and without specific characteristics described), **abscesses and haematomas**, which present heterogeneous echogenicity.

Abnormalities of the gallbladder and bile ducts

Biliary tract obstruction

Ultrasonographic changes indicating biliary tract obstruction include:

- Distension of the gallbladder
- Thickened and hyperechogenic gallbladder wall
- Common bile duct dilation (> 5 mm)
- Biliary sludge
- Dilation of intrahepatic bile ducts.

The distended intrahepatic ducts appear as tubular structures with echogenic walls, which are sometimes tortuous, and do not show vascular flow when evaluated with Doppler. Their luminal content can be anechogenic,

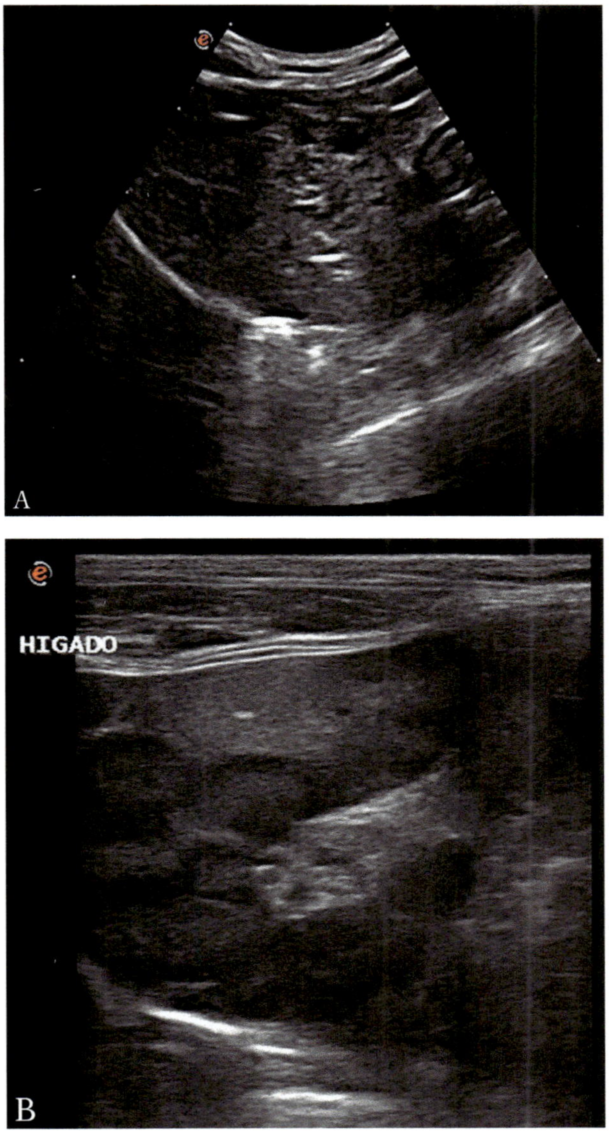

Figure 77. Image of a patient with a cystadenoma where a hyperechogenic lesion with multiple small-sized cystic structures (A) are seen. Another patient, in this case with cholangiocarcinoma where multiple nodules of mixed echogenicity and a target like appearance are seen (B).

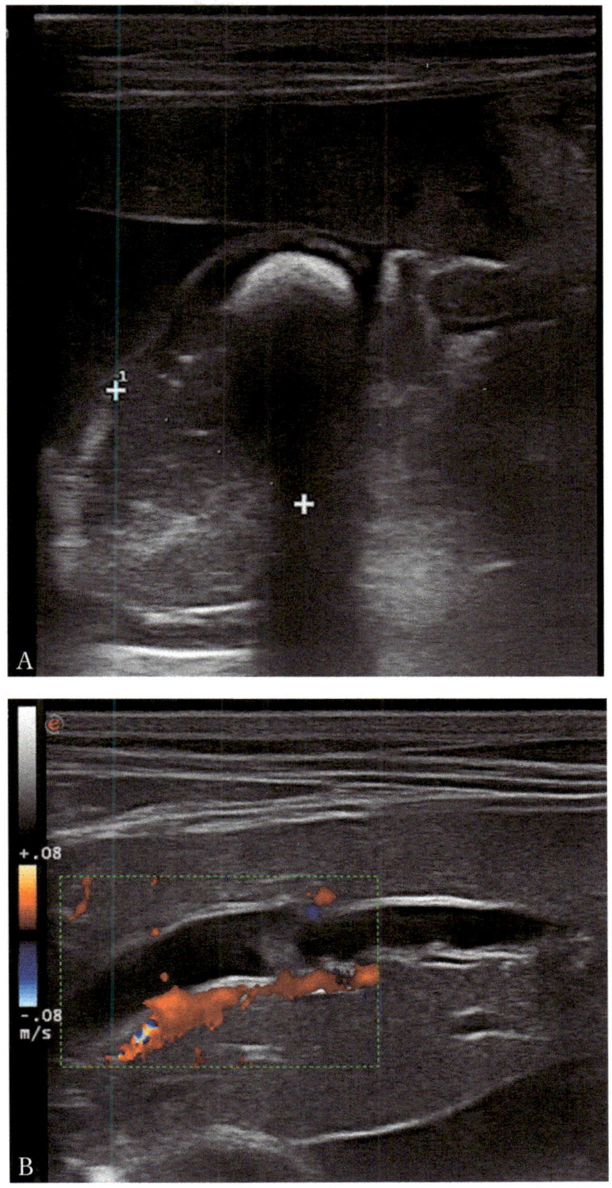

Figure 78. Sagittal section of the caudal aspect of the liver where the presence of a calculi can be seen in the common byle duct, visible as a hyperechoic structure with acoustic shadow and marked distension of the common byle duct (A). A more cranial section where distension of an intrahepatic bile duct can be seen (B).

echogenic and amorphous or hyperechogenic with acoustic shadow (mineralization) (Figure 78). The common bile duct may remain distended after resolution of a previous obstruction, as the elasticity of the wall may decrease due to chronic inflammation or obstruction.

Gallstones can be fortuitous findings, although an underlying inflammatory cause, such as cholecystitis or cholangitis, is more frequently identified in cats. They can cause intra or extrahepatic biliary obstruction, but can also be a consequence of an obstruction.

Neoplasia of the gallbladder

Gallbladder polyps and neoplasms are rare but may be associated with biliary obstruction. Polyps usually present as hyperechogenic masses that protrude into the lumen of the gallbladder. Several cases of **lymphoma** in which the gallbladder was affected have been described, although the ultrasonographic appearance is different in each case.

Portosystemic shunts

Ultrasonographic changes associated with the presence of portosystemic shunts include:

- Small liver.
- Reduced visualization of the intrahepatic portal vessels.
- Renomegaly.
- The presence of urinary calculi.

All these changes appear to be less frequent in cats than in dogs.

The most frequently described type of shunt in cats is the **portocaval extrahepatic shunt**, which connects the portal vein or its tributaries (splenic, right gastric, left gastric, gastroduodenal veins) with the vena cava. An **abnormal, tortuous vessel is** typically observed, originating from a portal branch and typically ending in the vena cava or azygos vein. Intrahepatic shunts occur less frequently and, in this case, those on the left side are more common.

Acquired portosystemic shunts are rare in cats compared to dogs. They develop secondarily when there is chronic liver disease with portal hypertension. Typically, an abnormal vessel that runs from the splenic vein and that is directed caudally towards the renal region can be observed, although it may be difficult to follow its path. Small tortuous vessels can also be observed in the mesentery around the vena cava, especially near the kidneys.

Gastrointestinal tract

The aspects of the gastrointestinal tract which should be assessed include **overall wall thickness, echogenicity, wall layering, relative thickness of each layer, organ lumen pattern, and peristalsis** (Figure 79).

The **wall thickness varies** in each gastrointestinal segment. The ileum is generally considered the segment with the thickest walls. However, a recent study indicates that this is only valid if the measurement is taken over the folds, and not between folds. The thickest mucosa is found in the duodenum and ileum, while the muscularis is thicker in the ileum and other segments. In contrast, the colon is the segment with the thinnest wall. The mucosa layer is thicker than all the other layers in the rest of the segments, the muscularis is thicker than the submucosa and the serosa, and the submucosa is thicker than the serosa in all segments.

The lumen of the gastrointestinal tract may contain **mucous, gas, liquid, food and faecal** content. All of these elements create different ultrasound patterns.

- The **mucous pattern** is seen as an echogenic line without acoustic shadow.
- The **gas** produces a hyperechogenic surface at the interface between the gas and the wall of the stomach or intestine, with acoustic shadow and reverberations.
- The **liquid content** is seen in the lumen of the stomach or intestine as being between anechoic and hypoechoic. The echogenicity varies depending on the type of liquid and the presence of food particles or small gas bubbles in suspension.
- **Food particles** may have a variable appearance but do not usually generate significant acoustic shadows, although there are exceptions.
- **Faeces** are normally associated with acoustic shadows.

Some cats have fatty tissue accumulated in the submucosa of the stomach and it can be detected by ultrasound in some patients as a thicker submucosa.

The pylorus can be seen between the pyloric antrum and the duodenum and has a prominent muscularis layer (Figure 80). The duodenum can be followed caudally to the pylorus. The major duodenal papilla is usually located near the pylorus and is a small nodular area located in the mesenteric border of the wall.

The terminal ileum is located medial to the descending duodenum. The ileocolic junction is found in the final part. In addition, the existence of a prominent submucosa and muscularis layers is characteristic of the terminal ileum, which gives it a cartwheel appearance. With high frequency probes, Peyer's patches can be visualized in the terminal jejunum and ileum, as an hypoechoic and asymmetric additional layer in the submucosa.

Foreign bodies

Many foreign bodies have a hyperechoic surface with **marked acoustic shadow**; however, this is not always the case and less echogenic foreign bodies can be seen with mild acoustic shadow or without acoustic shadow. Visualisation of a **focal or regional distension of the small intestine with gas or liquid** is an indicator of obstruction.

Linear bodies are seen as linear hyperechogenic structures in the intestinal lumen, and the **intestinal walls around them typically look plicated.** They can cause a strong acoustic shadow, especially when they are thick, but when they are thin (fine strings, threads) the acoustic shadow can be minimal or non-existent (Figure 81).

Intussusception

Intussusceptions have a multi-layered ultrasonographic appearance or can appear as a target-shaped lesion of the intestinal wall. The multiple layers are formed by the overlapping walls of the intussusceptum and the intussuscipiens. In cross sections, the multilayer appearance is visualized as **concentric rings**. Any of the gastrointestinal segments can be involved and the distension of the intestinal loop cranial to the intussusceptum is normally observed (Figure 82).

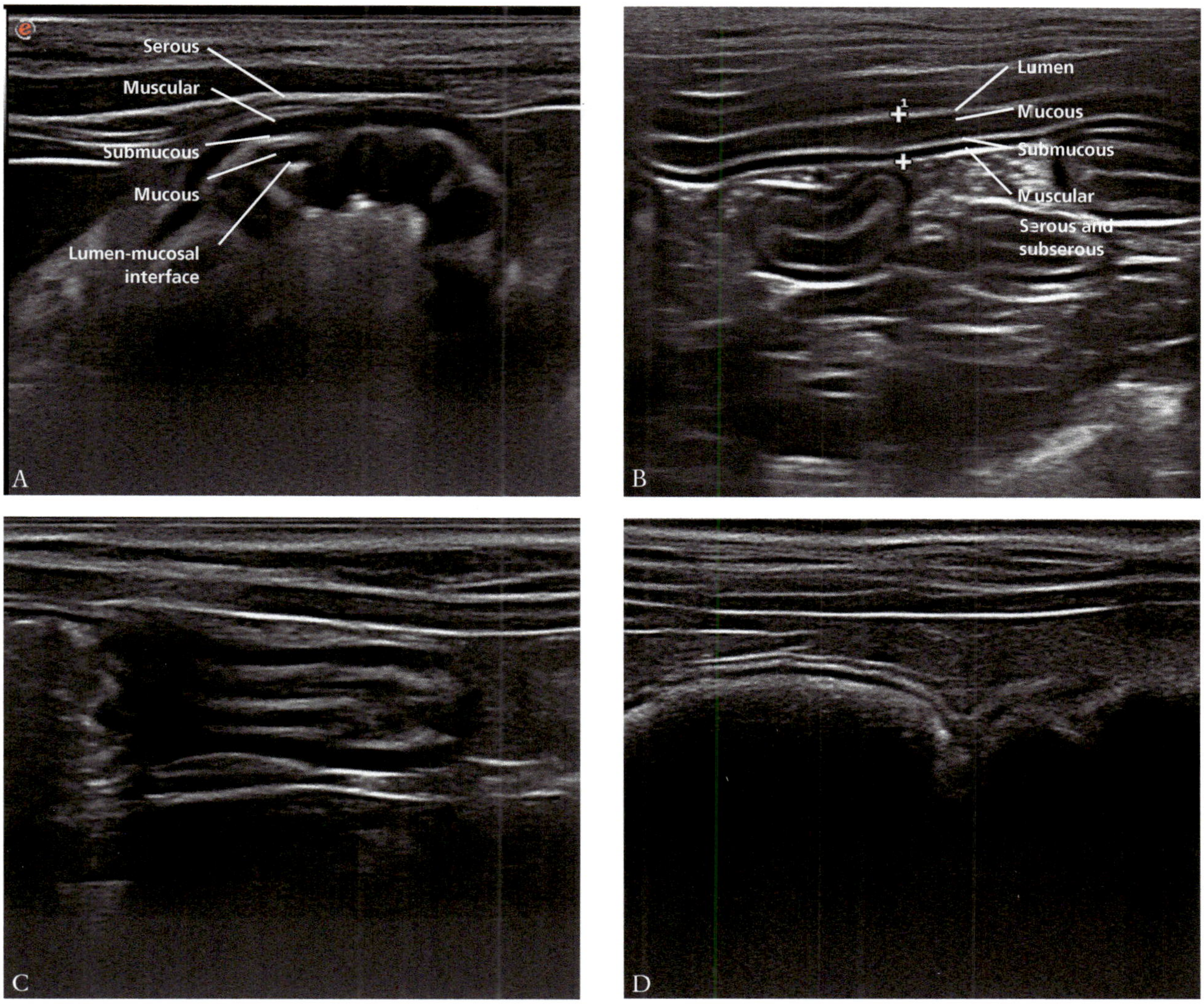

Figure 79. Normal appearance and layering of the stomach (A), jejunum (B), ileum (C) and colon (D).

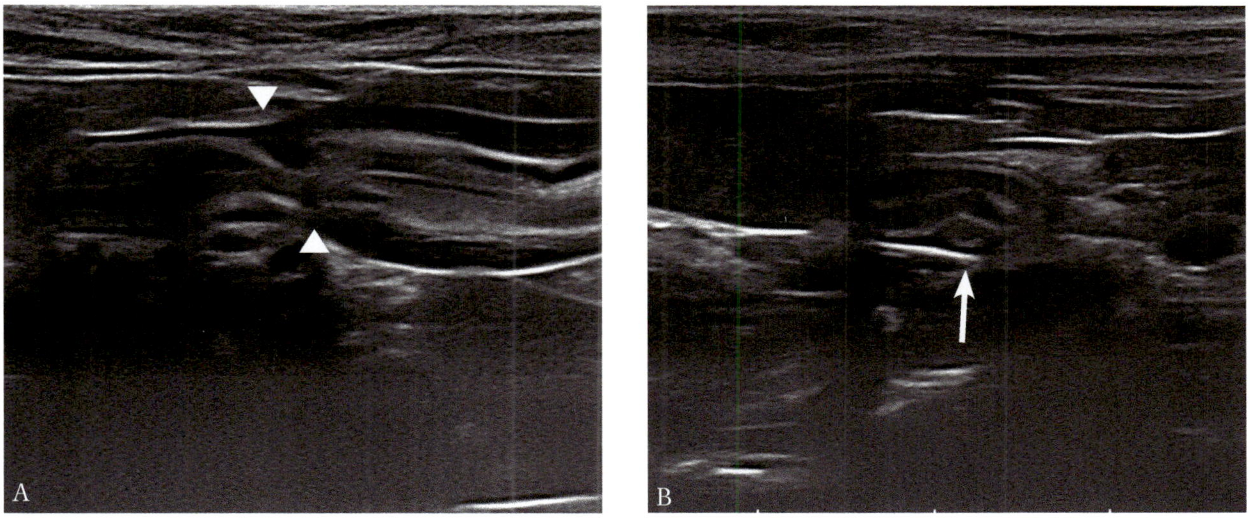

Figure 80. Longitudinal section of the pyloric region (between the arrowheads) (A) and short longitudinal section of the duodenum showing the duodenal papilla (arrow) (B).

Inflammatory diseases

Gastritis and enteritis may not show significant ultrasonographic changes. In cats with inflammatory bowel disease, such as **eosinophilic or lymphoplasmacytic enteritis,** the reported ultrasound findings **include increased wall thickness, thickening of the muscularis** layer, hyperechogenic mucosa, and a visible hyperechogenic band on the mucosa. In one study, cats

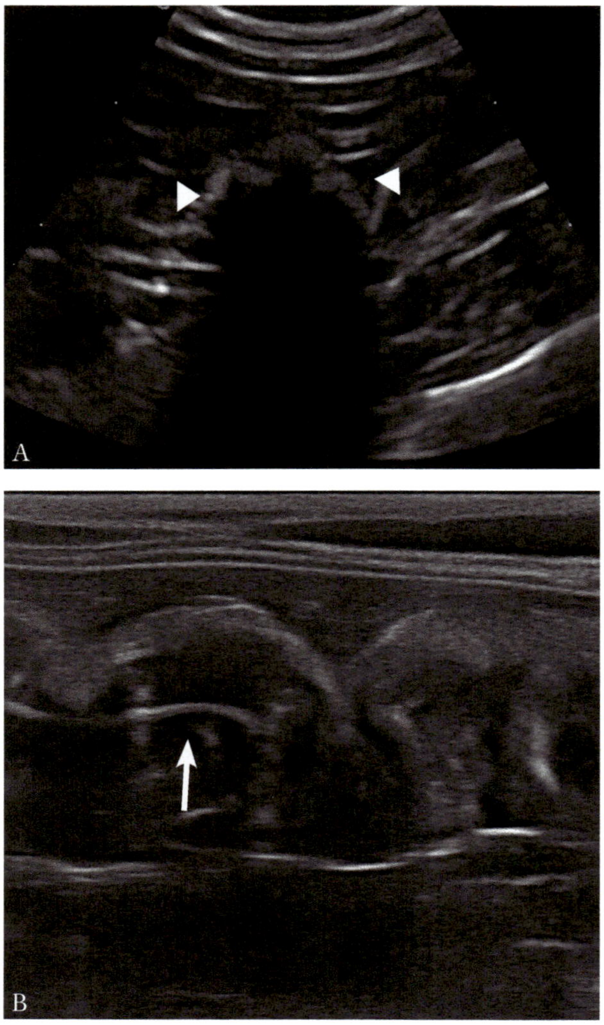

Figure 81. Section of the stomach where a rounded foreign body can be seen (arrowheads), which is causing marked acoustic shadow (A). Section of intestinal loops showing a linear foreign body (arrow) in the small intestine, with corrugated intestinal walls surrounding it (B).

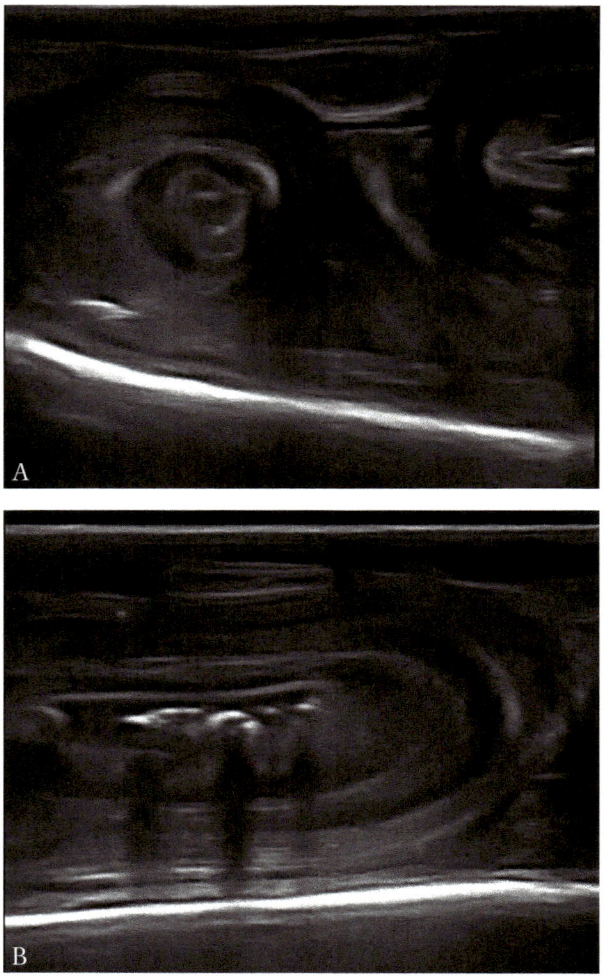

Figure 82. Transverse and longitudinal sections of an invagination where the multi-layer appearance of the invaginated segment can be seen.

with eosinophilic enteritis had an increased jejunal wall thickness and a higher incidence of thickening of the muscularis layer compared to cats with lymphoplasmacytic enteritis (Figure 83).

In **feline infectious peritonitis**, focal masses may appear in the intestinal wall. Lymphadenopathy, free fluid, and/or granulomas may also be seen in the mesentery or other organs.

Feline eosinophilic sclerosing fibroplasia is a non-neoplastic lesion produced by the inflammatory response by eosinophils and mast cells organized in a dense proliferative nodular structure. Ultrasonographically, masses appear with **thickening of the wall and loss of stratification**. These lesions show mixed echogenicity with hyperechogenic regions believed to correspond to areas of fibrosis. They have been described in the stomach, duodenum, jejunum, and colon.

Micronodular ultrasonographic lesions have been described in the submucosa of the colon, with a round or oval shape, measuring between 1 and 3 mm and with hypoechoic or anechoic ultrasound appearance. These changes have been proposed as **representing reactive intraparietal lymphoid follicles** and may be indicative of inflammation of the colon.

Neoplasia

The most common gastrointestinal neoplasias in cats are **lymphoma, adenocarcinoma, and mastocytoma.**

Large B or T cell lymphomas typically produce single or multiple masses in the stomach, small intestine, or colon. Associated ultrasound changes include wall thickening with diffuse loss of layering, decreased wall echogenicity, and regional lymphadenopathy (Figure 84a). Lesions may appear as focal masses, with marked wall thickening, and may ulcerate.

Gastrointestinal small T-cell lymphoma shows echographic and histological features similar to inflammatory bowel disease (IBD). Both IBD and lymphoma are characterized by having a diffuse or regional distribution in the small intestine, with ultrasound

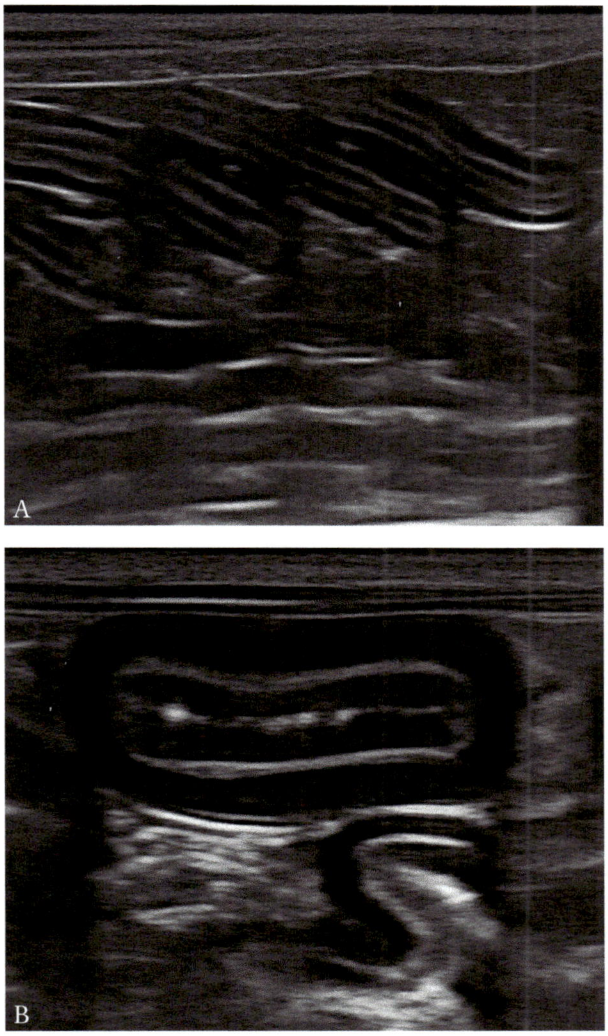

Figure 83. Longitudinal images of the small intestine of two cats with lymphoplasmacytic enteritis. Thickening of the muscular layer is more marked in image B and a slight increase in mucosal echogenicity can be seen.

features including thickening of the intestinal wall due to thickening of the muscularis propria and maintenance of the wall layers without mass formation (Figure 84 b and c). In one study, it was observed that in elderly cats with a thickened intestinal muscle layer, the diagnosis was more likely to be T-cell lymphoma than IBD.

Intestinal adenocarcinoma is usually focal and often causes partial or complete obstruction. It presents a circumferential thickening of the intestinal wall, which can be asymmetric or symmetrical.

The most frequent ultrasound pattern for **feline mastocytoma** is a hypoechogenic focal thickening of the wall that can be non-circumferential and eccentric, or circumferential, asymmetric and eccentric. Less frequently, it may appear as a diffuse infiltration of the submucosa. Alterations in wall stratification may also occur, but without complete loss of the layering. The muscularis propria is the layer most frequently affected on ultrasound examination.

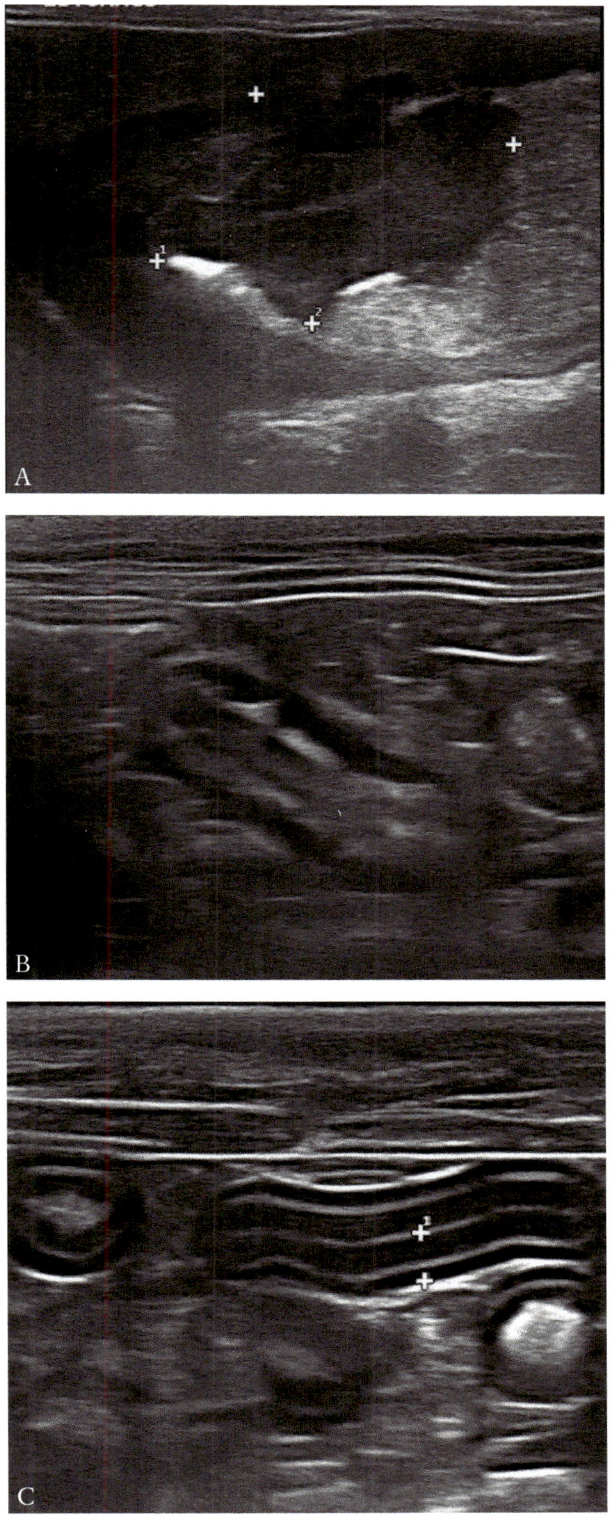

Figure 84. Patient with gastric lymphoma where a thickened gastric wall can be seen, with loss of normal layering and the presence of a hypoechogenic mass which protrudes into the lumen (A). The ileum and jejunum of another patient, with small T cell lymphoma where layering is maintained but a thickening of the muscularis can be seen (B and C).

The presence of an obstructive pattern due to the mass seems to be more frequent in adenocarcinomas than in mastocytomas.

Ulcers

When there are ulcerations in the gastrointestinal wall, **focal defects** are observed in the mucosa with the appearance of a crater and delineated by **hyperechogenic microbubbles**. In some cases, small hyperechogenic spots can be seen on the wall due to the presence of gas.

They can be associated with both inflammatory diseases and neoplasms.

Pancreas

The pancreas is divided into three parts:

1. Right lobe
2. Left lobe
3. Body

It is approximately **0.5–1 cm thick**. The left lobe and body are thicker than the right lobe, and therefore easier to identify (Figure 85).

The **right lobe** is located in the mesoduodenum, dorsomedial to the descending duodenum, ventral to the right kidney and ventrolateral to the portal vein. The **body** is found in the pyloroduodenal angle, located approximately in the midline, craniomedial to the right kidney and ventral to the portal vein. The angle that the pancreatic lobes make with the body is smaller than in the dog. In the **right lobe**, a central tubular structure is visualized that corresponds to the **pancreaticoduodenal vein**.

The **left lobe** originates from the pancreatic body and is located dorsocaudal to the pyloric antrum, then continues towards the midline, caudal to the stomach and cranial to the transverse colon. Finally, it goes to the left of the abdomen, cranially to the left kidney. The anatomical reference of the triangle delineated by the stomach, spleen and cranial pole of the left kidney can be used to locate the left pancreatic lobe.

The **pancreatic duct** is observed in the left pancreatic lobe as a tubular structure with hyperechogenic walls and an anechoic lumen located in the central region of the pancreatic parenchyma, measuring between 0.5 and 2.5 mm. Some studies have observed a tendency for the diameter of the pancreatic duct to increase with age.

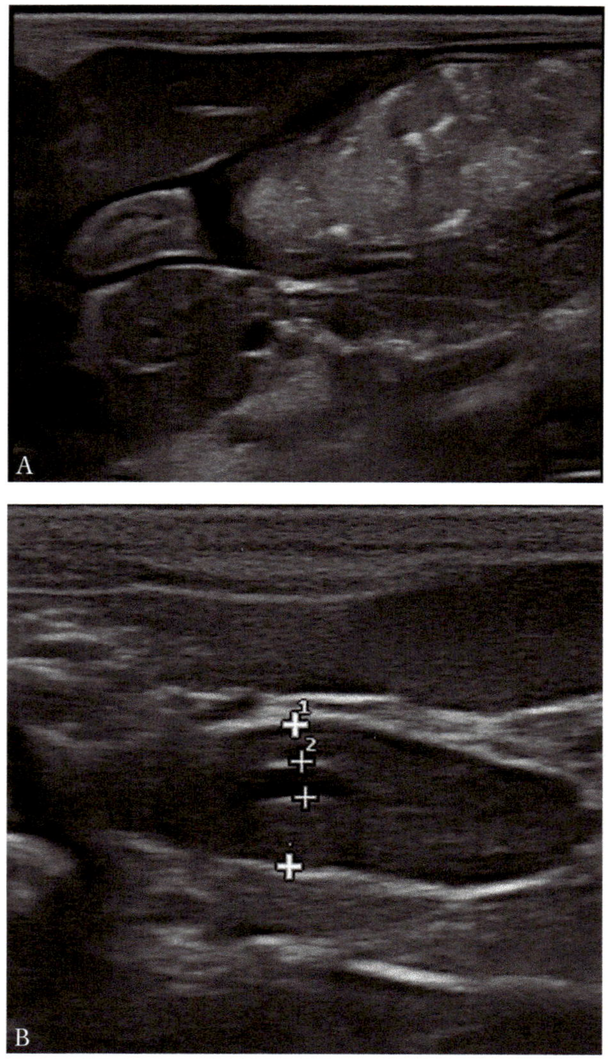

Figure 85. Image of the pylorus where the body of the pancreas can be seen (A). The left lobe of the pancreas and the pancreatic duct between the fundus and spleen can be appreciated (B).

Pancreatitis

In cats, the sensitivity of ultrasound for the diagnosis of pancreatitis varies from low (11–35%) to higher (78%) according to studies, although the specificity is low (22%). Several studies have observed a **relationship between the presence of pancreatitis, inflammatory bowel disease, cholangitis and lipidosis**, so concomitant changes can be observed in these organs.

In **acute pancreatitis** the ultrasound changes may be similar to those described in dogs, with a hypoechogenic pancreas or with mixed echogenicity, with a diffuse increase in size, accompanied by greater echogenicity of the peripancreatic fat due to the saponification process and with free liquid (Figure 86). However, these changes are usually less obvious in cats.

In cases of **acute haemorrhagic or necrotizing pancreatitis**, irregular regions with hypoechoic content may be observed due to necrosis and haemorrhage of the pancreas and peripancreatic tissue. The edges of the pancreas may be poorly defined.

In **chronic pancreatitis** the ultrasonographic changes are more subtle or non-existent. The pancreas may be well defined and hypoechoic, or with hyperechoic regions that may represent areas of fibrosis (Figure 87). Sometimes the edges are irregular, and the parenchyma can have mineralized foci.

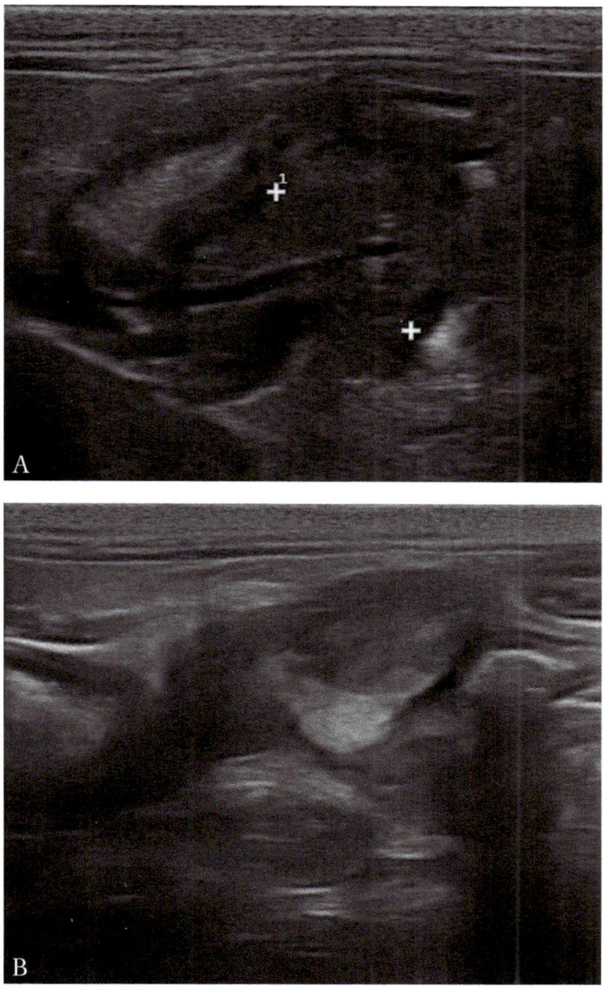

Figure 86. Patient with pancreatitis. The right lobe is enlarged (1.1cm) with irregular edges and poorly defined with a heterogeneous appearance to the peripancreatic fat with markedly hyperechogenic areas.

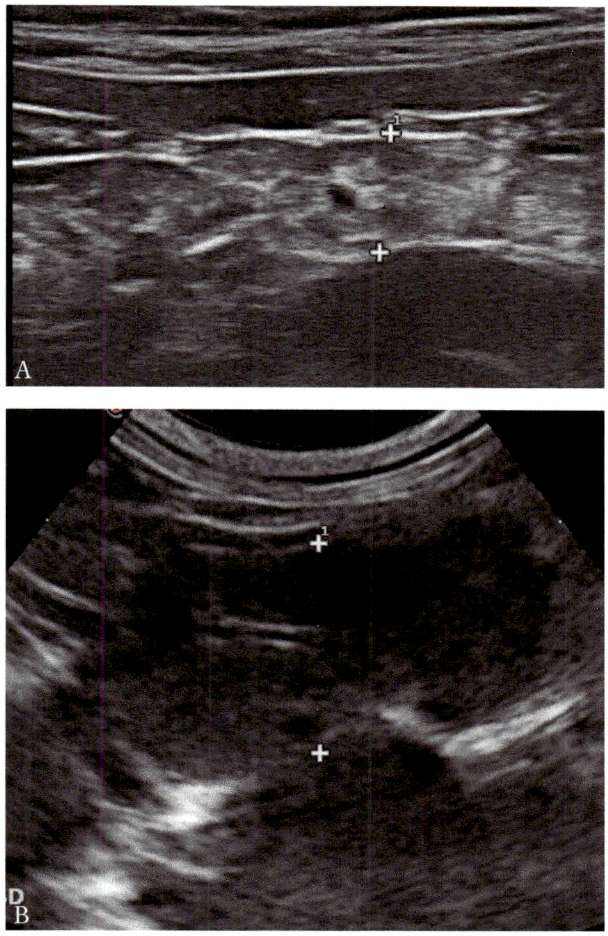

Figure 87. Images of two patients with chronic pancreatitis. In the patient image A the pancreas is hyperechoic and slightly heterogeneous meanwhile in image B it is enlarged and heterogeneous.

In cats with **acromegaly**, a significant **thickening of the left lobe** of the pancreas occurring with diffuse hypoechogenicity or presence of nodules or cysts has been seen.

The pancreatic duct can be distended in acute and chronic pancreatitis or in elderly cats (without evidence of pancreatic disease) so this is **not a specific finding** for pancreatitis.

Cystic lesions

Different types of cystic lesions can be found including pseudocysts such as sequelae of pancreatitis, congenital cysts (associated with PKD), and retention cysts, but it is **not possible to distinguish between the different types ultrasonographically**. It is also difficult to distinguish ultrasonographically between true cystic lesions and abscesses.

Neoplasms

Pancreatic neoplasms are uncommon in the cat. Adenocarcinoma is the most frequent neoplasm and some sarcomas have also been described. Other neoplasia described in the literature includes adenoma, squamous cell carcinoma, lymphoma, lymphangiosarcoma, and carcinosarcoma. The most frequent ultrasound appearance is that of a **hypoechogenic focal mass or nodule** or, less frequently, with mixed echogenicity, which may present mineralised foci (Figure 88).

A diffuse irregular thickening of the pancreas with multiple hypoechoic nodules has also been seen with adenoma and adenocarcinoma. Diffuse infiltration of the pancreas can also be observed in cases of lymphoma.

Nodular hyperplasia

It is a **frequent incidental finding in old cats.** Ultrasonographically, multiple well-defined nodules of **less than 1 cm** are seen, which are usually iso or hypoechoic. They may be associated with an increased thickness of the pancreas. Its appearance is similar to that described in cases of pancreatic neoplasms, although hyperplastic nodules tend to be multiple and smaller than exocrine neoplasms.

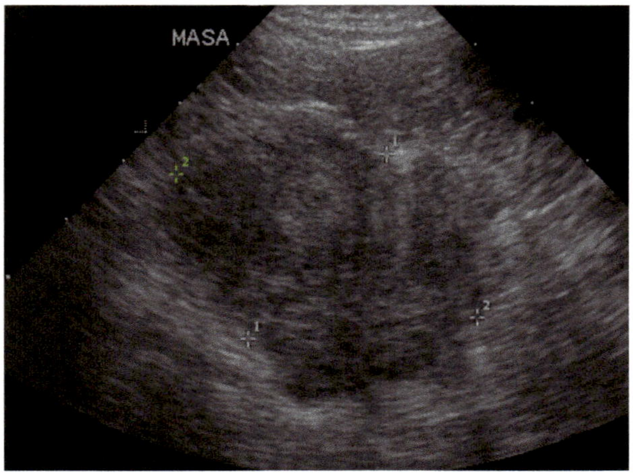

Figure 88. A heterogeneous mass with irregular edges in the pancreatic region can be seen which corresponds with a pancreatic carcinoma.

Spleen

In healthy patients, the spleen has **a thin, smooth, hyperechogenic capsular surface with sharp, well-defined margins** (Figure 89). The visceral surface has a more irregular contour due to the presence of small indentations through which the veins emerge. In a transverse plane the **spleen is triangular** in shape. This organ has a dense, homogeneous, fine granular texture. The splenic parenchyma has been reported to be more echogenic than that of the liver and kidney. However, in other studies, it has been shown that in cats the normal renal cortex is much more echogenic than the spleen due to the presence of lipids in the tubules of the renal cortex.

Diffuse splenomegaly

The thickness of the spleen can be used to determine the presence of splenomegaly. **A spleen measuring more than 9.1 mm is compatible with splenomegaly**.

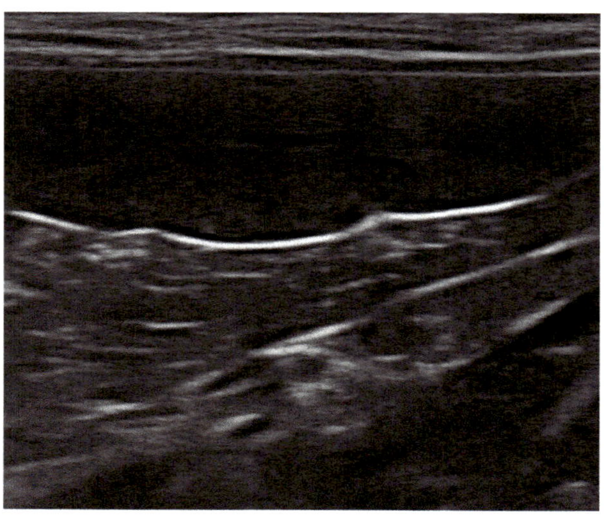

Figure 89. Images of a normal spleen. The hyperechoic capsule and homogenous granular parenchyma can be seen.

This finding, along with other ultrasonographic findings and patient examination, requires a more in-depth study of the spleen or fine-needle aspiration of the spleen to obtain a diagnosis. Visualisation of a **spleen folded in on itself** is also a sign of splenomegaly in cats.

The causes of splenomegaly (Figure 90) in the feline species include:

- Extramedullary haematopoiesis
- Chronic anaemia
- Immune-mediated haemolytic anaemia
- Infections (feline leukaemia virus, feline infectious peritonitis, mycobacteriosis, bacterial splenitis, leishmaniosis, etc.)
- Fungal diseases such as histoplasmosis
- Nodular hyperplasia
- Neoplastic infiltration (mastocytoma, lymphoma, plasmacytoma)
- Acromegaly

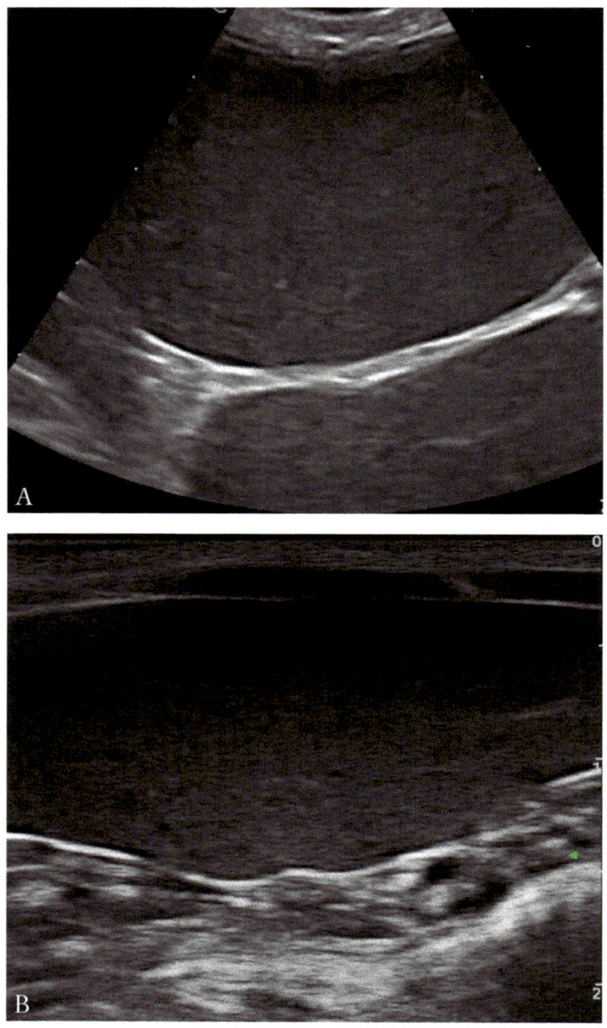

Figure 90. Images showing splenomegaly. Cat with lymphoma where clear splenomegaly can be seen, with a markedly rounded spleen which is folded over on itself (A). Cat with chronic anaemia where diffuse splenomegaly and a slightly heterogeneous parenchyma can be seen (B).

- Hypereosinophilic syndrome
- Haematomas
- Erythroid leukaemia
- Myelodysplastic syndrome
- Myeloproliferative diseases
- Vascular compromise
- Venous congestion

Neoplasia

The most frequent splenic tumours in the cat are **mastocytoma and lymphoma** (Figure 91) with **splenomegaly being a common finding with lymphoma.** The appearance of the splenic parenchyma is variable, from diffusely hypoechoic with a mottled texture and/or the presence of several small hypoechogenic foci, to unique hypoechogenic masses. Splenic masses or decreased parenchymal echogenicity can also be observed without splenomegaly. The ultrasound changes observed in cats with splenic mastocytoma are similar to those described in cases of lymphoma.

Visceral haemangiosarcoma is rare in cats and are usually multifocal, with splenic lesions in approximately 23% of cases. Ultrasonographically, they have been described as heterogeneous or hypoechogenic lesions, with anechogenic foci in some of them, accompanied by abdominal effusion (Figure 91).

Target like lesions (hyper or isoechogenic centre with hypoechoic periphery) are generally associated with malignant conditions, such as metastasis. However, they have also been described in benign lesions, such as in hyperplasia.

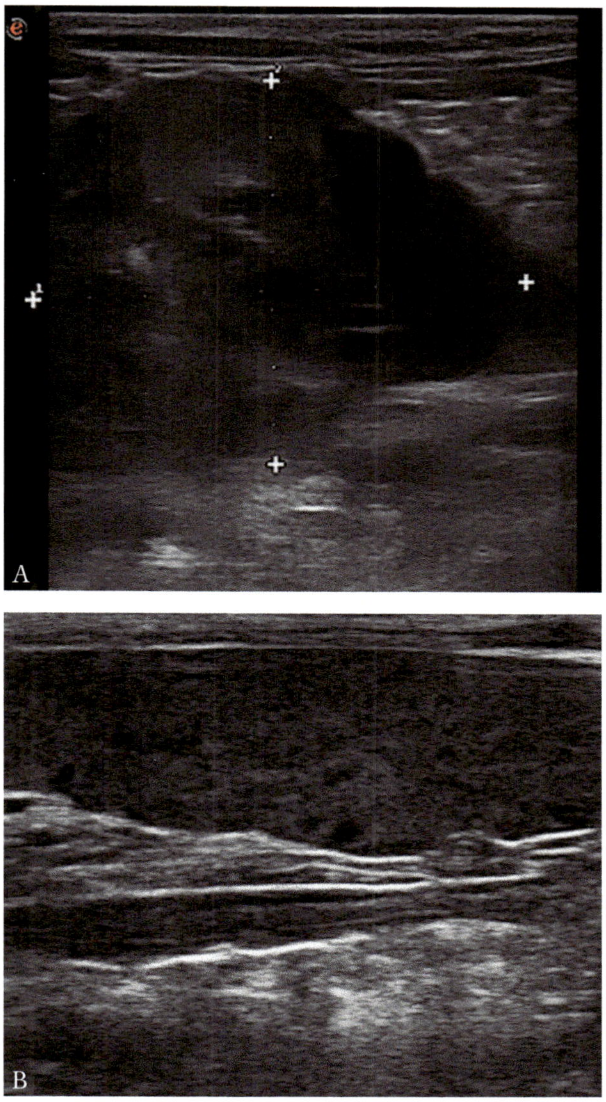

Figure 91. Heterogeneous splenic mass with cavitated appearance in a female cat with splenic haemangiosarcoma (A). Image of a spleen of a female cat with splenic lymphoma. The parenchyma appears heterogeneous and there are multiple hypoechogenic foci present (B).

Myelolipomas

Occasionally, focal and nodular areas can be seen, which are hyperechogenic in the splenic parenchyma and in contact with the vessels along the visceral surface. These areas are compatible with fat accumulation and are called lipomatosis or myelolipomas.

Haematomas

Haematomas can be seen as focal or multifocal lesions, of **variable echogenicity** (from hypo to anechogenic or of mixed echogenicity). In some cases, they can deform the splenic capsule or have a **subcapsular location** (Figure 92).

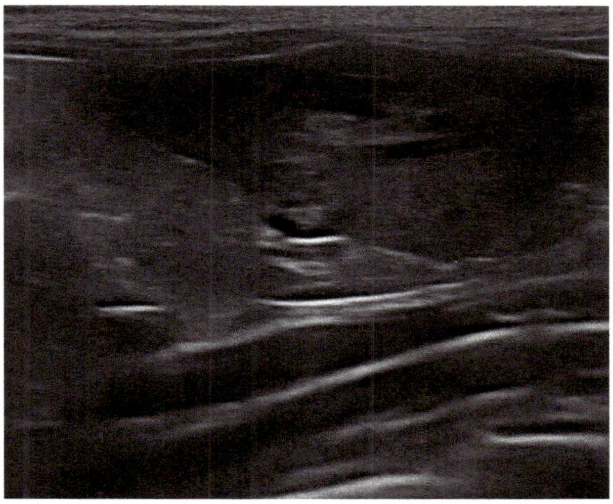

Figure 92. Heterogenous lesions deforming the surface of the splenic capsule in a patient with a splenic haematoma due to polytrauma.

Adrenal glands

The left adrenal gland is located between the origin of the cranial mesenteric artery and the left renal artery, **near the cranial pole of the left kidney.** The caudal vena cava, just cranial to the right kidney, serves as an anatomical reference, since the right adrenal gland is located slightly dorsolateral to the vein (Figure 93).

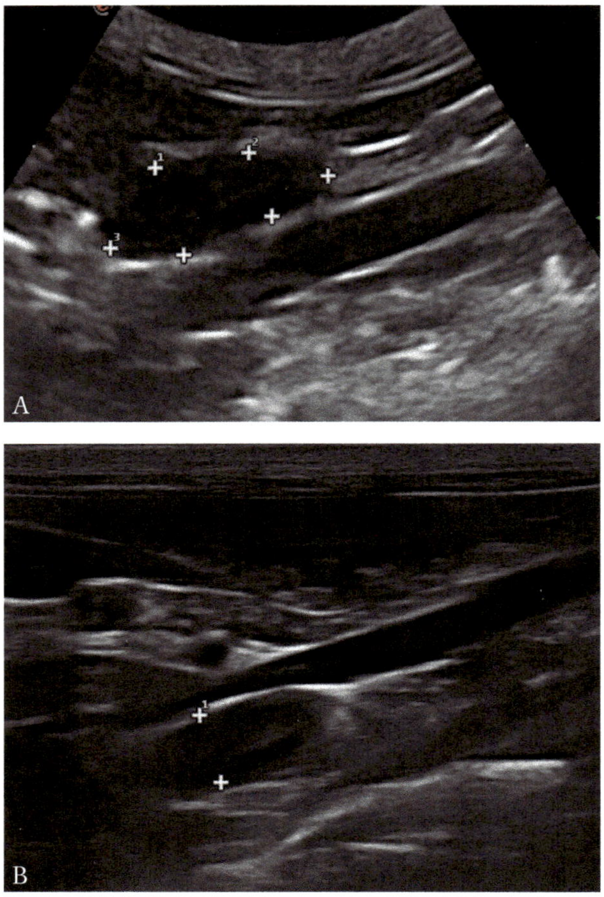

Figure 93. Left adrenal gland (between cursors) in close relation to the aorta (A). Right adrenal gland in direct contact with the caudal vena cava (B).

The feline adrenal glands are **well-defined, bilobed, hypoechoic structures** surrounded by a hyperechogenic halo of fat. In some patients, it is possible to differentiate two areas in the parenchyma: a more hyperechogenic **central region** and a more hypoechogenic **peripheral region.** Both adrenal glands are similar in size, shape, and contour, with an **oval or bean-like** appearance. In some cats, internal foci with distal acoustic shadow can be seen in the adrenal parenchyma. These areas may represent **foci of mineralization**, which have been described in up to 30% of healthy cats.

The reference values for adrenal gland thickness vary according to different studies, with means and standard deviations of **4.3 ± 0.4 to 3.7 ± 0.9 mm.**

Neoplasia

Adrenal neoplasms are **rare in the cat**. They are classified into cortical tumours (adenomas or adrenocortical carcinomas) or medullary tumours (pheochromocytomas).

Cases of cats suffering from primary hyperaldosteronism are mostly a consequence of the presence of unilateral adenomas or adrenal carcinomas (Figure 94), although cases of bilateral adrenal hyperplasia have also been described.

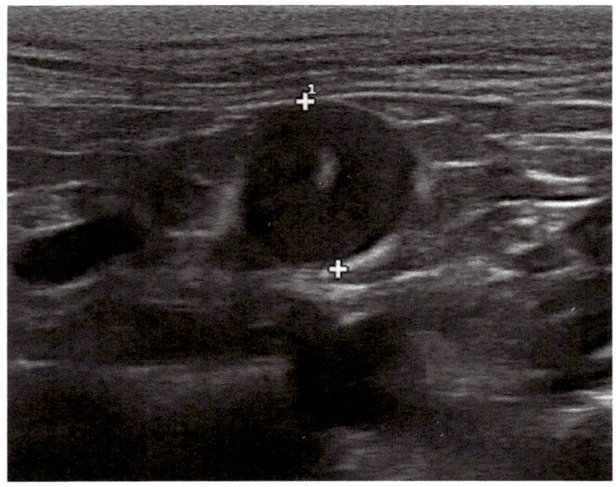

Figure 94. A hypoechogenic adrenal mass measuring 1 cm in diameter with a central hyperechogenic region can be seen. There was no definitive diagnosis available but the clinical signs, blood test results and diagnostic imaging tests were compatible with primary hyperaldosteronism.

Ultrasonographic signs of adrenal neoplasia include adrenal masses, calcification, and changes in normal echogenicity. However, it is important to remember that finding a larger adrenal gland or adrenal mass does not mean that excess aldosterone is being secreted. These masses can range from adrenal masses of no clinical importance ("incidentalomas"), through to masses that secrete other types of hormones such as cortisol or progesterone, to pheochromocytomas.

The combination of primary hyperaldosteronism with hyperprogesteronism has been described in cats with adrenal masses. Furthermore, there are also several published clinical cases that describe functional adrenal malignancies with excess production of sex hormones.

Hyperthyroid cats have been found to have larger adrenal glands than healthy cats of a similar age, with a greater number of hyperechogenic foci in the parenchyma. A similar finding has been observed in **acromegalic cats**, in which the thickness of the adrenal glands is significantly greater than that of control cats.

Kidneys and ureters

The **right kidney** is located in the renal fossa of the caudate lobe of the liver. Its anatomical references are the right adrenal gland and the caudal vena cava medially, and the abdominal wall as the lateral limit. As the kidneys are very mobile in the cat, the liver is not always visualized at the same time as the kidney on ultrasound. The **left kidney** is located caudal to the gastric fundus and caudomedially to the head of the spleen. The left adrenal gland and the aorta are its medial landmarks, with the descending colon ventral to it.

The anatomical relationships with the spleen and the liver allow **comparison of the renal echogenicity with the neighbouring organs**. In general, the renal cortex is iso or hypoechogenic compared to the liver and hypoechogenic compared to the spleen, although this relationship may vary in obese cats with fatty infiltration that increases the echogenicity of the kidney. The increased echogenicity of the **renal cortex** in healthy cats is caused by the increase in fat present in the epithelial cells of the proximal tubule, especially in male cats. There is a clear difference between the medulla and the cortex: the medulla is hypoechoic compared to the cortex. The **pelvis** is seen as a hyperechogenic line about 1–2 mm wide. The renal crest is the continuation of the **medulla** that is in contact with the pelvis. This is surrounded by the renal sinus, which contains fat, is hyperechogenic and is particularly prominent in obese cats. The renal capsule is visualized as a hyperechogenic line in the outermost part of the kidney (Figure 95).

The ureters run ventrally to the psoas muscles and 1–2 cm laterally to the median plane, very close to the aorta and caudal vena cava. At the level of the pelvis, they run through the base of the broad ligament or the genital fold until reaching the ureteral papilla in the bladder trigone. This **ureteral papilla is seen as a small bump on the bladder wall**. In a healthy cat, the ureters have a **luminal diameter of 0.4 mm** and it is not normally possible to visualize them on ultrasound.

Diffuse parenchymal diseases

Increased cortical echogenicity

It is the most frequent finding in cases of kidney failure, although it is a **non-specific lesion. Acute renal failure** is one of the pathologies in which it occurs and renomegaly and sometimes retroperitoneal fluid can also be seen. Initially, there is usually an increase in cortical echogenicity, but corticomedullary differentiation is maintained. As the disease progresses, the echogenicity of the medulla increases, with loss of definition and its normal ultrasonographic structure. In **ethylene glycol poisoning** (Figure 96), the deposition of oxalate crystals in the cortex and the medulla produces cortical hyperechogenicity 5–8 hours after ingestion, with the differentiation between cortex and medulla being lost as time passes. In advanced cases, a thin hypoechoic zone can be observed around the corticomedullary junction, which is an indicator of a poor prognosis.

Ultrasonographic changes consistent with **chronic kidney disease include small kidneys** with an **irregular kidney contour**, poor corticomedullary definition,

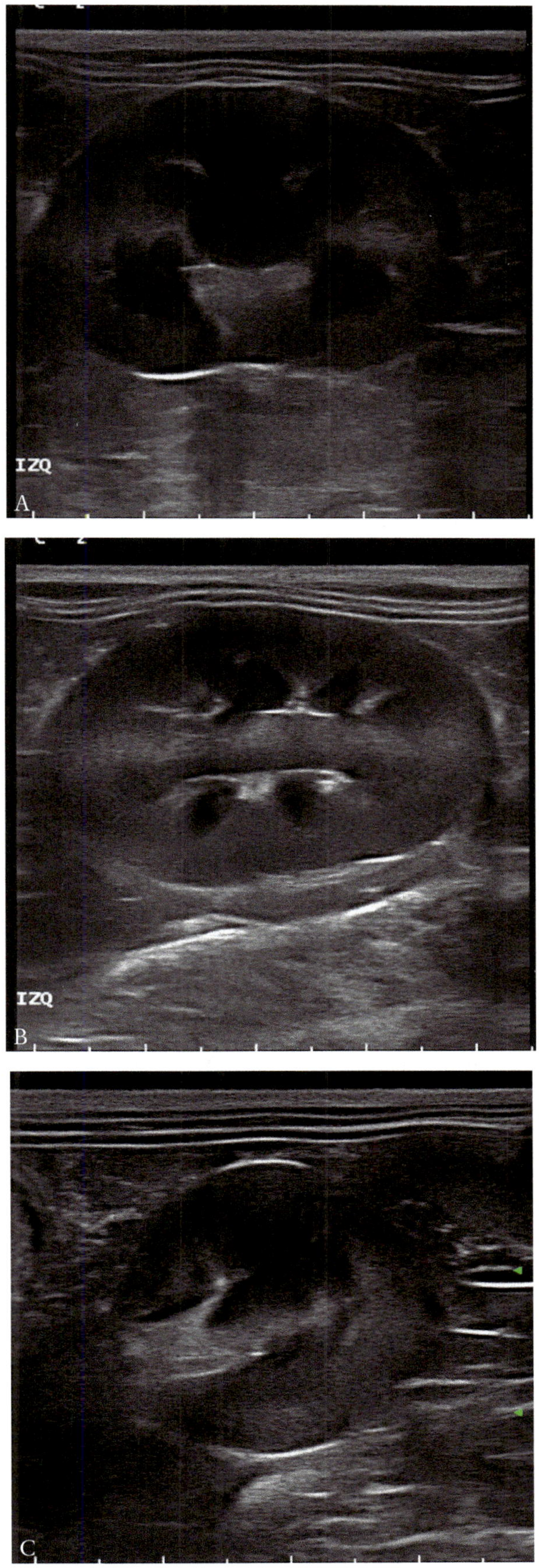

Figure 95. Longitudinal (A and B) and transverse (C) sections of the kidney in a healthy cat, where the hyperechogenic cortex, hypoechoic medulla, pelvis and pelvic diverticula are seen as hyperechoic lines. The hilar region of the kidney appears slightly hyperechogenic due to the presence of fat.

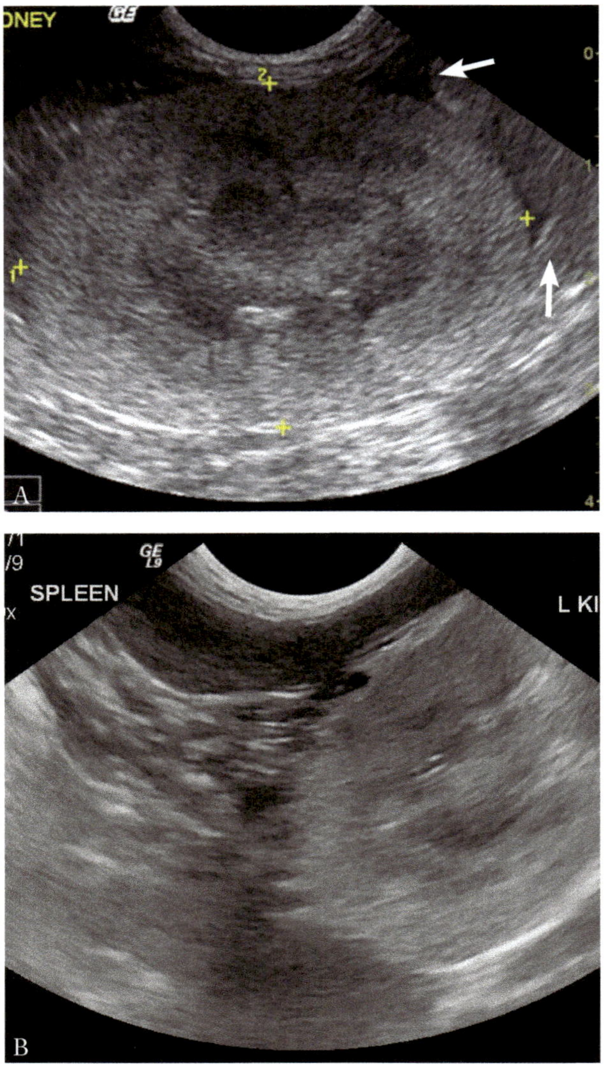

Figure 96. Kidneys from two cats with acute renal failure due to ethylene glycol poisoning. A marked increase in renal echogenicity can be seen (comparable with the spleen in image B) and in image A the presence of a small quantity of free retroperitoneal liquid can be seen (arrows).

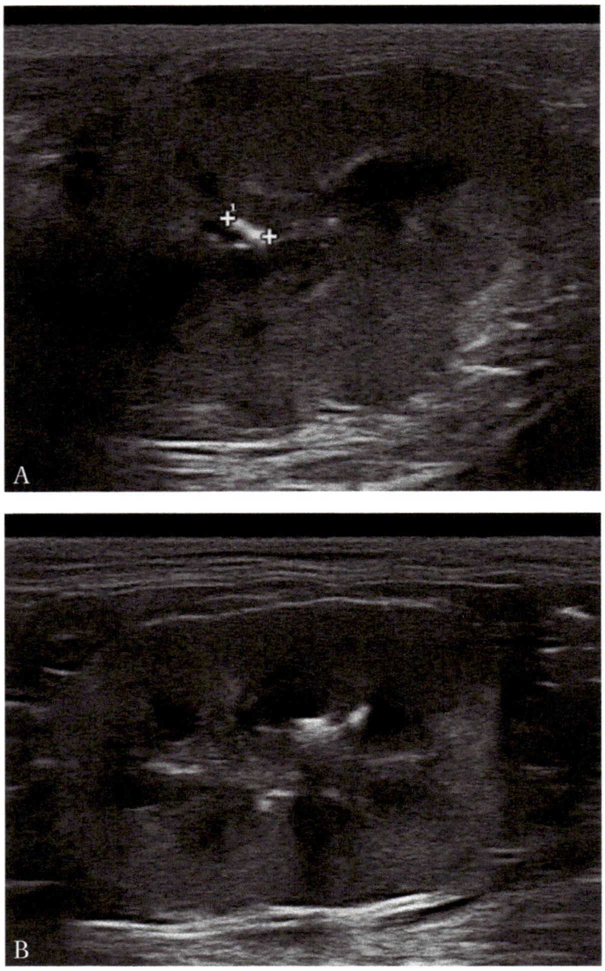

Figure 97. Kidneys from two patients with chronic renal disease. In image A the renal contour is notably irregular and an increase in cortical echogenicity can be seen with loss of definition between the cortex and medulla, as well as a calculi (between cursors). In image B similar, less marked changes can be seen.

heterogeneous renal parenchyma, focal or diffuse medullary hyperechogenicity, the medullary rim sign, infarcts, and/or mineralization of the renal parenchyma (Figure 97).

In the **terminal phases**, very small, irregular kidneys are observed, with a completely altered echostructure and which may present hyperechogenic foci with or without acoustic shadow that corresponds to **deposits of calcium and phosphorous.** Sometimes the so called "big kidney, small kidney" syndrome can be seen, in which one kidney is markedly reduced in size and the other kidney is enlarged.

Dysplastic kidneys are also usually hyperechogenic and smaller, with poor corticomedullary definition, and may have cysts and a **hydroureter.**

Alterations in echogenicity also occur in **feline infectious peritonitis**, both in its wet and dry forms. In the wet form, the presence of **subcapsular fluid** is observed, while in the dry form, **pyogranulomatous inflammation** develops that causes renomegaly, an irregular contour and increased echogenicity with a medullary rim sign. Occasionally, a subcapsular hypoechoic margin may be seen.

Neoplasms such as **lymphoma** (Figure 98) and **metastatic squamous cell carcinoma** may occur with increased echogenicity and with good corticomedullary differentiation. Renomegaly is usually present, although normal sized kidneys can also be seen. The presence of a hypoechoic halo around the cortex has been described in lymphoma. This halo differs from perinephric fluid in that it is only observed around the cortex and not in the rest of the retroperitoneal space.

Medullary rim sign

This sign can be seen both in cats without clinical signs and in cats with kidney disease. It is described as a **thin hyperechogenic line** at the outer limit of the medulla, parallel to the corticomedullary junction. It can be **both**

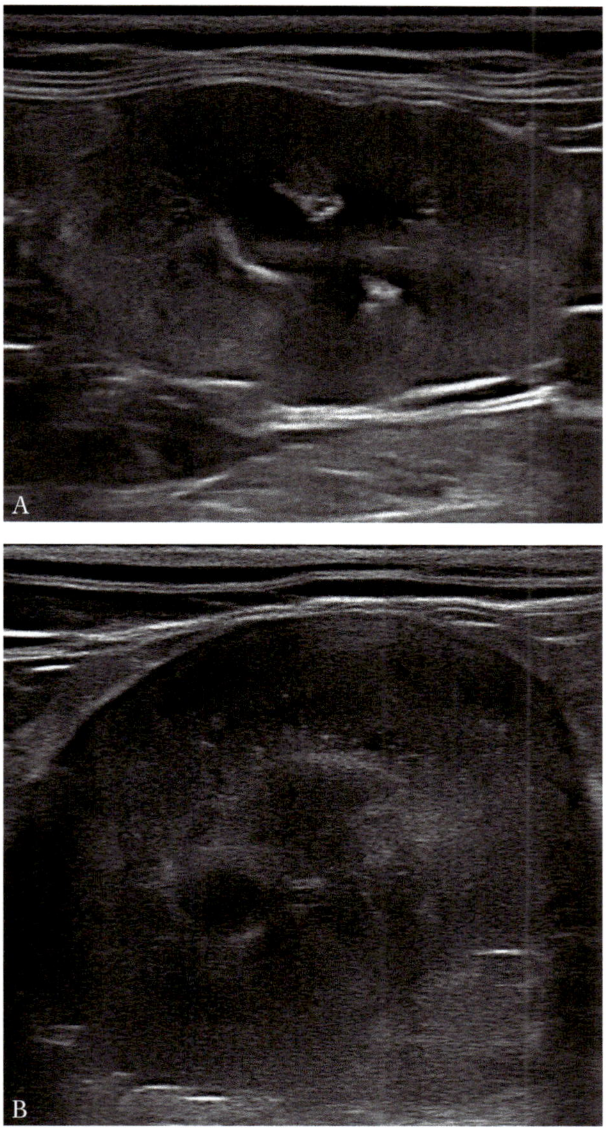

Figure 98. Kidneys from two patients with renal lymphoma. In image A irregular edges and a decreased corticomedullary differentiation can be seen. The patient in image B shows increased echogenicity, reduced corticomedullary definition and a hypoechogenic subcapsular halo.

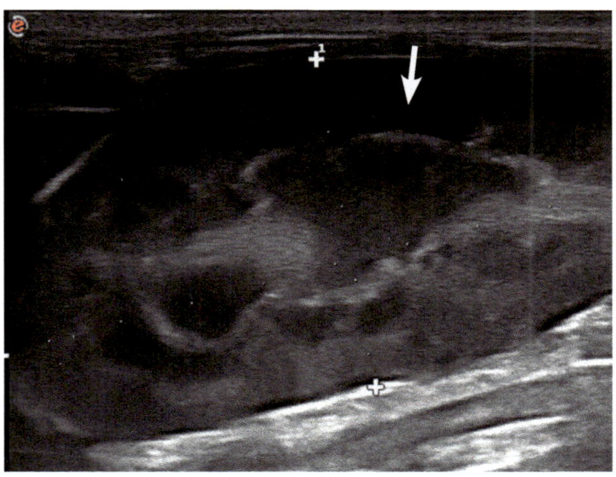

Figure 99. 2-year-old patient with FIP. Renomegaly, an increase in cortical echogenicity, with a mildly irregular contour, medullary rim sign (arrow) and hypoechoic subcapsular halo can be seen.

an incidental and secondary finding to a wide variety of kidney lesions, such as ethylene glycol poisoning, pyogranulomatous vasculitis due to FIP (Figure 99), interstitial nephritis and renal calcification secondary to hypercalcaemia.

Perinephric pseudocysts

These usually occur in **older cats** and may accompany chronic kidney disease lesions (Figure 100) or may occur as a consequence of surgery or neoplasm with venous congestion. On ultrasound, an **accumulation of anechogenic fluid** is observed between the **renal capsule and the parenchyma**. One or both kidneys may be affected. The kidney usually occupies an eccentric position and presents an altered echostructure, with less corticomedullary definition and a hyperechogenic cortex.

Focal diseases

Infarctions

Chronic renal infarction in the renal cortex is seen as a **hyperechogenic triangular section**, with a broad base towards the renal capsule (Figure 101). Acute infarction presents decreased or mixed echogenicity. Upon chronification, echogenicity increases, and atrophy of the periphery occurs, causing indentation in the capsule.

Cysts

Polycystic kidney disease (PKD) is common in **Persian cats** and their crossbreeds. It is characterized by the presence of cysts in the renal cortex or medulla, although the presence of cysts in the liver and pancreas have also been described.

Cysts are visualized as **anechogenic or hypoechogenic rounded cavities**, most often located in the cortex or in the renal medulla, well differentiated from

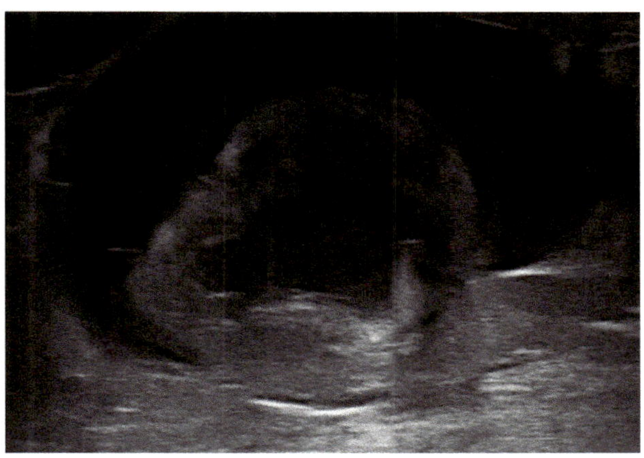

Figure 100. Patient with chronic renal disease and a perinephric pseudocyst. A small, irregular kidney with an echogenic cortex and a large amount of subcapsular liquid surrounding it can be seen.

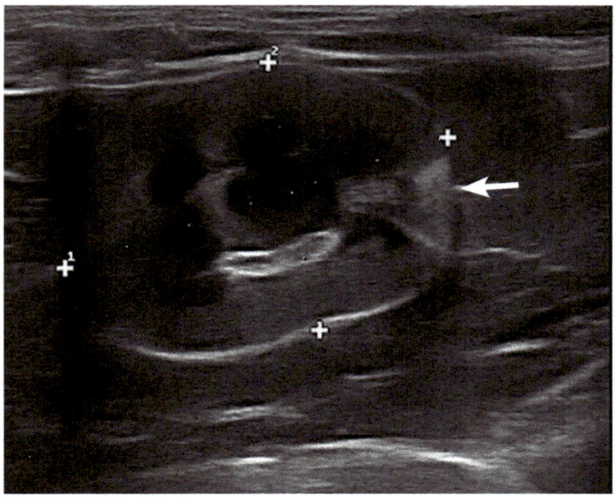

Figure 101. Patient with a renal infarction in the caudal pole of the kidney. A triangular hyperechoic region can be seen in the renal cortex.

the parenchyma, with a thin wall. The number and size of cysts is highly variable and increase with age until, on occasion, they completely replace the normal renal parenchyma and cause renal failure.

In old animals, cysts can be observed as an incidental finding and not associated with PKD.

Neoplasia

The different neoplasms that can affect the kidneys (Figure 102) usually cause **renomegaly** and produce **hypoechoic nodular areas**, as in the case of lymphoma, or masses.

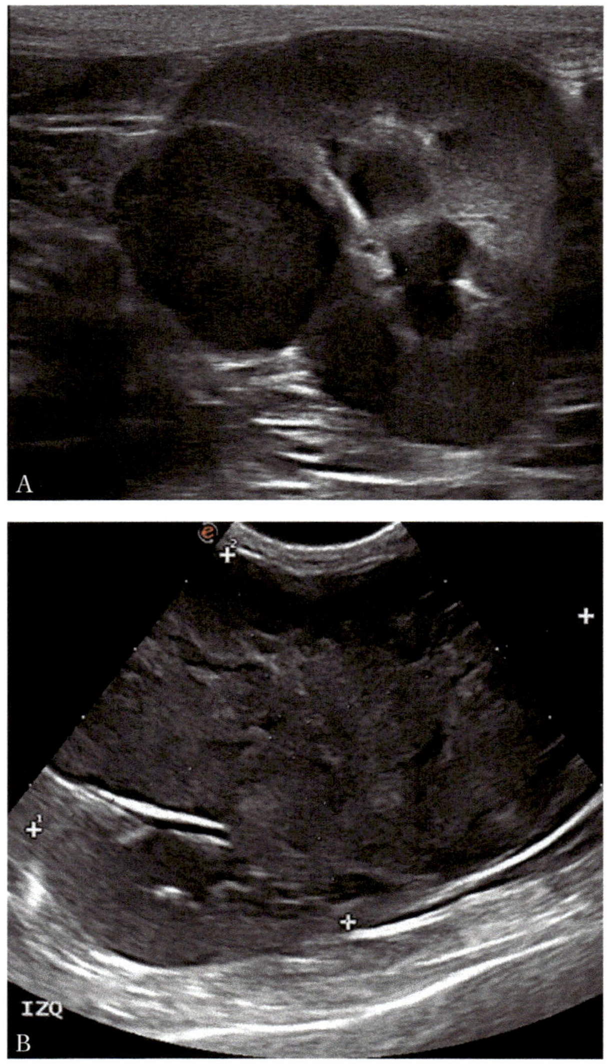

Figure 102. Patient with renal lymphoma (A), causing a well-defined hypoechoic nodule on the cranial pole and a patient with renal carcinoma (B) with a more heterogeneous mass.

In lymphoma with focal lesions, as well as in the diffuse form, the presence of a **subcapsular hypoechoic halo** around the kidney can be observed, although this halo is also visible in cats with **FIP and renal carcinoma**. Renal carcinoma usually affects one of the renal poles and produces hyperechoic lesions.

Abscesses and haematomas

Abscesses and haematomas are **uncommon in cats**.

Abscesses are seen as **cavitated masses, of mixed echogenicity**, with a thick and irregular wall and anechogenic or hyperechogenic content. They may have echogenic septa inside. If there is gas production, this is seen as echogenic spots with acoustic shadow.

Haematomas are usually hypoechoic and are usually located in the **subcapsular region** in cats that have suffered severe trauma or after a biopsy (Figure 103).

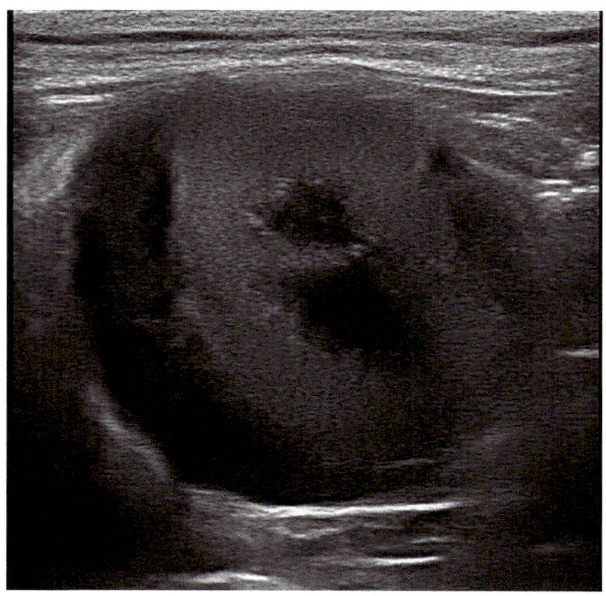

Figure 103. Subcapsular haematoma, visible as a hypoechoic region in a patient after a biopsy for acute kidney failure.

Diseases of the renal pelvis and collecting system

Distension of the renal pelvis

This can be seen in healthy cats (with fluid therapy, diuretics) and cats with different types of kidney disease or

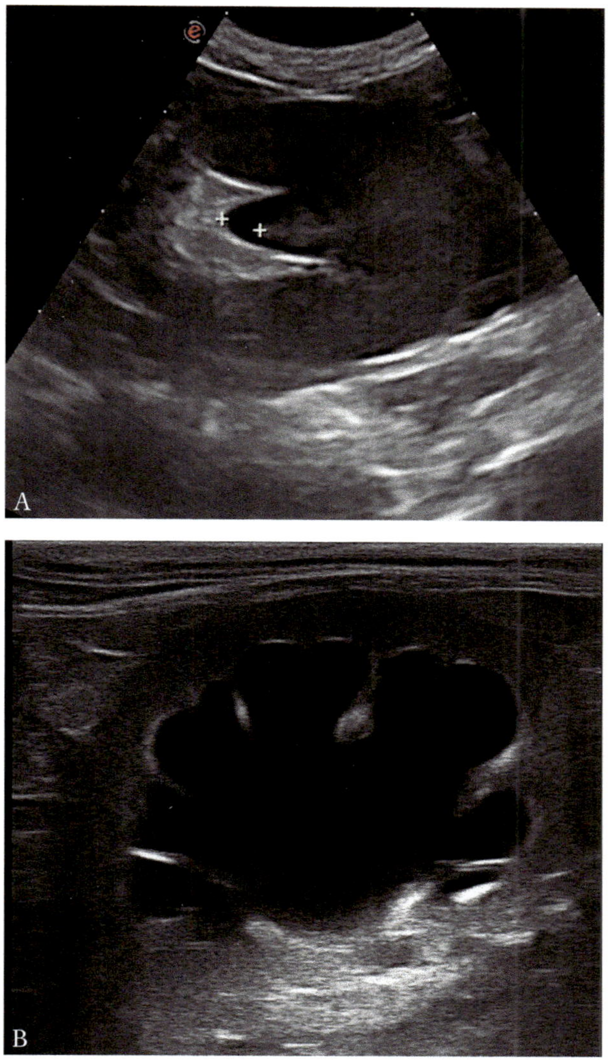

Figure 104. Transverse section in a cat with mild pyelectasia due to polyuria (A) and a patient with market hydronephrosis due to a ureteral obstruction (B).

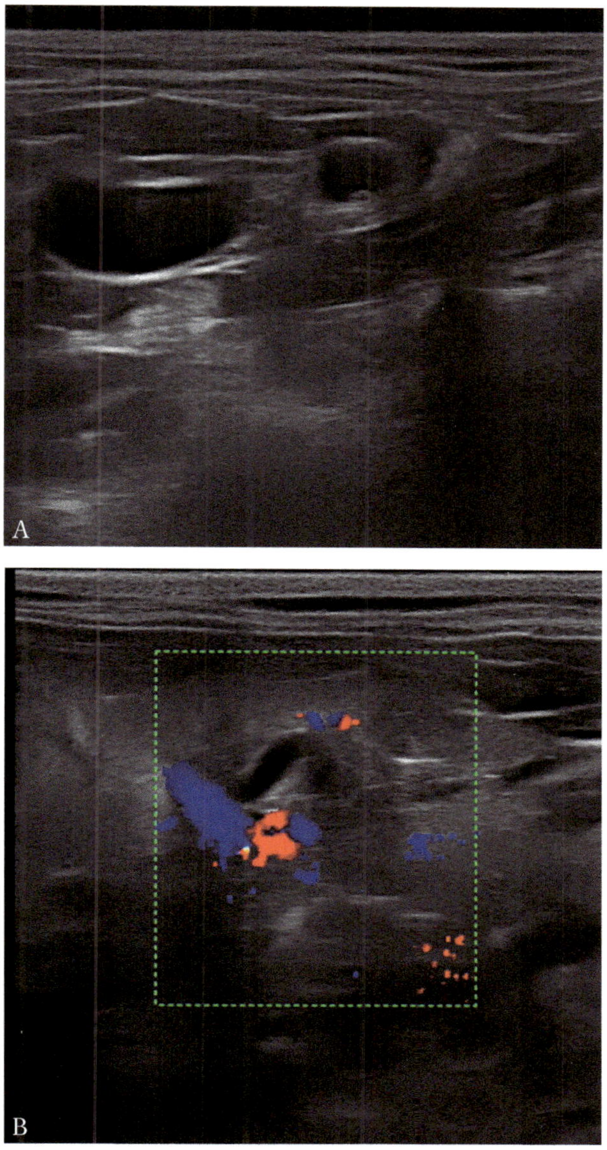

Figure 105. Patients with hydroureters due to ureteral calculi. Colour Doppler can be useful to distinguish the ureter from nearby vascular structures.

obstruction (Figure 104). In cats with clinically normal renal function, **a 1.6 mm distention** has been described, and progressively increases in the presence of renal failure, pyelonephritis and obstruction. The term **pyelectasis is used to describe mild to moderate distension of the renal pelvis.** In cats with **obstructions,** distention of the pelvis is usually much greater than that described in other pathologies, reaching up to **13 mm,** although they can also be reduced in size.

Marked distention of the pelvis is identified as hydronephrosis and there are also various grades. As the distention increases, the **cortex atrophies** until, in the most extreme cases, a very thin cortex is seen surrounding a large cavity with fluid, leaving the pelvic diverticula as echogenic lines perpendicular to the cortex.

Hydroureter

Distension of the ureter along its path with urine inside that allows it to be visualised with ultrasound. Cat's ureters are often not markedly distended, as can be seen in dogs, but even in the presence of calculi that obstruct the ureter and associated hydronephrosis, the ureter might be only slighlty distended and difficult to follow in some sections (Figure 105). The distension of the ureter is usually due to an obstructive cause, including stones, abdominal masses causing compression, and bladder neoplasms.

Renal and ureteral lithiasis

Mineralisations and uroliths appear on ultrasound as hyperechogenic structures with **acoustic shadow.** The acoustic shadow can be marked, but sometimes, especially if the calculi are small, the shadow can be very subtle or practically non-existent. Another feature that can help confirm their presence is the twinkling artefact when examined with colour Doppler (Figure 106).

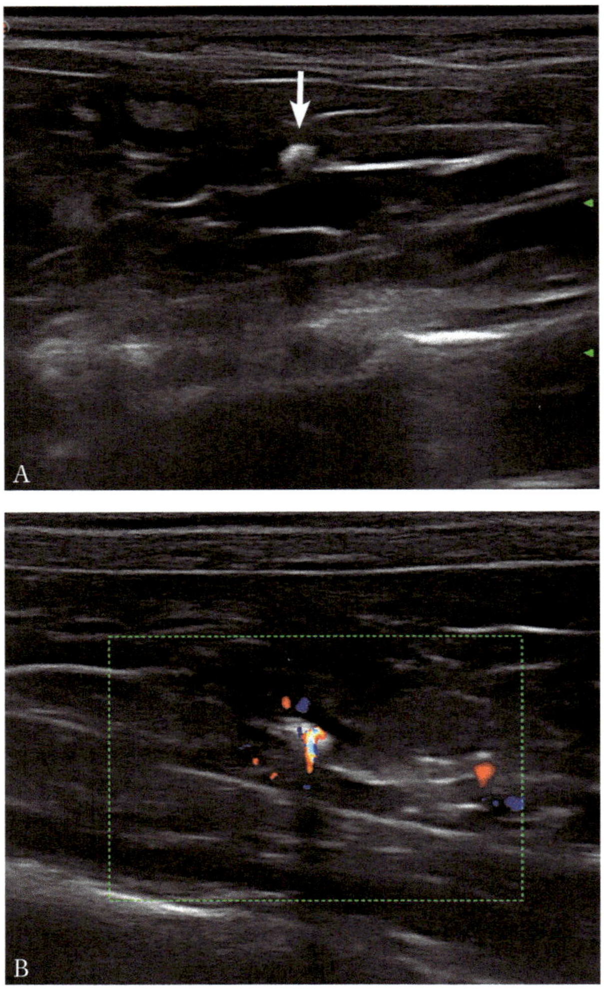

Figure 106. Patients with ureteral calculi, with a mild acoustic shadow in the first case (A). A twinkling artefact with the appearance of a colour mosaic superimposed on the calculi and part of the acoustic shadow can be seen (B).

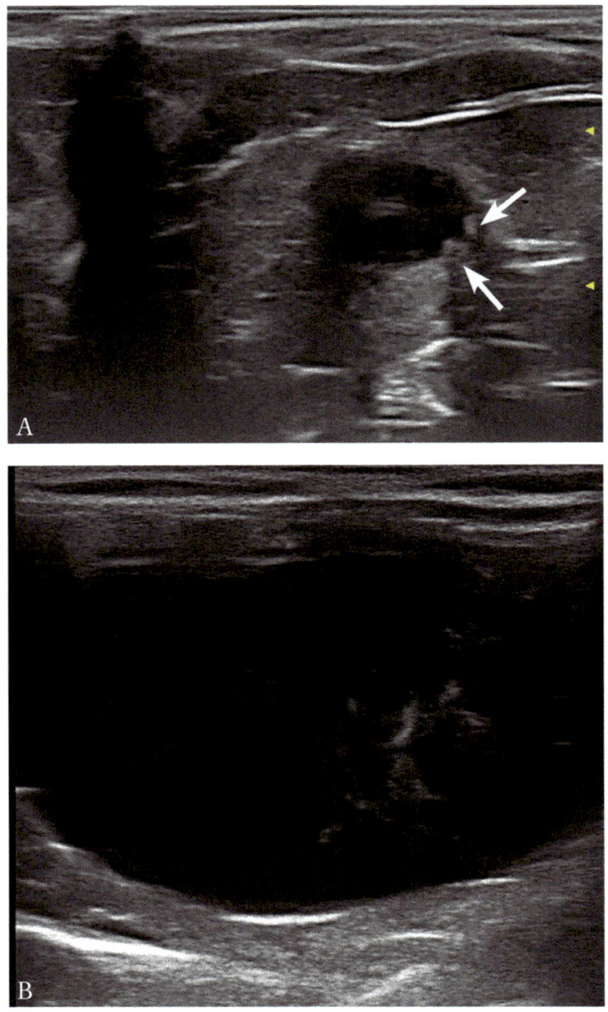

Figure 107. Area of the trigone where the ureteral papillae are visualised (A, arrows). A moderately distended bladder with echoes in suspension compatible with lipiduria (B).

Ectopic ureters

Congenital ureteral anomalies in the cat are not frequent. Generally, affected cats have **urinary incontinence**, although this may not necessarily be present. The presence of an ectopic ureter is usually accompanied by **hydroureter and hydronephrosis**, and sometimes also by ureterocoele. Although, if these are not present, resorting to other diagnostic techniques for their detection may be necessary.

Bladder

The thickness of the bladder wall varies depending on the degree of bladder filling; as the bladder distends the thickness decreases. In cats the **normal thickness range is 1.3–1.7 mm.**

The bladder trigone or neck of the bladder is not clearly delineated from the rest of the bladder. The trigone corresponds with the bladder's caudal border, which has a more conical shape, before continuing with the urethra. The **ureteral papillae** can be seen on the dorsal border of this area, identifiable as **small protrusions in the wall**, which should not be confused with focal lesions (Figure 107 A). Occasionally, urine can be visualized entering through the papilla, visualized on ultrasound as a small, hyperechogenic, jet-like ultrasonographic movements. Colour Doppler aids visualisation.

Normal urine is anechoic in appearance, but artefacts can often occur in the bladder region, such as lateral lobe artefacts, which simulate the presence of more echogenic sediment or urine. Many cats present **physiological lipiduria, manifested as hyperechogenic pinpoint echoes** in suspension in the urine, which are occasionally seen grouping together (Figure 107B). The position of these echoes does not depend on gravity and they do not present acoustic shadow, reverberations or twinkling artefacts.

Cystitis

The presence of inflammation or infection of the bladder does not always cause obvious ultrasonographic changes. When present, an **irregular thickening of the bladder wall** is observed, often on the cranioventral aspect, but it can also be diffuse. The changes may be accompanied by increased urine echogenicity, and the presence of calculi or clots in the bladder lumen.

Ultrasonographic changes to the content of the bladder lumen in cases of FLUTD include **echogenic urine**, with a swirling effect due to the presence of cells or high protein content. In cases of obstruction, distension of the bladder and urethra can be observed, and there may also sometimes be inflammation of the mesenteric fat around the urethra and a small amount of free periurethral fluid (Figure 108).

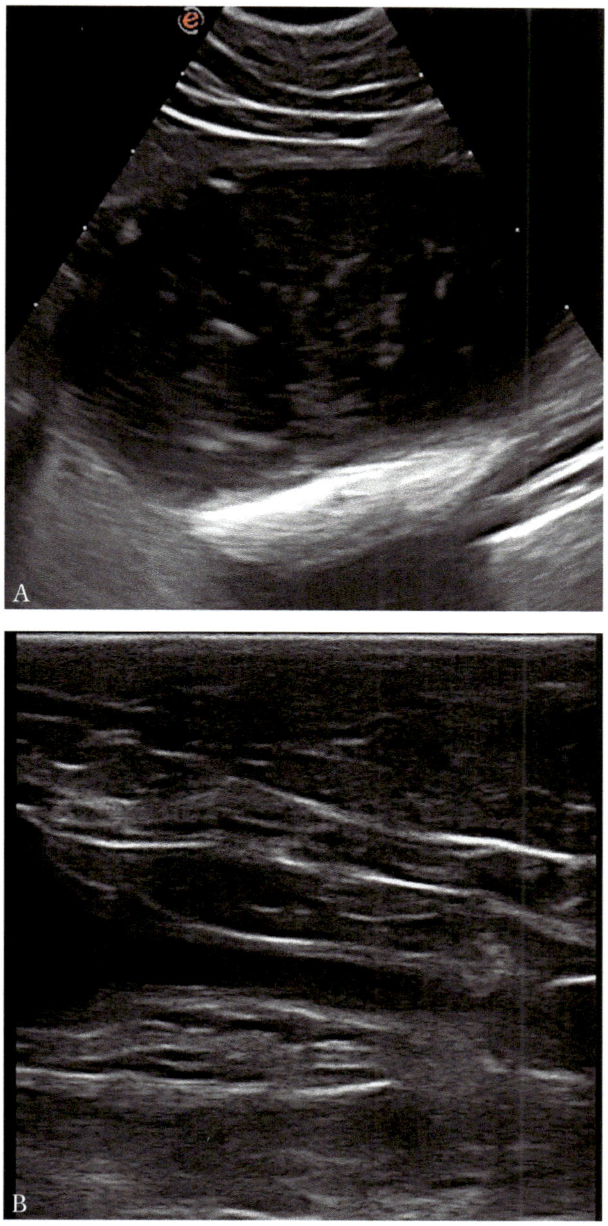

Figure 108. Image of the bladder of a patient with FLUTD. The bladder is distended with markedly echogenic urine and mineralised sediment is present with acoustic shadow (A). Patient with urethral obstruction. The periurethral mesenteric fat has an oedematous, striated appearance with alternations of hyperechogenic and anechogenic regions (B).

The development of pseudomembranous cystitis associated with urinary tract obstruction has been described in some cats. Ultrasonographically, these cases have a thickened bladder wall with **hyperechogenic septa** (histologically formed by fibrinohaemorrhagic material) which divides the bladder into compartments.

Chronic cystitis may result in **mineralization of the mucosal surface of the bladder** (Figure 109).

Neoplasia

Bladder neoplasms (Figure 110) are rare in cats. Transitional cell carcinoma is the most frequent neoplasm that can be found, and it is an aggressive disease

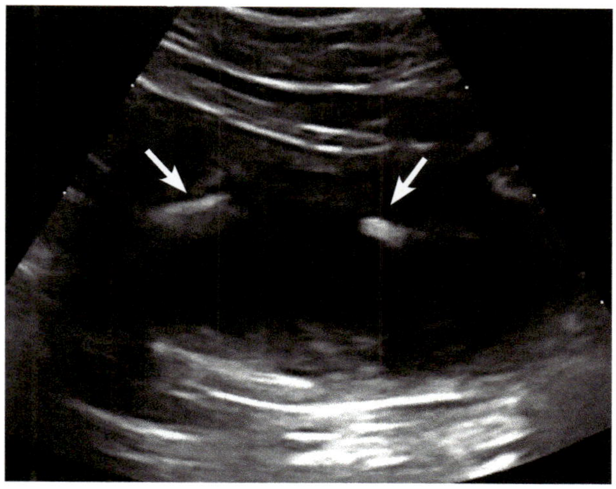

Figure 109. Sagittal section of the bladder. Two hyperechogenic linear regions can be seen which delineate the surface of the ventral mucosa and cause a slight acoustic shadow.

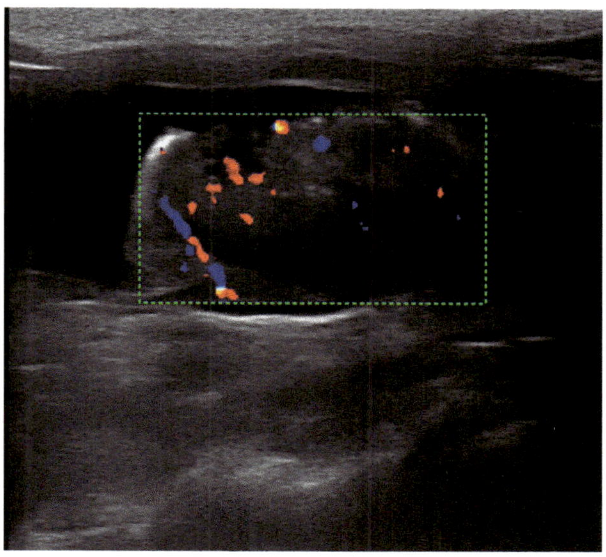

Figure 110. A wide-based mass with heterogeneous echogenicity can be seen on the medial and caudal aspect of the bladder which reaches the trigone region. It was highly vascularised upon evaluation with Doppler.

that, contrary to in the dog, is frequently located in **regions distant to the bladder trigone**. It can also extend into the urethra and be associated with a urinary obstruction.

Other neoplasms that can be found in the bladder are mesenchymal tumours, sarcomas, and lymphoma. The cases of feline lymphoma described in the literature have a variable appearance.

Calculi

Bladder or urethral calculi are seen as **hyperechogenic structures**, which often have a rounded shape, but their shape and size may vary. In the bladder, calculi accumulate in **dependent regions.** Acoustic shadow is commonly associated with stones, however, this is variable and small calculi may not show shadowing.

Haemorrhage and clots

Blood in urine appears on ultrasound as an increase in echogenicity, with **pinpoint echoes in suspension,** these form a sediment if the patient remains in one position for a sufficient length of time. The presence of clots in the bladder lumen are normally seen as variably shaped, heterogeneous structures, simulating the presence of a mass (Fig 111A). Colour Doppler evaluation (with absent signal) and demonstration of mobility within the bladder when the patient changes position help to differentiate clots from neoplasms or other inflammatory wall lesions.

Bleeding or bruising to the bladder wall is more difficult to distinguish sonographically from inflammatory or neoplastic lesions. The clinical history and performing follow up ultrasounds to assess the evolution of the lesion are very useful to distinguish between the two (Figure 111B).

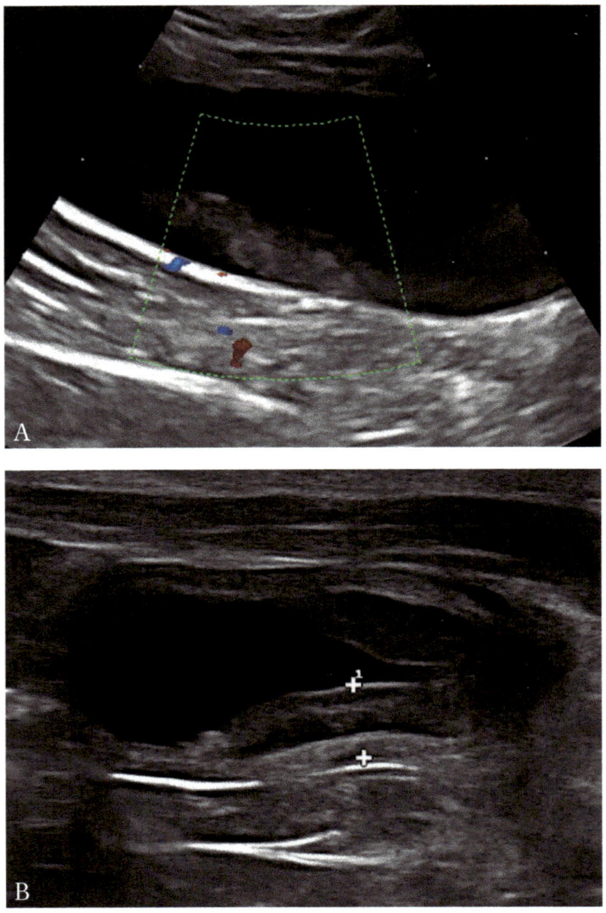

Figure 111. Intravesicular clot in a cat with polytrauma. An echogenic structure with a more or less fusiform shape is moderately defined in the dependent region of the bladder lumen and does not show a Doppler signal (A). Haematoma in the bladder wall in a cat which has suffered a road traffic accident. A thickening of the wall in the neck area of the bladder with a heterogeneous echogenicity can be seen (B).

Reproductive system

The **testes have a medium echogenicity** with a fine, homogeneous ultrasound texture and a fine, more hyperechogenic margin that represents the tunica albuginea. In sagittal section a hyperechogenic central line (the testicular mediastinum) can be seen, which appears as a central hyperechogenic focus in the transverse plane. The epididymis is more hypoechoic and thicker in texture than the testicles, although it is smaller and more difficult to visualize than in dogs.

The **prostate is not visualized** under normal conditions due to its intrapelvic position.

The **ovaries** are located caudally and laterally to the caudal poles of the kidneys. They are rounded to oval in shape and **less than 1 cm in size in cats** (Figure 112 A). Their appearance varies throughout the oestrous cycle. With high-frequency probes, observation of sub-millimetre anechogenic structures in the ovaries is possible, corresponding to primordial follicles and are usually located on the periphery.

The **uterus** is seen as a tubular structure located between the bladder and the colon (uterine body) and on the dorsolateral wall of the caudal abdomen (uterine horns). In cats, it is difficult to identify the cervix, since the characteristics described in other species, such as a focal thickening of the uterine body or the typical "bull's eye" appearance, are not seen. Ultrasonographically, the uterus presents a thin external hyperechogenic halo (serosa), which is easier to see in sagittal than transverse planes (Figure 112B).

Gestation

In a recent study, using high-frequency probes, it was observed that **from day 11 of gestation the embryonic vesicles were already visible** as anechogenic cavities in the lumen of the uterus with a 1.2 mm (± 0.1) diameter. Little by little, the vesicle grows and changes shape

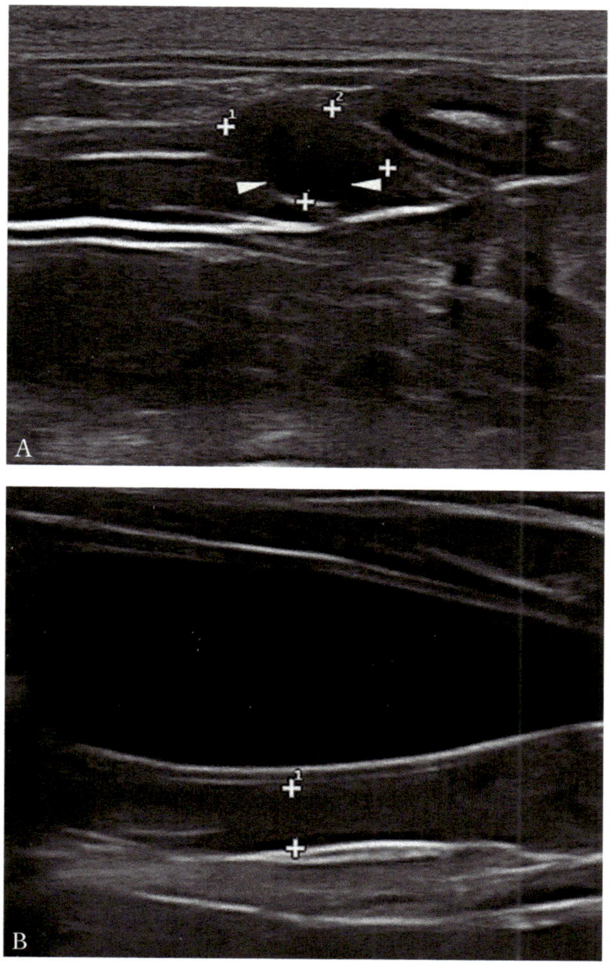

Figure 112. Ovary (between cursors) in a female in oestrus. An anechoic structure (between arrowheads) in the periphery can be seen (A). Sagittal section of the body of the uterus of a 7-year-old healthy female visible dorsal to the bladder (B).

until day 15, when its diameter measures an average of 5.3 mm (± 0.6).

The **embryo is usually visible around day 16** as a hyperechogenic structure in the lumen of the embryonic vesicle.

- The **heart is visible between days 16–18**.
- Heart rate can be detected between 16–20 days of gestation.
- From day 19 of gestation it is possible to differentiate the head of the foetus, although it can be more easily identified on day 20.
- On day 20 it is possible to observe the formation of the extremities, although these can be observed better from the 24th day of gestation, the anterior limbs show somewhat earlier development than the posterior limbs.
- The stomach can be seen from day 26.
- From day 27–28 of gestation, the symmetry of the head starts to become evident with the development of the cerebral hemispheres, which are slightly hyperechogenic structures, while the amount of anechogenic content in the head decreases. At this time, the heart, liver, and stomach are clearly visible, and the embryo is similar in shape to what it will be at birth (Figure 113).

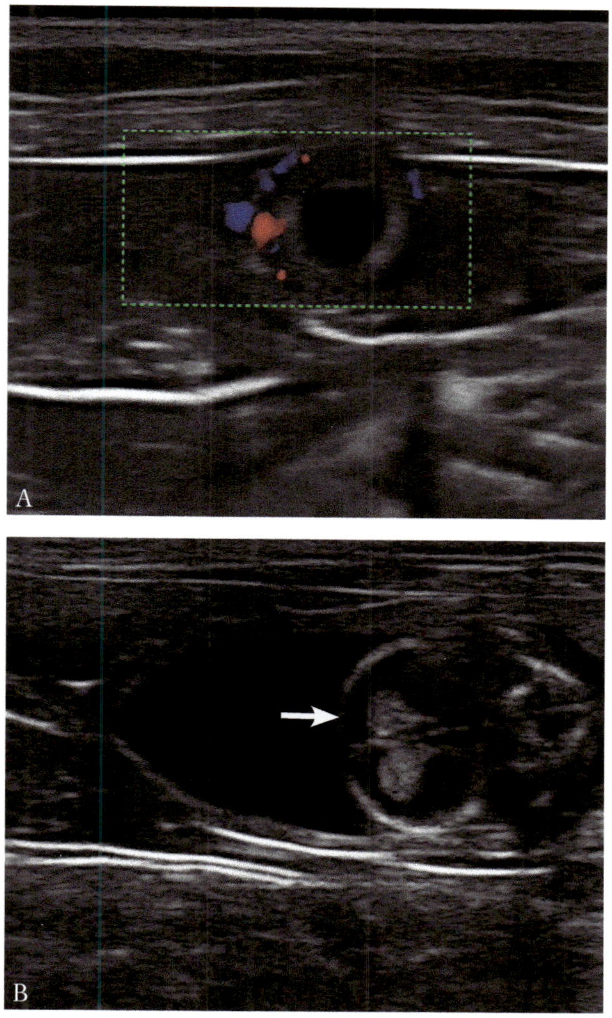

Figure 113. Embryonic vesicle prior to day 16. The embryo is not yet visible (A). Cranium of the foetus after day 28. The cerebral hemispheres can be seen as hyperechogenic structures (B, arrow).

In cats, **uterine involution takes about 24 days.** During this period of time, the thickness of the uterine walls and the volume of intraluminal fluid decrease, so that gradually the uterus becomes less evident.

Cryptorchidism

The testes can be located in the abdominal cavity (in any position from the caudal pole of the kidneys to the inguinal region), in the inguinal canal or in an ectopic subcutaneous location between the superficial inguinal ring and the scrotum.

Prostate abnormalities

Prostate disease is rare in cats. Some cases of prostatic neoplasia and other non-neoplastic lesions have been

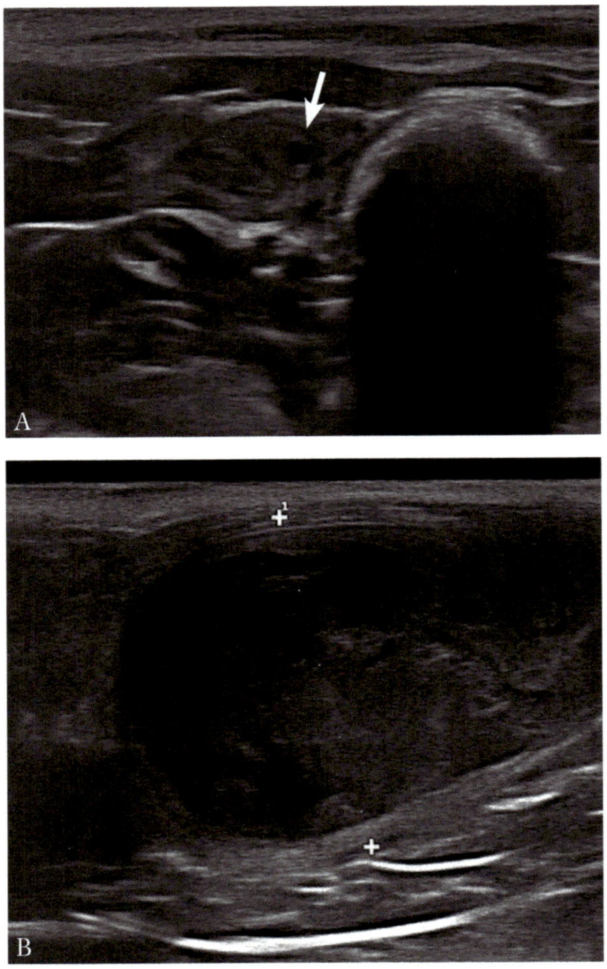

Figure 114. Images of the uterus of the same cat. Uterine region near to the body where a cystic structure in the uterine wall (arrow) compatible with endometrial hyperplasia can be seen (A). The left horn (between cursors) is notably distended with echogenic liquid content, compatible with a pyometra (B).

described (periprostatic cysts, prostatic hyperplasia, bacterial prostatitis, and prostatic metaplasia).

Ovarian abnormalities

Ovarian cysts are usually incidental findings (anovulatory follicular ovarian cysts), especially in nulliparous adult-geriatric females. Ultrasonographically, they are seen as one or more anechogenic structures between 1–5 cm in diameter, well defined with a thin hyperechogenic wall and posterior enhancement. Differential diagnoses includes ovarian tumours, especially granulosa cell tumours.

Uterine abnormalities

In the cystic endometrial hyperplasia (CEH) -pyometra complex, cystic dilation of the endometrial glands, non-inflammatory accumulation of aseptic viscous fluid in the uterine lumen with subsequent bacterial contamination, endometrial inflammation with the presence of blood and pus is observed. When the **pyometra** has become established, the typical appearance of a dilated uterus with the presence of liquid content can be observed on ultrasound (Figure 114).

Gestation abnormalities

The most frequent pathologies are **embryonic resorption** (embryonic death before 25 days of gestation) and **abortion** (foetal death after 35 days of gestation).

In cases of embryonic resorption, the embryonic vesicle appears deformed, loses its spherical shape, appears wrinkled with a less defined wall, and an accumulation of hyperechogenic material is observed in the lumen. Loss of heartbeat, disintegration, and finally collapse of the embryonic vesicle are observed.

In cases of foetal death, the heartbeat and movements of the foetus are no longer appreciated, abnormal foetal posture, increased echogenicity of the fluid surrounding the foetus, and even the presence of gas in the foetus or inside the uterus may be observed.

Bibliography

Aarsvold S, Reetz JA, Reichle JK, Jones ID, Lamb CR, Evola MG, Keyerleber MA, Marolf AJ. *Computed tomographic findings in 57 cats with primary pulmonary neoplasia.* Vet Radiol Ultrasound. 2015 May-Jun;56(3):272–7.

Atlas of Small Animal ultrasonography. Eds; Penninck D, d'Anjou MA. Wiley-Blackwell 2015.

BSAVA Manual of Canine and Feline Abdominal Imaging. Eds: O'Brien R, Barr F. 2009 British Small Animal Association, Gloucester, UK.

BSAVA Manual of Canine and Feline Thoracic Imaging. Eds: Schwarz T, Johnson V. 2008 British Small Animal Association, Gloucester, UK.

Byron JK, Shadwick SR, Bennett AR. *Megaesophagus in a 6-month-old cat secondary to a nasopharyngeal polyp.* J Feline Med Surg. 2010 Apr;12(4):322–4.

DeSandre-Robinson DM, Madden SN, Walker JT. *Nasopharyngeal stenosis with concurrent hiatal hernia and megaesophagus in an 8-year-old cat.* J Feline Med Surg. 2011 Jun;13(6):454–9.

Diagnostic Ultrasound in cats. Novellas R. Domínguez E, Espada Y, Martínez Y, Tobón M. Ed Novellas et al. Servet, Zaragoza, Spain, 2015.

Diagnóstico por imagen en pequeños animales. Eds: Agut, A. 2014 Multimédica, Barcelona.

Evola MG, Edmondson EF, Reichle JK, Biller DS, Mitchell CW, Valdés-Martínez A. *Radiographic and histopathologic characteristics of pulmonary fibrosis in nine cats.* Vet Radiol Ultrasound. 2014 Mar-Apr;55(2):133–40.

Forrest LJ, Graybush CA. *Radiographic patterns of pulmonary metastasis in 25 cats.* Vet Radiol Ultrasound. 1998 Jan-Feb;39(1):4–8.

Fujita M, Miura H, Yasuda D, Hasegawa D, Orima H. *Tracheal narrowing secondary to airway obstruction in two cats.* J Small Anim Pract. 2004 Jan;45(1):29–31.

German AJ, Cannon MJ, Dye C, Booth MJ, Pearson GR, Reay CA, Gruffydd-Jones TJ. *Oesophageal strictures in cats associated with doxycycline therapy.* J Feline Med Surg. 2005 Feb;7(1):33–41.

Geyer NE, Reichle JK, Valdés-Martínez A, Williams J, Goggin JM, Leach L, Hanson J, Hill S, Axam T. *Radiographic appearance of confirmed pulmonary lymphoma in cats and dogs.* Vet Radiol Ultrasound. 2010 Jul-Aug;51(4):386–90.

Goldfinch N, Argyle DJ. *Feline lung-digit syndrome: unusual metastatic patterns of primary lung tumours in cats.* J Feline Med Surg. 2012 Mar;14(3):202–8.

Guglielmini C, Diana A. *Thoracic radiography in the cat: Identification of cardiomegaly and congestive heart failure.* J Vet Cardiol. 2015 Dec;17 Suppl 1:S87–101.

Keenihan EK, Lynch S, Priestnall SL, Harrington NT, Benigni L, Lamb CR. *Unusual rib metastasis in two cats with pulmonary carcinoma.* J Feline Med Surg. 2013 Dec;15(15):1145–8.

Lacava G, Zini E, Marchesotti F, Domenech O, Romano F, Manzocchi S, Venco L, Auriemma E. *Computed tomography, radiology and echocardiography in cats naturally infected with Aelurostrongylus abstrusus.* Feline Med Surg. 2016 Mar 9. pii: 1098612X16636419.

Le Boedec K, Roady PJ, O'Brien RT. *A case of atypical diffuse feline fibrotic lung disease.* J Feline Med Surg. 2014 Oct;16(10):858–63.

McGrotty YL, Knottenbelt CM. *Oesophageal stricture in a cat due to oral administration of tetracyclines.* J Small Anim Pract. 2002 May;43(5):221–3.

Norris CR, Samii VF. *Clinical, radiographic, and pathologic features of bronchiectasis in cats: 12 cases* (1987–1999). J Am Vet Med Assoc. 2000 Feb 15;216(4):530–4.

Oura TJ, Young AN, Keene BW, Robertson ID, Jennings DE, Thrall DE. *A valentine-shaped cardiac silhouette in feline thoracic radiographs is primarily due to left atrial enlargement.* Vet Radiol Ultrasound. 2015 May-Jun;56(3):245–50.

Schmierer PA(1), Schwarz A(2), Bass DA(2), Knell SC(2). *Novel avulsion pattern of the left principal bronchus with involvement of the carina and caudal thoracic trachea in a cat.* J Feline Med Surg. 2014 Aug;16(8):695–8.

Sleeper MM, Roland R, Drobatz KJ. *Use of the vertebral heart scale for differentiation of cardiac and noncardiac causes of respiratory distress in cats: 67 cases* (2002–2003). J Am Vet Med Assoc. 2013 Feb 1;242(3):366–71.

Textbook of Veterinary Diagnostic Radiology. Eds Thrall, D. 2013. Elsevier, Missouri.

Trumble C. *Oesophageal stricture in cats associated with use of the hyclate (hydrochloride) salt of doxycycline.* J Feline Med Surg. 2005 Aug;7(4):241–2.

Wilson HE, Jasani S, Wagner TB, Benigni L, Milne JR, Stokes AL, Luis-Fuentes V. *Signs of left heart volume overload in severely anaemic cats.* J Feline Med Surg. 2010 Dec;12(12):904–9.

Winter MD, Giglio RF, Berry CR, Reese DJ, Maisenbacher HW, Hernandez JA. *Associations between 'valentine' heart shape, atrial enlargement and cardiomyopathy in cats.* J Feline Med Surg. 2015 Jun;17(6):447–52.

Zambelli AB. *Pneumomediastinum, pneumothorax and pneumoretroperitoneum following endoscopic retrieval of a tracheal foreign body from a cat.* J S Afr Vet Assoc. 2006 Mar;77(1):45–50.

Zwicker LA, Matthews AR, Côté E, Andersen E. *The effect of dexmedetomidine on radiographic cardiac silhouette size in healthy cats.* Vet Radiol Ultrasound. 2016 May;57(3):230–6.

Test

1. A normal vertebral heart score in the cat is:

A) 10.5 in a DV projection.
B) 8.1 in a lateral projection.
C) 9.5 in a DV projection.
D) 9.5 in a lateral projection.

2. In the cat, regarding the cranioventral mediastinum:

A) If it exceeds the width of a vertebral body this is always indicative of a mediastinal mass.
B) It should not exceed the width of two vertebral bodies.
C) It can exceed the width of a vertebral body in obese patients, without being pathological.
D) Is where the tracheobronchial lymph nodes are found.

3. Which are among the characteristics of an alveolar lung pattern?

A) Lobar sign.
B) Air bronchogram.
C) Silhouette effect with structures adjacent to the lung.
D) All of the above.

4. Among the radiographic signs of left cardiomegaly which of the following can be found:

A) Increased convexity or bulging of the caudal edge in a lateral view.
B) Elevation of the cardiac apex in a lateral view.
C) Displacement of the apex cranially and to the left in the DV/VD projection.
D) Increased convexity or bulging of the cranial aspect of the heart in a lateral view.

5. Bronchiectasis:

A) It is part of the alveolar pattern.
B) Is only a thickening of the bronchial wall.
C) It is a sign of chronic bronchial disease and is irreversible.
D) All of the above.

6. In a pleural effusion:
A) Pericardial fat can help visualize the heart.
B) The rounded margins of the lung lobes indicate an acute or poorly reactive effusion.
C) Air opacity is observed in the pleural space.
D) All of the above.

7. Radiographically:
A) Linear foreign bodies often cause signs of obstruction with marked intestinal distension.
B) The normal colon should not exceed 12 mm in diameter.
C) Distension of the colon greater than 1.5 times the length of L5 is indicative of megacolon.
D) Distension of the colon greater than 1.5 times the length of L2 is indicative of megacolon.

8. Causes of microhepathy visible radiographically include:
A) Peritoneopericardial diaphragmatic hernia.
B) Diaphragmatic rupture.
C) Portosystemic shunt.
D) All of the above.

9. Perirenal retroperitoneal effusion can be observed in cases of:
A) Urethral obstruction.
B) Chronic renal failure.
C) Hydronephrosis.
D) Any of the above.

10. Regarding the radiographic characteristics of the bladder:
A) The presence of mineralization in the wall is always synonymous with neoplasia.
B) Double contrast cystography is used to diagnose bladder rupture.
C) Diverticula in the bladder apex may be incidental.
D) Loss or reduction of serosal detail around the bladder neck occurs only due to rupture of the bladder or urethra.

11. When oesophageal perforation is suspected, the imaging technique of choice for diagnosis is:
A) Ultrasound.
B) Oesophagogram with iodinated contrast.
C) Barium contrast oesophagogram.
D) Double contrast oesophagogram.

12. Regarding cystography:
A) Atmospheric air is recommended if severe cystitis is suspected.
B) If severe cystitis is suspected, the positive contrast of choice is ionic iodine contrast.
C) It is only advisable to perform cystography with non-ionic iodinated contrast in any case.
D) None of the above.

13. Regarding ultrasound of the liver:
A) Visualization of the common bile duct is indicative of pathology.
B) Visualization of intrahepatic bile ducts is indicative of pathology.
C) A septate gallbladder is abnormal in feline patients.
D) Visualization of the cystic duct is indicative of pathology.

14. A hyperechoic renal cortex:
A) Can be normal due to the presence of fat.
B) Is always indicative of kidney disease.
C) Only occurs in chronic kidney disease.
D) None of the above.

15. A thickening of the muscularis layer in the small intestine:
A) May be due to inflammatory bowel disease (IBD).
B) May be due to lymphoma.
C) May be due to a mastocytoma.
D) All of the above.

16. The twinkling artefact:

A) Is seen with Doppler and is due to the presence of small gas bubbles.

B) Is seen with Doppler and is due to the presence of calculi.

C) Occurs with B mode and is due to the presence of small gas bubbles.

D) Occurs with mode B and is due to the presence of calculi

Clinical cases

Case 1

Signalment: 9-month-old neutered male domestic shorthair (DSH) cat.

History: acute vomiting, apathy and anorexia.

Diagnostic tests: findings compatible with dehydration, without other significant changes.

Imaging tests available: abdominal radiography and ultrasound.

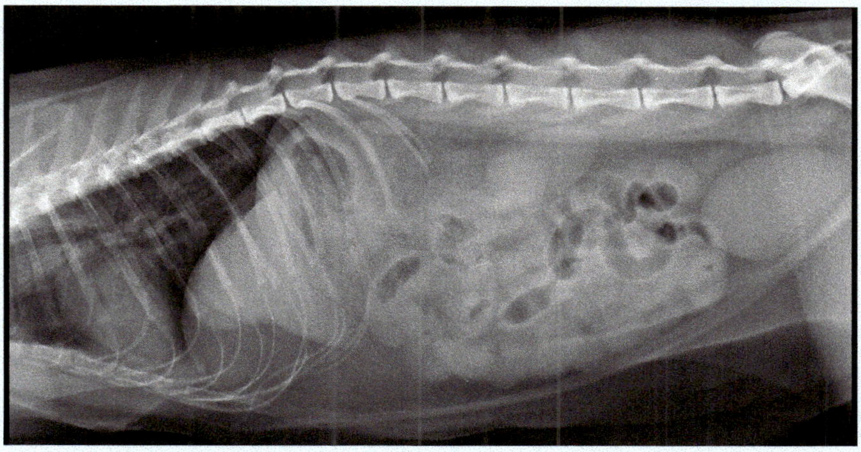

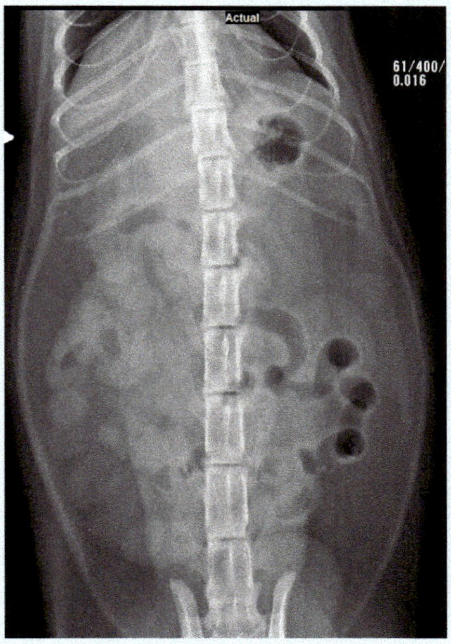

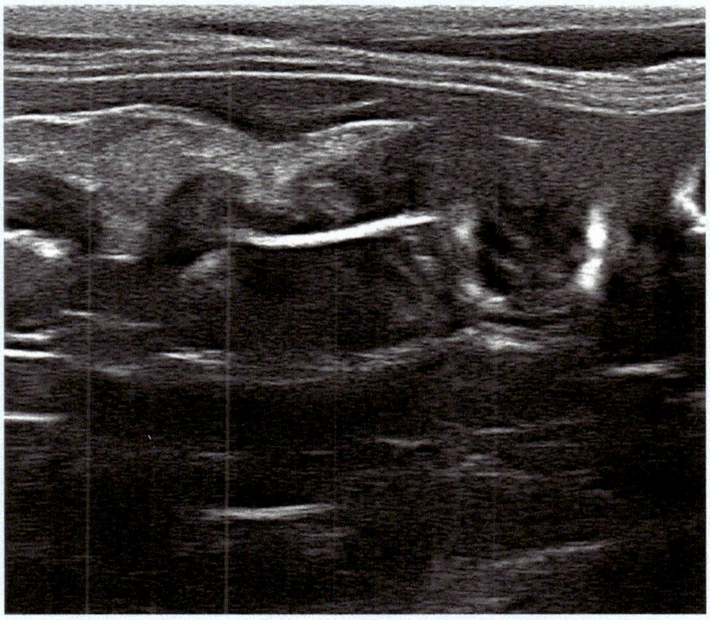

Answer the following questions:

1. **The abdominal radiograph shows:**

A) Marked generalised intestinal distension.

B) Marked distension with gas from the colon.

C) Bunched-up small intestine, with some triangular gas bubbles.

D) Loss of serosal detail and lymphadenopathy.

2. **The radiographic changes are therefore suggestive of:**
   A) Pancreatitis.
   B) Enteritis.
   C) Linear foreign body.
   D) Feline infectious peritonitis.
3. **The ultrasound shows:**
   A) A hypoechoic pancreas.
   B) An intestine with a plicated appearance and a linear structure in the lumen.
   C) An intestine with a plicated appearance and a focal structure and marked acoustic shadow in the lumen.
   D) An intestine distended with fluid.
4. **Which of the following can also be seen on the ultrasound image:**
   A) Hyperechoic peritoneum around part of the intestine.
   B) Free gas.
   C) Free liquid.
   D) All of the above.
5. **Ultrasonography confirms diagnosis of:**
   A) Pancreatitis.
   B) Enteritis.
   C) Linear foreign body.
   D) Feline infectious peritonitis.

Case 2

Signalment: 3-year-old DSH neutered male cat.
History: outdoor cat, who returns home with dyspnoea.
Diagnostic tests: without significant abnormalities.
Imaging tests available: lateral and ventrodorsal thoracic radiographs and lateral abdominal radiography.

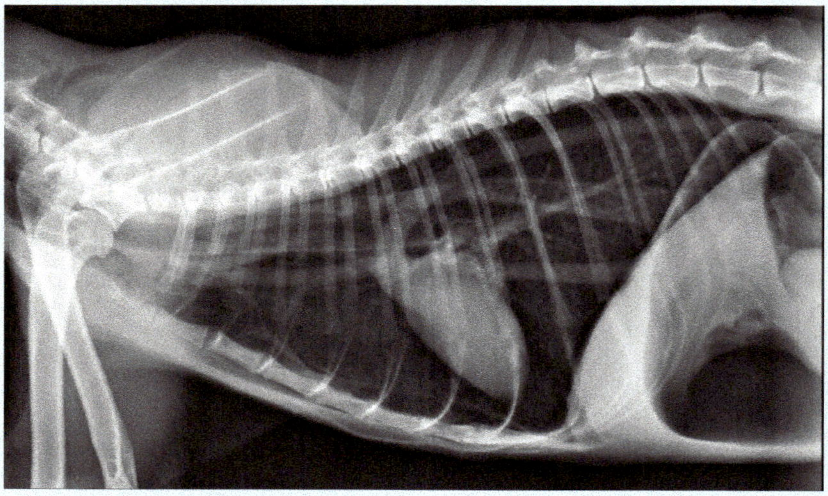

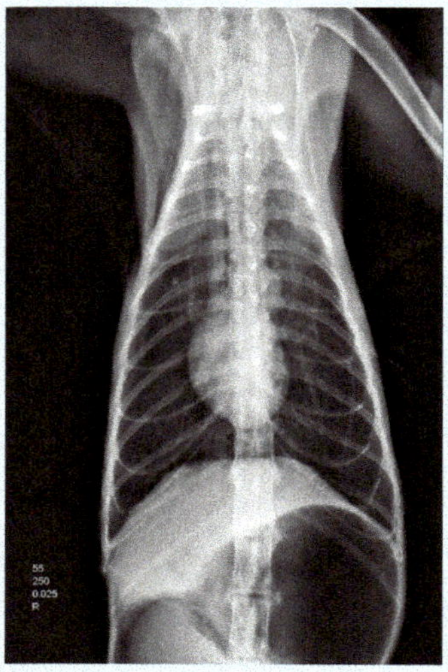

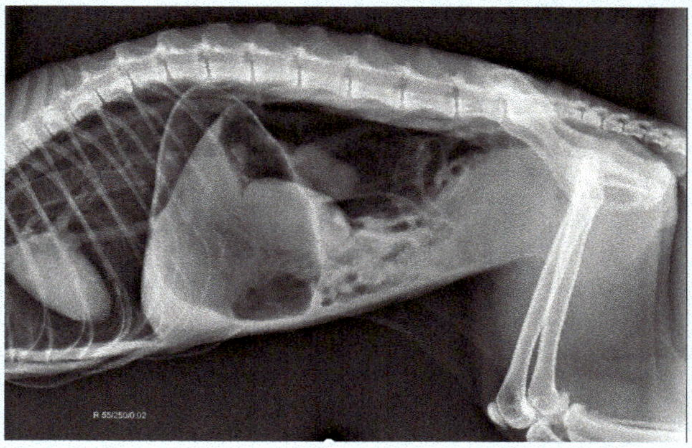

vAnswer the following questions:

1. **Which of the following can be seen in the thoracic radiographs:**
   A) Pneumomediastinum.
   B) Pneumothorax.
   C) Pleural effusion.
   D) All of the above.
2. **Which of the following can also be seen on thoracic radiographs:**
   A) Subcutaneous emphysema.
   B) Oesophageal distension.
   C) Overdistension of the rib cage.
   D) All of the above.
3. **In the abdominal projection which of the following are visualized:**
   A) Pneumoperitoneum.
   B) Pneumoretroperitoneum.
   C) Abdominal effusion.
   D) All of the above.
4. **Possible differential diagnoses for the set of changes include:**
   A) Tracheal rupture.
   B) Neck injury.
   C) Thoracic trauma.
   D) Any of the above.

Answers

Test

1. B	7. C	13. B
2. C	8. D	14. A
3. D	9. A	15. D
4. A	10. C	16. B
5. C	11. B	
6. A	12. D	

Case 1

1. C
2. C
3. B
4. A
5. C

Case 2

1. A
2. D
3. B
4. D

In this case, the cause was unknown, although trauma was suspected due to the sudden onset and the fact that the animal was an outdoor cat.

Feline dermatology

3

Giordana Zanna

Contents

Introduction

In the context of feline dermatology it is salient to apply the old maxim "**The cat is not a small dog.**" Looking back to their earliest ancestors, we find feline domestication has influenced their anatomy, which in turn impacts the symptoms of skin disease and secondary complications as seen in the cat.

The story of the domestication of cats began thousands of years ago. When early man stopped following herds of wild animals to establish the first rural settlements, this agricultural lifestyle brought its own needs. When human survival depended on adequate grain reserves, it was imperative to protect these valuable supplies from rodents. So began a mutually beneficial relationship where **wild cats were encouraged to predate on vermin** in grain stores. These animals were **selected for their hunting prowess**, rather than physical characteristics such as face shape or colour, and so to a large extent these animals retained their **original physical and behavioural characteristics.** Even today, despite cats being hugely popular pets worldwide, there are still relatively few breeds (80 cat varieties versus more than 300 for dogs).

From the perspective of the cat's skin and coat, the species has a number of **behavioural and anatomical traits** different to dogs. As outlined below the veterinarian is wise to keep in mind when considering differential diagnosis and treatment of the feline dermatology patient.

Grooming

Grooming is a physiological behaviour, also known as "preening". It consists of licking (Figure 1), rubbing the nose with the medial part of the forelimbs, and occasionally biting (to remove ectoparasites). Other functions of grooming include thermoregulation (via the evaporation of saliva from the coat) and to stabilize social relationships within a group of cats.

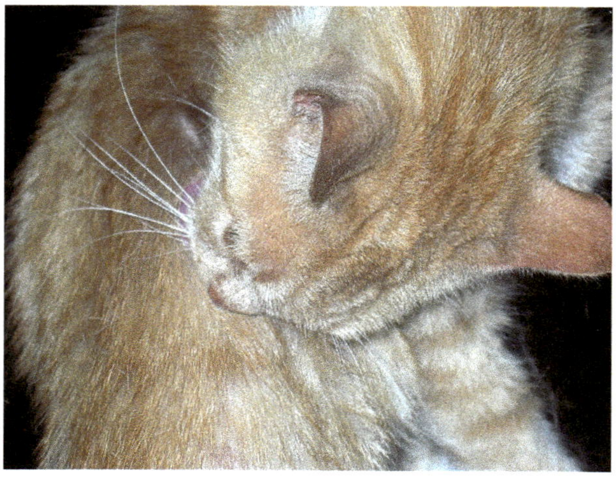

Figure 1. A cat licks the dorsal area of body as part of normal grooming behaviour.

Normal cat behaviour is to spend up to 50% of their awake time oral and scratch grooming, equivalent to around 15% of a 24-hour cycle. Therefore, it is valuable to recognize that an itchy stimulus (such as ectoparasites or allergens) leads to an increase in grooming activity, whilst a disease causing systemic failure can lead to a decrease in such activity and a loss of coat condition.

Nails

Cat claws are very sharp (Figure 2a) and are a unique atavistic characteristic of the feline species, perfectly designed to climb, grip prey, and for defence. Claws are also an important communication tool, used for scratching and marking territory.

In the cat, **scratch grooming** is considered part of the usual repertoire of behavioural patterns. Indeed the act of scratching eliminates scale that forms on the nails. When, a cat is deprived of the ability to scratch for several days, when this ability is restored the individual shows a 200% increase in normal scratching behaviour for the next 12 hours. Due to the sharp nature of feline nails, the consequences of excessive scratching due to a dermatological problem are potentially more serious in cats than in dogs.

Teeth

Cat teeth are much sharper (Figure 2b) than their dog counterparts, and along with their atavistic hunting behaviour, are designed to deliver maximum impact on their prey. When grooming, the incisors are used mainly for tugging out burrs. Although less common, a pruritic stimulus that causes the cat to bite the body has the potential to cause greater self-trauma than in the dog.

Tongue

This organ serves to firmly hold food in the mouth during hunting activity, scrape meat from the bones of prey and, naturally, for oral grooming. The tongue has a **bristled surface** due to the presence of numerous filiform papillae (Figure 2c), which are hook-like and give the tongue its characteristic rough texture. It follows that any increase in frequency or intensity of licking behaviour can result in **skin damage due to self-trauma**.

Curling up to sleep

Cats like to sleep curled up, which is atavistic behaviour designed to warm the body and

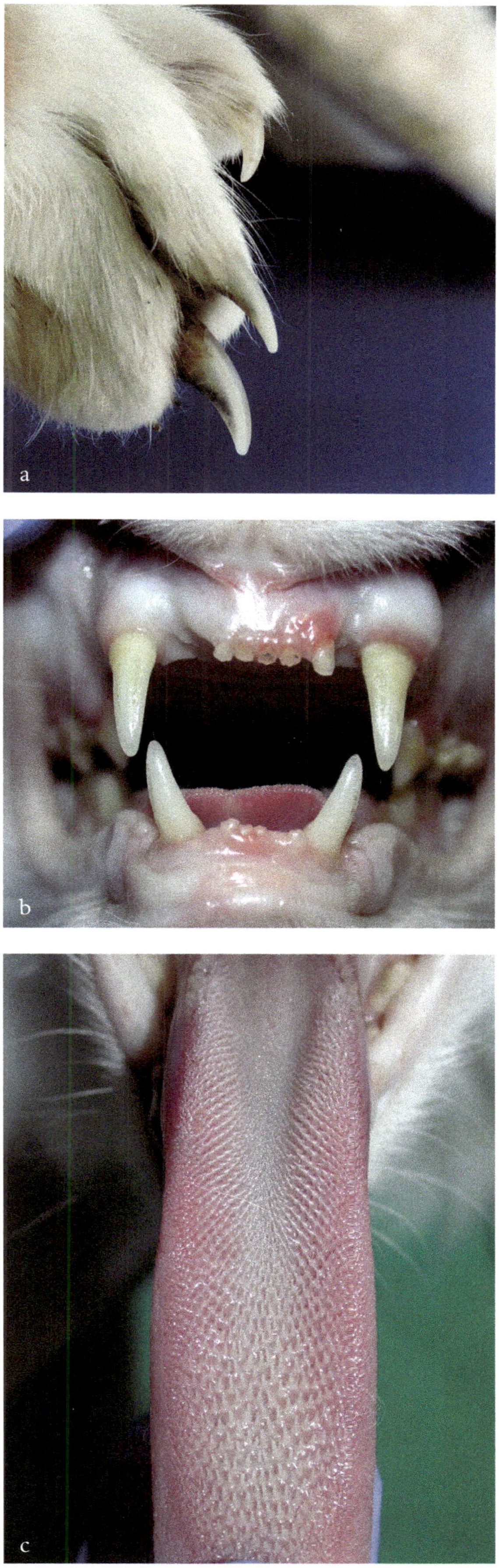

Figure 2. Anatomical characteristics of cats: (a) nails with sharp points (b) pointed canine teeth (c) filiform papillae on the tongue (images B and C conceded by Margherita Gracis).

facilitate thermoregulation, especially in outdoor cats. Consequently this behaviour favours the **transmission of ectoparasites between cats**, or the transference of otoacariasis infestations from the ear canal to the rest of the body.

Dermatology problems

The **general principles** of clinical dermatology are the same for cats as for dogs; however there are **significant differences** to bear in mind when approaching the feline dermatology case.

In general, felines respond to a large variety of initiating factors with the following clinical presentations:

1. **Pruritus**: the four main reaction patters are associated with:
   A) Miliary dermatitis (MD), often referred to as papular-crusting dermatitis.
   B) Self-induced alopecia (SIA).
   C) Face, head, neck pruritus (FHN), characterised by erosions or ulcers to the face, head and neck.
   D) Eosinophilic granuloma complex (EGC).
2. Focal-multifocal alopecia.
3. Exfoliative dermatosis.
4. Erosive-ulcerative dermatosis.
5. Nodular dermatosis.
6. **Symmetrical, diffuse alopecia** (not self-induced).

In contrast to dogs, **pustular dermatitis is rare in cats** and most commonly associated with an autoimmune disease such as *foliaceous pemphigus*. (Figure 3).

Superficial pyoderma is considered a common dermatological disease in dogs, but in the feline species relatively little is known about the condition. In fact, in cats there is little information available regarding the predisposing causes, prevalence, clinical characteristics, diagnostic criteria or therapeutic indications for superficial pyoderma. In general, (as in dogs) **superficial pyoderma is considered secondary to a predisposing condition** such as allergic dermatitis or parasitic disease. Commonly feline cases **present with pustular and crusted dermatitis** (with yellowish scabs), affecting the **head and neck**, most probably because scratching is concentrated in these areas.

Regarding otitis in cats, it represents a dermatological problem which is normally secondary to parasitic disease (such as otoacariasis causing pruritus and associated lesions) (Figure 4), or more rarely **inflammatory polyps**, or **ear canal tumours** such as adenoma-adenocarcinoma of the ceruminous glands.

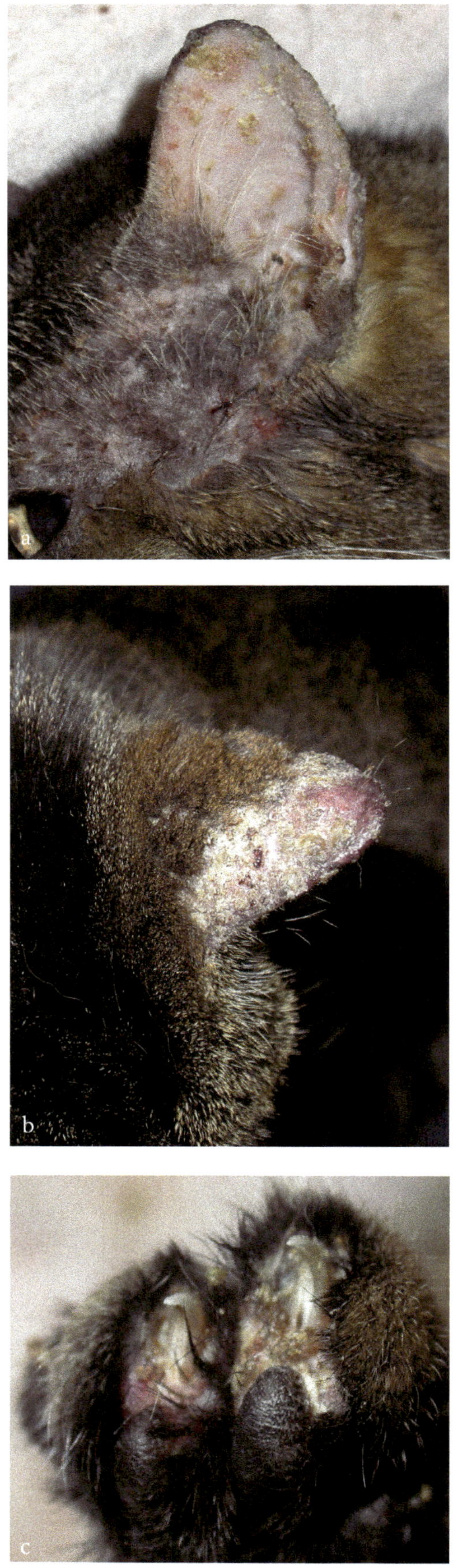

Figure 3. Cat with scabby-pustular dermatitis due to pemphigus foliaceous: (a) yellow scabs on the inner surface of the pinna (b) yellow scabs and some erosions/ulcers on the external surface of the pinna (c) paronychia (with yellow scabs and erosions).

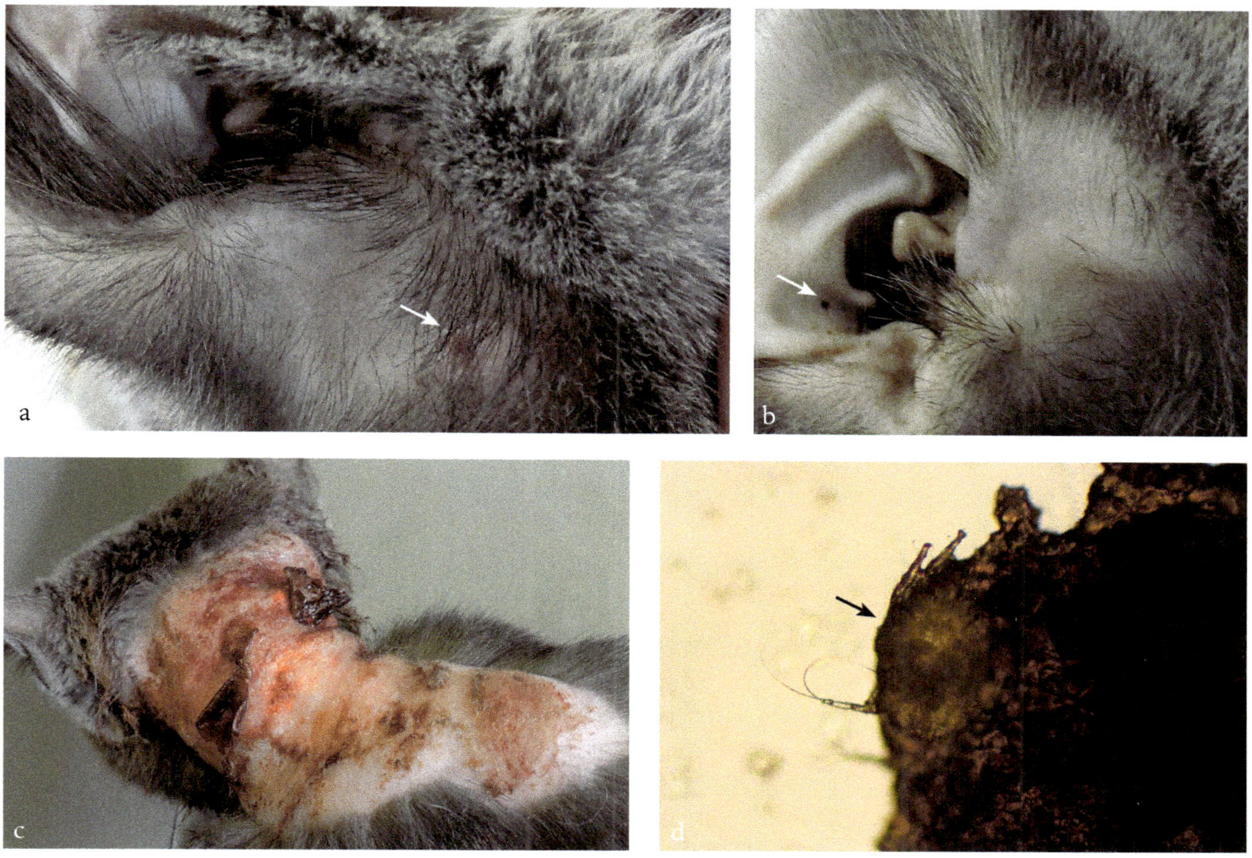

Figure 4. The same cat with *Otodectes cynotis* as a cause of: (a) miliary dermatitis (white arrow); (b) bilateral ceruminous otitis externa: dark coloured wax (white arrow) in the ear canal (c) pruritus in the dorsal area of the neck with erosion-ulcer lesions and bloody scabs (d) presence of the mite in the wax in the ear canals (black arrow).

Pruritus

Pruritus is not a disease but as an **unpleasant skin sensation** it triggers the energetic motor response known as **scratching** (Figure 5).

With recent progress into knowledge regarding the **neurophysiology of pruritus**, it has been discovered that nerve receptors located in the dermo-epidermal junction, transmit the sensation of pruritus through free myelin nerve fibres, which then run through the spinal cord in the spinothalamic bundle, which is contralateral to the pruritus centre in the thalamus, and from it to the frontal cortex (Figure 6).

Within the topic of pruritus, the cat represents an enigma because in this species the same pruritic disease can be characterized by phenotypic variability or, conversely **different diseases can manifest themselves with the same reaction pattern.**

In general, the main dermatological diseases that cause pruritus in cats are shown in Table 1.

In most cases, the cat responds to this variety of diseases with one or more of **four main reaction patterns**

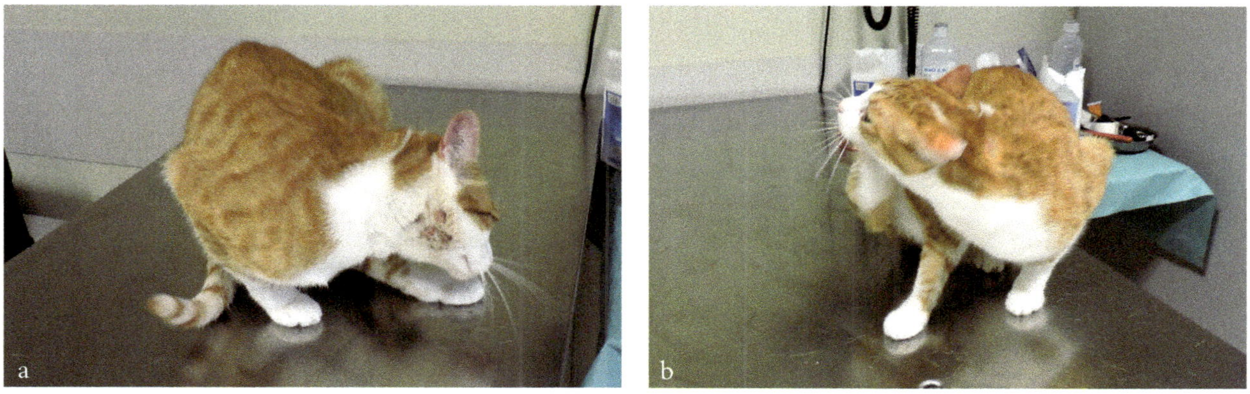

Figure 5. Cat energetically scratching the side of the neck causing lesions in this area.

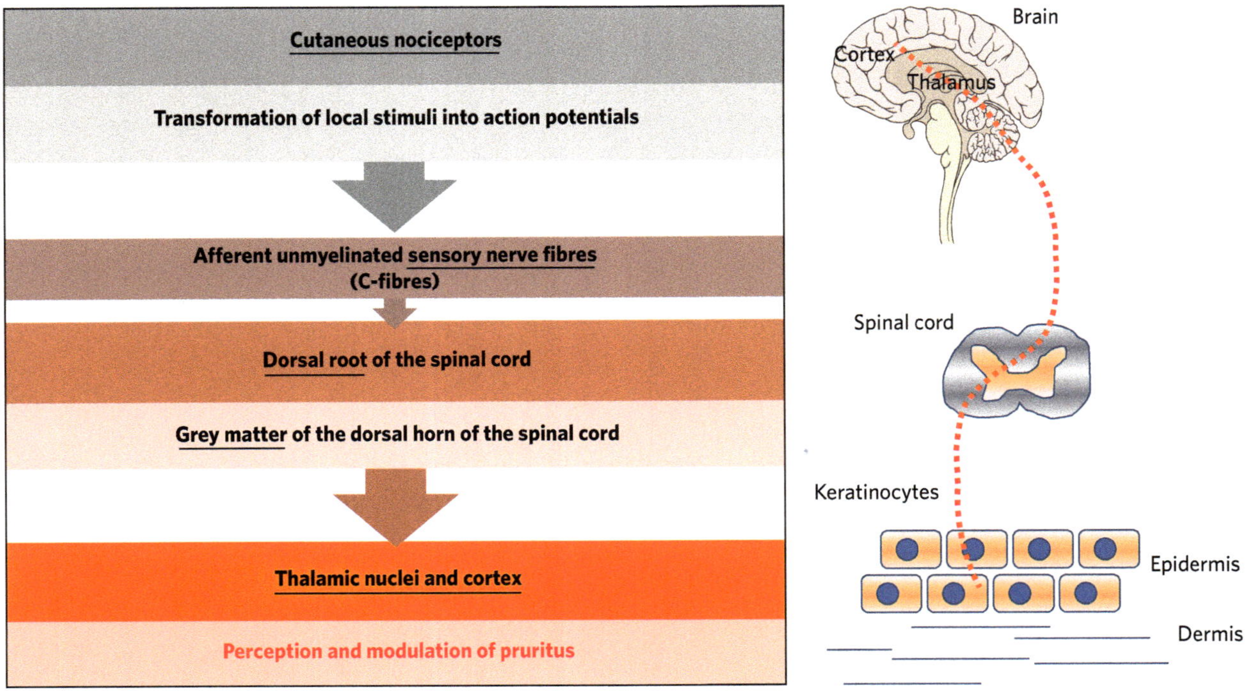

Figure 6. The neurophysiology of pruritus.

Table 1. Main skin diseases in cats which cause pruritus.

Parasitic diseases	Otoacariasis Cheyletiellosis Trombiculosis Pediculosis Pulicosis Demodicosis
Cutaneous hypersensitivity reactions	Flea allergy dermatitis (FAD) Food Allergy (FA) Feline Atopic Skin Syndrome (FASS)* Reactions to insect bites
Neoplasia	Cutaneous epitheliotropic lymphoma (fungal mycosis)

* Newly proposed terminology according to ICADA (International Committee on Allergic Diseases of Animals. DOI: 10.1111/vde. 12933) – Veterinary Dermatology 2021: Feline atopic syndrome (FAS) is the newly-proposed terminology encompassing allergic diseases of the skin, gastrointestional and respiratory tract in the cat. Feline atopic skin syndrome (FASS) describes allergic skin disease.

(Figure 7). Therefore, lesions associated with pruritus include:

1. Miliary dermatitis (MD). Papules and scabs in the head or trunk region.
2. Self-induced alopecia (SIA). Diffuse hair loss in the abdominal or flank region as a result of an increase in oral grooming.
3. Face, head, neck pruritus (FHN), characterised by erosions or ulcers to the face, head and neck.
4. Eosinophilic granuloma complex (EGC). Ulcers, plaques and nodules in nodular plaque dermatitis.

Therefore a methodical clinical approach is important when working up a feline dermatology case in order to reduce the possibility of making interpretive errors.

1. A **thorough signalment and history**. For example, in cats that live together or in overcrowded conditions, flea reservoirs may exist such that continuous reinfestation occurs. Also, for other parasitic diseases (such as notoedric mange or otoacariasis) transmission is mainly by direct contact so recognizing the opportunity for spread is essential.
2. This should be followed by the **exact identification of primary lesions** such as papules or plaques and **secondary lesions** such as excoriations, erosions, ulcers or scabs, later defining them within the main reaction patterns and making a corresponding list of different differential diagnoses for each.
3. Subsequently, appropriate **complementary examinations** should be carried out, such as a Wood lamp's examination, superficial and deep skin scrapings, back-combing, scotch®test and the earwax exam.
4. If the clinical presentation, for example of facial ulcers, also suggests other differentials such as epitheliotropic viruses or neoplasms, **additional tests such as skin biopsy**, in some cases associated with immunohistochemistry, are required. It is also important to **rule out infections** or overgrowth by bacteria and yeasts.

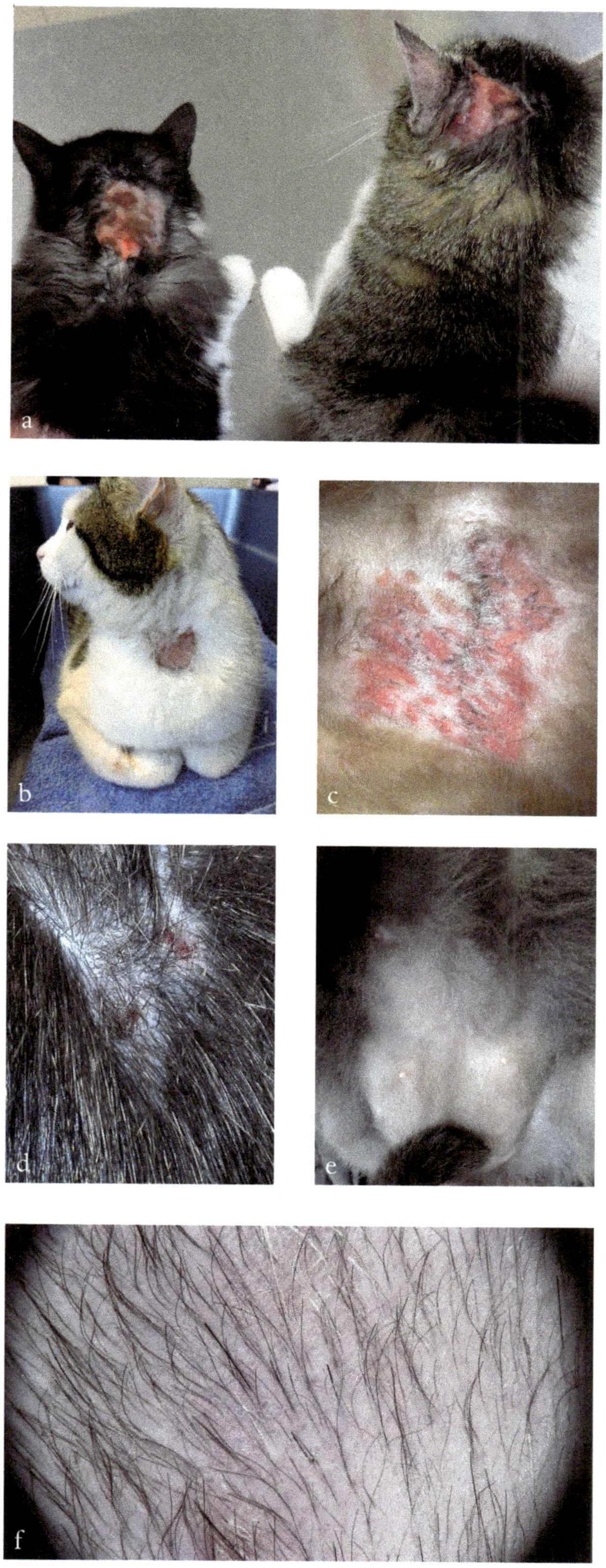

Figure 7. The four main reaction patterns: (a-b) face, head, neck pruritus (FHN), characterised by erosions or ulcers to the face, head and neck. (c) plaques in the abdominal region of a cat with nodular plaque dermatitis (feline eosinophilic granuloma complex (EGC)) (d) papules in the dorsal trunk area in a cat with miliary dermatitis (e) diffuse hair loss in the abdominal region in a cat with symmetrical alopecia (self-induced) (f) dermoscopic image from the same area (hairs with broken tips) (20×).

Investigating the pruritic cat

Table 2 is a summary of the **main diseases associated with pruritus**, their reaction patterns, and suggested tests to reach an appropriate diagnosis.

However, even if tests performed give a negative result, and after the exclusion of other non-allergic diseases previously mentioned, an appropriate **anti-parasitic treatment** (including the environment) should be administered and the clinical response evaluated. For example, evidence of flea exposure such as the presence of faeces or adults, is not always apparent even when infestation has occurred.

Non-flea induced feline hypersensitivity

If the previously mentioned anti-parasite therapeutic trial does not cause clinical improvement, the problem is part of the group of **non-flea induced hypersensitivity dermatitis** (NFHD). The clinical criteria are documented in Table 1.

This approach has a **sensitivity of 90% and a specificity of 83% when 6/10 criteria** are met.

Therefore, the patient should be:

- Carefully re-examined.
- Lesion identified and distribution noted.

Then in a **second level of diagnostic-therapeutic exclusion**, in cats with **non-seasonal pruritus,** the possibility of **food allergy** should be considered as a differential diagnosis. The incidence of food allergy is debatable, but even so an elimination diet should be undertaken.

An **elimination diet** (**food restriction test**) involves feeding the cat a diet based on a **unique, new protein source** they have not previously ingested, or a **commercial diet of hydrolysed protein**. This diet is fed for a minimum of **eight consecutive weeks** during which time the cat does not have access to any other food sources.

If the **pruritus disappears** or is considerably reduced, with the consequent reduction in related lesions, a **provocation test** (or challenge) should be carried out. The objective is to reintroduce, at regular intervals, a previously eaten protein source, with the aim of seeing if clinical lesions recur (usually this happens within hours or days of the challenge). Consequently, the aetiology of the lesions is confirmed as a food allergy.

Box 1. Clinical criteria for non-flea induced hypersensitivity dermatitis.

1. Presence of **pruritus** right from the start of the problem.

Table 2. Description of non-allergic causes of pruritus and complementary tests within each reaction pattern.

Reaction pattern	Main differential diagnoses	Complementary tests
Face, head, neck pruritus (FHN)	Ectoparasites	Back combing, skin scraping, scotch®test, microscopic hair examination, examination of ear wax
	Dermatophytes	Wood's lamp, microscopic hair examination, fungal dermatophyte culture, PCR
	Epitheliotropic viruses (calicivirus/herpesvirus)	Skin biopsy, immunohistochemistry, PCR
	Neoplasia (lymphoma, EGC)	Skin biopsy, immunohistochemistry
Miliary dermatitis (MD)	Ectoparasites	Back combing, skin scraping, scotch®test, microscopic hair examination
	Dermatophytes	Wood's lamp, microscopic hair examination, fungal dermatophyte culture, PCR
Self-induced alopecia (SIA)	Ectoparasites (including Demodex gatoi)	Skin scraping, scotch®test, microscopic hair examination, examination of ear wax
	Dermatophytes	Wood's lamp, microscopic hair examination, fungal dermatophyte culture, PCR
Eosinophilic granuloma complex (EGC)	Ectoparasites	Back combing, skin scraping, scotch®test, microscopic hair examination, examination of ear wax
	Deep bacterial and fungal disease	Cytological examination, tissue culture, skin biopsy with special stains
	Neoplasia (mastocytoma, lymphoma, EGC)	Skin biopsy

(Adapted from: Favrot C. Feline non-flea induced hypersensitivity dermatitis: clinical features, diagnosis and treatment. Journal of Feline Medicine and Surgery 2013; 15:778–84).

2. Presence of, as a minimum two of the following reaction patterns:
   A) **Miliary dermatitis (MD)**, often referred to as papular-crusting dermatitis.
   B) Self-induced alopecia (SIA).
   C) Face, head, neck pruritus (FHN), characterised by erosions or ulcers to the face, head and neck.
   D) Eosinophilic granuloma complex (EGC).
3. At least **two body locations** affected.
4. Presence of **papular crusted dermatitis** or miliary dermatitis as the predominant reaction pattern.
5. Presence of **eosinophilic dermatitis** or self-induced symmetrical alopecia or erosions/ulcers on the head, face, ears or neck.
6. Presence of **non-symmetrical alopecia** in the dorsocaudal region, tail or hind limbs.
7. Presence of self-induced alopecia in the **abdominal region**.
8. **Absence of erosions/ulcers** on the forelimbs.
9. **Absence of lesions** in the armpits or sternum.
10. **Absence of nodules** and tumours.

(Adapted from: Favrot C et al. Establishment of diagnostic criteria for feline non flea-induced hypersensitivity dermatitis. Veterinary Dermatology 2012; 23:45–50).

One of the **most frequent errors** in this diagnostic protocol is **not performing the dietary provocation** with a previously ingested protein. For example, if a cat stops scratching during the period of the elimination diet, this could be due to seasonal hypersensitivity which resolved spontaneously due to the time of year and absence of triggering environmental allergens.

In the majority of cases that **do not show a response to the elimination diet, are most likely suffer from hypersensitivity to environmental allergens**. Therefore, in the third part of the diagnostic-therapeutic process, once the presumed diagnosis of hypersensitivity to environmental allergens is reached, there are two options:

1. Investigate using **intradermal or serological tests** for the allergens responsible and then desensitize the animal with allergen-specific immunotherapy.
2. Administer **symptomatic treatments** such as glucocorticoids or cyclosporine.

However, the role of **IgE is controversial in felines** since it can also be positive in serological or intradermal tests in healthy cats and in general, although pruritus is a distinctive feature, the distribution pattern of lesions is very variable in a cat affected by FASS (feline atopic skin syndrome).

Symptomatic treatment of pruritus

Drugs that manage the symptoms are widely used in clinical practice, but it should be kept in mind that, in the long term, these are high-risk treatments.

For example, **glucocorticoids** can cause serious **side effects** such as **polyuria-polydipsia**, iatrogenic **hypercortisolism** with cutaneous atrophy, and **diabetes mellitus**. In general, whenever possible, **oral dosing** is preferred to parenteral administration and slow release products should be avoided. For example, **methylprednisolone at a dose of 1.4 mg/kg** or **triamcinolone at 0.18 mg/kg every 24 hours for 1 or 2 weeks** until the onset of remission, seems to be well tolerated. Topical corticosteroids may be helpful, but the frequency of application and area of the skin to be treated should be carefully evaluated since cats appear to be more sensitive than dogs to skin atrophy which may follow the application of these treatments.

Good therapeutic responses are obtained with the administration of **cyclosporine at a dose of 7 mg/kg once a day for at least 4 weeks** and, once the therapeutic effect has been achieved, it can be **administered every 2 or 3 days**.

There are also other treatment approaches including the use of **fatty acids**, **antihistamines**, and a targeted therapy that selectively inhibits JAK-1 dependent cytokines involved in allergy such as oclacitinib. To date, the latter has only been reported in a few studies and a dosage of approximately 1 mg/kg once or twice daily is considered as an effective treatment option for FASS.

In conclusion, the diagnostic-therapeutic protocol in a cat with pruritus often involves a process which is long and frustrating even for the owner, and always depends on the correct identification of the problem, its main reaction patterns, and recognition of the underlying diseases they indicate.

Focal-multifocal alopecia

The term **alopecia** is understood to mean the **lack of hair in a region where its presence is considered normal.** Alopecia is not strictly speaking a lesion, and can be both **primary and secondary.**

In general the clinical appearance of alopecia is similar in the dog and the cat; however the underlying causes are usually different. For example, **in dogs** the triad of diseases associated with infection that present with alopecia are: bacterial folliculitis, demodicosis, dermatophytosis.

In contrast, **in cats alopecia is commonly caused by self-trauma** as shown by broken ends to the hair shafts and patchy alopecia, and more rarely follows diseases such as dermatophytosis or demodicosis.

In fact, **feline dermatophytosis is often accompanied by small, whitish scales** which may adhere to the skin surface, generally indicating a problem within the desquamative dermatoses (See Exfoliative Dermatosis).

In the few cases described with **feline demodicosis**, there are a variety of associated lesions including:

- Focal and multifocal alopecia.
- Papules.
- Scabs on the head, neck, extremities.
- Ceruminous otitis externa (Figure 8), linked with *Demodex cati.*
- Symmetrical (self-induced) alopecia, linked with *Demodex gatoi.*

In general, while **localized demodicosis is self-limiting**, the development of a **generalized demodicosis presupposes or is triggered by an underlying condition** such as diabetes mellitus, feline immunodeficiency or neoplasia.

A diagnosis of demodicosis is established by performing **microscopic** hair examination, a **deep skin scraping** or an **earwax examination** for the mite *Demodex cati* that resides in the hair follicle. Whilst in the case of the shorter *Demodex gatoi*, mite with a more superficial location, tests such as the **scotch®tape test** are indicated.

There is **no consensus** on the most effective and safe treatment for feline demodicosis. Protocols consist of 2% calcium polysulphide baths, the use of amitraz (consider toxicity) at a dose of 0.0125–0.025% weekly or subcutaneous ivermectin injections. Recently, the use of **isoxazolines** in the treatment of generalized feline demodicosis has been described.

Desquamative dermatosis

Scales represent aggregates of corneocytes that have become detached from the skin's surface.

To aid interpretation of this clinical sign, the morphology of the scales (Figure 9) should be considered:

- **Small, thin, whitish grey scales** that are easily collected with combing. They are seen in cats with **dermatophytosis, cheyletiellosis or in obese cats** unable to groom adequately.
- **Largish, whitish scales** that adhere to the skin's surface. They can be observed in **thymoma-associated paraneoplastic syndrome**, in erythema multiforme and in **epitheliotropic cutaneous lymphoma.**
- **Yellowish-brown scales attached to the skin surface** and hair. They can be observed in **feline allergies with *Malassezia spp.* overgrowth.**
- Scales attached to the hairs forming "**follicular casts.**" They are observed in cats with **sebaceous adenitis** or idiopathic **follicular keratinization** disorders such as chin acne and also in cats with dermatophytosis.

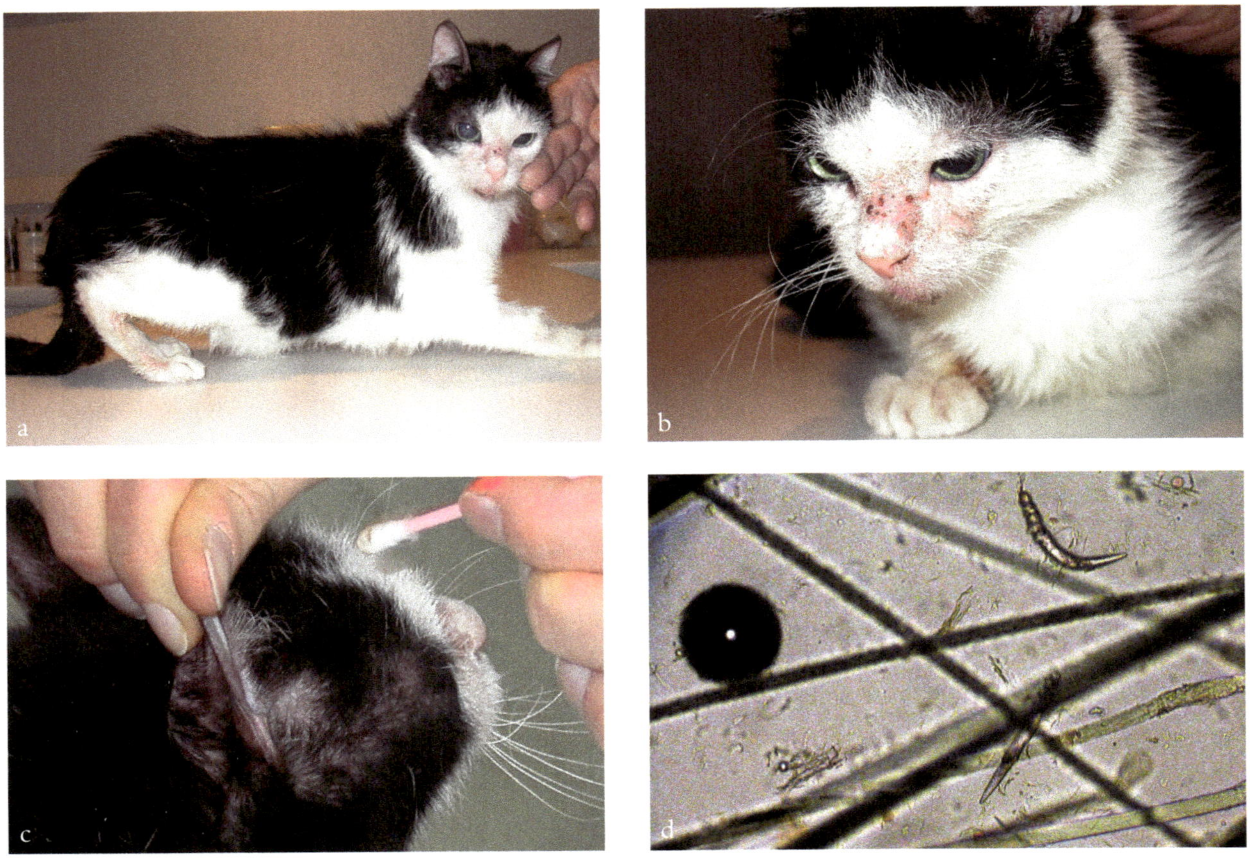

Figure 8. Cat with demodicosis caused by *Demodex cati*. (a) multifocal alopecia in the facial area and on the limbs, erythema and red scabs; (b) close-up image of the facial lesions (c) bilateral ceruminous otitis externa (d) *Demodex cati* (10x).

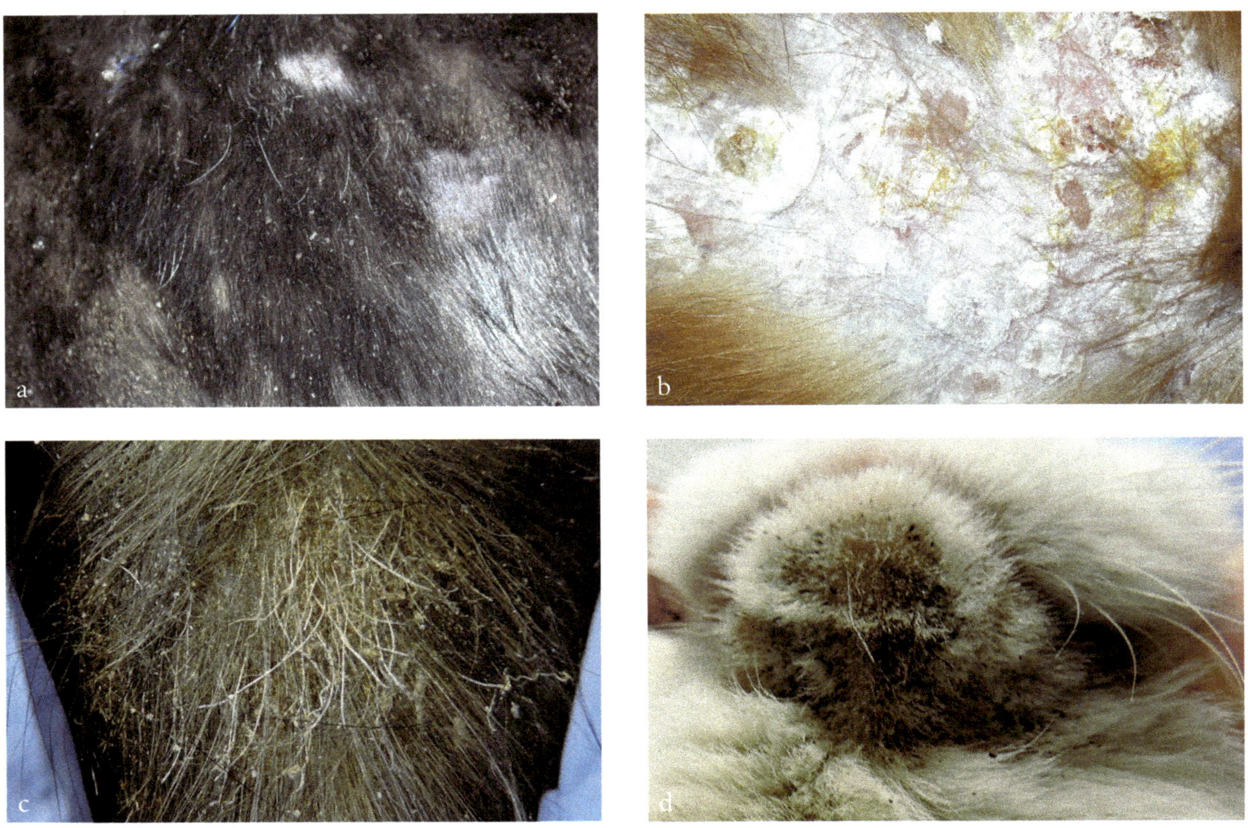

Figure 9. Types of scales: (a) small, fine, white scales on the back area of an obese cat (b) large white scales which stick to the skin surface on the trunk area of a cat with cutaneous lymphoma (c) scales stuck to the skin and hairs of a cat with dermatophytosis (d) scales stuck to the hairs forming "follicular casts" in a cat with chin acne.

Dermatophytosis

Among desquamative diseases, **dermatophytosis is especially important**. Due to the **pleomorphic clinical signs** and its **infectious nature** in cats (and zoonotic potential), dermatophytosis is considered one of the most important diseases in the feline species.

Among the species of zoophilic dermatophytes, ***Microsporum canis* mainly affects cats**, with evidence of a **breed predisposition in Persian cats**. It is transmitted mainly by **direct contact with infected animals** or by **contaminated fomites** (combs, hairbrushes). The clinical signs reflect the pathogenesis of the disease, that is, the **fungal invasion of keratinized structures** (Figure 10).

The most common clinical signs are:

- Annular or irregular alopecia with whitish grey exfoliation sometimes likened to "cigarette ash".
- Erythema.
- Papules.
- Scabs.
- Deposits in the form of keratin casts attached to the base of the hair.
- Itching is variable, but often minimal.
- In rare cases, on the dorsal trunk and at the base of the tail, ulcerated and draining subcutaneous nodules attributable to what is defined as dermatophytic pseudomycetoma can be observed. However, due to its clinical appearance, it is usually included in nodular dermatoses.

Currently, **no diagnostic test is considered gold standard** for dermatophytosis. In fact, it is diagnosed using various complementary tests, which include **Wood's lamp and microscopic hair examination** to document active infection; **fungal culture** for the identification of the fungal species involved and monitoring the response to treatment; as well as **skin biopsy** with special stains to detect nodular or atypical fungal infections.

The treatment of dermatophytosis involves combinations of topical, systemic and environmental therapies:

- Among the topical treatments, enilconazole or **miconazole/chlorhexidine shampoo,** twice a week, represents effective treatment and are currently recommended.

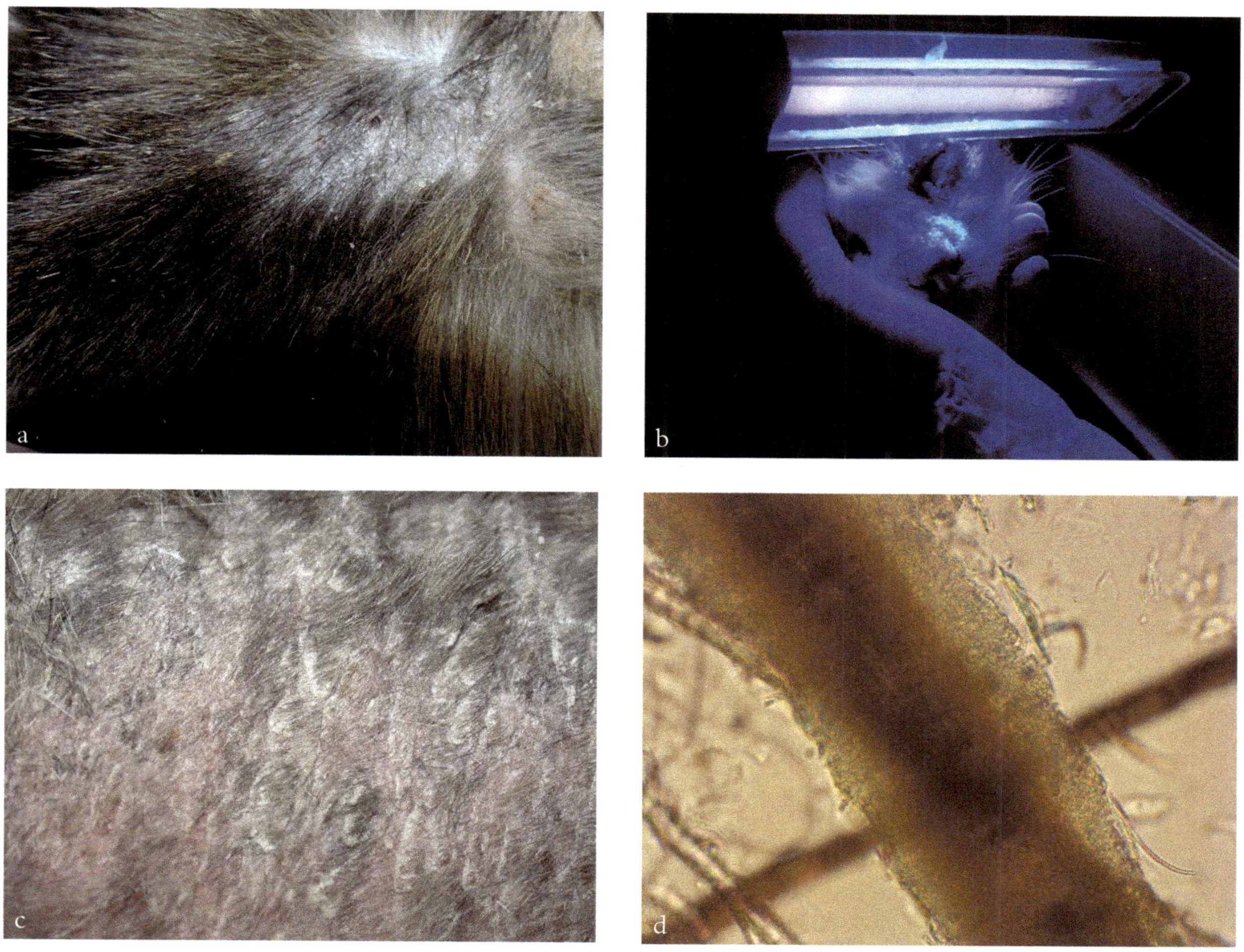

Figure 10. Dermatophytosis caused by *Microsporum canis* and its diagnosis: (a) ring alopecia with whitish-grey exfoliation similar to "cigarette ash" in the dorsal area (b) Wood's lamp (positive in the facial area); (c) alopecia, erythema and fine, white scales on one of the distal limbs (d) fungal spores which de-structure the hair shaft.

- Among systemic treatments, **itraconazole at 5–10 mg/kg** or terbinafine at a dose of 10–30 mg/kg is recommended.

Environmental treatment can reduce the spread of the disease and involves vacuuming up hairs and scales (with careful disposal of the resulting dust), plus disinfection of surfaces with sodium hypochlorite (household bleach) which is proven to be effective when used in concentrations ranging from 1:10 to 1:100, even with short environmental contact times.

Epitheliotropic cutaneous lymphoma

Another uncommon scaly disease in cats is **epitheliotropic cutaneous lymphoma or fungoid mycosis** (Figure 9b), which occurs mainly in **elderly cats**. One variation takes the form of large dry, whitish scales, attached to regions such as the trunk and head; and is usually associated with mild to **severe pruritus**.

On histology, epitheliotropic cutaneous lymphoma is characterized by lymphoid neoplastic infiltration of the epidermis and attached structures. Also, **specific immunohistochemical tests** can help identify cells such as CD3+ (T cells). Treatment is subject to advice from an oncologist.

Paraneoplastic syndrome

Paraneoplastic syndrome is a rare disease associated with thymoma. To be defined as such, it should not be attributable to local or metastatic spread but to the indirect or **"remote" effects of the thymoma** resulting in synthesis or release of active molecules.

In general, the pathogenesis is poorly understood, despite a theory that the clinically visible lesions are the consequence of cell-mediated autoimmunity. In fact, the thymus, is responsible for the maturation and selection of T lymphocytes and in thymomas some immature T lymphocytes could enter the cycle as **self-reactive T cells** and be responsible for **direct attack against keratinocytes**.

Dermatological clinical signs such as **erythema and exfoliation** (Figure 11) are initially located on the **head, neck and ears** until they progressively extend to the entire body and usually precede systemic symptoms such as anorexia, lethargy, weight loss, cough, and dyspnoea. Pruritus is absent, unless bacterial

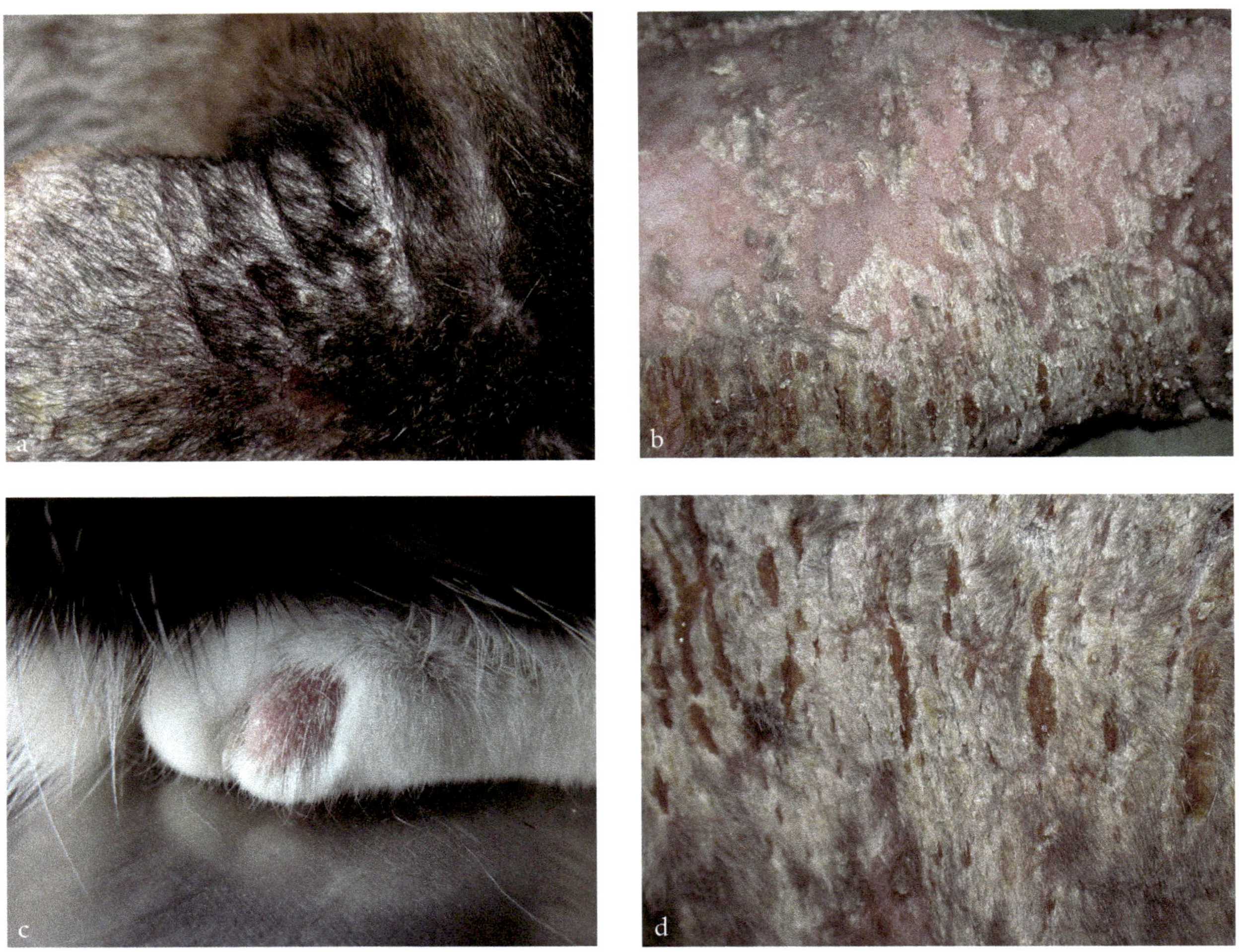

Figure 11. Cat with paraneoplastic syndrome associated with a thymoma. Whitish scales of varying size which stick to the skins surface can be seen on the pinna and on the entire trunk region. (Image conceded by Dr. F. Albanese).

infections or ***Malassezia spp.*** **present as secondary complications.**

The diagnosis requires a dermatopathological examination of **skin biopsies** and diagnostic imaging methods (radiology, CT scan) to determine the **presence of a thoracic mass**.

Although the **primary tumour is usually benign** and its surgical excision leads to resolution of the dermatological clinical signs, in most cases the problem is identified at an advanced stage or the owner refuses surgery and the patient is euthanized.

Erosive-ulcerative dermatosis

Erosions are defined as a loss of skin tissue up to the dermo-epidermal junction to form a moist, smooth and shiny excavation. **Ulcers extend beyond this to the middle and deep dermis** and are characterized by a **haemorrhagic base**. As a result, erosions heal without a scar, while ulcers heal with scar formation.

Those diseases mainly connoted by erosions and ulcers include (Figure 12):

- Infectious diseases.
- Adverse drug reactions.
- Immune diseases.
- Neoplasms.
- Vasculitis.

In most cases, **epidermal-dermal tissue destruction is due to self-induced trauma** (allergic-based pruritus). However, in the cat other diseases also occur with erosions and ulcers as the main lesion, as seen in Table 3 (excluding allergic dermatitis).

In all these cases, it is important to **identify the associated systemic clinical signs** (for example, in cats with extensive burns or toxic epidermal necrolysis), the **site and distribution of the lesions** (for example, feline herpesvirus with facial distribution) and to conduct an appropriate **diagnostic therapeutic protocol**.

This begins with **cytological examination of material from a direct impression** of erosions or ulcers. However, in most cases these lesions are excellent substrate for colonization and bacterial growth, and results indicate degenerate polymorphonuclear neutrophils and abundant intra and extracellular bacteria (such as cocci). Therefore, the main problem should **not simply be interpreted as pyoderma, but the underlying causes should be investigated** further. Thus, blood tests and, above all, the **dermatopathological examination** are essential, and depending on the case and clinical suspicions, additional tests such as immunohistochemistry may be needed. In all cases, successful **treatment depends on identifying and addressing the underlying disease.**

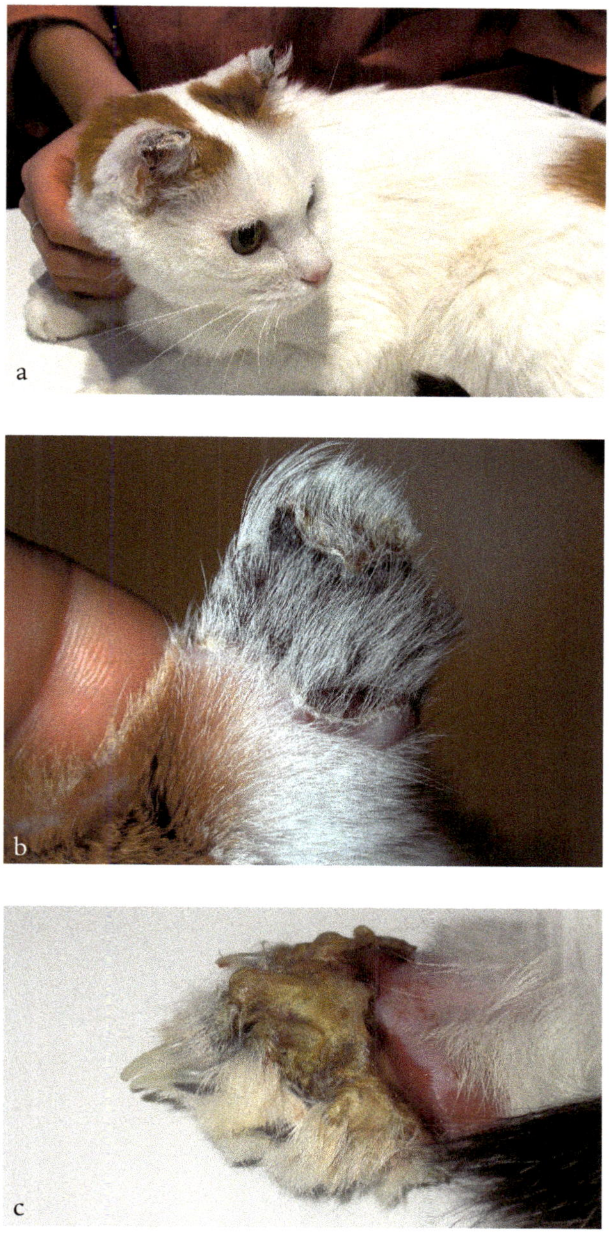

Figure 12. Cat with idiopathic vasculitis: In this case despite diagnostic tests the triggering cause was not identified. Ulcerous lesions and necrosis with formation of localised eschars can be seen on the tips of the ears and the skin detachment on the distal limbs

Some **feline eosinophilic granuloma complex (EGC) lesions**, such as indolent ulcers, (Figure 13) can also be ascribed to the erosive-ulcerative dermatosis group, although normally attributed to eosinophilic granuloma complex and therefore, **the diagnostic approach is different.** Indolent ulcers are typically yellowish-brown, rounded lesions, a few centimetres in diameter, which are almost always (although not exclusively) located on the upper lips, uni or bilaterally.

Table 3. Main dermatological diseases (and their anatomical locations) as a cause of erosions/ulcers in cats.

Disease	Lesion distribution
Chemical or heat burns	Localised and extensive
Erythema multiforme – toxic epidermal necrolysis	Extensive and oral mucosal involvement
Epitheliotropic viral infections (herpesvirus-calicivirus)	Localised (facial) and bilateral conjunctivitis, severe corneal ulceration (herpesvirus) and buccal ulceration (calicivirus)
Vasculitis	Limbs, tip of the tail, tips of the ears
Dystrophic epidermolysis bullosa	Oral cavity, plantar pads
Pemphigoid bullous	Oral cavity, mucocutaneous junctions
Squamous cell carcinoma (cutaneous)	Nasal septum, eyelids, ears

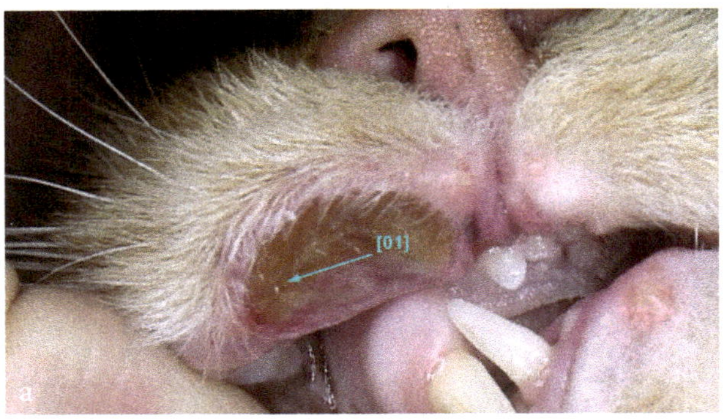

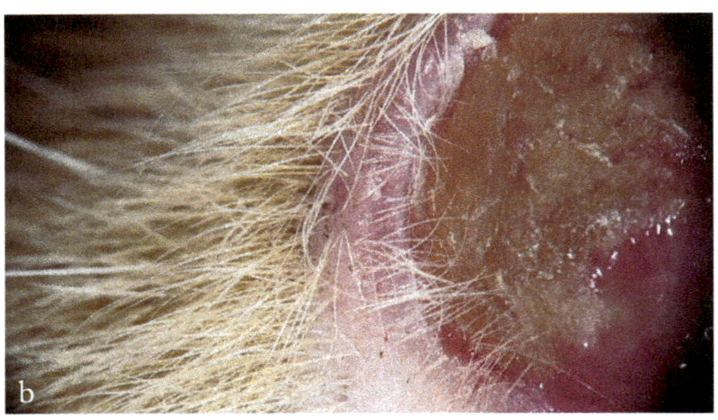

Figure 13. (a) Cat with indolent ulcer (within EGC); (b) Dermoscopic image of the same lesion (20x).

Nodular dermatosis

A nodule is defined as a **prominent, solid, circumscribed, lesion** (of variable size); and, depending on its anatomical location, it can be **epidermal, dermal or subcutaneous**. They are usually **related to infectious, sterile, neoplastic diseases** (with tissue deposition of substances) or increasingly frequently with **leishmaniosis** (depending on geographical area).

The key to diagnosis of a nodular dermatosis **is cytological examination to differentiate an inflammatory condition from neoplasia**. Samples can be obtained by **fine needle aspiration** or by **scraping the ulcerated surface** of the mass. This is followed by a **dermatopathological examination**, as appropriate, with special stains and/or immunohistochemistry, fungal or bacterial culture, serologies or PCR.

In general, on cytology:

- In the presence of granulomatous/pyogranulomatous inflammation:
  - The presence of **clear filaments or free yeasts** in the macrophage cytoplasm, attributable for example to infections by **atypical bacteria or cryptococcosis**, should be ruled out.
  - The presence of **intracytoplasmic particles** suggestive of *Leishmania spp*. amastigotes, should be ruled out.
- Large numbers of eosinophils suggests lesions such as **eosinophilic granuloma**.
- **Lymphocytes and plasma cells** may indicate **feline plasmocytic pododermatitis**:
- In the case of **cutaneous tumours** and according to the cell line from which they are derived:
  - **Round cells** can be distinguished, with delimited borders and with purple metachromatic granules in the cytoplasm, as occurs in mastocytomas.
  - Or **mesenchymal cells**, with diffuse borders and traits of malignancy (anisokaryosis, evident nucleoli, mitosis) in fibrosarcomas.

In all cases, **the definitive diagnosis is obtained by dermatopathological** examination and auxiliary tests

Table 4. List of diseases associated with nodular dermatitis.

Infectious diseases	Bacterial: Feline leprosy Botryomycosis Actinomycosis
	Fungal: Dermatophytic pseudomycetoma Pheohyphomycosis Cryptococcosis Sporotrichosis Histoplasmosis
Neoplasias	Mastocytomas Fibrosarcoma Melanoma Haemangiosarcoma Histiocytic disorders
Sterile	Eosinophilic granuloma (within EGC) Feline plasmocytic pododermatits Insect bite reactions (in the form of papular nodular dermatitis)
Substance deposits	Cutaneous xanthoma
Parasitic diseases	Leishmaniasis

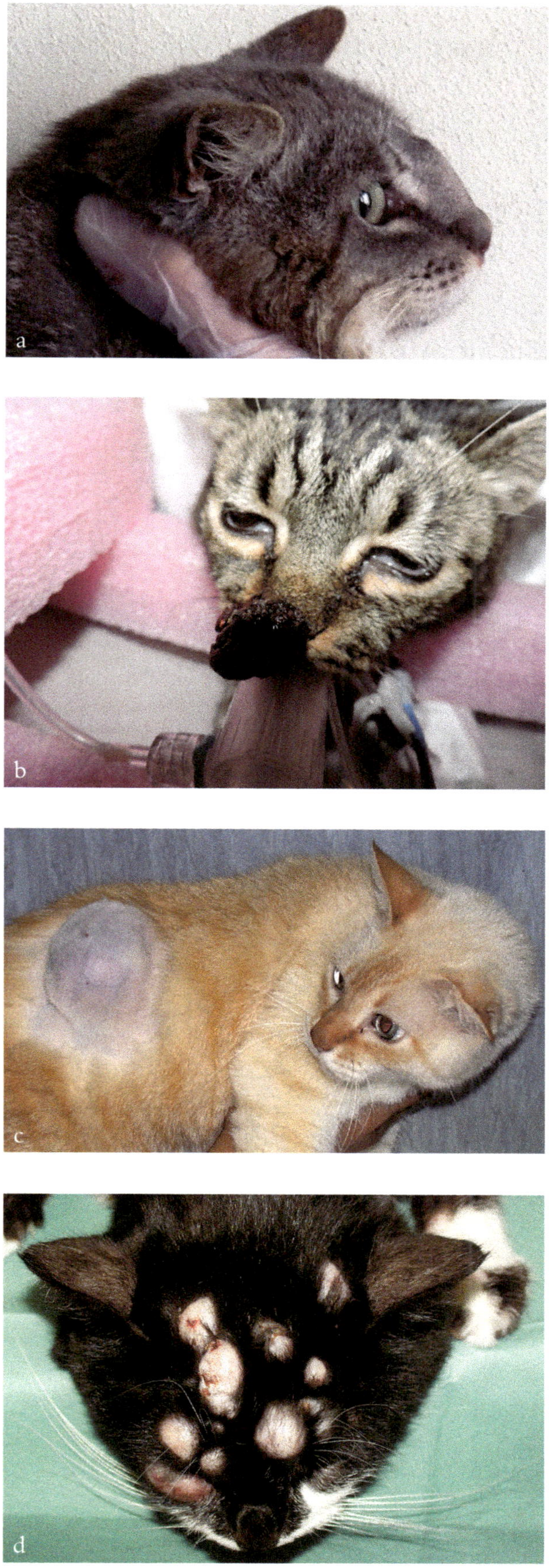

Figure 14. Example of nodular diseases in cats: (a) cryptococcosis with deformity of the top of the nose; (b) cat with melanoma; (c) cat with fibrosarcoma (image conceded by Dr. F.Albanese); (d) cat with mastocytoma (image conceded by Dr. F. Leone).

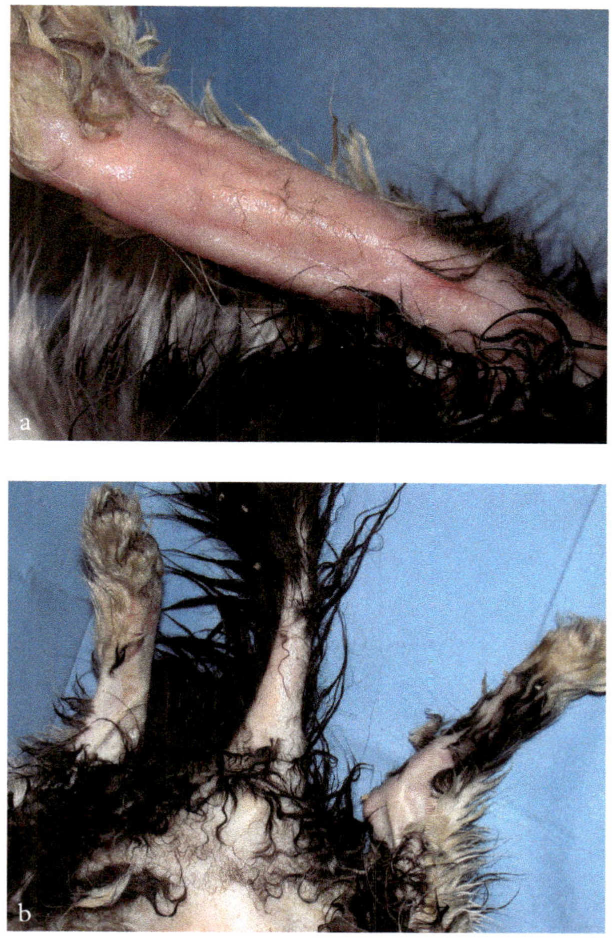

Figure 15. Paraneoplastic alopecia associated with pancreatic carcinoma (shiny skin with waxy appearance) (image conceded by Dr. F. Albanese).

as described above. Treatment is dependent on the disease identified.

Some examples of nodular diseases in cats can be seen in Figure 14.

Symmetrical alopecia (not self-induced)

This is **rare in cats** and associated with an **endocrinopathy** such as hyperadrenocorticism, **paraneoplastic alopecia** associated with pancreatic carcinoma, cholangiocarcinoma, hepatocellular carcinoma and metastatic intestinal carcinoma or **defluxions** (telogen/anagen effluvium).

Apart from alopecia, cats with **hyperadrenocorticism** also have **very thin skin** with cutaneous fragility, while in **paraneoplastic alopecia** the ventral region of the body (from the thorax to the abdomen, limbs) appears **bright, thin, waxy** and hair comes out easily (Figure 15).

To diagnose these conditions, auxiliary tests such as blood tests, hormone tests, ultrasound imaging or computed tomography are necessary to reach a definitive diagnosis and provide, whenever possible, a targeted therapy.

Bibliography

Introduction

Dobney K, Larson G. *Genetics and animal domestication: new windows on an elusive process.* Journal of Zoology. 2006; 269:261–271.

Lipinski MJ, Froenicke L, Baysac KC et al. *The ascent of cat breeds: genetic evaluations of breeds and world wide random-bred populations.* Genomics. 2008; 91:12–21.

Vigne JD, Guilaine J, Debue K, Haye L, Gerard P. *Early taming of the cat in Cyprus.* Science. 2004; 304:259.

Pruritus

Colombini S, Hodgin EC, Foil CS et al. *Induction of feline flea allergy dermatitis and the incidence and histopathological characteristics of concurrent indolent lip ulcers.* Veterinary Dermatology. 2001; 12:155.

Diesel A. *Cutaneous hypersensitivity dermatoses in the feline patient: A review of allergic skin disease in cats.* Veterinary Science 2017; 4(2).

Diesel A. *Feline Atopic Syndrome: Pathogenesis, Epidemiology, and Clinical Presentation in Feline Dermatology.* Springer, Cham. 2020; pp 451–464.

Favrot C, Steffan J, Seewald W et al. *Establishment of diagnostic criteria for feline nonflea-induced hypersensitivity dermatitis.* Veterinary Dermatology. 2012; 23:45-e11.

Favrot C. *Feline nonflea induced hypersensitivity dermatitis. Clinical features, diagnosis and treatment.* Journal of Feline Medicine and Surgery. 2013; 15:778–784.

Foster AP, Roosje PJ. *Update on feline immunoglobulin E (IgE) and diagnostic recommendations for atopy.* In: August JR, ed. Consultation in Feline Internal Medicine, 4th edn. Philadelphia: W.B. Saunders. 2004; pp 229–38.

Ganz EC, Griffin CE, Keys DA et al. *Evaluation of methylprednisolone and triamcinolone for the induction and maintenance treatment of pruritus in allergic cats: a double-blinded, randomized, prospective study.* Veterinary Dermatology 2012; 23:387-e7.

Halliwell R, Banovic F, Mueller R.S et al. *Immunopathogenesis of the feline atopic syndrome.* Veterinary Dermatology. 2021; 32:13-e4.

Halliwell R, Pucheu-Haston CM, Olivry T et al. *Feline allergic diseases: introduction and proposed nomenclature.* Veterinary Dermatology. 2021; 32: 8-e2.

Hobi S, Linek M, Marignac G et al. *Clinical characteristics and causes of pruritus in cats: a multicentre study on feline hypersesnitivity-associated dermatoses.* Veterinary Dermatology. 2011; 22:406–413.

Mueller R.S., Olivry T., Prélaud P. *Critically appraised topic on adverse food reactions of companion animals (2): Common food allergen sources in dogs and cats.* BMC Veterinary Research 2016; 12:9.

Mueller RS, Nuttall T, Prost C et al. *Treatment of the feline atopic syndrome – a systematic review.* Veterinary Dermatology. 2021; 32:43-e8.

Mueller RS, Olivry T, Prélaud P. *Critically appraised topic on adverse food reactions of companion animals (2): common food allergen sources in dogs and cats.* BMC Veterinary Research 12:1–4, 2016.

Mueller RS, Olivry T. *Critically appraised topic on adverse food reactions of companion animals (6): prevalence of non-cutaneous manifestations of adverse food reactions in dogs and cats.* BMC veterinary research. 2018; 14: 1–5.

Noli C. *Feline Fleas and Flea-Bite Allergy in Cats.* In: Feline Dermatology, Springer, Cham. 2020; pp 437–449.

Olivry T, Mueller RS, Prélaud P. *Critically appraised topic on adverse food reactions of companion animals (1): duration of elimination diets.* 2015; BMC Veterinary Research 11:225.

Olivry T, Mueller RS. *Critically appraised topic on adverse food reactions of companion animals (3): prevalence of cutaneous adverse food reactions in dogs and cats.* BMC Veterinary Research. 2016; 13: 1–4.

Roberts ES, Speranza C, Friberg C et al. *Confirmatory field study for the evaluation of ciclosporin at a target dose of 7.0 mg/kg (3.2 mg/lb) in the control of feline hypersensitivity dermatitis.* Journal of Feline Medicine and Surgery, 2016; 18:889–897.

Santoro D, Pucheu-Haston CM, Prost C et al. *Clinical signs and diagnosis of feline atopic syndrome: detailed guidelines for a correct diagnosis.* Veterinary Dermatology. 2021; 32: 26–e6.

Scholz FM, Burrows AK, Griffin CE et al. *Determination of threshold concentrations of plant pollens in intradermal testing using fluorescein in clinically healthy nonallergic cats.* Veterinary Dermatology. 2017; 28: 426–455.

Scott DW, Miller WH, Erb HN. *Feline dermatology at Cornell University: 1407 cases (1988–2003).* Journal of Feline Medicine and Surgery. 2013; 15: 307–316.

Focal-multifocal alopecia

Beale K. *Feline demodicosis: a consideration in the itchy or overgrooming cat.* Journal of Feline Medicine and Surgery 2012; 14:209–13.

Matricoti I, Maina E. *The use of oral fluralaner for the treatment of feline generalised demodicosis: a case report.* Journal Small AnimPractice. 2017; 58:476–479.

Desquamative dermatosis

Cavalcanti JV, Moura MP, Monteiro FO. *Thymoma associated with exfoliative dermatitis in a cat.* Journal of Feline Medicine and Surgery. 2014; 16:1020–3.

Linek M, Rüfenacht S, Brachelente C et al. *Non thymoma-associated exfoliative dermatitis in 18 cats.* Veterinary Dermatology. 2015; 26:40–5.

Moriello KA, Coyner K, Paterson S et al. *Diagnosis and treatment of dermatophytosis in dogs and cats.* Clinical Consensus Guidelines of the World Association for Veterinary Dermatology. Veterinary Dermatology 2017; 28:266-e68.

Erosive-ulcerative dermatosis

Hosie MJ, Addie D, Belák S et al. *Feline herpesvirus infection. ABCD guidelines on prevention and management.* Journal of Feline Medicine and Surgery. 2009; 11:556–64.

Yager JA. *Erythema multiforme, Stevens-Johnson syndrome and toxic epidermal necrolysis: a comparative review.* Veterinary Dermatology 2014; 25:406-e64.

Nodular dermatosis

BERNHARDT A, VONBOMHARD W, ANTWEILER E et al. *Molecular identification of fungal pathogens in nodular skin lesions of cats.* Medical mycology 2015; 53:132–44.

PENNISI MG, HARTMANN K, LLORET A et al. *Leishmaniosis in cats: ABCD guidelines on prevention and management.* Journal of Feline Medicine and Surgery. 2013; 15:638–42.

Symmetrical non-self-induced alopecia

BOLAND LA, BARRS VR. *Peculiarities of feline hyperadrenocorticism: Update on diagnosis and treatment.* Journal of Feline Medicine and Surgery 2017; 19:933–47.

CAPORALI C, ALBANESE F, BINANTI D et al. *Two cases of feline paraneoplastic alopecia associated with a neuroendocrine pancreatic neoplasia and a hepatosplenic plasma cell tumour.* Veterinary dermatology 2016; 27:508-e137.

Test

1. With which of these disease groups is symmetrical (self-induced) alopecia in cats not related?
A) Allergic diseases.
B) Endocrine diseases.
C) Parasitic diseases.
D) Behavioural problems.

2. Within the reaction pattern of papular-crusted dermatitis or miliary dermatitis, which of these diseases would you not consider?
A) Cheyletiellosis.
B) Dermatophytosis.
C) Otoacariasis.
D) Erythema multiforme.

3. In which of these diseases is pruritus is not normally seen?
A) Epitheliotropic cutaneous lymphoma (fungoid mycosis).
B) Otoacariasis.
C) Cryptococcosis.
D) Flea allergy dermatitis (FAD).

4. Which of the following is not one of the clinical criteria for NFHD (non-flea induced hypersensitivity dermatitis)?
A) Presence of nodules or tumours.
B) Presence of pruritus from the start of the problem.
C) At least two body regions affected.
D) Presence of papular-crusted or miliary dermatitis as a predominant reaction pattern.

5. To detect the *Demodex gatoi* mite, what diagnostic technique is recommended?
A) Microscopic examination of the hair.
B) Deep skin scraping.
C) Sellotape or scotch®test.
D) Back combing.

6. In the case of a cat with dermatophytosis, Wood's lamp and microscopic hair examinations are used to:
A) Document active hair infection.
B) Identify the fungal species involved.
C) Monitor the response to treatment.
D) Detect nodular or atypical fungal infections.

7. Within the pustular dermatitis group, which of these diseases would you include?
A) Epitheliotropic lymphoma.
B) Erythema multiforme.
C) Pemphigus foliaceous.
D) Dystrophic bullosa epidermolysis.

8. The paraneoplastic syndrome associated with thymoma is considered as part of which group diseases:
A) Pustular.
B) Erosive-ulcerative.
C) Desquamative.
D) Nodular.

9. Epitheliotropic cutaneous lymphoma is characterized by:
A) Scales attached to the hairs forming "follicular casts."
B) Small, thin, grey-white scales, that are easily collected by combing.
C) Yellowish-brown scales attached to the skin surface and hair.
D) Whitish scales, of largish size and that adhere to the skin's surface.

10. Yellowish-brown scales attached to the skin surface and hair can be seen in:
A) A cat with focal-multifocal alopecia due to *Demodex cati*.
B) An allergic cat with *Malassezia spp*. overgrowth.
C) A cat with papular-nodular lesions due to insect bites.
D) A cat with facial ulcerative lesions due to herpesvirus.

11. How is an ulcer defined?
A) Loss of cutaneous tissue up to the middle and deep dermis.
B) Aggregates of corneocytes that detach from the skin's surface.
C) Loss of cutaneous tissue up to the dermo-epidermal junction.
D) A solid, circumscribed, prominent, variable sized lesion.

12. In a cat with facial ulcerative lesions, which of these diseases would you not consider as a differential diagnosis?
A) Herpesvirus.
B) Food allergy.
C) Cheyletiellosis.
D) Squamous cell carcinoma.

13. Which of the following diseases causes deformation of the top of the nose in cats?
A) Calicivirus.
B) Toxoplasmosis.
C) Cryptococcosis.
D) Mycoplasmosis.

14. What dose of cyclosporine is considered most effective in cats with allergic dermatitis?
A) 7 mg/kg.
B) 10 mg/kg.
C) 5 mg/kg.
D) 3 mg/kg.

15. In a cat with dermatophytosis, which systemic treatment would you advise?
A) Lufenuron 80–100 mg.
B) Iodide 20 mg/kg.
C) Amphotericin B 0.1 mg/kg.
D) Itraconazole at 5–10 mg/kg or terbinafine at a dose of 10–30 mg/kg.

Clinical cases

Case 1

"Luna", a 2-year-old neutered common European cat, weighing 3.5 kg.

Three months ago, she presented with lesions located on the head, neck and base of the tail.

She was scratching the facial region insistently and licking the base of the tail. She has been treated with injectable corticosteroids with apparent clinical improvement, but over the last 15 days the pruritus has become unmanageable and has had to wear a Buster collar.

She is vaccinated and several months before the visit she received treatment for ectoparasites-endoparasites with a product containing fipronil, (S)-methoprene, eprinomectin and praziquantel.

The owners do not show evidence of skin lesions and the cat lives in a flat and has outdoor access.

1. **Which of these main reaction patterns can you see?**
   A) Papular-crusting dermatitis or miliary dermatitis + symmetrical (self-induced) alopecia.
   B) Erosions or ulcers to the face, head and neck (FHN) + eosinophilic granuloma complex (EGC) lesions.
   C) Erosions or ulcers to the face, head and neck (FHN) + miliary dermatitis (MD or papular-crusting dermatitis).
   D) Erosions or ulcers to the face, head and neck (FHN) + self-induced alopecia (SIA).
2. **Which of these diseases would you not include on your list of differential diagnoses, considering these reaction patterns?**
   A) Flea allergy dermatitis (FAD).
   B) Food allergy (FA).
   C) Sebaceous adenitis.
   D) Imitation atopic dermatitis.

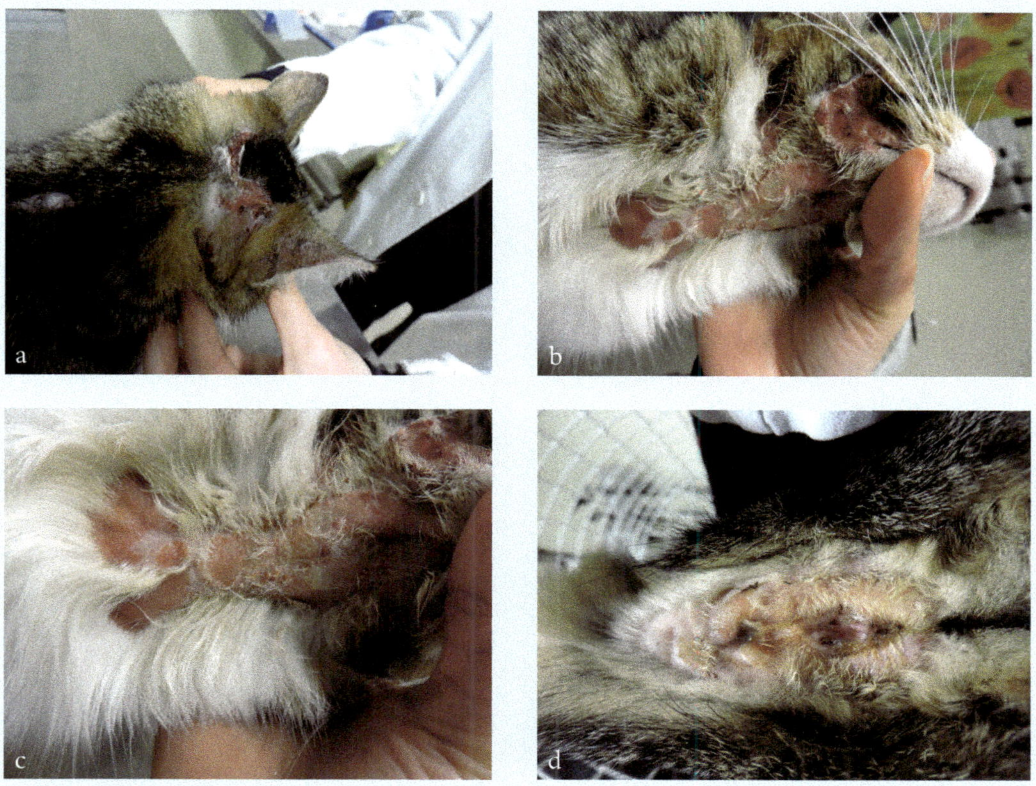

3. **Which of these complementary tests would you do first?**
   A) Blood tests (blood chemistry test).
   B) Fine need cytology.
   C) Skin biopsy.
   D) Microscopic examination of the hair, apposition cytology.

4. Given the history, which of these diseases do you think is the most likely?
- A) Flea allergy dermatitis (FAD).
- B) Food allergy (FA).
- C) Imitation atopic dermatitis.
- D) None of the answers are correct because it is essential to follow an appropriate diagnostic-therapeutic procedure with progressive exclusion of the aforementioned diseases.

5. What would you propose to the owner?
- A) Treat secondary infections with topical products (if the animal allows it) + broad spectrum product against all ectoparasites + restriction to indoors only, if possible, for a while and then follow, depending on the response, with an elimination diet.
- B) Investigate the allergens responsible using intradermal or serological tests and then desensitize the animal with allergen-specific immunotherapy.
- C) Administer cyclosporine at a dose of 7 mg/kg once daily for at least 4 weeks.
- D) Try again with just injectable glucocorticoids as they have worked previously.

Case 2

"Soffio", 3-year-old neutered male Persian cat, which weighs 5 kg. The cat has been suffering from facial pruritus for a couple of months.

He has been treated with a topical chlorhexidine solution (10-day intervals on average) and with injectable antibiotic (cefovecin sodium, only one administration), with improvement observed with relapse a few days after treatment was discontinued.

He is treated with selamectin every month for ectoparasites. He is vaccinated and dewormed, is FIV-FeLV negative, eats commercially available food and lives in a flat with a dog that has no dermatological problems.

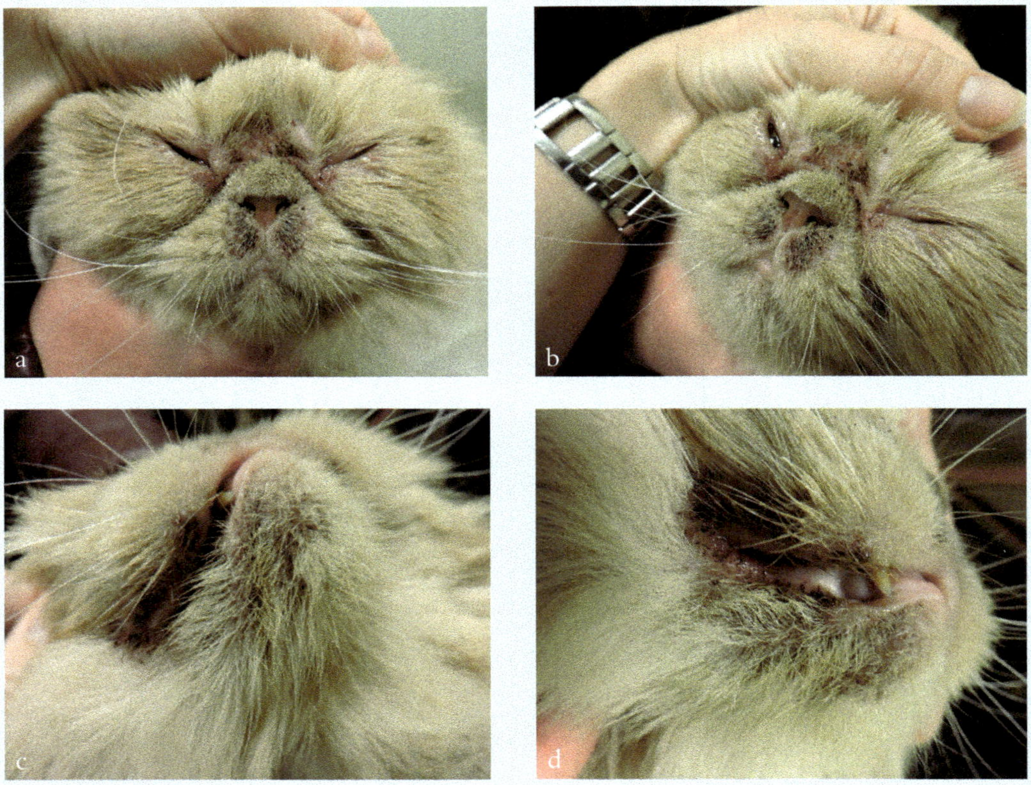

1. Study the first photo. To which dermatological problem would you attribute the injuries that you can see?
- A) Nodular dermatosis.
- B) Symmetrical (self-induced) alopecia.
- C) Erosive-ulcerative dermatitis.
- D) Pustular dermatitis.

2. **Look at the second and third photos. Especially on the facial, perilabial and chin folds, what can you see?**
   A) Wax like, dark scales that surround the hair shafts.
   B) Yellowish crusts that are closely adhered to the skin's surface.
   C) Partial alopecia and erythematous papules.
   D) Multiple erythematous nodules.
3. **Given the signalment and history, which of these diseases do you think is the most likely?**
   A) Flea-allergy dermatitis (FAD).
   B) Idiopathic facial dermatitis.
   C) Calicivirus.
   D) Squamous cell carcinoma.
4. **What is normally associated with the severity of these injuries?**
   A) Infection by epitheliotropic viruses.
   B) Fungal infection by *Microsporum canis*.
   C) Secondary bacterial infection (*Staphylococcus spp*.) and *Malassezia spp*. overgrowth.
   D) Infection with primary or secondary nasal pathogens such as *Mycoplasma spp*. or *Bordetella spp*.
5. **Once secondary infections have been treated, what treatment can be prescribed?**
   A) Cyclosporin 6–7 mg/kg/day.
   B) 0.1% Tacrolimus every 12 hours.
   C) Prednisolone 2.2 mg/kg/day.
   D) All the treatments mentioned above have been documented as effective.

Answers

Test

1. B	7. C	13. C
2. D	8. C	14. A
3. C	9. D	15. D
4. A	10. B	
5. C	11. A	
6. A	12. C	

Case 1

1. B
2. C
3. D
4. D
5. A

Case 2

1. C
2. A
3. B
4. C
5. D

4

Ophthalmology

Kerry Smith

Contents

The ophthalmic examination

It is a common misconception that ophthalmic examinations are difficult. However, with practice, patience, and some basic equipment the first opinion clinician can glean much vital information from an eye exam (Figures 1 and 2).

The following are prerequisites for a good ophthalmic examination.

- A room which can be darkened.
- A bright light source.
- Minimal, gentle restraint.
- Sufficient time.

Allow plenty of time for the exam, initially 30–35 minutes (which includes 20 minutes for mydriasis).

A bright light source is essential. Many normal animals demonstrate abnormal pupillary light reflexes purely because an insufficiently bright light is used to elicit them. A battery-operated pen torch is adequate but a **Finhoff transilluminator**, the head of which fits onto a direct ophthalmoscope base, offers more versatility as it has a rheostat for variable brightness.

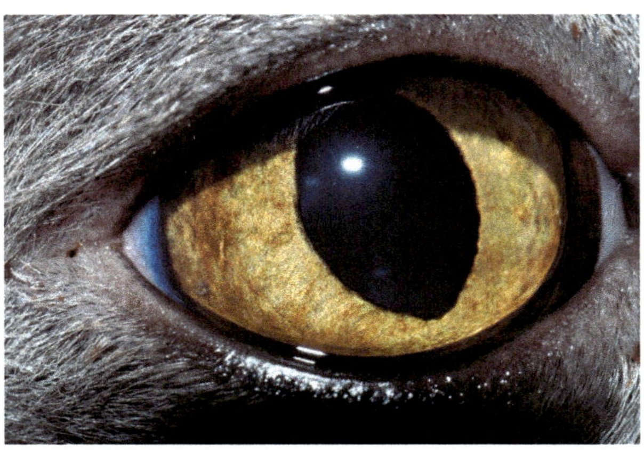

Figure 1. The normal feline eye. © Rachel Lockhart.

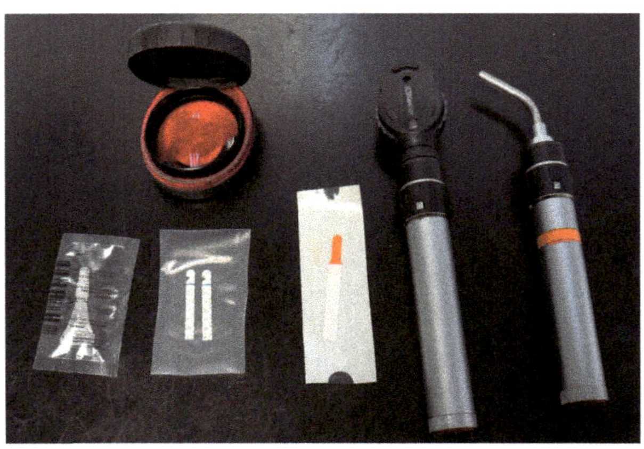

Figure 2. Minimum equipment required for a good ophthalmic examination. © Kerry Smith.

With cats, it is beneficial to adopt a **'less is more' approach with regards to restraint**. The patient is often calmer when held by their owner, so always try this first with the cat seated on the consulting table gazing straight ahead facing the examiner. Ideally, if the cat carrier has a removable top half, leave the cat sitting in the bottom half which helps reduce their stress. The best ophthalmic exams are obtained conscious, so fractious cats should be gently wrapped in a towel (ideally spritzed with feline pheromone spray).

Sedation or general anaesthesia are seldom rewarding since the globes tend to rotate downwards and the third eyelids elevate which prevents a full inspection. In additon, many sedative or anaesthetic agents alter the tear film, change pupil size, and prevent examination of the ophthalmic reflexes.

The basic equipment and consumables required to perform a good examination include:

- bright light source
- direct ophthalmoscope
- condensing lens (ideally 20 dioptres)
- Schirmer Tear test (STT) strips
- topical anaesthetic e.g. proxymetacaine 0.5%
- fluorescein
- mydriatic i.e. tropicamide 1.0%.

Always **follow a logical system** for the examination to make best use of equipemnt and prevent interference with tests which may later be required (e.g. moistening the eye with a topical preparation before performing a Schirmer tear test). Sticking to a system increases proficiency and confidence, but also helps avoid omissions. All observations should be recorded.

The exam is broadly divided into the:

1. Hands-off examination.
2. Hands-on, lights on.
3. Hands-on, lights off.
4. Ancillary tests.
5. Post-mydriatic examination.

Hands-off examination

Observing the patient from a distance should not be underestimated as a means of gathering information. If practical, allow the cat out of the basket to wander free in the consulting room whilst a history is taken. Observe the cat's behaviour such as their ability to negotiate obstacles, if they circle, hug the wall, bump into things, or just sits and is reluctant to move. Once the history is complete, have the owner sit the cat on the consulting table and **assess it from a distance for signs of photophobia**, blepharospasm (blinkiness), increased blink rate, asymmetry of the globes or orbits, anisocoria (unequal pupil size) and the presence of ocular discharge.

Hands-on, lights-on examination

The following tests assess **vision and cranial nerve function**.

Menace response

This is a learned response which is not present until 12 weeks of age, and many cats can **voluntarily suppress it making the menace test unreliable in felines**. It is elicited by briskly moving a flat hand or pointed finger towards one eye whilst covering the other. Care should be taken to avoid excessive air movement or touching the whiskers or vibrissae. It should be performed both **medially and laterally**. In a sighted patient a blink reflex should occur. The afferent arm of the response is the Optic nerve (CN II) and the efferent is the facial nerve (CN VII).

Dazzle reflex

A **bright light shone in each eye in turn should result in a blink**. The afferent arm of the reflex is the Optic nerve (CN II) and the efferent arm is the Facial nerve (CN VII). Even patients with a dense cataract should have a positive dazzle reflex if a sufficiently bright light is used.

Pupillary light reflexes (direct and consensual)

A bright light shone into the eye results in a **constriction of the same pupil (direct) and of the contralateral pupil (consensual).** The latter is particularly useful to assess retinal function in an eye with an opaque anterior chamber due to glaucoma, extensive keratitis or trauma (i.e. the direct PLR cannot be assessed). The afferent arm of the reflex is the optic nerve (CN II) and the efferent arm is the parasympathetic fibres which run with the oculomotor nerve (CN III).

Palpebral reflex

This tests the **sensory innervation to the lids** and is evaluated by gently tapping the medial and then the lateral canthus. It should elicit a blink in response, and retraction of the globe. The afferent arm is either the ophthalmic (medial and lateral canthi and centre of upper lid) or maxillary (centre of lower lid) branch of the trigeminal nerve (CN V) and the efferent arm is the facial nerve (CN VII) and the abducens nerve (CN VI) which innervates the retractor bulbi muscle.

Corneal reflex

This tests the **sensory innervation to the cornea**. It is evaluated by touching the peripheral cornea gently with a wisp of cotton wool. A positive response results in a blink. The efferent arm of the reflex is the ophthalmic branch of the trigeminal nerve (CN V), and the afferent arm is the facial nerve (CN VII) and the abducens nerve (CN VI) which innervates the retractor bulbi muscle.

Vestibulo-ocular or oculocephalic reflex

This **assesses eye movement in relation to changes within the vestibular apparatus**, thereby indirectly assessing cranial nerves III, IV and VI which innervate the extraocular muscles, and the vestibular nerve (CN VIII). The cat's head is moved from side to side and up and down. During this movement the cat's eyes attempt to stay looking in the direction they were before the test was started; resulting in a slow movement of the eyes away from the direction of head movement. As head movement continues, the eyes then move quickly in the direction of head movement. The eyes should move in unison and stop moving when the head stops.

Whilst still holding the head, the **orbital rims should be palpated**, the **globes retropulsed** and the resultant movement of the third eyelids observed. Behavioural testing of vision which can be especially useful in cats (due to the unreliability of the menace response in this species) is assessed at this stage:

Visual tracking	Examiner drops a cotton wool ball in front of cat and observes visual tracking. Can also use a laser pointer.
Visual placing	Examiner picks up cat and covering one eye brings it to edge of consulting table. See if cat reaches out a paw as it approaches surface. (Figures 3a, 3b).
	Perform straight on and laterally, covering each eye in turn.

Hands-on, lights-off examination

Pupil sizes, dazzle and pupillary light reflexes should always be reassessed in the dark to obtain accurate results which is vital to achieving a diagnosis.

The following structures should then be examined using a focal light source:

- adnexae – lids, third eyelid, lacrimal punctae, conjunctiva
- cornea
- anterior chamber
- iris
- lens.

Check for masses, aberrant hairs or eyelashes, colour change, opacities, presence or absence of blood vessels, at all levels. It is important to observe from all angles and make use of the phenomenon of parallax

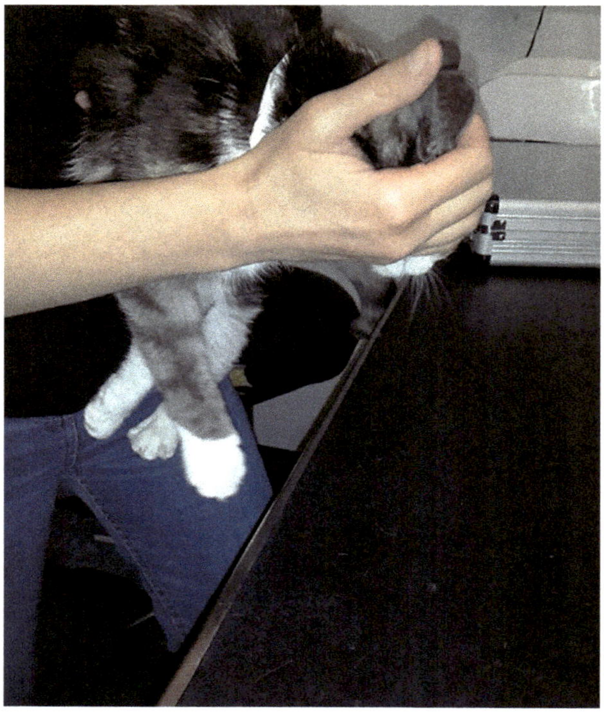

Figure 3a. The visual placing test. The cat is brought to the edge of the table with one eye covered. © Kerry Smith.

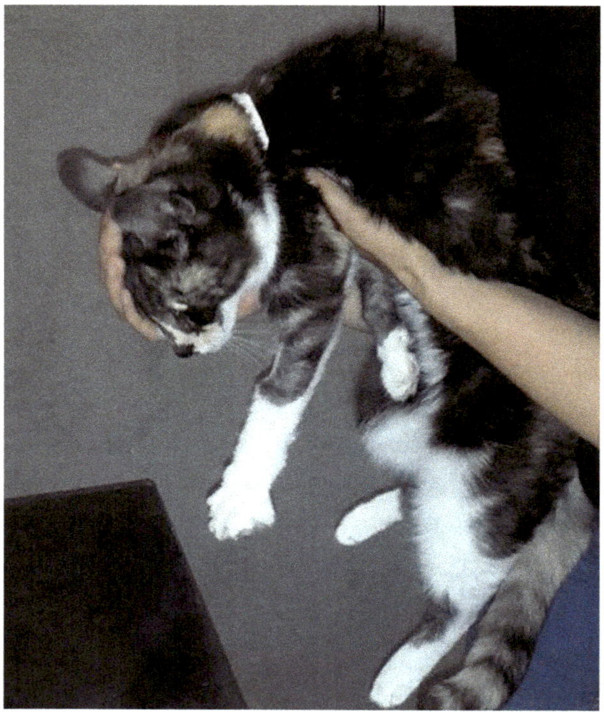

Figure 3b. If the cat is visual in the uncovered eye, it will reach out a paw to the table. © Kerry Smith.

(Lowe, 2014) to best localize lesions. The Purkinje images on the cornea (the reflection of light) should be assessed; this gives information about the health of the cornea and tear film.

The Schirmer Tear Test (STT)

STT should be performed before any topicals are instilled into the eye. This is done without local anaesthetic, and **measures baseline and reflex tearing**. The strip is placed in the lower conjunctival fornix, about two-thirds of the way along the lid from the medial canthus. The value of STT in cats is hugely variable and repeatability often low, but one recent study reported a range from **9–34mm/min in healthy cats** with a median value of 18mm/min (Sebbag et al., 2015).

Bacteriology swabs

Swabs from the conjunctival sacs are taken after STTs but before the instillation of topical anaesthetic or fluorescein, both of which may affect bacterial growth.

Ocular cytology

This can be informative, particularly for **conjunctivitis or keratitis**. Samples are taken from the locally anaesthetised eye (a couple of drops of 0.5% proxymetacaine from a single-use vial a few minutes apart) using a kimura spatula, the blunt end of a Bard-Parker blade or a cytobrush; the latter may give a smaller cellular harvest but excellent cell preservation. Once the sample is smeared on a microscope slide, it can be stained with Diff-Quik, and examined in-house, or submitted to an external laboratory.

Fluorescein staining

This **checks for corneal ulceration** (Figure 4) and should be a part of every routine eye examination. Fluorescein is available either in a single use vial of 2.0% alkaline sodium fluorescein solution, or impregnated paper strips. The strips are more versatile and the fluorescein is more concentrated. The strips are moistened with a drop of sterile saline and gently touched on the bulbar conjunctiva. They should not touch the cornea as this can leave a staining pattern that is easily misinterpreted as pathology. Fluorescein is highly lipophobic and hydrophilic and turns from **orange to green when in contact with the tear film**. It is therefore repelled by the lipid containing cell-membranes of the epithelium, but retained by any hydrophilic exposed stroma. When evaluating ulcers, it is important to thoroughly **irrigate the corneal surface with sterile saline** or balanced saline solution following application to flush away excess fluorescein which may give misleading results: it can pool, both in healed stromal deficits and descemetocoeles.

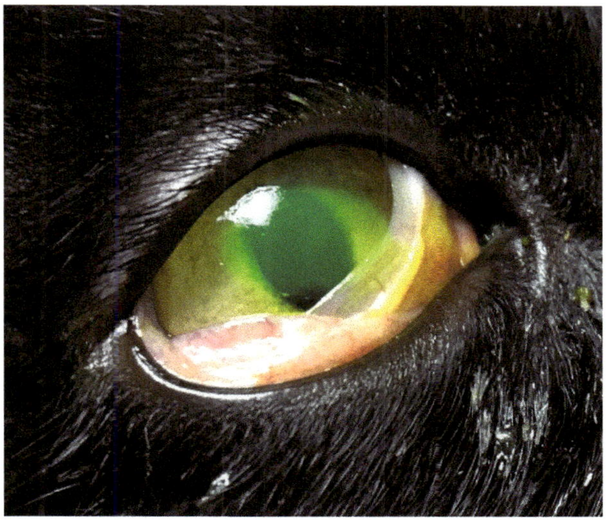

Figure 4. Fluorescein staining of a superficia ulcer. © Agata Tsvetanova.

Illumination with a blue light source will enhance any fluorescein-positive lesions, particularly useful if you want to demonstrate them to the client.

Fluorescein can be used to check for **leakage of aqueous humour from corneal lacerations**: the **'Seidel test'**. Fluorescein is applied to the cornea in the location of the lesion without flushing. It instantly turns green upon contact with the tear film, but if an aqueous leak is present, this will be seen running as a clear rivulet through the green dye: 'Seidel positive'. A further use of fluorescein is the 'Jones test'; fluorescein is applied to the eye without rinsing and is then timed to see when it appears at the ipsilateral nares. The reported values for normal passage vary widely, but in a cat it should be expected to be present within ten minutes.

The cornea behind the third eyelid should also be assessed for lesions immediately after fluorescein staining; a sterile cotton bud can be used to reflect it for inspection, and then swept behind it to check for the presence of foreign bodies. It can also be used to explore the dorsal and ventral conjunctival sacs.

Intraocular pressure (IOP)

When the means to measure IOP are available, this should be done after the application of topical anaesthetic, but prior to dilating the pupils which can affect IOP readings and may be contraindicated if they are high. There are a variety of devices available for the purpose, ranging in price.

The Schiotz indentation tonometer is the cheapest but takes some practice to use. **Correct positioning of the animal is essential** (nose pointing upwards, neck gently extended and corneas horizontal), as is minimal restraint. With any method of measuring IOP it is paramount not to restrain the animal around the neck, as pressure on the jugular veins will give a falsely elevated reading. A conversion chart, which comes with the Schiotz tonometer, will convert the numerical reading obtained to a pressure in mmHg, whilst readings from applanation (e.g. Tonopen) (Figure 5) and rebound (e.g. Tonovet) (Figure 6) digital tonometers are already in mmHg. **Normal IOP for a cat, using an applanation tonometer is reported as 9–31 mmHg** (Miller et al., 1991) and a more recent study using a rebound tonometer gave a mean value of 21mmHg (Rusanen et al., 2010). If no tonometer is available, a very limited amount of information can be obtained by digital tonometry (pressing the globes with forefinger through closed lids). In practice, this is only useful if the IOP is markedly different in each eye, and there is one normal eye with which to make the comparison. If you have any concerns about IOP, but no means of measuring it, **swift referral to a specialist is the best option for the cat.**

The pupils can now be dilated (Figure 7) using 1% tropicamide. Single-use vials should be employed to avoid contamination and wastage. **Atropine is not an appropriate mydriatic** for diagnostic purposes; it has

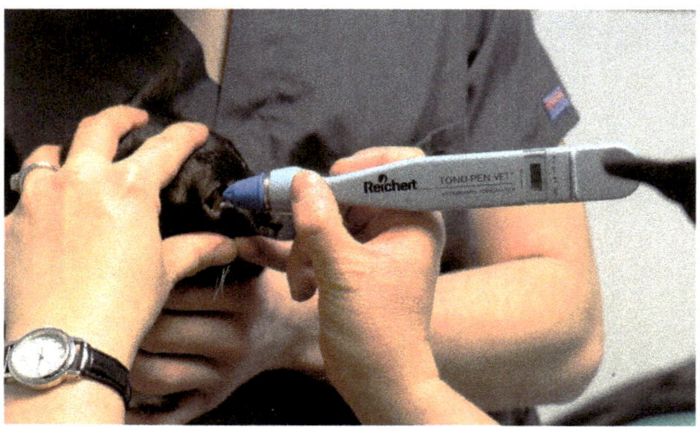

Figure 5. Measuring IOP with a Tonopen™. © Kerry Smith.

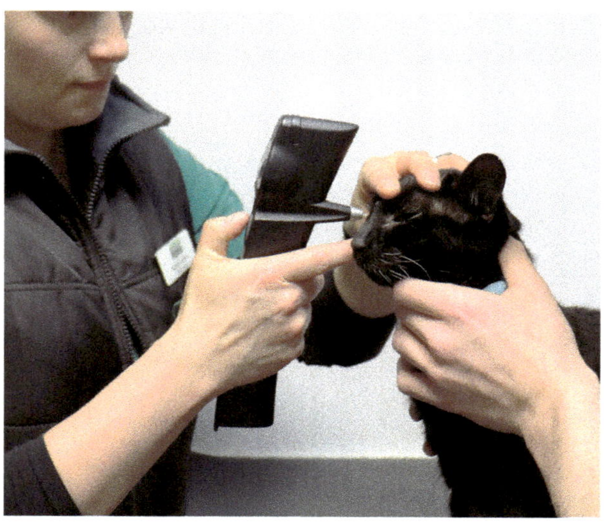

Figure 6. Measuring IOP with a Tonovet™. © Kerry Smith.

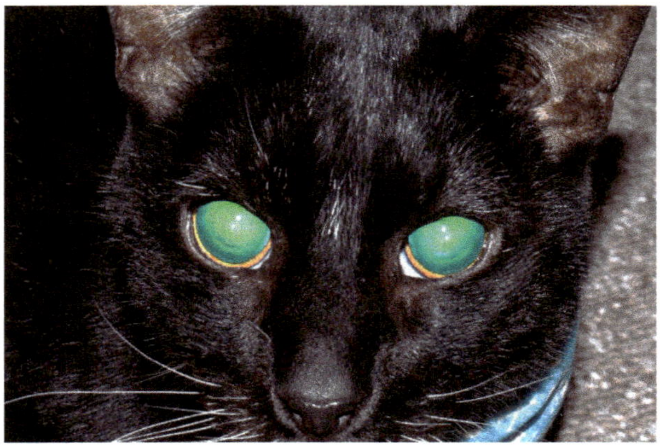

Figure 7. Maximally dilated pupils. © Ioannis Tzouganakis.

a long duration of action (several days in the normal eye), is contraindicated in certain conditions (e.g. glaucoma), and causes salivation which can be alarming to the owner. Even **1% tropicamide lasts approximately eight hours**, and clients should be warned to keep their pet away from bright lights after the examination. Its peak action occurs approximately 45 minutes post-application in the cat but the pupil should be adequately dilated after 15–20 minutes.

Post-mydriatic examination

Once the pupils are fully dilated, perform both direct and indirect ophthalmoscopy to examine the internal structures of the eye (Figures 8, 9 and 10). The advantages of each include:

	Direct ophthalmoscopy	Indirect ophthalmoscopy
Image type	Real	Virtual
Image orientation	Upright	Inverted and back to front
Magnification	Up to 15x	1–3x
Field of View	Narrow	Wide

For a complete examination both direct and indirect methods should be used. To avoid discomfort for the animal, the light level should be the minimum needed for each piece of equipment to achieve examination.

The **direct ophthalmoscope is used for both close and distant examinations**. For both, the eyepiece of the instrument is held as close to the examiner's face as possible, with the rest at the top in apposition with the brow. Close examination is performed with the instrument in close proximity to the animal's cornea, whilst distant direct ophthalmoscopy is performed at arm's length.

- Close direct ophthalmoscopy gives a highly magnified view of the fundus, and the examination performed in

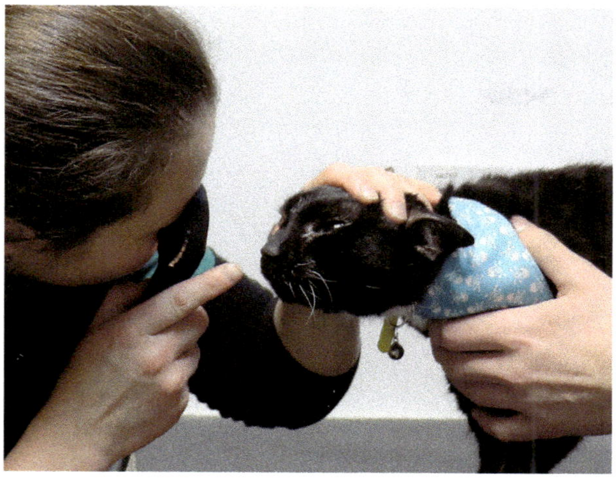

Figure 8. Close direct ophthalmoscopy. © Kerry Smith.

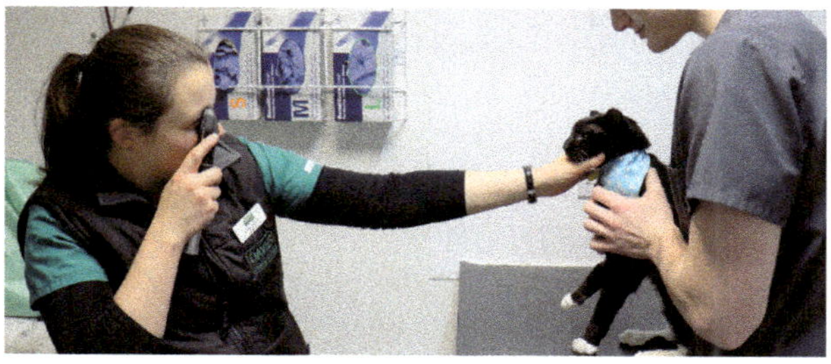

Figure 9. Distant direct ophthalmoscopy. © Kerry Smith.

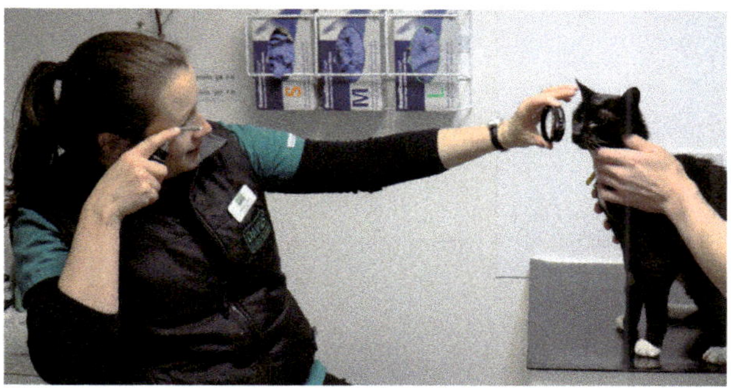

Figure 10. Indirect ophthalmoscopy. © Kerry Smith.

sectors or quadrants, moving in a systematic way so as not to miss anything.

- Distant direct ophthalmoscopy is an invaluable tool for detecting opacities in the ocular media (e.g., cataracts), which appear as black silhouettes against the colour of the tapetal fundus.

Indirect ophthalmoscopy can be performed using a head-mounted indirect ophthalmoscope, which gives a stereoscopic view, but the best results are obtained using a handheld Finhoff transilluminator with the 20 dioptre lens. Again the fundus should be examined in sectors. For examiners with little experience of fundic examination it is initially useful to focus on just one aspect of the fundus (e.g. trying to locate the optic nerve head in every cat examined) before moving onto performing the full examination.

Normal ophthalmoscopic appearance of the feline eye

The fundus comprises (Figure 11):

- the tapetal fundus
- non-tapetal fundus
- retinal vasculature
- optic nerve head.

Viewed ophthalmoscopically, the **tapetal fundus is roughly triangular**. It is located dorsally with the base of the triangle lying just above or below the optic nerve head. This coloured reflective structure is responsible for the 'eyeshine' seen in cats and is composed of layers of polyhedral cells or 'iridocytes' containing reflective riboflavin. Its function is to reflect light back through the photoreceptors to restimulate them. It may appear orange, yellow, green or blue, and in colour-dilute cats may be absent. Multiple small dark spots may be observed throughout the tapetum; these are small blood vessels within the choroid connecting the medium–sized vessel and choriocapillaris layers viewed 'end on' and known as Stars of Winslow. These are more obvious in cats than in dogs. Tapetal development commences at about six weeks in the cat and is usually complete by about three months of age. Prior to this the whole fundus has a greyish or lilac appearance.

Typically, the **non-tapetal fundus is heavily pigmented**: dark brown or grey and generally homogeneous. This is the Retinal Pigment Epithelium (RPE) being observed. In colour-dilute animals this area may be lightly or non-pigmented and the choroidal vasculature is seen through it (Figure 12). Cats possess a 'holangiotic' retina in which the whole of the inner retina receives a direct blood supply.

Typically **three to five major veins are visible** converging at the periphery of the optic disc. In the cat

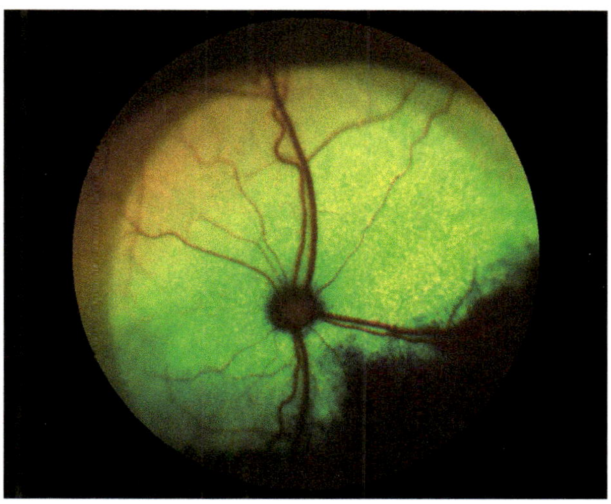

Figure 11. The normal feline fundus. © Rachel Lockhart.

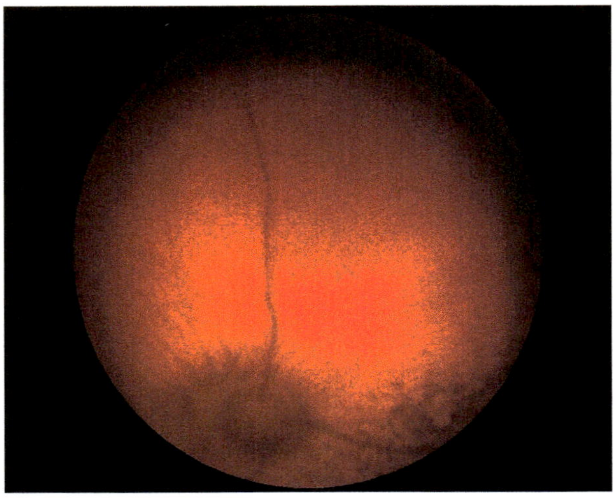

Figure 12. The normal colour-dilute or 'tigroid' feline fundus. © Rachel Lockhart.

three or four arterioles radiate from the periphery of the optic disc. The vessels arc around a clear area 3–4 mm lateral to the optic disc known as the area centralis, which is an area of high cone density, roughly equivalent to the fovea in humans. This is most obvious in the cat. Apart from the lack of vessels in this area, it is ophthalmoscopically indistinguishable from the rest of the fundus.

The optic disc or **optic nerve head** (**ONH**) is the beginning of the optic nerve which is composed of retinal ganglion cell axons. The disc is generally grey in colour in cats due to lack of myelination and is roughly circular.

General pathological changes of the fundus

Although histologically composed of ten cell layers the neurosensory retina is transparent so its health is judged on the appearance of deeper structures (whether they are more or less obvious), and its blood vessels. Our ability to visualise the tapetum, or the RPE/choroid in the non-tapetal fundus, through the retina provides important information about it.

Ophthalmic conditions of the cat

Conditions of the eyelids

Eyelid agenesis

Eyelid agenesis or coloboma of the eyelids is a congenital defect often occurring bilaterally. In the main, it affects the lateral aspect of the upper eyelids. The absence of the eyelid margin, together with a greater or lesser degree of eyelid tissue, can lead to **exposure keratitis and trichiasis.** In turn this has the possible sequelae of neovascularisation, fibrosis and desiccation

Fundic Change	Appearance
Hyperreflectivity	Brighter/shinier tapetal reflex. Indicates atrophy or degeneration of the retina which may be inherited or the result of a previous toxic, infectious or inflammatory insult.
Hyporeflectivity	Dull greyish areas. Indicates retinal detachment, choroidal effusion, inflammatory exudates or neoplastic infiltrate.
Pigmentary changes	Pigmentation or colour changes of the tapetum, and loss of pigmentation, hyperpigmentation or pigment clumping in the non-tapetal area.
Vascular changes	Retinal vessels may exhibit attenuation in degenerative conditions, dilation, 'sausaging', or colour changes in certain systemic conditions, and perivascular cuffing in inflammatory ones.
Haemorrhages	Bleeding can occur above, below or within the retina; the appearance of haemorrhage varies according to its location: • Subretinal haemorrhages are often large and have a dark appearance. • Intraretinal haemorrhages tend to be smaller and lighter in colour – 'dots and blots'. • Superficial retinal haemorrhages classically have a 'flame' shaped appearance as they follow the nerve fibres of the ganglion cells. • Vitreal haemorrhages have a classic 'keel-boat' appearance. NB Retinal haemorrhages can resemble pigment especially when present for some time; can be distinguished from pigment using the red-free filter (green light) on the direct ophthalmoscope. Haemorrhage appears black, but pigment will remain brown.
Retinal detachments	Vary in size from focal to total or 'infundibular' detachments. Focal detachments – greyish and dull with a well-demarcated border. Vessels crossing the detachment will appear elevated. Larger detachments – a membrane hanging from the ora serrata or optic disc, immediately behind posterior lens capsule. Infundibular-retina remains attached only at the ora serrata and around the optic nerve head (takes on the appearance of the inside of a marquee roof).
Optic nerve head changes	Colour-pale/grey if atrophic, pinker if swollen Also size and profile changes

of the cornea, corneal ulceration and sequestrum formation. Depending upon the size of the defect and clinical signs, treatment may vary from long-term corneal lubrication, cryoepilation of misdirected hairs, simple surgery involving conversion of the defect to a four-sided wedge with primary closure in two layers, to more complex multi-stage reconstructive procedures where the defect is especially large. The latter include the sliding H-plasty, modified Mustardé technique, or a modified lip to lid technique (Whittaker et al., 2010).

Entropion

Entropion (Figure 13) occurs far less frequently in cats than dogs. **Primary entropion is unusual** but is reported in the Persian. **Secondary entropion can occur as a result of chronic painful corneal conditions** (beginning as a spastic entropion but becoming permanent) or in older cats as a result of enophthalmos due to loss of orbital fat and muscle. A modified Hotz-Celsus skin muscle resection is generally recommended to treat feline entropion. Removal of a greater amount of tissue than one would anticipate in the dog is necessary in order to avoid recurrence. Overlength of the lids is often a feature of feline entropion and the Hotz-Celsus procedure may need to be combined with full thickness wedge resection to shorten the lid.

Lipogranulomatous conjunctivitis

This is a condition of **middle-aged to older cats** involving the development of **white/cream subconjunctival swellings in the palpebral conjunctiva adjacent to the eyelid margin** (Figures 14a, 14b). It is thought to be an inflammatory response to sebaceous material released in the tissue from ruptured Meibomian glands. The lesions are termed 'chalazia'. White or light-coloured cats appear to be predisposed and a link to UV-light induced damage has been proposed (Read and Lucas, 2001). Small focal lesions may not cause any clinical signs, but if there is ocular discomfort, surgical curettage via a conjunctival approach is recommended.

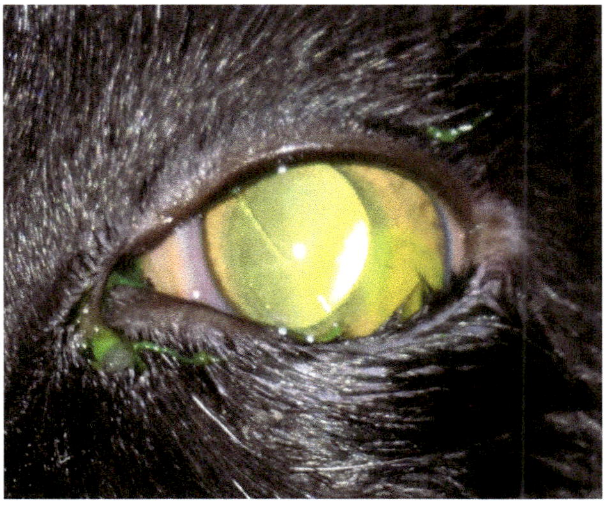

Figure 13. Entropion of the lower lid leading to corneal ulceration. © Agata Tsvetanova.

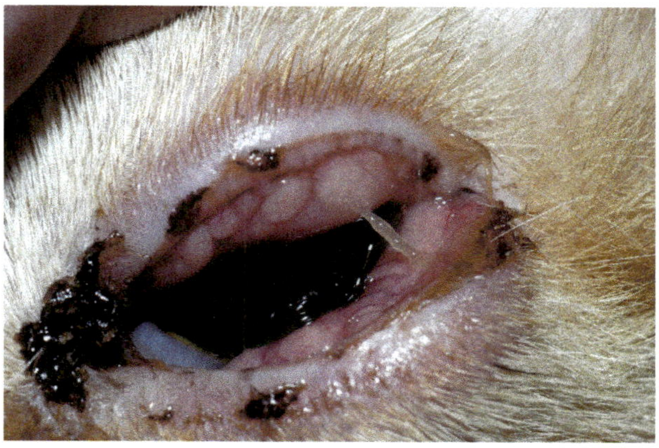

Figure 14a. A severe case of lipogranulomatous conjunctivitis, upper lid. © Rachel Lockhart.

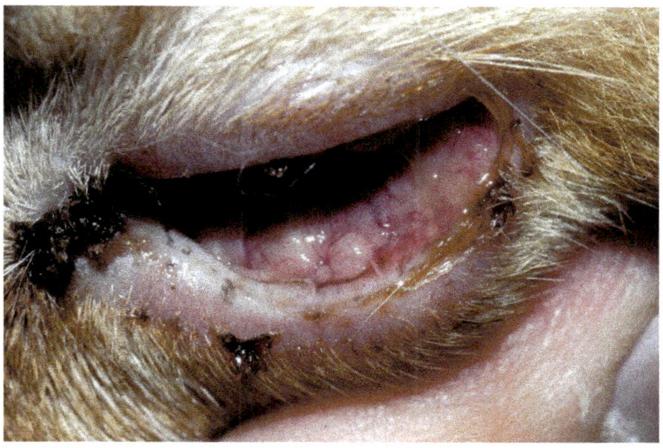

Figure 14b. Lower lid of the same case. © Rachel Lockhart.

Eyelid tumours

In cats the vast majority (up to 90%) of **eyelid neoplasms are malignant** (McLaughlin et al., 1993, Newkirk and Rohrbach, 2009); they include squamous cell carcinoma (Figure 15), mast cell tumour, haemangiosarcoma, adenocarcinoma, lymphoma, peripheral nerve sheath tumours (Figure 16), and the benign apocrine hidrocystoma (Figure 17).

The average age at presentation is over 10 years. **Removal of any eyelid mass is recommended** as lesions can cause local irritation manifested by blepharospasm, lacrimation or ocular discharge, conjunctival hyperaemia and corneal neovascularisation or ulceration. But because of the **high propensity for malignancy**, surgical removal of feline lid masses should be approached with particular care. Removal of lid masses is generally by surgical excision, although cryotherapy, hyperthermia, and laser CO_2 ablation have also been used.

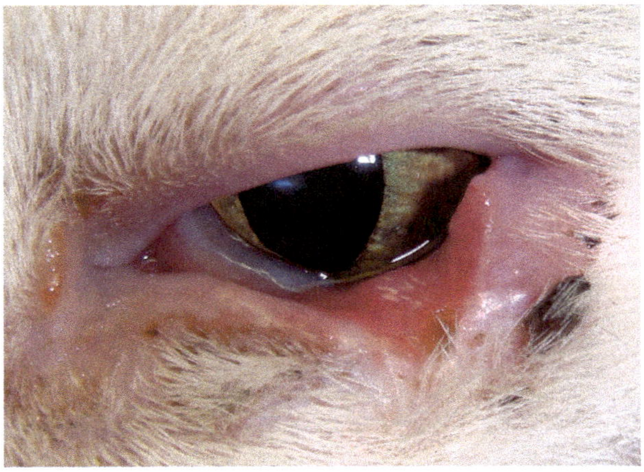

Figure 15. Squamous cell carcinoma of the lower lid – a typically erosive lesion. © Rachel Lockhart.

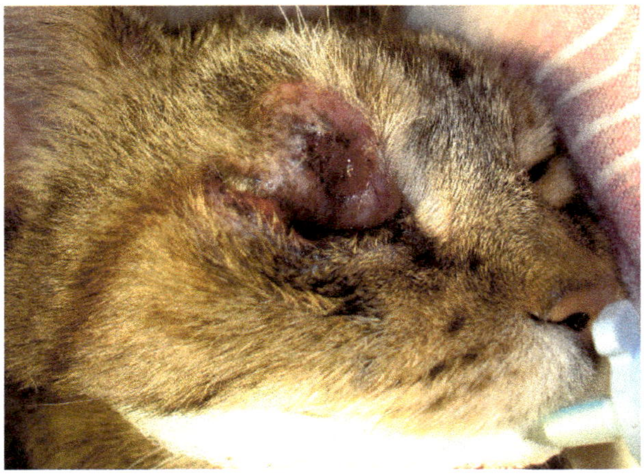

Figure 16. Peripheral nerve sheath tumour of the upper lid. © Rachel Lockhart.

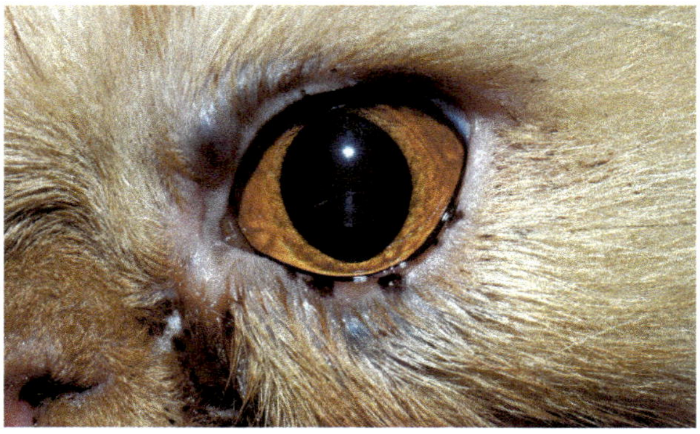

Figure 17. Benign apocrine hidrocystomas in the Persian. © Rachel Lockhart.

The surgical approach depends upon the size, location and most importantly nature of the mass. For this reason ideally an **FNA or snip biopsy should be obtained prior to surgery to enable optimal surgical planning**, obtain adequate margins and thereby avoid the need for repeated procedures.

Because of high likelihood of malignancy, staging (chest radiographs, abdominal ultrasound) should be performed prior to excision. Eyelid masses are best removed at the earliest opportunity so as to leave the smallest possible surgical defect. Benign masses up to one-third eyelid length can be removed by four-sided full thickness wedge resection followed by primary closure in 2 layers of simple interrupted 6–0 polyglactin with a figure of eight suture at the lid margin. The upper eyelid is more mobile and is less forgiving of poor wound apposition at closure; the aim is to have a smooth, continuous eyelid margin with no 'step' at any point. Removal of masses greater than one-third eyelid length or those which are malignant and require wide margins of excision involve the need for some form of reconstructive procedure. **Referral is the best option in these cases**. All excised masses should be submitted for histopathology preferably by a specialist ocular histopathologist. Adjunctive treatments such as radiation, cryotherapy or chemotherapy may be required depending on the pathology results.

Conditions of the third eyelid

Bilateral third eyelid protrusion or Haw's syndrome

This is **self-limiting syndrome of bilateral third eyelid protrusion** (Figure 18) which is occasionally seen in young cats (often <1 year old) accompanied by diarrhoea. The cause is unknown but is thought to be related to **torovirus infection**. No treatment is required as the condition resolves by itself.

Dysautonomia

Dysautonomia is associated with bilateral third eyelid protrusion, dilated pupils, the absence of pupillary light reflexes, and a lack of tear production. Affecting both dogs and cats, this uncommon condition results in widespread autonomic nervous system dysfunction. The cause has never been determined but histological studies show degeneration of neurons within autonomic ganglia.

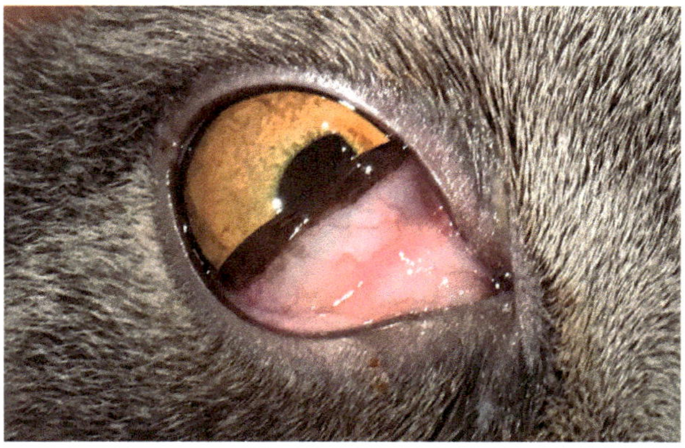

Figure 18. Third eyelid protrusion. © Agata Tsvetanova.

Non-ocular clinical signs include anorexia, vomiting or regurgitation, dysphagia, constipation, distention of the bladder, dehydration and dry mucous membranes. The prognosis for such animals is extremely guarded, but some with the milder form may survive after a prolonged period of supportive therapy.

Tumours of the third eyelid

Although **uncommon in the cat**, neoplasms of the third eyelid include: mast cell tumour, squamous cell carcinoma, haemangiosarcoma, fibrosarcoma, adenocarcinoma and melanoma. Lymphoma of the third eyelid is also seen (Figure 19), either as part of a generalised systemic neoplastic process or occasionally as a solitary lesion. **Biopsy of the lesion is essential** and depending upon its nature excision of the third eyelid may be required. Neoplasia of the third eyelid is the only indication for its removal.

Prolapse of the nictitans gland

This is reported in the cat, but is very rare and must be distinguished from a neoplastic change (Figure 20). Treatment is surgical replacement as for dogs.

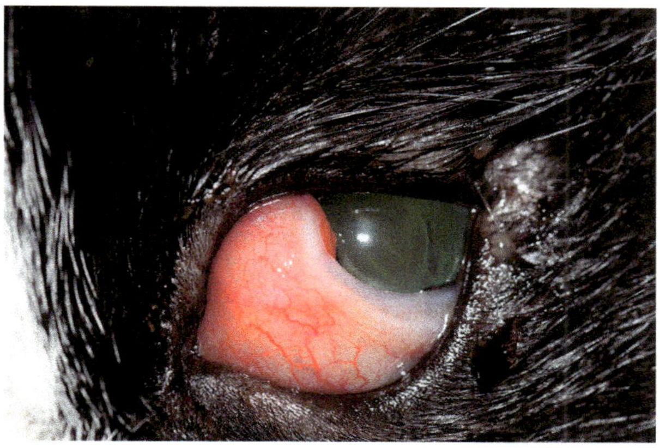

Figure 19. Lymphoma of the third eyelid. © Kerry Smith.

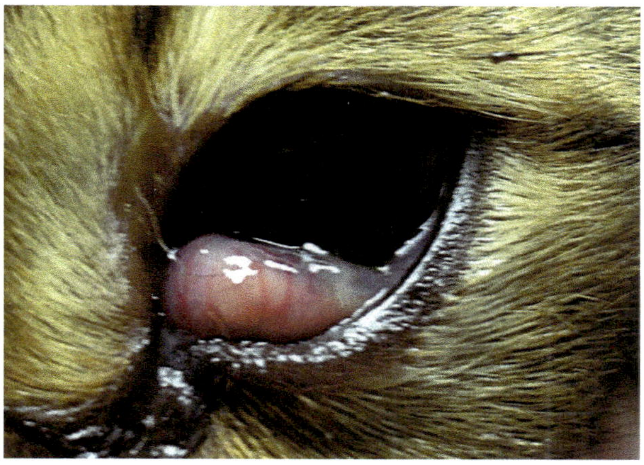

Figure 20. Prolapse of the nictitans gland in a 5 month old kitten. © Agata Tsvetanova.

Conditions of the conjunctiva

Conjunctivitis

Conjunctivitis is a common condition in cats. Clinical signs include hyperaemia, chemosis, and serous, mucoid or purulent discharge. The vast majority of cases of feline conjunctivitis are caused by **bacterial or viral infections.**

Non-specific bacterial conjunctivitis can be treated with broad spectrum topical antibiotics: fusidic acid or **chloramphenicol. The latter is preferred as a first line treatment in cats as it has efficacy against both Gram-positive and Gram-negative bacteria.** It should be applied TID in ointment form or QID as a drop, and for no longer than ten days without making a specific diagnosis. Specific infections should be treated accordingly.

Chlamydiosis

Caused by *Chlamydia felis* (a Gram-negative bacterium with a predilection for the conjunctiva) this typically affects young cats (Figure 21). The gastro-intestinal, genital and respiratory tracts are also infected but clinical signs are usually minimal with acutely infected cats suffering a mild rhinitis, sneezing and nasal discharge with the predominantly ocular signs.

Ocular signs, which are confined to the conjunctiva, may begin as unilateral but involve the contralateral eye within a couple of days: hyperaemia, chemosis, and blepharospasm and serous followed by mucopurulent discharge. These ocular signs occur as a result of host cell lysis as the *Chlamydia spp* release elementary bodies. ***C. felis* does not cause corneal lesions**. Asymptomatic carrier states can occur with the organism persisting in genital or GI tracts, leading to problems with control in

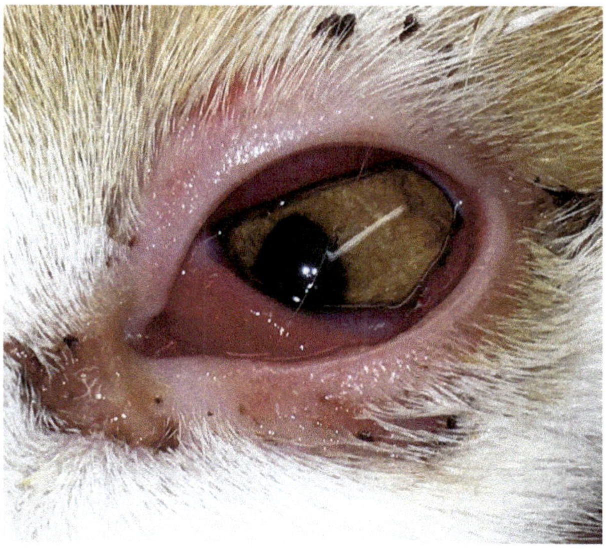

Figure 21. Conjunctivitis and chemosis caused by *Chlamydia felis* infection. © Agata Tsvetanova.

multicat households/breeding colonies. **Vaccination is available; it does not prevent infection but leads to milder symptoms** and reduces the duration of organism shedding and may be of use in such situations.

Diagnosis was previously based on the identification of characteristic cytoplasmic inclusion bodies in conjunctival smears. However these are easily missed, reduce in numbers two weeks post-infection, and must also be differentiated from 'blue bodies' which arise due to application of topical ointments. **A PCR test is now the principal method of diagnosis**. Systemic treatment is recommended to eliminate latent infection. **Doxycycline at 10 mg/kg/day for 3–4 weeks** (Dean et al., 2005) with food or followed by a water bolus in order to avoid oesophagitis, or potentiated amoxycillin clavulanate for the same period (Sturgess et al., 2001) have been shown to be effective. The latter is preferable in young kittens to avoid discolouration of the teeth by tetracyclines.

Mycoplasmosis

Mycoplasma spp. (prokaryotes) are a potential cause of feline conjunctivitis. Low et al., (2007) showed that *Mycoplasma spp*. were significantly more prevalent in cats with conjunctivitis compared with healthy animals, but other studies involving experimental infection have been more equivocal. It is thought prior infection of cats with FHV-1 or *Chlamydia felis* may create an environment in which *Mycoplasma* can thrive (Cullen and Webb, 2013). **Diagnosis is via PCR testing**. *Mycoplasma spp*. are sensitive to many topical antibiotics.

Feline Herpes Virus-1 (FHV-1)

FHV-1 is an alphaherpesvirus; double stranded DNA viruses which exhibit a short replication cycle, tendency to induce cell lysis, and persistence in host sensory ganglia (Gould, 2011). Primary infection usually occurs in kittens or juvenile cats as maternal antibodies begin to wane at eight weeks of age. Ocular signs at this stage are acute conjunctivitis and keratitis, in conjunction with rhinotracheitis. **Vaccination confers only partial immunity against clinical disease** and no protection against reactivation/shedding of virus.

Up to 97% of all cats worldwide have been exposed to FHV-1 (Maggs et al., 1999). Following exposure upwards of 80% of cats will become persistently infected (Gaskell et al., 1977) with 45% of these shedding virus spontaneously in response to stress and 70% shedding virus in response to administration of corticosteroids. **The virus remains in a latent state in the trigeminal ganglion.**

There are several ocular manifestations of FHV-1 including primary disease, recrudescence of latent infection, and immune-mediated disease directed at viral antigenic material trapped within the cornea. The corneal manifestations are discussed later.

When kittens are infected before the time of eyelid opening (Ophthalmia neonatorum), a mucopurulent discharge can build up behind them. This can cause significant corneal damage and even rupture of the globe in severely affected cases. Treatment involves surgical opening of the eyelids and irrigation of the cornea.

Acute conjunctivitis is the main presenting sign of primary FHV-1 infection typically occurring in kittens which are 8–12 weeks old. It occurs in conjunction with rhinotracheitis following an incubation period of two to six days. It is usually bilateral, with hyperaemia and a degree of chemosis +/– conjunctival ulceration (due to viral-induced epithelial necrosis).

Symblepharon occurs when severe conjunctivitis in young cats leads to the development of adhesions of the conjunctiva, either to itself, to the cornea, or across the nasolacrimal punctae or within the duct (Figure 22). This can lead to significant problems including blindness due to conjunctivalisation of the cornea caused by the loss of the local limbal stem cell population, keratoconjunctivitis sicca due to damage to lacrimal gland ductules, or permanent epiphora due to blockage of the nasolacrimal duct/s.

Fluorescent antibody testing (FAT), virus isolation (VI) and polymerase chain reaction (PCR) tests are available to detect viral antigen, live virus or viral DNA respectively. **PCR is recommended as the test with the highest sensitivity and specificity.** It can be performed on dry conjunctival or corneal swabs without the need for viral transport medium. Samples for PCR testing should be taken prior to the application of local anaesthetic or fluorescein. Testing for FHV-1 infection is problematic with both false positive, and false negative results arising from the various tests available (Gould, 2011). Therefore diagnosis is based on a

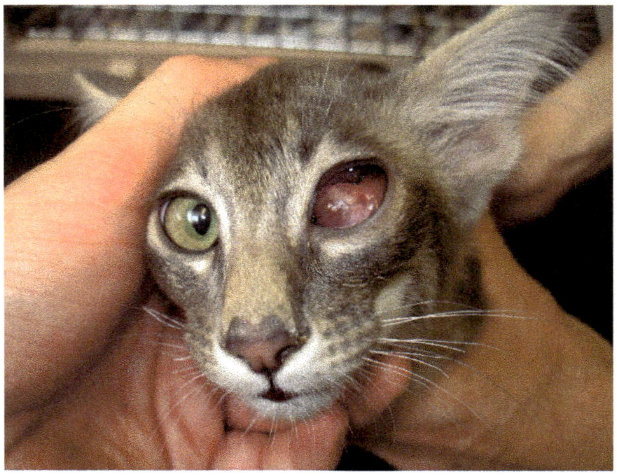

Figure 22. Severe, blinding symblepharon in the left eye of a young Oriental cat. © Rachel Lockhart.

combination of testing, clinical signs and response to treatment. The latter is discussed in the cornea section.

Feline Calicivirus

FCV, a single-stranded RNA picornavirus, is a minor cause of conjunctivitis in cats. It **primarily causes respiratory disease** but also oral ulceration and polyarthritis. Most cats eliminate the infection, but some remain persistently infected and shed virus. Vaccination does not prevent infection or the development of the carrier state but reduces disease severity. **Antivirals are ineffective against FCV** because they disrupt DNA rather than RNA replication. Secondary bacterial infection may require topical antibiotics.

Conjunctival tumours

In the cat the most common conjunctival mass is squamous cell carcinoma which occur either by extension from eyelid masses, or affect the conjunctiva of the third eyelid. Conjunctival melanoma can also occur and in this species and has a predilection for the bulbar conjunctiva. Whilst the majority are pigmented, a proportion are amelanotic. Their behaviour is relatively aggressive with both local recurrence and metastasis reported (Figure 23).

Conditions of the cornea

Ulcerative keratitis

A corneal ulcer in its simplest form is the **loss of an area of surface epithelium leading to exposure of the corneal stroma**. The causes of ulcerative keratitis are less numerous in the cat than the dog. The most likely being as follows:

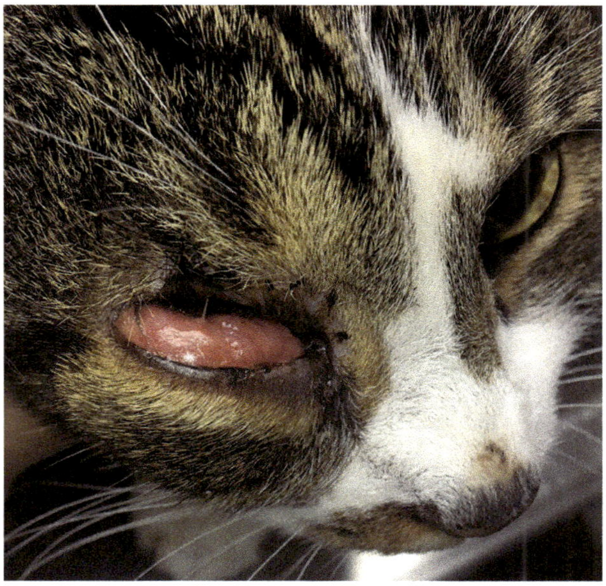

Figure 23. Extensive conjunctival tumour in an elderly cat, the owner declined investigation. © Agata Tsvetanova.

- feline herpesvirus-1 (FHV-1) infection
- entropion
- trauma.

Treatment of superficial ulcers involves **removal/correction of the inciting cause** (i.e. surgical correction of entropion, reduction of stress, antiviral treatment in cases related to FHV-1), and **prophylactic topical antibiosis** whilst the cornea remains fluorescein-positive. **Superficial ulcers should heal within seven days.** Broad spectrum prophylactic therapy in the form of fusidic acid BID or chloramphenicol drops QID is recommended until healing is effected.

Any superficial ulcer which has remained for more than about ten days is described as 'indolent'. These ulcers are trying to heal unsuccessfully; epithelium fails to adhere adequately to the underlying exposed stroma, and this is manifested clinically by a rim of non-adherent epithelium through 360° around the ulcer. When fluorescein is applied and rinsed off with sterile saline, a 'halo' of lighter staining around the ulcer is seen where the dye seeped under the poorly adhered epithelium. In this situation, **gentle debridement of the loose epithelium under topical anaesthesia with a cotton bud,** speeds up healing. This procedure should be repeated no more than twice and no more frequently than 10 days apart. **A grid keratotomy should NEVER be performed on a cat** as this rapidly leads to the development of a corneal sequestrum: a far more challenging and costly problem to treat.

Specialist referral for a superficial keratectomy is recommended for any superficial ulcer which has not healed in 3–4 weeks. Protracted healing of an ulcer is also a risk factor for corneal sequestrum development. The procedure involves the removal of the anterior one third of the corneal stroma (with the aid of an operating microscope) in the ulcerated area to leave a healthy bed of stromal tissue into which epithelial cells can better adhere. The procedure has a high success rate (upwards of 90%) and healing is usually effected within seven to ten days, although may take up to three weeks.

Regardless of the cause, **secondary bacterial infection of any superficial ulcer can progress to a deeper one with significant stromal loss**. The development of melting ulcers (**keratomalacia**) (Figure 24) occurs when certain bacteria, inoculated into the corneal stroma, release collagenase enzymes. This has a knock-on effect on corneal stromal cells known as keratocytes, and on neutrophils attracted to the site; both are induced to produce collagenases which compound the damage.

Treatment of melting ulcers involves appropriate antibiosis, ideally based on culture and sensitivity. Studies on bacterial keratitis in cats have revealed

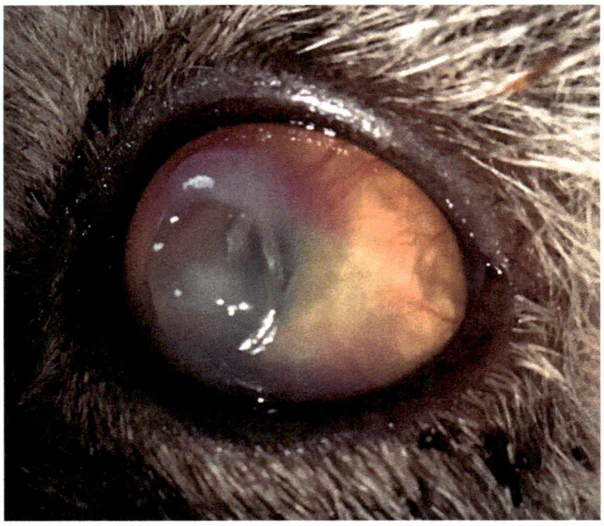

Figure 24. Melting ulcer. © Agata Tsvetanova.

between 55 and 66% of isolates to be *Staphylococcus species*, followed by *Streptococcus* or *Pasteurella species* (Goldreich et al., 2020, Suter et al., 2018). Unlike in dogs, *Pseudomonas species* are a less frequently isolated from cases of keratomalacia. The Staphs and other aerobic bacteria isolated were **mostly sensitive to chloramphenicol, ofloxacin, and gentamycin**.

Whilst awaiting results, one of the former two should be **applied every two hours as a loading frequency for the first 24–48 hours** then reducing to QID. Although gentamycin is the only licensed alternative (in the UK) this can be irritant and is epitheliotoxic so should only be used a maximum of QID.

Aggressive treatment is required to halt the keratomalacia, with **topical antibiotics accompanied by two-hourly autologous serum or an alternative anti-collagenase treatment.** Autologous serum contains both serine protease and matrix metalloproteinase (MMP) inhibitors as well as growth factors and vitamins and is the anticollagenase of choice. Serum is preferable to plasma as it contains higher levels of epithelial growth factor, platelet-derived growth factor and vitamin A. Serum must be prepared in an aseptic manner with strict attention to handling and storage.

- A **fresh blood sample** should be drawn from the patient, into a plain or serum gel tube, **allowed to stand for 30 minutes, centrifuged and the supernatent harvested.**
- It should be decanted into a **sterile dropper bottle** or a sterile tube, drawn up and applied using single-use sterile pipettes or 1 ml syringes.
- **Storage should be in the refrigerator** and it should be discarded after 48 hours as it has no preservatives and is an excellent growth medium for bacteria.
- Because of the risk of serious viral cross-infection, **donor cat serum should never be used.**
- If it proves impossible to bleed the cat or to obtain sufficient serum then alternatives include acetylcysteine (I-lube™) or a solution of EDTA which can be made up by filling an **EDTA blood tube with sterile saline and mixing well.** These should be applied up to q4hrs.

Immediate referral to a specialist ophthalmologist is indicated if:

- Corneal melting progresses in spite of intensive medical treatment for 12–24 hours.
- The ulcer's depth remains the same in spite of intensive medical treatment for 12–24 hours.
- The ulcer is greater than half stromal depth on presentation.
- There is a descemetocoele on presentation.

The latter is a **deep corneal ulcer which has progressed down to Descemet's membrane**, the basement membrane of the corneal endothelium (i.e. the whole of the corneal stroma is gone). A descemetocoele can be diagnosed following fluorescein staining of the cornea followed by thorough but gentle flushing with sterile saline; the walls of the ulcer will stain green, but the base does not. The base of the ulcer may have a clear or even black appearance, and because Descemet's membrane in the cat is highly elastic, it may bulge outwards, even beyond the contour of the cornea. It does not take up fluorescein. An eye is this condition is extremely fragile and great care should be exercised in handling the patient in the consulting room.

In these situations, immediate referral is recommended for surgical treatment: a conjunctival pedicle (Figure 25), amnion or corneoconjunctival transposition graft (Figure 26).

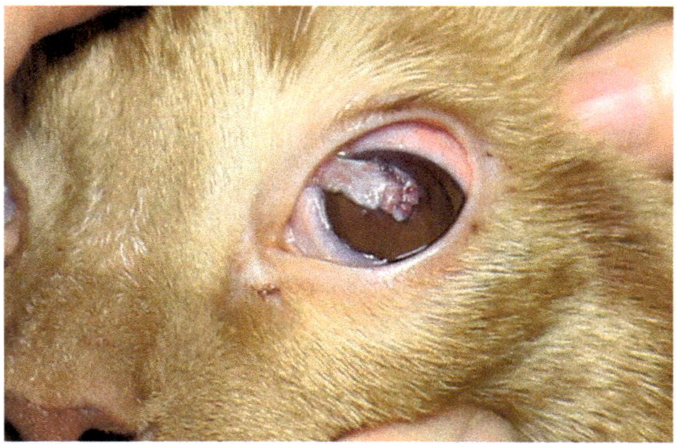

Figure 25. Conjunctival pedicle graft, 1 day post-operatively. © Kerry Smith.

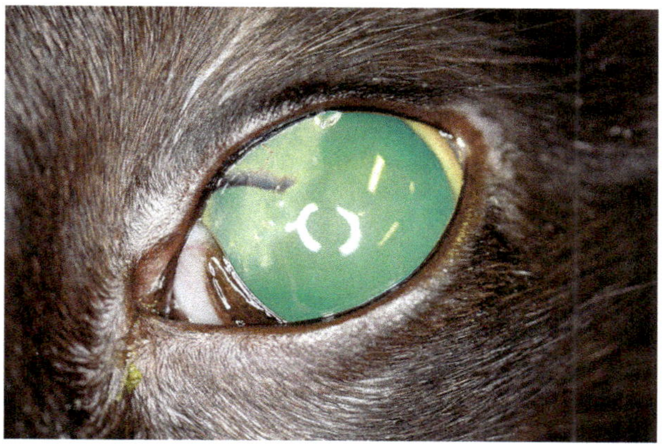

Figure 26. Corneo-conjunctival transposition graft, 6 weeks postoperatively. © Kerry Smith.

Corneal manifestations of FHV-1 infection

FHV-1 keratitis can take several forms:

- **Dendritic ulceration**: fine branching linear superficial ulcers are considered **pathognomonic for FHV-1 infection** (Nassisse et al., 1989). They can occur both in primary infection and in recrudescent disease. They are identified by fluorescein staining the cornea and examination with a cobalt blue light. Rose Bengal stain is an alternative; thorough flushing out following application is recommended as this stain is irritant.
- **Geographic ulceration**: large irregular areas of superficial ulceration (with the appearance of countries on a map of the world, hence the name) (Figure 27) can occur both in primary or recrudescent infection.
- **Stromal keratitis**- this is a chronic phenomenon which occurs as a result of an inappropriate ocular immune response directed at viral antigen sequestered within the cornea (Figure 28). Corneal pathology includes **neovascularisation, inflammatory cellular infiltrate, and corneal fibrosis.** It often occurs after bouts of recrudescent disease or chronic ulceration; active viral disease is usually absent.

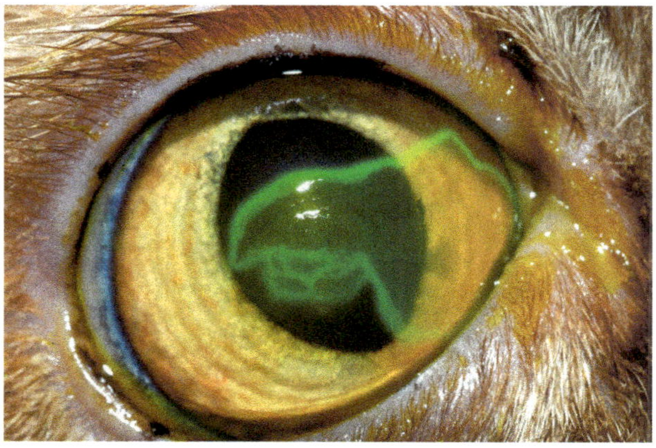

Figure 27. Geographic corneal ulceration. © Rachel Lockhart.

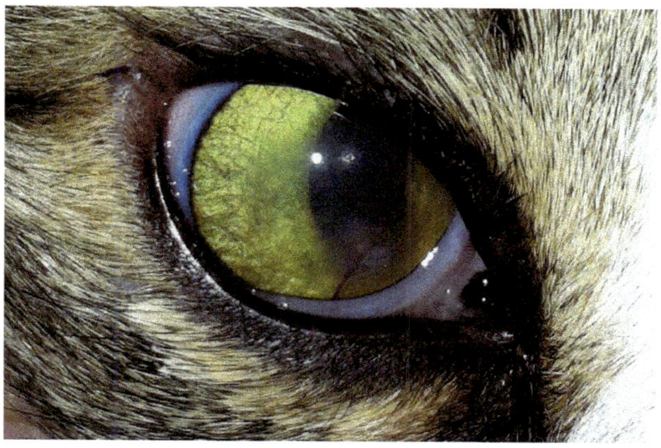

Figure 28. Stromal keratitis. © Agata Tsvetanova.

Treatment of FHV-1 manifestations

Most useful topical anti-viral drugs are **nucleoside analogues** which competitively inhibit DNA polymerase triggering chain termination of replicating DNA (Galle, 2004). In vitro studies have shown efficacy in the following order from most to least efficacious: trifluorothymidine, idoxuridine, ganciclovir, cidofovir, penciclovir, vidarabine, acyclovir.

In spite of this a prospective trial of acyclovir in cats has suggested it is clinically effective (Williams et al., 2005). Only acyclovir and cidofovir have undergone clinical trials in cats. As all of these agents are virostatic frequent application to the ocular surface is required (between four and six times daily is recommended). Only acyclovir (3%) ointment and ganciclovir (0.15%) gel are currently available in an ophthalmic form in the UK, although trifluorothymidine can be compounded by ophthalmic hospital pharmacies. However the latter is expensive and can be irritant. **Ganciclovir is currently the topical of choice being both efficacious and well-tolerated.**

Famciclovir is an orally administered guanosine analogue which is converted to the active penciclovir following absorption in the gastrointestinal tract. Although doses between 40–90 mg/kg TID have been shown to reduce viral shedding and conjunctivitis scores (Thomasy et al., 2011, 2016a), anecdotally much lower doses have been reported to be efficacious. 62.5 mg per os BID is a recommended starting dose. It is metabolised by the liver and excreted by the kidneys. No clinical trials have been performed on cats with renal failure so it should be avoided in cats which may be renally compromised. An oral famciclovir paste has recently become available in the UK.

Interferons which may stimulate the host antiviral response, and L-lysine which may decrease viral replication have both been postulated as adjunctive antiviral treatments against FHV-1 infection, but clinical trials for both medications (reviewed extensively by Gould, 2011) have produced mixed results so they **cannot be recommended for treatment**. A review of drugs with activity against feline herpesvirus-1 is presented by Thomasy and Maggs (2016b), amongst whose recommendations are that antiviral drug dosages should not be tapered, and that a hyaluronate-based mucinomimetic should be used as an adjunctive treatment due to FHV-1's long-term and marked reduction in goblet cell density.

Corneal sequestrum

This is a condition unique to cats in which a **focal area of corneal stromal degeneration occurs leaving a plaque of devitalised cornea with a characteristic brown/ black colour** (Figures 29, 30 and 31). It may be accompanied by a rim of peripheral superficial ulceration, corneal neovascularisation and variable discomfort.

The cause is unknown, but predisposing factors include **overexposure of the corneal surface** and chronic corneal irritation. **Brachycephalic breeds** are more likely to be affected: Persian, Himalayan, Birman and Burmese. However it can also occur as a secondary phenomenon following chronic corneal ulceration

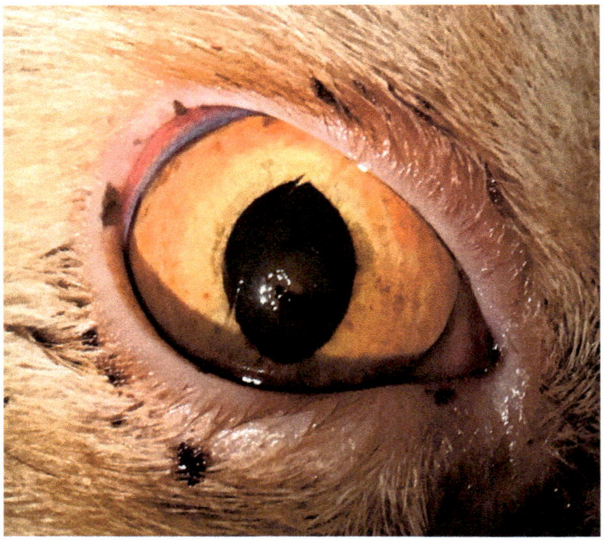

Figure 29. Early corneal sequestrum. © Agata Tsvetanova.

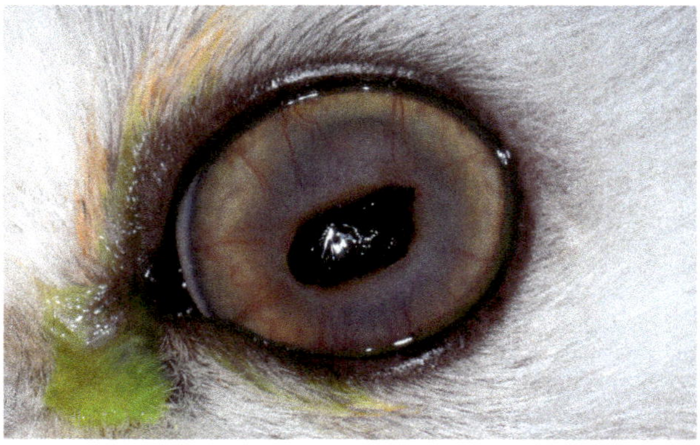

Figure 30. Denser/ more established corneal sequestrum. © Rachel Lockhart.

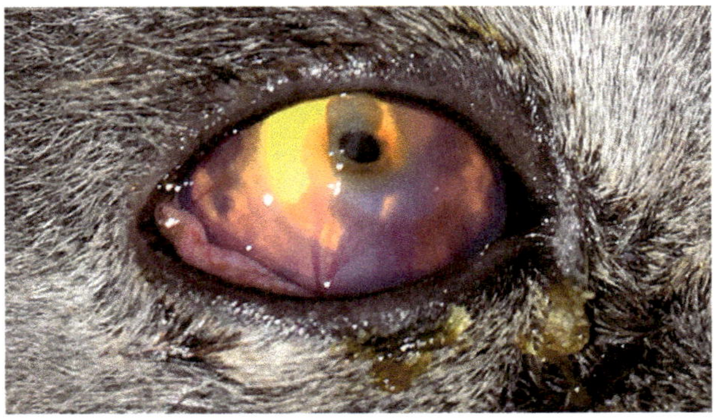

Figure 31. Perforated corneal sequestrum. Note the 'blob' of clotted aqueous dorsal to the pigmented lesion © Agata Tsvetanova.

in any breed of cat; many of these cases will have had **FHV-1 infection** as the initial cause of ulceration. Studies have shown between 18 and 55% of corneal sequestrum samples to contain FHV-1 according to PCR analysis (Stiles et al., 1997, Nassisse et al., 1998).

Treatment is always surgical: a lamellar keratectomy performed with the aid of an operating microscope, and depending on the depth of the lesion, placement of a conjunctival pedicle graft or corneoconjunctival transposition graft in the defect. Grafting is recommended to reduce the risk of recurrence. **Sequestra should not be allowed to slough**, which can take months during which time the cat is in chronic pain and because some are full thickness through the stroma, their loss can lead to a significant corneal defect or even perforation.

Eosinophilic keratoconjunctivitis

Eosinophilic keratoconjunctivitis is an **immune-mediated condition** in which eosinophils infiltrate the cornea and conjunctiva. It manifests as superficial raised pink/whitish plaques on the surface of, or infiltrates within, the cornea and conjunctiva, accompanied by neovascularisation and sometimes depigmentation and erosion of the eyelids, uni- or bilaterally (Figures 32 and 33). Diagnosis is made by identifying any eosinophils

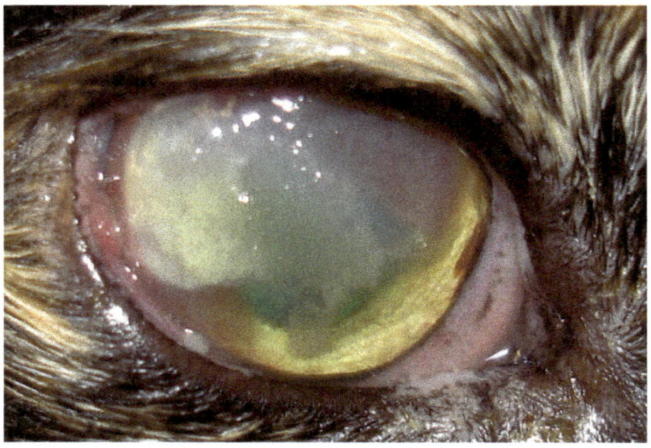

Figure 32. A severe case of eosinophilic keratoconjunctivitis. © Rachel Lockhart.

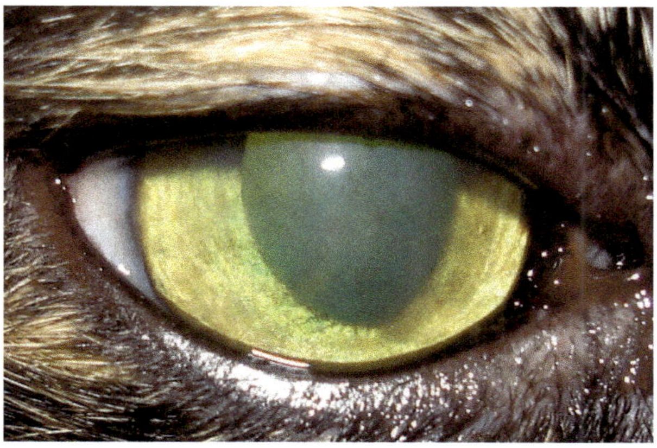

Figure 33. Eosinophilic keratoconjunctivitis (same case as Fig. 32) 6 weeks post treatment with dexamethasone phosphate QID. © Rachel Lockhart.

on a corneal/conjunctival scrape. The role of FHV-1 in this condition is unknown, but it has been identified in 85.7% of cases in one study (Volopich et al., 2005). Care must be exercised in treatment which involves local immunosuppression as latent virus may be induced to recrudesce.

Treatment modalities for different manifestations of FHV-1

Manifestation	Treatment
Primary infection	Antivirals-either topical or oral, antibiosis for secondary bacterial infection, fluids, supportive treatment.
Recrudescent infection	Antivirals-either topical or oral.
Stromal keratitis	Topical immunosuppressives +/– antivirals
Eosinophilic keratoconjunctivitis	Immunosuppressives (topical +/– oral)+/– antivirals
Corneal sequestrum	Surgical removal +/– corneal/ conjunctival grafting

Stromal keratitis and eosinophilic keratoconjunctivitis both involve immune-mediated pathology. Local and, if intractable, systemic immunosuppression is indicated. A good first line treatment for either is **cyclosporin ointment BID**, but if this is not sufficient topical steroids (dexamethasone phosphate (Maxidex™)) starting at an initial frequency of QID, may be required. The two can be started in tandem with the aim of withdrawing the steroid once the condition is in abatement and maintaining on cyclosporine alone.

Be aware that although both of these conditions can occur in the absence of **FHV-1 infection, recrudescence of latent disease is a real possibility** and treatment can be a juggling act. The owner should be warned of the potential difficulties from the outset, so as to reduce expectations. Because stromal keratitis often involves a significant vascular response, the non-steroidal anti-inflammatory, ketorolac trometamol (Acular™) can be effective in improving the appearance of the cornea. This is not immunosuppressive so will not be beneficial in all cases, but it also does not have the same potential to cause recrudescence of FHV-1 as steroids. **Eosinophilic keratoconjunctivitis is often relatively intractable and systemic prednisolone may be required.** Older textbooks suggest the use of megestrol acetate, which was effective in very stubborn cases but is no longer readily available.

Because FHV-1 is shed by cats in response to stress, **elimination of stress is an essential part of treatment** and cannot be overestimated, particularly in multicat households. Eliciting information from the owner about the environment in which the cat is kept and acting to make any changes required, is therefore a very important part of a holistic approach to treatment. Frequent topical administration is in itself a stressor to the cat, and sometimes a hands-off approach, withdrawing all treatment will achieve better results, particularly when the course of a bout of recrudescent disease has become intractable.

Acute bullous keratopathy

This is an **uncommon condition affecting mostly young cats,** but also older individuals with a history of chronic topical or systemic steroid administration (Figure 34). The **cause is unknown.** The clinical presentation is **acutely developing corneal oedema** (a bluish steamy haze to the cornea) followed by the development of **large fluid-filled bullae** which may rupture, and if sufficiently deep within the cornea, may lead to corneal perforation. It can occur uni- or bilaterally.

Early surgical intervention is recommended to prevent loss of the globe. Grafting procedures such as conjunctival pedicle or corneoconjunctival grafts can work well, but in most cases a third eyelid flap to tamponade the cornea works equally (Pederson et al., 2016) and may even be preferable as the condition resolves with less corneal scarring and a less invasive procedure for the cat. However, referral is recommended to ascertain the diagnosis as the appearance can resemble a descemetocoele for which a third eyelid flap would not be an appropriate procedure.

Conditions of the uvea

The uvea comprises the iris ciliary body and choroid. Being rich in both blood vessels and lymphatic tissue, the uvea is an important site for both inflammation and neoplasia.

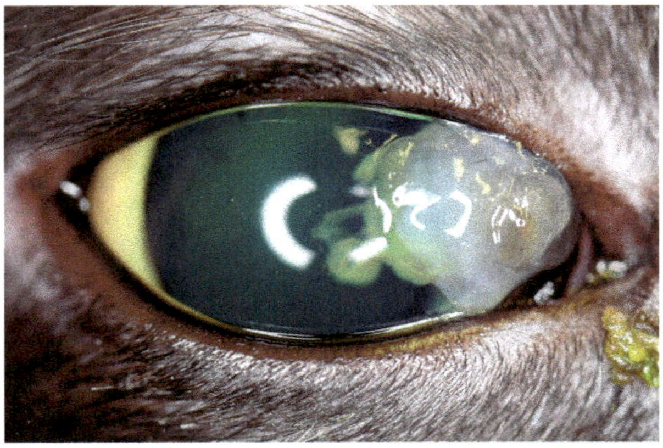

Figure 34a. Acute bullous keratopathy. © Kerry Smith.

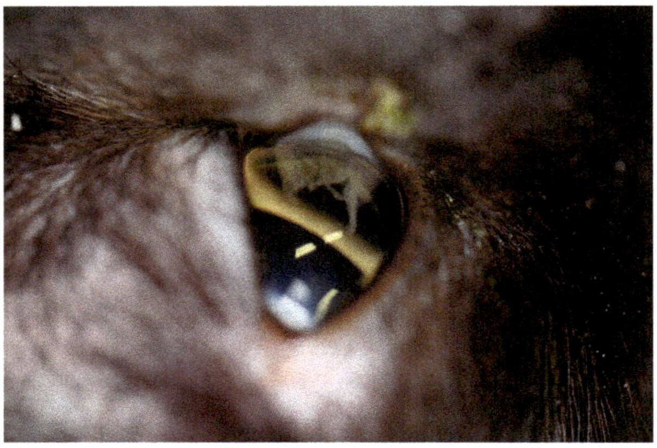

Figure 34b. Lateral view of same case showing intraocular fibrin, indicating a full-thickness rupture. © Kerry Smith.

Uveitis

Inflammation of the anterior uvea (iris and ciliary body) is a relatively common presentation in the cat. There are **many potential causes for uveitis** including blunt or penetrating trauma, infectious (including sepsis or bacteraemia from infections elsewhere in the body e.g. dental disease, abscess, pyometra), immune mediated, neoplastic (primary ocular or metastatic) and idiopathic. Potential infectious causes in the cat are as follows:

Viral	Feline immunodeficiency virus (FIV)
	Feline leukaemia virus (FeLV)
	Feline infectious peritonitis (FIP)
Bacterial	Bartonellosis
Protozoal	Toxoplasmosis
	Leishmaniasis
Fungal	Cryptococcosis
	Histoplasmosis
	Coccidiomycosis
	Blastomycosis
	Candidiasis
Parasitic	Ophthalmomyiasis interna (Dipteran larvae)

Clinical manifestations of acute anterior uveitis (Figure 35) include:

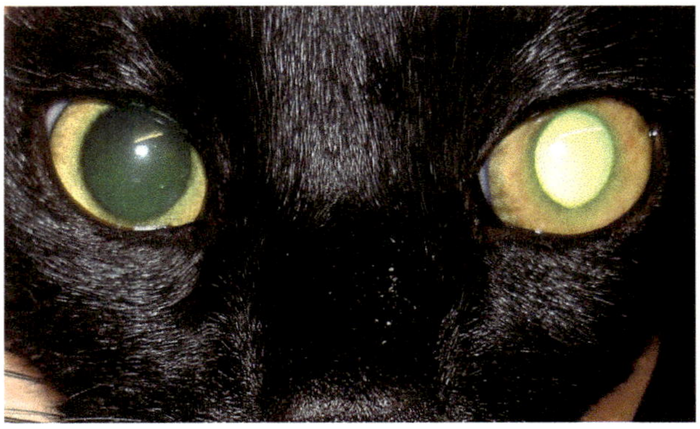

Figure 35. Uveitis affecting the left eye. Note the miosis and subtle rubeosus iridis. © Rachel Lockhart.

- miosis: constriction of the pupil
- aqueous flare: a cloudiness to the anterior chamber best appreciated by passing a slit beam of light across it
- rubeosus iridis; a reddening of the peripheral iris due to inflammation of blood vessels including the major arterial circle (Figure 35)
- corneal oedema
- lowered intraocular pressure.

Signs of chronic uveitis include:

- darkening of the iris,
- iris rests: clumps of pigment on the anterior lens capsule)
- posterior synechia (Figure 36): adhesions of the pupillary margin to the anterior lens capsule
- keratic precipitates: pale yellow/brown aggregates of inflammatory cells adherent to the corneal endothelium). (Figure 37).

A thorough work-up to elucidate the cause is always indicated, finance permitting. The following is the 'gold standard' uveitis work-up, but a diagnosis may well be made before the full list has been worked through.

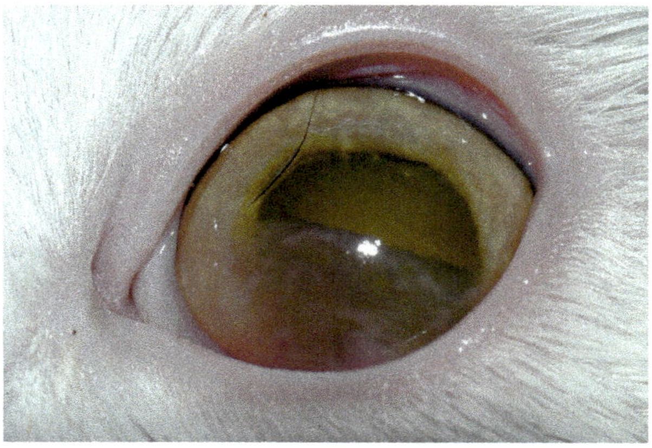

Figure 36. Uveitis with fibrinous exudate in the anterior chamber, swollen thickened iris and pupillary dyscoria due to posterior synechiation. © Rachel Lockhart.

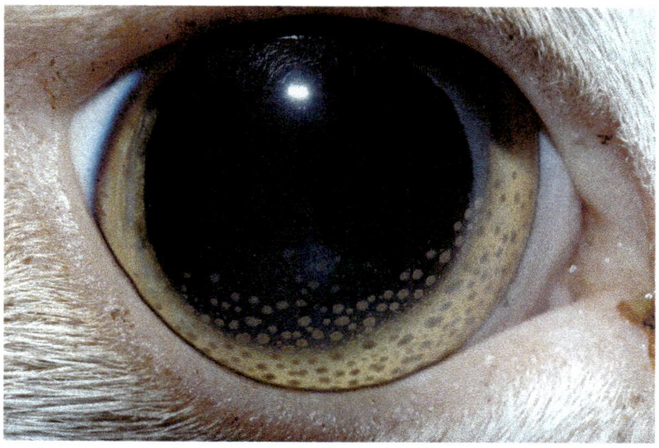

Figure 37. Keratic precipitates. © Rachel Lockhart.

- **History** – where and how acquired (e.g. breeder, farm, rescue centre), ill-health of litter mates, travel history, where and how housed (i.e. multicat household, indoor or outdoor), hunting behaviour, concurrent systemic signs or pre-existing illness, vaccination status, antiparasiticide treatment, and concurrent medications.
- General **clinical** examination.
- Thorough **ophthalmic examination**.
- **Haematology and biochemistry** including total protein and albumin: globulin ratio.
- ELISA for **FIV and FeLV**.
- Serology for **coronavirus and toxoplasma**.
- Other serology dependent on country of origin/travel history.
- **Ocular ultrasound** (if intraocular exam limited due to opacity of the cornea or anterior chamber e.g. hyphaema/oedema) particularly if a primary ocular cause suspected e.g. intraocular neoplasia.
- Chest radiographs.
- Abdominal ultrasound.
- **Aqueocentesis**: sampling of the aqueous humour via a fine needle inserted at the limbus. The resultant fluid is submitted for cytology, culture and even PCR. The procedure is not without risk as it may stimulate further inflammation, and there is a chance of both intraocular haemorrhage and lens damage. However it can be very useful, especially in making a diagnosis of lymphoma (Linn-Pearl et al., 2015).

If the work-up reveals a specific infectious cause then this should be treated.

- **Bartonellosis**: doxycycline 10 mg/kg q12–24 hours for two to six weeks. The tablets should be given whole and followed by a water 'chaser' to minimise the risk of oesophagitis. Flea control is essential to minimise the risk of infection.
- **Toxoplasmosis**: clindamycin 12.5 mg/kg q12 hours for at least four weeks but total clearance of infection is unlikely and recrudescence may occur.

Whilst awaiting infectious disease serologies, topical treatment can be commenced with **ketorolac trometamol** (**Acular™**), a non-steroidal anti-inflammatory, q4–6 hours. For non-infectious, presumed immune-mediated uveitis and FIP-induced uveitis, topical prednisolone acetate 1% (Pred Forte™) can be used q4–6 hours for the first few days, then gradually titrating down the dosage frequency according to the response to treatment. It should not be stopped suddenly or 'rebound uveitis' may occur, and may be required at a low dosage frequency long-term to keep clinical signs in abatement.

When using topical or systemic steroids in cats, be aware of the **potential for recrudescence of latent FHV-1 infection**. The owners should be apprised of signs which could indicate corneal ulceration, and asked to re-present the cat if they occur. In this situation the prednisolone acetate should be swapped for ketorolac trometamol, and any systemic prednisolone withdrawn.

Where **posterior segment inflammation is present** (i.e. pars planitis) (Figure 38), systemic prednisolone is likely to be necessary. This should be started at a dose of 0.5–1 mg/kg q24 hours and titrated down over a period of a few weeks according to response to treatment. It is possible to use prednisolone in FIV positive cats long-term without any problems, but the owner should be warned about the risks in an already immunocompromised cat.

It is not known whether systemic steroids induce reactivation of toxoplasmosis, but oocyst shedding does not seem to occur.

All cats with **acute onset uveitis, where miosis is a feature**, will benefit from topical atropine sulphate 1%

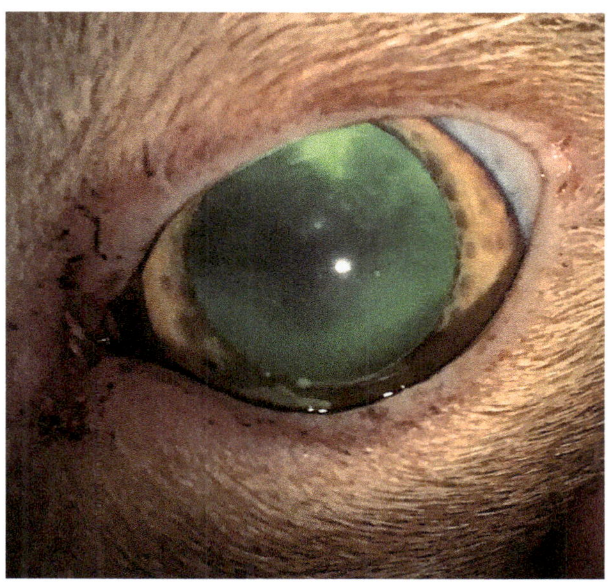

Figure 38. Uveitis affecting both the anterior and posterior segments. There are raised lymphoid follicles on the anterior iris face, and 'pars planitis' – white clumps of inflammatory cells behind the posterior lens capsule at the equator. © Agata Tsvetanova.

q4 hours to effect, ceasing once the pupil is fully dilated. This has the two-fold effect of abolishing painful irido-ciliary spasm, and stabilizing the blood ocular barrier. It can cause quite dramatic salivation in cats and atropine ointment is preferable if available. The pupil may stay dilated for several days; the owner should be warned and bright lights avoided. **Care should be taken if there is a suspicion of raised intraocular pressure as atropine will cause further elevations in IOP potentially worsening glaucoma.**

Uveal tumours

The feline eye is associated with three types of tumour, two of which are highly malignant and are indications for enucleation.

Feline diffuse iridal melanoma (FDIM)

FDIM is the most common intraocular tumour of the cat. This presents as **progressive pigmentation in several areas of the iris** over a period of months to years (Figures 39 and 40). As it progresses **the iris becomes thicker**, loses its surface architecture to take on a velvety appearance, and there may be changes in pupil shape or mobility. If there is infiltration into the drainage angle functional obstruction of aqueous occurs, leading to **secondary glaucoma**. In contrast to melanocytic tumours in dogs, the **metastatic rate is up to 63%** (Cullen and Webb, 2013). Metastasis is usually to the liver, other abdominal organs, or lungs and can occur as late as one to three years post-enucleation.

Because most eyes are visual and comfortable at first presentation, it can be difficult to decide when to enucleate the eye. **Attempting to biopsy the lesions by FNA is pointless** as even benign lesions can transform to malignancy at a later stage.

The salient features which may indicate malignancy (Figure 41) include:

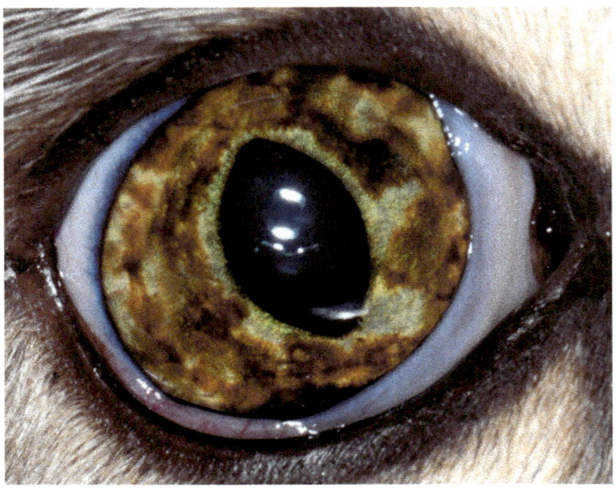

Figure 39. Melanosis or melanoma? © Rachel Lockhart.

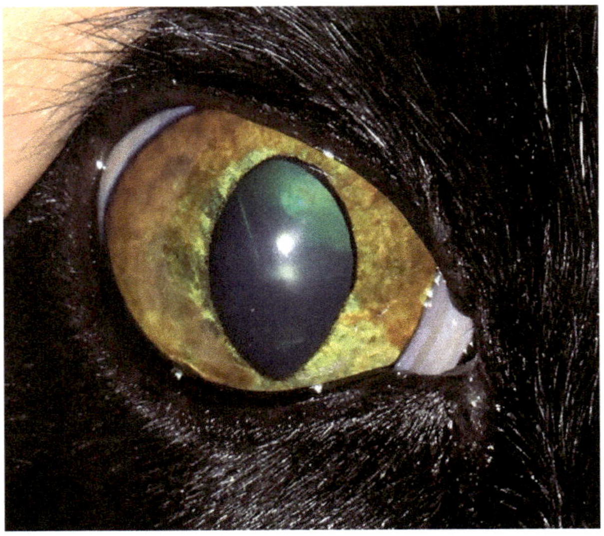

Figure 40. FDIM:Diffuse but subtle colour change of the iris extending to the periphery. Ectropion uveae occurring from 12 o'clock to 3 o'clock. FDIM was confirmed histopathologically following enucleation. © Agata Tsvetanova.

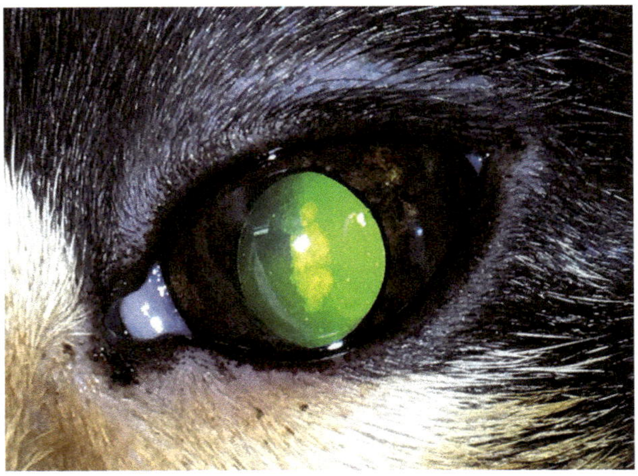

Figure 41. FDIM features highly suggestive of malignancy: total colour change of the iris and change of architecture, ectropion uveae through 360° and pigmented cells on the anterior lens capsule. © Agata Tsvetanova.

- changes in iris architecture
- the presence of free-floating pigmented cells in the anterior chamber
- pupil abnormalities including dyscoria, anisocoria or ectropion uveae
- a mass lesion
- total colour change of the iris
- the presence of uveitis or secondary glaucoma
- on gonioscopy, the presence of tumour within the drainage angle.

The latter is extremely important as once tumour cells enter the drainage angle and scleral venous plexus there is a high risk of metastasis.

If the lesions are flat, discrete, and light in colour then a 'watch and wait' approach can be adopted.

Owners should be informed of the potential risks both of leaving the eye in situ and of prematurely enucleating a normal but pigmented eye. Re-examination to check the lesions, measure intraocular pressure, perform gonioscopy, and dilate the pupil are recommended every three to four months. Serial photography to document the lesions is useful.

Screening for metastatic disease with **chest radiography** prior to enucleation is recommended (ideally three views) and **abdominal ultrasound.** If tumour extends through the sclera, then exenteration is recommended but the prognosis is poor. Enucleated globes should be submitted to a specialist ocular histopathologist.

Lymphoma

Lymphoma is the **second most common intraocular tumour in the cat**. Although generalised lymphadenopathy may be present, feline lymphoma may present ocularly (Figure 42). Signs include uveitis, nodular masses or diffuse infiltration of the iris. Hyphaema may occur as part of a paraneoplastic phenomenon. Fundic examination may reveal subretinal infiltrates.

Diagnosis is by identifying the neoplastic cells on cytology or histology. Samples can be taken from lymph nodes, organs, or the aqueous humour by aqueocentesis. The latter is particularly useful in making the diagnosis of lymphoma (Linn-Pearl et al., 2015). **Note that prior administration of topical steroids can mask the diagnosis** – something to be aware of if considering treating uveal changes symptomatically. A variety of treatment protocols are available for lymphoma.

Feline ocular post traumatic sarcoma (FOPTS)

Whilst not strictly a uveal tumour, this is a **highly malignant intraocular tumour of cats** associated with previous ocular trauma that occurs in a similar location. The average time from trauma to detection of the tumour is 6.2 years (Wood and Scott, 2019) but can occur earlier. Damage to the lens capsule is a major risk factor and thought to arise from **a malignant transformation of the lens epithelium** (Zeiss et al., 2003). Other risk factors include chronic uveitis, intraocular surgery, and intravitreal gentamycin injections (Duke et al., 2013).

Clinically FOPTS may present as an intractable uveitis, glaucoma, intraocular haemorrhage, or enlargement of a previously phthitic globe. Occasionally a pink or white mass may be visible. Early enucleation with exenteration of the orbit is recommended as extension through the sclera and into the nerve can lead to distant metastasis. Many cats die of metastatic disease even after enucleation. This is a **persuasive argument for the early enucleation of blind traumatised eyes in cats**, and those which remain visual and comfortable should be closely monitored.

Conditions of the lens

Cataracts

The majority of cataracts in cats occur secondarily to other ocular disease. There are only **sporadic reports of primary inherited cataracts**; which are bilateral, symmetrical, and occur in the absence of other ocular disease. The vast majority of these appear to be congenital (Figure 44). The author has operated on presumed inherited cataracts in the Maine Coon (Figure 43) and British Shorthair breeds.

Feline cataracts usually occur secondary to uveitis, trauma, glaucoma or lens luxation, with the former being most common.

Previously **'milk replacer' cataracts** were reported in kittens fed commercial or homemade milk formulas.

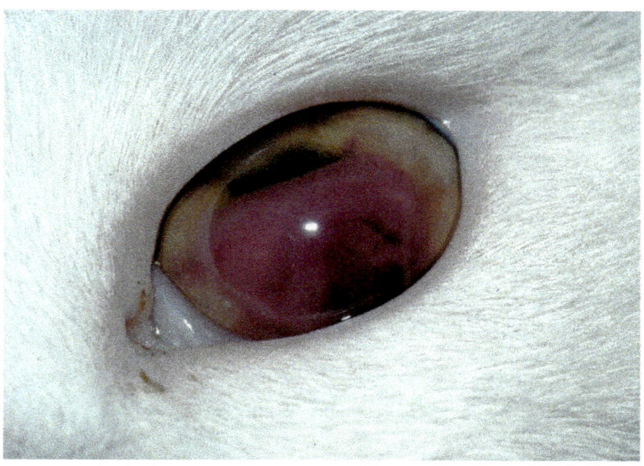

Figure 42. Intraocular lymphoma, diagnosed by aqueocentesis. © Rachel Lockhart.

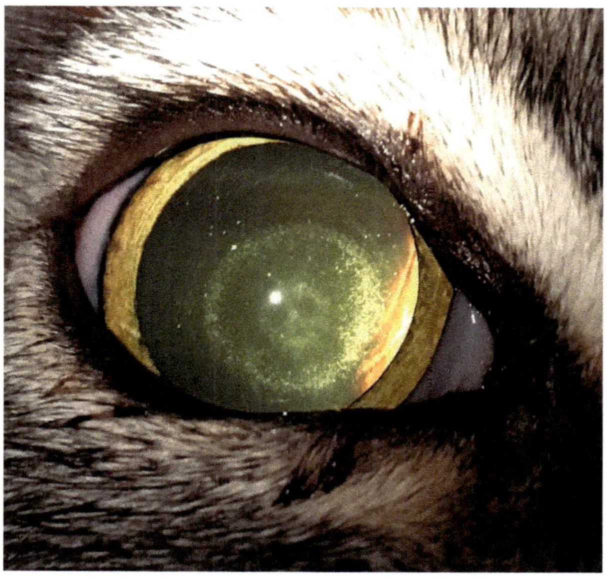

Figure 43. Congenital perinuclear cataract in a Maine Coon. Changes were apparent bilaterally. © Agata Tsvetanova.

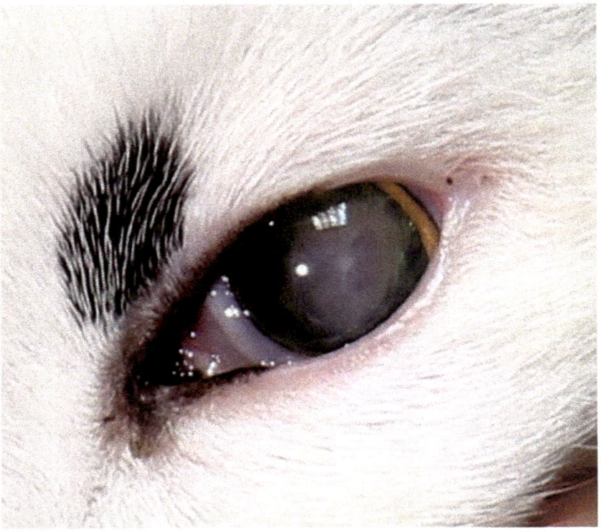

Figure 44. Congenital nuclear cataract in a Domestic Shorthair. Changes were apparent bilaterally. © Kerry Smith.

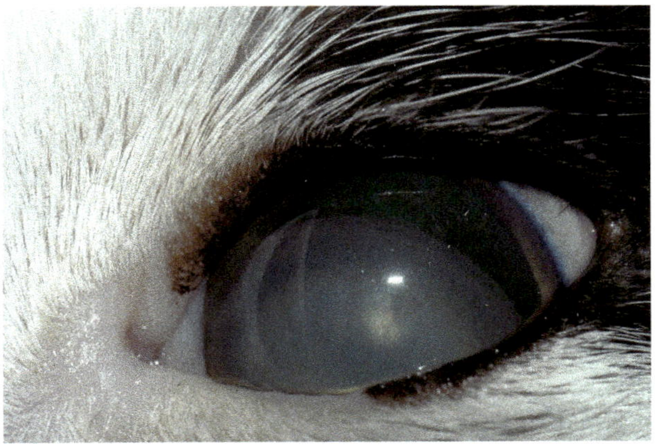

Figure 45. Anterior lens luxation, secondary to uveitis. © Rachel Lockhart.

The effect is thought to be due to a deficiency of arginine which is less likely in modern formula products. Cataracts developed when the kitten was fed milk-replacer in the first week after birth, with spheroidal or ring-shaped opacities located in the foetal lens nucleus first noted at the age of three weeks. The cataracts did not progress and rarely caused blindness.

Diabetic cataracts do not usually occur in cats, due to low levels of the lenticular enzyme 'aldose reductase' in older cats (i.e. those most likely to develop diabetes) (Richter et al., 2002).

***Encephalitozoon cuniculi* has been identified as a potential cause of feline cataracts** (Benz et al., 2011).

Cataract removal by phacoemulsification is relatively straightforward in cats with primary cataracts as they do not have the same tendency to post-operative inflammation as dogs, although post-operative hypertension in the first few days after surgery is common.

When cataracts have occurred secondarily to uveitis, **surgical removal should only be considered if the cause of uveitis has been identified and treated,** and the eye is completely quiet. The risk of recrudescence of uveitis is high in these cases and may adversely prejudice the surgical outcome.

Lens luxation

Lens luxation in the cat usually occurs secondarily to uveitis (Figure 45) or glaucoma where the lens zonules have been damaged by ongoing inflammation, or stretched and torn due to enlargement of the globe. **Lens luxation in the cat does not always cause secondary glaucoma** (as occurs in the dog) as the feline anterior chamber is deeper and relatively better able to accommodate the presence of the lens. Lens removal surgery (intra-capsular lens extraction or ICLE) can be undertaken but is not always necessary for comfort and can be problematic in the face of ongoing uveitis.

Conditions of the retina

Retinal dysplasia

Genetically inherited retinal dysplasia, common in dogs, is **not recognised in the cat** but can occur as a result of infectious disease. It has been described in kittens experimentally infected with FeLV infection in the foetal or neonatal period (Albert et al., 1977). Histologically it causes full thickness retinal folds which appear ophthalmoscopically as **grey/green rosette structures within the tapetal fundus**. Retinal dysplasia is also seen in kittens which have been infected in utero or neonatally by the parvovirus, feline panleukopaenia virus (FPV). The fundic lesions are accompanied by cerebellar hypoplasia which becomes evident when the kittens start to walk (hypermetria and ataxia).

Feline progressive retinal atrophy

Inherited retinal degenerations are seen in some pedigree cat breeds. These are bilaterally symmetrical degenerations of the photoreceptors which occur at a given age range for each genetic mutation and lead to untreatable blindness. The ophthalmoscopic appearance is of increasing tapetal hyperreflectivity and vascular attenuation, culminating in an 'end-stage retina': widespread tapetal hyperreflectivity, total absence of retinal vessels and atrophy of the optic nerve head (Figure 46). Several forms of PRA have so far been recognised in the cat (see table at the bottom of the page).

Enrofloxacin toxicity

The **antibiotic enrofloxacin is associated with an acute irreversible retinal degeneration** in cats. The phenomenon has also been reported experimentally

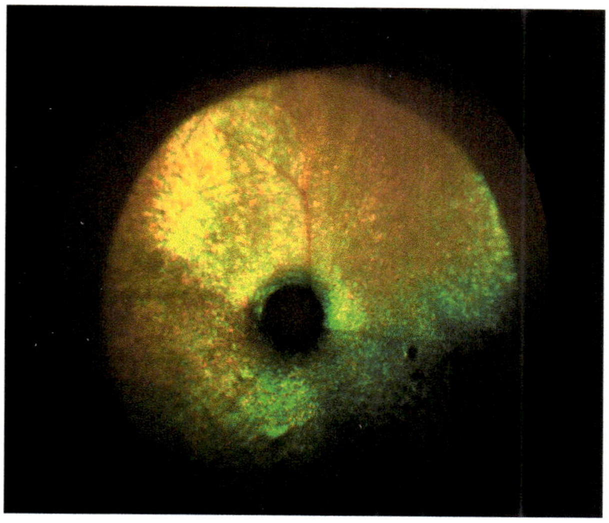

Figure 46. Progressive retinal atrophy (PRA): diffuse tapetal hyperreflectivity and vascular attenuation. © Rachel Lockhart.

with the fluoroquinolones marbofloxacin and orbifloxacin at high doses. Degeneration of the outer retinal layer is observed on histopathology, and electroretinograms are extinguished (Gelatt et al., 2001).

The manufacturer's recommended dose is 5 mg/kg/24 hours based on studies on young cats, but reported cases had been receiving anywhere from 4.6 mg/kg to 27 mg/kg when they developed retinal changes. Cats have been found to have differences in the ABCG2 binding protein (a transport molecule which normally restricts passage of fluoroquinolones across the blood-retinal barrier) (Ramirez et al., 2011).

Ocular signs include blindness and mydriasis. Early fundic signs are granularity of the tapetum, with increased reflectivity and moderate attenuation of the retinal vasculature, progressing to diffuse tapetal hyperreflectivity, vessel loss, and pigment loss and clumping within the non-tapetal fundus.

Current recommendations for enrofloxacin use in cats are to **only to administer if there is no other suitable antibiotic**, to dose for the cat's exact bodyweight, to consider split dosing (i.e. 2.5 mg/kg q12 hours) and to avoid rapid i/v infusion and administration to elderly cats.

Taurine deficiency retinopathy

Taurine is a sulphur-containing amino acid and an essential nutrient in cats. **Lack of taurine in the diet causes a characteristic retinopathy.** Lesions begin with a granular appearance to the tapetal fundus, which progresses to a hyperreflective lesion in the area centralis. A similar lesion will then develop on the nasal side and the two foci will coalesce to form a horizontal streak dorsal to the optic disc. Further degeneration occurs eventually involving the entire retina. Taurine is found at high concentrations in the inner and outer segments of photoreceptors and is thought to protect them from light and chemical damage. Lesions remain lifelong so their presence does not necessarily indicate current taurine deficiency.

Measurement of plasma taurine is necessary to confirm the diagnosis, with normal plasma levels being 80–120 nmol/ml (Cullen and Webb, 2013); less than 40 nmol/ml is indicative of a problem and dietary change is recommended. Currently available commercial cat foods are unlikely to be taurine deficient. Only cats fed an inappropriate diet or those suffering from malabsorption problems are likely to be affected.

Chorioretinitis

Due to their close anatomical involvement, inflammation of the choroid and retina usually occurs simultaneously. Chorioretinitis may have a traumatic, neoplastic, immune-mediated, or infectious cause.

Potential infectious causes of feline chorioretinitis include:

Viral	Feline infectious peritonitis Feline panleucopaenia Feline leukaemia virus Feline immunodeficiency virus
Bacterial	Mycobacteriosis Bartonellosis
Protozoal	Toxoplasmosis
Parasitic	Ophthalmomyiasis interna (Dipteran larvae)
Mycotic	Blastomycosis Cryptococcosis Coccidiomycosis Histoplasmosis

Condition	Breeds affected	Mode of inheritance	Defective gene	Genetic test available
Rod-cone dysplasia (Rdy)	Abyssinian	Autosomal dominant	Crx	Yes
rdAc	Abyssinian, Somali, Siamese, Ocicat	Autosomal recessive	CEP290	Yes
Rod-cone dysplasia	Persian	Autosomal recessive	AIPL1	Yes
Early onset primary photoreceptor disorder	Bengal	Autosomal recessive	Elucidated but not yet published	Yes

The effects may be restricted to the eye or the condition may be part of a wider systemic disease. The appearance of lesions may hint at the aetiology. Inflammatory lesions can be uni- or bilateral and are usually irregular in shape. In contrast to inherited retinopathies, the two eyes are rarely bilaterally symmetrical. The ophthalmoscopic appearance is very different depending on whether the inflammation is acute or inactive.

Ophthalmoscopic changes in chorioretinitis

	Acute chorioretinitis	Inactive chorioretinitis
Tapetal fundus	Areas of retinal oedema/cellular infiltration: greyish areas of hyporeflectivity with an indistinct border.	Irregular well-demarcated areas of hyperreflectivity which may have heavily pigmented centres due to hypertrophy/ hyperplasia of the RPE.
	Haemorrhages: appearance depends on location Increased pigmentation due to hypertrophy of the RPE	Colour change or destruction of the tapetum exposing choroidal vessels and sclera.
Non tapetal fundus	Grey or white areas with indistinct borders	Well demarcated areas of depigmentation with exposure of choroidal vessels, Areas of pigment clumping
Retinal vasculature	Perivascular cuffing: grey or white accumulations of inflammatory cells around the vessels	Attenuation, tortuousity or delineation with pigment.
Optic nerve head	Swelling and haemorrhages	Atrophy
Other changes	Retinal detachments: greyish areas of elevation with a distinct border. Granulomatous changes in some forms of chorioretinitis especially those of fungal origin Vitreal 'haze', syneresis (liquefaction) or clumps of inflammatory cells	Atrophy of choroidal vessels

Glaucoma

Glaucoma is defined as **the final common pathway of a group of diseases resulting in elevation in intraocular pressure and loss of vision.**

Primary glaucoma, associated with a genetically inherited abnormality of the iridocorneal drainage angle, **is rare in the cat**. It has been reported in the Burmese (Hampson et al., 2002) and Siamese (McLellan and Miller, 2011).

Secondary glaucoma, where the rise in intraocular pressure is **associated with antecedent ocular disease, occurs far more commonly** and may result from uveitis, intraocular neoplasia, trauma or intraocular haemorrhage. Glaucoma comes on slowly in cats, often without pain initially, and consequently presents much later. Because **the ocular tunics of the cat are more elastic than those of the dog**, the feline eye is initially able to accommodate a rise in intraocular pressure without pain or loss of vision. The initial presenting signs may therefore be a **dilated pupil, buphthalmos (enlarged globe) or visual deficits.**

Glaucoma can arise in older cats due to **'aqueous misdirection'**. This occurs when aqueous flows into the vitreous leading to anterior displacement of the iris and lens and subsequent occlusion of the drainage angle. It can be diagnosed clinically by the observation of a shallow anterior chamber in combination with a raised intraocular pressure and in the absence of any other ocular disease. Surgical treatment for aqueous misdirection involves **phacoemulsification** to remove lens contents (increasing the size of the anterior chamber), combined with an **extensive vitrectomy**, however many cases will respond to medical management.

For the rare cases of **primary glaucoma and aqueous misdirection glaucoma**:

- Topical **carbonic anhydrase inhibitors**, dorzolamide and brinzolamide, can be used TID.
- Studies involving the beta blocker, timolol, have been equivocal and it can have unwanted cardiovascular side effects in small patients.
- Prostaglandin analogues, latanoprost and travoprost, will cause miosis in treated cats but have minimal long term effects on intraocular pressure. This is thought to be due to the fact that these drugs mediate a reduction in IOP via prostaglandin F receptors which cats lack.

In cats with **secondary glaucoma, the underlying cause should be treated where possible, and carbonic anhydrase inhibitors used as an adjunct to reduce IOP**. If medical treatment is ineffective or if the cat shows signs of chronic pain, enucleation is indicated.

Orbital conditions

Orbital abscess/cellulitis

This is a relatively common presentation in cats, caused by **bacterial infection which enters the orbit by a variety of routes** such as a penetrating injury or foreign body through the conjunctival sac or eyelids, via the oropharynx, or haematogenously from elsewhere in the body. Whereas an abscess suggests a focal collection of purulent material, cellulitis is a more diffuse inflammation of the tissues.

Clinical signs generally present acutely and include:

- exophthalmos
- pain on opening the mouth
- increased resistance to retropulsion
- protrusion of the nictitans membrane
- chemosis
- conjunctival hyperaemia
- lagophthalmos
- inability to blink
- exposure keratitis.

Work-up includes examination of the oral cavity under GA and ocular ultrasound. A CT or MRI scan gives more information which is invaluable for surgical planning if an orbital foreign body is suspected.

Examination of the mouth may reveal a reddening or 'pointing' of the oral mucosa caudal to the last molar tooth. If so this area can be gently opened up by blunt dissection using a pair of haemostats. Sometimes this establishes a route for drainage and yields purulent material which can be swabbed for bacterial culture and sensitivity.

Ultrasonography of the retrobulbar space can reveal the presence of a fluid pocket, or diffuse inflammatory changes. Comparison with the contralateral normal eye is useful. Depending upon location, any fluid pockets may be amenable to **drainage or sampling via an ultrasound guided approach** but this should only be undertaken by operators with a very sound knowledge of periorbital anatomy as there are many vital structures behind the globe which could be easily damaged.

Both orbital abscessation and cellulitis can place traction on the optic nerve which can result in permanent visual deficits if not treated quickly. If the nature of the bacterial infection cannot be established then a **four week course of broad spectrum antibiotics with sensitivity against both aerobes and anaerobes** (e.g. potentiated amoxicillin and metronidazole) is indicated. This is also appropriate interim treatment whilst awaiting culture and sensitivity results. Because the presentation can be similar to that of orbital neoplasia, referral should always be considered, particularly if the cat is older or if there is no clear history of a potential source of infection.

Orbital tumours

In cats 90% of orbital tumours are malignant. They often present late and have a guarded prognosis from the outset. Tumours may be primary, arising from orbital structures, or secondary arising as a result of extension from adjacent structures e.g. nasal or oral cavity, brain or globe, or metastasis from distant sites. Orbital neoplasia (Figure 47) generally affects patients greater than eight years of age. (Attali-Soussay et al., 2001).

In cats most orbital tumours are secondary and include lymphoma, squamous cell carcinoma, melanoma, adenocarcinoma, cerebral meningioma or metastatic disease.

Affected cats exhibit a **slowly progressive unilateral exophthalmos** and resistance to retropulsion of the globe is increased on the affected side. In contrast to cases of orbital cellulitis or abscessation, pain on opening the mouth or palpation of extraocular tissues is usually absent. However some orbital neoplasms can mimic the clinical signs (including pain) of acute orbital inflammatory disease. (Hendrix and Gelatt, 2000). Tumours involving destruction of bone are particularly associated with pain. There is often a **lagophthalmos** (inability to blink over the protruding globe) leading to exposure keratitis with desiccation of the cornea and corneal ulceration. Menace response and pupillary light reflexes are variable. The exophthalmos may be accompanied by an ipsilateral nasal discharge, haemorrhage or crusting of the nostril, and reduced airflow on the affected side.

Diagnosis is principally by imaging. Skull radiography (including intraoral views) can be useful, demonstrating soft tissue densities of the nasal cavities, destruction of nasal turbinates, pathological fractures, osteoproliferation, or bone lysis (which is highly

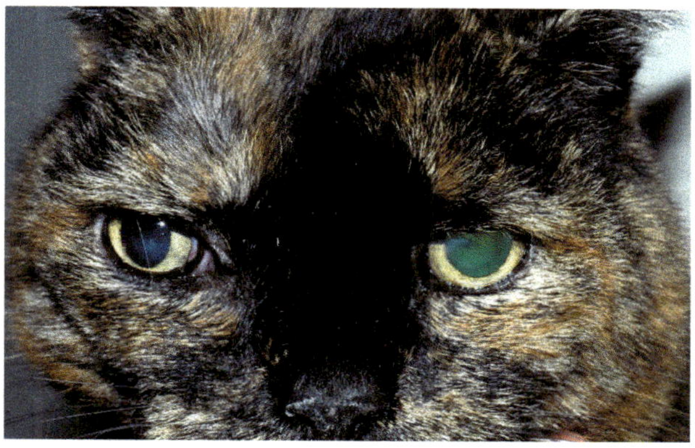

Figure 47. Orbital tumour affecting the right hand side. Note the obvious facial asymmetry, lateral deviation of the globe and protrusion of the third eyelid. © Rachel Lockhart.

suggestive of malignancy.) Ultrasonography can be employed but the depth of penetrance is a problem when evaluating the retrobulbar space. **The gold standard imaging modalities are CT or MRI scans**. Finance permitting, these give the most information about the extent of the lesion and to a degree can identify the type (Armour et al., 2011). Depending on the location biopsy of the lesion may be possible via ultrasound guided FNA or even via the nose. **Survey imaging in the form of chest radiographs and abdominal ultrasound is recommended** for staging purposes, and if neoplasia is suspected in an animal showing compatible clinical signs (e.g. cough or respiratory distress), may be performed first to look for metastasis and spare the patient an expensive, lengthy investigation.

Treatment depends upon the tumour type. For malignant types only **palliation** may be possible. Some are amenable to radiotherapy or surgical excision including exenteration or orbitotomy. The latter involves considerable pre-operative planning and should be undertaken by a specialist. **Palliative enucleation** may be considered if the globe is likely to become damaged, providing the patient is deemed to have sufficient survival time to benefit. In many cases euthanasia is the only reasonable option.

Feline restrictive orbital myofibroblastic sarcoma (FROMS)

This is an unusual condition unique to the cat which involves **an insidiously progressive fibrosis of the orbital tissues resulting in fixation of the globe and eyelids**. It affects mainly older cats, with no obvious breed predisposition. Commencing unilaterally, involvement of the contralateral eye usually follows. Clinical signs include:

- exophthalmos
- progressive restriction of movement of globe and eyelids
- thickening and retraction of the eyelids
- lagophthalmos
- exposure keratitis
- corneal desiccation
- corneal perforation.

Diagnosis is made on biopsy of eyelid or thickened haired skin with subcutis. Although this was previously thought to be a non-neoplastic condition, a recent study has shown infiltration of the orbit, eyelid and periorbital skin with **neoplastic spindle cells which spread along fascial planes but did not form discrete masses** (Bell et al., 2011). Treatment in the form of immunosuppressive drugs has been attempted but has not been successful; enucleation may buy a little more time, but most cats are euthanased eventually.

Ocular manifestations of systemic disease

Systemic hypertension

Systemic hypertension is defined as a **repeatable systolic blood pressure of > 160 mmHg, and/or diastolic of > 100 mmHg in a calm animal** (Stepien, 2010) Systemic hypertension may be **primary** (essential) or more likely, **secondary to other disease processes** e.g. renal disease, hyperthyroidism, primary aldosteronism, or diabetes mellitus.

The **eye is a target organ for damage** by prolonged high blood pressure. The sequence of events by which hypertension damages the eye is as follows:

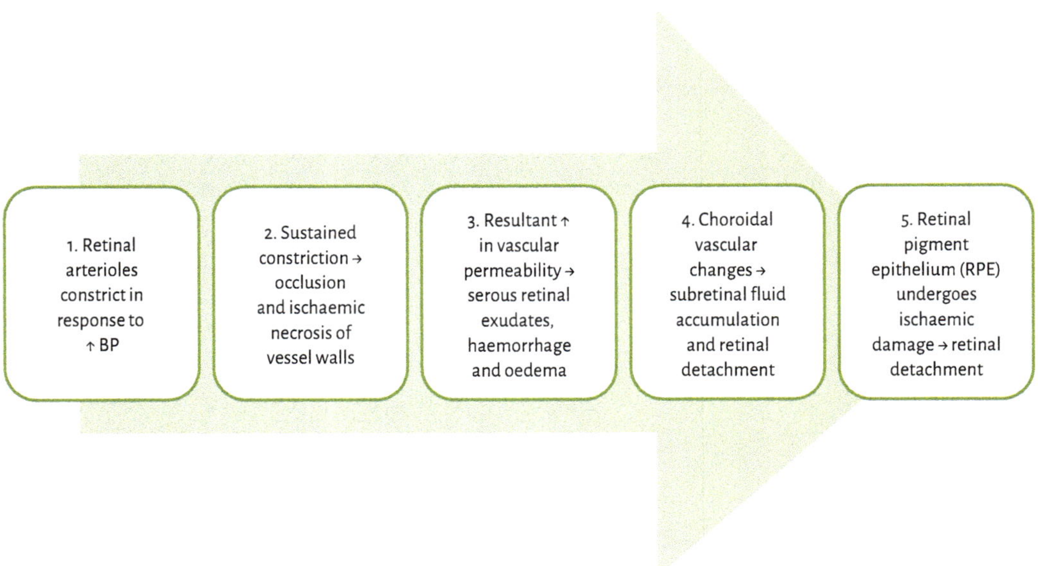

(Crispin and Mould 2001)

Most hypertensive cats are ten years old or over, and **acute blindness** is a common presenting sign. Hypertensive chorioretinopathy is seen in 40–65% of all cats with systemic hypertension (Stepien, 2011). Ocular findings include:

- arterial tortuosity
- variations in calibre of retinal vessels
- retinal oedema
- pre-, intra- and sub-retinal haemorrhage
- partial or total retinal detachment (Figure 48)
- papilloedema and haemorrhage in the vitreous or anterior chamber (hyphaema) (Figure 49). The latter was seen in 30% of affected cats in a recent study by Linek (2020) who also showed 14% of cats to have aneurysms of the iridal vessels.

Diagnosis and treatment of hypertension are discussed elsewhere in this book.

Cats can regain vision even after the retinas have detached **providing treatment is begun swiftly;** retinal reattachment can occur although some level of degeneration is inevitable. The best prognosis for return of vision is in cats whose retinas have been detached for less than a week, however a recent study suggested vision could be recovered in cats which had been blind for much longer (Young et al., 2019).

As the best outcome is always achieved the earlier in the course of the disease that the diagnosis is made, it is recommended that all cats over ten, and certainly those already diagnosed with chronic renal failure or hyperthyroidism should have a **fundic examination and BP measurement every 12 months.**

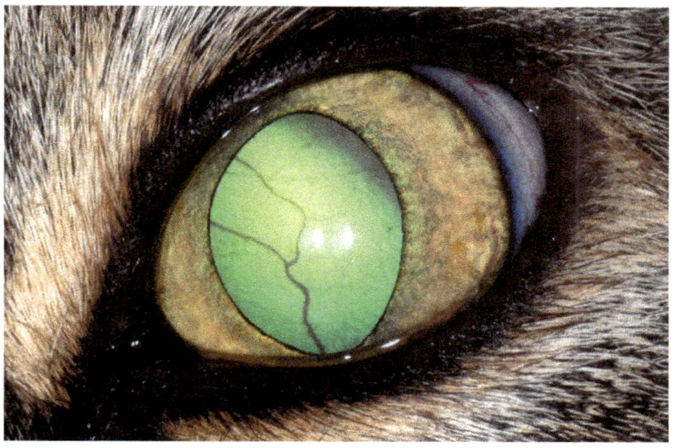

Figure 48. Retinal detachment. The retina can be seen hanging immediately posterior to the lens with the naked eye. © Rachel Lockhart.

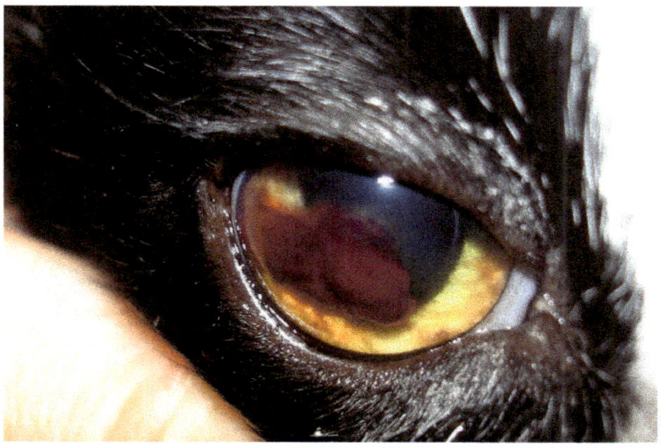

Figure 49. Hyphaema caused by systemic hypertension. © Rachel Lockhart.

Taurine deficiency

Discussed previously.

Thiamine deficiency

This deficiency can occur in cats fed diets with **large amounts of raw fish** which contains thiaminases or in cats with **severe gastrointestinal disease** which prevents thiamine absorption. As well as progressive neurological signs, affected cats exhibit fixed dilated pupils, papilloedema, optic nerve head vascularisation and peripapillary retinal haemorrhage. Clinical signs and blood thiamine levels are diagnostic: normal feline blood thiamine levels are approximately 32 μg/dl.

Bartonellosis

B. henselae (the cause of 'cat scratch fever' in humans) is transmitted among cats by the cat flea (*Ctenocephalides felis*). It is thought transmission is not via flea saliva, but flea excrement is involved. Ocular signs including **anterior uveitis and chorioretinitis** have been reported in cats in the USA (Lappin and Black, 1999), but the condition has thus far not been reported in the UK. More recent studies have been equivocal (Fontanelle et al., 2008, Powell et al., 2010) and the role of the organism in uveitis is currently unclear (Stiles, 2011).

Feline coronavirus (FIP)

Ocular signs include:

- **fibrinous anterior uveitis** (Figure 50)
- chorioretinitis with perivascular cuffing
- signs of hyperviscosity ('box-carring' of retinal vessels).

A definitive diagnosis is only possible post-mortem via histology and immunohistochemistry. In the live cat, a combination of coronavirus titre, serum total protein levels, serum albumin and globulin ratios, and clinical signs are most helpful. Treatment of FIP with remdesivir is possible but very expensive. Without treatment the disease is usually fatal with the 'dry' form usually having a more protracted course. Within a cattery/breeding colony situation, elimination of chronic FECV

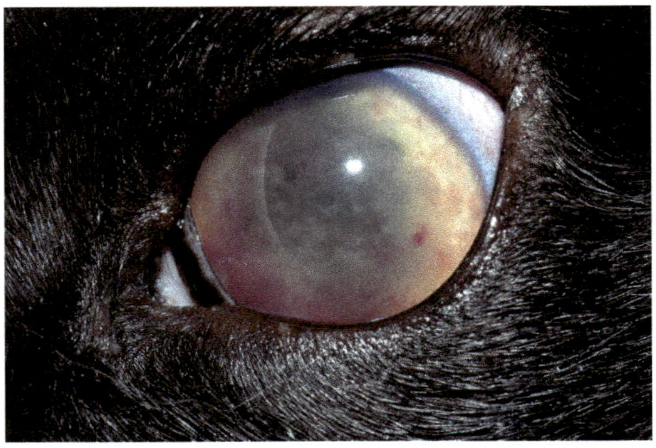

Figure 50. Fibrinous uveitis in FIP. © Rachel Lockhart.

(feline enteric coronavirus) shedders is the most important way of reducing FECV infection (Addie, 2009).

Feline immunodeficiency virus (FIV)

FIV causes ocular signs by direct damage of ocular tissues, secondary immune-phenomena, and allowing opportunistic infections (English et al., 1994). **Uveitis is the most important manifestation** and may be anterior, or intermediate uveitis/'pars planitis' (Figure 51) which is an inflammation of the posterior ciliary body manifested by white opacities (inflammatory cells) with a '**snowstorm**' appearance within the anterior vitreous immediately behind the lens. Neuro-ophthalmic signs e.g. anisocoria or nystagmus are likely to be related to CNS disease rather than direct ocular disease. FIV infection predisposes to secondary infections e.g. with *T. gondii* or *Chlamydia felis*.

Feline leukaemia virus (FeLV)

Infection of **foetal or newborn kittens can result in retinal dysplasia or panuveitis** (Albert et al., 1977). In adult cats the 'D-shaped' or '**reverse D' pupil**, or anisocoria are direct manifestations of the **neurological effects of FeLV infection on the malar or nasal branches of the short ciliary nerves.** Cats remain visual and other ocular signs are not usually noted. However **FeLV- induced lymphoma** may also manifest ocularly: usually with uveitis or iridal masses. FeLV effects on the haemopoetic system (i.e. anaemia or thrombocytopaenia) can also manifest ocularly producing pallor of conjunctival or retinal vessels, hyphaema, or retinal haemorrhages (Brightman et al., 1991).

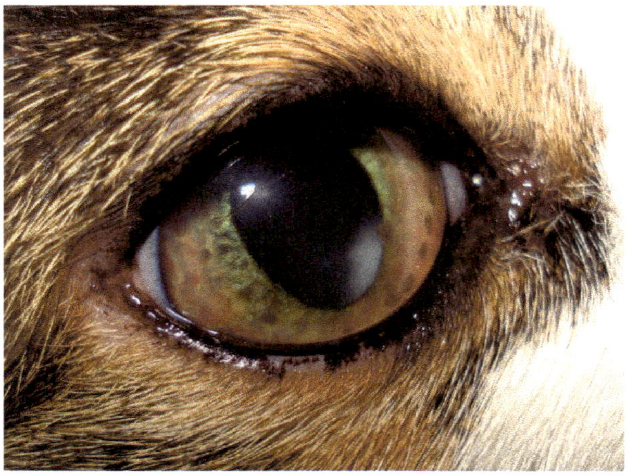

Figure 51. Pars planitis or 'snow-banking' seen beyond the posterior lens capsule, associated with FIV infection. © Rachel Lockhart.

Toxoplasmosis

Ocular signs include:

- uveitis
- chorioretinitis
- optic neuritis.

Around 80% of cats with toxoplasmosis were observed to have ocular signs in one study (Aroch et al., 2013). Chorioretinitis is the most common manifestation (Davidson, 2000). **Histological demonstration of the parasite within tissues is the only definitive way of confirming diagnosis.** However in cats with uveitis serological testing is most commonly used. It is important to test for both *T.gondii* IgM and IgG antibodies in paired samples 2–4 weeks apart; the IgM class will rise and fall over approximately 3 months after infection, whereas IgG will rise more slowly and remain elevated in cats for years after exposure (Lappin et al., 1989). PCR testing on aqueous humour samples can indicate the presence of *T. gondii* within the eye but does not necessarily indicate active infection. **Toxoplasmosis is a zoonotic disease which poses risks to pregnant and immunocompromised individuals.**

Ocular trauma

The lifestyle and behaviour of cats means they are more likely than dogs to suffer ocular trauma (Figures 52 and 53).

Corneal foreign bodies

Potential foreign bodies (FBs) include plant material (e.g. seed husk or thorn) or fragments of cat claw (Figure 54). Organic FBs in the cornea stimulate a huge inflammatory response therefore even if the eye is comfortable, and a full blink can be achieved, **removal is indicated.**

FBs sitting on the corneal surface can often be removed in the consulting room. Apply several drops of **topical anaesthetic** at one minute intervals, and then gently prod the FB gently with a stick swab or cotton bud. Seed husks with a convex profile often lodge in

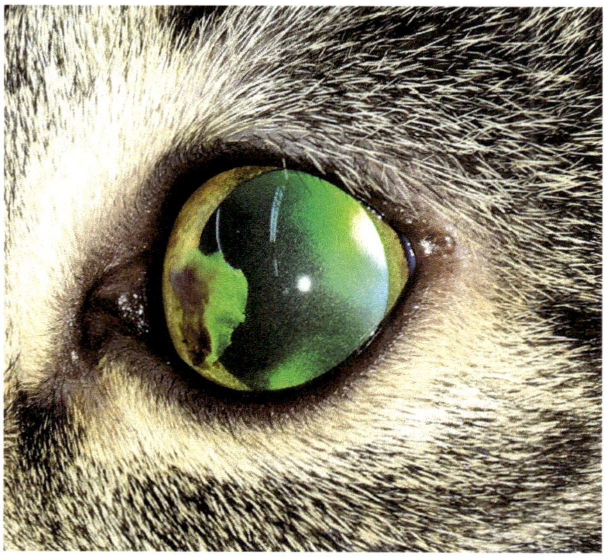

Figure 52. Penetrating corneal injury with haemorrhage and fibrin adherent to the corneal endothelium at the entry point, and diffuse cellular flare. © Agata Tsvetanova.

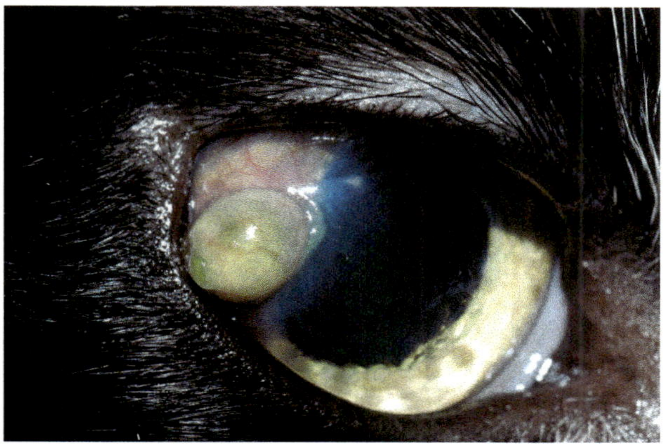

Figure 53. Larger corneal laceration with iris prolapse. © Rachel Lockhart.

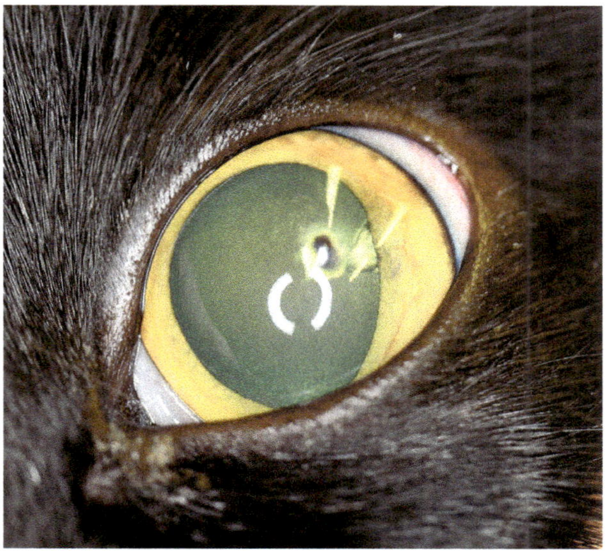

Figure 54. Penetrating corneal foreign body with an associated tear in the anterior lens capsule at the 3 o'clock position. © Kerry Smith.

the epithelium and may require a kimura spatula or FB spud to elevate them.

If a thorn is **lodged perpendicularly or obliquely within the corneal stroma** but is not full thickness through it, and still has a portion sticking proud from the corneal surface, it may be possible to remove it. **General anaesthesia is required**. The corneal surface is aseptically prepared with 1 in 50 povidone-iodine solution. The foreign body is approached with a FB spud or 23 gauge needle, **perpendicularly to the direction it entered the cornea**. It should be speared (gently) and withdrawn from the cornea in the reverse direction to how it entered. Grabbing the end of a FB with forceps to pull it out risks driving it further into the cornea, or even the anterior chamber.

Once removed, fluorescein should be applied to the eye without flushing, to perform a **Seidel test to check for aqueous leakage.** If leakage is present, a **Buster collar** should be placed **on the cat**, and it should be woken up and referred immediately. **If the thorn appears full thickness, or if you cannot tell whether it is full thickness, immediate referral should be sought**. An attempt should not be made to remove a full-thickness FB unless equipped to deal with the consequences: leakage of aqueous, a surgical-sized defect, or worse the FB entering the anterior chamber.

Corneal Lacerations

Lacerations usually occur due to cat fights. Whilst small deficits may self-seal, there is a danger of re-rupture when the fibrin clot, inside the eye, dissolves so referral is recommended. Most **defects greater than 2mm in length require direct suturing** and possibly a **conjunctival pedicle graft over the defect** for additional blood supply and strength, certainly if there is any infection or malacia. Even quite large corneal lacerations can be repaired if referred quickly. Emergency medical treatment for corneal lacerations is discussed later.

Lens trauma

Sometimes a laceration or **penetrating injury to the cornea**, particularly as a result of a cat fight, may involve the lens. If the anterior lens capsule is penetrated lens material leaks into the anterior chamber. Because of the way the lens develops embryonically (contained within its capsule) the body has never been exposed to lens protein and **perceives it as foreign material, mounting an aggressive inflammatory response: phacoclastic uveitis**.

Clinical signs include a **miotic pupil** (which may be resistant to mydriasis even with atropine), and a cloud or blob of whitish material adherent to the anterior lens capsule or protruding through the pupil. Although medical treatment for uveitis helps, the **lens material**

requires removal as it is the driver of the inflammation. This is done by **phacoemulsification**, the same procedure used to remove cataracts, so immediate referral is recommended. The owner has to be counselled as to the possible **future risk of FPTOS** before proceeding with lens removal.

Globe rupture

Globe rupture is most likely to be suffered following an **RTA**, but the cat may present with non-ocular injuries which should not be overlooked as they may be life threatening. Cats with suspected **skull fractures** often present with hyphaema (blood in the anterior chamber) which prevents intraocular examination. Whilst corneal damage can often be successfully repaired, damage to the posterior segment is more difficult to deal with. There are two ways to assess the damaged eye in order to establish a prognosis:

1. **Consensual pupillary light reflex**. Shine a bright light into the injured eye and watch the contralateral pupil. If it does not constrict or even dilates, this is a poor prognostic sign, probably indicating retinal detachment. Provided a sufficiently bright light has been used for the test you can confidently say there is no hope of recovering vision and the eye should be enucleated.(Lack of a dazzle reflex gives similar information, but may be less reliable as there may be other injuries which prevent blinking.)
2. **Ocular ultrasound**. If there is obvious corneal damage a stand-off (e.g. surgical glove filled with water) should be used. US examination gives an image of the posterior segment. There should be a smooth contour to the back of the eye filled with echogenically clear vitreous. **A 'seagull' sign within this space is pathognomonic for retinal detachment.** US may also reveal damage to the lens. If there are shape changes to the back of the eye, or an obvious breach in the ocular tunics, this may indicate a scleral rupture (Figure 55). Posterior scleral ruptures are not amenable to surgical repair, and even when the haemorrhage and swelling have subsided, they are likely to represent an ongoing source of intractable inflammation, therefore enucleation is indicated.

Emergency treatment for ocular trauma

Many of these cases will require immediate referral, but interim emergency medical treatment can make a huge difference to the ultimate outcome.

The immediate aims are to:

- provide pain relief
- facilitate intraocular examination
- prevent further deterioration in the condition of the eye.

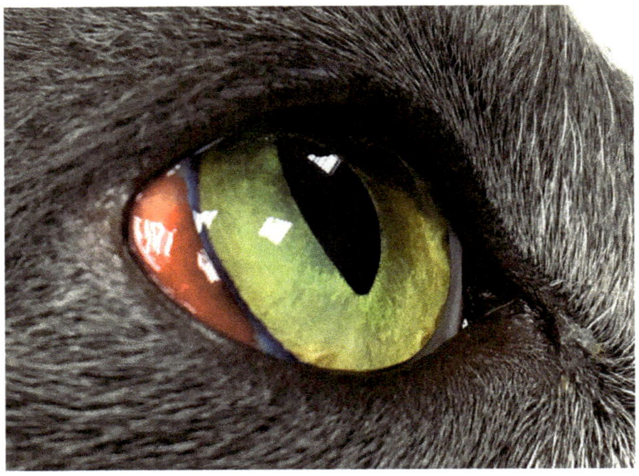

Figure 55. Subconjunctival/scleral haemorrhage can indicate a scleral rupture. © Agata Tsvetanova.

Pain relief should be administered in the form of **injectable opioids and nonsteroidals** unless there is a good pre-existing reason why they should not be given. The quantity and timing of the injections should be communicated to the referral centre to expedite surgical planning and minimise the risk of overdose.

In cases of corneal penetration, laceration and globe trauma, it is important to know whether the lens is involved in the pathological process. This can be greatly facilitated by the **application of topical atropine sulphate 1%** prior to leaving the practice. Tropicamide will not be sufficient as a mydriatic in these cases as all injury to the cornea is accompanied by a degree of 'reflex uveitis' leading to miosis which cannot be overcome by tropicamide. **Atropine should be applied every four hours** to effect and only stopped once the pupil is fully dilated. In addition to enabling inspection of the anterior lens capsule and further intraocular examination, it also stabilises the blood-ocular barrier, aiding the management of accompanying uveitis, and abolishes iridociliary spasm, contributing to pain relief.

Although cats generally have the good sense to leave their injured eyes alone, an Elizabethan collar should be considered to prevent self-trauma. However this should be avoided if the cat becomes distressed by the collar as this may lead to a rise in intraocular pressure or further trauma. If there is an obvious purulent discharge or other signs of infection then **chloramphenicol drops can be applied every four hours**. Ointments and gentamycin should be avoided as they can cause damage to the corneal endothelium, for the same reason use of topical anaesthetic should be limited.

Space precludes discussion of ophthalmic surgery here, however the following common procedure, which has serious implications in feline patients, must be mentioned.

Enucleation

This is sadly a commonly required procedure due to **irreparable trauma, intractable uveitis, intraocular neoplasia or glaucoma.** However the procedure must be approached with far more caution than in dogs because of the **risk of damage to the optic chiasm.** The feline optic nerve is very short and **traction on the globe during enucleation can lead to optic chiasm damage and blindness in the contralateral eye** which is a frighteningly common occurrence (Donaldson et al., 2014a). There is very little space in the feline orbit, so only small instruments should be used and the introduction of more than one instrument at a time into the orbit should be avoided. **Anterior traction should be avoided at all times.** Ligation of the optic nerve and its accompanying blood vessels is not recommended as it places excessive traction on the optic nerve and chiasm.

Removal of the eye can be achieved by either a **transconjunctival, or a transpalpebral approach**. A detailed description of each is provided by Donaldson (2014b). The former is a little more difficult and has greater potential for leaving conjunctival tissue in situ which can lead to subcutaneous cyst formation. It should not be performed in situations where there is a known infection, penetrating injury or neoplastic process involving the ocular surface; the transpalpebral approach is more appropriate in these situations.

The surgical site should be closed in three layers. A transorbital platform can be constructed with a simple continuous suture (e.g. 2 metric PDS) across the orbit vertically starting medially and working laterally. This leads to an improved immediate postoperative appearance, assists in haemostasis, and prevents sinking of the skin into the orbit post-operatively. This is followed by a simple continuous subcuticular layer with the same suture material, and finally cruciate, or simple interrupted sutures of 1.5m nylon in the skin.

Recommended reading

BSAVA Manual of Canine and Feline Ophthalmology Third edition (2014). Ed. Gould D. and McLellan G., BSAVA.

Slatter's Fundamentals of Veterinary Ophthalmology Fifth Edition (2012). Ed. Maggs D, Miller P. and Ofri R., Elsevier.

Veterinary Ophthalmology Fifth edition (2013). Ed. Gelatt K.N., Gilger B.C. and Kern T.J., Wiley-Blackwell.

Feline Ophthalmology: An Atlas and Text (1997) Barnett K.C. and Crispin S.M., Bailliere Tindall. (Out of Print).

Bibliography

Addie D.D. et al (2009) Feline infectious peritonitis. ABCD guidelines on prevention and management. Journal of Feline Medicine and Surgery, 11, 594–604.

Albert et al (1977) Retinal neoplasia and dysplasia 1. Induction by feline leukaemia virus. Investigative Ophthalmology and Visual Sciences, 16, 325–337.

Armour M.D. et al (2011) A review of orbital and intracranial magnetic resonance imaging in 79 canine and 13 feline patients (2004–2010), Veterinary Ophthalmology 14, 215–226.

Aroch I. et al (2013) Chapter 18 Ocular manifestations of Systemic Disease. In Slatter's Fundamentals of Veterinary Ophthalmology Fifth Edition (2013). Ed. Maggs, Miller and Ofri, Elsevier.

Attali-Soussay K. et al (2001) Retrobulbar tumors in dogs and cats: 25 cases. Veterinary Ophthalmology 4 (1), 19–27.

Bell C.M. et al (2011) Diagnostic features of feline restrictive orbital myofibroblastic sarcoma. Veterinary Pathology, 48, 742–750

Benz P., et al (2011) Detection of Encephalitozoon cuniculi in the feline cataractous lens. Veterinary Ophthalmology 14 Suppl. 1, 37–47.

Brightman A.H. et al (1991) Ocular disease in FeLV – positive cats: 11 cases (1981–1986). Journal of the American Animal Hospital Association, 198, 1049–1051.

Crispin S. and Mould J. (2001) Systemic hypertensive disease and the feline fundus. Veterinary Ophthalmology, 4, 131–140.

Cullen C.L. and Webb A.A. (2013) Chapter 35. Ocular Manifestations of Systemic Disease. Part 2: The Cat. In Veterinary Ophthalmology Fifth Edition. Ed. Gelatt, Gilger and Kern. Pp. 1978–2036.

Davidson M.G. et al (2000) Toxoplasmosis. Veterinary Clinics of North America: Small Animal Practice, 30, 1051–1062.

Dean R et al (2005) Use of quantitative real-time PCR to monitor the response of Chlamydophila felis to doxycycline treatment. Journal of Clinical Microbiology, 43, 1858–1864.

Donaldson D. et al (2014a) Contralateral optic neuropathy and retinopathy associated with visual and afferent pupillomotor dysfunction following enucleation in cats. Veterinary Ophthalmology 17, 373–384.

Donaldson D. (2014b) Chapter 8 The orbit and globe. In BSAVA Manual of Canine and Feline Ophthalmology. Third Edition. Ed. Gould and McLellan. Pp. 111–132.

Duke F.D. et al (2013) Feline ocular tumors following ciliary body ablation with intravitreal gentamicin. Veterinary Ophthalmology 16, 188–190.

English R.V. et al (1994) Development of clinical disease in cats experimentally infected with feline immunodeficiency virus infection. Journal of Infectious Diseases, 170, 543–552.

Fontanelle JP. et al (2008) Prevalence of serum antibodies against Bartonella species in the serum of cats with or without uveitis. Journal of Feline Medicine and Surgery, 10, 41–46.

Galle L.E. (2004) Antiviral therapy for ocular viral disease. Veterinary Clinics of North America: Small Animal Practice, 34, 639–653.

Gaskell R.M. et al (1977). Experimental induction of feline viral rhinotracheitis virus re-excretion in FVR-recovered cats. Veterinary Record, 12, 128–133.

Gelatt K.N. et al (2001) Enrofloxacin-associated retinal degeneration in cats. Veterinary Ophthalmology, 4, 99–106.

Goldreich J.E. Franklin-Guild R.J. and Ledbetter E.C. (2020) Feline bacterial keratitis: clinical features, bacterial isolates, and in vitro antimicrobial sensitivity patterns. Veterinary Ophthalmology, 23, 90–96.

Gould D.J. (2011) Feline Herpesvirus-1 Ocular manifestations, diagnosis, and treatment options. Journal of Feline Medicine and Surgery, 13, 333–346.

Hampson E.C.G.M. et al (2002) Primary glaucoma in Burmese cats. Australian Veterinary Journal, 80, 672–680.

Hendrix D. and Gelatt K. (2000) Diagnosis, treatment and outcome of orbital neoplasia in dogs: a retrospective study of 44 cases. The Journal of Small Animal Practice, 41 (3), 105–108.

Lappin M.R. et al (1989) Diagnosis of recent Toxoplasma gondii infection in cats by use of an enzyme-linked immunosorbent assay for immunoglobulin M. American Journal of Veterinary Research, 50, 1580–1585.

Lappin M.R. et al and Black J.C. (1999) Bartonella spp infection as a possible cause of uveitis in a cat. Journal of the American Veterinary Medical Association, 214, 1205–1207.

Linn-Pearl R.N. et al (2015) Validity of aqueocentesis as a component of anterior uveitis investigation in dogs and cats. Veterinary Ophthalmology, 18, 326–334.

Low et al (2007). Prevalence of feline herpesvirus1, Chlamydophila felis and Mycoplasma spp. DNA in conjunctival cells collected from cats with and without conjunctivitis. American Journal of Veterinary Research 68 (6), 643–648.

Lowe R. (2014) Chapter 16 The Lens. In BSAVA Manual of Canine and Feline Ophthalmology. Third Edition. Ed. Gould and McLellan. Pp. 297–321.

Maggs D.J. et al (1999) Evaluation of serologic and viral detection methods for diagnosing feline herpesvirus-1 infection in cats with acute respiratory tract or chronic ocular disease. Journal of the American Veterinary Medical Association, 214, 502–507.

McLaughlin S.A. et al (1993) Eyelid neoplasms in cats: a review of demographic data (1979–1989). Journal of the American Animal Hospital Association, 29, 63–67.

McLellan G.J. and Miller P.E. (2011) Feline glaucoma – a comprehensive review. Veterinary Ophthalmology 14 (Suppl. 1) 15–29.

Miller P.E. et al (1991) Evaluation of two applanation tonometers in cats. American Journal of Veterinary Research, 52, 1917–1921.

Nassisse M.P. et al (1989) Experimental ocular herpesvirus infection in the cat. Sites of virus replication, clinical features and effects of corticosteroid administration. Investigative Ophthalmology and Visual Sciences, 30, 1758–1768.

Nassisse M.P. et al (1998) Detection of feline herpesvirus 1 DNA in corneas of cats with eosinophilic keratitis or corneal sequestration. American Journal of Veterinary Research, 59, 856–858.

Newkirk K.M. and Rohrbach B.W. (2009) A retrospective study of eyelid tumours from 43 cats. Veterinary Pathology, 46, 916–927.

Pederson S. et al (2016) Use of a nictitating membrane flap for treatment of feline acute corneal hydrops-21 eyes. Veterinary Ophthalmology 19, Suppl 1, 61–68.

Powell C.C. et al (2010) Bartonella species, feline herpesvirus-1 and Toxoplasma gondii PCR assay results from blood and aqueous humour samples from 104 cats with naturally-occurring endogenous uveitis. Journal of Feline Medicine and Surgery, 12, 923–928.

Ramirez C.J. et al (2011) Molecular genetic basis for fluoroquinolone- induced retinal degeneration in cats. Pharmacogenetics and Genomics, 21, 66–75.

Read R.A. and Lucas J. (2001) Lipogranulomatous conjunctivitis: clinical findings from 21 eyes in 13 cats. Veterinary Ophthalmology 4, 93–98.

Richter M. et al (2002) Aldose reductase activity and glucose – related opacities in incubated lenses from dogs and cats. American Journal of Veterinary Research, 63, 1591–1597.

Rusanen E. et al (2010) Evaluation of a rebound tonometer (Tonovet®) in clinically normal cat eyes. Veterinary Ophthalmology, 13, 31–36.

Sebbag L. et al (2015) Reference values, intertest correlations, and test-retest repeatability of selected tear film tests in healthy cats. Journal of the American Veterinary Medicine Association, 246, 426–435.

Stepien R.L. (2010) Chapter 151 Blood pressure assessment. In Textbook of Veterinary Internal Medicine. Diseases of the Dog and Cat. 7th Edition. Ed. Ettinger and Feldman pp. 580–581.

Stepien R.L. (2011) Feline systemic hypertension: diagnosis and management. Journal of Feline Medicine and Surgery, 13, 35–43.

Stiles J. et al (1997) Use of nested polymerase chain reaction to identify feline herpesvirus in ocular tissue from clinically normal cats and cats with corneal sequestra or conjunctivitis. American Journal of Veterinary Research, 58, 338–342.

Stiles J. (2011) Bartonellosis in cats: a role in uveitis? Veterinary Ophthalmology 14 (Suppl1) 9–14.

Sturgess C.P. et al (2001) Controlled study of the efficacy of clavulanic acid-potentiated amoxicillin in the treatment of Chlamydia psittaci in cats. The Veterinary Record, 149, 73–76.

Suter A., Voelter K., Hartnack S., Speiss B.M., and Pot S.A. (2018) Septic keratitis in dogs, cats, and horses in Switzerland: associated bacteria and antibiotic susceptibility. Veterinary Ophthalmology 21, 66–75.

Thomasy S.M. et al (2011) Evaluation of orally administered famciclovir in cats experimentally infected with feline herpesvirustype-1. American Journal of veterinary Research, 72, 85–95.

Thomasy S.M. et al (2016a) Oral administration of famciclovir for treatment of spontaneous ocular, respiratory or dermatologic disease attributed to feline herpesvirus type 1:59 cases (2006–2013). Journal of the American Veterinary Medical Association, 249, 526–538.

Thomasy S.M. and Maggs D.J. (2016b) A review of antiviral drugs and other compounds with activity against feline herpesvirus-1. Veterinary Ophthalmology 19, Suppl. 1, 119–130.

Volopich S. et al (2005) Cytologic findings, and feline herpesvirus DNA and Chlamydophila felis antigen detection rates in normal cats and cats with conjunctival and corneal lesions. Veterinary Ophthalmology 8, 25–32.

Whittaker C.J. et al (2010) Lip commissure to eyelid transposition for repair of feline eyelid agenesis. Veterinary Ophthalmology 13, 173–178.

Williams D.L. et al (2005) Efficacy of topical acyclovir for the treatment of feline herpetic keratitis: results of a prospective clinical trial and data from in vitro investigations. Veterinary Record, 157, 254–257.

Wood C. and Scott E.M. (2019) Feline post-traumatic sarcomas: current understanding, treatment, and monitoring. Journal of feline medicine and Surgery 21, 835–842.

Young W. et al (2019) Visual outcome in cats with hypertensive retinopathy. Veterinary Ophthalmology 22, 161–167.

Zeiss C.J. et al (2003) Feline intraocular tumours may arise from transformation of lens epithelium. Veterinary Pathology, 40, 355–362.

Test

1. Which of the following pieces of ophthalmic equipment is the most appropriate to examine a lesion *in detail* in the tapetal fundus?

A) Slit lamp biomicroscope.
B) Direct ophthalmoscope.
C) Finhoff transilluminator with a 20D condensing lens.
D) Schiotz tonometer.

2. How long does tropicamide take to dilate the feline pupil?

A) 1–2 minutes.
B) 5–8 minutes.
C) 15–20 minutes.
D) 30–35 minutes.

3. The phenomenon of 'snow-banking' or *pars planitis* is commonly associated with which of the following infectious diseases?

A) FIP.
B) FeLV.
C) FIV.
D) Toxoplasmosis.

4. What is the range of normal feline intraocular pressure (IOP)?

A) 5–16 mmHg.
B) 10–29 mmHg.
C) 20–35 mmHg.
D) 15–40 mmHg.

5. What is the efferent arm of the *dazzle reflex*?

A) Optic nerve (CN II).
B) Oculomotor nerve (CN III).
C) Trigeminal nerve (CN V).
D) The facial nerve (CN VII).

6. Under what circumstances is the 'Seidel Test' performed?

A) To look for corneal ulceration.
B) To assess patency of the nasolacrimal duct.
C) To evaluate the quality of the tear film.
D) To test if a corneal lesion is leaking.

7. Which of the following fundic pathologies is most likely to result in tapetal hyperreflectivity?

A) Retinal detachment.
B) Choroidal effusion.
C) Retinal atrophy.
D) Neoplastic infiltrate.

8. Which of the following statements about feline eyelid neoplasia is true?

A) Masses affecting up to half the eyelid margin can be resected followed by primary closure.
B) The vast majority of feline lid tumours are benign.
C) The average age of an affected cat is 3–5 years.
D) When closing the defect, a figure of eight suture should be placed at the eyelid margin.

9. What is the main presenting ophthalmic sign of primary Feline Herpes Virus infection in kittens?
A) Conjunctivitis.
B) Symblepharon.
C) Dendritic corneal ulceration.
D) Anterior uveitis.

10. Following fluorescein staining, which of the following describes the appearance of an 'indolent ' ulcer?
A) Even fluorescein staining across the defect.
B) Strong fluorescein staining in the centre, with a halo of lighter staining around the periphery.
C) Strong fluorescein staining around the periphery of the lesion, with no staining in the centre.
D) No fluorescein staining.

11. Which of the following statements about the use of serum to treat melting corneal ulcers is true?
A) Plasma works just as well as serum.
B) It can be stored at room temperature for up to 48 hours.
C) It should be applied twice daily to the affected cornea in the early stages of a melt.
D) Donor cat serum should never be used to avoid the risk of viral cross-infection.

12. Which of the following is the best treatment for a corneal sequestrum?
A) A lamellar keratectomy followed by placement of a conjunctival pedicle graft.
B) Oral famciclovir and topical lubricants.
C) A third eyelid flap.
D) Benign neglect, it will slough off.

13. Which of the following is a sign of chronic uveitis?
A) Aqueous flare.
B) Miosis of the pupil.
C) Blepharospasm.
D) Keratitic precipitates.

14. A Persian cat breeder client wishes to have her new stud cat tested for inherited feline progressive retinal atrophy (PRA). Which of the following defective genes should he be tested for?
A) CEP290.
B) AIPL1.
C) PRCD.
D) Crx.

15. Which of the following statements about feline orbital tumours is true?
A) The vast majority are bengin.
B) Primary tumours are more common than secondary tumours.
C) Enophthalmos is an important presenting sign.
D) Computer-assisted tomography (CT) or magnetic resonance imaging (MRI) are the gold standard diagnostic tests.

16. You are presented with a cat with a full thickness corneal laceration and decide to refer it for treatment. Which one of the following options represents best treatment before the cat gets to the referral centre?
A) Injectable opioid, injectable meloxicam, and one application of topical fusidic acid.
B) Injectable opioid, injectable meloxicam, and one application of topical atropine.
C) An Elizabethan collar and one application of topical gentamicin ointment.
D) An Elizabethan collar and one application of topical prednisolone acetate.

Clinical case 1

1. **Describe the ocular findings**
2. **What is the name given to the intraocular condition?**
3. **What are the potential causes for this condition?**
4. **How would you work up this condition?**
5. **Assuming no infectious cause was found, how would you commence initial treatment of this presentation?**

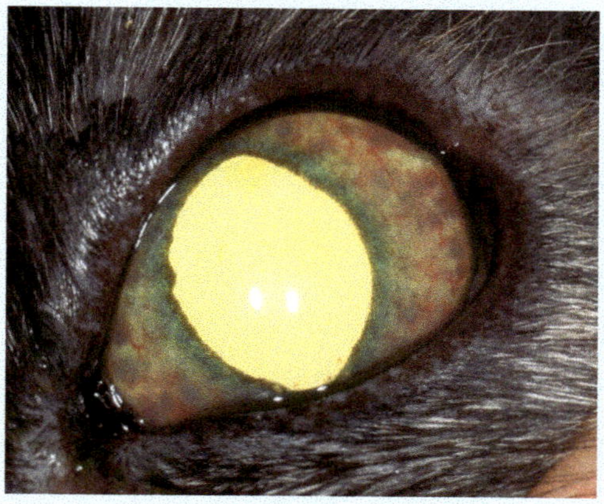

Correct answers

Test

1. B	7. C	13. D
2. C	8. D	14. B
3. C	9. A	15. D
4. B	10. B	16. B
5. D	11. D	
6. D	12. A	

Clinical case 1

1. A) Periocular alopecia and crusting.
   B) Mid-dilated pupil.
   C) Rubeosus iridis (prominent vessels around the iris periphery).
   D) Prominent iridal follicles.
   E) Loss of iris architecture/murky appearance to iris.
   F) Irregular pupillary margin with some areas of ectropion uveae (pupillary margin turning outwards).
   G) Iris rests (dots of pigment on the anterior lens capsule caused by the inflamed iris).
2. **Uveitis.**
3. **Blunt or penetrating trauma, infectious disease (including but not limited to, FIV, FeLV, FIP, bartonellosis, toxoplasmosis, leishmaniasis, cryptococcosis, histoplasmosis, coccidiomycosis, blastomycosis, candidiasis, ophthalmomyiasis interna), sepsis or bacteraemia from infections elsewhere in the body, neoplasia (primary ocular or metastatic), immune-mediated or idiopathic.**

4. A) Haematology and biochemistry including total protein and albumin: globulin ratio.
   B) ELISA for FIV and FeLV.
   C) Serology for coronavirus and toxoplasma.
   D) Other serology dependent on country of origin/travel history.
   E) Ocular ultrasound (if intraocular exam limited due to opacity of the cornea or anterior chamber e.g. hyphaema/oedema) particularly if a primary ocular cause suspected e.g. intraocular neoplasia.
   F) Chest radiographs.
   G) Abdominal ultrasound.
   H) Aqueocentesis- (the aqueous humour via a fine needle inserted at the limbus). Submission of resultant fluid for cytology, culture and PCRs.
5. **Topical ketorolac trometamol q4–6 hours, or prednisolone acetate 1% q4–6 hours (warn owner about possible recrudescence of FHV-1 infection if using the latter). If the posterior segment is involved then oral prednisolone at a starting dose of 0.5–1 mg/kg q24 hours.**

Oral diseases

5

Juanjo Vega Guerrero

Contents

Oral and dental disease are common in feline medicine and, unlike in other species, have **specific characteristics**. Prevalent pathologies include dental resorption, periodontitis, oropharyngeal inflammation, and maxillofacial cancer. All of these are painful conditions liable to cause eating difficulties which result in anorexia, weight loss, and behavioural changes.

Inflammatory oral lesions occur when the protective epithelial mechanisms (cellular and salivary) fail to work properly. Once the epithelium is damaged, this exposes the oral tissue to a medium rich in bacteria, which then **stimulates the local oral immune system** to react in the inflammatory manner so typical of feline oral lesions.

In addition, there is a **relationship between certain systemic diseases and oral pathology**. For example, chronic kidney disease is associated with gingivitis, whilst infectious agents can lead to significant inflammation of the oropharynx. Other causative conditions include degenerative, neoplastic, and traumatic diseases; and immune-mediated conditions.

Therefore every cat with clinical oral disease requires a **complete physical examination** to seek out contributing conditions. Oral disease is more frequent in older animals, but is also common in kittens and young adults. Thus, **all feline patients should have an oral examination** when visiting the vet. Due to the nature of the pathologies this exam may be painful, and **sedation may be required**, but this should not be considered a barrier to a proper assessment where pathology is suspected.

Clinical examination

Prior to a physical examination, it is important to obtain a **detailed clinical history**. The latter includes information regarding the **duration of the problem, previous investigations and treatments, and the response to these therapies**.

In addition a clinical history should include information on breed, age, sex, vaccination status, diet, number of cats in the household, where the cat was obtained from, whether it is an indoor or, outdoor cat or a combination of the two. Age should also be taken into account when drawing up a list of the most likely pathologies (Table 1).

The clinical signs most commonly associated with oral cavity disease in the cat are listed in Box 1.

Box 1. Common clinical signs of oral pathologies in cats.

- Halitosis.
- Hypersalivation.
- Bleeding from the mouth.
- Touching their mouths.
- Dental hypersensitivity.
- Facial swelling.
- Sneezing.

- Nasal discharge.
- Change in eating habits.
- Reduced food intake.
- Behavioural changes, such as reduced grooming activity.

Table 1. Most frequent pathologies according to age.

Age of cat	Most common diseases
Kitten (up to 12 months)	Viral and bacterial infections Juvenile gingivitis Juvenile periodontitis Malocclusion Breed related tooth resorption (Middle Eastern, Persian breeds)
Adult (1–7 years)	Periodontal disease Tooth resorption FIV infections (feline immunodeficiency virus) Chronic gingivostomatitis Eosinophilic granuloma complex Acute renal failure with oral ulceration
Senior (over 7 years)	Periodontal disease Tooth resorption Oral tumours (squamous cell carcinoma) Chronic renal disease with ulcers

The oral examination should be divided into several stages:

1. General examination of the cat.
2. Oral examination of the awake cat.
3. Intraoral examination of the sedated cat.

General examination

A complete physical examination should cover the following points:

- **Cardiopulmonary auscultation**: some heart murmurs occur as a consequence of periodontal disease that generates pericarditis.
- **Liver and kidney** diseases may be associated with advanced periodontitis.
- Assessment of joints for possible appearance of infectious arthropathy associated with oral problems.
- **Dermatological examination** to evaluate possible allergies, intolerances, or infections associated with oral disorders.
- **Assessment of facial symmetry**, zygomatic arches, eye sockets, eyeballs (Figure 1).
- **Palpation of the face** to rule out muscle atrophy, areas of skin softening, localized inflammation.

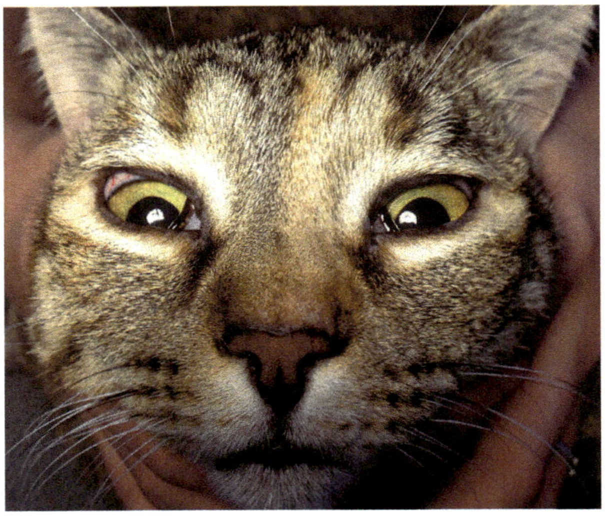

Figure 1. Evaluation of facial symmetry.

- **Examine the nostrils** for any unilateral or bilateral nasal secretions which may be related to maxillary teeth root abscesses that have caused an oronasal fistula.
- **Palpate the jaw and salivary glands**. The feline species has relatively large salivary glands compared to the dog. Paired glands include the parotid, mandibular, sublingual, and zygomatic glands; whilst some cats also have molar salivary glands. Part of the sublingual glands share common drainage with the mandibular salivary glands, at the base of the frenulum ligament.
- **Lymph nodes** should be palpated, although the salivary glands generally mask them.
- **Assess halitosis**, the main sign of oral disease, although it can also be associated with many other pathologies (Box 2).

Box 2. Pathologies that cause halitosis.

- Gingivitis, periodontitis.
- Dental resorption.
- Oral trauma.
- Bacterial infections (endodontic infections).
- Oral neoplasm.
- Viral diseases (Calicivirus, leukaemia virus and immunodeficiency).
- Oronasal fistulas.
- Upper respiratory tract diseases (chronic rhinitis, nasopharyngeal polyps, nasopharyngeal stenosis).
- Pharyngitis.
- Systemic oral ulcers secondary to kidney disease.
- Eosinophilic granuloma complex.
- Diabetes mellitus.
- Gastrointestinal problems that occur with vomiting and regurgitation.

Oral examination in the awake cat

The **entire oral cavity should be examined** including teeth and mucosa, internal structures, tonsils, oropharynx, and tongue. Sometimes it is difficult to perform this examination with the animal awake depending on its temperament or the pain associated with oral pathologies.

The following should be evaluated:

- **Dental occlusion of all teeth.** Assess whether dental occlusion is normal or abnormal. For the latter, assess if the malocclusion causes interference with the oral mucosa.
- **Number of teeth.** Kittens have 26 deciduous teeth and adults have 30 permanent teeth. Assess this number, assess their structure and the presence of possible pathologies or concurrent trauma. Also assess the positioning and placement of each tooth (Figure 2).
- **Internal structures** such as soft palate, mucoperiosteum of the hard palate, lips, tongue, caudal oral mucosa, and glossopalatine arch (Figure 3). Assess if there is inflammation of mucosa or any masses present. Where gingival mucosal inflammation is present assess if this is associated with contact with the teeth or other locations, which helps to differentiate between pathologies. Check also for ulcers and palatine fistula between the oral and nasal cavities.

At this point, it is essential to **record all findings in a detailed and orderly way**. For this a template with a detailed dentigram is very useful. This record should have a section to record the initial findings with additional sections to record how the lesions respond to treatment (Figure 4).

Examination of the sedated cat

To facilitate a thorough examination some patients require full anaesthesia with endotracheal intubation during the procedure. Should this be necessary, a **comprehensive pre-operative assessment** should take place.

As previously suggested, **evaluate the oral soft tissues** such as gingival mucosa, oral mucosa of the oropharynx and tongue; and the presence of **masses** (Figure 5).

A detailed **examination of each tooth** should be performed. A good knowledge of dental anatomy is necessary, in order to assess in detail what is normal and what is not. Special equipment (Figure 6) is required, such as a **curette and calibrated probe**, to study:

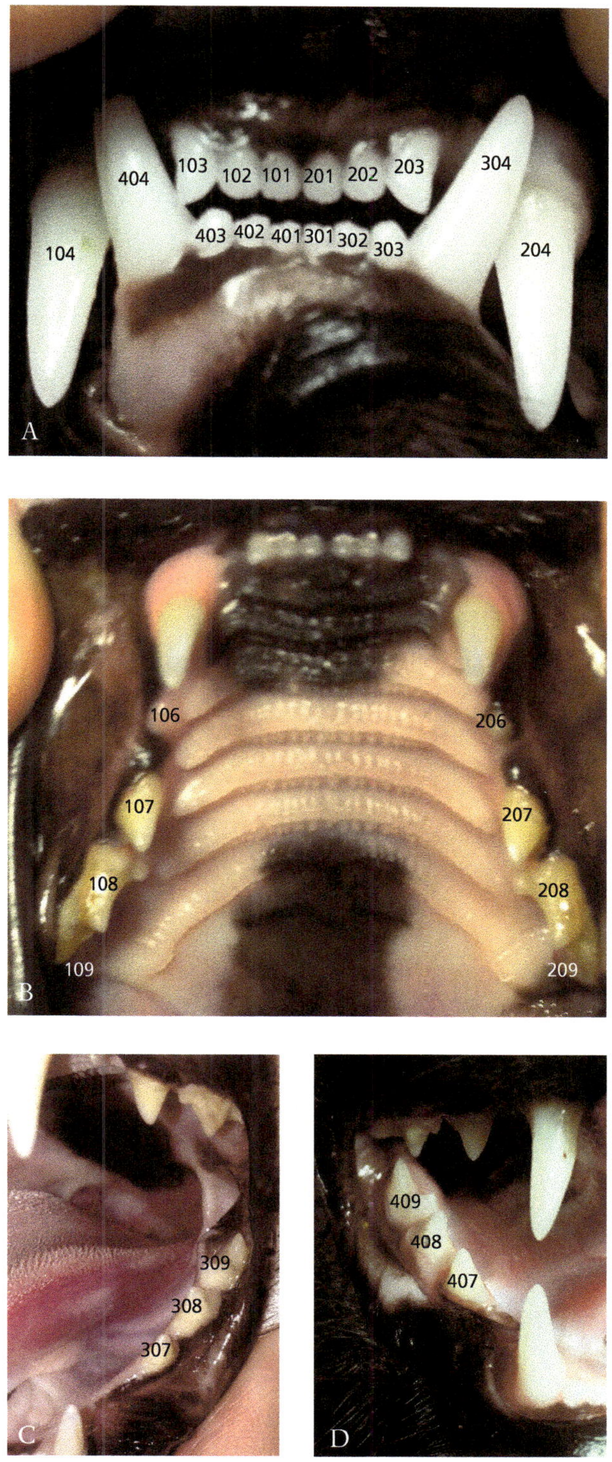

Figure 2. Teeth labelled according to the Triadan method adapted to cats.

- the **gingival margins** of each tooth
- the depth of any **gingival pockets**
- **retraction or hyperplasia** of the gingival mucosa
- the integrity of the **periodontal ligament**
- the possibility of **alveolar bone resorption**
- **Exposure of the furcation** (communication line between different roots in polyradicular teeth) and level of exposure
- **dental mobility**.

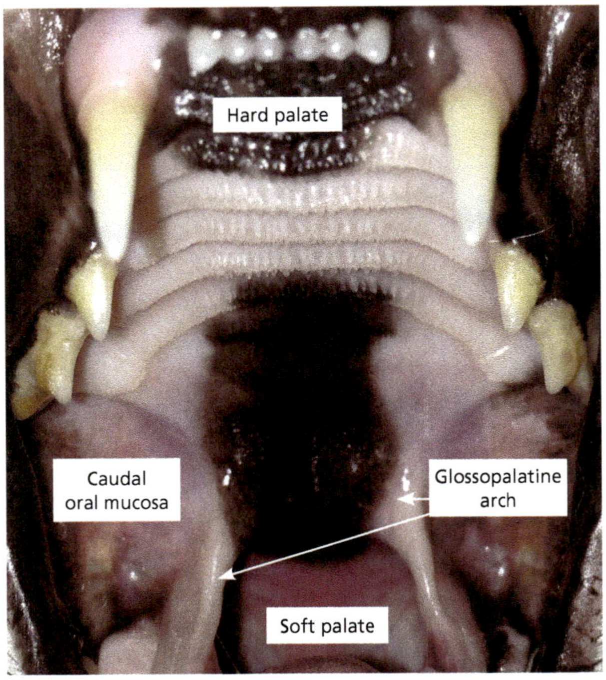

Figure 3. Areas of interest inside the mouth.

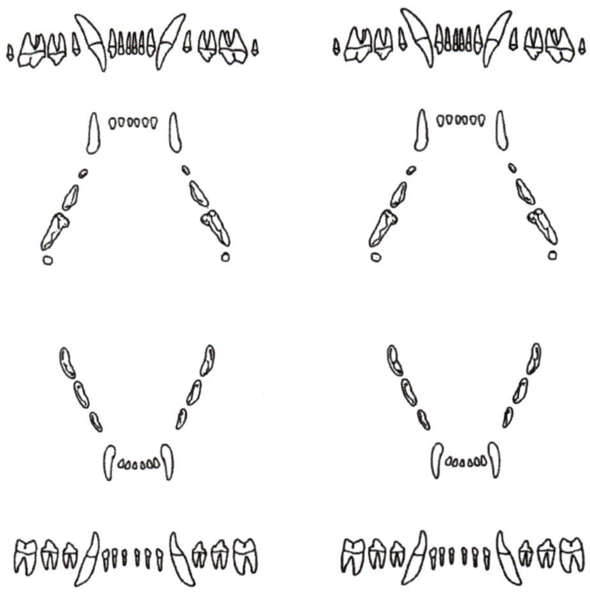

Figure 4. An example of a feline dental record for orderly annotation of findings on initial examination and progression after treatment.

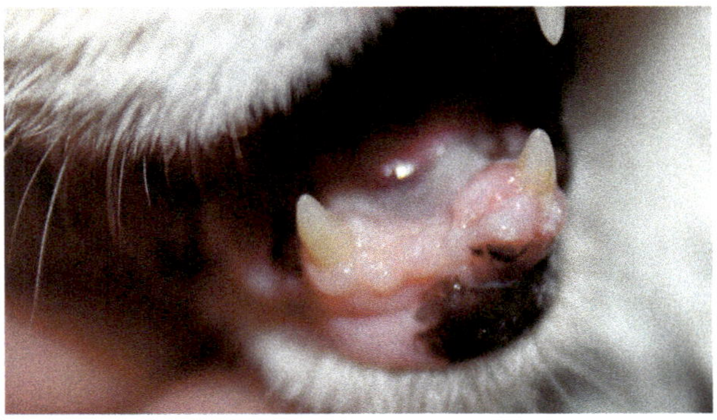

Figure 5. Rostral squamous cell carcinoma.

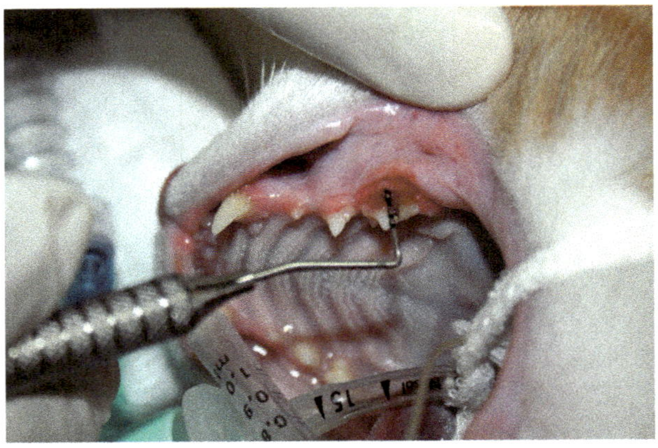

Figure 6. A graduated exploration probe.

This exam aims to determine the degree of progression of any pathological conditions and the viability of the tooth itself.

Advanced studies of the teeth are then performed, including intraoral radiographs (which are discussed in the next section).

If a mass or hyperplasia of the oral mucosa is detected, a sample should be taken for pathological examination.

All the information should be noted on the oral examination sheet along with any missing teeth. This allows for better re-evaluation when a treatment protocol is established.

Radiological examination

Radiography, including dental radiographs, is essential for both diagnosis and treatment. It allows for assessment of the nasal and frontal sinues, nasal cavity, and temporomandibular joint, along with assessment of the tooth roots and the alveolar bone in which they are encased.

Basic equipment consists of **conventional radiology equipment** which has the advantage of high image quality and safety levels due to less radiation dispersion. However, drawbacks include it being awkward to achieve good positioning and difficulty in interpreting images due to superimposed structures. Alternatively, **oral radiographic equipment** (Figure 7) offers the advantage of being comfortable to use with a **high range of movement** for superior positioning, and represents good value for money.

Radiographic films are screenless with different print speeds and are designated as D or E (Figure 8). There are several sizes, but in feline medicine the most widely used are size 0 for intraoral radiographs of premolars and mandibular and maxillary molars and size 2 for occlusal views of maxillary and mandibular canines, nasal sinuses and the temporomandibular joint (Figure 9).

Digital dental radiography devices can be used with radiological sensors of the appropriate size to perform

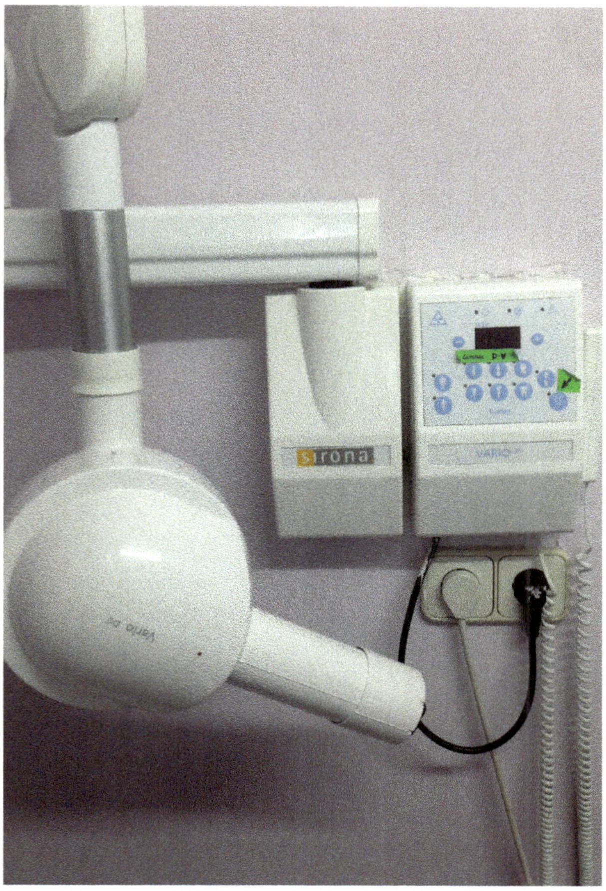

Figure 7. Specific dental radiology equipment.

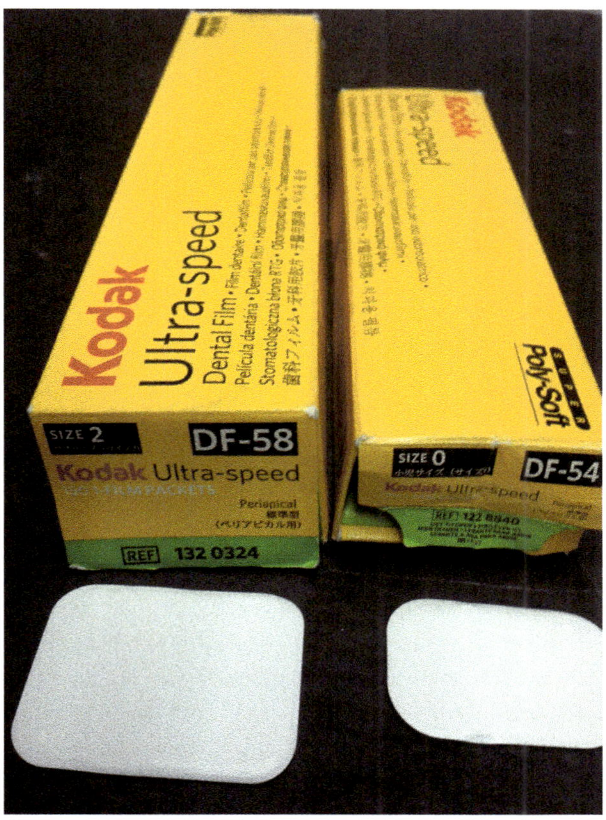

Figure 8. Radiographic films for manual development.

occlusal radiography. Drawbacks include difficulty obtaining intraoral premolar and molar radiographs, plus it is expensive equipment which is often double or triple the price of oral radiographic equipment. The author uses a combination of films with sizes such as those of conventional manual development, in a digital indirect radiography chassis which greatly reduces the cost of development (Figure 10).

Main oral diseases of the cat

In this chapter the main oral diseases in cats are described in order of frequency.

Periodontal disease

This is an **inflammatory condition affecting the periodontal ligament and the oral mucosa which covers the teeth** (gingival mucosa).

Aetiology and pathogenesis

In general, periodontal disease arises as a **consequence of dental plaque deposits**. In the natural state, dietary abrasion and the need to tear and cut animal protein delay plaque accumulation and therefore the development of periodontal disease. Currently, commercial feline diets are made to be convenient for both the cat and the owner and are thought to contribute to the development of the disease, although this has recently been questioned.

Dental plaque is initially an easily removable soft deposit, consisting of bacteria embedded in a biofilm made up of bacterial aggregates, food debris, inflammatory cell debris, and saliva. The **mineral composition of saliva** is responsible for plaque precipitating into a hard substance (tartar), which in turn favours further deposits of plaque.

Plaque formation can be induced by poor oral hygiene and other causes such as:

- poor occlusion
- loss of teeth
- inadequate diet
- decreased defences due to systemic disease (uraemia, diabetes, liver disease)
- viruses such as leukaemia, immunodeficiency, feline infectious peritonitis
- autoimmune diseases such as systemic or discoid lupus erythematosus
- the presence of other disorders in the mouth such as feline chronic gingivitis or feline eosinophilic complex.

Bacterial flora is a predisposing factor. The bacteria occupy all the structures of the mouth such as the tongue,

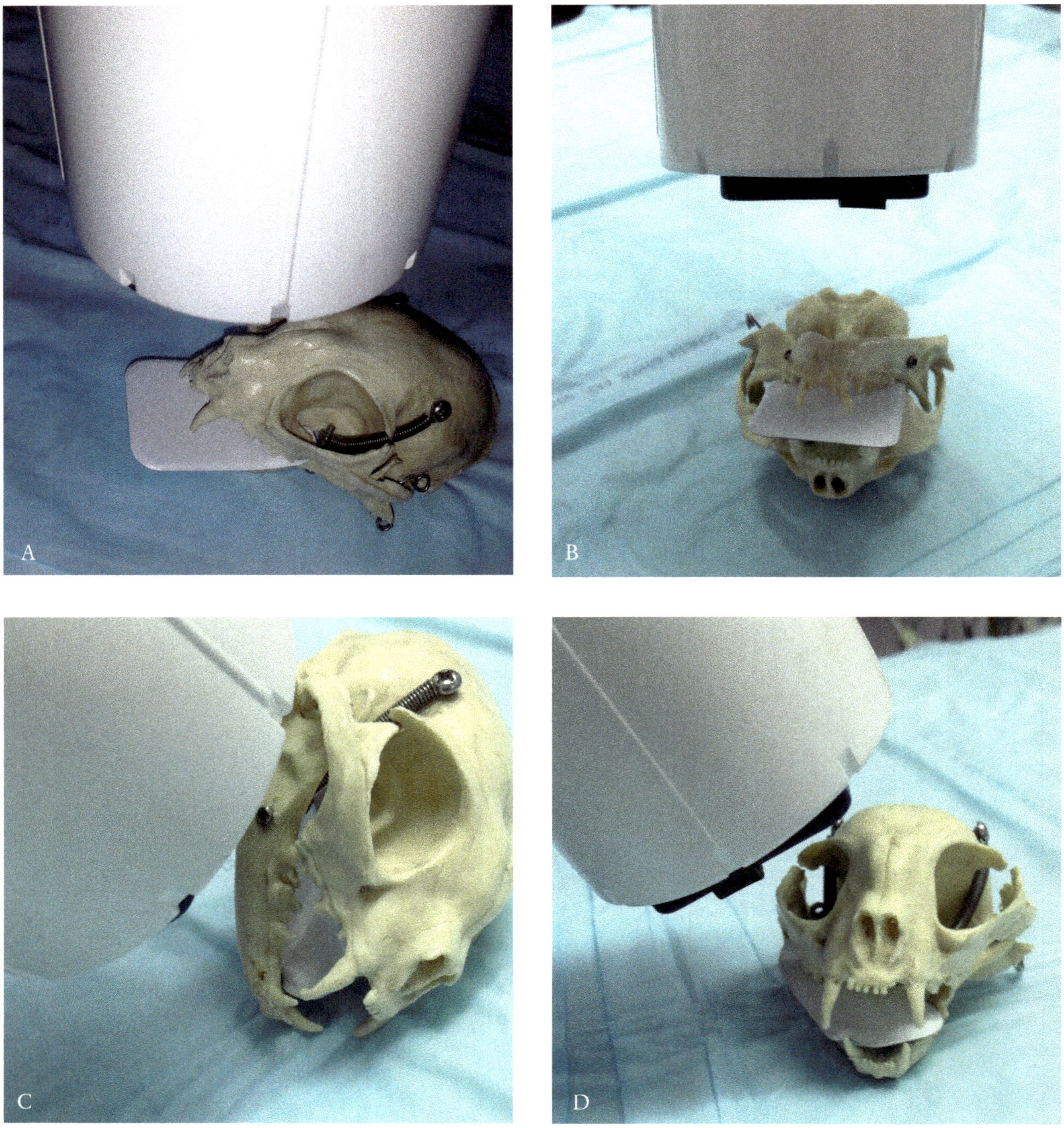

Figure 9. (A) Intraoral occlusal projection of maxillary incisors and canines.
(B) Intraoral occlusal projection of mandibular incisors and canines.
(C) Lateral intraoral projection of mandibular premolars and molars.
(D) Bisecting intraoral projection of maxillary premolars and molars.

gums, teeth and oral mucosa, although the greatest accumulation occurs on the surface of the teeth, especially at the gingival margin. This is where proteins from saliva and food first settle, forming an abundant film.

There are specific bacteria with properties that adhere to the film and these are responsible for perpetuating and causing the plaque to transform into calculus.

Some of the specific bacteria are those in the *Bacteroides spp.* group, *Pasteurella multocida*, but also *Streptococcus, Actinomyces, Lactobacillus, Clostridium porfphyromonas, Campylobacter* and *Fusobacterium*.

There is a gradation process for periodontitis:

1. **Gingivitis**: inflammation of the gum occurs (Figure 11), which is the oral mucosa that covers and protects the crown of the tooth. Swelling occurs with redness, bleeding and halitosis. It is evaluated as grade 0 if there is no bleeding after passing a cotton swab or grade 1, if there is bleeding. Gingivitis is reversible if plaque is removed and the animal has a normal immune response.

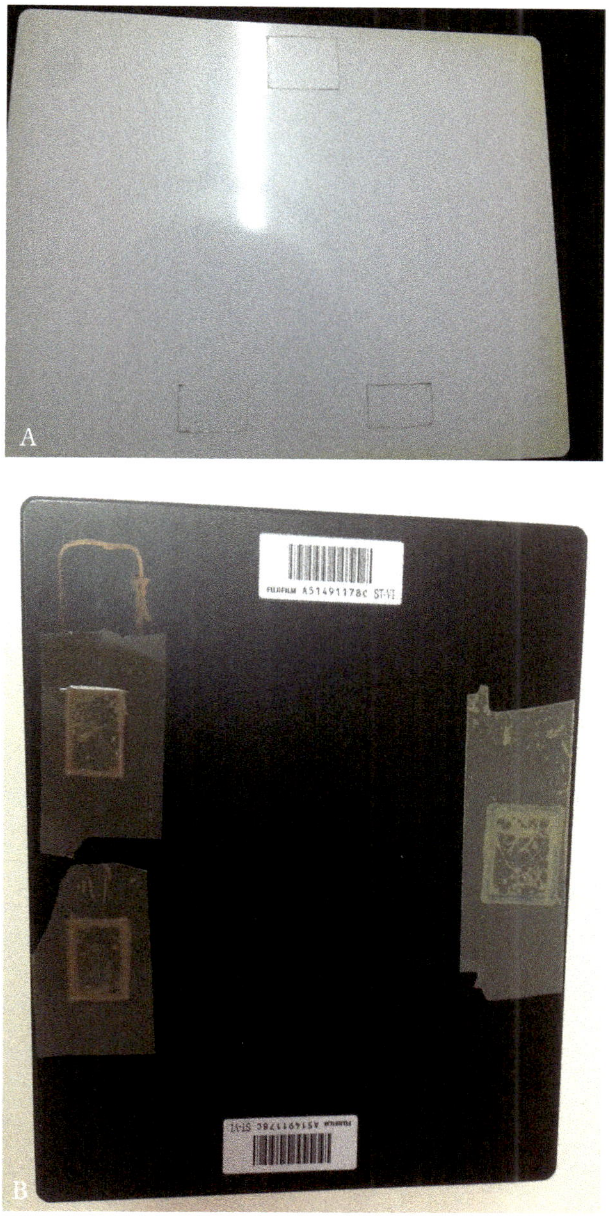

Figure 10. Developed film using indirect digital method where the appropriate size for intraoral radiographs has been marked out.

2. **Periodontitis**: the tooth is anchored in the jaw or maxilla by connective tissue called the periodontal ligament. Inflammation of this ligament weakens the attachment of the tooth to the alveolar bone and is called periodontitis.

   This causes a loss of bone and also of the gum, which leads to gingival retraction (Figure 12), and also the formation of gingival pockets between the tooth and the gum that enhances the accumulation of bacteria at the margin with the subsequent worsening of the disease, in addition to dental mobility.

In reality, these are similar conditions at different stages of development: **gingivitis is an inflammatory condition** induced by bacterial plaque at an early stage, while

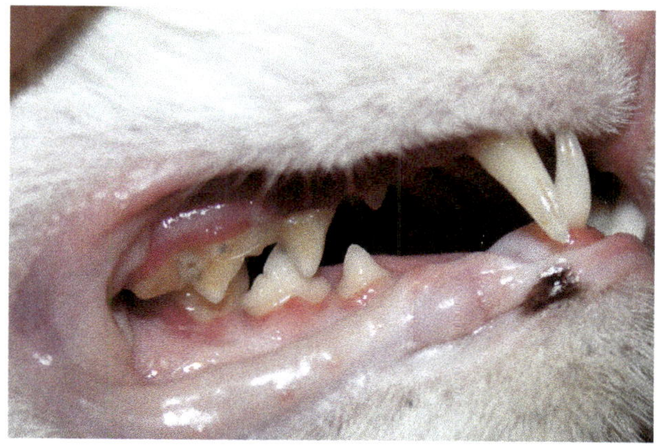

Figure 11. Mild gingivitis with minimum plaque accumulation which becomes tartar.

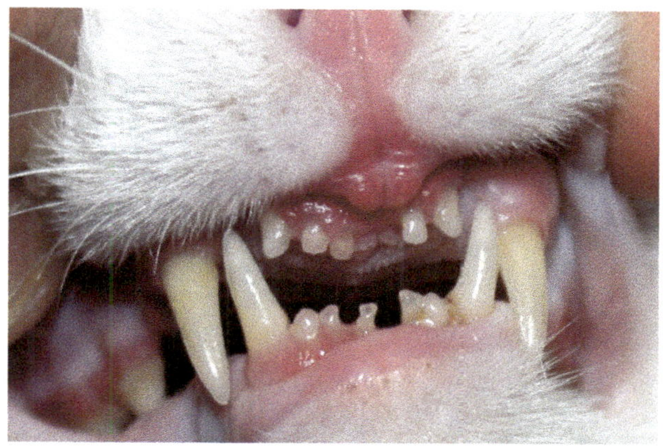

Figure 12. Advanced gingivitis around the incisors with the loss of some teeth.

periodontitis is a more established, chronic condition that indicates a more advanced phase and, on many occasions is irreversible.

Diagnosis

Furcation exposure is classified by various grades:

F1: On examination with a probe it is half the width of the tooth.
F2: Greater than half of the tooth.
F3: The probe crosses from the labial side to the lingual side of the tooth (Figures 13 and 14).

Dental mobility classification:

M0: less than 0.2 mm in any direction. Is physiological and not appreciable.
M1: 0.2–0.5mm.
M2: 0.5–1 mm.
M3: more than 1mm.

The greater degrees are visible to the naked eye.

Treatment

The first and most important step to managing the condition is to be aware of the **high incidence of**

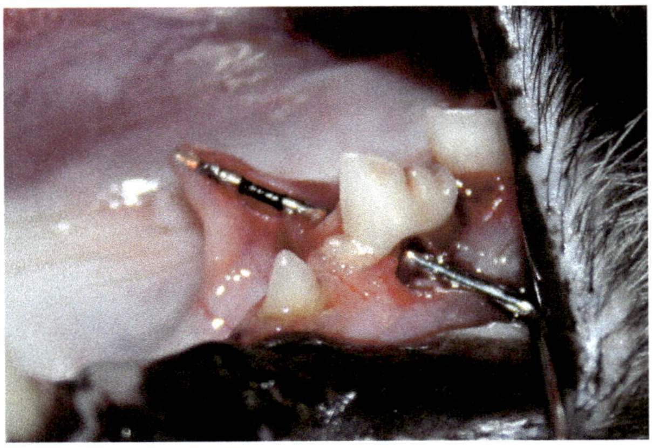

Figure 13. Maximum grade of furcation with severe gingival and alveolar retraction due to an advanced periodontitis.

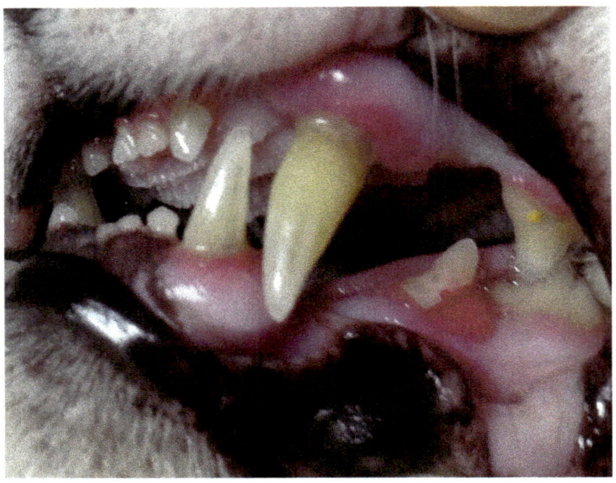

Figure 14. Severe periodontitis with gingival and alveolar retraction in a maxillary canine. A moderate dental resorption can also be seen in tooth 307.

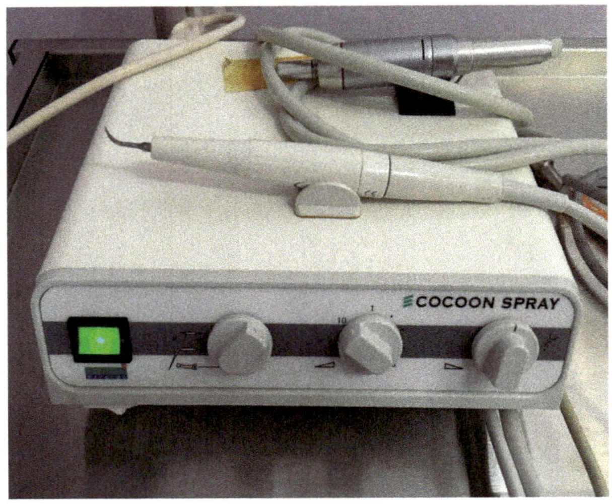

Figure 15. Basic dental equipment with ultrasound for dental cleaning and motor for polishing and cutting.

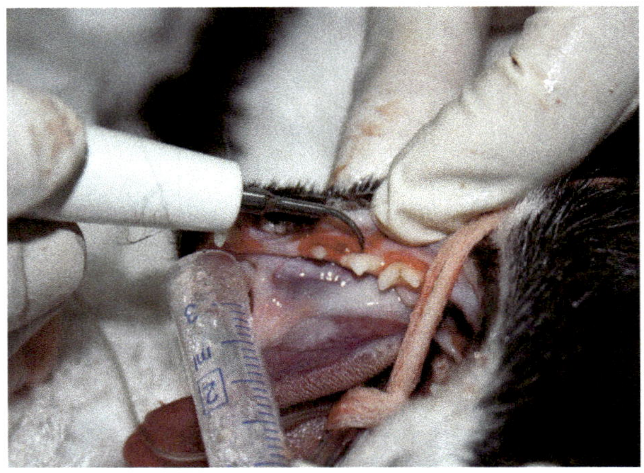

Figure 16. Professional dental cleaning with ultrasound.

periodontal disease in cats and check their mouths whenever there is the opportunity.

Tartar removal and buccal cleaning are essential for initial management of disease once present.

For ongoing oral care some cats tolerate the use of a toothbrush and brushing is effective if practiced regularly. **Pet toothpastes** must be used, as the fluoride content of human products is toxic to cats when swallowed. There are also commercial diets to help delay the accumulation of tartar, although their efficacy is controversial.

Application of **chlorhexidine gel** is the best possible antiseptic option to control bacterial colonization.

From a professional point of view, when the accumulation of tartar can no longer be removed by cleaning at home then dental cleaning with an **ultrasonic device** is required (Figure 15). **Subgingival curetting** is also performed (Figure 16) and subsequently polishing with abrasive substances at low speed is performed as a final step, cleaning the teeth. This polishing should always be performed.

Furthermore, if there is **gingival hyperplasia**, gingivoplasties or gingivectomies may be necessary.

The use of antibiotics is controversial. In principle antimicrobials should be useful to control the bacterial flora produced by the bacterial plaque, but their **continued use can produce resistance** and complicate matters.

Antibiotics such as ampicillin, amoxicillin or cephalosporins may be used prophylactically in teeth cleaning, oral surgery and dental extractions; but again their use is controversial with good technique preferred to prophylactic use. Therapeutic use must always be after a culture and antibiogram, however anaerobic microorganism cultures are difficult to grow. The most widely used antibiotics are clindamycin, metronidazole, and doxycycline.

However, if **gingival pockets of greater than 2 or 3 mm** are present, cleaning and removal of tartar will be insufficient, especially if there is bone loss and gingival retraction exposing the **dental furcation** (connection between the two roots of the same tooth).

These are both features that cause dental mobility. In these cases, **tooth extraction is appropriate**, before the teeth fall out by themselves with the risk of root retention and resulting pain.

Feline tooth resorption

Feline tooth resorption is described with other names, such as feline odontoclastic resorption. It used to be called "false feline caries" because of its radiographic and clinical similarity to human caries, but the difference is that in feline dental resorption, destruction of the hard part of the tooth by odontoclasts occurs, while human caries is produced by superficial bacterial toxins.

Destruction of the **dentin in permanent teeth occurs, especially at the cement-enamel junction, due to the activity of odontoclasts**. The latter are derived from haematopoietic stem cells from the bone marrow or spleen and migrate to the alveolar bone or periodontal ligament.

The incidence of the condition varies from **28% to 67%**, without a breed or sex predisposition, although it is known that resorption increases as cats age. In addition, there is a predisposition in certain teeth and, although it may be present in any, the most commonly affected teeth are **307 and 407** and it usually has a **symmetrical distribution**.

Aetiology and pathogenesis

The aetiology of this condition is not fully understood.

In the recent past it has been linked to excess vitamin D added to commercial diets, as the body is not able to synthesize this and formulation in the food is required. Several studies found cats with dental resorption to have elevated levels of 25 hydroxyvitamin D, compared to cats with no dental resorption. This was related to calcium metabolism, and the possibility of a relationship with chronic kidney disease was even raised. But in recent studies this relationship is not clear and **a link between excess vitamin D and dental resorption has not been established.**

Two types of resorption have been identified from a radiographic viewpoint:

- **Type 1**: in which the radiodensity of the root is normal and the periodontal ligament space can be appreciated.
- **Type 2**: in which there is radiolucency as a consequence of the loss of the periodontal ligament space.

This is of importance, as **type 1 is linked to a periodontal aetiology**, while type 2 is considered idiopathic.

A recent study (Thomas and Lappin, 2017) establishes a **clear relationship between the isolation of feline calicivirus by PCR**, the presence of chronic feline gingivitis, and feline dental resorption.

Diagnosis

Dental resorption gives rise to clinical symptoms such as **anorexia, ptyalism, and halitosis**. It can be very painful depending on the degree of involvement.

It is difficult to detect resorptive lesions by direct visualization until they have reached an advanced stage. This is because the initial areas of damage are often at the cement-enamel junction where inflamed gingival mucosa covers the tooth, which prevents the lesions from being visualized. Therefore, the ideal method when there are suspicions that tooth loss has occurred without just cause, are **dental radiographs** (Figure 17).

These allow us to assess all the structures of the tooth, but especially its root and its relationship with the alveolar bone that houses it, as well as structures such as the space between the tooth and the periodontal ligament. As degeneration progresses, the roots practically disappear.

Dental resorption can be classified according to stage, taking into account the clinical characteristics of the distribution of the lesions in combination with the radiological findings (Figure 18):

- **Stage 1**: slight loss of cement and enamel at the junction.
- **Stage 2**: moderate loss of enamel and cement. Dentin loss that does not reach the pulp cavity.
- **Stage 3**: profound loss of enamel and cement. Dentin loss that affects the pulp canal.
- **Stage 4**: extensive loss of enamel and cement. Dentin loss that affects the pulp canal. The crown may be affected as well as the root, or one or the other may be affected more.
- **Stage 5**: The destruction is such that there is a complete gingival covering. Remnants of cement, enamel, or dentin are visible radiographically.

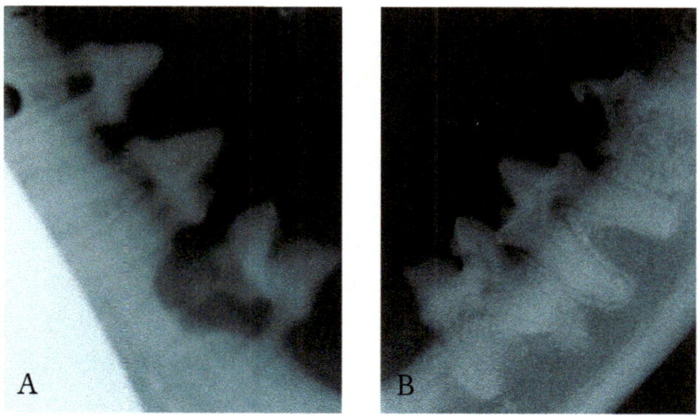

Figure 17. Radiographs of different teeth with dental resorption.

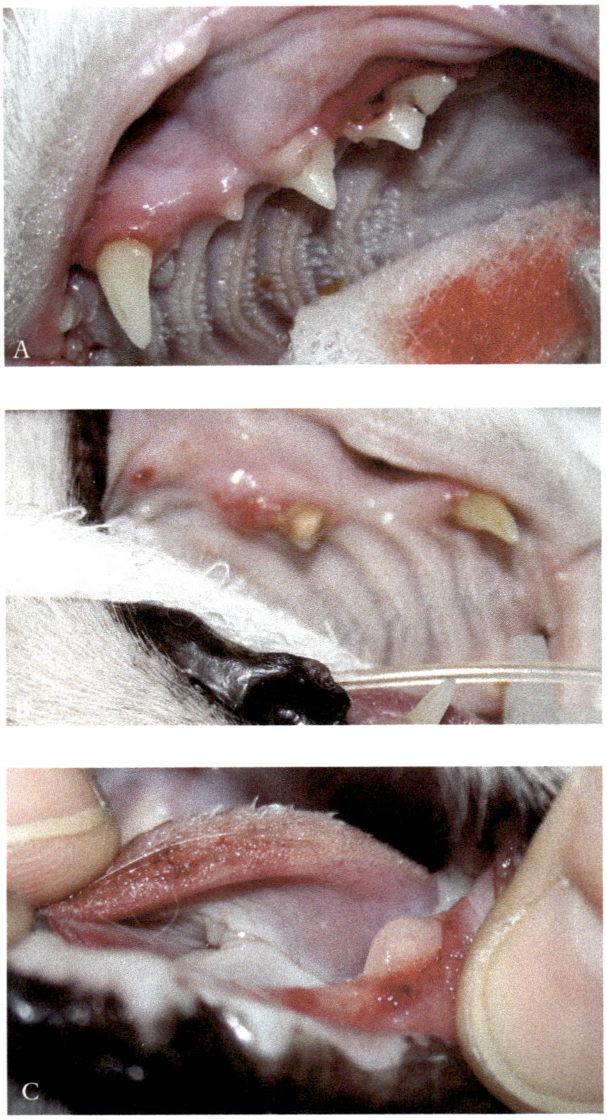

Figure 18. Dental resorption in various teeth and of different grades, even demonstrating their absence and different grades of recovering inflamed gums.

Treatment

Management of the condition should aim to relieve pain, halt the progress of resorption, and restore the tooth functionality. Fluorine and human medicine drugs for osteoporosis, such as alendronate have been used to attempt this, however, no significant improvements have been seen in the medium term. Reconstruction using endodontic methods has also been attempted, but resorption continues.

For type 2 resorptions, the possibility of crown amputation should be considered with a conjunctival covering flap. A possible complication of this is the appearance of root granulomas which then need additional procedures.

The treatment of choice is extraction, with this defined as the total extraction of the tooth, crown and root. It can be very difficult to extract the roots since sclerosis of the roots occurs with the alveolar bone.

Given that the cause of tooth resorption remains unknown, there is no clear recommendation that reduces the risk or prevents this disease, although good control of oral inflammation and periodontal disease is always recommended.

Feline chronic gingivostomatitis (FCGS)

Feline chronic gingivostomatitis is a disease that poses a therapeutic challenge on a day to day basis for the feline clinician. The condition has had many names, particularly describing the morphology of its lesions and pathological findings, leading to the following terms: chronic lymphoplasmacytic gingivitis, hyperplastic gingivostomatitis and proliferative ulcerative gingivostomatitis.

Aetiology and pathogenesis

FCGS is a multifactorial disease in which the host immune system responds inappropriately to stimuli created by antigens from different sources, both oral and non-oral.

Common findings associated with FCGS include **lymphocytic-plasmocytic infiltration and hypergammaglobulinaemia.** Associated dental problems such as periodontal disease and tooth resorption are chronic inflammatory conditions which may also play a role in the pathogenesis.

Factors involved in this complex condition include:

Infectious agents

Infectious agents play an important role, in addition to immune system abnormalities and the presence of periodontal disease.

Stress

In multi cat households and colonies, close contact between individuals facilitates the transmission of infectious agents and **stress contributes to lower levels of immunity**. In these environments the incidence of FCGS is higher.

Bacterial plaque and periodontal disease

This is probably the **most influential cause of FCGS**. The degree of oral inflammation is disproportionate to existing plaque deposition and periodontal disease, suggesting that factors related to the animal and immune system play an important role in FCGS.

Polyclonal gammopathy is due in part to the high load of oral anaerobic bacterial antibodies (Ab). Anaerobic bacteria found in oral cultures include *Bacteroides spp., Eikenella corredeus, Fusobacterium spp., Peptostreptococcus spp.* or *Clostridium spp.*, and aerobic flora include *Pasteurella multocida, Streptococcus spp. Lactobacillus spp., E. coli* and spirochetes.

Feline calicivirus (FCV)

According to various studies **70–80% of cats** with chronic inflammatory conditions (of more than 6 months of duration) in the oral cavity are **positive for FCV** isolated from the oropharynx. FCV has been shown to be a cause of ulcerative glossitis and palatine inflammation, in addition to acute upper respiratory tract diseases.

The role of FCV in FCGS is not fully understood, but it may facilitate the penetration of other agents causing damage to the cell membrane. However, other factors are necessary for FCGS to occur, since 30% of the population is estimated to be carrying FCV (Zicola, 2009).

Attempts have been made to induce caudal stomatitis with oropharyngeal samples from animals affected with caudal stomatitis, but this has not been reproducible in all animals.

With the development of PCR, it has been shown that only 30% of cats with calicivirus have FCGS.

However, a recent study at the time of writing this chapter (Rolim et al., 2017) found no relationship between FCGS and the presence of FCV.

Feline leukaemia and immunodeficiency viruses (FeLV-FIV)

Studies on the relationship of FCGS with FeLV/FIV are from 1989, when the incidence of retroviruses was higher and these indicated that 15% of cats with FCGS were positive for FeLV or FIV.

Currently, the levels are lower, although cats in the immunosuppression phase caused by **FIV may have secondary infections and medical management should be undertaken with this in mind**. Feline infectious leukaemia and immunodeficiency viruses (FeLV, FIV) contribute to the disease becoming established by preventing the immune system from responding appropriately to dental plaque.

Although feline leukaemia virus positive cats develop gingivitis or stomatitis (presumably due to immunosuppression secondary to infection), infection with FeLV is not associated with an increased prevalence of oral lesions. In addition to the immunosuppression that it causes, it can favour a hyper-reactive response by the immune system, leading to the presentation of immune mediated diseases with the formation of antigen-antibody complexes that possibly have a role in FCGS.

Evidence of feline immunodeficiency virus (FIV) as the causative agent or co-agent is also unclear, although epidemiological studies indicate a relationship. Some cats with chronic stomatitis are FIV positive, and oral inflammation is the most common clinical symptom in FIV positive cats. By contrast, **only 15% of cats with severe FCGS have FIV**.

Immune system

50% of cats with FCGS have polyclonal hypergammaglobulinaemia compared to normal cats. The immune response of animals that do not have FCGS is from T Helper type 1 (Th1) lymphocytes, whereas in animals with FCGS there is a mixed immune response with Th1 and Th2 that indicates that there is a poor cellular and humoral immune response.

On immunohistochemical tests performed on mucosal biopsies of animals affected with FCGS, it was found that the proportion of CD8+ is much higher than that of CD4+, which is indicative of a highly destructive cytotoxic immune system response, making it compatible with a viral aetiology.

Systemic diseases

The health of the oral mucosa depends on the balance between the bacterial flora of the mouth and the immune system. A systemic disease alters immunity and, in turn, the bacterial flora, a factor that contributes to the establishment, progression and persistence of bacterial plaque and therefore to periodontal disease with the appearance of oral inflammation.

Often these are animals that have had growth problems with respiratory infections and are below average litter size.

Diagnosis

The first thing that stands out is the incidence data. It is considered a common syndrome, but the documented incidence is 3% of all dental disease in cats, with a **breed predisposition in the Abyssinian, Somali and Persian cats.**

A 2007 study (Healey et al., 2007) showed that the prevalence of CFGS in veterinary first opinion centres was only 0.3% of the animals that came for consultations, with no sex, age or very marked breed predisposition.

Clinicians should be able to differentiate different dental pathologies in order to correctly address each problem.

CFGS is characterized by severe, persistent inflammation and/or ulceration, of more than 6 months duration, of the soft tissues in the oral cavity, including both the gingival mucosa that covers the teeth and non-gingival tissues and, occasionally, of the mucosa lateral to the **glossopalatine arch, pharynx, tongue, and caudal oral mucosa** (Figures 19 and 20).

Histologically, there is a polyclonal plasma cell infiltrate and a lymphocytic infiltrate in oral lesions, producing polyclonal hypergammaglobulinaemia with

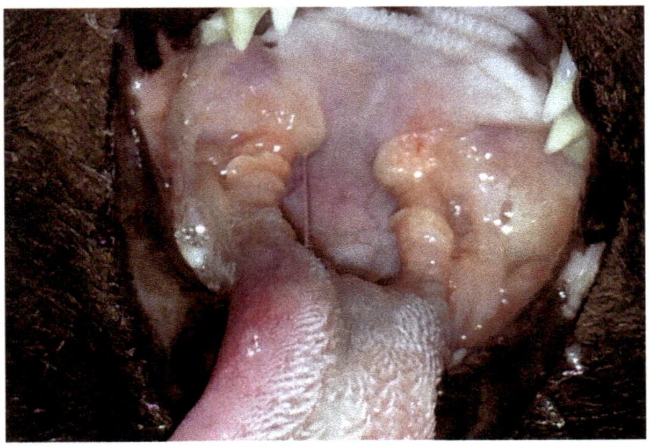

Figure 19. Cat with chronic feline gingivitis where severe mucosal inflammation can be seen that does not cover the teeth as in the case of caudal oral mucosa and the glossopalatine arch.

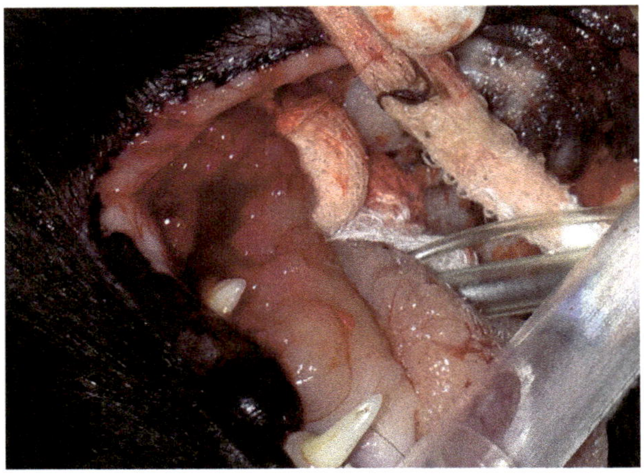

Figure 20. Severe inflammation and necrosis of the oral caudal mucosa in a cat with chronic feline gingivitis.

notable increases in immunoglobulins (Ig) IgM, IgG and also IgA.

This is an extremely painful condition.

Tests that assist the diagnostic approach

- The development and standardization of the polymerase chain reaction (PCR) technique has recently allowed easy detection of viruses such as **FeLV, calicivirus (FCV) and herpesvirus type 1 (FHV).** For FIV serology is used, since in Europe there is still no vaccination programme.
- As for the presence of bacteria, the test of choice is **aerobic and anaerobic culture**. A high proportion of *Pasteurella multocida* is recorded (Dolieslager, 2010).
- **Complete blood count and biochemistry** should be taken into account to detect any other systemic disease. 10% of cats with CFGS have chronic kidney disease. It is important to plan treatment based on underlying diseases, especially to decide on anaesthetic protocols or long-term treatments with NSAIDs.
- **Biopsy of the gingival mucosa** should be performed when the extent, appearance, or severity of the lesion is unusual. It is important to perform biopsies on non-symmetrical lesions, to rule out squamous cell carcinomas, lymphomas or other neoplasia. The result of the biopsy concludes with diagnosis of lymphoplasmacytic infiltration and this is absolutely non-specific, since it only indicates chronic inflammation of the mouth.
- A thorough **dental evaluation** must be undertaken, including**: dental examination and radiology of all teeth, present or not.**

Management of chronic feline gingivitis

There are no controlled efficacy studies of different treatments that can provide objective data on which to base standard therapeutic recommendations.

A gradual approach should be used that is implemented bit by bit, aiming to improve the cat's clinical signs.

A baseline treatment should be established to reduce oral antigen in all cases and an initial line of treatment should be established.

Most of the **treatments used in this disease aim to reduce inflammation and pain**, thus reducing discomfort and enabling the correct feeding of the animal.

Control of bacterial plaque

Tartar removal is beneficial, but only in the short term, unless it is followed by frequent and **effective home care**.

In patients with juvenile gingivitis, it is important that during their first years of life they have minimum exposure to bacterial plaque and any anatomical defects which promote plaque and tartar formation are resolved as soon as possible. This can involve **professional cleaning every three months** to minimize this exposure to bacterial plaque as much as possible and, as a result, there is less inflammation of the oral mucosa and the immune system is less active.

Control of other dental diseases

The clinical criteria (including partial extractions) should be followed for the management of dental diseases such as periodontal disease and dental resorption.

Analgesics

Opioids and non-steroidal anti-inflammatory drugs (NSAIDs) in the pre- and postoperative period: buprenorphine, meloxicam or gabapentin, among others.

Control of inflammation

For many years steroids have been widely used as an effective way of managing inflammation, but currently **steroid use is discouraged**. This is due to the existence of caliciviruses, since in the medium term steroids produce greater viral replication and eventual worsening of lesions.

The **use of NSAIDs in the short, medium and long term** is preferred.

Supportive treatment

Depending on individual needs vitamins, fatty acids and a special recovery diet can be administered. Placement of an oesophagostomy tube after surgery may be indicated in very weak cats to aid recovery after tooth extraction.

Antibiotics

Antibiotic treatment is recommended for a significant period of time, to reduce bacterial load in the mouth, and reduce inflammation and discomfort. Antibiotics should be used preoperatively and postoperatively for a minimum of 8–10 days. Common medications include:

- Clindamycin: 11–22 mg/kg once daily
- Amoxicillin/clavulanate: 12.5 mg/kg twice daily

The use of metronidazole at doses of 10–15 mg/kg every 12 hours, and fluoroquinolones such as marbofloxacin at doses of 2 mg/kg per day have also been documented.

Sometimes the use of pulse treatments is preferred for a certain timeframe followed by waiting periods.

Complete extraction and selective extraction

Complete tooth extraction is described as the treatment of choice and the trend is for this to be undertaken early and not left as a last resort treatment.

The statistics for this technique are (Girard, 2005):

- 50–60% of the cats were completely cured (Figure 21A).
- 27–33% improved markedly but required subsequent anti-inflammatory management.
- 7–13% were refractory to tooth extraction, with no improvement or only in the area of the gingival and oral mucosa in contact with the teeth and not in the caudal oral mucosa and glossopalatine arch (Figure 21B).

In these cases, it is important to carry out **post-extraction radiographic studies** since retained roots continue to cause an antigenic and inflammatory stimulus to the immune system, meaning lesions do not resolve satisfactorily.

Other anti-inflammatory or immunomodulatory treatments, evaluation of studies based on their safety and usefulness for CFGS

Recombinant feline omega interferon

Results from a three-year, double-blinded, randomized study (Hennet, 2010) with 39 cats positive for FCV and

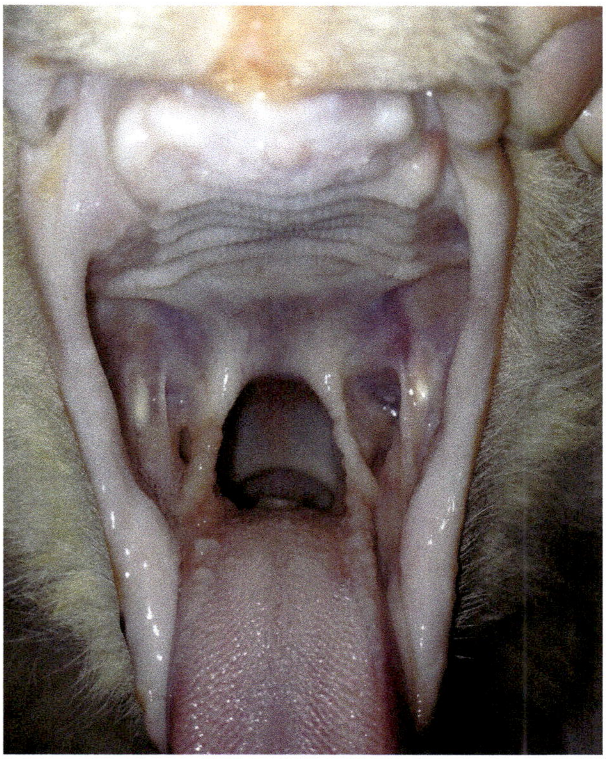

Figure 21. (A) Cat after complete exodontics where resolution of all the signs of inflammation in all areas of the mouth can be seen.

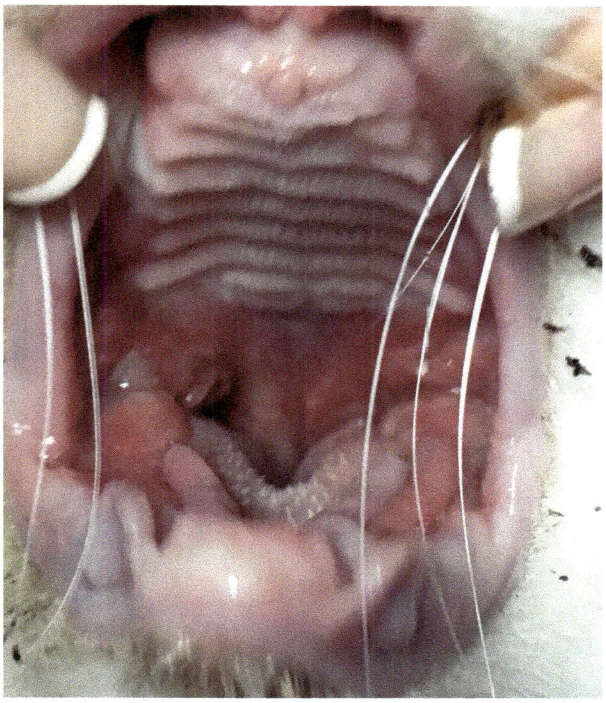

Figure 21. (B) Partial resolution of the signs of inflammation in a cat with chronic gingivitis after complete exodontics, where the resolution of signs can be appreciated in areas of mucosa which cover the teeth but not around the glossopalatine arch and in the caudal oral mucosa.

with an unfavourable response to selective extraction, found that **interferon therapy provided a better level of well-being** than other treatments, including corticosteroid treatment.

Oral use

- 10 MU (million units) are injected into 100 ml of 0.9% saline.
- This is divided into 10 ml aliquots and frozen. It can remain frozen for 1 year and in a refrigerator at 4°C for 21 days.
- Administer 1 ml/cat/day for three months orally.

Initial intralesional use

The consensus established in October 2010 by the European Veterinary Dental Society indicates that intralesional treatment is not necessary to initiate treatment, as was advised by the brand marketing the recombinant feline omega interferon.

In this study with calicivirus-positive cats suffering from FCGS with caudal stomatitis refractory to complete extraction, the results of interferon treatment was compared with that of oral or depot corticosteroids. Both treatments greatly decrease inflammation. However, cats treated with prednisolone had a reduction in inflammation followed by a rebound effect, while **animals treated with interferon were more stable and enjoyed a longer period without reappearance of symptoms.**

Hennet recommends a calicivirus test in cats with chronic gingivostomatitis refractory to complete tooth removal. In positive cats, treatment with feline omega interferon, antibiotics, and anti-inflammatories is advised.

Immunosuppressive therapy

Corticosteroids are the drug of choice, both for their anti-inflammatory and immunomodulatory effects, and are the treatment of choice in cases refractory to tooth extraction.

An alternative could be **chlorambucil or cyclophosphamide** although results of the studies are still inconclusive, as with the use of cyclosporin A.

Cellular treatments

The use of **mesenchymal stem cells (MSC)** is being implemented in both human and veterinary medicine. This is one of the mainstays in research for the management of immune-based diseases.

These **mesenchymal stem cells are mostly obtained from the patient's own fat**, where autologous MSCs (Arzi et al., 2016) are found. Their use in medicine is promising, although larger studies are still lacking.

Evaluation questionnaire for the management of the FCGS

Use of the FCGS activity questionnaire:

- It should be done regularly by the same person if possible and accompanied by photos.
- Any changes to the treatment protocol should be reported and re-evaluated within a week of starting the new treatment.
- The first two questions should be answered by the owner.
- The maximum score is 33, which corresponds to the worst clinical situation that can be found.

Patient information
Weight:
Diet:
Date:

CFGS activity index	Score (0–3)
Appetite[1]	
Activity[2]	
Grooming[3]	
Perception of comfort[4]	
Inflammation of buccal maxilliary mucosa[5]	
Inflammation of buccal mandibular mucosa[-5]	
Inflammation of maxilliary gums[5]	
Inflammation of mandibular gums[5]	
Inflammation lateral to the glosopalatine arch[5]	
Inflammation of the molar salivary gland[5]	
Oropharyngeal inflammation[5]	
TOTAL (maximum =33)	

1 Appetite: 0 = eats normally, 1 = eats dry food, but less than normal, 2 = only wet food, 3 = does not eat well, only when hand fed.
2 Level of activity: 0 = normal activity and plays, 1 = plays spontaneously, 2 = low level of activity, but plays occasionally when stimulated, 3 = not interested in people or other pets and spends most of the time asleep.
3 Grooming: 0 = normal grooming, 1 = overgrooming, 2 = occasional grooming but less than before, 3 = no grooming at all.
4 Comfort: score as 0 for maximum level of comfort and 3 for minimum.
5 Inflammation: 0 = none, 1 = mild, 2 = moderate, 3 = severe.

This questionnaire can be downloaded and printed for clinical use from:

http://publication.improveinternational.com

They have the ability to repair damaged tissues, as well as an immunomodulatory capacity. MSC inhibit the proliferation of T cells and alter the functionality of B cells.

The advantage is they have low immunogenicity, with **few side effects.** The disadvantage is the processing of the adipose tissue sample, which has to be extracted from the animal itself and has a culture and preparation time before treatment, which makes it expensive.

A 2016 study showed that MSC treatment of cases that were refractory to other treatments after complete tooth extraction had an **80% success rate**, with clinical sign free times of up to 48 months.

To do this, the same research group presented a study (Arzi et al., 2017) on the use of allogeneic MSC, which allowed for greater availability of cultures, with better quality control and at a much lower price. But the results were worse in terms of control of clinical signs, with only 50% of cats treated responding partially. It is thought that this was a consequence of immunogenic responses being initiated with antibody development, which disables stem cells.

New studies will appear in the near future which will further clarify the effectiveness of using MSC.

Dental extraction

As highlighted throughout this chapter, **tooth extraction is a treatment of choice** in some clinical situations and should not be considered as a rescue technique saved for when nothing else is working.

It is important to have visual 'before and after' materials to show owners so they can see the results of the extractions. On many occasions they have unwarranted fears, and it is important for them to see how the quality of life of these animals increases in the immediate postoperative period.

It is an aggressive surgical practice, which must be **carried out by experienced personnel**, since the small size of cats' mouths can cause a high percentage of complications, which will be detailed at the end of this section.

The indications for performing extraction include:

- severe periodontitis
- dental resorption
- FCGS
- complex dental fractures
- endodontic disease
- malocclusion.

Extractions are discouraged where local tumours are present due to the possibility **of spread of cancer cells** and in advanced and debilitating systemic diseases, also due to the possibility of haematogenous spread of microorganisms.

Equipment needed for dental extractions

The special equipment needed to perform extractions is not sophisticated or expensive.

Mouth openers are required, but many gag-type mouth openers designed for use in cats compress the flow of the maxillary artery with the consequent postoperative complication of the appearance of muscle weakness due to ischaemia and neurological disorders and may be permanent. A simple alternative is the use the cap of a needle as a mouthpiece between lower and upper canines on the same side (Figure 22).

Other instruments necessary for the extraction will be: different types of exploration probes, motor for cutting blade, which if possible, should be contra-angle, different types of drills and of different materials to fracture dental crowns, to drill in alveolar bone, to file alveolar bone, root elevators and dislocators for the periodontal ligament and extraction forceps for different sides, both angled and straight.

Anaesthesia and analgesia in exodontics

Exodontia has specific considerations for both anaesthesia and analgesia.

Any tooth extraction is a surgical procedure and requires appropriate protocols to achieve a deep anaesthetic plane and endotracheal intubation is always required. Some animals present in unfavourable circumstances, with a deteriorated body condition as a consequence of the dental pathology. For these patients a detailed pre-anaesthetic evaluation is essential and if necessary they should be managed conservatively to improve their health prior to the procedure.

Regardless of the general state of the animal, and because tooth extraction is a painful procedure,

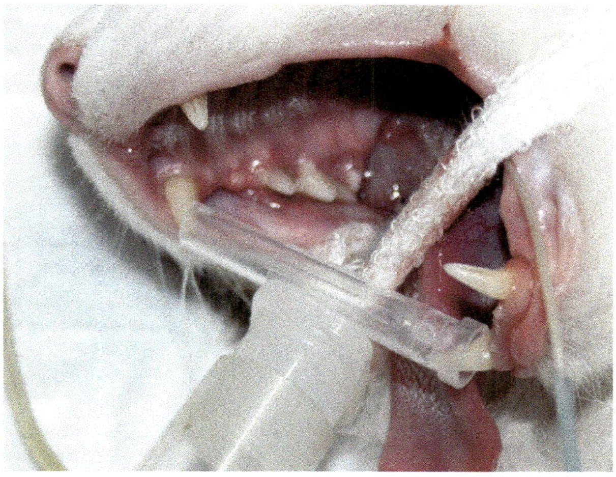

Figure 22. Home-made mouth opener using the protective cover from a needle.

multimodal anaesthetic and analgesic protocols should be considered, with the use of various drugs to achieve the following goals: hypnosis, muscle relaxation and analgesia, ideally using low doses to reduce the probabilities of complications during the procedure.

The use of **pure μ-receptor agonist opioid analgesics**, for both induction and maintenance, is highly necessary.

Anaesthetic blocks with local anaesthetic agents are essential in these cases. 2% lidocaine or 2% bupivacaine should be used, taking their toxic dose levels into account. Knowing the time each product needs to take effect and the duration of action is important.

For mandibular blocks:

- Rostrally, the middle mental foramen acting on the inferior alveolar nerve between 304 or 404 and 307 or 407 (Figure 23A) can be used.
- Caudally, the mandibular foramen on the lingual side of the body of the mandible (Figure 23B) can be used.

For maxillary blocks:

- The infraorbital foramen is used for the rostral and medial areas (Figure 23C).
- For caudal areas, the palatine foramen is used (Figure 23D).

Local anaesthesia can also be used in the mucosa and mucoperiosteum of each tooth.

Points of special attention with regards to anaesthesia for exodontia surgery include:

- **Fluid therapy** in general for surgeries should be prudent and not extrapolate rates of administration of dogs for cats. **It should not exceed 3–4 ml/kg/hour.**
- **Prevent movement of the endotracheal tube** in order to avoid trauma to the trachea. It must be fixed in the most effective way possible since it is easily moved when handling the structures of the mouth. Where it is foreseen that it is impossible to avoid tube movement then a **temporary tracheostomy** to maintain the airway should be considered.
- Never use endotracheal tubes without a Murphy hole, in order to avoid anoxia if the tube is bent.
- Prevent aspiration of material into the airway by **covering the pharyngeal inlet with soft material (cotton gauze, foam)** taking care to remove it at the end of the procedure.
- **Lubricate the balloon of the endotracheal tube** so that the airway can be sealed with less inflation of the balloon, thus preventing further trauma to the trachea.
- **Prevent hypothermia.** Oral procedures are accompanied by the use of irrigation fluids to perform continuous washing and dissipate heat when using cutting tools. Use surgical vacuum cleaners and keep animals as dry as possible in addition to providing heat by safe methods.

Surgical tooth extraction technique

With surgical extractions the first thing, as in any surgery, is to prepare a clean surgical field, which in this case is by **ultrasonic mouth cleaning**.

There are two different techniques for performing tooth extractions, each with different indications.

Closed extraction technique

A closed extraction technique may be used when only a few teeth require extraction.

For **single-root teeth,** the **periodontal ligament luxator** is inserted between the crown and the gum until the ligament is ruptured. Only when there is sufficient mobility should dental forceps be used for extraction. It should be remembered that single-rooted teeth are small and often anchored to the alveolar bone, but they are fragile and the use of excessive force may break the roots. Care and patience are required in order to cleanly extract the tooth without leaving root fragments in the bone.

For **polyradicular teeth the crown of the tooth is sectioned** with a high-speed diamond bur. Then each section of crown with its corresponding root is extracted, as for a single-root tooth.

For **canines**, an incision must be made in the vestibular mucosa to cut the alveolar bone that covers the root (Figure 24). Subsequently, the periodontal ligament is ruptured from the lingual side of the tooth with a luxator until there is movement and it can be extracted with forceps (Figure 25).

Open extraction technique

Open extraction techniques are used when extensive or total extractions are required. This is a more conventional surgery than simple tooth extraction.

The technique involves creating **mucosal flaps in order to expose the alveolar bone on the labial side** (Figure 26). A bur is used to cut the bone overlying each tooth root, which requires a detailed knowledge of anatomy and the number of roots for each tooth. Next, the periodontal ligament is mobilized for each tooth root with a luxator from the lingual side for subsequent extraction with forceps (Figure 27).

The open technique is controversial since large incisions are required which by definition will be contaminated. Although proper planning and good technique substantially reduce the risk of complications.

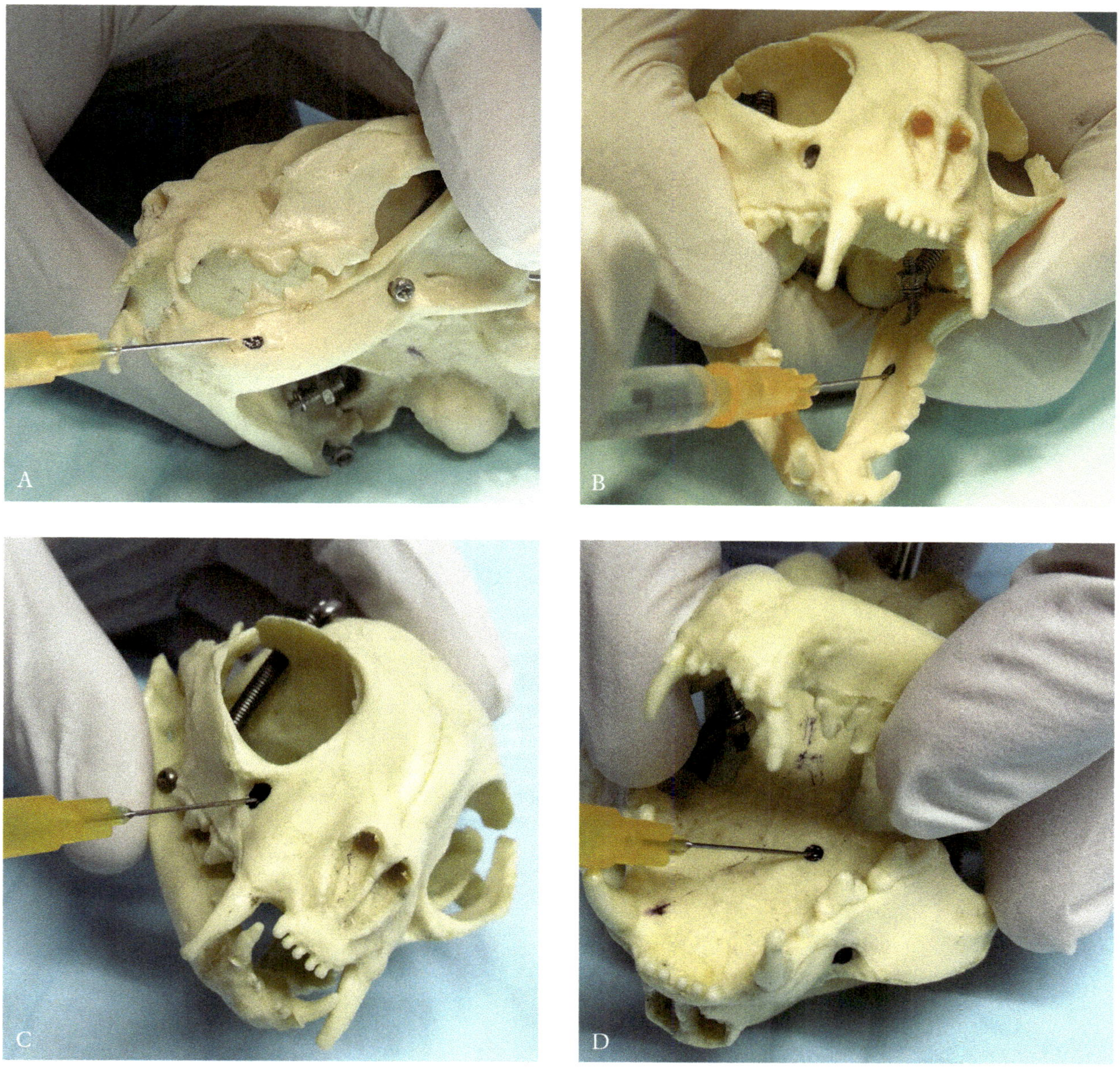

Figure 23. (A) Medial mandibular mental foramen. Site for injection of local anaesthesia for mandibular block. (B) Mandibular block on the lingual side of the mandibular foramen. (C) Rostral, medial maxillary block of the infraorbital foramen. (D) Palatine foramen for the caudal maxillary block.

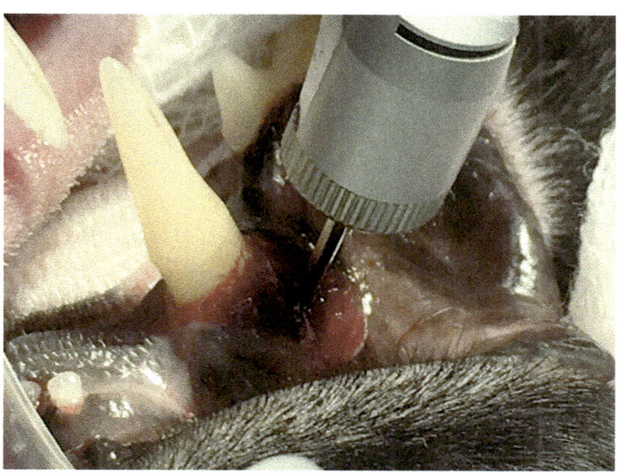

Figure 24. Cutting of alveolar bone on the labial aspect of a canine to allow visualisation of the root and better mobilisation of the periodontal ligament.

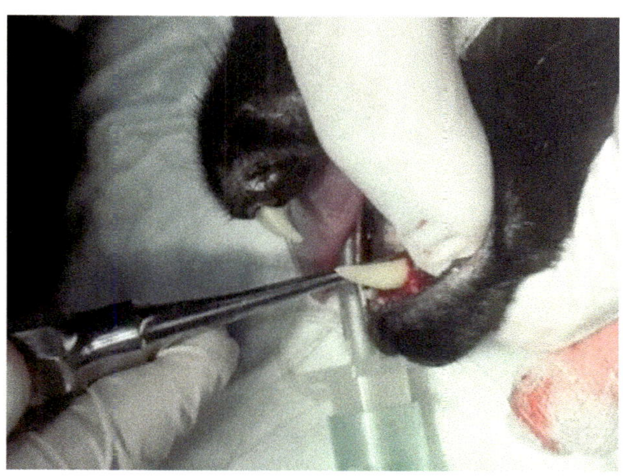

Figure 25 Video of the final process of extraction of the canine in the previous image. (Complete sequence at: http://publication.improveinternational.com).

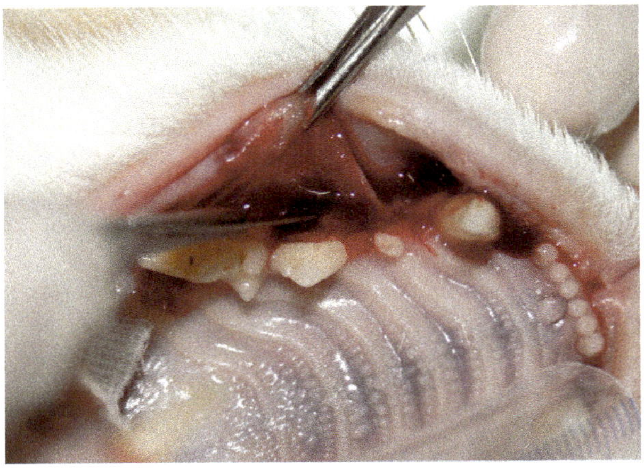

Figure 26. Creation of a flap using gingival mucosa to expose the labial aspect of the alveolar bone which covers the roots.

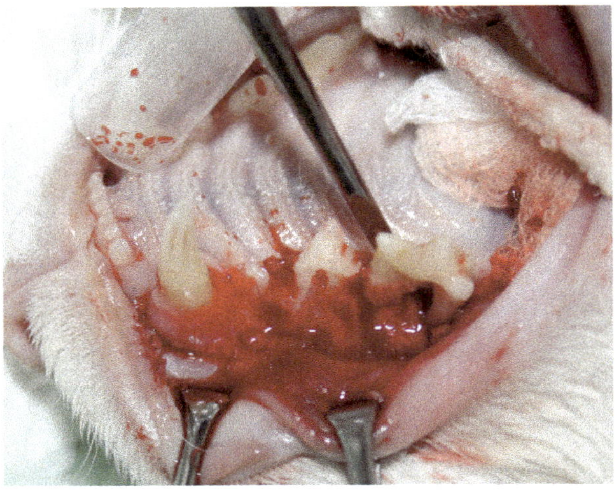

Figure 27. After cutting the alveolar bone each tooth is mobilised from the lingual aspect with a periodontal ligament luxator until it moves.

Although open extraction may appear a laborious technique, in truth surgical time is not increased, plus patients have much faster recoveries than with the closed technique.

When all extractions on the same side are finished, the bony projections where the teeth were housed are filed off and the flaps are sutured back in place with **absorbable 4–0 or 5–0 monofilament material** (Figure 28). The flaps must be handled very carefully so as not to devitalize them and thus avoid necrosis of the oral mucosa.

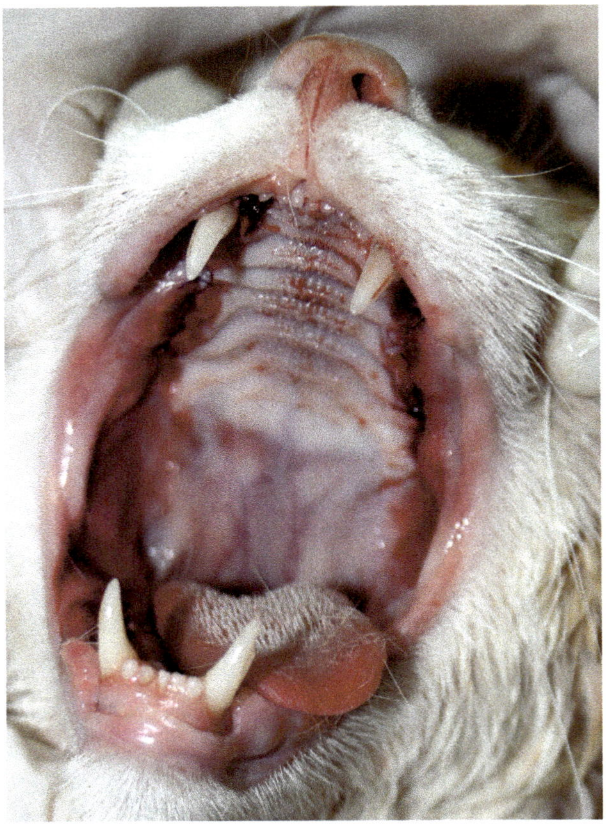

Figure 28. Final appearance after removal of teeth and suturing of the flaps.

Complications following exodontics

The possible complications that can be encountered when performing these extraction techniques include:

- **Root retention in bone.** If in doubt, a finger should be run across the surface of the root. If this surface is smooth, it is likely the entire root has been extracted, but if it has sharp edges, it may have fractured. When in doubt, an X-ray should be performed to verify this. If remnants of the root remain, it must be extracted and, if this is difficult, additional cutting should be performed until it has been removed.
- **Bleeding** if the mandibular or maxillary blood vessels are reached. If this occurs, pressure should be applied with a swab, soaked with adrenaline, or bone wax should be used to create a plug.
- **Iatrogenic trauma to oral structures** such as the tongue or salivary ducts, including perforation of the eyeball when using a luxator on the maxillary teeth. The mandibular symphysis can also be weakened or broken with consequent instability or any area of the mandible or maxilla broken or the temporomandibular joint dislocated.
- **Lingual oedema** if a salivary duct is obstructed.
- **Oronasal fistula.**
- **Subcutaneous or thoracic emphysema** if tracheal rupture occurs.

Therefore, although tooth extractions are a commonly performed procedure, **specific training and preparation is essential** to reduce and resolve any resulting complications.

Bibliography

Hennet P. *Chronic gingivostomatitis in cats: Long–term follow-up of 30 cases treated by dental extractions.* J Vet Dent 1997; (14) 15–21.

Harley R. Gruffydd-Jones TJ, Day MJ. *Salivary and serum immunoglobulin levels in cats with chronic gingivostomatitis.* Vet Rec. 2003 (5) 125–129.

Veterinary Clinics of North America. Volume 35, Dentistry, July 2005.

Girard N. Hennet P. *Retrospective Study of Dental Extractions Treatment of Chronic Caudal Stomatitis in 60 Positive Cats.* Proceedings 19 Veterinary Dental Forum 2005 p. 447.

Healey K.A. et al. *Prevalence of feline chronic gingivostomatitis in first opinion veterinary practice.* J of Fel Med and Surgery 2007; (5) 373–8.

Hosie MJ et al. *Feline immunodeficiency.* ABCD guidelines on prevention and management Review Article J of Fel Med Surgery, 2009 (11) 575–584.

Hosie MJ et al. *Feline calicivirus infection.* ABCD guidelines on prevention and management Review Article J Fel Med and Surgery, 2009 (11) 556–564.

Hennet P. Camy G. Privat V. McGahie D. *Comparative efficacy of a feline recombinant interferon omega in refractory cases of calicivirus positive cats with caudal stomatitis: a randomised, multicentric controlled double blind study of 39 cats.* Proceeding of 19 European Congress of Veterinary Dentistry Nice 2010 pp. 193–195.

Belows J. *Feline dentistry. Oral assessment, treatment and preventive care.* Ed. Wiley-Blackwell 2010.

Clarke and Caiafa. *Oral examination in the cat. A systematic approach.* J fel Med and Surgery. 2014 (16) 873–886.

Niemiec. *Feline Dental radiography and radiology. A primer.* J Fel Med and Surgery 2014 (16) 887–899.

Reiter and Soltero-Rivera. *Applied feline oral anatomy and tooth extraction techniques. An illustrated guide.* J Fel Med and Surgery 2014 (16) 900–913.

Gorrel C. *Tooth resorption in cats. Pathophysiology and treatment options.* J Fel Med and Surgery 2015 (17) 37–43.

Winer and Verstraete. *Therapeutic management of Feline Gingivostomatitis: A systematic Review of the Literature.* Frontiers in Veterinary Science 2016 (3) 1–10.

Arzi et al. *Therapeutic Efficacy of Fresh Autologous Mesenchymal Stem Cells for Severe Refractory Feline Chronic Gingivostomatitis.* Stem Cells Transnational Medicine 2016 (5) 75–86.

Arzi et al *Therapeutic Efficacy of Fresh Allogenic Mesenchymal Stem Cells for severe refractory feline Chronic gingivostomatitis.* Stem Cells Transnational Medicine 2017 (6) 1710–1722.

Test

1. Which of the following statements is false?

A) Oral disease is frequent in cats of any age.
B) The symptomatology of oral diseases is nonspecific, although pain and anorexia are usually present.
C) There is no relationship between oral pathologies in cats and other systemic diseases.
D) Examining the cat's mouth whenever the opportunity arises and not waiting for associated signs is highly recommended.

2. How many teeth do cats have?

A) 24 deciduous and 36 permanent teeth.
B) 28 deciduous and 30 permanent teeth.
C) 24 deciduous and 32 permanent teeth.
D) 26 deciduous and 30 permanent teeth.

3. Regarding oral radiology in cats, which statement is incorrect?

A) Oral radiology is a limited test for oral pathologies that does not offer much information.
B) There are many radiological abnormalities associated with different oral pathologies.
C) Oral radiological equipment is preferable because of its versatility, compared to conventional radiographic equipment.
D) In oral radiology, in addition to evaluating the teeth themselves, other adjacent structures that may be affected are also evaluated.

4. Which statement is correct?

A) Dental plaque is a deposit of substances at the gingival margin formed by bacteria from the mouth, food debris and inflammatory cells.
B) Dental plaque is mainly induced by a decrease in cleaning due to malocclusion and loss of teeth.
C) Bacteria in the mouth are the main predisposing factor in the initiation of dental plaque deposition.
D) All of the above are correct.

5. Regarding periodontal disease:

A) Gingivitis is an oral condition that has nothing to do with periodontitis.
B) Gingivitis is an inflammatory condition of the oral mucosa that covers the teeth.
C) Periodontitis is a more chronic condition than gingivitis, in which inflammation and weakening of the periodontal ligament occurs.
D) Answers b) and c) are correct.

6. Regarding the management of periodontal disease, the least appropriate treatment is:

A) Removal of dental plaque and tartar are the fundamental basis.

B) The use of specific antibiotics for the mouth may be necessary in some clinical situations.

C) No degree of periodontitis, even advanced cases, requires the need for dental extractions.

D) The use of chlorhexidine gel can replace daily cleaning with toothpaste to control dental plaque.

7. Regarding feline dental resorption:

A) Diagnosis, in addition to clinical signs, is mainly radiological.

B) It occurs mainly in deciduous teeth of very young animals.

C) The aetiology is very clear and is a consequence of the action of bacterial toxins that affect the dentin of the tooth.

D) All of the above are incorrect.

8. For the treatment of feline dental resorption, the most appropriate is:

A) Always be as conservative as possible, trying by all means to preserve the teeth.

B) To use drugs against osteoporosis in human medicine as a first choice.

C) The extraction of all affected teeth at the time of diagnosis and periodic re-evaluation in case more teeth are affected.

D) Reconstruct the affected tooth using endodontic techniques is the best treatment to control dental resorption.

9. The diagnosis of chronic feline gingivitis should be by which of the following:

A) Clinical examination of cats with chronic oral lesions in the mucosa that covers the teeth and in the caudal oral mucosa and glossopalatine arch, especially, in addition to performing an oral mucosa biopsy to determine the chronic inflammatory nature.

B) Dental radiography is the best method to identify the condition.

C) It is essential to establish whether feline calicivirus is present in the oral mucosa, since this virus is present in 100% of cats with this condition.

D) All of the above are correct.

10. The ideal treatment for chronic feline gingivitis is:

A) The use of corticosteroids only since it is an immune mediated process with a large local inflammatory component.

B) In the presence of calicivirus, the use of a specific antiviral such as feline omega interferon is the most appropriate.

C) As bacterial dental plaque influences the development of this condition, the use of antibiotics after a culture is the only valid recommendation.

D) As it is a multifactorial process, the ideal treatment does not exist. Some studies suggest that the extraction of premolars and molars produces the highest recovery rate, although some animals require additional treatments with antibiotics, pain relief and anti-inflammatories after it.

11. Regarding feline tooth extraction procedures:

A) It is a technique of last resort for any dental and oral pathology, which is only used when all other options fail.

B) It is a very simple procedure to carry out, since as cats are very small animals not much effort is required.

C) There are no significant complications associated with tooth extraction.

D) All of the above are incorrect.

Clinical case

Signalment

- 5-year-old castrated male cat, living indoors.
- Commercial food, majority which is dry.
- Eating normally.
- No vomiting.
- Stools which are well-formed and regular.

Reason for consultation

Second opinion consultation after going to two vets for the same problem.

The cat has been suffering from an oral problem for the last 3 years and has not improved with the different treatments that have been prescribed: previous diagnosis of chronic feline gingivostomatitis.

Previous treatments

- Antibiotic (cefovecin SC 8 mg/kg).
- Oral prednisone at a dose of 1 mg/kg at different moments in time.
- SC methylprednisolone at a dose of 2 mg/kg on different occasions. They cannot remember the number of times.
- Meloxicam at 0.05 mg/kg PO daily at different times.
- The response to the various previous treatments has been partial with frequent recurrences.

Examination

Weight of the animal: 3.2 kg. Body condition 3/9 (somewhat thin).
Vital signs within normal ranges. Some traces of saliva on the face. Hair which is dirtier than normal. Halitosis.

Oral examination

- Generalized periodontitis of varying severity in all the teeth present, with severe gingivitis in the oral mucosa that covers the teeth.

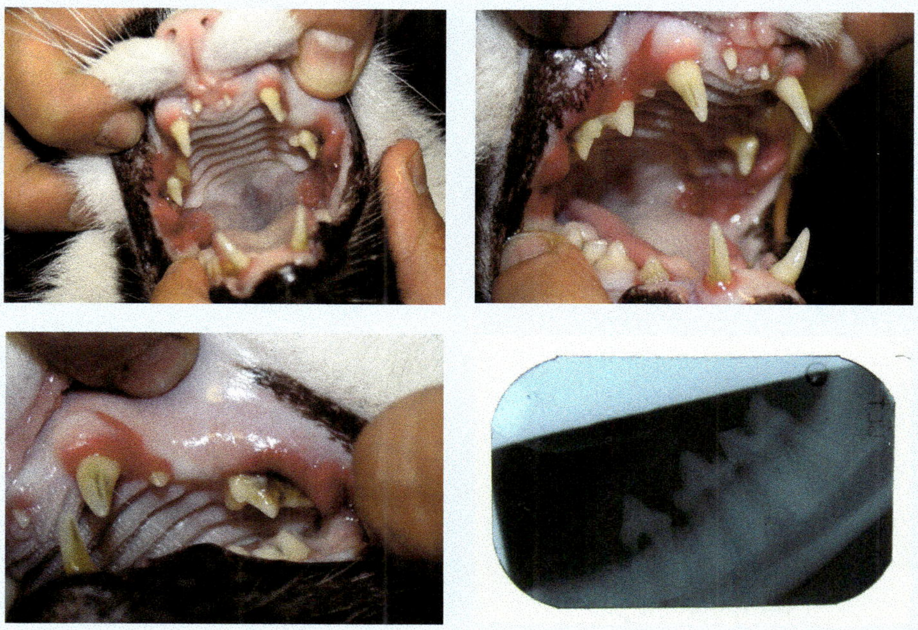

- Gingival and alveolar retraction of the four canines.
- Gingival retraction on maxillary and mandibular premolars and molars, with different degrees of furcation in parts of these areas.
- Severe inflammation with areas of necrosis and gingival hyperplasia in the caudal oral mucosa and the glossopalatine arch.
- Missing teeth: 101, 102, 202, 203, 208, 209, 301, 302, 303, 401, 402, 403.
- Intraoral radiograph showing dental resorption on tooth 407.

Further tests

The results of the CBC and blood biochemistry are shown in the tables below.
Moderate leukocytosis is observed due to marked neutrophilia in the first and moderate hyperproteinaemia due to hypergammaglobulinaemia in the second.

Table 1. Complete blood count.

Parameter	Result	Reference range
Erythrocytes	7.24 × 10^6/µl	5.00–10.00
Haematocrit	37%	30–45
Leukocytes	25.51 × 10^3/µl	5.50–19.50
Neutrophils	21.62 × 10^3/µl	2.50–12.50
Lymphocytes	3.00 × 10^3/µl	0.40–6.80
Monocytes	0.89 × 10^3/µl	0.15–1.70
Platelets	318 × 10^3/µl	175–600

Table 2. Biochemistry.

Parameter	Result	Reference range
Glucose	154 mg/dl	71–159
Creatinine	1.6 mg/dl	0.8–1.6
BUN	19 mg/dl	16–36
Total protein	9.3 mg/dl	5.7–8.9
Albumin	3.1 mg/dl	2.3–3.9
Globulins	6.2 mg/dl	2.8–5.1
ALT	77 U/l	12–130

1. What other complementary tests should be performed?
2. What would the diagnosis be, considering the blood tests and the results of the rest of the tests (see answer to question 1)?
3. What treatment would you recommend?

Answers

Test

1. C	5. D	9. A
2. D	6. C	10. D
3. A	7. A	11. D
4. D	8. C	

Clinical case

1. **What other complementary tests should be performed?**
   Retrovirus ELISA test (negative for feline leukaemia and FIV).
   PCR for calicivirus in caudal oral mucosa (tested positive for feline calicivirus).
2. **What would the diagnosis be, considering the blood tests and the results of the rest of the tests (see answer to question 1)?**
   As can be verified on oral examination, the radiograph and other complementary tests, there are three types of oral pathologies which appear to be present:
   - Gingivitis and periodontitis that have caused several teeth to be lost.
   - Dental resorption in one tooth.
   - Feline chronic gingivitis.
3. **What treatment would you recommend?**
   Complete extraction is performed using the closed technique on all the teeth.

Regional blocks with 2% bupivacaine should be performed in the preoperative period.
Radiography should be used to verify that there are no root remains from the teeth in areas where teeth are missing.
An oesophagostomy tube is placed after the procedure, to ensure proper feeding on the days immediately after surgery.
Recommended postoperative management includes:

- Meloxicam 0.02 mg/kg every 24 hours orally with food.
- Buprenorphine 15 µg/kg every 12 hours transmucosal.
- Clindamycin 15 mg/kg every 12 hours.

The patient needs a forced feeding tube for 10 days, which is removed after checking that they are able to feed on their own. Feeding wet food from now on is recommended.

- Buprenorphine is withdrawn after 6 days.
- Clindamycin is withdrawn after 14 days.
- Meloxicam is withdrawn after 35 days.

The decrease in the signs of inflammation in the gingival mucosa are gradual and constant.
Thirty days after tooth extraction, there is full recovery from the inflammation of the gingival mucosa that covered the teeth. Persistence of moderate inflammation in the caudal oral mucosa and no inflammation in the glossopalatine arch.
At 60 days after tooth extraction, there is still slight inflammation of the caudal oral mucosa.
At 120 days after the extractions, recovery is complete. No area of the oral mucosa is inflamed.
The animal is feeding normally. Its weight is 4.6 kg. The coat is normal.

Conclusions

- It is common to find more than one pathological process affects the oral cavity.
- Whenever there is the opportunity to examine a cat, opening its mouth is recommended to detect possible abnormalities.
- Routine oral hygiene is recommended in cats, oral chlorhexidine gel on the gums and teeth, once a day for the perfect control of dental plaque is preferred to dental cleaning with specialised toothpastes after each meal.
- Use of a systematic protocol to make an accurate diagnosis of the different oral problems that can occur in cats is advisable.
- When feline chronic gingivitis is diagnosed in the presence of calicivirus, corticosteroids may initially be very effective in controlling inflammation, however, with the passage of time, there is a greater replication of the virus and the causes a worsening of the condition.
- In the presence of teeth loss for no apparent reason, dental resorption should be considered. If diagnosed, the treatment of choice is always tooth extraction as it is a very painful condition.
- Complete extraction of premolars and molars for the management of chronic feline gingivitis should not be considered as a last resort treatment when medical management no longer improves the cat's clinical condition. It is the treatment of choice at the time of writing of this clinical case. The longer this management option is postponed, the longer the immune system is acting on the oral mucosa and the lower the chances of a full recovery being achieved when exodontics are carried out.

Gastrointestinal diseases

6

Valentina Aybar Rodríguez

Contents

Oesophageal disease

The following section details a clinical approach to the patient with oesophageal disease.

Oesophageal disease occurs less frequently in cats than in dogs, but if overlooked as differential diagnoses then oesophagitis or oesophageal strictures risk going undiagnosed.

Oesophageal disease is often linked to regurgitation as a symptom (German et al., 2005). **Regurgitation involves passive expulsion of food or liquid from the oesophagus**. This undigested food may contain mucus or saliva. If the oesophageal disease is located in the distal oesophagus or associated with motility problems (such as megaoesophagus) regurgitation **does not necessarily occur immediately after eating**. Indeed, it can be **difficult to differentiate vomiting from regurgitation**, in which case it is useful to ask the owner to video the cat eating at home or offer the patient food at the clinic to observe how they eat.

Clinical history

The first step in the diagnosis of oesophageal disease is to differentiate the clinical signs of regurgitation from vomiting or dysphagia. To do this the following factors should be assessed (Table 1):

Table 1. How to differentiate vomiting, regurgitation, and dysphagia in the cat.

Clinical sign	Vomiting	Regurgitation	Dysphagia
Swallowing	Before vomiting	–	++
Pain on swallowing	–	+/–	+/–
Nausea/prodromes	+/–	–	–
Persistent hypersalivation	–	+/–	+/–
Abdominal movement	++	–	–
Relation to food	Variable	After → Proximal oesophagus Variable → Distal or generalised	Associated with food
Content	Partially digested	Tubular, partially digested	Undigested
Bile	+/–	–	–
Fresh blood	+/–	+/–	+/–
Digested blood	+	–	–
Reingestion	+	+/–	+/–
Appetite	Variable	Normal	Poor

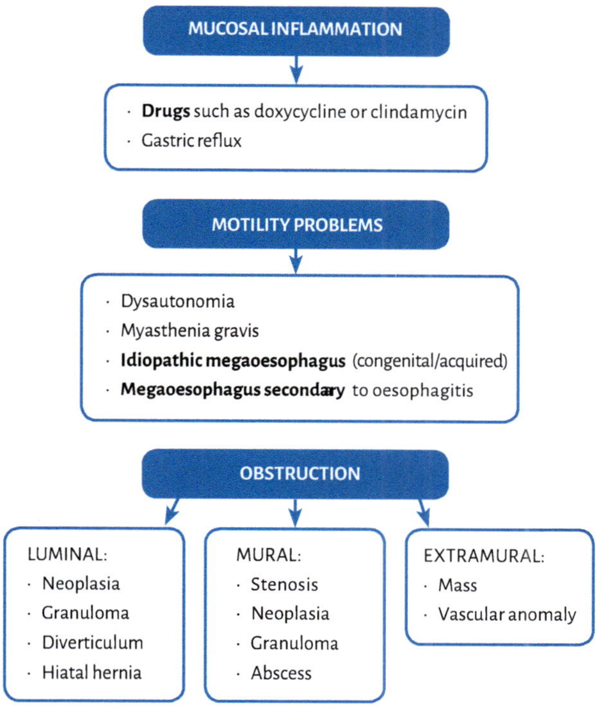

Figure 1. Differential diagnoses of oesophageal diseases.

Differential diagnoses

The second step in the process of diagnosis is to **establish list of differential diagnoses** (Figure 1).

Linking clinical history and physical examination with differential diagnoses

- **Age** at which the problem started. Clinical signs that occur after weaning are typical of vascular abnormalities or congenital megaoesophagus.
- **Breed**: Siamese and Middle Eastern breeds are associated with oesophageal motility problems, mediastinal lymphoma, and hiatal hernia. Persistence of the aortic arch and congenital megaoesophagus are more frequent in purebred cats.
- A history of **recent anaesthesia** may be associated with oesophagitis or oesophageal strictures.
- Recent administration of medication.
- History of possible ingestion of caustic agents.
- History of possible foreign body ingestion.
- An acute problem makes a foreign body more likely than neoplastic disease.
- A progressive problem makes oesophagitis and stenosis more likely.
- **Signs of pain** or difficulty swallowing are more likely to be associated with oesophagitis or a foreign body.
- Was all the food regurgitated? Was water also regurgitated? Regurgitation of food and water is more likely an obstructive problem than a motility problem.
- If there is **weight loss**, this indicates chronicity and severity of the clinical signs.
- If the oral examination shows **inflammation or ulceration**, it could be due to feline calicivirus (FCV) infections or caustic agents.
- Palpation of the neck may indicate pain due to oesophagitis, masses, or oesophageal dilation.
- Respiratory signs such as dyspnoea, tachypnoea, cough, fever, or nasal discharge may be due to aspiration pneumonia.

Diagnosis

The most appropriate diagnostic tests should be planned as guided by the most likely differential diagnoses.

Appropriate tests to investigate oesophageal diseases include plain and contrast radiographs, fluoroscopy, ultrasound, and endoscopy. Not all tests are necessary in all cases.

Radiography

Thoracic and neck radiographs are especially helpful for diagnosis of:

- Megaoesophagus.
- Focal pathologies such as those secondary to vascular ring abnormalities or obstruction.
- Diffuse, mild dilation or air in the oesophagus should be interpreted with caution because this may not be pathological.
- Anterior mediastinal mass.
- Oesophageal or peri-oesophageal mass.
- Radio-opaque foreign body.

Radiographs should be performed when the **cat is conscious or under light sedation**, because deep sedation and anaesthesia may dilate the oesophagus, and if the patient is not intubated this increases the risk of aspiration pneumonia.

The **normal oesophagus is not visible on plain radiographs**, but can be visualized when there is food, air, masses, or abnormalities present (Figures 2 and 3).

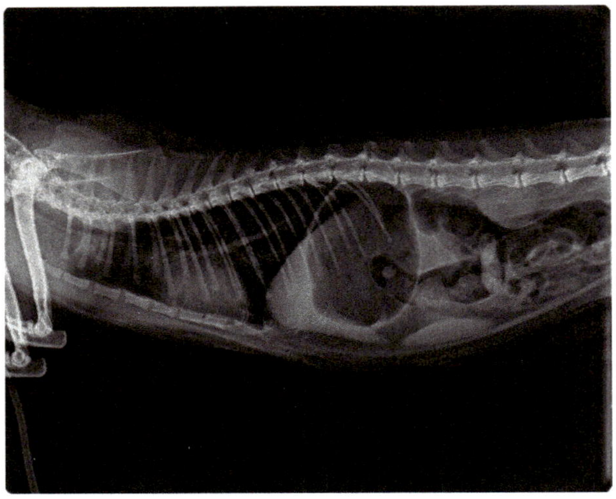

Figure 2. Plain lateral radiograph of a cat with regurgitation a week after being anaesthetised. The oesophagus is dilated and there is air in the stomach and the rest of the digestive tract.

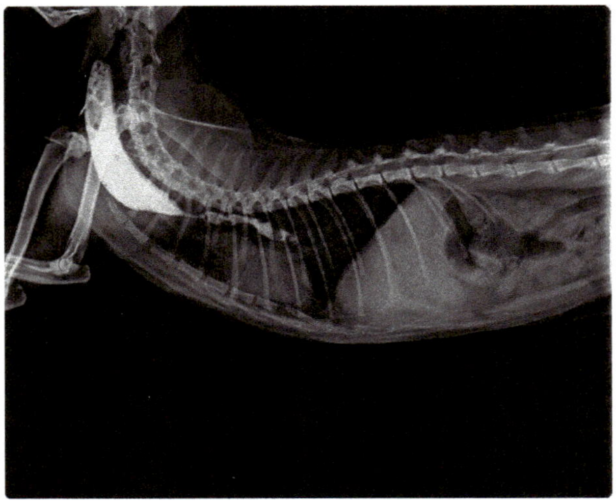

Figure 3. Contrast radiograph of the same cat from Figure 2. A narrowing can be seen in the cervical oesophagus.

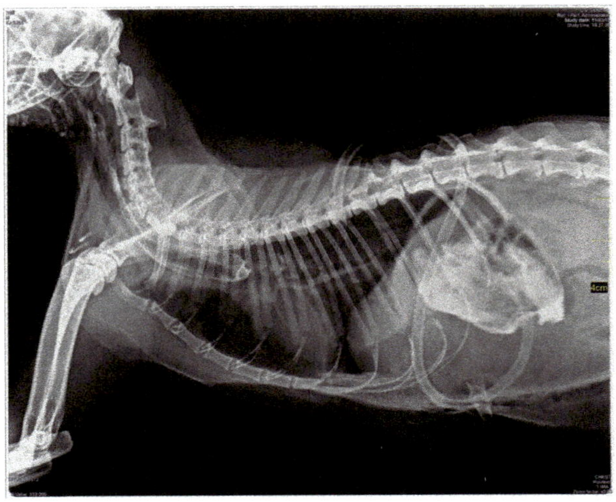

Figure 4. Contrast radiograph in a cat with oesophageal carcinoma.

In addition, radiographs facilitate **evaluation of possible complications** such as aspiration pneumonia or oesophageal perforations.

To perform contrast radiographs, contrast can be mixed with soft food and administered by syringe. Use of iodinated agents (iohexol, Gastrografin) is recommended, because in cases of perforation it is less irritating and absorbed faster. **Radiographs should be taken 10 seconds after the contrast is ingested.** If there is an abrupt break in the contrast, an obstruction should be suspected. If the contrast is retained throughout the whole oesophagus, muscular dysfunction should be suspected. Contrast is not necessarily reliable for the diagnosis of oesophagitis, as the agent may or may not be retained in areas of ulcerated mucosa.

After contrast radiography (Figure 4) at least 48 hours should elapse before endoscopy is performed.

Endoscopy

Endoscopy is a useful non-invasive method when a definitive diagnosis has not been established with plain and contrast radiographs. In addition, it allows extraction of foreign bodies, biopsy taking, and balloon dilation (in the case of oesophageal stenosis).

Endoscopy (Figure 5) is a sensitive method for diagnosing:

- Oesophagitis
- Oesophageal stenosis where balloon dilation can be used
- Oesophageal neoplasms/granulomas
- Foreign bodies
- Perforations

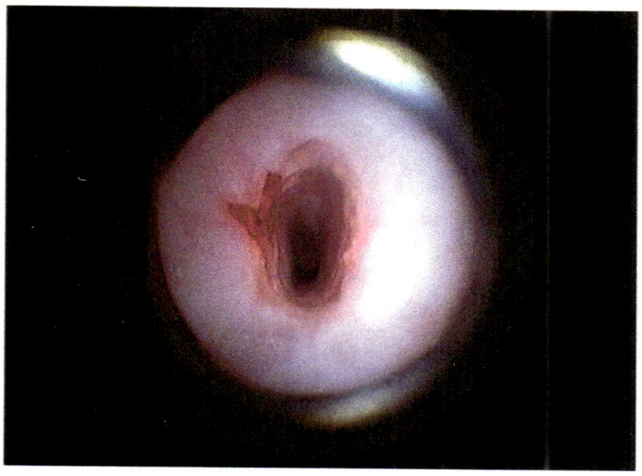

Figure 5. Endoscopy image showing oesophageal stenosis.

- Focal or generalized oesophageal dilations, although evaluating the degree of dilation is difficult with the cat anaesthetized

Treatment

Megaoesophagus

Symptomatic treatment of megaoesophagus

The patient should be fed frequently with small amounts of food and with their head elevated. Alternatively, the cat can be held in the owner's arms for 5–10 minutes after eating.

It is worth experimenting with different consistencies, sizes, and shapes of food. Although it seems logical that liquid or semi-liquid foods would pass along the oesophagus more easily, some cats with megaoesophagus better tolerate dry food. Ideally, high-end, high-calorie foods should be offered.

Prokinetic medications can be trialled, but in felines the response is often disappointing. However, some cases of congenital megaoesophagus do spontaneously resolve, without the cause ever being established.

Oesophagitis

Oesophagitis (Moses, 2000) often results from inflammation caused by foreign body irritation such as from hairballs, chemical irritants, medications, gastro-oesophageal reflux, persistent vomiting, hiatal hernias, and general anaesthesia. An important part of treatment is to identify and control the triggering cause (Kook, 2021).

Gastro-oesophageal reflux associated with general anaesthesia is one of the leading causes of severe oesophagitis in cats. There are some factors that increase gastro-oesophageal reflux, including:

- drugs that decrease oesophageal sphincter tone, e.g. atropine or xylazine
- handling the abdomen in a way that increases gastric pressure
- food in the stomach during surgery
- the position of the head during surgery or recovery.

Drugs given orally in the form of capsules or tablets can irritate the oesophagus and cause oesophagitis. Ingestion of a small amount of water or food after administering the drug, or the administration of capsules with butter or dietary gel helps to decrease this risk, because it increases the speed of transit and therefore reduces irritation. Special care should be taken in dehydrated sick cats that require the administration of oral medication.

When the cause is eliminated, mild oesophagitis usually resolves on its own with wet food. Severe cases may require gastrotomy tube feeding during the recovery period.

Feeding a low fat, high protein diet can improve gastric emptying.

Oesophageal stenosis

Oesophageal strictures (German et al., 2005) **occur due to injury to the submucosa and muscle, which results in connective tissue fibrosis.** The clinical signs associated with stenosis occur 5–14 days after the primary injury to the oesophagus.

In cases of oesophagitis and stenosis, radiographs may be normal but these are still useful to rule out other causes of the clinical signs, such as foreign bodies, masses, or complications such as aspiration pneumonia.

The treatment technique of choice is balloon dilation via endoscopy. Depending on the severity of the stenosis and the related damage, dilation should be repeated at an interval of 2–7 days. Supportive treatment after each dilation is very important and the appropriate treatment for oesophagitis should be administered (Table 2).

Although some cases require long-term treatment, aiming to maintain a good level of nutrition and reduce discomfort due to regurgitation, in most cases the clinical response is good or acceptable.

Vomition

This section covers a clinical approach to the vomiting patient.

In cats, after dermatological problems, vomiting is the second most common reason for presentation. Differentiating between possible diagnoses in a vomiting cat can be done in several ways e.g. acute versus chronic, or primary versus secondary due to systemic problems (Batchelor et al., 2012).

Gastrointestinal problems should be evaluated from a clinical point of view. **Mild, transient, self-limiting**

Table 2. Main pharmacological agents used in the treatment of oesophagitis and oesophageal stenosis.

Medication	Dose	Mechanism of action
Famotidine	0.5–1 mg/kg/12–24 hours oral	H_2 receptor antagonist, reduces gastric secretions
Metoclopramide	0.2–0.4 mg/kg/6 hours SC, oral	Prokinetic, promotes gastric emptying
Omeprazole	0.5–1 mg/kg/24 h oral	Proton pump inhibitor, reduces gastric secretions
Ranitidine	2.5 mg/kg/12 h IV or 3.5 mg/kg/12 h oral	H_2 receptor antagonist, reduces gastric secretions
Sucralfate	0.25 mg/cat/6–8 h oral	Mucosal protector
Buprenorphine	0.01–0.03 mg/kg/6–8 h transmucosal	Opioid, analgesic

vomiting is common in cats and resolves spontaneously without the need for specific treatment. In these cases, the triggering cause is usually not investigated but may be related to:

- Dietary changes
- Spoiled food
- Food hypersensitivity
- Ingestion of plants
- Ingestion of toxins/irritants

Infectious causes should be considered, especially in young cats. In these cases, **if the cat is clinically stable, then deworming and management with symptomatic treatment** based on a change in diet (high digestibility or hypoallergenic) and antiemetics is recommended. If the signs persist, a diagnostic protocol should be initiated (Figure 6).

A systematic diagnostic protocol is required when the vomiting is persistent, frequent, or accompanied by other clinical signs such as loss of appetite, weight loss, or change in stool consistency (Hauck et al. 2016).

It is helpful to remember that **vomiting can be due by primary gastrointestinal causes or the result of systemic disease.** To differentiate the two the clinical history, signalment, and clinical examination should be used to assess the most likely causes.

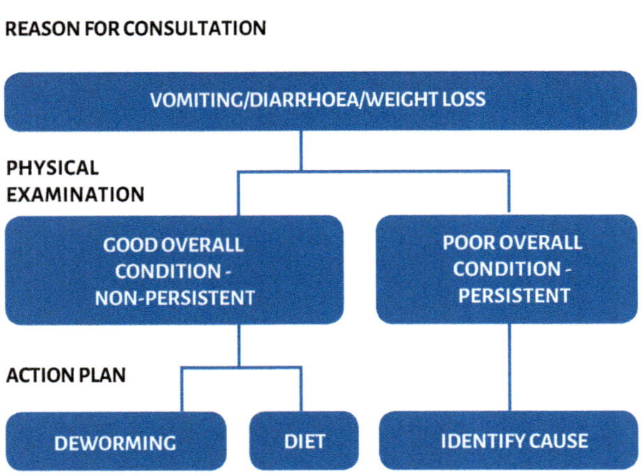

Figure 6. Management of gastrointestinal problems in cats.

Table 3. Decision making around gastrointestinal problems in cats.

When to act…	Very young/old patients Weight loss Frequent GIT signs Abdominal pain Haematemesis Dehydration Abdominal mass Ascites Depression, lethargy, inappetence Lack of response to symptomatic treatment Other signs: polyuria/polydipsia
When to wait…	GIT signs which have developed quickly Response to symptomatic treatment Normal clinical examination No other clinical signs Good appetite History of diet change

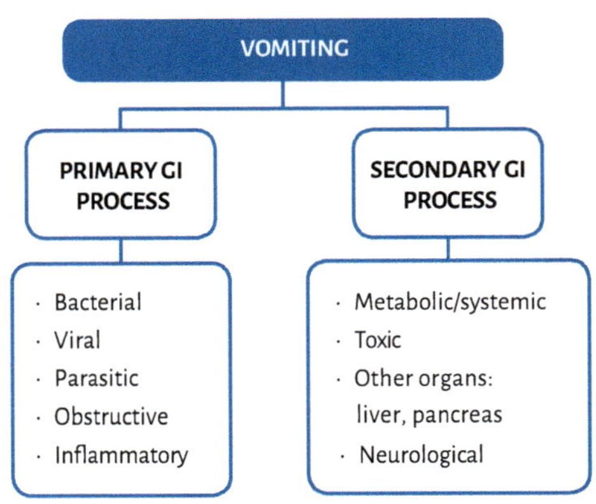

Figure 7. Diagram showing the diagnostic approach to the vomiting patient.

Signalment and clinical history

The **signalment and clinical history are key starting points**. For example, foreign body consumption is

Table 4. The main primary and secondary gastrointestinal conditions which cause gastrointestinal problems.

Primary GIT conditions	Bacterial	Helicobacter, intestinal bacterial overgrowth (SIBO), Salmonella
Secondary GIT conditions	Viral	Infection with feline panleukopoenia virus (FPV)
	Parasitic	Giardia, Ascaris
	Obstructive	Foreign body, neoplasia, intussusception
	Inflammatory	Diet, idiopathic
	Metabolic/ systemic	Renal disease, hyperthyroidism, diabetic ketoacidosis
	Toxins/ medications	Chemotherapy, toxic plants, NSAIDs, antibiotics (clindamycin, amoxicillin/ clavulanate)
	Other organs	Cholangitis, pancreatitis, neoplasms
	Neurological	

more likely in young cats, whilst in older cats, systemic or chronic diseases are more common (such as chronic kidney disease or hyperthyroidism).

In order not to miss information from the history, the use of questionnaires with closed questions is helpful (Figure 8), although it is also important to ask open-ended questions such as: "What would you attribute the sickness too?", "When did the clinical signs first start?"

As always, it is important to differentiate vomiting from regurgitation (Table 1). Sometimes this is not easy, especially if the caretaker does not witness the event but finds the vomit afterwards. **Vomiting is preceded by nausea**, which causes restlessness, hypersalivation, and lip licking. In the author's experience, abdominal contraction does not necessarily help with differentiation as it also occurs in regurgitation and can be confused with vomiting. **Bilious content is the result of vomiting** not regurgitation, whilst the content of regurgitation is usually food with a tubular shape and covered with saliva.

The presenting pattern of vomition is also relevant, because cats with acute gastritis usually show a sudden onset compared to chronic conditions, which present with vomiting spread out in time. The timing of vomiting in relation to feeding also aids diagnosis. Gastric emptying usually occurs 6–8 hours after eating, if it has food content 8 hours after food intake, this may be due to a motility problem or obstruction. **If the vomit is bilious, the pylorus is not obstructed** and the presence of blood (fresh or digested) indicates ulceration.

Obtaining a detailed history of everything that may be relevant to the investigation including diet, dietary changes, deworming, vaccination, and medications is essential.

Physical examination

Linear foreign bodies are a frequent cause of vomiting, therefore **the ventral area of the tongue should always be examined** where the foreign body itself or an injury caused by it may be visible. Abdominal palpation (Figure 9) allows evaluation of the presence of masses, the size and shape of the kidneys, pain, or thickening of intestinal loops (which in the author's experience corresponds to a thickening on ultrasound of about 0.5 cm.)

In all cats, palpation of the thyroid is also important and the clinician should be familiar with the technique.

Body condition and muscle mass scoring using scales (Table 5) help to assess the severity of the condition and how it is evolving.

Questions	Yes	No	Comments
HAVE THERE BEEN BEHAVIOURAL CHANGES? Interaction, grooming, activity, vocalisation, litter box use…	x		Over the last few months
IS HE/SHE EATING WELL? Fussy, change of habits, food falls from the mouth, gesticulates when eating…		x	Fussy, makes noise with teeth when eating
DOES HE/SHE DEFAECATE CORRECTLY? Number of times per day, consistency, smell, colour…	x		Not sure, goes outside
IS THERE VOMITING? NAUSEA? Frequency, relationship with food…		x	He/she has always vomited, but more so recently
CAN HE/SHE HEAR/SEE OK? Reduced response to stimuli, increased vocalisation…	x		He/she seems disorientated
HAVE YOU NOTICED ANY WEIGHT LOSS? Since when, what is the normal weight, what could this be due to…	x		Over the last few months

Figure 8. Example of history taking using closed questions.

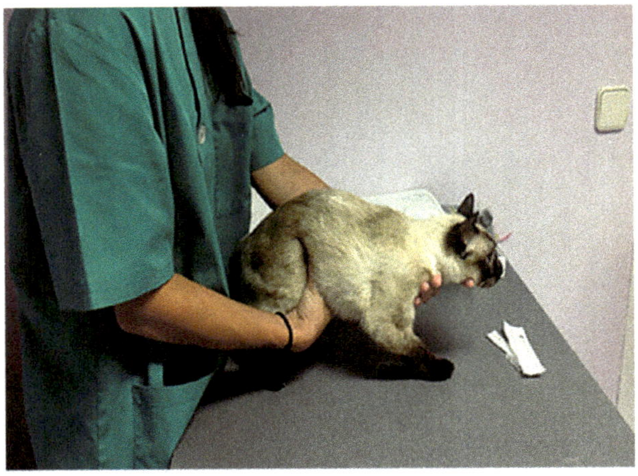

Figure 9. Abdominal palpation allows information about the kidneys, masses, bladder and size of the liver to be obtained.

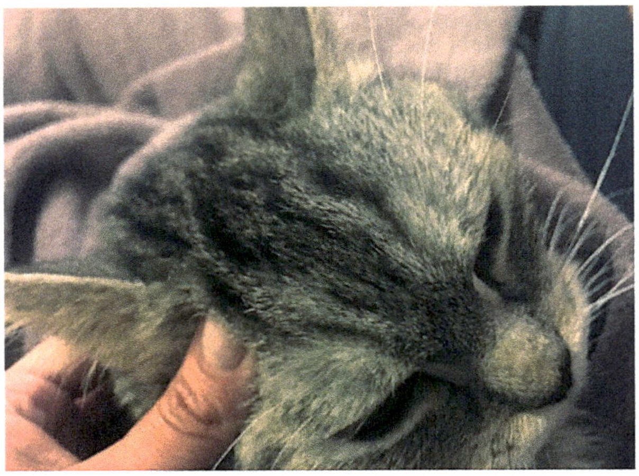

Figure 10. Measurement of muscle mass using palpation of the cranium.

Key points of the physical examination which should not be forgotten include:

- Weight/weight history/percentage change in weight/muscle mass (Figure 10).
- Mucous membranes: paleness, jaundice, capillary refill time.
- Hydration state.
- Appearance of the hair and coat.
- Oral examination.
- Palpation of the neck.
- Cardiopulmonary auscultation.
- Abdominal palpation.

Vital signs and other parameters should be assessed, such as:

- presence of pain
- hydration status
- heart rate
- respiratory rate
- temperature
- blood pressure
- mental state.

The following questions should be considered:

- Is the animal stable?
- Is supportive treatment needed?
- Are more diagnostic tests needed?

Diagnosis

Blood tests and urinalysis

Blood tests that include **complete blood count, biochemistry, and electrolytes** are important not only to differentiate a primary gastrointestinal condition from a secondary one, but also to assess the consequences of vomiting on hydration status and electrolyte levels.

Serum biochemistry analysis should include an assessment of kidney function (urea, creatinine, SDMA) **and liver function** (ALT, ALP, and bile acids), **glucose, electrolytes, and protein concentration.**

Care should be taken interpreting the results because cats can be severely azotaemic due to dehydration, and therefore renal functionality should always be interpreted together with urine density. **If urine specific gravity is greater than 1.035 then the azotaemia is likely to be prerenal.**

In cats, bilirubinuria is always pathological and appears prior to jaundice, which can help guide the diagnosis.

Table 5. Body fat and muscle mass scoring.

Score	Fat	Muscle mass
0	Absence of subcutaneous fat palpable over the ribs and abdomen	Severe muscle loss palpable over the scapula, cranium and wings of the ilium
1	Reduction in palpable subcutaneous fat over the ribs and abdomen	Moderate muscle loss palpable over the scapula, cranium and wings of the ilium
2	Normal amount of subcutaneous fat palpable over the ribs and abdomen	Mild muscle loss palpable over the scapula, cranium and wings of the ilium
3	Increase of palpable subcutaneous fat over the ribs and abdomen	Normal muscle mass palpable over the scapula, cranium and wings of the ilium

Table 6. Basic tests for the diagnostic approach to gastrointestinal problems in cats.

Complete blood count	Haematocrit, red blood cell count, white blood cell count, differential count, smear
Blood biochemistry	Total proteins, albumin, SDMA, globulin, ALP, ALT, glucose, creatinine, K, P, Na, Ca, cobalamin
Urinalysis	Density, sediment, glucose, ketone bodies, protein/creatinine ratio
Total T4	Diagnosis of hyperthyroidism
fPLI	Test alongside clinical signs and ultrasound helps in the diagnosis of pancreatitis

Unless the vomiting is associated with diarrhoea, then stool screening is not indicated in the investigation of chronic vomiting. **But in older cats total thyroxine (T4) should be used** to rule out hyperthyroidism as the cause of gastrointestinal signs.

Other specific tests for gastrointestinal and pancreatic diseases are: cobalamin, folates, fTLI and fPLI, which will be discussed later. The next step in the work-up depends on the results of the blood and urine tests.

Diagnostic imaging

Plain radiography is useful to identify intestinal obstruction or foreign bodies (Daniaux, 2014). (Figure 11).

Contrast radiographs can be helpful in the diagnosis of linear foreign bodies. The use of contrasts used for myelography is preferred, such as iohexol. This is because, in the event of perforation, the barium could irritate the peritoneum and oral iodinated contrasts are hypertonic and may alter the electrolyte balance.

Ultrasound is a very useful tool for the diagnosis of digestive diseases in cats (Figures 12, 13 and 14).

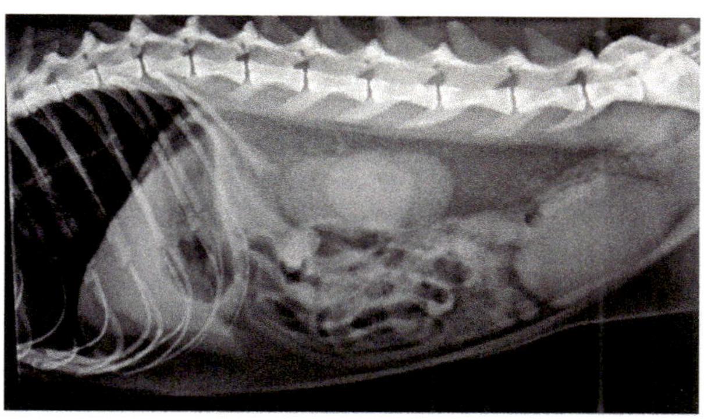

Figure 11. Lateral radiograph of a cat with chronic vomiting where intestinal loops containing gas and intestinal thickening can be seen.

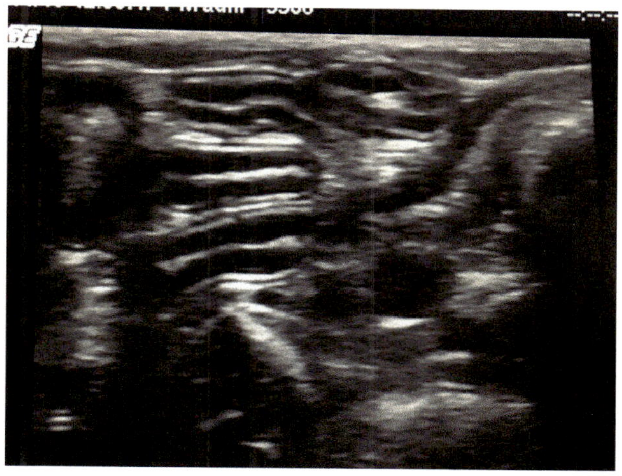

Figure 12. Ultrasound image of the small intestine where the integrity of layers, thickness, lymph nodes, and the rest of the abdomen can be assessed.

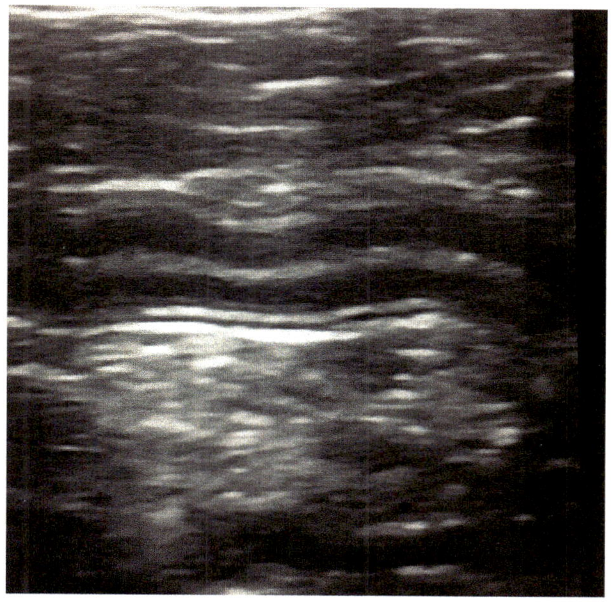

Figure 13. Five-layer structure of the small intestine: hyperechogenic lumen, hypoechogenic mucosa, hyperechogenic submucosa, hypoechogenic muscular layer and hyperechogenic serosa.

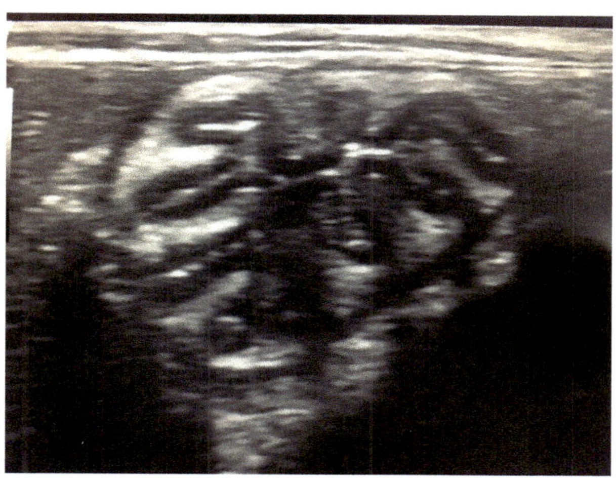

Figure 14. Ultrasound image of the stomach with the "cartwheel" appearance.

It allows location of thickenings in the walls of the stomach, intestine, lymphadenopathy, and foreign bodies, in addition to changes in size and echogenicity of the pancreas, liver, kidneys or spleen. **Ultrasound is also useful to aid fine needle aspiration of masses, the gallbladder and peritoneal fluid.**

The normal ultrasonographic appearance of a section of **small intestine shows the 5-layer structure in which hyper and hypoechoic layers alternate:**

- Serosal
- Muscular
- Submucosa
- Mucosa
- Lumen.

Published references indicate normal duodenal thicknesses of between 0.13 cm to 0.38 cm and **jejunal and ileal thicknesses of between 0.16–0.36 cm**.

Ultrasonography, does not provide a definitive diagnosis, but helps assess:

- Intestinal layer thickness.
- Thickened intestinal layer.
- Integrity of the stratification of layers.
- Location of the injury.

In one study of 100 cats with intestinal thickening greater than 0.28 cm, laparotomy biopsies in at least two locations were performed. It found the two most common diagnoses were inflammatory bowel disease (IBD) (n = 49) and lymphoma (n = 46). The jejunum and duodenum were affected in 90% of lymphomas, while the duodenum was affected in 70%. Distribution of the lesions was similar in IBD and lymphoma, except in the stomach, where IBD was more frequent.

This information is useful when biopsy by endoscopy or laparotomy is required to make a definitive diagnosis.

Biopsy of the intestines and other organs

In some cases, a histological study of the affected tissues is needed. Sampling can be performed by endoscopy, exploratory laparotomy, or laparoscopy (Kleinschmidt et al., 2010).

Endoscopy is a relatively non-invasive procedure, but it has some important limitations.

For example the **samples are small, and only contain mucosa, which may not be diagnostic**.

Endoscopy allows for visualisation of the proximal small intestine and the colon. A study showed that 27% of cats do not have pathologies in the proximal intestine. In addition, nine out of ten cats with inflammatory bowel disease also had pathologies in other organs, and seven out of eight cats with intestinal lymphoma also had pathologies in other organs. Ultrasound is a useful means to select suitable cases for endoscopy, but even so the latter may not provide a definitive diagnosis.

Exploratory laparotomy is an invasive procedure, but highly useful from both a diagnostic and sometimes therapeutic perspective e.g. removal of a foreign body (Figure 15). Biopsy of multiple organs should be performed including the intestine, pancreas, liver and lymph nodes, plus biopsy samples taken of the gallbladder and liver parenchyma to carry out cultures and antibiograms.

Laparotomy should only be performed when the cat is stable and by expert surgeons. **Administration of vitamin K before taking the biopsies is recommended.** In the author's experience, the cat's recovery is much better when adequate nutrition is ensured at the time of surgery, with the placement of an oesophagostomy tube. (Figure 16).

Laparoscopic biopsy is less invasive and has fewer complications than laparotomy, but is not yet a technique routinely available to most clinicians.

Sometimes clearly differentiating severe IBD from lymphoma is not easy, even on the basis of histopathological criteria.

Immunophenotyping by flow cytometry differentiates between a monomorphic population of

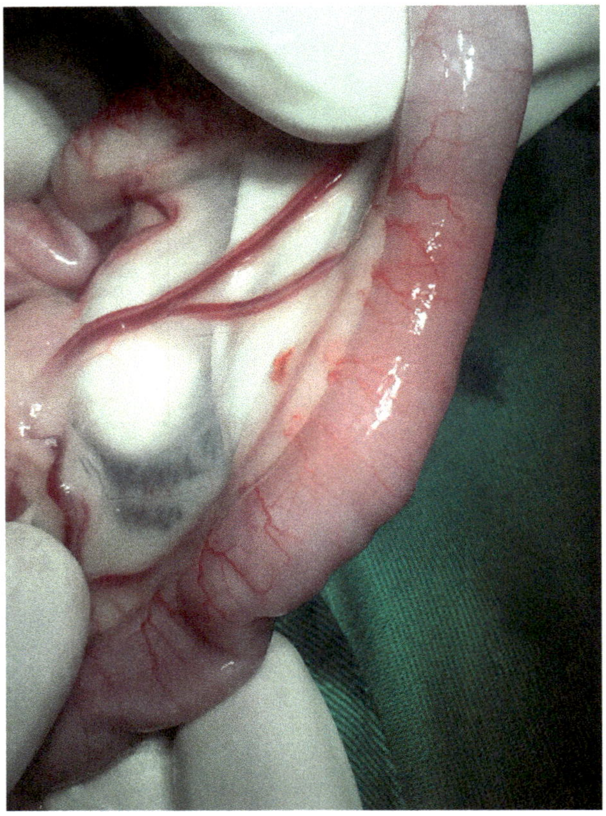

Figure 15. Macroscopic appearance of the thickened small intestine on laparotomy. On histological examination IBD was diagnosed with lymphocytic infiltrate.

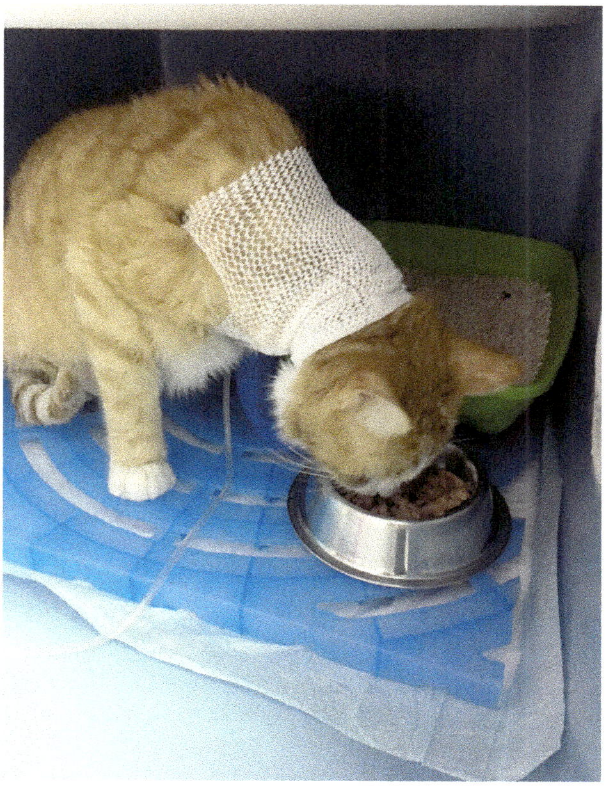

Figure 16. Cat recovering from exploratory laparotomy with oesophagostomy tube and eating simultaneously.

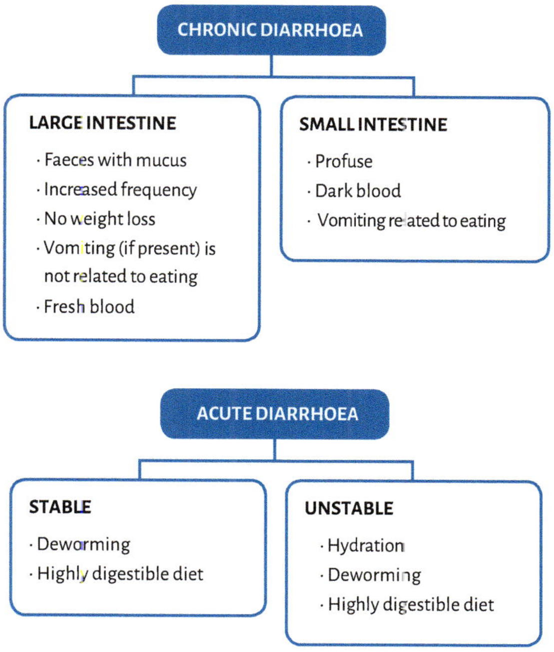

Figure 17. Cases of chronic diarrhoea require a diagnostic and treatment protocol, as do unstable cats with cases of acute diarrhoea or those which do not respond to treatment.

lymphocytes that is suggestive of lymphoma, and a lymphoplasmacytic population linked to IBD. Another useful diagnostic test in these ambiguous cases is the PARR (PCR for antigen receptor rearrangement) to differentiate clonality of T and B cells. Cells from the neoplastic population are clonal or oligoclonal, while inflammatory cells are polyclonal.

A combination of these diagnostic systems helps differentiate IBD from lymphoma.

Diarrhoea

This section details the clinical approach to the cat with diarrhoea.

Diarrhoea is another frequent reason for consultation in feline practice. **Diarrhoea is defined as an increase in the liquid content of the stool which is reflected by changes in consistency.**

Differentiation is important between acute diarrhoea (less than 3 weeks in duration) and chronic diarrhoea (more than 3 weeks) (Figure 17), also whether it is **small or large intestinal diarrhoea**, although in many cases the signs are mixed.

Investigation of the **presence or absence of systemic signs** is important because diseases such as hyperthyroidism, chronic kidney disease, pancreatic disease, neoplasms or toxaemias can present with diarrhoea.

In addition, if the cat presents vomiting, increased or decreased appetite, weight loss, dehydration or fever this should be taken into account when establishing the diagnostic and treatment plans.

Although the list of possible differential diagnoses is long, most cases are the result of:

- Idiopathic inflammatory bowel disease
- Diet-responsive enteropathy
- Lymphoma.

IBD is characterized by inflammation of any section of the gastrointestinal system, although it most commonly affects the small intestine. The cause of IBD is unknown, although some articles suggest the influence of genetic factors which affect the immune system of the intestinal mucosa, factors related to diet, and the role of bacterial flora.

Lymphoma is characterized by the proliferation of a monoclonal population of malignant lymphocytes.

Signalment and clinical signs

Age, breed, history of deworming, vaccination, diet, type of diarrhoea, etc. are important in the management of chronic diarrhoea.

Physical examination

Before starting the diagnostic protocol, a **preliminary examination** should be undertaken to assess

Table 7. Comparison of inflammatory bowel disease (IBD), diet responsive enteropathy and lymphoma.

	IBD	Diet responsive enteropathy	Lymphoma
Signalment	Middle aged	Young	Middle aged and geriatric
Clinical signs	Lethargy, weight loss, hyporexia, vomiting, diarrhoea	Diarrhoea +/– weight loss +/– cutaneous lesions	Lethargy, weight loss, hyporexia, vomiting, diarrhoea, +/– jaundice
Clinical course	Recurrent or progressive	Recurrent or progressive	Progressive
Physical examination	Normal, thickening of intestinal loops, abdominal pain if the pancreas or liver is affected	Normal, may present with skin signs	Normal or thickening of intestinal loops +/– palpable masses
Diagnosis	Rule out non-intestinal causes, lymph node cytology, masses, biopsy	Rule out parasites, dietary trial	Rule out non-intestinal causes, lymph node cytology, masses, biopsy

Table 8. Collection of information focused towards digestive conditions.

Clinical history of a cat with diarrhoea	
Age	Young: dietary, infectious, parasites Geriatric: inflammatory, neoplastic
Vaccination status	Panleukopoenia, FeLV
Diet	Dietary changes, adverse reactions, if diarrhoea when not eating may be osmotic diarrhoea
Environment	Plants, chemicals, toxins, outdoor cats …
Medications	Antibiotics, NSAIDs …
Medical problems	Response to previous treatments
Appearance of diarrhoea	Differentiate if small or large intestine
Other clinical signs	Vomiting (can be due to inflammation of the small intestine), anorexia, weight loss (due to reduced ingestion or maldigestion/ malabsorption)

the severity of the condition and **whether supportive treatment is necessary.** The mental state, degree of dehydration, body condition, abdominal tenderness or the presence of fever help to answer the following questions:

- Are more diagnostic tests needed?
- Is supportive treatment needed?
- Is medication needed?

A cat in good general condition with diarrhoea of a few days' duration can be **dewormed and prescribed a low-residue, highly digestible diet, and the diet administered for 7 days.** Following this previous diet can be reintroduced little by little.

On palpation of the abdomen, **masses associated with the intestinal tract** may correspond to intussusception, tumours, foreign bodies, or focal inflammation and thickening of the wall of the small intestine may be appreciated. **Palpation of intestinal wall thickening can be confused with increased muscle tone due to pain.** Repeating palpation if the cat is sedated or anaesthetized is recommended as information can be obtained that was not appreciable before with the cat able to defend its abdomen.

Chronic diarrhoea syndrome associated with protrusion of the nictitating membrane is seen frequently. The cause is unknown, although it appears to be associated with infectious conditions in which toroviruses (a coronavirus-related virus) may be involved and is more common in multi-cat households. The type of diarrhoea associated with protrusion of the third eyelid is small intestinal and there are often no systemic signs or weight loss. Associated with this syndrome, temporary anal incontinence can also be present. There is no treatment that improves symptoms, which resolve spontaneously (although it can take months).

Diagnosis

Faecal analysis

The most common ways to carry out a stool test are:

- **Direct analysis** of the sample: Collecting a small sample of fresh faeces (collected directly or within less than an hour) with 0.9% saline solution. The sample should be examined for trophozoites like *Giardia spp.* and *Tritrichomonas foetus*.
- **Faecal smear**. Can be stained with methylene blue and bacteria and internal structures of some protozoa can be observed.
- **Flotation**, preferably with centrifugation to search for cysts, oocysts and eggs of parasites.

In **young cats with chronic diarrhoea**, especially those:

- from a breeder or multi-cat households
- with small intestinal diarrhoea which does not respond to diet changes or deworming
- with a negative stool analysis

then PCR tests for the diagnosis of *Tritrichomonas foetus* should be carried out and also tests for *Giardia spp.*

Faecal cultures do not provide useful clinical information.

Blood tests and urinalysis

Blood tests and urinalysis help diagnose systemic diseases that can cause diarrhoea and assess the consequences of diarrhoea, such as dehydration and electrolyte abnormalities.

If the cat is suffering from chronic diarrhoea, but is in good general condition without weight loss, they can be **managed with a diet consisting of a novel or hypoallergenic protein** while obtaining test results and monitoring to assess the response to the diet.

Cobalamin and folates

These are water **soluble vitamins whose absorption can be decreased in gastrointestinal diseases.** These vitamins need specific receptors from different parts of the small intestine. Chronic gastrointestinal diseases can damage these receptors and decrease their concentration. Folate and cobalamin levels may also decrease in cases of exocrine pancreatic insufficiency.

The handling of blood samples is important. Folate is unstable at room temperature and needs to be frozen and protected from light so that results are not altered. Furthermore, samples can be affected by haemolysis.

Hypocobalaminaemia does not always occur with intestinal disease, but in one study was present in 78% of cats with intestinal lymphoma. However, hypocobalaminaemia is also found in other non-gastrointestinal diseases. If **hypocobalaminaemia is detected on tests, cobalamin should be supplemented to improve clinical signs** (Toresson et al., 2017).

fTLI (feline trypsin-like immunoreactivity) and fPLI (feline pancreatic lipase immunoreactivity)

fTLI and fPLI help in the diagnosis of pancreatic diseases

- fTLI for the diagnosis of exocrine pancreatic insufficiency
- fPLI for pancreatitis.

Severe lipaemia alters fTLI and fPLI results.

Elevated fPLI indicates pancreatic disease but not its pathological nature.

Diagnostic imaging

Plain radiography helps identify foreign bodies and masses.

Ultrasonography is useful for detection of thickenings, integrity of the intestinal layers, masses, lymph nodes and abnormalities in other organs. Likewise, it allows fine needle aspirations of the abnormalities identified. Ultrasonography also helps the clinician decide which is the best biopsy sampling technique: endoscopy or laparotomy.

Constipation

This section details the clinical approach to the patient with constipation.

Constipation is defined as difficulty defaecating due to the retention of faeces in the colon and rectum. When constipation is prolonged and stools are impacted and hardened, this results in obstipation. If constipation and obstipation are chronic and recurrent megacolon occurs, an increase in intestinal diameter develops that does not respond to treatment. **Megacolon is not a specific disease but indicates an advanced stage of chronic constipation.**

In most cases it is managed by treating the primary cause, which can be attributed to (Byers et al., 2006):

- Stool retention due to colorectal pain or anal pain.
- Difficulty defaecating:
  - Faeces-related factors: hard stools due to dehydration.
  - Colon related factors: decreased peristalsis.
- Physical obstruction:
  - Masses.
  - Injuries that decrease the size of the pelvic canal (Figure 18).

It is common for **multiple factors to combine which then favour stool retention**. For example, a cat with CKD and mild dehydration, plus arthritis in the hips may be at increased risk of constipation (Thanaboonnipat et al., 2021).

Clinical signs

The clinical signs of difficulty urinating and dysuria can be confused with those of straining to pass faeces. Also, some cats with constipation may have intermittent diarrhoea due to irritation by hard stools in the colon. **Cats can also exhibit anorexia, lethargy, weight loss, and**

vomiting (which are caused by stimulation of vomiting receptors in the colon) (Whitehead et al., 2016).

Physical examination

Physical examination and abdominal palpation can confirm the presence of stools, but it can be difficult to differentiate faeces from masses or lymph nodes. In case of doubt, **to confirm the diagnosis abdominal radiography is advisable**. Musculoskeletal examination should pay particular attention to signs of recent trauma (Figures 18 and 19), pain in the hips, or in the lumbosacral area. Geriatric cats with loss of muscle mass may show clinical signs associated with arthritis.

Neurological examination is important: proprioception, reflexes, gait and lesions in the lumbosacral area should be evaluated.

Rectal palpation with a lubricated glove allows the anal sacs to be emptied and the perineal area to be assessed. If it is painful, it is preferable that the anal examination be carried out under sedation.

Dehydration is a frequent cause of constipation. In the case of cats with underlying diseases that cause

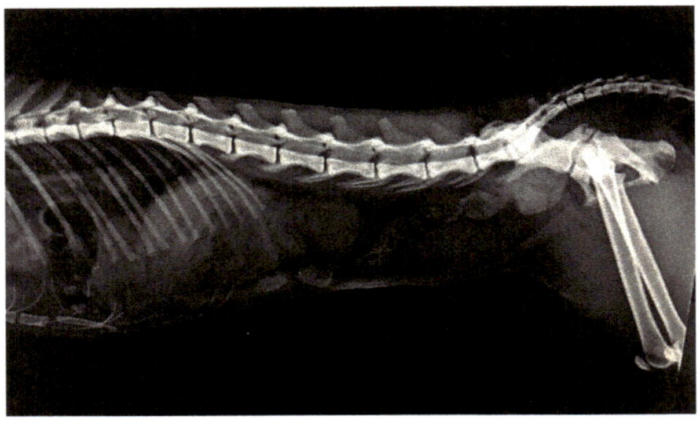

Figure 18. Constipation in a cat with a hip fracture and diaphragmatic hernia due to trauma.

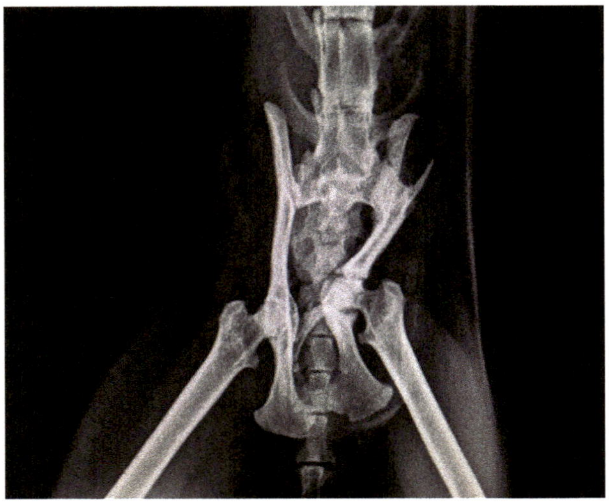

Figure 19. Hip fracture due to trauma.

Box 1. Differential diagnoses for constipation in the cat.

- Mechanical obstruction:
  Intraluminal: foreign body, neoplasia, stenosis, perineal hernia, rectal diverticulum.
  Intramural: neoplasia, granuloma.
  Extraluminal: pelvic fractures (23%), neoplasia, prostatic disease
- Aetiological: changes in sand used in litterbox, environmental changes, hospitalisation, inactivity.
- Inflammatory: sacculitis, abscesses, proctitis, perineal fistula, arthritis.
- Metabolic-endocrine:
  Obesity, dehydration, hypokalaemia, hypercalcaemia, CKD.
  Endocrine: hypothyroidism, hyperparathyroidism.
- Neuromuscular abnormalities:
  Spinal diseases: lumbosacral disease, spinal deformities such as in the Manx.
  Pelvic or hypogastric nerve abnormalities: trauma, dysautonomia.
  Myenteric or submucosal plexus neuropathy.
  Muscular abnormalities in the colon: idiopathic megacolon (62%), age.
- Medications: opioids, anticholinergics, diuretics, phenothiazines, barium sulphate.

dehydration, first it should be corrected and then reassessed.

Hypokalaemia and hypocalcaemia reduce the muscular functionality of the colon, so electrolyte abnormalities should be corrected first.

Treatment

Treatment of constipation should follow the following outline (Benjamin and Drobatz, 2020):

1. Elimination of obstructed faeces
2. Improvement of colonic motility
3. Reduction of the faecal bolus
4. Improvement of hydration status
5. Management of primary causes.

Management of a constipation episode in a healthy cat with mild obstruction

The first step is for stools to be eliminated. **In uncomplicated cases, paediatric glycerine suppositories or micro enemas (Microlax)** can be used. These products work by lubricating the walls of the colon to facilitate the passage of stools. The author prefers to use micro enemas in the consultation and then observe defaecation. If the micro enema cannot be easily applied and

Table 9. Use of laxatives in cats.

Laxative classification	Example	Observations
Hyperosmotic	Lactulose	Start with 2 ml/cat/12 h
Emollient	Docusate	50 mg/cat/12 h PO
Stimulants	Bisacodyl	5 mg/cat/24 h PO

sedation is necessary, the procedure in the next section should be followed.

After the obstruction has been removed, **colon motility and colon contractibility must be improved.** Medical management of constipation can be done with laxatives.

Medical management of constipation

Faecal bolus reduction is an important part of long-term treatment. Traditionally, a high fibre diet has been recommended that stimulates colonic contraction and motility, but these diets increase faecal volume, which can worsen constipation.

To prevent megacolon from occurring, which is believed to be the end result of chronic colon dilation, it is advisable to **reduce the stool bolus with a low-residue diet**.

The increase in wet diet reduces recurrences and maintains hydration status, which is especially important in constipation secondary to chronic kidney disease, along with subcutaneous fluid therapy and potassium control.

Pain management is critical in cats with arthritis, as is the repair of traumatic injuries that reduce pelvic diameter.

Management of cats with repeated episodes of constipation and obstipation

In cases of obstipation (Figure 20), some cats may be in poor general condition and need to be stabilized before they are anaesthetised to resolve the obstruction. **Dehydration status and electrolyte disturbances must be corrected.**

Micro enemas do not usually work in these cases. **Enemas of a warm isotonic solution and soap** should be used. Administration must be slow, to avoid the dilation of the colon causing vomiting. A **volume of about 5 to 10 ml/kg** is required. Mineral oil (5–10 ml/cat) can be added as a lubricant or emollients like docusate (5–10 ml/cat), but never together. **Enemas containing sodium phosphate should not be used** because they can induce severe hypernatraemia, hyperphosphataemia, and hypocalcaemia in cats.

Sometimes manual removal of the stool is required, by breaking it up with a finger and massaging to extract

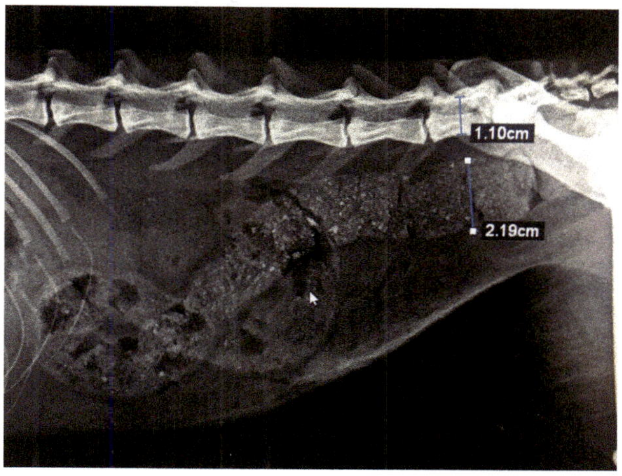

Figure 20. Obstipation in a cat with sacrocccygeal luxation.

it, but care should be taken because the colon is already weak and can be perforated. It is a painful procedure and **strong analgesia must be administered with opiates**, even assuming that as in humans' opioids reduce peristalsis: evacuation is more important.

Cats need to be maintained with medical treatment with **2 ml lactulose/cat/12 hours orally**.

Megacolon

Megacolon can be defined as a serious and irreversible dilation of the colon with hypomotility and faecal retention.

On a lateral radiograph, the **colon should be less than the width of the L7 vertebral body.** There are no guidelines and diagnosis is subjective, but some authors suggest that if it measures more than 1.5 and an average of 2.4 times more than L7 it may indicate chronic dilation. If it is also refractory to medical treatment and dietary management, it may be a megacolon.

A case review shows that 62% of megacolons are idiopathic, 23% due to a reduced pelvic canal, 11% due to neurological damage.

Megacolon management

By definition, megacolon is **refractory to medical therapy**, so the treatment is surgical and **consists of a subtotal colectomy**. The prognosis is usually good. At first, stools may be poorly formed, but they usually improve in 1 to 6 weeks after surgery (Grossman et al., 2021).

Inflammatory bowel disease

Inflammatory bowel disease (IBD) in cats is characterized by recurrent gastrointestinal signs, such as diarrhoea. This is due to a chronic form of immune-mediated enteropathy with histologically demonstrable inflammation. Affected cats often have concurrent inflammation of the pancreas and liver, which worsens the severity of clinical signs.

The **aetiology of inflammatory bowel disease is not fully understood**, but clinical studies suggest disease development is due to an interaction between genetic factors and the presence of bacteria.

Diagnosis is one of exclusion and requires biopsy of the intestinal mucosa to characterize the type and severity of the inflammatory infiltrate, as well as to differentiate inflammatory bowel disease from other conditions, such as alimentary lymphoma.

The term "inflammatory bowel disease (IBD)" is applied to chronic enteropathies with infiltration of the intestinal mucosa by inflammatory cells. In cats, the cell infiltrate is made up of a variable population of lymphocytes, plasma cells, eosinophils, and neutrophils that are distributed in the gastrointestinal wall. This produces serious changes in the wall affecting the mucosal architecture, intestinal villi atrophy, fibrosis and lymphangiectasis.

The World Small Animal Veterinary Association (WSAVA) Gastrointestinal Standardization Group created diagnostic guidelines and defines inflammatory bowel disease with the following criteria:

1. **Chronicity**. Cat with gastrointestinal signs of more than 3 weeks duration.
2. **No response to symptomatic treatment**. Clinical symptoms do not resolve with a hypoallergenic diet and antiparasitic treatment.
3. **No known cause**. To diagnose it, other intestinal or extraintestinal conditions that may cause gastrointestinal signs must be excluded.
4. **Histological evidence.** Biopsy without signs associated with a neoplastic condition. The presence of an inflammatory infiltrate in the gastrointestinal tract is not in itself diagnostic, because there are other causes such as bacteria, protozoa, allergies and food intolerances that can cause this infiltrate. In some cases of diffuse lymphosarcoma, an increase in inflammatory cells can also be found.
5. **Clinical signs improve with immunosuppressive treatment** (Washabau, 2010).

Clinical presentation

IBD is more common in middle-aged cats, although it can even occur in cats younger than two years of age. There is a **breed predisposition in Siamese cats and other Middle Eastern breeds** to suffer from this inflammatory syndrome.

The main clinical signs are:

- **Vomiting**: this is not always related to eating; and can be mucoid or bilious.
- **Small intestinal diarrhoea**.
- **Weight loss with or without appetite loss**: Weight loss in cases where body condition records are not available can be a subjective parameter and difficult to assess. Weight variations are very important as a warning sign in the health of the cat and in chronic conditions weight loss is accompanied by loss of muscle mass over the ribs, pelvis, scapula and neck.

These symptoms may be present intermittently, over a long period of time, or resolve spontaneously. Clinical signs may be exacerbated by dietary changes, drugs (e.g. antibiotics, NSAIDs, steroids) or exposure to transient intestinal pathogens.

On abdominal palpation (Figure 21) **thickening of the intestinal loops and enlarged mesenteric nodes may be found**. It can be considered subjective, but when thickening and intestinal rigidity is felt this corresponds to an ultrasound thickness of about 0.5 cm.

Key to the physical examination is to **determine whether the clinical signs correspond to an intestinal**

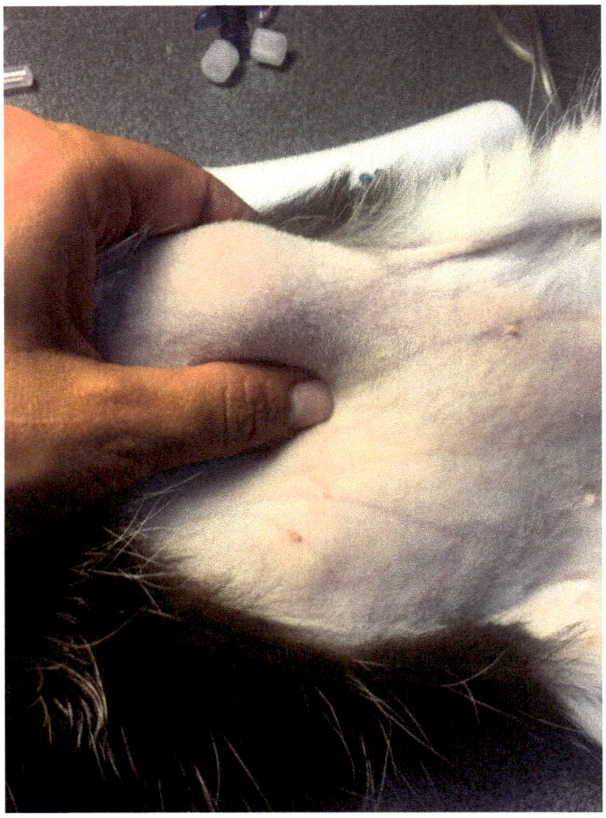

Figure 21. Abdominal palpation in a cat while preparing for ultrasound.

or non-intestinal condition. For example, weight loss may be due to poor digestion associated with exocrine pancreatic insufficiency, increased metabolism associated with hyperthyroidism, or poor energy utilization as a result of diabetes mellitus. It is important to **palpate the neck and look for thyroid nodules** in addition to taking a detailed history. There are other conditions that may be related: for example in **20% of cases diagnosed as inflammatory bowel disease, dermatological problems such as miliary dermatitis, alopecia, or pruritus were found.**

Pathophysiology

Inflammatory bowel disease has traditionally been viewed as an immune-mediated disease. The local immune system of the intestinal mucosa plays an important role, but recent work shows **alterations of the gut bacterial population can initiate the inflammatory process**. The most probable theory regarding the pathogenesis of inflammatory bowel disease is **hypersensitivity of the mucosa to antigens in the lumen such as bacteria, parasites, and dietary antigens**. The gastrointestinal flora causes an increase in proinflammatory cytokines which alter the mucosal immune response. The practical importance of these studies is to understand that the **management of intestinal dysbiosis plays a key role in the prognosis of inflammatory bowel disease.**

Although it is not specifically described in cats, clinical experience indicates that **chronic intestinal inflammation causes changes in motility** and if a detailed history is taken, the cat's owners usually comment that they vomit "normally" and bring up "fur balls" frequently. It is important to make the most of every occasion available to obtain information on the habits and behaviour of the cat, and assemble a detailed clinical history.

Diagnostic approach

A diagnosis is made by integrating the clinical history, physical examination, laboratory tests, diagnostic imaging and histopathology of intestinal biopsies, with the exclusion of other conditions.

Obtaining a basic data profile of the cat including **complete blood count, biochemistry, serum T4, urinalysis, and abdominal radiography** is important to rule out systemic and metabolic diseases (kidney disease, hyperthyroidism, liver disease) which can cause chronic gastrointestinal signs in cats.

There are **no typical laboratory findings** for inflammatory bowel disease, and many cats may have completely normal complete blood counts and blood biochemistry. Others may have:

- A **moderate increase in liver enzymes** (with or without associated signs) produced by secondary cholangitis or by dissemination of inflammatory intestinal cells through the portal circulation
- **Azotaemia or haemoconcentration caused by dehydration**
- Chronic inflammation reflected on the blood count by neutrophilia, monocytosis, and hyperglobulinaemia
- **Hypocobalaminaemia** may be a consequence of inflammation in the ileal area and a drop in folate due to inflammation of the proximal intestine.

After excluding infectious or parasitic diseases, non-gastrointestinal diseases, exocrine pancreatic insufficiency, and intestinal structural abnormalities requiring surgery, the most common chronic small intestine diseases are:

- Diet-responsive enteropathy
- Inflammatory bowel disease
- Alimentary lymphoma.

Diagnostic imaging

Abdominal radiography is not very specific, but helps rule out other conditions such as a foreign body and allows dilated intestinal loops, gas loops, or paralytic ileus (Figure 22) to be visualised.

Intestinal ultrasound is a useful method for evaluating the intestinal tract. In inflammatory **bowel disease, the intestinal wall may be focally or diffusely thickened,** but **loss of architecture of the intestinal layers is not common** (Figure 23).

The normal thickness of the intestinal wall in the duodenum is less than or equal to 2.8 mm and less

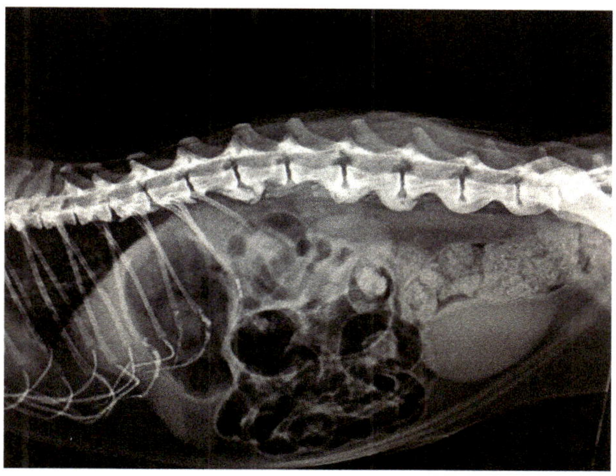

Figure 22. Lateral abdominal radiograph of a cat with IBD. Reduced intestinal transit, the presence of gas in intestinal loops and the stomach can be seen.

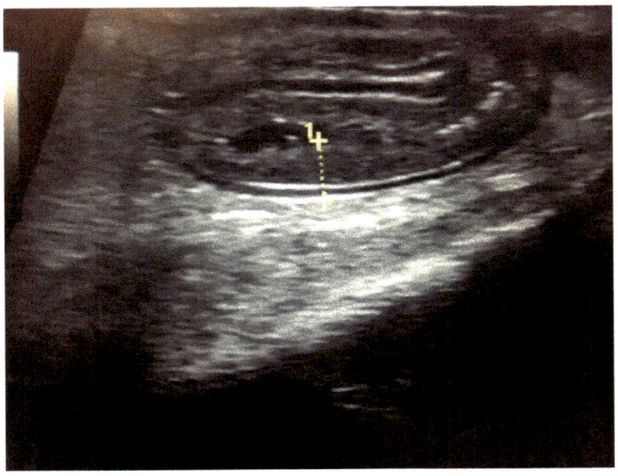

Figure 23. Abdominal ultrasound of the small intestine where thickening of the mucosa without loss of structure can be seen in a cat with IBD.

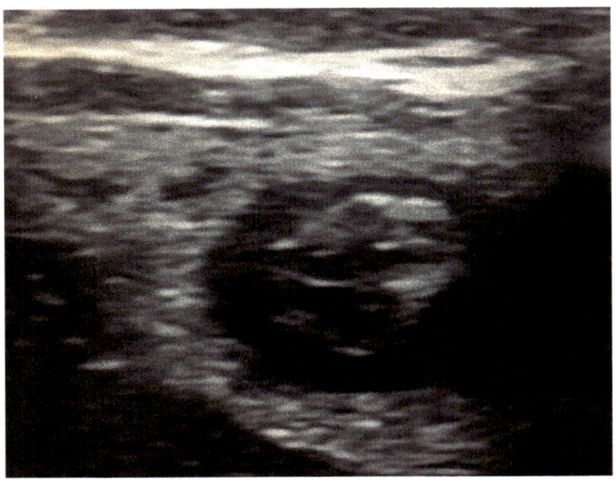

Figure 24. Abdominal ultrasound where thickening of the ileocaecal valve structure is seen in a cat with clinical signs of IBD.

than or equal to 3.2 mm in the ileum. Thickening of the mucosa is more frequent in inflammatory bowel disease. **In neoplastic conditions, the muscular layer is usually thickened.** Evaluation of the ileocaecal valve is important, to rule out a loss of structure that could be indicative of a neoplastic infiltrative process (Figure 24). Mesenteric lymph nodes can be enlarged, and their shape can help differentiate between inflammatory and neoplastic lymph nodes.

It is important to work together with the histopathologist. A good quality histological sample should be provided, and a dialogue indicating the clinical history and morphological findings observed when the sample was taken, as well as the location of the lesions, changes in architecture, thickening of the villi, oedema or erosion of the epithelium. Sometimes the characterization of histological findings as mild, moderate or severe does not correspond with the clinical symptoms and vice versa. Concurrent inflammation of

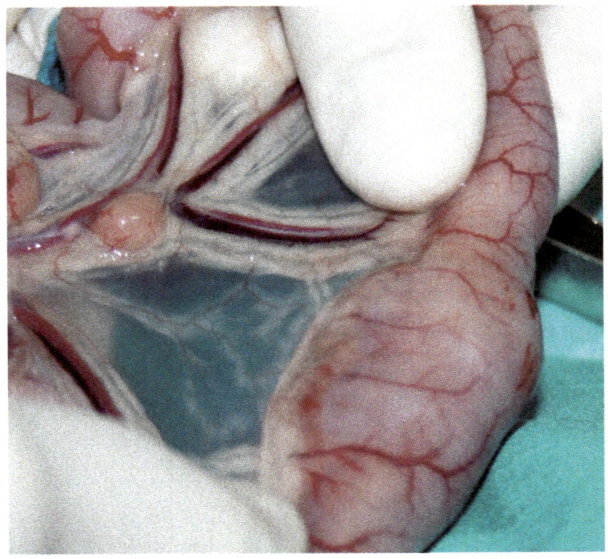

Figure 25. Loss of structure and thickening can be seen in the small intestine upon exploratory laparotomy. Histologically dietary lymphocytic lymphoma was diagnosed.

the pancreas and liver with intestinal inflammation has been described: tests that help approximate a diagnosis of pancreatitis or cholangitis should be carried out, as will be seen in other sections.

Histological diagnosis will be required to determine if there is an inflammatory or neoplastic intestinal infiltrate, and even then, there are cases where **it can be difficult to differentiate inflammatory intestinal lesions from low-grade lymphoma**. If a laparotomy is performed for sample taking, it is preferable that they be of full thickness (Figure 25). If the sample is obtained using endoscopy, indications regarding the number of samples should be followed and the limitations of partial thickness biopsies considered.

Diagnosis based on clinical criteria

The following points should be addressed:

- **Duration of more than 3 weeks of gastrointestinal signs** such as vomiting, diarrhoea, or weight loss with or without appetite
- There is **no positive response to symptomatic treatments** such as deworming, dietary changes or antibiotics
- Without other known causes. Exclusion of hyperthyroidism, and FeLV/FIV
- Histological confirmation of the non-existence of a neoplastic condition.

In between 70 and 100% of cases the infiltrate is lymphocytic/plasmocytic but can also be eosinophilic, findings with a neutrophilic or granulomatous infiltrate often show a worse response to treatment.

Treatment of inflammatory intestinal disease

Treatment is based on:

- Diet
- Immunomodulators
- Treatment of concurrent diseases.

Dietetic procedures

Many cases of intestinal disease in which an inflammatory infiltrate is found are related to diet.

A high percentage of cats with gastrointestinal clinical signs and structural inflammatory changes in the intestinal mucosa improve with a **hypoallergenic diet** alone. In addition, **improvement occurs in less than 4 days**, not in 8 weeks, as occurs in dermatological conditions due to food hypersensitivity.

Cats with inflammatory bowel disease show an improvement when their diet is changed because **fewer residues mean a decrease in the substrate necessary for bacteria growth** and this decreases osmotic potential.

To try to objectively evaluate the clinical improvement that occurs in cats when the diet is changed or medication is added, the disease activity index can be used combined with an evaluation of how this evolves.

When planning dietary therapy for a cat with inflammatory bowel disease, there are three critical aspects to consider:

1. Effect of diet on flora: dysbiosis or destruction of flora.
2. Dietary intolerance as a non-immunological effect.
3. True food allergy.

To find out which of the three situations is most likely, a change in diet should be made and the therapeutic effect quantified on the evolution of the disease. In general, there is **no one diet that suits all cats** and a suitable diet should be established on an individual basis.

In cats with mild inflammatory bowel disease, with moderate inflammatory cell infiltration and no weight loss, diets with **protein hydrolysates or with a single source of protein,** low levels of carbohydrates and few additives and flavourings may be indicated. Protein digestibility must be greater than 87% and in normal diets it is around 78–81%. This factor may be key to the therapeutic success of the treatment for inflammatory bowel disease, because **non-digestible proteins are the necessary resource for bacterial growth** and for toxic products to be generated in the gastrointestinal system that increase damage to the flora.

It is important to recognize when a diet is not well accepted by a cat or does not improve clinical signs, it should not be assumed this will be the same in another cat. If the cat does not improve with the dietary change in 2 weeks, **trying a different type of diet from another manufacturer in the same category** or considering the possibility of natural diets is advisable.

The **addition of prebiotics and probiotics** should be considered to prevent destruction of the microflora (Box 2).

Although dietary therapy is the key to normalizing intestinal microflora, it can be difficult to decrease pathogenic species that are overpopulating the intestinal lumen. In addition, in cases of concurrent pancreatitis, an antibiotic must be administered to avoid infections in the bile duct and intestine.

Metronidazole therapy is effective not only for its antimicrobial action but also as an immunomodulator, but the dose administered, and the time of administration must be taken into account to avoid adverse effects. Neurotoxicity and damage to the DNA of intestinal cells can occur, therefore it must be administered with certain considerations (Box 3).

Box 2. Role of probiotics in the prevention and treatment of gastrointestinal disease in cats.

Act on three levels:

1. **Metabolic effect**: effect on the digestion of lactose and other disaccharides and on the production of intestinal gas.
2. **Protective effect:** seem to have a protective therapeutic effect on acute diarrhoea caused by antibiotics or gastrointestinal infections and prevent systemic infections due to bacterial translocation.
3. **Trophic effect**: effect on the immunity of the mucosa and the growth of epithelial cells.

Situations where **probiotic supplementation can be considered**:

- Acute idiopathic diarrhoea.
- Diarrhoea in groups of puppies.
- Chronic diarrhoea where a traditional approach is unsatisfactory.
- In situations of stress, dietary change, medications, or travel.
- Antibiotic associated diarrhoea: probiotics can be used at the same time as antibiotics because they are resistant.
- Diarrhoea associated with intestinal parasites (*Tritrichomonas foetus*).

Box 3. Management recommendations for metronidazole

- Metronidazole should not be administered for more than 10 consecutive days and a period of another 10 days should elapse before re-administering.
- Adverse effects are caused by dose or administration times.
- Dose should be calculated carefully. Administration of liquid formats orally means dose can be easily adjusted to weight, although in some cats it can cause salivation due to its unpleasant taste (this should not be confused with an adverse effect).

Pharmacological treatment

This is based on oral corticosteroids at immunosuppressive doses.

In cats with very marked weight loss or severe clinical signs, the author prefers to **start treating with corticosteroids** even if no change in diet has been made: the cat needs to be stabilised before therapeutic tests are carried out. When the signs resolve and the corticosteroid dose has been decreased, a stimulation test can be performed with the old food, observing for food hypersensitivity.

There is no consensus regarding the use of corticosteroids. Prednisolone is used orally, and the dose depends on the severity of the clinical signs:

- Treatment with prednisolone can be started at **doses of 2 mg/kg/orally once daily**. If a sample has been taken for histopathology, prednisolone treatment should not be started for at least a week to avoid postoperative complications.
- The disease activity index should be analysed and if there is improvement after two weeks, the dose should be maintained for a further 2 to 4 weeks.
- When the cat regains weight and shows no clinical signs, the dose is lowered to 1 mg/kg/orally once a day.
- Treatment can take months to reach the minimum effective dose.

If hypocobalaminaemia is confirmed, cobalamin should be supplemented parenterally at a dose of 250 µg/cat subcutaneously once a week for 6 weeks, then every 2 weeks for 6 weeks and monthly after this. The owner can be taught to inject and thus avoid the stress of clinic visits.

Some cats do not improve with conventional treatment. In these cases, the diagnosis should be reconsidered, the patient re-evaluated, and the pathologist contacted to review the sample again. Before increasing the dose of corticosteroids or adding other immunosuppressants such as chlorambucil at a dose of 2 mg/cat orally every 2 days, infectious conditions must be ruled out.

Table 10. Medications used to treat inflammatory intestinal disease.

Medication	Dose
Prednisolone	5 mg/cat/12–24 hours oral
Budesonide	0.5–1 mg/cat/24 hours oral
Cyclosporine	5 mg/kg/12–24 hours oral
Chlorambucil	2 mg/cat/48–72 hours oral
Cobalamin	250 µg/cat SC 1 weekly injection for 6 weeks, 1 injection every 2 weeks for 6 weeks and 1 injection per month

Studies in cats with chronic lymphoplasmacytic enteropathy show good responses to treatment with diet, antibiotics, and immunosuppressants. Sequential treatment helps determine which treatment is most effective for each cat:

- **Hypoallergenic diet for 7 days** and with subsequent evaluation of response with the IBD activity index.
- **Metronidazole** (15 mg/kg/24 hours PO) for 10 days. If the IBD activity index improves, the dose should be reduced by 25% every 2 weeks until withdrawal.
- If there is no response to diet or metronidazole, the animal should be treated with **prednisolone (2 mg/kg/24 h PO)** or in combination with metronidazole. The dose should be reduced by 25% every 2 weeks until the minimum dose that controls symptoms is reached.

In summary

- Feline inflammatory bowel disease (IBD) is **an immunologically mediated gastrointestinal inflammatory disorder**.
- The exact **aetiology is unknown**, but studies indicate that there may be an interaction between genetic factors, enteric bacteria, and host-related immune factors.
- **Clinical signs** in cats include vomiting, weight loss, diarrhoea, and inflammatory histopathologic lesions in the stomach, small intestine, or colon. Affected cats may have concurrent inflammation in the pancreas and liver, worsening clinical signs.
- There is **controversy regarding the method by which intestinal biopsies are obtained:** endoscopy, laparoscopy or laparotomy. It is important that the sample is full thickness and from the ileal area to differentiate IBD from alimentary lymphoma
- **Treatments are empirical and should be administered sequentially**: they are based on the combination of diet, immunosuppressive drugs and antibiotics, without forgetting effective deworming.

Feline pancreatitis

Feline pancreatitis is a difficult disease to diagnose, especially in chronic cases that have intermittent clinical signs. This section aims to review the diagnostic and therapeutic approach to both acute and chronic forms of pancreatitis (Brazelle et al., 2014).

In cats, reaching a diagnosis of pancreatitis requires different indicators to be considered, including:

1. Compatible **clinical signs**
2. **Physical exam** with detection of abdominal pain
3. **Ultrasound**
4. Laboratory tests:
    a. Serum elevation of **immunoreactive feline pancreatic lipase** (fPLI).
    b. **Serum amyloid A (SAA).** Acute phase protein is useful for diagnosis and treatment monitoring.

The specificity and sensitivity of the diagnosis of pancreatitis is high when these different methods are combined, although they are reduced for chronic pancreatitis.

Treatment is symptomatic, but should focus on:

- Maintaining fluid volume
- Controlling pain, vomiting and nausea
- Preventing secondary infections.

Classification of feline pancreatitis

Histologically feline pancreatitis can be classified into 3 types:

- Acute necrotizing pancreatitis:
    - Acute pancreatitis with neutrophilic infiltrate without fibrosis is less frequent and affects younger cats.
- Acute suppurative pancreatitis (feline only).
- Chronic non-suppurative pancreatitis (the most frequent):
    - This is the most frequent form characterised by lymphocytic inflammation with loss of structure and fibrosis.

From a clinical perspective, pancreatitis can be **classified as acute and chronic**, although it is not easy to differentiate between them because most cats display symptoms of pancreatitis as the result of an **exacerbation of a chronic condition** (called acute in chronic).

It is important to recognize when the **acute condition is present because it is reversible** and 2/3 of cats with acute pancreatitis have another **concurrent disease which needs to be diagnosed and treated** to correctly manage the pancreatitis.

The incidence of pancreatitis in cats

Determining the exact prevalence of feline pancreatitis is difficult and varies greatly depending on whether the diagnosis is made before or after death. Clinical evidence suggests the prevalence of feline pancreatitis is 0.6%, whereas post-mortem results indicate a prevalence of up to 67%. However, the true incidence of feline pancreatitis is unknown and possibly underestimated, due to the difficulties of diagnosis. (Figure 26).

In clinical studies, the actual prevalence of pancreatitis is likely to be underestimated since there are usually no clinical suspicions of this disease and limited diagnostic tests. On the other hand, post-mortem studies probably overestimate the prevalence of clinically relevant feline pancreatitis since clinical signs may appear only in the presence of concurrent diseases.

The actual prevalence of pancreatitis in cats has not been determined conclusively, but it has been defined as **clinically important and a common disease in this species. Chronic pancreatitis is more common** than acute pancreatitis, accounting for 65% to 89% of all cases of pancreatitis, while the acute form represents 9% to 33% of cases. However, acute and chronic pancreatitis can be found in the same pancreas in 10% to 44% of cases.

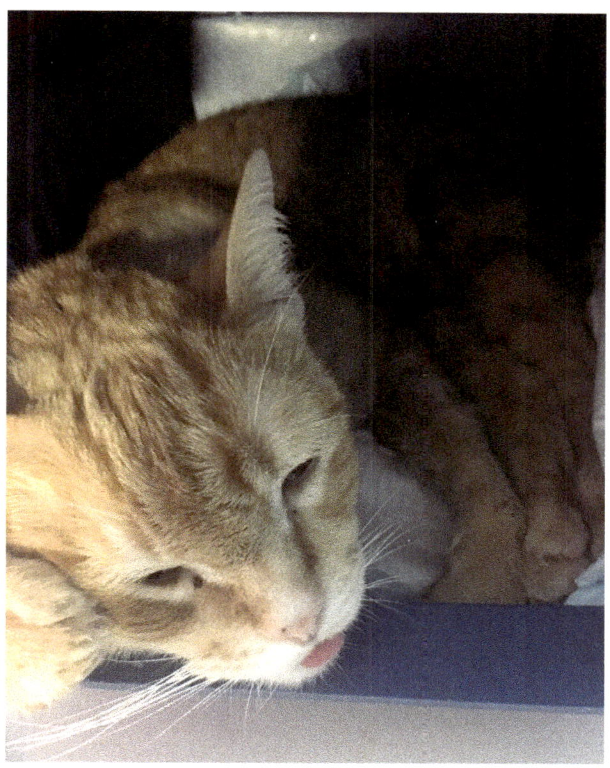

Figure 26. Cat with signs of acute pain due to pancreatitis. Pain management is key, even before examination and performing diagnostic tests.

Aetiology

Contrary to humans where an aetiology is identified in more than 90% of pancreatitis patients, in the vast majority of cats it is not possible to identify an underlying cause and the pancreatitis is considered idiopathic.

An association between **pancreatitis, inflammatory bowel disease (IBD), and liver diseases**, (mainly cholangitis) has been shown in various studies. However, it remains unclear which disease occurs first and whether there are cause and effect relationships between them. Viral and parasitic agents are occasionally associated with feline pancreatitis, but none have been shown to be a major, common cause of pancreatitis in this domestic species (Cerná et al., 2020).

Other reported or **suspected causes of feline pancreatitis** include:

- abdominal trauma in road traffic accidents and high-rise syndrome
- ischaemia with hypotension secondary to poorly compensated anaesthetics
- acute hypercalcaemia
- organophosphate poisoning
- pharmacological substances
- pancreatic tumours
- pancreatic duct obstruction.

Risk factors

There are several recognized risk factors for feline pancreatitis:

- **Hypoperfusion**: this is the most important determining risk factor for pancreatitis, which in addition to triggering, worsens the condition, so the cat must be kept hydrated and normovolaemic during sedation or anaesthesia.
- **Diet**: in canine medicine, diets rich in fat, obesity, and hyperlipidaemia are known to be risk factors for pancreatitis, but there are no studies confirming this in cats. One study linked pancreatic inflammation to hyperglycaemia, but not hyperlipidaemia.
- **Breed**: Siamese cats appear to be overrepresented.
- **Infectious agents**: pancreatitis has been related to toxoplasmosis in some publications, but it depends on the prevalence in each area. There are also studies linking it to feline infectious peritonitis (FIP) and feline panleukopenia virus (FPV), but these are isolated cases.
- **Medications**: there is no evidence that steroid administration is related to the appearance of pancreatitis, although the administration of azathioprine, chlorothiazide, hydrochlorothiazide, oestrogens, furosemide, tetracyclines, and sulphamides do affect the pancreas. The pancreas is an organ which is very sensitive to drugs, stress, metabolic disorders and ischaemia.

It is thought the action of harmful stimuli may cause a decrease in pancreatic enzyme secretion with the consequent formation of cytoplasmic vacuoles. By lowering the pH, the intracytoplasmic activation of trypsinogen occurs, which triggers the self-digestive actions of pancreatic enzymes.

The following can occur secondary to pancreatitis:

- Interstitial nephritis (42%)
- Third spacing (47%)
- Lipid accumulation in the liver (47%)
- Intestinal lesions (32%).

When examining a cat with inflammatory bowel disease, possible abnormalities of adjacent structures should be considered such as the pancreas and common bile duct. **20% of cats with histologically confirmed pancreatitis have concurrent inflammatory bowel disease,** so inflammatory bowel disease is probably the biggest risk factor for feline pancreatitis.

There are factors specific to cats that increase the risk of pancreatitis.

Inflammatory bowel disease is a common cause of gastrointestinal disease, and pancreatitis can overlap. Clinically differentiating a cat with pancreatitis or inflammatory bowel disease can be tricky.

Due to the anatomy of the pancreatic duct and bile duct, duodenal content may rise due to reflux during vomiting or abnormal duodenal motility (Figure 27). In dogs this is unlikely, but in cats the pancreatic biliary sphincter is common to the duodenal papilla. As a consequence, both **duodenal and biliary branch reflux can affect the pancreatic ductal system**. In a cat with inflammatory bowel disease, the content that penetrates the ductal system has a greater number of

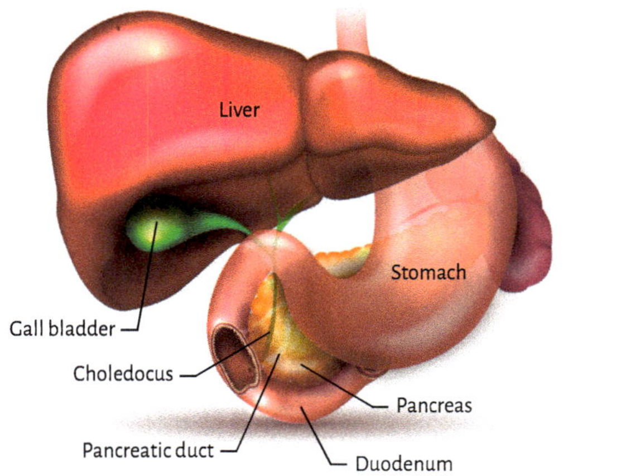

Figure 27. Anatomy of the liver, pancreas and duodenum.

pathogenic bacteria, bile salts and activated pancreatic enzymes that cause tissue damage, infection and inflammation in the pancreas. In addition, reflux from vomiting, impaired intestinal motility, and dysregulation of the immune system cause gastrointestinal reflux in the pancreatic duct causing clinical signs to worsen.

More studies are needed to understand the pathogenesis of inflammatory bowel disease and lymphoplasmacytic pancreatitis, but it seems clear that they are **closely related pathologies and that the clinician should think about them together.** Therefore, when considering a pancreatic biopsy, liver and small intestinal biopsies should also be performed, if possible, to determine the extent of the problem and may be important in determining subsequent treatment.

Clinical signs

Acute or chronic pancreatitis presents with a wide range of clinical signs of varying severity. The mildest cases may be clinically undetectable, with the severest suffering from cardiovascular shock and multi-organ failure. **The presentation of pancreatitis ranges from mild and almost asymptomatic to acute and necrotizing,** with the latter requiring intensive treatment and may be fatal. In chronic pancreatitis, the clinical signs may be present for a long period of time or appear intermittently.

Acute and chronic pancreatitis cannot be differentiated from a clinical perspective alone. However, mild cases of pancreatitis are often subclinical or associated with mild clinical signs. When **clinical signs are present they are non-specific** and may not even be suggestive of gastrointestinal disease.

The most frequently reported clinical signs are:

- anorexia and lethargy
- vomiting
- weight loss
- diarrhoea
- **Abdominal discomfort**: although the main clinical sign of human pancreatitis, it is less frequently reported in feline cases. However, it should be kept in mind that cats cannot express abdominal pain as obviously as humans, and the author believes abdominal discomfort should be assumed in all cats with pancreatitis.

The most frequent findings on **physical examination** are:

- dehydration
- pallor
- jaundice
- tachypnoea or dyspnoea
- hypothermia or fever
- tachycardia
- abdominal pain
- palpable abdominal mass
- In cats with severe pancreatitis, significant systemic complications may occur, such as disseminated intravascular coagulation, cardiovascular shock, and multiple organ failure.

Clinical signs in cats are difficult to recognize:

- **Abdominal pain**. Detected less often than in the dog, but whenever pancreatitis is suspected, pain should be assumed and treated because it exists in 100% of cats, although only appreciated in 25% of cases due to lack of recognition by clinicians. In other studies, using cat-specific scale systems, abdominal pain was detected in 75% of cases.
- **Anorexia and lethargy** are the most frequent clinical signs.
- **Vomiting**, although this is less frequent than in the dog.

Many patients with **chronic pancreatitis have vague clinical signs and concurrent diseases** such as gastrointestinal, liver disease, or poorly controlled diabetes. Fibrosis of the pancreatic acini due to chronic pancreatitis can also lead to the not uncommon complication of **exocrine pancreatic insufficiency**.

Diagnosis

Pancreatitis should be considered in any cat with anorexia, lethargy, or vomiting of unknown cause. A diagnosis of pancreatitis also requires investigation of any possible concurrent disease and complications such as anaemia, hypalbuminaemia, and hepatic lipidosis.

Blood tests

Haematology may show leukocytosis or leukopoenia. Leukopoenia, decreased haematocrit, and thrombocytopaenia imply a negative prognosis for pancreatitis.

Biochemistry may show:

- elevated liver enzymes and bilirubin
- azotaemia
- hypoalbuminaemia
- hypercholesterolaemia
- hyperglycaemia
- hypocalcaemia should be considered a negative prognostic factor, even in the absence of associated clinical signs
- hypokalaemia should be identified and corrected.

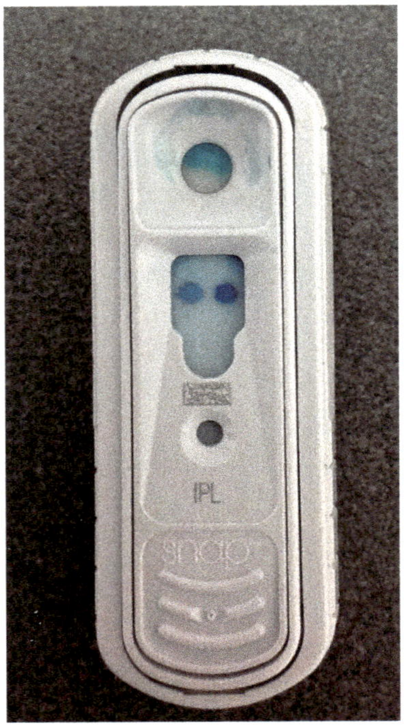

Figure 28. Test for fPLI (Idexx) showing a positive diagnosis of feline pancreatitis.

Liver function should be assessed (ALT, ALKP, GGT, bile acids) along with **gastrointestinal function** (folate and cobalamin). The diagnosis must be differentiated from hepatic lipidosis, inflammatory liver disease, interstitial nephritis, and diabetes mellitus.

The most frequent changes in blood biochemistry are:

fPLI

Feline pancreatic lipase (fPLI) immunoreactivity has a sensitivity and specificity of 100% for acute pancreatitis, but in chronic pancreatitis the degree of sensitivity is 54% (Figure 28). The level of fPLI is related to a negative prognosis for pancreatitis. fPLI is more useful in diagnosing moderate and severe pancreatitis, but in mild cases may not be increased.

fTLI

Feline trypsin-like immunoreactivity (fTLI) is useful for the diagnosis of **exocrine pancreatic insufficiency (EPI)** but is not sensitive for pancreatitis. It has a sensitivity of 80% in acute pancreatitis, but only 8% in chronic pancreatitis. Levels can also be increased by other gastrointestinal diseases such as inflammatory bowel disease or lymphoma.

Serum amyloid A

Serum amyloid A (SAA) is an **acute phase protein that increases in pancreatitis**. It is useful to monitor evolution, which helps adjust treatment accordingly and thus avoid recurrences.

Diagnostic imaging

The use of abdominal radiography for the diagnosis of feline pancreatitis is limited. Its main use is that **it allows other differential diagnoses to be ruled out** in patients with similar clinical signs. The abdominal radiograph lacks sensitivity and in most cases of feline pancreatitis abdominal radiographs are normal. In cases of abnormal radiographic results, these are non-specific and may be associated with other systemic diseases or abdominal organ diseases.

Therefore, it is not possible to establish a definitive diagnosis or rule out pancreatitis based solely on abdominal radiography.

In cats in which pancreatitis is suspected, **radiography should be performed in conjunction with other more sensitive and specific tests.** Possible radiographic findings in cats with pancreatitis are decreased detail and contrast in the cranial abdomen, dilatation of the small intestine (due to fluid or gas), hepatomegaly, and the presence of a cranially positioned abdominal mass.

A normal abdominal ultrasound does not definitively rule out pancreatitis, and an enlarged pancreas is not always indicative of pancreatitis but may be due to pancreatic oedema.

The usefulness of abdominal ultrasound for the diagnosis of feline pancreatitis largely depends on the operator's skills, the equipment used, and severity of the lesions. The most significant **changes on abdominal ultrasound that suggest pancreatitis are changes in echogenicity**, including hypoechogenicity of the pancreas (Figure 29) and hyperechogenicity of peripancreatic fat. Occasionally, hyperechogenic areas of the pancreas can be identified, possibly indicating the presence of pancreatic fibrosis. Other possible ultrasound findings include abdominal effusion (Figure 30), enlargement of the pancreas, hepatomegaly, cavitary lesions of the pancreas such as pseudocysts, and calcification of the pancreas.

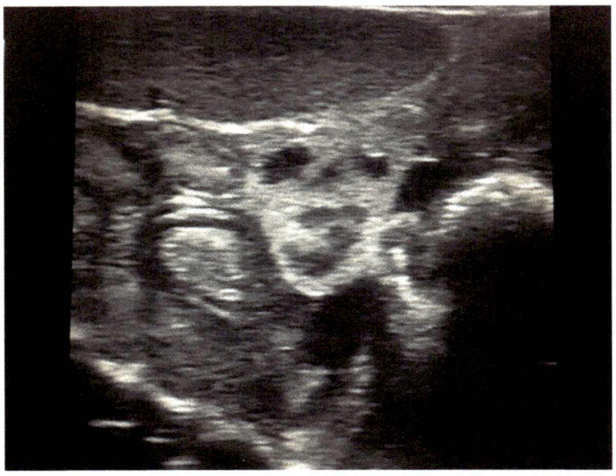

Figure 29. Abdominal ultrasound showing image of an enlarged heterogeneous pancreas with hypoechogenic areas.

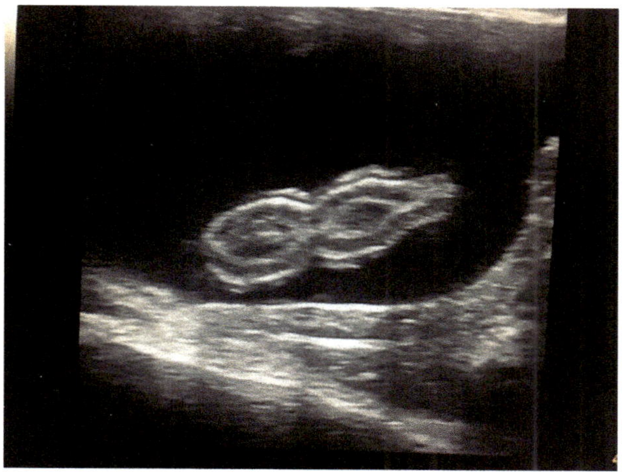

Figure 30. Abdominal ultrasound image of the same cat as in Figure 29 showing free fluid in the abdomen.

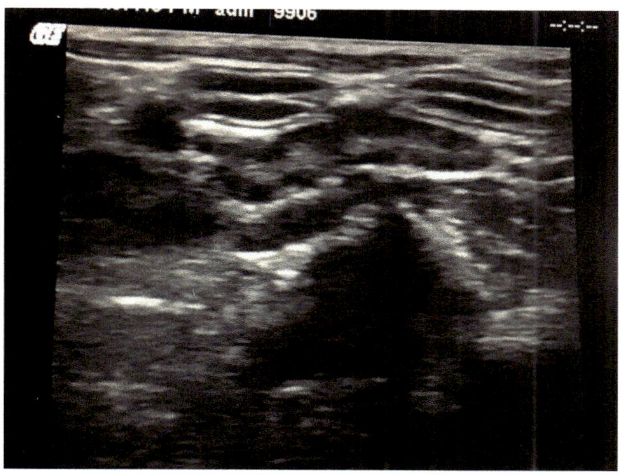

Figure 31. Abdominal ultrasound image of a cat with pancreatitis and concurrent IBD.

It should be emphasized that certain **pathologies of the pancreas** (neoplasms, hyperplastic nodes, oedema due to portal hypertension or hypoalbuminaemia) **may be associated with similar ultrasound findings** and these abnormalities can be difficult to differentiate from pancreatitis (Figure 31).

Abdominal ultrasound is also useful for investigation of possible pathological causes of clinical signs similar to those of pancreatitis.

Ultrasound patterns vary:

- hypoechoic pancreas in pancreatic necrosis
- hyperechogenic pancreas due to fibrosis or pancreatic masses
- hyperechogenic peritoneum due to necrosis of mesenteric fat
- hypoechogenic region around the pancreas
- mass effect: in pancreatic abscesses or pancreatic pseudocysts
- dilatation of the pancreatic duct.

The normal pancreas measures less than 9.5 mm on the left side, the body less than 8 mm and less than 6mm on the right side with the pancreatic duct measuring less than 2.5 mm. The pancreas is isoechoic with respect to the liver.

A pancreatic diameter of more than 2 cm indicates a probable neoplasm in this organ. The most frequent finding in acute pancreatitis is hyperechogenicity of the peripancreatic fat. Other changes are less specific. In cats with suspected acute pancreatitis, ultrasound should be repeated 48 hours later to observe any changes.

Cytology using fine needle aspiration of the pancreas is considered relatively safe. The presence of inflammatory cells is specific to pancreatitis. However, as can occur with histopathology, localized lesions may go unnoticed. Therefore, negative results are not enough to rule out pancreatitis (Crein et al., 2015).

In human medicine, the non-invasive technique of choice in the diagnosis of pancreatitis is CT, but the cost, availability, and difficulty of image interpretation mean this is not a useful technique in first opinion clinical practice. Furthermore, the combination of ultrasound and fPLI has a greater sensitivity than CT.

Histopathology

Histopathology is the technique of choice for the diagnosis of pancreatitis, but requires stabilization of the patient to perform surgical sampling. It is important to note that the distribution of the lesions may be focal and its is possible that no abnormalities are detected in the sample obtained.

When an exploratory laparotomy is performed for biopsy, **macroscopic pancreatic lesions are not always seen**, especially in mild cases, but in other cases necrosis of the peripancreatic fat, pancreatic haemorrhage and congestion, and an opaque granular capsular surface are observed. **A definitive diagnosis, as well as differentiating acute from chronic pancreatitis, can only be made by histopathological examination of pancreatic tissue.**

Since pancreatitis in cats often occurs simultaneously with inflammatory liver or intestinal diseases, **liver and intestinal biopsies should also be considered** when pancreatitis is suspected.

Histologically, **pancreatitis is classified as acute necrotizing, acute suppurative, and the chronic non-suppurative form** which is the most frequent (characterized by a mononuclear infiltrate and fibrosis).

The combination of clinical history, fPLI, ultrasound, cytology and/or histopathology (when possible) is key to the diagnosis of pancreatitis in cats (Figure 32).

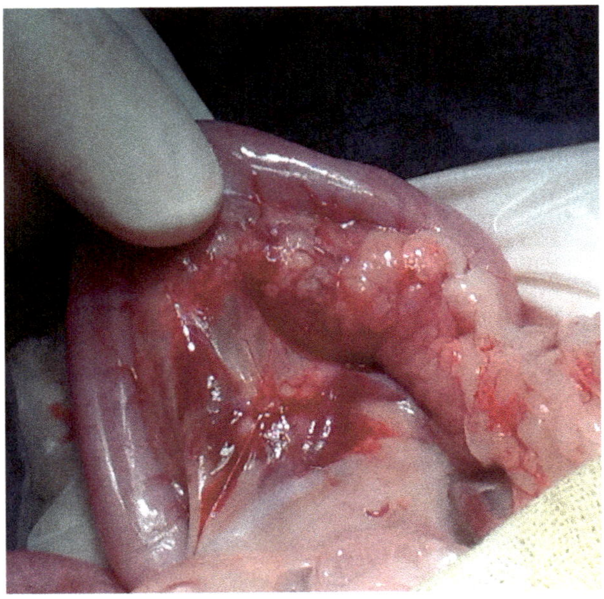

Figure 32. Macroscopic appearance of the pancreas in a cat with signs compatible with pancreatitis where it can be seen to be swollen, oedematous along with peritoneal reaction.

Treatment

Fluid therapy

Cats with pancreatitis are often **dehydrated** due to vomiting, diarrhoea, or lack of water intake. In severe cases, rapid and significant fluid loss can lead to hypovolaemia or even hypovolemic shock. In order to maintain general tissue perfusion and pancreatic perfusion in particular, **intravenous fluid therapy with replacement crystalloids** should be started as soon as possible, usually with a compound sodium lactate (Ringers) or 0.9% NaCl solution, depending on the simultaneous electrolyte abnormalities.

Electrolyte abnormalities are usually seen in cats with more severe forms of pancreatitis. The most frequent are hypokalaemia, hypocalcaemia, hyponatraemia and/or hypochloraemia. Therefore, in cats with pancreatitis, electrolytes should always be measured and corrected appropriately. **Aggressive fluid therapy with crystalloids and colloids** can prevent pancreatic ischaemia which triggered the systemic inflammatory response syndrome (SIRS) cascade.

Plasma administration helps restore oncotic pressure by providing albumin and other high molecular weight proteins, as well as clotting factors.

Nutrition

Nutrients must be provided to prevent hepatic lipidosis, malnutrition, intestinal atrophy, and dysbiosis. **Enteral nutrition is preferred** over parenteral nutrition because a central venous catheter is required and complications such as thrombosis or sepsis can occur.

In cats with pancreatitis that have been without food for more than two to three days at diagnosis, **placement of a nasoesophageal, oesophagostomy, or gastrostomy tube** should be considered. In patients with vomiting that does not cease, partial or total parenteral nutrition can be used.

The cat should not be forced to eat because optimal daily calorie levels cannot be achieved in this way and often results in food aversion. If the cat is anorexic, placement of an enteral feeding tube is the best option. If the cat eats alone, **highly digestible hydrolysed protein diets** used to treat inflammatory bowel disease are suitable for treating pancreatitis.

Analgesia

It is well known that **acute pancreatitis is painful**, however, lymphoplasmacytic pancreatitis is a chronic disease that presents with focal or a low degree of inflammation. Low-grade pain in cats is difficult to detect. Humans with chronic pancreatitis show similar clinical signs, with low-grade pain in the right upper quadrant and loss of appetite with a general malaise that does not resolve with anti-inflammatories but does with opiates. Cats with low-grade pain hide, have little appetite, and occasionally vomit, in which case **opioid is indicated.**

- Cats with mild to moderate pain can be effectively controlled with **buprenorphine** (0.01–0.03 mg/kg/h IV or IM).
- Cats suffering with severe pain can be controlled with **fentanyl** (0.005–0.01 mg/kg/2 h IV, IM or SC or by constant continuous infusion 0.002–0.004 mg/kg/hour).
- In severe cases, **multimodal analgesic treatment** in the form of a constant continuous infusion can be attempted because it appears more effective than monotherapy analgesia and is associated with fewer side effects, due to the lower dose needed of each component.
- The use of **ursodeoxycholic acid** decreases pain because it increases bile and pancreatic flow.
- **S-adenosyl methionine (SAMe)** increases glutathione concentrations and improves pancreatic enzyme levels.
- The author has observed that supplementation with **pancreatic enzymes** given with food reduces postprandial pain.

Occasionally, appetite stimulants must be administered, or the placement of an enteral feeding tube is necessary.

Antibiotics

Secondary bacterial colonization damages intestinal epithelium and causes dysbiosis. The microorganisms that most frequently colonize the pancreas are Gram negative, anaerobic ones from the gastrointestinal system: *E. coli, Klebsiella spp., Enterobacteriaceae* and *Clostridium spp.*

Antibiotics should be administered when there is **evidence of pancreatic abscess or systemic inflammation** e.g. leukocytosis, fever, or hypoglycaemia. They must be **broad-spectrum antibiotics** with good pancreatic penetration such as marbofloxacin, amoxicillin-clavulanic acid, or clindamycin.

Control of vomiting and nausea

Treatment with antiemetics should be given to all vomiting cats suffering from pancreatitis.

- **5-HT$_3$, antagonists** can be used, such as dolasetron (0.6 mg/kg/12 h IV, SC or PO) or ondansetron (0.1–0.2 mg/kg/6–12 h slow IV infusion), but they are expensive and difficult to source.
- Maropitant is an antiemetic that acts as an **NK$_1$ receptor inhibitor,** which is very effective in cats, and can be used at doses of 0.5–1.0 mg/kg/24 h IV, SC. Use of maropitant can be useful even if the cat does not vomit to avoid the feeling of nausea, which is very uncomfortable and hinders the cat's recovery.
- **Dopaminergic antagonists** such as metoclopramide (0.2–0.5 mg/kg/6–8 h IV, IM, SC, PO, or 0.3 mg/kg/h IV as a constant infusion) are considered less effective in cats. As a prokinetic metoclopramide is favoured for symptoms in cats with gastroduodenal ileus.

Treatment of thromboembolic complications

Heparin prevents coagulopathies secondary to SIRS, but there are no published studies of its benefits in cats. Low molecular weight heparin (100 IU/kg/24h SC) can be used.

Treatment of exocrine pancreatic insufficiency

In some cases, exocrine pancreatic insufficiency (EPI) occurs and administration of pancreatic enzymes is necessary. **Cats in the recovery phase with pancreatitis can also benefit from the administration of pancreatic enzymes since there is negative feed-back and reduced post-prandial pancreatic secretion, decreasing pain.**

Vitamin B12, cobalamin supplementation

Cobalamin levels should be monitored since, although they are not altered at the time of diagnosis, during the course of the disease they can decrease and must be supplemented (Trehy et al., 2014) (250 µg once a week for 6 weeks SC).

Corticoids

The most effective anti-inflammatory and immunomodulatory treatment for inflammatory bowel disease (and presumably for pancreatitis) are **corticosteroids.**

The authors commence corticosteroid therapy for pancreatitis after 2 weeks of antibiotic treatment, but there are no studies that support its efficacy. Prednisolone is metabolized more rapidly than prednisone in cats and is administered in doses of 0.5–1 mg/kg/12–24 h PO.

Prognosis

Prognosis is variable and depends on the promptness with which intensive therapy is implemented, but **in acute pancreatitis a mortality rate of 41% is documented** (Dias C. et al. 2015).

If the following is observed, the **prognosis is poor**:

- hyperkalaemia
- dyspnoea
- arrhythmias
- fPLI concentrations > 20 µg/l.
- hypocalcaemia.

Summary

Assessment of a combination of clinical history, abdominal pain, minimal test data, fPLI, SAA, and ultrasound changes are necessary to confirm a diagnosis of pancreatitis.

Treatment is supportive, feeding must be enteral, and when this is not possible, parenteral.

Feline liver diseases

Liver diseases are common in cats. The most frequent diseases are hepatic lipidosis, cholangitis and its various forms, neoplasms and hepatocellular necrosis associated with toxins or drugs. Other liver diseases can be reactive liver diseases and other inflammatory liver diseases associated with various infections (FIP, toxoplasmosis, and virulent calicivirus) and portosystemic vascular abnormalities.

In the case of a cat with clinical-pathological signs of liver disease, there is a high probability of **hepatic lipidosis (HL), neutrophilic cholangitis (NC) or lymphoplasmacytic cholangitis (LC)**, these being the three most common conditions to affect the feline liver.

Diagnosing feline liver disease

The clinical signs of liver disease are usually non-specific. The most frequent clinical signs are usually **gastrointestinal** (anorexia, vomiting, diarrhoea, weight loss), **urinary** (polyuria-polydipsia, stranguria, dysuria), and **central nervous system signs** (depression and apathy).

In some cases, the clinical signs are more specific due to the presence of jaundice (ruling out pre and post-hepatic causes), ascites (rare in cats), coagulopathy and bleeding, or signs of hepatic encephalopathy (ptyalism, blindness, head-pressing, stupor, and coma).

Given the liver's large functional reserve capacity **the most specific signs of liver disease usually appear late in the course of the disease.**

Markers of liver disease

The most widely used liver disease markers in laboratory tests are:

- **ALT and AST** (which indicate cell damage):
  - Both highly specific but less sensitive
  - Normal values do not rule out liver disease due to the short half-lives:
    - ALT half-life 6 hours
    - AST half-life <1 hour
- **ALP and GGT** (which indicate damage to cell membranes of the biliary and canalicular epithelium):
  - ALP: Highly specific due to a short half-life (6 hours) and lower enzyme levels in the cells, but low sensitivity:
    - Cats lack the corticosteroid-associated isoenzyme therefore ALP elevations are more specific in the cat than the dog
  - GGT elevations have a high sensitivity and low specificity compared to ALP.

These **liver enzymes** (with their provisos) are markers of liver disease, but are **not indicators of liver function.**

Liver function tests

The classic markers of liver functionality (**hyperbilirubinaemia, hypoglycaemia, hypoalbuminaemia, hyper or hypocholesterolaemia, increased coagulation times**) are very specific, but not very sensitive since they are **only altered when liver dysfunction is advanced.** An increase in bilirubin (Figure 33) in the absence of anaemia, pancreatic disease, or extra-hepatic biliary obstruction is a good indicator of liver disease and failure.

Bilirubinuria (Figure 34) precedes bilirubinaemia and is **always pathological in cats** (Figure 35).

Table 11. Specificity and sensitivity of ALT, AST, ASP and GGT for diagnosis of feline hepatic pathologies.

Test	Specificity	Sensitivity	Half-life
ALT	High	Low	6 hours
AST	High	Low	<1 hour
ALP	High	Low	6 hours
GGT	Less	Greater	Greater

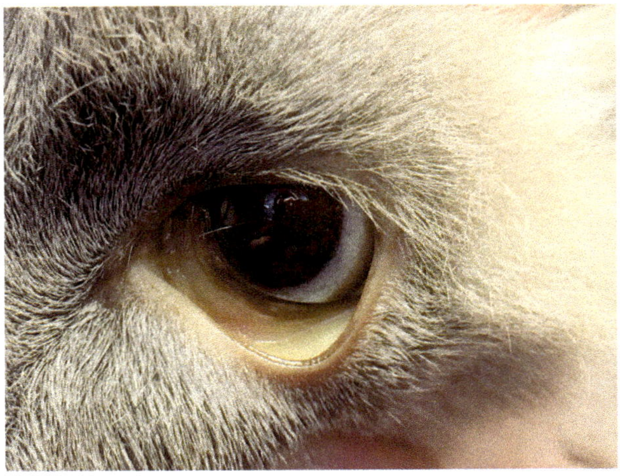

Figure 33. Icteric mucous membranes in a cat with liver disease.

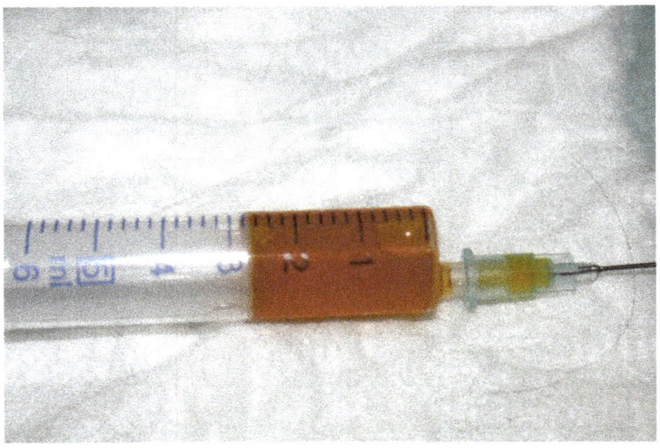

Figure 34. Bilirubinuria.

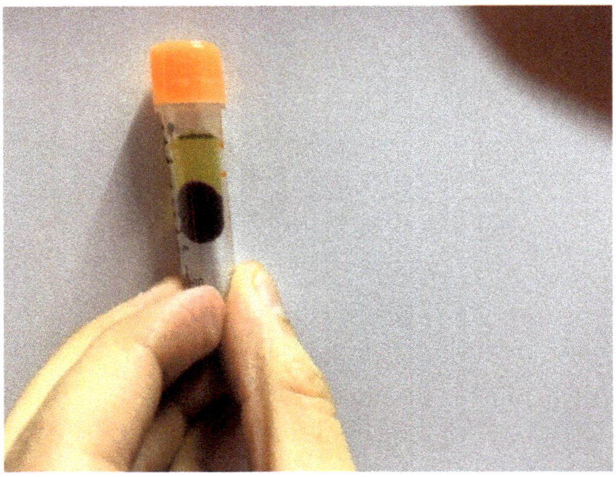

Figure 35. Icteric serum from a cat with liver disease.

When bilirubin is normal, the **most sensitive and specific marker of liver functionality is a bile acid stimulation test**, where the bile acids are measured on an fasting stomach and then two hours after food intake.

The following laboratory parameters help focus on differential diagnoses (Figure 36), along with clinical signs, history, and diagnostic tests.

Ultrasound

All cases of feline liver disease should have an ultrasound exam, which is often helpful when reaching a diagnosis. However, a normal result is not unusual and does not rule out liver disease.

Ultrasonography is diagnostic in some cases with focal lesions such as liver cysts or neoplasms. In other cases, it acts as a good guide; for example, in hepatomegaly with diffuse hyperechoic parenchyma, where suspicions of hepatic lipidosis should be very high, while dilatation of intrahepatic bile ducts suggests cholangitis

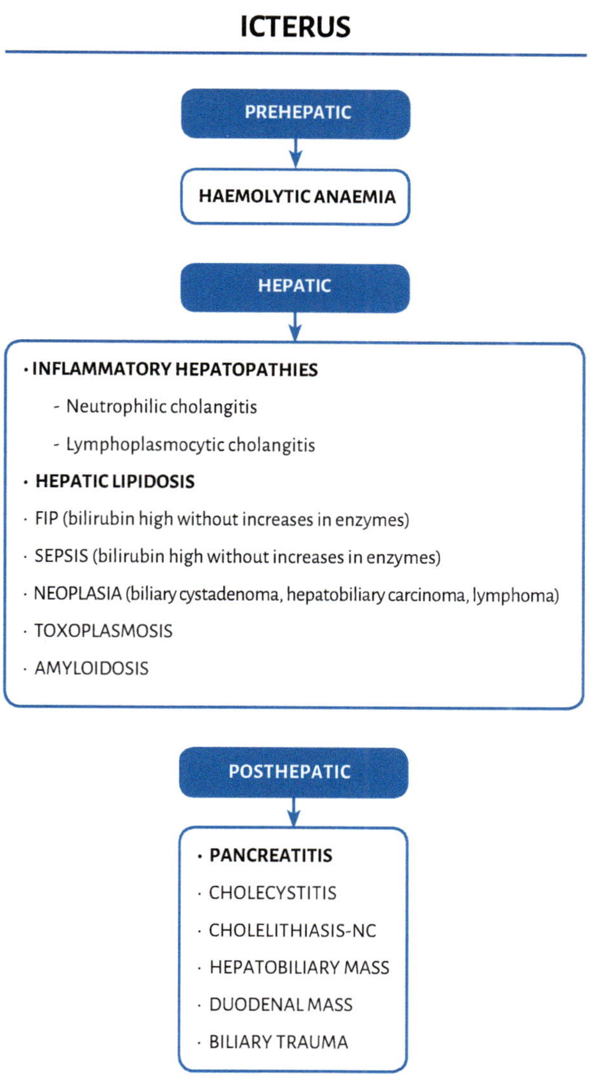

Figure 36. Differential diagnoses in a cat with jaundice.

Table 12. Most probable differential diagnoses according to information obtained from the complete blood count and blood biochemistry.

	Neutrophils	ALKP	GGT	BIL	GLOB
FIP	↑	–	–	↑	↑↑↑
Sepsis	↑↑	↑	↑	↑	+/–
NC	↑↑	↑	↑	↑	+/–
LC	+/–	↑	↑	↑	↑↑↑
HL	–	↑↑↑	–	↑↑↑	+/–

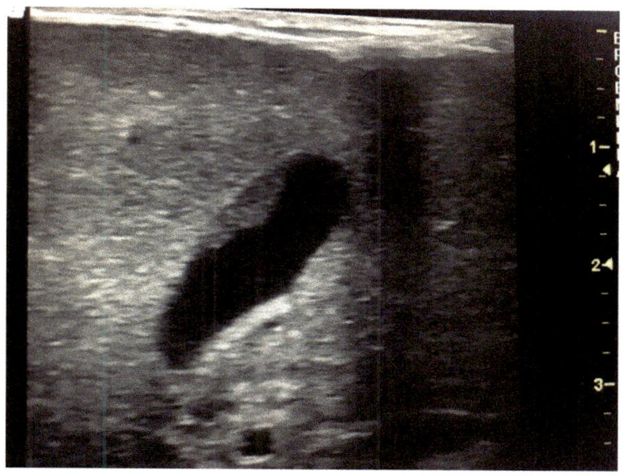

Figure 37. Liver ultrasound image showing a dilated common bile duct.

(Figure 37). Ultrasonography is also useful for the evaluation of extrahepatic bile ducts and the gallbladder, in addition to assessing hepatic vascularization for the diagnosis of portosystemic shunts. Ultrasound guided fine needle aspirates can also be of benefit.

Liver biopsy

Liver biopsy and histology provide a definitive diagnosis. However, sometimes a conclusive diagnosis can be reached without the need for biopsies.

In many cats a diagnosis of hepatic lipidosis can be reached with a correct interpretation of the history, clinical signs, liver enzyme patterns, ultrasound, and cytology of fine needle aspirations (FNA).

However, **liver cytology using FNA is not highly sensitive or specific**, especially with inflammatory liver disease, and the correlation with histological biopsy studies is rather low.

In addition, hepatic lipidosis can coexist with other liver, gastrointestinal, or endocrine diseases, so the presumptive diagnosis of lipidosis is not always a definitive diagnosis.

In cats with suspected cholangitis, **cholecystocentesis** is a useful and safe technique for obtaining bile samples for cytology and culture. In cats with suspected neutrophilic cholangitis if the response to antibiotic treatment is good, then biopsy is not always necessary.

Feline cholangitis

Inflammatory liver disease in cats develops mainly in the bile ducts (cholangitis) and in rare cases spreads to the portal space and liver parenchyma (cholangiohepatitis) (Gunn-Moore and Reed, 2010).

There are **different forms of this disease depending on the histological pattern**: neutrophilic (acute and chronic), lymphocytic, and cholangitis associated with parasitic flukes. There is significant **clinical overlap** between the different forms of cholangitis, and it is not possible or necessary to carry out a histological study in all cases, therefore it is not always possible to reach a definitive diagnosis regarding the type of cholangitis.

Cats with neutrophilic cholangitis often present with gastrointestinal clinical signs, **fever**, jaundice, abdominal pain, and hepatomegaly.

Diagnosis

The **CBC is usually inflammatory, and all liver enzymes are elevated**, especially GGT. Normal liver enzyme values do not rule out the diagnosis and, in fact, this occurs with some frequency. The presence of neutrophilia and a left shift suggests a higher likelihood of the acute forms (mainly neutrophilic inflammation), but in many cases the clinical distinction between acute and chronic forms (mixed neutrophilic, lymphocytic, and plasmocytic inflammation) is impossible unless a biopsy is taken.

The most common **abnormalities on ultrasound** are hepatomegaly, hyperechogenicity, dilation of the common bile duct, and gallbladder abnormalities.

If cholangitis is suspected, it is essential to perform ultrasound guided cholecystocentesis to obtain bile for culture and cytology (Figure 38). Bile cultures have been shown to be more useful than liver sample cultures in some studies. However, sensitivity of bile culture is poor (less than 50%) and in addition there is not a strong correlation between positive culture and observation of bacteria on cytology (Byfield et al., 2017).

Other techniques for detecting bacteria using PCR or FISH (florescence in situ hybridization), although not readily available these are more sensitive and allow detection of bacteria in 1/3 of cats with cholangitis.

Treatment

Consequently, when cholangitis is suspected, **treatment with antibiotics** (cephalosporins, amoxicillin-clavulanate, fluoroquinolones, and metronidazole) should be **administered for 4 to 6 weeks**. If there is not

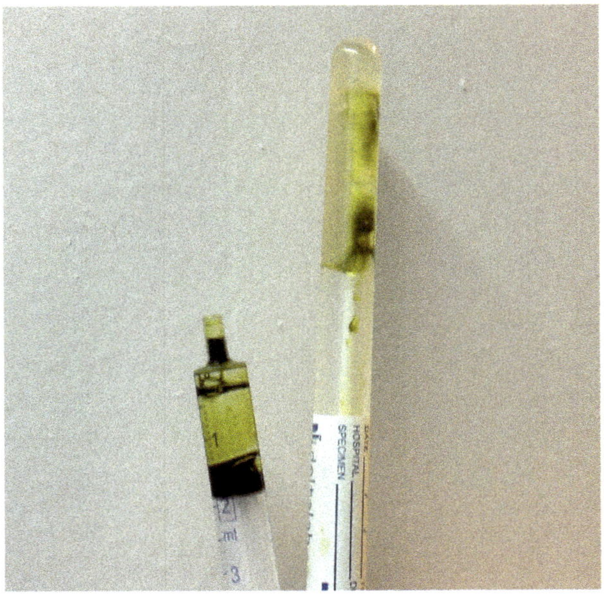

Figure 38. Sample taken from the gallbladder by cholecystocentesis for culture and cytology.

a good response after a few weeks, a biopsy or the addition of corticosteroids should be considered.

Depending on the severity and clinical state of each cat, treatment is supportive (fluids, enteral nutrition) and symptomatic (analgesia, antiemetics). Some clinical studies show that **ursodeoxycholic acid** as a complementary treatment in cholangitis can be of use due to its anti-inflammatory, immunomodulatory, antifibrotic and choleretic actions. Nutritional supplements (SAMe and silymarin) and vitamins are also frequently prescribed, although there are no clinical studies regarding their benefits.

Due to the association of the condition with infection, **antibiotics should be administered in conjunction with symptomatic treatment.** Antibiotics may need to be administered for 1–3 months. *E. coli* is the most frequently isolated organism, but mixed infections are common. Ideally, antibiotics should be administered based on the culture and antibiogram of bile and liver samples, but the empirical options are as follows:

- Amoxicillin/clavulanate (11–22 mg/kg/8–12 h PO).
- Cephalexin (10–35 mg/kg/8–12 h PO) and a fluoroquinolone (good concentration in bile). The authors prefer marbofloxacin (2 mg/kg/24 h PO) to enrofloxacin because of the risk of irreversible blindness in cats.
- Metronidazole, due to its anaerobic efficacy and immunomodulatory effect (7.5–10 mg/kg/12 h PO). **Higher doses should not be used** as they can be hepatotoxic, neurotoxic, and potentially teratogenic.
- Clindamycin (5.5 mg/kg/12 h PO) is effective against anaerobes and Gram-positive microorganisms, but not against Gram negative ones. It is concentrated

in the bile, but care must be taken in cases of liver deterioration, since this is the main pathway for its metabolism.

In very severe cases, treating to "cover the 4 quadrants" via IV administration is necessary (that is, to cover Gram positive and negative, aerobic and anaerobic, for example, with amoxicillin/clavulanic acid plus clindamycin or metronidazole).

Supportive treatment may be needed to control pancreatitis (e.g. intravenous fluid therapy, analgesia, antibiotics), and if inflammatory bowel disease is present, concurrent treatment may be necessary.

Supportive treatment

- antiemetics: maropitant 1 mg/kg/24 h IV SC
- vitamin K1: 0.5 mg/kg /1 h IM
- hepatoprotectants: SAMe 20 mg/kg/24 h PO
- ursodeoxycholic acid: 10 mg/kg/24 h PO.

If concurrent pancreatitis is suspected, **pain should be managed with opioids.** Buprenorphine may be a good option at a dose of 0.01 to 0.03 mg/kg/6–8 hours via oral mucosa or SC.

Lymphocytic cholangitis

Lymphocytic cholangitis is a chronic progressive immune-mediated disease with a lymphocytic inflammatory pattern. Clinically, the presentation is similar to chronic neutrophilic cholangitis and only histology allows differentiation between the two diseases.

Interestingly, the cases of lymphocytic cholangitis documented in North America and Europe show important clinical differences: when described in cats in Europe the presence of hyperglobulinaemia and ascites is frequent, and a greater predisposition has been observed in the Persian and Norwegian Forest breeds.

Treatment

Treatment is based on the administration of antibiotics and prednisolone at high doses (2 to 3 mg/kg/24 h) and reducing the dose depending on the clinical-pathological response and, ideally, according to the information obtained on the repetition of biopsies, which is rarely done. In some cases, if the response to prednisolone is insufficient, an immunosuppressant such as chlorambucil can be added.

Hepatic neoplasia

Primary liver neoplasia is rare in cats. The most frequent primary liver tumours are hepatocellular tumours and cholangiocellular carcinomas. Hepatic lymphoma is usually the result of lymphoma that developed elsewhere, rather than primary.

Diagnosis is based on imaging tests and histological confirmation. **For primary liver tumours the treatment is surgical resection,** where possible with adjuvant chemotherapy.

Amyloidosis

Amyloidosis is caused by amyloid deposits in the liver and/or other organs, possibly in response to chronic inflammation. It has been described more frequently in the Abyssinian cat, but also in other breeds.

The most common clinical sign is spontaneous rupture of the liver, causing haemoabdomen (Figures 39, 40 and 41).

There is no specific treatment, only supportive treatment with vitamin K and transfusions.

Feline hepatic lipidosis

Hepatic lipidosis (HL) is a common and potentially life-threatening condition. The prognosis for patients with HL is reserved with a survival rate of 50%, which drops to 20% when concurrent pancreatitis is present. Key to improving survival is early recognition of clinical signs and rapid implementation of appropriate treatment (Webb CB. et al. 2018).

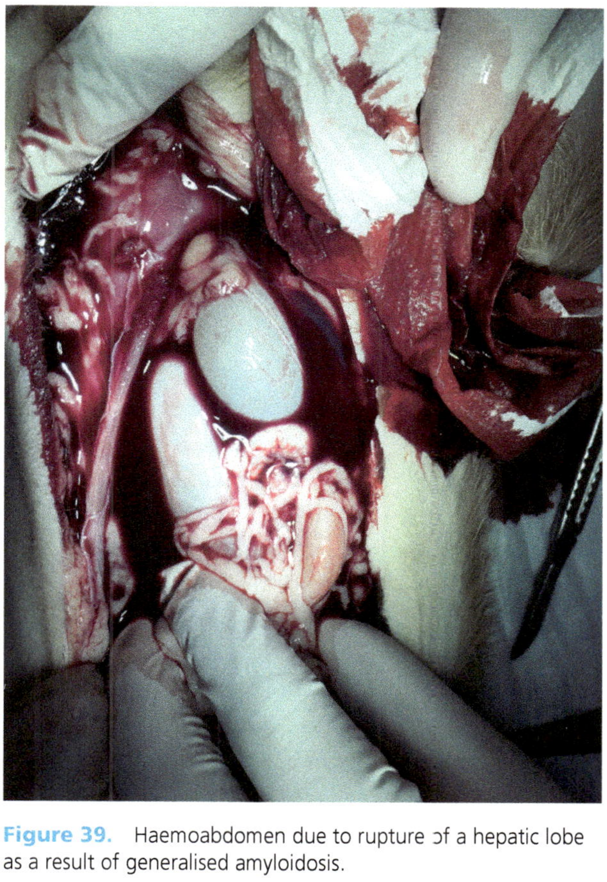

Figure 39. Haemoabdomen due to rupture of a hepatic lobe as a result of generalised amyloidosis.

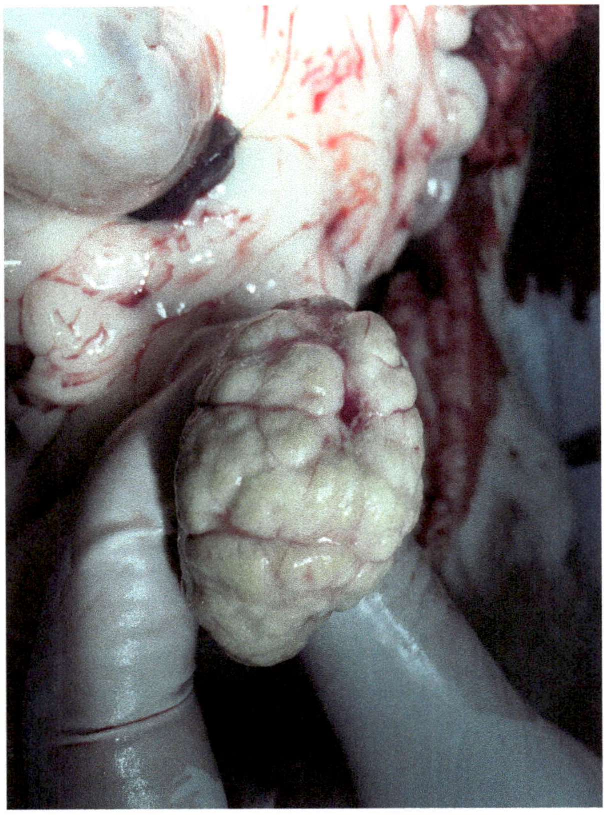

Figure 40. Renal amyloidosis.

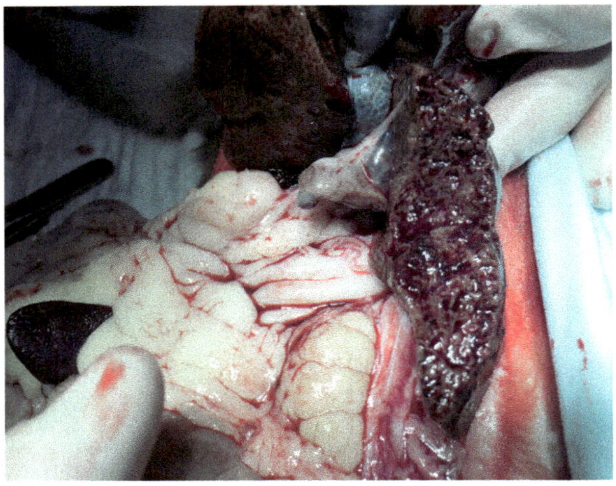

Figure 41. Liver rupture due to generalised amyloidosis.

HL occurs as a consequence of a prolonged period of anorexia which triggers lipolysis. Once described as an idiopathic disease, it has now been shown that in 95% of cases an underlying cause is responsible for triggering the initial catabolic state. This ultimately result is an imbalance between the amount of fat stored in the liver, the availability of fatty acids for energy production, and the hepatic elimination of triglycerides. The latter is illustrated by data showing a healthy feline liver contains 1% triglyceride, compared to 43% in a cat with HL, which has a direct impact on hepatocyte functionality.

Treatment is aimed at establishing nutritional support, correcting metabolic disorders and correcting the primary trigger.

Aetiology

Obesity is a predisposing factor to suffering from HL, since if a period of reduced food intake occurs, fats from peripheral deposits are mobilized and accumulate in the liver. In addition, obese cats are more resistant to the action of insulin, which also helps the process.

HL can affect cats of any age, although it is more common in **middle-aged cats.**

Clinical signs

Vomiting, lethargy, weight loss, and decline are the most common clinical signs.

On physical examination cats often have a history of a body condition score of 4/5 and weigh over 4.5 kg. Owners usually report a period of inappetence of between two and seven days, with weight loss due to dehydration and abdominal fat loss.

Gastrointestinal signs are variable:

- vomiting (38% of patients)
- diarrhoea
- constipation
- jaundice (70% of patients)
- palpable and non-painful hepatomegaly
- electrolyte disturbances, when severe, may present cervical ventroflexion and marked ptyalism when stressed or offered food.

Other clinical signs may be associated with concurrent diseases (Box 4).

Box 4. Main concurrent diseases with HL in order of prevalence.

- Gastrointestinal diseases.
- Inflammatory bowel disease.
- Dietary lymphoma.
- Hepatic diseases:
  - Cholangitis: acute neutrophilic, chronic lymphoplasmacytic.
- Pancreatitis:
  - Acute necrotizing.
  - Chronic.
- Lower urinary tract:
  - Urethral obstruction.
  - Idiopathic inflammation.
- Endocrinopathies:
  - Diabetes mellitus.
  - Hyperthyroidism.

- Renal disease:
  - Chronic kidney disease.
  - Ureterolithiasis.
  - Neoplasms (non-alimentary).
- Stress:
  - Dietary changes, environmental changes.

Diagnosis

Complete blood count

63% of cats with HL present poikilocytosis and predisposition to Heinz body formation.

Anaemia is present in 22% of blood counts in cats with HL and is usually mild to moderate and non-regenerative. Care should be taken with the number of blood samples taken and the possible **bleeding as a result of coagulopathies**, for procedures such as placement of feeding tubes, cytology and biopsies.

When suspicions of HL are confirmed, administering **vitamin K at a dose of 0.5–1 mg/kg IM or SC is advisable.**

Biochemistry

The most frequent findings on blood biochemistry are increased activity of liver enzymes:

- alkaline phosphatase (ALP) increases in more than 80% of cases
- alanine aminotransferase (ALT) increases in 72% of cases
- aspartate aminotransferase (AST) increases in 89% of cases
- blood urea nitrogen (BUN) decreases in 58% of cases
- total bilirubin increases in more than 95% of cases.

Cats with concurrent inflammatory liver disease (cholangitis, bile duct occlusion, bile duct carcinoma) pancreatitis, or pancreatic adenocarcinoma may show an increase in γ-glutamyl transpeptidase (GGT) in 48% of cases, presenting with two or three times the reference value.

- Albumin may be low, associated with gastrointestinal disease.
- ALP elevations occur prior to bilirubinaemia, and can be an early indicator to aid early intervention. Marked elevations of ALP are indicative of HL.
- Bile acids are elevated in cases of bilirubinaemia, so it is not necessary to measure them if the cat is jaundiced.
- If liver disease without jaundice is suspected, bile acids may be an early indicator of disease that allows early action.
- Globulin, cholesterol and glucose concentrations may be decreased or increased if the primary cause is diabetes mellitus or pancreatitis.
- Electrolyte abnormalities are responsible for the high mortality rate that this condition can present:
  - hypokalaemia (30%)
  - hypophosphataemia (17%)
  - hypomagnesaemia (28%) may occur initially or when fluid therapy is instituted, or abnormalities due to refeeding syndrome may appear. These abnormalities are responsible for the decline, intestinal atony, vomiting, behavioural changes and increased risk of haemolysis due to hypophosphataemia
  - **hypokalaemia is considered a negative prognostic factor.**

Bilirubinuria can be found on urinalysis, in addition to a lipid layer when the sample is centrifuged.

Clotting times may be affected, therefore vitamin K1 (0.5–1 mg/kg/12 h IM) should be administered to prevent complications. In case of considering the need to perform an invasive procedure such as biopsy or oesophagostomy (OT) placement, coagulation tests must be performed. Complications and the need for transfusion should be assessed in cats with less than 80,000 platelets/ml and activated partial thromboplastin times more than 1.5 times the reference range.

57% of cats with HL have vitamin B12 deficiency, so measurement and supplementation are recommended.

Diagnostic imaging

On abdominal radiography hepatomegaly or other signs of primary disease may be found, but abdominal effusion is rare. Radiography is a subjective and not very specific method for diagnosing HL.

Abdominal ultrasound shows homogeneous hyperechogenic parenchyma with an echogenicity similar to that of falciform fat, a finding with a positive predictive value of 100%.

Cats without associated cholangitis show no abnormalities of the gallbladder, common bile duct,

Table 13. Significant laboratory parameters in hepatic lipidosis.

Parameter	Variation
ALP	↑↑↑
ALT	↑
GGT	–
Bilirubin	↑↑↑
Potassium	↓
Phosphorus	↓
Magnesium	↓
Triglycerides-cholesterol	↑
Glucose	+/–
Coagulation times	Altered

or other biliary structures. The **right lateral quadrant should be carefully evaluated for associated pancreatitis or neoplasia.** Pancreatic disease can be identified as changes in echogenicity, mass lesions, enlargement, dilatation of the pancreatic duct, and increased echogenicity of peripancreatic fat.

In most cases, the ultrasound and cytology by **fine needle aspiration of the liver parenchyma are sufficient for the diagnosis** of HL. This is performed with local anaesthesia, without the cat sedated. At least 80% of hepatocytes are observed with lipid vacuoles. Several aspirations are recommended to avoid samples of falciform fat.

It is important to bear in mind that cats with HL are in an unstable metabolic state where the anaesthetic and surgical complication risks are increased.

Cats recovering poorly after 10 days of treatment may be candidates for biopsy to determine the cause of hepatobiliary disease (Figure 42).

Treatment

Success in treating cats with HL is directly related to **early diagnosis and treatment** of the underlying primary disease in secondary HL, along with **early enteral nutritional treatment.**

In the author's opinion forced oral feeding increases stress levels in the patient and the use of appetite stimulants (such as benzodiazepines) can cause acute fulminant liver necrosis.

The treatment of cats with HL is divided into two phases: an initial stabilization phase, followed by a long-term treatment phase.

Stabilization phase (1–2 days)

In the stabilization phase, **dehydration must be corrected by intravenous fluid therapy** with isotonic crystalloid solutions. Since **many of these cats are hypokalaemic** as a consequence of anorexia, the blood potassium levels should be measured and the deficit corrected with fluid therapy. In turn, it is advisable to **supplement the fluids with thiamine** (vitamin B1) 100 mg/day for 3 days. Many cats with HL have **vitamin K1 deficiency**, which manifests itself as a tendency to bleed: vitamin K1 SC (0.5–1 mg/kg) should be administered, repeating the dosage 1 and 12 hours later.

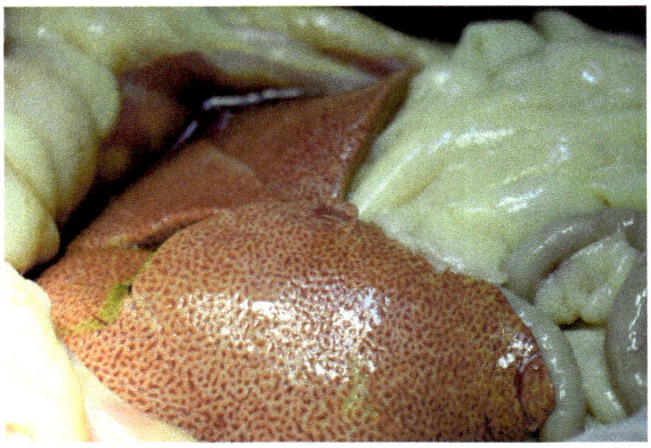

Figure 42. Macroscopic appearance of hepatic lipidosis during exploratory laparotomy.

Cats with severe liver disease suffer from rapid depletion of their liver stores of glutathione, the main protective agent against oxidizing agents, so **administration of N-acetylcysteine is recommended** by a slow IV route (140 mg/kg followed by 70 mg/kg/12 h) to replenish these reserves.

In the **presence of symptoms of hepatic encephalopathy** and if the cat is able to tolerate the oral administration, lactulose PO (0.3–0.5 ml/kg/8 h) should be administered along with antibiotics (amoxicillin 22 mg/kg/12 h; metronidazole 7.5 mg/kg/12 h).

Vomiting must also be controlled by using antiemetics such as maropitant (Cerenia, Zoetis) 1 mg/kg/24 h IV, SC.

In cats with secondary HL, treatment for the underlying disease should be commenced.

Even in this first stabilization phase, **the cat must be fed enterally**: if the clinical state allows it, an oesophagostomy tube should be placed or, even better, a nasogastric tube where placement is minimally invasive. It is advisable not to perform any invasive techniques (such as laparotomy, liver biopsy). in this stabilization phase.

The average duration of a patient's stabilization period is approximately one to two days. Prolonged nutrition through a nasogastric tube is not recommended due to the risk of rhinitis and the fact that the lumen of these small tubes limits feeding to a liquid diet.

Symptomatic treatment is aimed at:

- reduce vomiting:
  - Maropitant at a dose of 1 mg/kg/24 h IV, SC
  - Omeprazole, which some authors use if nausea persists. But cats do not have "acidic stomachs," so routine use of proton pump inhibitors or H_2 receptor antagonists is not recommended
- appetite stimulants:
  - Mirtazapine 1.875 mg/cat/24 h PO. This is the general dose, but if the cat also suffers from CKD, this dose would be administered every 48 hours. There are cats that present with vocalizations, tremors and hypersalivation as a side effect
- pain control. It is important in cats with associated pancreatitis:
  - Buprenorphine at a dose of 0.01–0.03 mg/kg/6–8 hours, transmucosally.

Long-term treatment

The long-term treatment phase begins once the patient is stable and can endure sedation or anaesthesia which allows placement of a long-term enteral feeding tube. The author uses an oesophagostomy tube.

Oesophagostomy tubes are inserted quickly under anaesthesia, are painless, easy to care for and use, and are rarely complicated by infection or retroflexion during vomiting. Proper placement of the tube, cranial to the gastric cardia, should be verified using thoracic radiography. Inserting the tip of the tube into the stomach increases the risk of reflux oesophagitis. The cutaneous entrance of the tube should be appropriately secured with a Roman sandal suture and cleaned daily. In addition, a small amount of antiseptic ointment should be applied and the area covered with a protective bandage.

Diet and feeding

The best clinical results are obtained using a **diet rich in proteins, of high nutritional value, with a high caloric density.** If the cat presents signs of hepatic encephalopathy, protein in the diet should be reduced and a renal diet can be administered, but this is rare (Brenner et al., 2011).

Once a diet has been chosen, the daily calorie requirement (approximately 70–80 kcal/kg/day) should be calculated and, using this information, the amount of food to be administered calculated. **On the first day, 25% of the daily energy requirements are administered**, increasing this each day by 25% until reaching, on the fourth day, 100% of the maintenance energy requirement.

Administration of food should cause the least possible stress to the patient until the cat wants to voluntarily eat adequate amounts of food, since the tube does not prevent this (Cook et al., 2021).

The total amount of daily **food is administered in six feeds on the first two days** and subsequently in four feeds, to avoid vomiting. After each intake, the tube should be cleaned with 10–15 ml of warm water. The most frequent complication is vomiting after food administration, which can be avoided by decreasing the administration rate (10–15 minutes/feed), the volume of food in each intake (not more than 25 ml) and warming the food until it reaches body temperature.

Subsequently, the number of feeds is progressively decreased, so that when the cat returns home, the owner must administer three feeds per day. This may take three days.

Hospital discharge should be given as soon as possible to reduce the stress of hospitalization for the cat: when it is not vomiting, is stable, and not dehydrated. Appropriate instructions should be given to the owner about the handling of the feeding tube, and they should contact the clinician immediately if the patient coughs when the food is administered, vomits food or the tube, pus is detected at the entrance of the tube, or the tube has been torn off.

It is necessary to examine and evaluate the evolution of the patient in the first few weeks by physical examination, a complete blood count, and a biochemical profile. If the evolution is favourable, it should be confirmed whether the cat ingests food by itself. In order to do this the owner must offer the cat their favourite food. It should be noted that the tube does not prevent eating. The enteral feeding tube should be removed when the cat ingests its daily calorie requirements on its own. In most cases, the **duration of enteral feeding is 3 to 6 weeks.**

Monitoring

The total serum bilirubin concentration is the best predictive value of the evolution of cats with HL. Bilirubin concentrations decrease by 50% during the first 7–10 days of treatment in cats which survive.

Monitoring changes in liver enzymes does not work, but cats in which total serum bilirubin does not decrease usually die within the first 7 days of treatment.

Box 5. Management of cats with HL.

1. Sedation, anaesthesia, jugular catheters, feeding tubes, cystocentesis, or liver aspiration should be avoided until 12–24 hours have elapsed since vitamin K1 administration.
2. General anaesthesia should avoided until electrolyte abnormalities and dehydration have been controlled.
3. The primary causes that have triggered HL should be identified.
4. Cytology of fine-needle aspirations, clinical signs, and ultrasound imaging provide enough diagnostic information to establish intensive treatment. Liver biopsy is not necessary to plan treatment.
5. Fluids containing lactate should be avoided and should not be supplemented with dextrose, as it can increase accumulation of triglycerides in the liver.
6. Electrolyte abnormalities should be corrected.
7. Complications that may occur when feeding begins should be anticipated so that feedback syndrome does not occur.
8. A diet high in protein should be used except in cases of hepatic encephalopathy. Placement of feeding tubes increases the chances of survival of cats with HL. The diet should provide a

caloric intake of 70–80 kcal/kg/day and a protein content of between 33–45%. Enteral nutrition guidelines should be followed and administration of small amounts in several feeds to facilitate gastric emptying and avoid vomiting is preferable. Liquid foods should be used when feeding using the nasoesophageal tube, while other commercial recovery preparations can be used with oesophagostomy tubes or orally. These diets cover nutritional deficiencies, of trace elements (amino acids, magnesium, phosphates, taurine) and vitamins (thiamine, cobalamin, vitamins K, C and E).

9. Glucagon (GSH) and S-adenosylmethionine (SAMe) reserves are depleted due to lack of appetite, so can be supplemented with acetylcysteine (initially 140 mg/kg, followed by 70 mg/kg/12 h SC) 2–4, 12, 16 and oral SAMe. This prevents oxidative damage to the liver and promotes recovery.
10. If there is ventroflexion of the neck, electrolyte disturbances and thiamine (vitamin B1) deficiency should be considered. Thiamine should be administered at a dosage of 100 mg PO or slow IV diluted in one litre of crystalloid fluids. IM or SC administration should be avoided because anaphylaxis can occur.

Bibliography

Oesophageal disorders

Beatty JA, Swift N, Foster DJ et al. *Suspected clindamycin associated oesophageal injury in cats: five case.*, J Feline Med Surg 8:412, 2006.

German AJ, Cannon MJ, Dye C et al. *Oesophageal strictures in cats associated with doxycycline therapy*, J Feline Med Surg 7:33, 2005.

Glazer A, Walters P. *Esophagitis and esophageal strictures.* Comp Contin Edu Pract Vet 30:281, 2008.

Kook PH. *Esophagitis in cats and dogs.* Vet Clin North Am Small Anim Pract. 2021.

Vomiting

Batchelor DJ, Devauchelle P, Elliott J, Elwood CM, Freiche V, Gualtieri M, et al. *Mechanisms, causes, investigation and management of vomiting disorders in cats: A literature review.* J Feline Med Surg. 2013; 15(4):237–65.

Hauck SR, Gisselman K, Cordner A, Nicholson AG. *Chronic Vomiting in Cats: Etiology and Diagnostic Testing.* J Am Anim Hosp Assoc. 2016 Sep-Oct;52(5):269–76.

Kleinschmidt S, Harder J, Nolte I, Marsilio S, Hewicker-Trautwein M. *Chronic inflammatory and non-inflammatory diseases of the gastrointestinal tract in cats: diagnostic advantages of full-thickness intestinal and extraintestinal biopsies.* J Feline Med Surg. 2010; 12(2):97–103.

Diarrhoea

Daniaux LA, Laurenson MP, Marks SL, Moore PF, Taylor SL, Chen RX, et al. *Ultrasonographic thickening of the muscularis propria in feline small intestinal small cell T-cell lymphoma and inflammatory bowel disease.* J Feline Med Surg. 2014; 16(2):89–98

Toresson L, Steiner JM, Olmedal G, Larsen MB, Suchodolski JS, Spillmann T. *Oral cobalamin supplementation in cats with hypocobalaminaemia: a retrospective study.* J Feline Med Surg 2017; 19(12):1302–6.

Washabau RJ: 2005 Report from: WSAVA Gastrointestinal Standardization Group. Available at http://www.wsava.org/GIStandards1.htm. Accessed January 17, 2010.

Whitehead K, Cortes Y, Eirmann L. *Gastrointestinal dysmotility disorders in critically ill dogs and cats.* J Vet Emerg Crit Care (San Antonio). 2016 Mar-Apr;26(2):234–53.

Constipation

Byers C, Leasure C, Sanders NA: *Feline idiopathic megacolon.* Comp Contin Edu Pract Vet 28:658, 2006.

Grossman RM, Sumner JP, Lopez DJ, Dornbusch JA, Singh A, Lux CN, Sample SJ, Liptak JM, Grimes JA, Upchurch DA, Blumenthal MS, Traverson M, Buote NJ, Marvel SJ, Steffey MA, Arai S, Little JP, Atilla A, Huck JL, Pitt KA. *Evaluation of outcomes following subtotal colectomy for the treatment of idiopathic megacolon in cats.* J Am Vet Med Assoc. 2021 Nov.

Thanaboonnipat C, Kumjumroon K, Boonkwang K, Tangsutthichai N, Sukserm W, Choisunirachon N. *Radiographic lumbosacral vertebral abnormalities and constipation in cats.* Vet World. 2021 Feb.

White R: *Surgical management of constipation.* J Feline Med Surg 4:129, 2002.

Inflammatory bowel disease

Benjamin SE, Drobatz KJ. *Retrospective evaluation of risk factors and treatment outcome predictors in cats presenting to the emergency room for constipation.* J Feline Med Surg. 2020 Feb; 22(2):153–160.

Gunn-Moore D, Reed N. *Feline inflammatory liver disease – an overview.* Vet Focus. 2010; 20(3):2–8.

Jergens AE. *Feline Idiopathic Inflammatory Bowel Disease: What we know and what remains to be unravelled.* J Feline Med Surg. 2012; 14(7):445–58.

Feline pancreatitis

Bazelle J, Watson P. *Pancreatitis in cats: Is it acute, is it chronic, is it significant?* J Feline Med Surg. 2014; 16(5):395–406.

Černá P, Kilpatrick S, Gunn-Moore DA. *Feline comorbidities: What do we really know about feline triaditis?* J Feline Med Surg. 2020 Nov; 22(11):1047–1067.

Crain SK, Sharkey LC, Cordner AP, Knudson C, Armstrong PJ. *Safety of ultrasound-guided fine-needle aspiration of the feline pancreas: a case-control study.* J Feline Med Surg. 2015; 17(10):858–63.

Dias C, Carreira LM. *Serum ionised calcium as a prognostic risk factor in the clinical course of pancreatitis in cats.* J Feline Med Surg 2015; 17(12):984–90.

Feline liver disease

Brenner K, KuKanich KS, Smee NM. *Refeeding syndrome in a cat with hepatic lipidosis.* J Feline Med Surg. 2011; 13(8):614–7.

Byfield VL, Callahan Clark JE, Turek BJ, Bradley CW, Rondeau MP. *Percutaneous cholecystocentesis in cats with suspected hepatobiliary disease.* J Feline Med Surg 2017; 19(12):1254–60.

Cook S, Whitby E, Elias N, Hall G, Chan DL. Retrospective evaluation of refeeding syndrome in cats: 11 cases (2013–2019). J Feline Med Surg. 2021 Oct; 23(10):883–891.

Daniel AGT, Lucas SRR, Júnior AR, Monteiro PRG, Ramos D, Pires CG, et al. *Skin fragility syndrome in a cat with cholangiohepatitis and hepatic lipidosis.* J Feline Med Surg. 2010; 12(2):151–5.

Gunn-Moore D, Reed N. *Feline inflammatory liver disease – an overview.* Vet Focus. 2010; 20(3):2–8.

Trehy MR, German AJ, Silvestrini P, Serrano G, Batchelor DJ. *Hypercobalaminaemia is associated with hepatic and neoplastic disease in cats: A cross sectional study.* Vol. 10, BMC Veterinary Research. 2014.

Webb CB. *Hepatic lipidosis: Clinical review drawn from collective effort.* J Feline Med Surg. 2018; 20(3):217–27.

Test

1. Cats with oesophageal disease:

A) Regurgitate immediately after eating undigested content.
B) Regurgitation does not always occur after eating if the oesophageal disease is located in the distal area of the oesophagus.
C) Vomit digested content after eating.
D) Vomiting can be easily differentiated from regurgitation because there is abdominal effort and persistent saliva in the vomit.

2. The treatment of choice for a cat with severe oesophageal stenosis with weight loss is:

A) Oesophageal surgery.
B) Medical treatment with famotidine, sucralfate and omeprazole.
C) Balloon dilation via endoscopy.
D) Feeding a semi-liquid diet and with the head elevated.

3. Intestinal ultrasound:

A) Is a non-invasive technique that allows the integrity of the stratification of the intestinal layers to be evaluated. If there is loss of structure this is suggestive of lymphoma.
B) It is a technique that allows the thickness of intestinal layers to be evaluated. If the muscle is thickened, this is suggestive of lymphoma.
C) Allows the presence of mesenteric adenopathy to be evaluated. If the mesenteric lymph nodes are rounded and enlarged, this is suggestive of lymphoma.
D) All of the above are correct.

4. What are the 3 main differential diagnoses in a cat with chronic diarrhoea?

A) Intestinal bacterial overgrowth, parasitosis and inflammatory bowel disease.
B) Cholangitis, lymphoma and inflammatory bowel disease.
C) Pancreatitis, inflammatory bowel disease and dietary responsive enteropathy.
D) Inflammatory bowel disease, diet-responsive enteropathy, and lymphoma.

5. Protrusion of the membrane of the third eyelid is a non-specific clinical sign associated with:

A) Feline dysautonomia syndrome.
B) Chronic diarrhoea of the small intestine.
C) Infectious eye conditions.
D) All three are correct.

6. Regarding specific blood tests for digestive diseases:

A) Hypercobalaminaemia is associated with small intestinal disease.
B) fTLI is helpful in the diagnosis of pancreatitis.
C) Elevated fPLI indicates pancreatic disease but not the type of pathology.
D) fPLI is helpful in the diagnosis of exocrine pancreatic insufficiency.

7. A cat with IRIS stage 4 chronic kidney disease may develop constipation from:
A) Hypokalaemia.
B) Dehydration.
C) Hyperparathyroidism.
D) They can all be correct.

8. In cases of severe obstipation, which of the following treatments should be considered:
A) Treatment with fibre.
B) Prokinetics.
C) Lactulose.
D) Subtotal colectomy with excision of up to 98% preserving the ileocaecal valve.

9. Treatment of chronic lymphoplasmacytic enteropathies is based on:
A) A low residue diet for digestive problems.
B) Sequential treatment with metronidazole, prednisolone and a hypoallergenic diet.
C) Chlorambucil is the first-choice treatment.
D) Cyclosporine is the first-choice treatment.

10. The most common type of pancreatitis in cats is:
A) Acute necrotizing pancreatitis.
B) Acute suppurative pancreatitis.
C) Chronic non-suppurative pancreatitis.
D) Pancreatitis in cats is rare.

11. The most likely differential diagnoses for hepatic jaundice are:
A) Pancreatitis and inflammatory liver disease.
B) Lipidosis and inflammatory liver diseases.
C) Haemolytic anaemia and pancreatitis.
D) Inflammatory liver disease and hepatic lipidosis.

12. Regarding abdominal ultrasound in cases of hepatic lipidosis:
A) It is diagnostic in cases where hyperechogenic and isoechogenic parenchyma with respect to falciform fat are found.
B) It does not provide information for the diagnosis of hepatic lipidosis.
C) It is diagnostic in cases in which a hypoechoic parenchyma is found.
D) Diagnosis of hepatic lipidosis requires fine needle aspiration and biopsy.

13. When should an intestinal biopsy be performed in a cat with signs of inflammatory bowel disease?
A) When there is no response to treatment with a hypoallergenic diet.
B) Performing a biopsy is not necessary, other tests provide a definitive diagnosis.
C) Laparotomy is not necessary because it is a very invasive test.
D) A biopsy is necessary if there is hypoalbuminaemia, ultrasound signs of loss of stratification of the intestinal layers, presence of enlarged lymph nodes, chronicity of the condition without response to treatment.

14. Regarding pancreatic biopsy ...
A) An fPLI test should be done first because if it is negative, there is no pancreatitis and biopsy is not warranted.
B) A single branch biopsy is taken, and a small amount of sample is taken to avoid complications.
C) If done via laparotomy, and a healthy pancreas is seen with no signs of abnormalities, it is best not to take a sample.
D) The macroscopic appearance of the pancreas does not determine the severity of the condition, biopsies should still be done even if the appearance is normal or misdiagnosis should be considered with a poor macroscopic pancreatic appearance.

15. Regarding refeeding syndrome ...
A) It always occurs when commencing force-feeding, although it may not cause significant clinical signs.
B) In malnourished animals, the amount of insulin is low and energy levels in the form of ATP are minimal. After carbohydrate administration, insulin is initially insufficient for these new glucose levels, inducing hyperglycaemia and cellular processes such as ATP synthesis, which cause depletion of phosphorus, fundamentally causing severe hypophosphataemia with signs such as muscle weakness, haemolysis, severe neurological signs, hypoventilation, heart failure and death.
C) It is easy to manage, in any case.
D) None of the previous answers are correct.

16. Regarding inflammatory bowel disease ...

A) There is a known cause, there is no response to symptomatic treatment, it is a chronic condition, there must be histological evidence and the specific treatment involves the use of immunosuppressants.

B) There is usually no known cause, it is a chronic condition and the specific treatment involves the use of immunosuppressants.

C) The previous two answers are incorrect.

D) None of the above are correct.

Clinical case

Lashmi, a 5-year-old cat, comes to the practice because she has vomited 2 or 3 times a day for a week and has not eaten for 3 days. The owners' reasons for consultation are:

- Anorexia
- Vomiting
- Apathy
- Behavioural changes

Clinical history

A month ago, they adopted another cat and they do not seem to get along as they snort when they meet each other at feeding time.

The owners mention that two weeks ago they have changed the food to a "light" version so that they would lose weight and they believe that from that moment Lashmi began to eat less. They have noticed that she drinks water in different places and that they have to change the sand in the litter box more frequently. When they "force" her to eat and bring her food closer, she begins to "dribble."

She is not a cat that usually eats strings or other things that she should not.

Physical examination

A can of Lashmi's favourite wet food is opened to see her reaction and she is nauseous (in cats nausea can be seen as hypersalivation or swallowing movements). She shows no interest in food and turns her face away.

On physical examination it is important to be systematic:

- Weight / weight history / percentage change in weight / muscle mass index. Lashmi's history was revisited and the previous weight records compared with the current one: 1 year ago, she weighed 5.5 kg with a body condition of 4 out of 5, while at the time of the examination her weight was 4.7 kg. The owners mention that a month ago they weighed her at home, and she weighed 4.9 kg, but they did not think it was significant because they thought it was due to the "light" food. There is no loss of muscle mass.
- Mucous membranes. Severe jaundice that can be seen in the ears and conjunctival mucosa.
- Mental state. Stuporous. She is normally a cat that does not like being handled at the vet and she shows no resistance. She is recumbent.
- Hydration status. She has sunken eyes and skinfolds remain when checking for dehydration. 6% dehydration is calculated.
- Appearance of hair. Poor coat, in separate tufts.
- Skin examination. Petechiae on abdomen, peripheral oedema.
- Oral examination. No abnormalities or signs of the presence of foreign bodies. Jaundiced palate.
- Neck palpation. Does not present abnormalities. A jugular pulse and jugular engorgement can be seen.
- Cardiopulmonary auscultation. Heart and lung auscultation without abnormalities. Heart rate of 150 bpm. Respiratory rate of 28 bpm.
- Abdominal palpation. Kidneys reduced in size and not painful. Distended urinary bladder. Pain on abdominal palpation.
- Temperature 38.7°C

Questions

1. **What is the problem list?**
2. **What is the most likely diagnosis?**
3. **What would your diagnostic plan be?**
4. **What information can be obtained from urinalysis? (The results of Lashmi's CBC and biochemistry can be seen on the next page.)**
5. **With this information, what pathology could be suspected as the cause of jaundice?**
   A) Prehepatic jaundice can be ruled out as she is not anaemic.
   B) Suspect hepatic lipidosis due to high liver enzymes and jaundice.
   C) Suspect neutrophilic cholangitis.
   D) Suspect post hepatic jaundice from pancreatitis.
6. **What would a possible interpretation of the results be?**
7. **What would be an appropriate treatment?**
   A) Performing a biopsy as there is not a definitive diagnosis.
   B) Supportive treatment: oesophagostomy tube, antibiotic and fluid therapy **without** corticosteroids.
   C) Supportive treatment: oesophagostomy tube, antibiotic and fluid therapy **with** corticosteroids.
   D) She is not stable enough to anaesthetize

CBC

Parameters	Results	Reference
Erythrocytes	5.62 M/µl	5.00–10.00
HCT	**23.0%**	**30.0–45.0**
HGB	9.6 g/dl	9.0–15.1
MCV	**40.9 fl**	**41.0–58.0**
MCH	17.0 pg	12.0–20.0
MCHC	-.- g/dl	29.0–37.5
RDW	20.1%	17.3–22.0
%Reticulocyte	0.9%	
Reticulocytes	49.7 K/µl	3.0–50.0
Leucocites	**34.35 K/µl**	**5.5–19.5**
% Neutrophiles	76.5%	
% Lymphocytes	9.6%	
% Monocytes	8.9%	
% Eosinophiles	5.0%	
% Basophils	0.0%	
Neutrophiles	**26.28 K/µl**	**2.50–12.50**
Lymphocytes	3.30 K/µl	0.40–6.80
Monocytes	**3.06 K/µl**	**0.15–1.70**
Eosinophiles	**1.71 K/µl**	**0.10–0.79**
Basophils	0.00 K/µl	0.00–0.10
Platelets	205 K/µl	175–600
MPV	22.5 fl	
PDW	34.5%	
PCT	0.46%	

Biochemistry
(September)

Parameters	Results	Reference	Biochemistry (March)
Glucose	88 mg/dl	74–159	213 mg/dl
Creatinine	1.8 mg/dl	0.8–2.4	1.6 mg/dl
BUN	**10 mg/dl**	**16–36**	**27 mg/dl**
BUN/CREA	6		16
Phos	4.6 mg/dl	3.1–7.5	4.6 mg/dl
Ca	10.2 mg/dl	7.8–11.3	9.4 mg/dl

Parameters	Results	Reference	Biochemistry (March)
TP	8.3 g/dl	5.7–8.9	7.0 g/dl
Alb	3.1 g/dl	2.2–4.0	3.0 g/dl
Glob	**5.2 g/dl**	**2.8–5.1**	**4.0 g/dl**
Alb/Glob	0.6		0.7
ALT	**137 U/l**	**12–130**	**40 U/l**
ALKP	**662 U/l**	**14–111**	**40 U/l**
GGT	**8 U/l**	**0–4**	**2 U/l**
Tbil	**7.7 mg/dl**	**0.0–0.9**	**0.1 mg/dl**
Chol	150 mg/dl	65–225	175 mg/dl

Answers

Test

1. B	7. D	13. D
2. C	8. D	14. D
3. D	9. B	15. B
4. D	10. C	16. B
5. D	11. D	
6. C	12. A	

Clinical case

1. **What is the problem list?**
   Stupor, dehydration, jaundice, peripheral oedema and ptyalism.
2. **What is the most likely diagnosis?**
   Lashmi is jaundiced and a differential diagnosis of jaundice is made (see Figure 36 in the chapter).
3. **What would your diagnostic plan be?**
   Liver diseases are common in cats. The most frequent diseases are hepatic lipidosis, cholangitis and its different variations, neoplasms and hepatocellular necrosis associated with toxins or drugs.
   Other liver diseases can be reactive liver diseases and other inflammatory liver diseases associated with various infections (FIP, toxoplasmosis, virulent calicivirus) and portosystemic vascular abnormalities. In the case of a cat with clinical-pathological signs of liver disease, there is a high probability of lipidosis or cholangitis since these two are the most frequent.
4. **What information can be obtained from urinalysis?**
   Bilirubinuria in cats is always pathological.
   Bilirubinuria is detected before jaundice. Bilirubinuria occurs when there are more than 2 mg/dl bilirubin
5. **With this information, what pathology could be suspected as the cause of jaundice?**
   Answers a, c and d are correct.
6. **What would a possible interpretation of the results be?**
   Interpretation:
   - Mild anaemia → rules out haemolytic anaemia.
   - Leukocytosis-neutrophilia-monocytosis-eosinophilia → neutrophilic cholangitis?
   - Hypoglycaemia.
   - Hyperglobulinaemia → lymphoplasmacytic cholangitis?
   - Marked bilirubinaemia.
   - ALP markedly high, GGT and ALT high.
   - Positive fPLI → associated pancreatitis.

   Blood test data indicates possible inflammatory liver disease associated with pancreatitis.

7. What would be an appropriate treatment?

B) Supportive treatment: oesophagostomy tube, antibiotic and fluid therapy **without** corticosteroids.

Lashmi is considered too unstable to perform a laparotomy with biopsy. She presented with peripheral oedema and petechiae due to coagulopathy.

It is preferable to stabilize her and observe the response to supportive treatment. In case a biopsy is needed, administering vitamin K a few days before is recommended.

- Hospitalization with antibiotic treatment with marbofloxacin and IV metronidazole.
- Rehydration, electrolytes (K, Mg, P).
- Proper nutrition:
  - Oesophagostomy tube. 60/kcal/kg/day;
    200–300 kcal/cat/day.
  - Danger of refeeding syndrome. Start feeding very gradually.

Feline urology

7

Susana Silva

Contents

Diagnostic tests

Patients with urinary tract disease do not always present with obviously suggestive symptoms, especially when the problem lies in the upper urinary tract. The **clinical signs can be non-specific** and a minimum database (haematology, biochemistry, and urinalysis) is required to narrow down the differential diagnoses.

Routine haematology and biochemistry are important for diagnostic purposes, monitoring, and to help eliminate the possibility of concurrent or precipitating disease. In addition, **urinalysis is an important tool** in any patient, but essential in the investigation of all urinary tract problems.

Haematology

Kidney disease is frequently associated with a non-regenerative, normocytic, normochromic anaemia, which is suggestive of chronicity. This is rarely associated with clinical signs of anaemia since the problem is mild and compensatory mechanisms occur. However, in the later stages of chronic kidney disease, more severe and clinically significant anaemia is relatively common due to a multitude of factors, including a lack of erythropoietin.

In cases with severe haemorrhage originating from the upper or lower urinary tract, a variable degree of anaemia is expected, which may be regenerative or non-regenerative depending on the duration of the blood loss. In these cases, **gross haematuria** is usually obvious, although the cause or origin might be difficult to identify. It is important to remember **generalized**

haemostatic disorders, especially thrombocytopaenia, as a differential diagnosis and rule these out before investigating urinary tract disorders.

Changes in white cell number or differential counts are frequently encountered too similarly to other pathologies; we will look in more detail into this in the context of specific disorders.

Biochemistry

Urea and creatinine

Urea is synthesised in the liver, via the urea cycle, (Figure 1) from protein catabolism (exogenous from food and endogenous from muscle protein.)

Serum urea levels are influenced by protein intake, hepatic disease, endogenous protein catabolism, and glomerular filtration rate. Serum urea is inversely proportional to glomerular filtration rate (GFR), but also passively reabsorbed by the renal tubules. **A higher percentage of urea is absorbed at slower tubular flow rates**, such as with hypovolaemia or dehydration. This can explain the, sometimes disproportionate, increase in urea (compared to creatinine) in pre-renal azotaemia and the increase in urea alone in some cases of dehydration.

Serum creatinine is a breakdown product of muscle phosphocreatine and almost entirely excreted by glomerular filtration, which means it can provide an estimate of GFR. Large reductions in GFR early in the course of the disease may not increase creatinine but, at a late stage, when most of the renal function is lost, a small decrease in GFR will result in a large "jump" in serum creatinine (Figure 2).

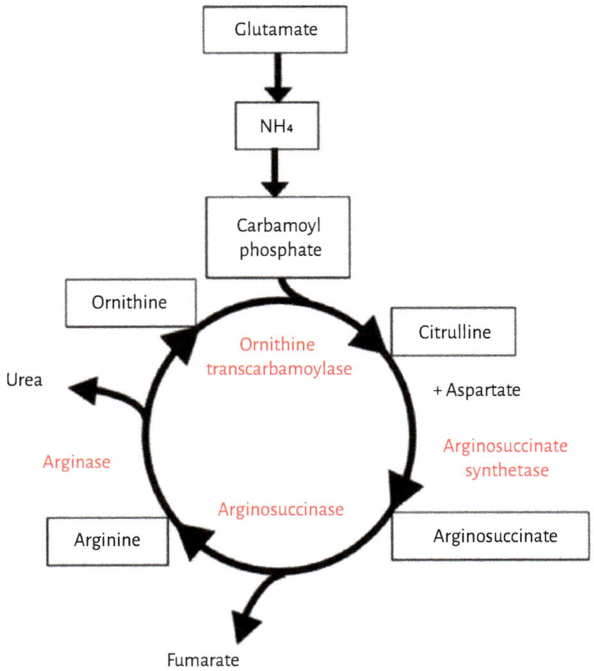

Figure 1. Simplified urea cycle.

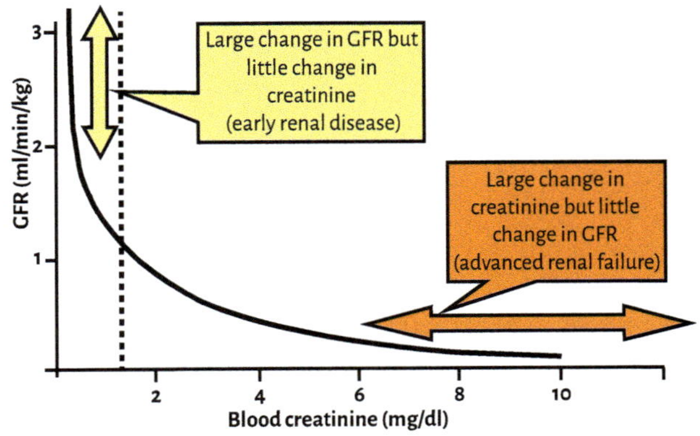

Figure 2. Relationship between blood creatinine concentrations and GFR.

Other potential **influences on serum creatinine** include:

- **Muscle mass**: decreased muscle mass can lead to decreased serum creatinine levels.
- **Age**: lean body mass (a source of creatinine) declines with age, which leads to a decline in serum creatinine. However, once a critical level of nephron damage occurs, serum creatinine levels will rise.
- **Dehydration and hypovolaemia**: these decrease GFR and creatinine clearance, potentially leading to an increase in serum creatinine.

Symmetric dimethylarginine (SDMA)

SDMA is a methylated form of arginine, which is produced by all cells in the body and then released into the circulation. **SDMA is almost exclusively excreted by the kidneys**, which makes it a good marker of renal function.

SDMA levels are not affected by muscle mass, which is advantageous in chronic renal disease where patients tend to lose muscle mass leading to lower than expected serum creatinine levels.

Studies confirm SDMA can detect kidney disease when an average of only 40% of GFR is lost (versus 70–75% for creatinine) and some cases were detected when only 25% of the GFR was lost.

SDMA is also arguably more reliable that creatinine as a marker for renal function before and during treatment of hyperthyroidism.

A recent study documented that in hyperthyroid cats, a high serum SDMA (> 14 μg/dl) with a normal creatinine is very sensitive in predicting the development of azotemia after treatment with radioiodine (sensitivity 97.7%). However, the presence of normal SDMA does not rule out the development of azotemia after treatment as the specificity was low (33%). A more recent study reported normalization of SDMA in a significant percentage of patients treated with radioactive iodine.

Other factors that influence GFR and consequently SDMA include:

- sepsis
- neoplasia
- diabetes mellitus
- pyelonephritis
- nephrolithiasis and ureterolithiasis.

Phosphate

Hyperphosphatemia is a risk factor for progression of chronic renal disease (CKD) and is associated with shorter survival. Multiple studies have documented beneficial effects of serum phosphate reduction by feeding diets restricted in phosphate.

Secondary renal hyperparathyroidism is a familiar term for most veterinarians, but this term has now been replaced by a more encompassing one: mineral and bone disorders in CKD (MBD-CKD). While the term secondary renal hyperparathyroidism is still in use, MBD-CKD acknowledges that factors other than parathyroid hormone are involved in phosphate homeostasis. The role of fibroblast growth factor-23 (FGF-23) and magnesium in phosphate homeostasis and MBD-CKD are some of the most important recent discoveries.

MBD occurs due to adaptative changes in hormones that regulate calcium and phosphate and its prevalence increases with the IRIS (http://www.iris-kidney.com) Stage of CKD. In early stages, the serum phosphate and calcium are maintained within normal limits through elevation of fibroblast-growth factor-23 (FGF-23) and parathyroid hormone (PTH) (Figure 3). Hyperphosphatemia is usually not observed until later stages of CKD. As such, MDB occurs from very early stages in CKD with increases in FGF-23 and PTH being indicators of this while phosphate is still normal.

The role of FGF-23 is incompletely understood but further information can be found within the references provided. A recent study documented that plasma FGF-23 is an independent predictor of survival time and progression over 12 months.

As the glomerular filtration rate (GFR) decreases the excretion of phosphate will decrease, leading to an increase in serum phosphate levels. In turn, the increase in serum phosphate will cause activation of the hormones that regulate calcium and phosphate homeostasis with the aim of controlling phosphate levels. In earlier stages of CKD, this is achieved by the action of FGF-23 which has a phosphaturic action, decreases calcitriol and inhibits PTH formation. In very late CKD, the presence of end-organ resistance to PTH and FGF-23 leading to hyperphosphataemia and calcitriol deficiency.

FGF-23 secretion from bone osteocytes acts on the kidney to induce phosphaturia via NaPi 2a/c

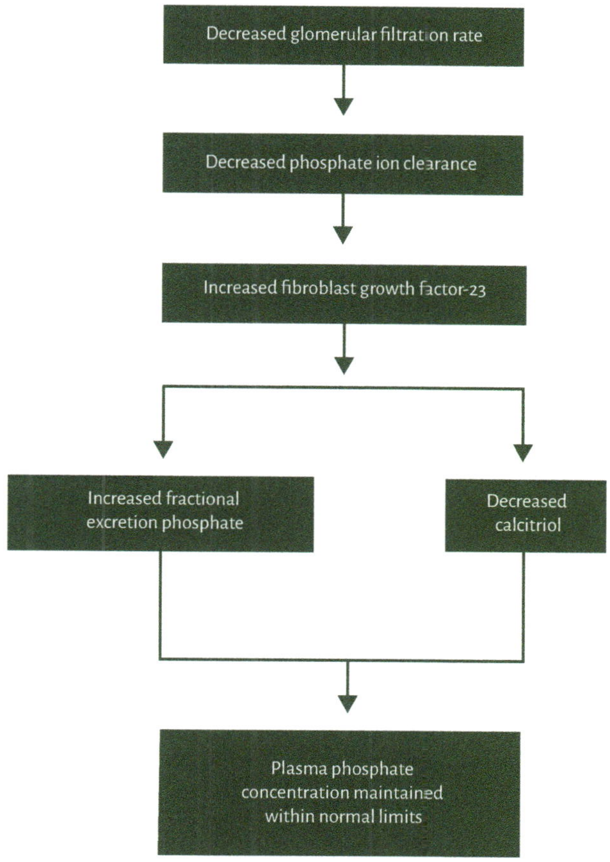

Figure 3. Mechanisms to maintain phosphate within normal limits at early stages of GFR loss.

transporters, similar to PTH, which acts via the PTH receptor. However, in contrast to the action of PTH to induce 1α hydroxylase, the enzyme that hydroxylates 25 vitamin D to 1,25-D, FGF23 acts to suppress 1α hydroxylase. 1,25-D is responsible for increased calcium and phosphate absorption from the gut and supports bone mineralization. The action of FGF23 on the parathyroid gland has been reported to suppress PTH secretion in vitro and in rodent models (Figure 4).

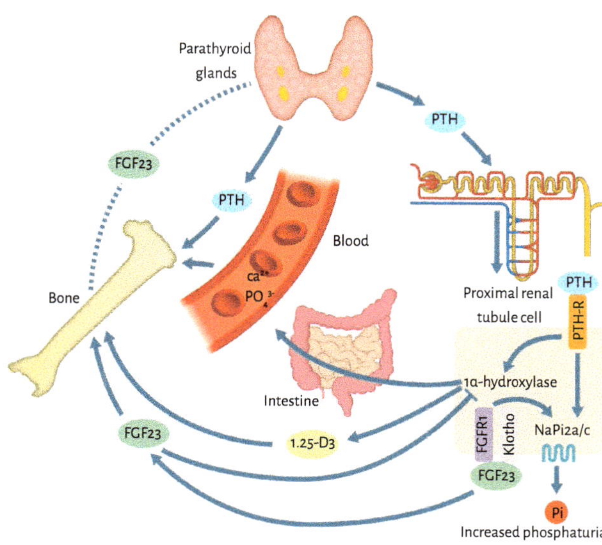

Figure 4. The PTH-Vitamin D-FGF-23 axis.

The prevalence of hyperparathyroidism is estimated to be as high as 84% in cats with CKD with a much larger proportion of cats in IRIS Stage 2 having hyperparathyroidism than hyperphosphatemia (47% vs 20%).

In cats with CKD, hyperphosphatemia is associated with shorter survival times and according to one study, plasma phosphate can predict the progression of feline CKD. Additionally, reducing phosphate intake by feeding a renal diet has been shown to increase survival in CKD.

Although it is possible to measure PTH, due to practical difficulties in assessment of PTH and its high cost this is very uncommonly performed in clinical circumstances.

As discussed above, measurement of phosphate as a surrogate marker of CKD-MBD would be inaccurate and would underestimate it. As such the goal should be to maintain phosphate towards the low end of normal or within the IRIS recommended range with an aim to prevent and reverse MBD.

Measurement of FGF-23 is commercially available and has been introduced in the IRIS treatment recommendations. FGF-23 assessment, in IRIS stage I and II cats with serum phosphate within the recommended levels, may help direct phosphate reduction measures. FGF-23 is expected to be elevated in IRIS stage III and IV, as a consequence of CKD, therefore there are no known clinical benefits of its measurement in these cases.

The IRIS recommendations for serum phosphate in CKD is in the table below.

IRIS Stage	Target phosphate (mmol/l)
Stage I	0.9 – 1.5 mmol/l
Stage II	0.9 – 1.5 mmol/l
Stage III	0.9 – 1.5 mmol/l (more realistic 0.9 – 1.6 mmol/l)
Stage IV	0.9 – 1.5 mmol/l (more realistic 0.9 – 1.9 mmol/l)

Potassium

Hypokalaemia occurs in approximately 20–30% cases of CKD and, depending on the severity, can lead to inappetence, gastrointestinal dysmotility, cardiac arrthythmias, impairment of urine concentration ability and generalised muscle weakness. Potassium is lost into the urine at higher tubular flow rates and cats with CKD often have a poor appetite, which results in even lower intake of potassium from the diet. In addition, diets too low in sodium will also activate the renin-angiotensin-aldosterone system resulting in further potassium wasting.

CKD patients that are dehydrated and already hypokalaemic may show a disappointing response to intravenous fluid therapy (due to muscle weakness and inappetence) unless their serum potassium levels are corrected. Crystalloids such as Hartmann's solution contain very little potassium and therefore supplementation is required.

Patients with hyperaldosteronism tend to have hypertension and hypokalaemia and, frequently have concurrent CKD. In a patient with CKD and hypokalemia, particularly if the hypokalemia is marked and poorly responsive to adequate supplementation, hyperaldosteronism should be considered as a differential diagnosis.

Hyperkalaemia is most frequently seen in post-renal azotaemia, acute kidney injury and acute-on-chronic kidney disease, particularly if the cat is oliguric or anuric. Significant hyperkalaemia can result in arrhythmia and death so it is a priority to identify and manage.

Calcium

The kidneys play a crucial role in calcium homeostasis and calcium disturbances form part of the syndrome mineral and bone disorder in chronic kidney disease (MBD-CKD). As such, it is not surprising that around 12–21% of cats with chronic renal disease have elevated total calcium. However, cats frequently have idiopathic hypercalcemia which can complicate matters further.

There is ongoing debate whether it is necessary or not to assess hypercalcemia with ionised calcium in cats. The current thinking is that ionised calcium should be assessed for great accuracy. If a cat with CKD has total hypercalcemia then the likelihood is that there is ionised hypercalcemia as the specificity is close to 100%. However, the sensitivity of total calcium for detection of ionised hypercalcemia is low and therefore ionised calcium should be measured in cats with CKD.

Acid-base status in renal disease

Metabolic acidosis is common in cats with severe renal disease but seen less frequently in cases with mild CKD. It occurs as renal function declines due to a failure of reabsorption of bicarbonate and the reduced excretion of hydrogen ions.

Severe metabolic acidosis occurs in problems such post-renal azotemia (e.g. urinary tract rupture or obstruction) and also in acute kidney injury (AKI), especially if this is caused by ethylene glycol toxicity (due to the formation of toxic metabolites).

In cats with CKD, chronic acidosis may cause increased protein catabolism and therefore most renal diets are designed to be less acidifying and have increased buffering capacity than normal feline diets.

Measurement of Glomerular Filtration Rate (GFR)

Assessment of GFR was traditionally used in patients with unexplained pu/pd and in cases where renal disease is suspected but serum creatinine remains normal. However, with the most recent wide availability of SDMA the measurement of GFR is seldom indicated.

The iohexol clearance test can be used in clinical practice; it is easy to perform and does not require specialized equipment or collection of urine; more information can be found within the references provided. However, it is recommended to consult with the specialist laboratory prior to running the test.

Urinalysis

Urinalysis is vital in the investigation of urinary tract disease. It can help localise azotaemia, identify complicating factors (e.g. infection), identify treatment targets (proteinuria) and suggest acute renal injury (casts).

The urine sample should be collected into a sterile container and should ideally be analysed at room temperature, within 1 hour of collection; potentially even sooner if looking for crystals.

Complete urinalysis requires the assessment of the chemical and physical properties of the urine and should include the following:

- Gross inspection of urine
- Specific chemical testing of urine
- Microscopic examination of urine sediment
- +/– Bacterial culture

Normal urine may be of various shades of yellow due to the natural pigments (uropigments) and it should be clear or just slightly cloudy. The normal colour of urine can be affected by the presence of excess of bilirubin, haemoglobin or myoglobin.

Collection method

There are pros and cons to each collection method.

- Free catch
  - **Suitable for urine chemistry** provided not contaminated after voiding
  - Not the best choice for bacteriology as can be contaminated by distal genital tract, perineal flora and/or organisms on the litter tray
- Transurethral catheterisation
  - Not normally recommended unless a catheter already is in place for another reason
  - **Risk of trauma, iatrogenic infection** and will also be contaminated by genital tract
- Cystocentesis
  - With practice this is an easy technique to master. It is the **collection method of choice for bacterial culture**

Urine specific gravity (USG)

Urine SG primarily reflects renal tubular concentration ability and the capability of producing concentrated urine in face of antidiuretic hormone (ADH).

There is no such thing as a normal urine SG range. Results need to be interpreted in light of age, hydration status, concurrent diseases, renal parameters, urine glucose and protein concentrations, along with any recent therapeutic interventions (e.g. fluid therapy, diuretics, corticosteroids).

There is some controversy whether human refractometers give a true representation of feline urine SG, which has lead to the development of a formula for more accurate results (but the use of this formula is also subject to debate.) It is **preferable to use a veterinary refractometer** with different scales for dogs and cats.

Classification of feline urine according to specific gravity.

Well concentrated	> 1.035
Range of minimal concentration	1.013–1.034
Isosthenuria	1.008–1.012
Hyposthenuria	< 1.008

Interpretation of urine dipsticks depends on **observing the colour change of the test pad after a specific time.** The colour change continues after this ideal time, and the results can be invalid if read late. Cold urine also interferes with the reaction in the dipstick pads, and therefore previously refrigerated urine should be allowed to **warm to room temperature before testing**. Additionally, the presence of pigments in the urine, e.g. severe haemoglobinuria prevents the reading of the dipstick.

The presence of a positive haem reaction on the dipstick can be secondary to the presence of either **haemoglobin or myoglobin**. The most accurate way to assess haematuria vs haemoglobinuria is to **examine the sediment for the presence of red blood cells.** Haemoglobinuria can be differentiated from myoglobinuria by spinning the blood and **evaluating the colour of the supernatant**.

Urine dipstick evaluation of proteinuria is only loosely semi-quantitative and estimates albumin only – it measures albumin concentration >0.3 g/l (+1 reaction). Assessment of proteinuria on the dipstick should be **made in light of the urine pH and SG** as alkaline urine (pH> 7.5) and urine with SG >1.030 can cause a false-positive dipstick. Additionally, the significance of +1 urine in an isosthenuric urine can be different from the same +1 in a urine with SG>1.030.

The sensitivity and specificity of using a dipstick for assessment of proteinuria are thought to be relatively low with results of 90% and 11% respectively and, in some circumstances, both the positive and negative predictive value are around 50%.

Proteinuria should be quantified whenever a disease predisposing to proteinuria is detected or whenever proteinuria is present in a screening test such as a dipstick.

Although there are other methods of measuring proteinuria, the **urine protein: creatinine ratio** (**UPC**) is the most accurate and comparison of the results allows assessment of the patient over time.

Persistent proteinuria is defined as positive test results on three or more occasions, on samples obtained two or more weeks apart. Changes in proteinuria should be **interpreted in light of the serum creatinine** as proteinuria may decrease in progressive renal disease as the number of functional nephrons decreases.

The **urine UPC can be elevated due to pre-renal and post-renal** causes and those should be ruled out before assuming that the proteinuria is renal in origin.

- **Pre-renal proteinuria** is characterised by increased protein in the blood overwhelming renal reabsorptive mechanisms and is generally excluded by measuring total serum protein.
- **Post-renal proteinuria** occurs when a source of protein enters the urine after the kidneys, i.e. in the bladder or genital tract. Cystitis and urinary tract infection are the most common cause consequently a UPC should be interpreted in conjunction with sediment exam +/– culture results and re-measured following resolution of any lower urinary tract inflammation/infection.
- **Renal proteinuria:** persistent proteinuria that results in a UPC > 0.4 for which pre-renal and post-renal causes have been excluded is consistent with renal proteinuria, which usually results from glomerular or tubulointerstitial disease.

According to the IRIS guidelines, patients with UPC< 0.2 are considered non-proteinuric. If the UPC is between 0.2 and 0.4 the patients are considered borderline proteinuric. Patients that have a **UPC > 0.4 are proteinuric**.

In non-azotemic, persistently proteinuric patients, further investigation and treatment of potential concurrent infectious, inflammatory disorders or neoplastic diseases is necessary. In cats, viral diseases, neoplasia, immune-mediated diseases and systemic hypertension are some of the most common causes of renal proteinuria. Unfortunately, in a significant percentage of cases an underlying disease cannot be identified. **When an underlying disease cannot be identified or treated specifically, non-specific treatment for proteinuria should be considered**.

A **positive dipstick for bilirubin is always abnormal in a cat** as the renal threshold for excretion is 9 times greater than in the dog. This should prompt further investigation into its cause.

Glucosuria can occur due to either hyperglycaemia, or secondarily to diseases preventing the renal proximal tubules from removing glucose from the filtrate. If the glucosuria is persistent and/or severe, appropriate tests should be considered. It is important to remember that **patients with glucosuria are predisposed to urinary tract infections** due to concurrent immunosuppression.

Dipsticks detect acetone and acetoacetate but not beta-hydroxybutyrate which is the most common ketone in DKA; this can lead to false-negative or falsely lowered results.

The use of the pads to test for urobilinogen and leucocytes is not recommended.

Microscopic evaluation of the urine sediment is used to detect an increased concentration of cells, casts, microorganisms or crystals. Multiple factors can affect the examination of the sediment and therefore this should be performed by experienced clinicians/nurses to avoid potential errors.

- **White blood cells**: the presence of **white blood cells is an indicator of inflammation and/or infection**
- **Renal casts**: if casts are seen this suggests that there is renal pathology as casts are formed when moulds of the tubules form due to aggregates of proteins or cells.
- **Crystals**: crystalluria is not synonymous with urolithiasis and urolithiasis can occur without observable crystalluria. Nonetheless, crystalluria might represent a potential risk factor for urolith formation. To correctly assess crystalluria a sample should be collected and examined within 15 to 20 minutes; immediately if the urine sample is going to be refrigerated. Delays in assessing urine can lead to false-positive crystalluria due to *ex vivo* formation.
- **Bacteria**: bacterial urinary tract infections (UTI) are extremely unusual in healthy, young cats.

A **cystocentesis sample should be used whenever a urine culture is needed.** Although there are guide values for the number of pathogens (CFU/ml) of what represents a significant amount of bacteria when collected by different methods, its use is increasingly discouraged.

Differentiating pre-renal, renal and post-renal azotaemia

It is **essential to distinguish between the types of azotaemia** as they have different pathologies and treatment.

There is always a possibility of pre-renal azotaemia and renal azotaemia/post-renal azotaemia co-existing (e.g. the dehydrated CKD cat) so a **true measure of renal azotaemia can only be made once volume deficits have been corrected**. This must be combined with a full physical examination to assess hydration status and post-renal issues (e.g. large, painful bladder) to make the distinction.

In some cases, an **assessment of urine SG is helpful** to determine if the azotaemia is pre-renal or renal, as a urine SG > 1.035 in a dehydrated patient is mostly consistent with pre-renal disease.

Differentiating AKI from CKD

Differentiating acute from chronic kidney disease is important for treatment and prognostic reasons. The table below may help with the differentiation.

In a significant percentage of cases, it **is impossible to discriminate between AKI and acute deterioration of CKD** (acute-on-chronic renal disease). This occurs when factors precipitate a crisis, resulting in an acute progression of the existing renal disease. Factors causing this progression include:

- Any condition causing **volume deficits** (vomiting, diarrhoea, inappetence)
- A **urinary tract infection/pyelonephritis**
- Any other disease (remember geriatric cats often have multiple co-morbidities)

AKI	CKD
History	**History**
Healthy until episode	Indicators of previous disease might exist (e.g. PU/PD, weight loss)
History of toxin/drug exposure	
Clinical examination	**Clinical examination**
Good body condition	Loss of body condition
Painful kidneys, possibly enlarged	Kidneys firm and small
Very unwell for level of azotaemia	Surprisingly well for the level of azotaemia
Possibly small bladder	Urine present in bladder
Clinicopathological findings	**Clinicopathological findings**
Hyperkalaemia	Hypo or normokalaemia
Metabolic acidosis (marked, particularly in ethylene glycol toxicity)	Non-regenerative anaemia
Anuria or oliguria	Polyuria
Cylindruria	Isosthenuria
Proteinuria	Sediment usually unremarkable
Isosthenuria	

Acute Kidney Injury (AKI)

Acute kidney injury is characterized by **an abrupt and sustained injury to the renal parenchyma**. This can be clinically undetectable or lead to failure of the renal function (acute renal failure – ARF) with inherent loss of the ability to excrete waste products, regulate acid-base, and electrolyte balance.

AKI is a term adopted from human medicine and includes a continuum of functional and parenchymal damage, from the milder to more severe forms of damage.

In humans, AKI is recognised primarily as hospital-acquired rather than community-acquired, while in veterinary medicine non-hospital acquired causes seem more common. In human medicine, the incidence of AKI is reported to be 2 to 7% of all patients and nearly 15% in critical patients with a mortality rate around 50%. In veterinary medicine less studies are available but the reported mortalities are 23–78% in dogs and around 47% in cats.

It is important to remember that **patients with AKI may have normal creatinine levels**. Remember that creatinine is poorly correlated with glomerular filtration rate (GFR) at low levels of dysfunction, a small change in creatinine (despite within the normal reference range) may represent a dramatic decrease in renal function.

Commonly recognised **risk factors for hospital-acquired AKI** include pre-existing renal disease, dehydration and volume depletion, decreased cardiac output, advanced age, fever, hypotension, hypoalbuminemia, sepsis, electrolyte imbalances, acidosis, hyperviscosity syndrome, liver disease, nephrotoxic drugs, administration of radiocontrast media, pancreatitis, diabetes mellitus, anaesthesia and surgery.

The **development of hospital-acquired AKI has a negative impact on** prognosis with one study documenting a 30-day survival rate for cats developing AKI within 2 days of hospitalization to be 48% versus 85% survival for those not developing AKI. The survival difference was not significant for cats developing mild AKI but it was significant for cats with more severe AKI (creatinine > 140 µmol/l and a rise > 26 µmol/l). In this scenario, it is clear to see that hospitalised patients considered at risk of AKI should be closely monitored and proactive intervention implemented if needed.

Negative prognostic indicators include:

- Lack of urine output
- Low body temperature
- Low serum albumin
- Elevated potassium: one study documented each unit increase in potassium was associated with a 57% decrease in survival

AKI classification

Acute kidney injury is classically divided into three categories:

- pre-renal
- renal
- post-renal

However, in most cases, there is an overlap of the different categories.

Pre-renal AKI

Pre-renal or haemodynamic causes include those bringing about a decrease in renal perfusion or excessive vasoconstriction. If the inciting cause is eliminated, these are rapidly reversible. However, prolonged ischaemia can contribute to renal parenchymal injury.

Intrinsic AKI

Intrinsic causes of AKI include ischemia (e.g. shock, anaesthesia), infectious diseases (e.g. pyelonephritis), renal lymphoma, toxins or systemic diseases with renal manifestations. Removal/treatment of the inciting cause of injury is often the only way of directly addressing this type of injury.

In the cat, the most common nephrotoxins are ethylene glycol, lilies, and NSAIDs.

The kidneys receive around **20% of the cardiac output**, and of this the renal cortex receives about 90% of the flow, which makes them (and particularly the renal cortex) very **susceptible to ischaemia and blood-borne toxic damage**.

Potential causes of intrinsic renal failure
Toxic
Ethylene glycol (EG)
NSAID's
Aminoglycosides
Lilies
Heavy metals
Amphotericin B
Phosphate enemas
Intravenous contrast agents
Tetracyclines
Doxorubicin
Platinum agents
Infectious
Pyelonephritis
Glomerulonephritis
Feline infectious peritonitis
Obstruction
Neoplasia
Urolithiasis
Other causes of obstruction
Others
Shock
Systemic hypotension
Burns/Heatstroke
Post-cardiac arrest syndrome
Thromboembolic disease
Sepsis
Anaphylaxis
Prolonged GA
Transfusion reaction
Traumatic injury

Post-renal AKI

Post-renal AKI is due to obstruction or diversion of urine flow, including urethral obstruction, bilateral ureteral obstruction or unilateral obstruction with a non-functional contralateral kidney, and also rupture of the urinary tract. In these patients, restoration of the urine flow (allowing urine to leave the body) may rapidly reduce the concentrations of uremic toxins. However, prolonged obstruction may lead to parenchymal renal injury.

Phases of AKI

There are **four recognised phases of AKI** and this "division" makes understanding AKI and it's progression easier (see table below from www.iris-kidney.com).

Depending on the degree and extent of AKI, the condition can progress through the different phases. Once the maintenance phase is reached **one of three outcomes** is possible (Figure 5):

1. recovery with CKD IRIS Stage 1
2. CKD with IRIS Stage 2 to 4
3. death

Diagnosis of AKI

The diagnosis of AKI is based on history, physical examination, and documentation of azotaemia +/– oliguria or anuria in advanced cases.

Acutely uremic patients can present with systemic signs of illness such as lethargy, vomiting, and diarrhoea and, on occasions, neurological signs.

Urinalysis findings may reveal isosthenuria or minimally concentrated urine (SG < 1.035), proteinuria, and glucosuria. Casts on the urine sediment suggest ongoing renal damage; casts are very fragile therefore the urine should be examined swiftly. The presence of **calcium oxalate crystals may suggest ethylene glycol toxicity.**

It is important to remember **AKI can be present even if serum creatinine is normal**, with increases as small as ≥ 26.4 µmol/l (≥ 0.3 mg/dl) in 48 hours being significant.

Radiographs may demonstrate normal to enlarged kidneys and/or uroliths within a different section of the urinary tract.

Table from IRIS kidney (www.iris-kidney.com)

AKI phases	
Initiation	Begins without clinical signs and is secondary to an ischaemic or nephrotoxic insult, and continues until there is a perceived change in renal function such as decreased urine output or increased creatinine. The length of time necessary for these changes to occur depends on the nature and severity of the insult. During this phase, early intervention may prevent progression of AKI.
Extension	During this phase continued hypoxia and an inflammatory response propagate kidney damage. Structures in the cortex are predisposed to toxic and ischaemic damage due to the high blood flow and also their high metabolism. Hypoxia leads to a decrease in ATP levels, reduction in function of Na/K pump with subsequent cell swelling and death. In this phase intervention may not be successful.
Maintenance	It generally lasts for 1 to 3 weeks. The urine output may be increased or decreased, and the urine resembles the ultrafiltrate as there is little modification by the tubules. At this stage, a critical amount of damage has occurred.
Recovery	This phase is associated with an increase in urine output that may or may not be accompanied by a decrease in urine sodium. During this period, extreme sodium losses can occur which can lead to volume depletion, therefore it is very important to monitor and replace the sodium and water. Renal recovery depends on recovery of sub-lethally injured cells, removal of necrotic cells and intra-tubular casts, and regeneration of renal cells. The regeneration and repair of the renal tissue may take weeks to months.

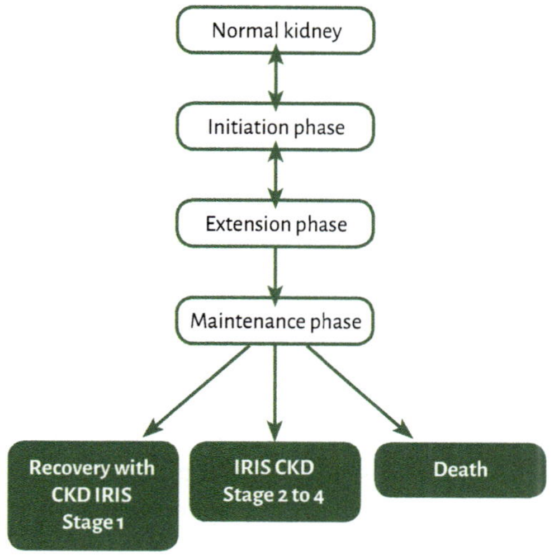

Figure 5. Progression of acute renal injury.

On ultrasound, the kidneys may be normal or enlarged (see below the most common differential diagnoses for renomegaly). In cases with **ethylene glycol toxicity, the kidneys may be hyperechoic.** The presence of **hydronephrosis may be indicative of obstruction** or **pyelonephritis** but it important to remember that mild to moderate renal pelvis dilation can occur due to aggressive diuresis. In some cases, it is possible to identify a dilated ureter and to trace it to an obstructive ureterolith. A recent study documented that 70% of cats with AKI have renomegaly and that pyelectasia was present in around 60% of cases and therefore ultrasound, alongside other findings, can help diagnose AKI.

If **renal lymphoma** is suspected cytology of the kidneys often helps achieve a diagnosis.

Any critically ill pet is at risk of developing AKI and those patients with additional specific risk factors may need to be monitored more closely than normal.

Most common differentials for renomegaly

- FIP
- Lymphoma (other neoplasia)
- Hydronephrosis
- AKI
- PKD
- Perinephric pseudocysts
- Trauma and haemorrhage
- Amyloidosis
- Pyelonephritis
- Acromegaly

IRIS Grading for AKI

The **IRIS (International Renal Interest Society)** recently adapted a systematic approach to classify and grade the severity of AKI in dogs and cats (see table below).

Unlike the IRIS staging system for CKD, for the grading of AKI, the **kidney disease does not need to be stable** as the grade represents a moment in the progression of the disease and is likely to change as the condition gets worse or improves.

According to IRIS, grading for AKI may provide data for earlier recognition, therapeutic stratification, and outcome assessment in dogs and cats. However, studies are still needed to make this relevant on a day-to-day basis.

Animals caught in the early stages (AKI I and II) and managed appropriately may **regain adequate renal function within two to five days**. In general, patients with higher grades of AKI at diagnosis or that progress to higher grades during hospitalisation may require weeks of treatment before the renal repair starts.

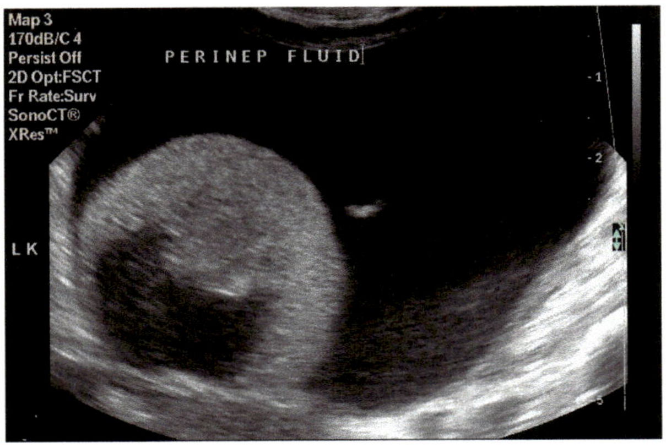

Figure 6. Ultrasound of a perinephric pseudocyst which was detected when investigating a renomegaly case with elevated renal parameters.

There is also evidence that patients with AKI grade IV and V may die within a matter of days if renal replacement therapy is not implemented.

IRIS AKI Grade I

- Defines **non-azotaemic animals** with historical, clinical, laboratory (biomarkers such as glucosuria, cylindruria, inflammatory sediment, microalbuminuria, etc), and imaging evidence of AKI; and/or those with clinical oliguria/anuria.
- IRIS AKI Grade I includes animals with **progressive (hourly or daily) increases in blood creatinine of ≥ 26.4 μmol/l (≥ 0.3 mg/dl)** within the non-azotemic range during a 48-hour interval.
- IRIS AKI Grade I also includes animals whose decreased urine production is readily fluid volume-responsive. **Fluid volume responsiveness represents an increase in urine production to > 1 ml/kg/h within 6 hours**; and/or decrease in blood creatinine to baseline over 48 hours.

IRIS AKI Grade II

- Defines animals with **documented AKI characterized by mild** azotemia in addition to other historical, biochemical, anatomic, or urine production characteristics of AKI (as for grade I), and similarly includes those whose oliguria and/or azotaemia is readily fluid responsive.
- Fluid volume responsiveness represents an **increase in urine production to > 1 ml/kg/h within 6 hours**; and/or decrease in blood creatinine to baseline over 48 hours.
- IRIS AKI Grade II also includes animals that have an **increase from their baseline creatinine concentration of ≥ 26.4 μmol/l (≥ 0.3 mg/dl) during a 48-hour interval** associated with pre-existing CKD.

IRIS AKI Grading Criteria (from www.iris-kidney.com)

AKI Grade	Blood Creatinine	Clinical Description
Grade I	< 140 μmol/l < 1.6 mg/dl	Non-azotemic AKI Documented AKI (historical, laboratory or imaging evidence of AKI, clinical oliguria/anuria, volume responsiveness* and or Progressive non azotemic increase in blood creatinine ≥ 26.4 μmol/l (≥ 0.3 mg/dl) within 48 h Measured oliguria (< 1 ml/kg/h) or anuria over 6 h
Grade II	141 – 220 μmol/l 1.7 – 2.5 mg/dl	Mild AKI Documented AKI and static or progressive azotemia Progressive azotemic increase in blood creatinine ≥ 26.4 μmol/l (≥ 0.3 mg/dl) within 48 h or volume responsiveness Measured oliguria (< 1 ml/kg/h) or anuria over 6 h
Grade III	221 – 439 μmol/l 2.6 – 5.0 mg/dl	Moderate to severe AKI Documented AKI and increasing severities of azotaemia and functional renal failure
Grade IV	440 – 880 μmol/l 5.1 – 10.0 mg/dl	
Grade V	> 880 μmol/l > 10.0 mg/dl	

* volume responsiveness is an increase in urine production to > 1 ml/kg/h over 6 hours; and/or decrease in serum creatinine to baseline over 48 h

IRIS AKI Grade III, IV and V

- Defines animals with documented AKI **and progressively greater degrees of parenchymal damage and functional failure** (uraemia).

Each grade of AKI is further **sub-graded on the basis of current urine production** and and on the requirements for renal replacement therapy (RRT).

- oligoanuric (O; oliguria, <1 ml/kg/h) or
- anuria, (no urine produced over 6 hours) or
- nonoliguric (NO; >1 ml/kg/h)

The inclusion of sub-grading by urine production is due to the importance of the relationship between urine production to the pathological or functional contributions to the renal injury and its influence on the clinical presentation, therapeutic options, and outcome of AKI.

Sub-grading based on the **requirement for renal replacement therapy (RRT)** is established on the need to correct life-threatening iatrogenic or clinical consequences of AKI including:

- severe azotaemia
- hyperkalaemia
- acid-base disorders
- overhydration
- oliguria or anuria
- elimination of nephrotoxins.

Sub-grading based on the requirements for RRT has similar clinical, therapeutic, and prognostic implications, as for urine production, to categorize the severity of the renal injury and its influence on outcome.

Management of AKI

Treatment goals for patients with AKI are aimed at limiting further renal damage by identifying the underlying cause (and whenever possible treating it) and maximising the possibility of enhancing cellular recovery. Treatment is most successful during the induction and extension phases, and success decreases in later phases.

The management of AKI depends largely on the underlying cause. However, the ultimate goal in all cases is to optimize haemodynamic status, restore adequate perfusion to the kidneys, promote and maintain diuresis and address secondary complications of AKI.

If there is suspicion of toxin ingestion, the Veterinary Poisons Information Service should be contacted for information on management of the case; this service is available 24 hours a day.

In cases with suspected pyelonephritis, due to the presence of an active sediment +/- suggestive ultrasonographic features, antibiotics should be started while results of culture and sensitivity are pending. More information on the topic is available on the section on urinary tract infection.

Imaging of the urinary tract is often pivotal in helping to establish a diagnosis or ruling out differential diagnoses.

Renal biopsies may be able to help determine the extent of the insult, whether the disease is truly acute or acute-on-chronic and can also help with prognosis. However, they are not often used in patients with AKI as usually they don't alter the management and are associated with risks and potential complications. Neoplasia such as lymphoma is frequently diagnosed with fine needle aspirates.

One of the pillars of treatment of AKI is to try to promote diuresis and reverse azotaemia using fluid therapy. This however should be performed judiciously as fluid overload has a significant negative impact on survival.

AKI patients may present with hypovolemia, normovolemia, or even with fluid overload and this will have a huge impact on the fluid therapy plan. Hypovolemia is a decreased fluid volume in the vascular compartment, and it can occur with or without depletion of whole-body fluid (dehydration).

Clinical signs of over-hydration include wet mucous membranes, shivering, nausea, vomiting, restlessness, with serous nasal discharge, chemosis, tachypnoea, ascites, diarrhoea, and subcutaneous oedema being present in later stages of fluid overload.

Fluid deficits can lead to reduced renal blood flow, decreased GFR (with consequent reduction in urine production) and cause further renal injury. As such fluid balance should be address as a matter of priority and, if the cause of AKI is pre-renal it may be reversible if addressed swiftly.

Renal perfusion should be optimised before determining whether the oliguria is physiological or pathological. Correction of hypovolaemia should be a priority and replacement of other fluid deficits should be performed within a few hours.

Hypovolaemia should be corrected with isotonic crystalloids, with Hartmann's solution being often the most appropriate. The use of synthetic colloids is not recommended in patients with AKI.

A fluid bolus of 10–15 ml/kg should be administered over a 10-to-15-minute period and, if the required end-points have not been met, further fluid boluses (usually of 5–10 ml/kg) can be administered until the patient is haemodynamically stable.

Critically ill cats frequently present with hypothermia which, until corrected, can lead to overestimation of the fluid deficit. As such, warming should be performed at the same time as addressing fluid deficits to avoid inadvertently causing a fluid overload in those patients.

Once the haemodynamic status is corrected, hydration should be addressed considering the estimated dehydration present. If the patient has AKI, it is often advised to correct dehydration within a shorter time frame than in most other cases (usually a few of hours rather than 12–24 h), provided other co-morbidities allow it.

Dehydration can only be detected clinically when above 5% therefore it would be fair to assume that any oliguric patient that does not appear dehydrated could have up to 5% dehydration. In this setting, a volume of fluids of up to 5% of the body weight should be administered to those patients provided there is no evidence of overhydration.

Measurement of urine output is essential in the monitoring of patients with AKI and the response to fluid therapy. It is also pivotal in the implementation of the method "Ins and Outs" of fluid administration, which aims to help maintain an adequate fluid balance by matching the volume administered to the volume excreted, therefore trying to avoid underperfusion and overhydration.

Urine output should be monitored as accurately as possible. Ideally, an indwelling urine catheter should be placed aseptically and should be attached to a closed collection system. The collection bag should be lower than the patient to allow urine drainage and should be kept on a clean surface like a clean tray (rather than on the floor!).

It is necessary to consider the pros and cons of placing urinary catheters in patients with evidence of an active urinary tract infection, in diabetic patients, in immunocompromised patients and in patients with coagulopathies. Ascending nosocomial infections are also a concern, especially in patients already on systemic antibiotic therapy.

If placement of a urinary catheter is not possible then calculating urinary output by weighting litter trays and/or bedding pre- and post-urination can be used by assuming 1 g = 1 ml of urine.

In cats with urinary tract obstruction or rupture, providing a method of urinary diversion out of the body (e.g. urinary catheter or cystotomy tube) is essential.

Once fluid deficits are corrected, patients with normal renal function and adequate renal perfusion, would be expected to be producing a minimum of 1–2 ml/kg/h. However, AKI patients may be oliguric (urine production <1 ml/kg/h) or anuric (no urine production). Conversely, in some cases, significant polyuria and solute loss is present and this should be taken into account for calculation of maintenance fluid therapy regimens.

In cases with apparent oligo-anuria it is important to rule out urinary tract obstruction, urinary catheter obstruction or leakage of urine (SC, intraperitoneal, retroperitoneal) prior to considering the oligo-anuria is real. Additionally, all fluid deficits should be corrected before reassessing the urine output.

Once fluids deficits are corrected, ongoing losses such as vomiting, diarrhoea and polyuria should be taken into account when calculating maintenance fluid needs. At this stage, the type of fluids used must be adjusted based on the patient's fluid and electrolyte status.

Anuric patients should receive only replacement of insensible losses to avoid overhydration.

Once the patient is stable and the azotaemia has resolved or improved significantly, fluid therapy may be able to be slowly weaned (by around 20% a day) while making sure there is a proportionate decrease in urine output without worsening of the azotaemia or without any other evidence of dehydration. If the urine output does not decrease accordingly the fluid rate should be increased back to the previous rate and the weaning of fluid therapy will need to be tried at another time.

Monitoring of AKI patients

Clinical examination is critical in the assessment of the fluid volume status and measurement of other relevant parameters such as blood pressure also plays a vital role in assessing perfusion status. The most commonly used parameters in the assessment and monitoring of AKI are in the table below.

Clinical parameters that may help with patient assessment and monitoring

Pulse rate and quality	Urine output and specific gravity
Capillary refill time	Blood pressure
Mucous membrane colour	Oxygen saturation (SpO_2)
Respiratory rate and effort	PCV/total solids
Pulmonary sounds	Serum lactate
Skin turgor	Renal parameters
Rectal temperature	Electrolytes
Extremity temperature	Venous/ arterial blood gases
Mental status	

Evaluation of renal parameters should be done one or twice daily while other blood test parameters such as serum electrolytes, acid base status and glucose might need to be repeated more often depending on the case.

Patient with AKI should be weighted 3 to 4 times a day on the same scales to monitor fluid balance as rapid changes in body weight primarily reflect a change in body water; the expected daily decrease in weight due to anorexia is usually negligible. When weighting patients, it is important to make sure that this is done always in the same conditions (e.g. with an empty bladder, prior to feeding) to avoid introducing confounding variables.

Measurement of central venous pressure (CVP) is a very useful tool to help monitor fluid balance. A CVP $<$ 0 cm H_2O is suggestive of volume depletion while a CVP $>$ 10 cm of H_2O is consistent with volume overload or right-sided congestive heart failure. Overall, monitoring the trend in CVP is more clinically relevant that assessment of numbers independently.

Use of diuretics

If pathological oliguria or anuria persist despite correcting the pre-renal component, most clinicians would consider using diuretics to convert oliguria to non-oliguria. There is no evidence that diuretics improve the outcome of acute renal failure, and it is suggested that the ability to respond to diuretics may be a marker of less severe renal injury.

In human medicine the use of diuretics for AKI is no longer recommended when dialysis is available. In veterinary medicine dialysis is only very seldom used due to its very limited availability, high cost and intensive management required and therefore we still reach to diuretics despite the lack of evidence that it improves renal recovery or mortality.

If used indiscriminately and without balancing the pros and cons, diuretics may lead to worsening of kidney injury and severe electrolyte imbalances amongst others.

Some of the drugs used are:

- Frusemide
  - Frusemide is usually the drug of choice to promote diuresis and to try to convert patients onto a non-oliguric state. Frusemide acts on the ascending loop of Henle and induces diuresis and natriuresis and, although it does not increase the GFR, it may help address or prevent fluid overload. There are very few studies of the use of frusemide in cats. Frusemide is contraindicated in patients with aminoglycoside-induced AKI.
  - If frusemide is used a bolus of 1–5 mg/kg IV is expected to lead to an increase in urine production around 20–60 minutes after administration. If a positive effect is seen it can be administered every 6–8 hours or as a continuous rate infusion (CRI) at 0.25–1 mg/kg/h.
  - CRI administration of frusemide is thought to provide a more sustained diuresis with lower cumulative doses. However, a recent study on the use of frusemide in congestive heart failure in dogs and cats identified a higher risk of possible side-effects in the CRI group when compared to the intermittent doses.
  - It is important to remember that continued frusemide administration may lead to fluid and electrolyte imbalances and therefore monitoring is important.
- Mannitol
  - Mannitol is an osmotic diuretic that causes extracellular volume expansion, which can improve GFR and inhibit sodium reabsorption in the kidney by inhibiting renin. Amongst other potential beneficial effects, mannitol increases tubular flow, which may relieve intratubular obstruction from casts and debris. Mannitol should not be used in anuric patients due to the risk of volume overload, and it also should not be given to patients that are dehydrated, as it will exacerbate intracellular dehydration. In addition, the use of mannitol is contra-indicated if there is already over-hydration or cardiac disease.
  - The use of mannitol in cats with AKI has not been proven beneficial.
- Dopamine
  - Dopamine is a catecholamine that has an agonist effect on dopaminergic receptors. Historically, low-dose dopamine was used, in human and veterinary medicine, in patients with oliguric or anuric AKI. More recent data shows lack of proven benefit and potential severe detrimental effects and therefore its use in human and veterinary medicine is no longer recommended.
- Fenoldopam
  - Fenoldopam is a selective dopamine-1–receptor (DA-1) agonist, inducing vasodilatation, and selectively increasing both renal cortical and outer medullary blood flow and GFR, similar to dopamine but without some of its side-effects.
  - There is controversial data regarding the benefit of fenoldopam in human AKI and a retrospective study found no beneficial effects of its use in dogs and cats with AKI.

Secondary complications and supportive treatment

- Hypertension
  - Healthy kidneys can auto-regulate their perfusion with blood pressures between around 80 to 180 mmHg therefore the systolic blood pressure should be maintained within these levels (preferably below 160 mmHg) to try to avoid further damage.
  - Hypertension is reported to occur in 38% of cats with AKI and will need to be addressed. In cases with AKI, ACE inhibitors should be avoided as they cause afferent arteriolar constriction which can lead to further reduction in renal perfusion. Hypertension is discussed in more detail in the section on chronic renal disease.
- Hyperkalaemia
  - Hyperkalaemia is frequently encountered with AKI due to decreased excretion in cases of anuria/oliguria or urinary tract obstruction. Severe hyperkalaemia can lead to cardiac arrhythmia and should be managed by decreasing the heart sensitivity to the arrhythmogenic potential of hyperkalaemia +/− reducing serum potassium while addressing the underlying cause (re-establishing diuresis and/or relieving obstruction). More information on the topic is available on the section on urethral obstruction.

- Metabolic acidosis
  - Metabolic acidosis is expected to occur in AKI due to:
    - reduced bicarbonate production in the kidneys
    - reduced ability to excrete hydrogen ions
    - increased concentration of uraemic acids
  - Consequences of metabolic acidosis include disruption of cellular metabolism, exacerbation of hyperkalaemia due to extracellular shift of potassium, with intracellular shift of hydrogen ions and increased protein and bone turnover. Frequently the acidosis is compounded by concurrent fluid deficits and hypoperfusion.
  - Treatment of metabolic acidosis should start by focusing on the correction of deficits of perfusion and ideally addressing of the underlying cause of AKI. Specific treatment of metabolic acidosis with bicarbonate will be discussed at a later stage.
- Gastrointestinal signs
  - Vomiting and anorexia are commonly seen with AKI and, frequently are the reason for the initial presentation by the owners. Uremic toxins and electrolyte and acid-base disturbances are amongst some of the reasons for the development of these signs. Medications such as maropitant, ondansetron, omeprazole and famotidine can be used as part of the supportive treatment.
- Nutrition
  - Patients with AKI are in a negative nutritional balance at a time when nutrition is essential for repair of cellular damage. In addition, most patients will remain inappetent or with reduced food intake for a significant period of time.
  - Enteral feeding such as with nasoesophageal feeding tubes can be used to provide caloric requirements when vomiting is controlled. If vomiting is not controlled parenteral feeding should be considered.
  - Feeding tubes can also be used for administration of additional fluids in patients recovering from AKI.

Intoxication with ethylene glycol (EG)

Intoxication with EG is usually caused by ingestion of anti-freeze either accidentally or due to malicious poisoning of food. In cats the minimum lethal dose is much lower than in dogs (1.5 ml/kg vs 4.4–6.6 ml/kg in dogs). The mortality rate in cats is around 96–100% whilst in dogs it ranges from 59–70%.

EG is not toxic, but its metabolites can cause severe AKI. Absorption of EG is rapid and peak blood levels occur within 1 hour after ingestion. It is almost totally metabolized and excreted within 24 hours. EG is metabolised by alcohol dehydrogenase onto several acidic metabolites such as glycoaldehyde and oxalic acid, which cause severe metabolic acidosis and contribute to the neurological signs.

Serum calcium and oxalic acid bind and form calcium oxalate crystals which then lead, alongside the toxic metabolites and the metabolic acidosis, to acute kidney injury.

Clinical signs of intoxication can develop within 20 to 30 minutes and are caused by both unmetabolized EG and its toxic metabolites. EG causes clinical signs similar to those seen with ethanol intoxication such as gastrointestinal signs (nausea, hypersalivation, vomiting), polyuria/polydipsia and neurological signs (ataxia and mentation changes).

These clinical signs occur very quickly after ingestion and last for about 12 hours. The development of oliguric renal failure occurs about 12–24 hours after ingestion in cats.

The most common laboratory findings in patients with EG toxicity are in the table below.

Laboratory Findings Following Ethylene Glycol Toxicity

- Metabolic acidosis
- Increased anion gap
- Hypocalcaemia
- Calcium oxalate crystalluria
- Azotaemia
- Isosthenuria
- Hyperphosphatemia (due to phosphate containing 'rust prevention' additives)
- Increased serum osmolarity
- Ethylene glycol detectable in the blood (test available for humans)

Most studies on cage-side tests have shown these to have questionable sensitivity, especially at low (but still nephrotoxic) levels of EG, and also have potential for false positive results with compounds such as glycols and alcohols.

Some countries may have available a bedside test that reportedly has a low detection threshold of 20 mg/dl of EG, on plasma of both dogs and cats, from 30 minutes until 12–24 h post ingestion, depending on amount ingested and size of patient.

Some EG products contain fluorescein and therefore fluorescence with the Wood's lamp may be present in the paws, fur, stomach content and for the first few hours on the urine too.

Emergency treatment of EG intoxication includes decontamination via induction of emesis if ingestion is very recent. Emesis is contra-indicated if the patient is already showing GI signs such as vomiting or if neurological signs are present given the increased risk of aspiration of the gastric contents.

Decontamination using activated charcoal is of little use as EG is not significantly adsorbed by charcoal.

Treatment of EG intoxication involves inhibiting the metabolism of EG into its toxic metabolites and promoting the excretion of unmetabolized EG by promoting diuresis. Treatment with either 4-methylpyrazole or ethanol must be started within a short time after ingestion to maximise survival; if azotaemia is present this is unlikely to be successful. Treatment prior to clinical signs is the most effective way to ensure the best possible prognosis.

Ethanol is used as a competitive substrate that is capable of binding to the enzyme ADH therefore preventing the metabolism of EG. Ethanol can be administered IV with several different protocols and different concentrations being described in the literature. The risks of using ethanol include exacerbation of the neurological signs, hypoglycaemia and worsening of the serum hyperosmolality induced by EG. When it is not possible to source ethanol, 40% alcohol such as vodka can be used instead with protocols for administration available in the reading list.

The drug 4-methylpyrazole (4-MP or fomepizole) is a direct inhibitor of ADH preventing the metabolism of EG. The dose of fomepizole that has been reported as effective in cats is significantly higher than the dose used in dogs. Fomepizole is almost impossible to obtain in Europe.

Haemodialysis is recommended for cases with EG intoxication to help address the AKI and remove the circulating metabolites and toxins.

Supportive care similar to the one used in all cases of AKI is also essential.

Toxicity by lilies

All species of the genera *Lilium* (true lily) and *Hemerocallis* (day lily) are toxic to cats and can lead to AKI. Other plant species whose common name include the word lily can also be toxic with different effects. Animals other than cats tend to exhibit gastrointestinal signs but not nephrotoxicity.

Lilies have an unknown water-soluble toxin, and all parts of the plant are toxic, including the flower, the pollen, the stems, and the leaves. However, one study identified the flowers as much more toxic than the leaves. The ingestion of even minute quantities of toxin such as licking a small amount of pollen from the coat may lead to fatality in cats.

Clinical signs usually start minutes after ingestion with salivation and vomiting and tend to abate after a few hours. The second phase of clinical signs occurs around 12–24 hours after ingestion with the development of AKI, central nervous system signs, hypothermia, etc.

Some patients may develop seizures which seem to be unrelated to the presence of azotaemia.

Unlike patients with EG toxicity, severe metabolic acidosis very early on is not a feature, crystalluria is not common and serum calcium is usually normal.

If treatment with decontamination (induction of emesis and use of activated charcoal) and fluid therapy is started within a few hours after ingestion the probability of survival is high. If treatment is started more than 12–18 hours post ingestion the prognosis is extremely guarded. General treatment for acute kidney injury is also needed in most patients.

The mortality rate in cats with AKI secondary to lily intoxication is estimated to be 50–100% according to an early study while other studies report a much higher survival rate despite some cats being left with CKD as a consequence.

Renal replacement therapy (RRT)

RRT is the treatment of choice for patients that fail to respond to medical management, and it is a global term that encompasses different forms of dialysis. The exact timing is controversial, but it is indicated in patients with unresponsive hyperkalaemia, life-threatening volume overload and persistent uremic symptoms. Dialysis and therapeutic plasma exchange (plasmapheresis) can also help remove some toxins from circulation.

Peritoneal dialysis (PD) is rarely used for acute uraemia in critically ill people, but in animals it is a lot more readily available than haemodialysis. PD uses the peritoneum as a semi-permeable membrane, which allows shift of solutes and water between the blood stream and the fluid infused into the abdominal cavity (dialysate) and are later removed when the dialysate is drained out. In cats, there are few studies looking at the use of PD in AKI.

Peritoneal dialysis requires intensive specific treatment and nursing given the high risk of complications such as retention of the dialysate, catheter blockage, leakage around the catheter site, peritonitis, and electrolyte abnormalities. Peritoneal dialysis is possible to be performed in most larger hospital/clinics with adequate facilities.

Haemodialysis is only very rarely available in Europe.

Chronic kidney disease (CKD)

From five to six years of age, the incidence of chronic kidney disease starts to increase and, in referral populations of geriatric animals CKD is estimated to affect **30–50% of cats over 15 years of age**.

The main role of the kidneys is to excrete nitrogenous waste and excess acid alongside maintaining fluid and electrolyte homeostasis.

Measurement of the **glomerular filtration rate (GFR) is a useful measure of the kidneys' excretory capacity**. When inadequate filtration occurs nitrogenous products accumulate in the body and as kidney disease progresses the GFR declines. In practical terms, measurement of serum creatinine and more recently SDMA is often used as a surrogate marker of GFR.

Most of the cases of CKD are acquired but some breeds are prone to heritable CKD, such as the Abyssinian (medullary amyloidosis) and the Persian (polycystic kidney disease).

Risk factors for the development of CKD include diseases such as cystitis, urolithiasis, diabetes mellitus and hyperthyroidism. A multitude of other pathologies has been associated with renal disease in cats including pancreatitis, FeLV +/– FIV infection, and neoplasia.

Possible causes of CKD

Congenital disease
- Amyloidosis (Abyssinians, Siamese and Oriental Shorthair)
- Polycystic kidney disease (Persian and Himalayans)

Acquired disease
- Pyelonephritis
- FIP
- Neoplasia
- Hypercalcemia
- Hydronephrosis (urethral obstruction)
- Primary glomerulonephropathies
- Results of acute kidney injury
- Renal ischaemia
- FIV-related nephropathy
- Immune-mediated (rare)

The majority of cases of feline CKD are caused by chronic tubulointerstitial disease and the **inciting cause cannot be identified**. The difficulty of finding a cause is often the result of the kidneys response to injury being the same, regardless off the inciting cause.

Factors thought to influence the progression of CKD include intra-glomerular hypertension, glomerular hypertrophy, hypertension, and proteinuria.

When part of the renal mass is lost, compensatory hypertrophy and intra-glomerular hypertension occur in the remaining nephrons, resulting in an **increase in single nephron GFR (SNGFR)**. This adaptive process initially maintains GFR but these mechanisms lead to in cell damage and disease progression. **Arterial hypertension** may also cause proteinuria, which causes further damage. Also, transmission of hypertension to the glomerulus is detrimental to renal function, which makes **controlling hypertension a priority**.

Patients with CKD are categorized into stages along a continuum of progressive disease. This staging facilitates application of appropriate clinical practice guidelines for diagnosis, prognosis, and treatment.

IRIS CKD staging system

According to the IRIS (International Renal Interest Society System) CKD patients are classified into **1 of 4 stages based on serum fasting creatinine and, more recently, SDMA**; this measurement should be performed at least **twice in a period of a few weeks**. It is also important to remember that **only stable CKD patients can be staged** and, in those animals, a change in serum SDMA and creatinine < 20–25% is expected in order to assume a stable GFR and therefore stable disease.

SDMA is a more sensitive marker and less impacted by loss of lean body mass. In cases of persistent discrepancy between creatinine and SDMA, IRIS recommends **adopting the higher stage of the two** and treating the patient as such.

The IRIS staging system only applies to cats with **stable CKD**. Cases with acute renal disease or decompensated chronic renal disease might need **four to eight weeks to stabilize** and be accurately staged.

This staging system recognises that a large proportion of kidney damage occurrs before a rise in creatinine is seen therefore patients with stage I and early stage II have normal or top-normal creatinine.

In addition to staging, IRIS recommends to substage patients based on:

Criteria for a patient to be classified as CKD IRIS Stage I

Persistent renal proteinuria
Abnormal shape/size of the kidneys confirmed by imaging
Increasing, despite within normal, serum creatinine and/or SDMA documented with serial blood samples in and adequately hydrated patient.
Persistently elevated SDMA between 14–17 μg/dl.

IRIS Staging for CKD

IRIS Staging CKD for cats	Serum creatinine	SDMA
IRIS CKD Stage I	< 140 μmol/l < 1.6 mg/dl	< 18 μg/dl
IRIS CKD Stage II	140–250 μmol/l 1.6–2.8 mg/dl	18–25 μg/dl
IRIS CKD Stage III	251–440 μmol/l 2.9–5.0 mg/dl	26–38 μg/dl
IRIS CKD Stage IV	> 440 μmol/l > 5.0 mg/dl	> 38 μg/dl

- **Proteinuria** by measurement of urine protein: creatinine ratio – UPC
- **Systolic arterial blood pressure**

Sub-staging based on proteinuria

To sub-stage a patient, pre-renal and post-renal proteinuria must be ruled out. Persistent proteinuria is ideally documented by **measurement of UPC** in at least three urine samples, two or more weeks apart.

In cats with CKD, proteinuria is an independent risk factor for all-cause mortality.

After documenting the **proteinuria is of renal origin**, feline patients should be sub-staged based on proteinuria according to the IRIS guidelines (Figure 7).

Once the proteinuria is addressed, the sub-staging will need changing and a reference to treatment "(treating)" placed alongside the new sub-staging.

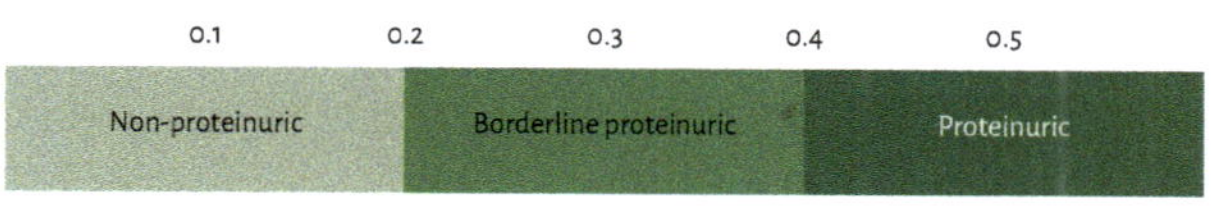

Figure 7. IRIS substaging of CKD according to proteinuria.

Sub-staging based on arterial blood pressure

Hypertension is estimated to occur in a significant percentage of cats with CKD, with some studies suggesting 66% of CKD cats are hypertensive.

High blood pressure (BP) is detrimental to the kidneys and kidney disease can lead to problems in blood pressure regulation and therefore hypertension. In addition, hypertension damages other organs (end-organ damage) such as the heart, eye, and brain.

The most common changes seen in these organs are:

- **Left ventricular hypertrophy** which can be confused with hypertrophic cardiomyopathy.
- **Hyphaema**, hypertensive retinopathy with retinal haemorrhage, retinal detachment, and blindness.
- **Brain vascular accidents** leading to lethargy, changes in mentation, and seizures.

The pathophysiology of hypertension as a complication of kidney disease is not completely understood. Some of the changes that are thought to contribute are:

- Dilation of the afferent glomerular arteriole reduces the ability to protect the glomerulus from fluctuations in arterial blood pressure.
- Affected nephrons have reduced filtration and sodium excretion capacity, and increased renin secretion, which is resistant to feedback mechanisms.
- The increase in renin secretion leads to increased production in angiotensin II and subsequently aldosterone. Angiotensin II has a direct stimulatory effect on the sympathetic system leading to increased vascular tone and, in the diseased kidney, preferential vasoconstriction of the efferent arteriole.
- Activation of the renin-angiotensin-aldosterone system (RAAS) action concurrent to activation of the sympathetic system and the reduced renal inability to compensate with increased sodium excretion can lead to increased blood pressure.

Indirect/non-invasive blood pressure measurement in cats is widely used in general practice. Using indirect techniques can **indicate systolic blood pressure**, although this technique is not as accurate as direct methods. Experience of the equipment will improve the ability to achieve accurate results. The ISFM Consensus Guidelines on the Diagnosis and Management of Hypertension in Cats has extremely useful information on how to minimise "white coat" hypertension, and how to perform and interpret blood pressure monitoring.

Avoiding 'White Coat' Hypertension

- Avoiding stress prior to entering the consult room is very important. It helps to have a separate cat room or area, alongside other cat-friendly techniques
- Wear earphones when using Doppler, to prevent noise upsetting the cat
- If not using headphones then keep volume off until the probe is in position
- Keep owners present if possible
- Use minimal restraint
- Inflate the cuff gently rather than suddenly
- Ignore the first couple of readings
- If the readings are not consistent, have a break, leave the cuff on, reassure the cat and start again
- Take at least five readings and then take their average
- Check heart rate corresponds with readings from machines
- If contact is not great with Doppler, then use more gel
- Clean area with surgical spirit before using gel and Doppler probe
- Avoid clipping as this can stress the patient.

The ACVIM Consensus Statement: Guidelines for the identification, evaluation and management of systemic hypertension has been updated at the end of 2018 and is recommended reading.

IRIS CKD Substaging based on blood pressure

Systolic blood pressure	IRIS CKD Substage – likelihood of target organ damage
< 140 mmHg	Normotensive – minimal risk of target organ damage
140 mmHg – 159 mmHg	Prehypertensive – low risk of target organ damage
160 mmHg – 179 mmHg	Hypertensive – moderate risk of target organ damage
> 180 mmHg	Severely hypertensive – high risk of target organ damage

If no known target organ damage (e.g. retinal changes) is present then blood pressure measurement is recommended over a period of time (usually one to two weeks) to document a persistent elevation. If there is evidence of target organ damage, treatment should be started without the need to document persistent increase in blood pressure.

After treatment the patient's staging needs updating for sub-staging as the proteinuria and/or hypertension are corrected. For example, a previously hypertensive patient that is now controlled would be classed based on the current actual blood pressure/UPC and marked as such with a "treating" after the sub-staging.

Management of Chronic Kidney Disease

The IRIS board has developed empirical recommendations for the management of CKD according to stage. These represent suggested starting points and **should be adjusted to the individual case**, which often implies frequent monitoring. The likelihood of complications increases with the stage.

All patients with CKD should have potentially **nephrotoxic drugs discontinued** (or at least used with care) and **reduce the risk of dehydration** by always having fresh drinking water available, and in more advanced stages parenteral fluid supplementation.

In a clinical setting, CKD is more commonly diagnosed as part of a sick patient's investigation, rather than after routine blood tests. In this instance, it is common for **patients to present with dehydration, which needs correction prior to IRIS staging**. In addition, some patients might not be in stable CKD and therefore it will be four to eight weeks before staging is possible. Meanwhile staging for AKI is indicated.

The use of **fluid therapy** in animals with CKD includes the **correction of dehydration and supplementation of ongoing losses**, not forgetting to factor in that polyuria/polydipsia increases fluid requirements.

The common approach of "loading the patients with fluids to flush the kidneys" is unnecessary provided the fluid requirements outlined above are met. **Excess of fluid creates haemodilution, which artificially lowers the renal parameters** and may create problems. Additionally, once the excess fluid therapy is withdrawn the renal parameters will increase again.

It is extremely important to **identify the primary cause of the CKD**. This is of special importance in patients with **stage I and early stage II** as the amount of irreversible change is smaller than in advanced stages and treatment of the primary cause may halt disease progression. This could be attempted using tests such as urinalysis and urine culture, imaging +/– renal biopsy where appropriate. Known causes of CKD diagnosed with this approach include acquired disease and some heritable causes.

Although specific therapy directed at eliminating or controlling the primary cause of CKD does not usually reverse the existing renal damage, it is important to minimise further damage. Often, it not possible to identify a cause of CKD therefore it is not possible to institute appropriate specific treatment.

Overall, the main points to consider in patients diagnosed with CKD include:

- Stop nephrotoxic drugs (or use with caution)
- Identify and treat potential inciting causes
- Identify mechanisms of progression and use renoprotective therapies
- Symptomatic therapy

Assessment of progression and renoprotective measures

Some of the mechanisms activated during CKD which contribute to renal damage include:

- Systemic and glomerular hypertension
- Mineral imbalance
- Proteinuria
- Renal fibrosis

Renoprotective measures are those that may slow the progression of kidney disease and are listed in the table below.

Renoprotective measures to consider for CKD
Dietary phosphorus restriction
Anti-hypertensive agents in patients with high blood pressure
Treatment of proteinuria (including diet)
Dietary fish oil supplementation

Dietary Phosphorus restriction

Management of hyperphosphatemia is important in the management of CKD. Studies demonstrate hyperphosphatemia is common in CKD along with **elevated PTH**. It is widely accepted that PTH elevations contribute to the pathogenesis and clinical signs of CKD. **Renal secondary hyperparathyroidism is common** in cats with later stages of CKD (87% of cats with clinical signs of CKD in one study). In the same study cats eating a renal diet had a reduction in PTH and significantly longer survival times (median 633 days vs 264 cats eating a maintenance diet).

Normal commercially available maintenance food contains a high amount of phosphate and therefore the use of phosphate-binders is unlikely to achieve the treatment target.

In recent years, there has been some controversy on the use of renal diets due to concerns over protein malnutrition. However, the IRIS recommendations suggest **starting a renal diet in IRIS stage II cats and recommends its use in IRIS stage III and IV**.

Alongside with lower protein content, **renal diets** have lower phosphorus and sodium content and they also contain increased caloric density, increased Vitamin B, and more soluble fibre than normal diets. Also, they are usually designed to have a neutral effect on acid-base and provide supplementation of omega-3 fatty acids.

Feeding a renal diet, preferably wet to help maintain hydration, can prevent or delay the onset of uraemia and premature death due to complications of CKD. In addition, these diets also help ensure adequate nutrition, which is essential as malnutrition is a major cause of morbidity and mortality. **The goal is a body condition of 4 to 5 out of 9**. In this setting, the use of appetite stimulants, anti-emetics, and feeding tubes might be appropriate to maintain nutrition and hydration. The recently published 2022 ISFM Consensus Guidelines on Management of the Inappetent Hospitalised Cat have extremely useful information for patient management.

Some patients are reluctant to eat a new diet, so **consider a slow transition over a few weeks**, trying more than one brand, and consider **using appetite stimulants may help with the transition**. The introduction of the new diet during hospitalisation or periods of inappetence or vomiting/nausea should be avoided as this can lead to food aversion.

Reduction of dietary phosphate may not cause significant changes in serum phosphate for several weeks. If after one to two months of diet introduction, serum phosphate is still above the therapeutic target, phosphate binders should be used. In animals with late-stage III and IV, dietary management alone is frequently not effective and therefore phosphate binders are often used from the start.

The current IRIS guidelines include assessment of FGF-23 in cats with IRIS stage I and II with serum phosphate levels below 1.45 mmol/l as this can help direct the use of phosphate-restricted diets as outlined in the picture below. (Figure 8).

Intestinal phosphate binders need to be given at mealtimes to bind the dietary phosphate present in the food and must be mixed in every meal. In addition, if calcium-based products are not given with food they act as calcium supplements. Some of the commercially available formulations contain lactose and should be used with caution in diabetic patients.

The most common intestinal phosphate binders are aluminium-based products and calcium-based products.

In recent years, **aluminium-based phosphate binders** such as aluminium hydroxide have been removed from the market in some countries due to toxicity in humans. Although aluminium based products appear to be relatively safe in small animals, there are reports of dogs with advanced CKD that have developed toxicity in cases where high doses were being used; there are no reports in cats.

Calcium-based phosphate binders should be used with caution, especially in patients being administered calcium carbonate, as hypercalcemia is a known side effect.

Lanthanum carbonate is a phosphate binder that has been shown to be effective, well accepted and tolerated by cats. However, at high doses may lead to vomiting assumed due to gastric irritation. Currently, no veterinary licensed product is available.

Phosphate binding agents of different groups can be combined to minimise the risk of overdosage. However, calcium-citrate should not be used in combination with aluminium-based products as it increases absorption of aluminium increasing the risk of toxicity.

Cats with serum phosphate within the IRIS target may be at increased risk of developing hypercalcemia when fed renal diets. If there is an increase of serum calcium above 3.0 mmol/l the IRIS recommendations are to switch to a normal commercial senior diet or mix renal diet with senior diet on a 50:50 by volume.

Dietary fish oil supplementation

There is some evidence to support the use of omega 3-polyunsaturated fatty acids in CKD and most commercial diets have supplementation.

Treatment of proteinuria

Proteinuria is predictive of survival and an independent risk factor i.e. independent of other significant factors such as creatinine level.

Hypertension also has a relationship with proteinuria. Hypertensive patients are more likely to be

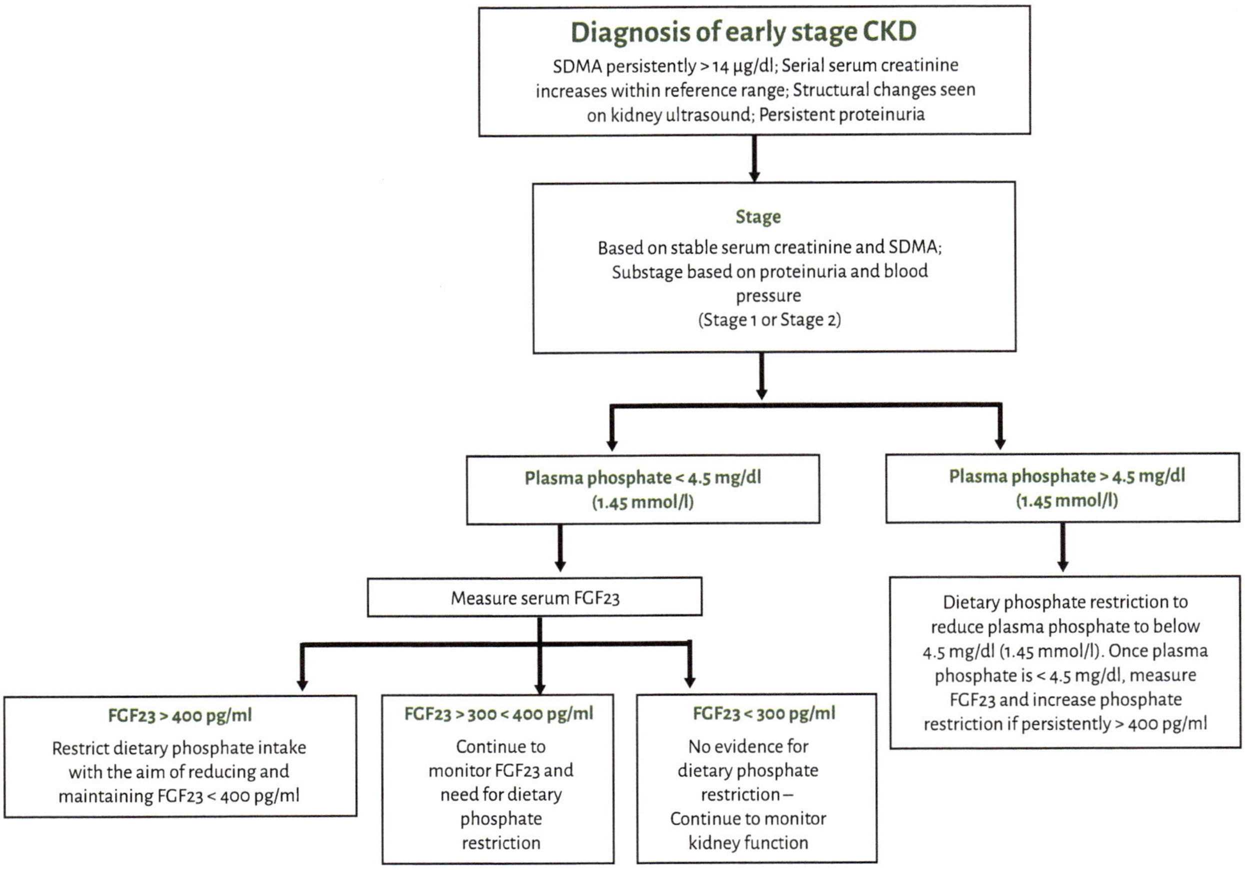

Figure 8. Flowchart indicating the utility of serum FGF23 in guiding treatment of early-stage CKD cats. From IRIS kidney (www.iris-kidney.com).

proteinuric than normotensive ones, probably due to glomerular hypertension. The **control of hypertension may help to reduce proteinuria** and slow the progression of the disease.

Angiotensin-converting enzyme inhibitors (**ACEi**) may reduce proteinuria by decreasing efferent arteriolar resistance leading to reduction of intra-glomerular pressure and therefore reducing proteinuria. Other possible mechanisms of action include decreasing the size of glomerular endothelial pores.

Typically enalapril or benazepril (0.5 mg/kg PO SID) are used. The dose may need to be escalated or increased to twice-daily dosing if there is no improvement in proteinuria after two to four weeks.

More recently, **angiotensin receptor blockers** (**ARBs**) such as telmisartan (Semintra®) are licensed for the treatment of proteinuria and hypertension in cats. ARBs ameliorate the negative effects of the RAAS in a different way to ACE inhibitors. They work by directly targeting the AT1 receptor and by blocking the binding of angiotensin II to this receptor. However, ARBs do not bind to the AT2 receptor. The latter modulates Angiotensin II action, which are renoprotective such as vasodilation, natriuresis, inhibition of renin secretion, anti-inflammatory, anti-ischaemic and antifibrotic. This overall means that **the harmful effects of the RAAS are blocked but the protective effects are preserved.** Additionally, since ARBs mediate their effect at the receptor level there is no potential for ACE escape, which may occur with ACE inhibitors.

ACEi or ARBs should not be started in dehydrated or hypovolemic patients as this can lead to a dramatic decrease in GFR with devastating consequences.

In humans, aldosterone receptor antagonists (e.g. spironolactone) reduce proteinuria and stabilise kidney function acting in an additive manner with ACE inhibitors and ARB's; there are no published studies for this use in cats.

IRIS recommends patients with persistent proteinuria (UPC > 0.4) be investigated for an underlying cause and antiproteinuric medication started in a stepwise approach:

- ACEi or ARB alongside renal diet
- Monitor response to treatment and disease progression:
  - Stable creatinine and decreasing UPC – good response
  - Progressive increase in creatinine and/or increase in UPC – disease progression.

Although evidence is lacking, it is likely that, similarly to dogs, proteinuric cats may have an increased tendency for thromboembolic disease. As such, IRIS suggests the use of clopidogrel (10–18.75 mg/day) with aspirin (1 mg/kg every 72 h) as an alternative.

According to some studies, even borderline proteinuria (UPCs of 0.2–0.4) had a significant effect on survival compared to UPCs of < 0.2. However, there is insufficient evidence that anti-proteinuric drugs slow the progression of disease in this subset of patients. As such, currently, the **IRIS guidelines state anti-proteinuric treatment could be offered in patients with borderline proteinuria despite the lack of evidence**.

Treatment of hypertension

The goal of treatment with anti-hypertensives is to **maintain the systolic blood pressure below 160 mmHg** to minimise the risk of end-organ damage.

If systolic blood pressure is persistently > 160 mmHg the treatment should be started.

If there is evidence of target organ damage treatment is indicated without the need to prove persistent hypertension.

Patients without target organ damage should be reassessed to confirm persistent blood pressure > 160 mmHg:

- Hypertensive patients (moderate risk of end organ damage) – document persistency (160–179 mmHg) in a 1–2 week period
- Patients with marked hypertension (high risk of end-organ damage) – document persistency (> 180 mmHg) in a 1–2 week period

The aim is to **reduce the blood pressure gradually** without sudden drops. The treatment of hypertension should be done in a step-by-step manner and is different in dogs and cats.

In cats, IRIS recommends:

1. Gradual reduction of dietary salt (despite lack of evidence that it reduces blood pressure) **in combination with medication**
2. CCB (amlodipine 0.125–0.25 mg/kg SID) or ARB (telmisartan 2 mg/kg SID)
3. Double the dose of amlodipine (0.25–0.5 mg/kg SID) if this is being used. Please note that the datasheet does not recommend increasing the dose of telmisartan above 2 mg/kg SID
4. Combine amlodipine with telmisartan if none of them individually controls hypertension.

Hypotension (systolic blood pressure <120 mmHg) or clinical signs suggestive of it (e.g. weakness and tachycardia) should be avoided as it can have detrimental effects in renal perfusion and function.

It is also important to remember that there are currently no studies on the use of telmisartan in cases with severe hypertension > 200 mmHg and therefore in such cases it may be preferable to start using amlodipine.

Treatment of hypertension can lead to a small persistent increase in creatinine (< 45 µmol/l) and SDMA (< 2.0 µg/dl) but a marked increase can suggest a drug adverse effect or disease progression.

Common complications and co-existing conditions

As kidney disease progresses so the prevalence of complications increases, for example metabolic acidosis, bacterial urinary tract infection, anaemia and potassium imbalances.

Dehydration

CKD patients frequently have difficulty in maintaining hydration especially as, if there is reduced water intake, they are unable to concentrate their urine accordingly. This can lead to a pre-renal component of the azotaemia and may cause further reduction in food and water intake, which can then spiral out of control with worsening of the CKD.

Clean water that is regularly replaced should always be available, preferably in wide enough containers to avoid the whiskers touching the sides when drinking as some cats dislike that. The use of cat fountains and flavoured water can help encourage drinking and feeding canned food rather than dry can also contribute favourably to hydration.

Recently, a liver flavoured, nutrient enriched fluid with higher viscosity than water, has become available commercially to be used in a separate bowl (alongside regular water and food) with current reports documenting an increase in fluid intake with associated decrease in urine specific gravity and urine osmolality in the population tested. Further studies are needed to study its effect in cats with CKD and other diseases that might benefit from increased water intake.

Dehydration will worsen renal blood flow and contribute to the clinical signs of CKD.

If there is dehydration, regardless of the cause, it should be addressed promptly with replacement fluids intravenously as needed in order to avoid clinical deterioration and potentially worsening of the CKD or an acute-on-chronic episode.

In some cases, particularly in later stages of CKD, administration of subcutaneous fluids can be helpful in preventing dehydration and improve the patient's quality of life and is often well tolerated by owners and patients alike. The frequency and volume administered is dependent on multiple factors, but twice weekly administration of 100–150 ml warmed to body temperature is common. More information including guidelines for owners can be found in the iCatcare.org website.

Most frequently clinicians use Hartman's solution, albeit the IRIS treatment recommendations suggest using maintenance fluids for this purpose, which have low sodium (30–40 mmol/l) and that ideally have supplemented potassium (around 13 mmol/l).

In more advanced cases of CKD (later stage III and stage IV), placement of a feeding tube may be indicated in some cats to help provide meet nutritional demands, provide extra fluid orally and they can also be used to administer medication.

Clinically significant anaemia

Anaemia is a common abnormality affecting 32–65% of cats with CKD.

The main cause for anaemia in chronic kidney disease is **reduced erythropoietin (EPO) production**, however other factors such as blood loss, iron deficiency, poor nutrition and renal secondary hyperparathyroidism also play a role.

Cats can adapt to slow developing anaemia and may exhibit minimal clinical signs. Additionally, some of the clinical signs of anaemia such as lethargy, anorexia and weakness are also seen because of the CKD itself. In cases with severe anaemia, the decreased oxygen tissue delivery can affect the kidneys (and all other organs) with further progression of the renal disease.

If the anaemia is affecting the patient' quality of life (usually when the haematocrit is below 20%) treatment should be considered and the risks associated with the available options must be weighed against the benefit of improving the anaemia.

The most immediate way to treat anaemia is with the administration of an appropriately typed blood transfusion or, if available, packed red blood cells. However, its effect is short lived and even more so in patients with renal disease given the effect of uremic toxins in the red blood cell lifespan. Other factors that need to be considered include the possible development of immune reactions, donor-recipient incompatibility, and the limited availability of blood products.

In the past, anabolic steroids such as oxymetholone or nandrolone have been administered to stimulate RBC's production in animals that are anaemic, but their use cannot be recommended due to the lack of efficacy and the potential for hepatotoxicity.

Recombinant human erythropoietin (rHuEPO) and darbepoetin (DPO) have been used successfully for treatment of anaemia of CKD in humans, cats, and dogs. Darbepoetin is a modified form of EPO with longer duration of activity (allowing less frequent administration) and with a reduced risk of pure red cell aplasia (PRCA) when compared to rHuEPO (10% vs 25–30%). Darbepoietin is therefore most commonly used drug for treatment of anaemia secondary to CKD.

In addition to resolving the anaemia most patients treated with EPO-like drugs have improved appetite, weight gain, increased energy, etc. Adverse effects of the use of these drugs include PRCA, refractory anaemia, systemic hypertension, polycythaemia, seizures, vomiting, iron deficiency, injection discomfort, skins reactions, cellulitis, cutaneous or mucocutaneous reactions, fever, and arthralgia.

With the use of EPO-like drugs it takes 2–3 weeks to start seeing a positive response in the haematocrit and, in the interim, a blood transfusion may be needed for cases with severe anaemia. This would also allow assessment whether the anaemia is the main cause of the clinical signs as the patient would then expect to improve markedly after the transfusion. Additionally, a blood transfusion will also supplement iron to the patient.

Lack of available iron for erythropoiesis is a leading cause of treatment failure in humans receiving EPO. All patients treated with EPO should receive iron supplementation given the patients' higher demand with increased erythropoiesis. In addition, some authors recommend the evaluation of the iron profile (serum iron, transferrin saturation and serum ferritin) before and during treatment.

Refractory anaemia in patients on EPO therapy has many potential causes such as iron deficiency, ongoing blood loss, anaemia of chronic inflammatory disease or formation of anti-EPO antibodies, which causes PRCA. Pure red cell aplasia is characterized by severe non-regenerative anaemia with very marked decreased of red blood cells precursors in the bone marrow.

Currently there is no commercially available test for the presence of antibodies and diagnosis based on clinical suspicion +/− bone marrow examination.

Treatment should be stopped if development of anti-EPO antibodies is thought to have developed. The duration of antibody persistence is thought to be variable, and the patients become dependent on blood transfusions for management of the anaemia. This brings on concerns (ethical amongst others) regarding the use of multiple blood transfusions and can potentially culminate in euthanasia.

Metabolic acidosis

Intervention to correct metabolic acidosis is indicated in CKD when **serum bicarbonate falls below 16 mEq/l despite feeding a renal diet**. Clinical effects of metabolic acidosis include progressive renal injury and increased protein catabolism.

Treatment of metabolic acidosis involves the administration of sodium bicarbonate or potassium citrate (if concurrently hypokalemic).

Bacterial urinary tract infections

Urinary tract infections are common in CKD. For urine culture ideally the sample should be obtained by cystocentesis. The results of culture and sensitivity are crucial to guide antibiotic therapy.

Potassium imbalances

The therapeutic goal is to **maintain serum potassium between 3.5 to 5.5 mmol/l.**

The **clinical effects of hypokalemia are more common in cats** (especially Stage IV) than dogs and include **muscle weakness** and impairment of renal function.

Treatment of hypokalemia involves administration of potassium chloride parenterally and potassium gluconate or potassium citrate as oral supplementation.

Hyperkalaemia is of concern especially in dogs (rare in cats) with stage IV kidney disease as the excretory capacity of the kidney is insufficient to excrete the daily potassium load. In these cases, **home-cooked diets** may be of benefit as most commercial diets have supplemental potassium.

Hyperkalaemia higher than 5.5 mEq/l should be carefully monitored and if it reaches 6 to 6.5 mEq/l therapy should be adjusted, which may consist of reducing the dose of ACEi or ARB, stopping spironolactone, or feeding diets with low K content.

Cats with hyperaldosteronism (Conn's syndrome) often present with CKD and marked hypokalaemia which, in some cases, appears to be resistant to appropriate supplementation. Measurement of serum aldosterone should be considered in these circumstances.

Gastrointestinal signs

Patients with Stage III and IV of CKD often have complications such as reduced food intake, nausea, vomiting, uremic stomatitis, diarrhoea, colitis.

The use of anti-emetics and anti-nausea medication, such as maropitant, may help in these cases. **There is evidence that mirtazapine (1.88 mg/cat every 48 h for 3 weeks)** reduces vomiting, improves appetite and leads to weight gain in cats showing signs of inappetence and vomiting in IRIS stage III and IV patients.

The use of H2-blockers or preferably **proton-pump inhibitors** may be beneficial in some selected cases.

Overall, the IRIS staging system helps establish a treatment plan, according to the stage of CKD, with the main goal being slowing the progression of CKD, prevention of anticipated complications, and improve the quality of life of the patient.

CKD and hyperthyroidism

The existence of both diseases together is common, and practitioners are often unsure of how to manage the combination of conditions.

Usually, the diagnosis of hyperthyroidism can be made with a single measurement of serum T4. However, in early cases of hyperthyroidism and/or patients with concurrent non-thyroidal disease, serum T4 can be within normal limits. Measurement of free T4 can be helpful in cats with clinical signs with hyperthyroidism and total T4 within the top half of the reference range; in one study free T4 by equilibrium dialysis had a sensitivity of 98.5% in detecting hyperthyroidism. However, the specificity was low therefore free T4 should always be assessed in conjunction with assessment of total T4 and appropriate clinical signs.

Hyperthyroidism increases cardiac output, decreases peripheral vascular resistance, and therefore improves renal blood flow and glomerular filtration rate (GFR). This can lower the renal parameters and mean CKD is 'masked' by the hyperthyroidism.

After treatment, when the patient becomes euthyroid the true state of the renal function becomes visible. Unfortunately, it is very difficult to predict the development of azotaemia beforehand. However, the use of SDMA may help as previously discussed.

In cats, several studies have documented a deterioration in renal function after treatment of hyperthyroidism, regardless of whether the treatment is medical, surgical or with radioactive iodine.

The percentage of cats that develop azotaemia once euthyroid depends on many factors, but it is generally considered that between 15–49% of patients will do so. Unfortunately, it is very difficult to predict the development of azotaemia beforehand.

When treatment for hyperthyroidism is started, we anticipate a further decline in glomerular filtration rate (GFR) therefore it is generally recommended to start these patients on reversible medical therapy and assessing the true renal status once euthyroid and its impact on quality of life.

It is recommended, whenever possible, that hyperthyroidism is controlled. If hyperthyroidism is undertreated it may promote progression of renal disease via glomerular hypertension, hyperphosphatemia, and proteinuria amongst other mechanisms. Hyperthyroidism is also a catabolic process and can lead to heart disease with associated volume overload.

Patients with IRIS CKD stage 1 and 2 are usually started on routine doses of reversible medical treatment (e.g. methimazole) and the renal function is monitored while euthyroidism is achieved. In these patients an irreversible treatment approach could be considered if the patient has improved clinically with medical treatment.

For later stages of IRIS CKD, a more careful approach, with lower starting doses of medication, is often suggested. If there is a marked deterioration in renal parameters and worsening of clinical signs, some selected patients may benefit from a trade-off balance between level of azotaemia and control of hyperthyroidism.

Iatrogenic hypothyroidism is a well-recognised complication of hyperthyroidism treatment regardless of the type of treatment chosen.

Hypothyroidism has been detected in up to two thirds of cats with unmasked CKD after hyperthyroidism treatment. Hypothyroidism can lead to reduced GFR, and it has been associated with a worse prognosis. Unfortunately, in these patients there are frequently no clinical signs suggestive of its presence.

The diagnosis of hypothyroidism is unfortunately not as easy as documenting a low serum T4 as non-thyroidal disease can also cause serum T4 lower than the reference range. Additionally, up to 17% of cats with non-thyroidal illness can have flow free T4 by equilibrium dialysis. The combination of elevated TSH (using the canine assay) and low serum T4 may be useful in the diagnosis of iatrogenic hypothyroidism.

In cases with hypothyroidism, thyroxine supplementation can lead to an around 20% decrease in creatinine and about half of the patients will have the azotaemia disappear. Thyroxine supplementation has also been shown to improve survival time in cats with hypothyroidism and concurrent azotaemia.

CKD and Osteoarthritis

It is estimated that **osteoarthritis coexists in almost 70% of cats with CKD**.

NSAID's inhibit the expression of cyclooxygenase (COX) enzymes, the latter being essential to various biological functions and overall homeostasis. Both COX isoforms are expressed in the kidneys and have an important role in the maintenance of renal perfusion and auto-regulation. As such, there are concerns that inhibition of COX can lead to significant deleterious effects in patients with CKD. However, over the last decade a few studies, (two using meloxicam and one using robenacoxib) have **failed to demonstrate NSAID-associated renal side effects** and, in some studies there were no deleterious effects on survival times.

The World Small Animal Veterinary Association – Global Pain Council (WSAVA-GPC) recommends the administration of NSAIDs in cats with stable CKD as long as specific conditions are considered and discussed with the owners.

The recently licensed anti-nerve growth factor frunevetmab effectively decreases osteoarthritis pain in cats. Currently there are no studies regarding the safety and efficacy in IRIS CKD stage 3 or 4. However, the available data on earlier stages of CKD seem promising.

Prognosis of CKD

Recent studies have shown that the IRIS staging can help predict survival as multiple studies indicate that IRIS stage of kidney disease in cats is linked with survival time.

Overall the **mean age of diagnosis of CKD in all cats is 12 years** and the mean survival time from that point onwards is 2.3 years.

Studies report the mean survival time for cats with CKD to vary according to the IRIS staging as described below:

- Stage II – 490 to 1151 days
- Stage III – 154 to 778 days
- Stage IV – 20 to 103 days

Cats discharged with IRIS stage II CKD have only a 42% chance of dying of renal disease, compared to 68% for cats in stage III and 86% for cats in stage IV.

Nephrolithiasis and ureterolithiasis are found commonly in cats with CKD (up to 47%), and the incidence appears to have increased over the last two decades.

According to an older study, the presence of nephroliths in cats with IRIS Stage II and III CKD was not associated with an increase in mortality rate, change in rate of disease progression, the incidence of uremic crisis or death. However, a more recent study refutes this.

Renal transplant

Renal transplant is a method of treating end-stage CKD in cats. Peri-operative (one month) mortality is approximately 25%. The six-month survival rate is 60–70% and the three-year survival is around 40–50%.

Renal transplantation is not currently available in Europe.

Congenital and inherited renal disease

Congenital renal disease is present from birth regardless of the presence or not of clinical signs. Frequently patients present with clinical signs of chronic renal disease at an early age.

Animals with inherited renal disease usually have normal appearing and functioning kidneys at birth but progressive deterioration occurs early in life.

Congenital disease of the kidneys may manifest itself by lack of a kidney (aplasia) which is often found incidentally. However, it is possible to the kidneys to be abnormal in function (+/− macroscopic appearance) which would include hypoplastic and/or dysplastic kidneys.

The term renal dysplasia is a disorganization of the renal parenchyma which suggests abnormal differentiation. Renal dysplasia is very rare in the cat when compared to dogs.

If the kidneys are dysplastic their function is altered and often they have an abnormal appearance macroscopically and ultrasonographically. Nonetheless, renal dysplasia cannot be ruled out if the kidney appears to be normal as we cannot assess the microstructure.

Most animals with renal dysplasia will develop chronic renal disease very early in life.

Amyloidosis

Amyloidosis is characterised by the extracellular deposition of amyloid with the primary protein deposited in cats being amyloid-A which is formed by the polymerization of serum amyloid A protein (SAA) which is an acute-phase protein. Due to the association of amyloid-A with inflammation this type of amyloidosis is often called reactive or secondary.

It is relatively uncommon in cats with the exception of Abyssinian, Siamese and Oriental Shorthair cats with an inherited dominant pattern having been suggested in these breeds. There is evidence that the protein structure of the amyloid is different in the Abyssinians when compared to the Siamese. Currently, there is no test to predict the development of the disease.

In Abyssinians amyloid is deposited in several organs with the kidneys, especially the medulla, being the main target organ and these cats develop chronic renal disease very early in life. The mean age of affected cats is 7 years of age but many Abyssinians are diagnosed between 1 and 5 years of age.

Diagnosis of renal amyloidosis is based on a high-index of suspicion and exclusion of other causes of renal disease or at the endpoint on post-mortem examination. Pre-mortem renal biopsies containing renal medulla are associated with a high risk of complications and therefore generally not recommended.

In Siamese and Oriental shorthair cats amyloid deposition occurs most prominently in the liver with the subsequent development of severe hepatomegaly, hepatic rupture and haemoabdomen.

Amyloidosis is readily diagnosed with routine histopathological examination especially when the stain Congo red is used. Amyloid deposits stained with Congo red are seen as apple green in colour when examined under polarized light microscopy. There are some reports of cytological examination identifying material consistent with amyloid therefore increasing the degree of suspicion of amyloidosis.

There is no effective specific therapy for renal amyloidosis. The use of dimethyl sulfoxide (DMSO) and colchicine in cats with amyloidosis has not been studied.

The same treatment measures as for chronic renal disease should be implemented.

Polycystic kidney disease

Polycystic kidney disease (PKD) is the most common inherited disorder in cats, and it has been described most frequently in Persian cats with very varied prevalence across the globe. Nonetheless, it has been described in numerous other breeds.

A mutation in the PKD1 gene has been identified as the cause of PKD. However, occasionally cats without this mutation have been identified with PKD, leading to the suspicion that other mutations may exit in these cats. PKD is inherited as an autosomal dominant trait and therefore an affected cat has a 50% chance of passing it onto the offspring. Homozygous cats are thought to be rare with the possibility of the anomaly being lethal *in uterus* or leading to death at a very young age.

The number and size of the cysts is very variable amongst cats with cysts often being present in both the cortex and medulla. Cysts can often be seen in other organs such as the liver. Affected cats frequently don't have any clinical signs but will with time develop chronic renal disease.

Ultrasound is generally considered a sensitive and specific diagnostic tool when compared to genetic tests with figures of 96% and 91% respectively when performed at 10–14 weeks of age. Cysts are possible to be detected from 7 weeks of age but the number and size of the cysts increases with age with variable speed amongst cats.

PCR can be used to identify the genetic mutation causing PKD and the test is widely available through commercial laboratories.

There is no specific treatment for PKD with the same measures as for chronic renal disease being recommended.

Feline Glomerular disease and nephrotic syndrome

Clinical signs and physical examination findings in cats with glomerular disease are linked to the severity of proteinuria, stage of kidney disease, and histologic subtype of glomerular disease.

In a subset of patients with glomerular disease, hypoalbuminemia, and proteinuria are accompanied by hypercholesterolemia and extravascular fluid accumulation referred to as **nephrotic syndrome**, which is rare in cats.

Renal biopsy is required to determine the specific histological subtype of glomerular disease. However, this is **not indicated in every patient** and the risk/benefit balance carefully considered. Although more studies are needed to establish which patients would benefit from renal biopsies, it is thought patients with IRIS stage I and II (and possibly III) with severe proteinuria might benefit the most.

Renal biopsies should be examined with **light microscopy, electron microscopy and also immunofluorescent microscopy**. Although findings of light microscopy may be highly suggestive of a particular glomerular disease, electron microscopy is often required for definitive characterization of the histological subtype, and immunofluorescent microscopy to determine the specific nature of the immune deposits. Currently, there are two only laboratories worldwide that are recommended by the IRIS board for the assessment of renal biopsies.

Certain therapies are indicated in all patients with glomerular disease, regardless of the histologic diagnosis. These non-specific management recommendations can be divided into three categories:

1. Monitoring and treatment of non-infectious inflammatory disorders
2. Reduction of proteinuria
3. Management of uraemia and other complications of renal disease.

Proteinuria is common with renal disease and the magnitude of it depends to some extent whether the disorder is primary glomerular in origin or whether it is tubulointerstitial.

Glomerular disease is the consequence of abnormalities in the glomerulus or damage to the glomerular filtration barrier. While glomerular disease is common in the dog it is considered relatively uncommon in the cat. Conversely, in feline chronic renal disease, proteinuria (usually mild to moderate) is common and in this setting, it is secondary to tubular disease and glomerulosclerosis, whose severity tends to increase as the disease progresses.

A recent study suggests that, similarly to dogs, around 50% of the cats with proteinuria had immune-complex glomerulonephritis with membranous glomerulonephritis (MG) being the most common cause. MG which is a complement-driven disorder where the immune complexes are deposited in the basal membrane was the most common PLN.

The same study also describes the median-age as much lower than for cats with chronic renal disease (median 4.6 years versus 11–15 years). The magnitude of proteinuria due to glomerular disease is generally thought to be significantly higher than that due to tubulointerstitial disease and this was also seen in this study despite some overlap (median UPC 7.9 versus 1.1).

Although, in this study the cats with ICGN that received immunosupressive medication (varied drugs) had a higher median survival time that those that did not (244 days versus 17 days), currently there are no specific protocols.

The prognosis for cats with PLN is reported by the same study as guarded given that the medium survival time was below 14 months from the time of diagnosis.

Renal biopsies – indications, contra-indications, and possible complications

Renal biopsies are indicated when histological examination is likely to change patient management. As such, the most common indications are protein losing nephropathy (PLN) and potentially acute renal injury.

The results of histology are unlikely to alter the treatment and outcome of patients with IRIS CKD stage 4 and late stage 3.

Renal biopsies are performed either percutaneously or surgically with a wedge biopsy. Although ultrasound guided biopsies are the most common percutaneous technique for cats and dogs it is also possible to obtain renal biopsies via laparoscopy. Surgical wedge biopsies are usually collected when the patient is undergoing an exploratory laparotomy for another reason.

The patients should be anaesthetized for renal biopsies as immobilization is critical and, in most cases, at least 2 cortical samples should be obtained; the medulla should be avoided to reduce the risk of complications, and this should be considered when considering the type of needle to use. Frequently 16–18 G needles are used depending on the size of the patient.

Complications of renal biopsies are reported in up to 18% of cases. The most common is severe haemorrhage which is reported in up to 16% of cats in one study. Death is a very rare complication is less than 3% of patients.

Contra-indications for renal biopsy

- Metabolic acidosis
- CKD IRIS Stage 4 (and possibly late Stage 3)
- Severe azotaemia
- Severe anaemia
- Uncorrected coagulopathy
- Uncontrolled hypertension
- Hydronephrosis
- Renal cysts particularly if multiple or large
- Abscessation
- Pyelonephritis/ Pyonephrosis
- Inexperience operator

Renal cytology is it worth it?

The risk of significant bleeding with cytology is in general considered much smaller than with biopsy but this should still be kept in mind, as if it occurs there is the possibility that blood clots might obstruct the renal pelvis and/or ureter with its associated implications.

The patient should be under general anaesthesia for the procedure and the risk of an anaesthesia should be considered on a case-by-case approach.

The contra-indications for renal cytology are reasonably similar to the ones for renal tissue biopsy, such as uncontrolled hypertension and coagulopathy, pyonephrosis, renal abscess, and hydronephrosis.

Although when performing cytology, we lose the ability to evaluate organ structure, cytology can still be of help in cases where the main suspicion is renal lymphoma, and it can also help gather more supporting information in cases of possible feline infectious peritonitis.

Nephrolithiasis and Ureterolithiasis

Upper urinary tract uroliths are more frequent in cats than in dogs.

- **Nephroliths** are uroliths located in the renal pelvis and/or collecting diverticula of the kidneys.
- **Ureteroliths** usually stem from nephroliths that migrate onto the ureter and may then lead to ureteric obstruction.

This topic will be discussed in the section on lower urinary tract urolithiasis.

Renal neoplasia

Renal tumours are rare in cats. The most common tumours are lymphoma (most frequent), adenoma, adenocarcinoma, nephroblastoma, and haemangiosarcoma.

Treatment of neoplasia (other than lymphoma) is less rewarding and may involve nephrectomy (+/− chemotherapy) if unilateral disease is present.

Renal lymphoma is a high-grade disease and cats usually present clinically unwell. Bilateral renomegaly is a common finding, and an association with nasal and central nervous system lymphoma is discussed in the literature.

Clinical signs

Clinical signs usually are non-specific with lethargy, vomiting, weight loss and anorexia. PU/PD may be reported. The condition can occur in cats of any age, but usually middle-aged.

Diagnosis

Biochemistry may indicate azotaemia and AKI/CKD. Variable proteinuria may be documented; in some cases of renal lymphoma the cats are not azotemic.

Diagnosis of renal LSA may be made with imaging and fine-needle aspiration. Biopsy is not usually required as the tumour exfoliates easily. Often other organs are involved so assessment of the GI tract, etc is recommended.

Treatment

Treatment of renal LSA usually involves a **COP protocol**. Doxorubicin can be nephrotoxic so may not be advisable if the cat is azotaemic. If CNS involvement is present lomustine or cytosine arabinoside may be used in the protocol.

Cats with renal LSA may not have a long remission period with a median survival of 91 days in one study. As with all feline LSA the survival range is wide so treatment may be more successful in some cases with 20% of the cases being alive at 500 days in the same study.

Lower urinary tract disease

The term feline lower urinary tract disease includes a large group of **conditions which cause lower urinary tract signs**. Although **a common diagnosis** the condition known as **idiopathic cystitis or feline idiopathic cystitis** (**FIC**) is just one of these possible causes and is considered a diagnosed of exclusion after other causes of lower urinary tract disease have been eliminated, e.g. urolithiasis, bacterial UTI, anatomical abnormalities, and neoplasia.

The most common causes of lower urinary tract signs

Cats less than 10 years of age
Idiopathic cystitis is the most common diagnosis (60–70%)
Urolithiasis (10–20%) mainly secondary to struvite and calcium oxalate
Structural abnormalities (around 10%) such as urethral strictures
Behavioural abnormalities (around 10%)
Urinary tract infection (< 2%)
Bladder or urethral neoplasia (< 1%)
Other causes extremely uncommon

Cats over 10 years
Around 5% are idiopathic
Over 50% have a UTI, either alone or in combination with urolithiasis.

Physical examination may reveal a small painful bladder with some conditions and, if there is urinary obstruction, it is possible for severe signs of systemic disease to be present and the bladder to be overdistended or even ruptured.

Urinary tract obstruction

Urethral obstruction is a **common emergency** seen in small animals and much more **common in male cats** than females due to their narrower, longer, and more tortuous urethra.

Approach to the blocked cat

Urethral obstruction is a common emergency seen in small animals and is much more frequent in male cats than females due to the narrower, longer, and more tortuous urethra.

In cats, the most common cause of urethral obstruction is a mucous or mucocrystalline plug associated with feline idiopathic cystitis (FIC); urolithiasis is the second most common cause. Other less common causes of urethral obstruction are neoplasia, urethral stricture. In some patients, a physical obstruction may not be identified as the underlying cause is urethral spasm preventing normal urine outflow.

Urethral obstruction causes accumulation of urine in the bladder and increased intravesical pressure which, when severe, can lead to bladder damage and necrosis.

The intravesical pressure is transmitted upstream to the ureters and kidneys and will eventually exceed the glomerular filtration pressure, leading to decreased renal blood flow and a decline in glomerular filtration rate. In around 24–48 hours after complete urethral obstruction, uraemia will ensue which initially is post-renal but, with time, acute kidney injury occurs.

On top of the urethral obstruction *per se* and the difficulties of its resolution, patients with urethral obstruction may have severe acid-base and electrolyte abnormalities with the most important being hyperkalaemia and severe metabolic acidosis. A significant proportion of the patients will be reasonably stable, but many can present as real emergencies.

Hyperkalaemia

Hyperkalaemia results from a combination of decreased urinary excretion of potassium as well of shifting of potassium to the extracellular space secondary to the metabolic acidosis.

Muscular cells, including the myocardium are amongst the most sensitive to hyperkalaemia, which leads to a change in resting potential of the membrane with a consequent prolongation of the action potential and diminished ability of the myocardial cells to repolarize, ultimately leading to arrhythmia and even death. The common ECG findings associated with hyperkalaemia are in the table below.

Electrocardiographic (ECG) changes usually seen with hyperkalaemia

- Tall positive or large negative T-waves
- Diminished or absent P waves
- Prolonged P-R intervals
- Widened QRS complexes
- Ventricular tachycardia (rare)

The severity of arrhythmia is not predictable by serum potassium alone therefore monitoring and treatment should be based on ECG assessment as this represents the impact of the hyperkalaemia on the heart.

Very marked hyperkalaemia and/or severe metabolic acidosis are frequently the immediate cause of death in cats with urethral obstruction.

Initial **physical examination** should include assessment of mucous membrane colour, CRT, pulse quality and rate, temperature, and cardiac auscultation. Detection of an inappropriately low heart rate should alert the clinician for the possibility of severe hyperkalaemia and an ECG should be performed. It should be kept in mind that severe hyperkalaemia can be present in patients with a normal to rapid heart rate.

Fluid therapy plays an important role in correcting fluid deficits, re-establishing diuresis and favouring excretion of potassium. Traditionally, a potassium-free crystalloid like NaCl 0.9% was considered the ideal fluid therapy in cases with marked hyperkalaemia. However, any balanced isotonic solution, such as Hartmann's solution, can be utilised and it does not significantly contribute to the hyperkalaemia given the small amount of potassium present. Furthermore, the administration of NaCl 0.9% can contribute to the metabolic acidosis already present in cases of urinary obstruction.

During the initial stabilisation, an abdominal focus assessment with sonography for trauma (**AFAST**) can help determine the presence of free abdominal fluid which may impact the approach to the case. Imaging with standard ultrasound techniques and radiography are also invaluable to detect uroliths and other abnormalities; it should be performed as soon as possible but never in detriment of patient safety.

Treatment of hyperkalaemia involves a combined approach of decreasing the cardiac sensitivity to the hyperkalaemia and reducing serum potassium by resolving the underlying cause and shifting potassium into the intracellular space.

- Reducing cardiac sensitivity to hyperkalaemia
  - **Calcium gluconate** decreases the membrane threshold potential (antagonises the membrane effects of hyperkalaemia) and therefore is considered to have a cardioprotective effect, with the ECG changes improving almost immediately. Calcium gluconate (50–100 mg/kg) should be administered intravenously over 5–10 minutes while carefully monitoring the ECG as it can also lead to development of arrhythmias. Its administration "buys" time (around 20 to 30 minutes) for resolution of the underlying cause (e.g. urethral catheterization) and addition of measures to lower serum potassium.
- Reduction of serum potassium
  - Reduction of serum potassium can be achieved by a handful of methods such as administration of IV glucose, use of IV insulin and glucose or the use of sodium bicarbonate.
  - Regular insulin and glucose
    - The use of regular/neutral insulin (0.1–0.25 IU/kg) as a slow IV bolus promotes the intracellular movement of potassium. To avoid hypoglycaemia a slow bolus of 1 to 2 g of 25% glucose/unit of insulin should be given concurrently diluted in saline. This usually starts lowering the potassium within several minutes to 1 hour. It is advisable that glucose is regularly measured to monitor for potential hypoglycaemia. Supplementation of fluids with 2.5 to 5% glucose (adding 50% glucose to the crystalloids) can be considered if necessary.
    - In less severe cases, it is also possible to rely on the endogenous production of insulin after administration of 1–2 ml/kg of a 50% dextrose solution (diluted due to high osmolality). Please note that this approach does not work for diabetic patients.
  - Salbutamol
    - Salbutamol is a beta-2 agonist which can be administered via inhalation and can be used for emergency treatment of hyperkalaemia, **usually in combination with other measured described above**. It activates the Na^+/K^+ membrane ATPase pumps leading to lower serum potassium and has an onset of action of 15 to 30 minutes and the effects last 2–3 hours.
  - Sodium bicarbonate
    - Severe metabolic acidosis can predispose the heart to fatal arrhythmias, decrease the cardiac contractility, decrease the inotropic response to catecholamines and cause peripheral vasodilation, which contributes to hypoperfusion.
    - Sodium bicarbonate can help address the metabolic acidosis and lower serum potassium. Its effect begins within 30–60 minutes and may persist for a few hours.
    - Administration of sodium bicarbonate should be considered carefully as it can lead to significant complication such as paradoxical CSF acidosis and decreased ionised calcium. For more information on doses and administration protocols please consult a critical care textbook.
    - Sodium bicarbonate should be used judiciously and considered carefully as it can result in severe and difficult to reverse acid base abnormalities. The assessment (and frequent monitoring) of acid base balance and electrolytes is mandatory in these cases.

Severe hypocalcaemia (ionised) can occur in very ill patients, and it exacerbates the effects of hyperkalaemia on membrane excitability. Calcium gluconate can be used as described above to correct this problem.

Placement of a urinary catheter

In comatose patients, sedation might not be required for placement of a urinary catheter. However, most of the cats will require sedation or anaesthesia for the procedure.

Some of the drugs used in sedating patients with urethral obstruction are ketamine and diazepam or ketamine and midazolam. Ketamine should be avoided in patients with suspected cardiac problems. Analgesia should also be added trying to avoid drugs that cause hypotension or respiratory depression.

When sedation is insufficient, drugs such as IV propofol can be used in conjunction with the drugs above to achieve general anaesthesia and make catheterization easier due to appropriate urethral relaxation. Propofol as a single agent (in combination with analgesia) can be used for the procedure and a study comparing cats with urethral anaesthetised with either propofol or ketamine/diazepam documented that the cats receiving propofol recovered much faster from the anaesthesia.

Regardless of the drugs used, it is important to have all resources available for monitoring, intubation and maintenance of anaesthesia as required. The use of patient warming devices is extremely helpful as the patients are frequently hypothermic at presentation.

It is not best practice to relieve urethral obstruction and place a urinary catheter in a cat that is moving as this can lead to significant urethral damage/rupture and may also lead to failure in relieving the obstruction. Most cats will need general anaesthesia for the procedure.

A coccygeal epidural block can be used to help pass a urinary catheter and relieve urethral obstruction. It produces anaesthesia of the perineum, penis, urethra, colon, and anus without loss of hind motor function. There is minimal risk of complications with this procedure. Further information on the technique can be found in the American Animal Hospital Association Website. Anaesthesia is expected to start 5 minutes after injection.

Cystocentesis

The use of decompressive cystocentesis is controversial. Cystocentesis does not need to be performed in most patients but can be valuable in unstable patients and / or when relieving the obstruction is problematic.

If performed, cystocentesis should be done using a 22 G needle attached to an extension set and a 3-way tap so that the bladder is only entered once, and is emptied as much as possible, while reducing bladder wall trauma. While the bladder is stabilised with one hand, the needle should be angled at 45 degrees caudally towards the bladder neck when entering the bladder to minimise the risk of the needle tearing the bladder as it gets emptied.

Performing cystocentesis in a patient with a full bladder raises concerns about leakage of urine around the needle and into the abdomen; if the urine is sterile, it is usually rapidly reabsorbed and excreted.

It is possible that bladder rupture can occur in cases of severely damaged bladder wall (Figure 9) but, in this instance, the further increase in pressure with retrograde urohydropulsion could potentially also lead to bladder rupture.

Some of the potential benefits of cystocentesis are immediate reduction in intravesical pressure which can reduce pain and help kidneys relieve backflow pressure onto the kidneys. Additionally, it may help with the relieving of the obstruction via retrograde urohydropulsion as the pressure in the bladder is lower. Cystocentesis also allows collection of a urine sample

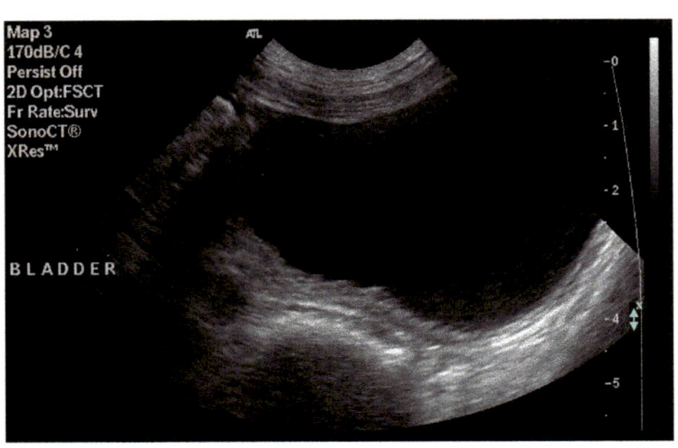

Figure 9. Ultrasound showing an abnormal thinning of the bladder wall in a cat with haematuria.

for analysis and culture that is not diluted with flush fluid and / or iatrogenically contaminated.

Cystocentesis should be decided on a case-to-case basis having in mind the pros and cons of this approach and should always be performed with appropriate technique to minimise the risk of complication. Repeated cystocentesis should be avoided due to the increased likelihood of problems.

Relieving urethral obstruction

For relieving urethral obstruction via retrograde urohydropulsion it is preferable to select and open-ended urinary catheter as the pressure from the retrograde flush will be directed forwards onto the obstruction.

This can be achieved with a urinary catheter or, for more distal obstructions, a lacrimal cannula, or a venous catheter (without needle) can also be handy. The lacrimal cannulas are quite stiff as they are designed to cannulate nasolacrimal ducts while the venous catheters are quite soft and tend to kink in the area where the catheter meets the hub.

Ideally the perineum should be shaved and, the skin aseptically prepared. Especially in cats with long hair, it may be easier to maintain sterility if the hair in the caudal part of the hind limbs is shaved and if, during the procedure, the tail is bandaged, from the base to the tip, with cohesive material.

The position in which to perform urethral catheterization is operator-dependent, with lateral recumbency, sternal recumbency or dorsal recumbency being possible. The author preference is to use dorsal recumbency with the patient placed at the edge of the table so that the tail hangs down and is immediately out of the way. With the patient in this position the penis is then retracted caudally and towards the table, to straighten out the urethra and make it parallel to the table.

The tip of the penis should be massaged to help dislodge any material present in that location, while attempting to massage it out rather than into the urethra.

Sterile lubricant should be placed on the tip of the catheter and sterile saline should be available, in prefilled syringes, to flush the urethra.

The tip of the catheter is placed in the urethra and advanced carefully until an obstruction is encountered. The catheter is then retracted a little bit and the catheter is used to flush sterile saline in an attempt to dislodge the obstruction onto the bladder. The catheter will then be advanced again, if possible, and the flushing repeated as necessary until it the balder is reached. If flushing alone is not dislodging the obstruction, the external urethral orifice can be held closed against the urinary catheter while further flushing is performed.

This step is easier if an assistant does the flushing and replacement of the pre-filled syringes, and the operator concentrates on holding the catheter in place and occluding the urethra.

In larger cats it may be possible to massage the urethra per rectum to help relieve urethral obstruction in conjunction with retrograde urohydropulsion

Some clinicians prefer using a mixture 3:1 or 4:1 of sterile saline and sterile lubricant to flush the urethra as they feel this may help to lubricate the urethra and help resolve the obstruction while decreasing urethral trauma. Acidic solutions, such as Walpole's solution, should not be used as it will cause more damage to the urethra and bladder.

"Pushing" against an obstruction with the catheter should not be attempted as this will lead to trauma of the urethra or even urethral rupture.

Once the obstruction is cleared the bladder should be flushed copiously with sterile saline, warmed to body temperature, until the fluid retrieved back is clear and without blood clots. While performing bladder lavage it can help to gently ballot it to suspend debris and crystals located in the dependent side, therefore aiding their removal.

If the catheterization has been challenging, provided the patient is stable, it is recommended to perform a retrograde urethrogram before to identify potential urethral rupture which can have devastating effects.

Patients that have needed multiple catheterizations over time are at risk of development of urethral strictures because of the repeated trauma of catheterization. A retrograde urethrogram is essential to investigate the presence of a stricture which would affect the ability to continue medical management in the patient.

After resolution of the obstruction a urinary catheter should be placed and secured in place with either surgical glue or sutures. An Elizabethan collar or similar device is essential to avoid the patient dislodging the catheter.

The urinary catheter should always be attached to a closed sterile collection system and not left draining freely as this will increase the likelihood of a urinary tract infection.

If collection system is attached to the base of the tail, there should be enough slack to ensure that tail movement doesn't elicit pulling of the stay sutures in the prepuce and therefore pain.

Which urinary catheter to use as indwelling catheter?

Not all catheters that are used for unblocking a cat should be used as indwelling urinary catheters.

In general, a 3.5Fr or 5Fr catheter is used as an indwelling catheter for feline patients. While it may be tempting to use the larger size catheter, to minimise kinking and catheter obstruction, in a large retrospective study the rate of re-obstruction was significantly lower when a 3.5Fr catheter was used compared to a 5Fr catheter (6.7% vs 19%).

Indwelling catheters should be made of soft, atraumatic material that doesn't elicit mucosal irritation or discomfort.

The length of catheter should be enough to allow the catheter to reach the bladder and not just sit at the transition bladder neck to proximal urethra. However, the catheter should not be so long that it can cause trauma to the cranial pole of the bladder or curl inside and potentially create a knot. If the catheter tip is in the proximal urethra, urine drainage may be intermittent and maintaining the bladder continuously drained may be impossible. At times, this can manifest itself as the catheter only draining urine when gentle pressure is applied onto the bladder but not when the catheter is aspirated.

There are numerous types, sizes, and lengths of urinary catheters available in the market which can be overwhelming. Below is a brief description of the relevant points of some of the available catheter types.

Catheters and their properties

- Polyprolylene catheters (e.g. Tom cat) are reasonably rigid catheters and can be made even stiffer with stylets. Use of these catheters, particularly with the stylet, can be associated with a higher risk of urethral trauma. They are not a good option as indwelling catheters.
- Nylon catheters (e.g. Portex® Jackson cat catheter) have side holes and are available with or without stylet and with a hub with suture holes. This catheter is not recommended to be used as indwelling.
- Polytetrafluoroethylene (PTFE) catheters (e.g. Slippery Sam®) are available as 3.5F 11 cm, 14 cm and, in some countries, 18 cm in length. They have an end-hole and are stiff enough that can be used for unblocking a cat. This brand of catheter has a hub with holes to allow the catheter to be secured to the patient. It can be very fiddly to connect a syringe or urine collection system to the hub and the hub is not luer lock. There are colleagues that reported the silicone hub disconnecting from the catheter itself and the catheter migrating into the urethra making retrieval a nightmare. This catheter is not recommended to be used as indwelling.
- Polyvinyl catheters (e.g. red rubber catheter or feeding tube) were traditionally used as indwelling urinary catheters after the obstruction as relieved. They are much less irritant that some of the older style catheters. Nowadays there are better options available, and they are rarely used.

- Polyurethane catheters (e.g Mila® Tomcat catheter) are available as 3.5Fr and 5Fr with lengths varying from 15 to 25 cm. It can be used to unblock the cat and as indwelling. This catheter can be obtained with or without an open core style, which makes the catheter more rigid for placement and relieving obstruction but also allows flushing via its open core. This catheter has various length markers and a moveable suture device to allow selection of the appropriate length for the patient. The catheter hub is luer lock allowing for ease of connection to the collection bag.
- Teflon-type catheters (Vygon® Katkath) is available as 3.5F in either fixed length of 11 and 14 cm and as 3.5F 18 cm with a moveable clip to adjust length to patient size. These catheters have a tapering open-end tip and have a rotating hub which allows the catheter to rotate around the hub while sutured. It is rigid enough to not need a stylet for placement but has good "bounce-back" properties and is therefore kink-resistant and does not tend to concertina.
- Silicone catheters (Surgivet® Tomcat) is available as 3.5F 12 cm in length with either side holes +/− end hole. It comes with a guidewire for ease of placement and the hub has suture holes for ease of attachment to the patient.

The monitoring of patients with urethral obstruction is very similar to that highlighted for acute kidney injury. At earlier stages, it is sensible to monitor the patient, electrolytes and renal parameters more frequently and then decrease the frequency of these as thought appropriate.

In patient with urethral obstruction, post-obstructive diuresis can be extremely severe in the first 24–48 hours therefore monitoring ins and outs is essential to adjust fluid therapy. In some instances, despite the initial presentation with hyperkalaemia, some patients may develop hypokalaemia within 24–36 hours and potassium supplementation of the intravenous fluid is necessary.

Once renal parameters have returned to normal it may be necessary to progressive reduce the rate of fluid therapy, while making sure that there is an equivalent decrease in urine output, to avoid iatrogenic diuresis.

The use of non-steroidal anti-inflammatories (NSAIDs) should only be considered in patients that do not have acute kidney injury and always after normalization of the renal parameters and haemodynamic status.

Analgesia plays a very important role in the management of these patients and often opioids are used during the hospitalization period to provide pain relief and ease patient discomfort with the urinary catheter.

Urethral relaxant drugs may be beneficial in some cases, especially those with idiopathic cystitis and cases with functional urethral obstruction due to urethral spasm. This topic will be discussed further in the section on idiopathic feline cystitis.

It is best not to use antibiotics unless it is absolutely essential as its administration while a urinary catheter is in place risks leading to development of resistant bacteria.

How long a urinary catheter is kept in place is extremely dependent on the case, reason for the obstruction and the presence/absence of systemic consequences of the obstruction.

In cats with a recent urethral obstruction, that don't present with azotaemia and electrolyte disturbances, and that don't have a physical cause to the obstruction, it may be appropriate to consider removal of the catheter after the bladder is emptied and lavaged.

Cats with azotaemia and severe electrolyte and acid base changes will likely benefit from having a urinary catheter for longer to allow urine output assessment and output of large urine volumes while renal parameters normalize. Ideally, the catheter would be maintained until the renal parameters have returned to normal and the urine doesn't have a strong haematuric appearance. If, after 24 hours, there is not a significant improvement of renal parameters, uroabdomen and/or acute kidney injury is suspected.

In cases where there are concerns about prolonged bladder distension and associated detrusor atony, some authors suggest urethral catheterization for 5 to 7 days to maximise the time the bladder is completely empty to try to promote detrusor stability. Bethanecol can be used in cases of detrusor atony and the presence of the urinary catheter ensures that there is no obstruction to urinary flow which is one of the contra-indications to its use.

Most cases of urethral rupture need to be treated surgically. However, in some cases of small urethral ruptures that are being addressed conservatively, the urinary catheter may have to remain in place for a significant period of time to ensure urine drainage and act as scaffolding while the urethra heals.

If urethral obstruction cannot be relieved, a **tube cystotomy** should be considered. These tubes can remain in place for a significant period of time allowing patient stabilization and a repeated attempt at relieving the urethral obstruction later when the patient is no longer in a critical state.

If after a few days, it remains impossible to relieve the obstruction, the patient is stable and the tissue trauma has very significantly reduced, increasing the likelihood of success of additional surgical procedures.

In patients with recurrent urinary obstruction non-responsive to medical treatment and/or cases of urethral stricture, a perineal urethrostomy (PU) may be indicated. However, a PU should not be seen as an emergency procedure or as an alternative to placement of a cystotomy tube.

Perineal urethrostomy is a technically demanding surgery, which is better performed when the patient is stable and when the urethra and peri-urethral tissue is not haemorrhagic or swollen. Performing surgery when there is extensive local trauma and often a distorted anatomy can lead to much higher risk of surgical complications.

Urolithiasis

Urolithiasis refers to stones anywhere within the urinary tract.

Over the last couple of decades, the incidence of calcium oxalate uroliths is increasing in proportion to struvite and their relative proportion is currently similar.

The most common uroliths in cats are struvite and calcium oxalate, which together represent over 90% of all feline urolithiasis.

Aetiology

Some of the known risk factors for development of uroliths include gender, age, anatomical and functional abnormalities of the urinary tract, metabolic abnormalities, urinary tract infection, diet, urine pH.

Minerals in uroliths may have been deposited in different layers or the urolith may be composed by a mixture of minerals without distinct layers but it is also possible for the urolith to be composed of a single mineral without visible layers.

Most frequently uroliths have different layers, which are denominated (from the inside to the outside):

- Nidus or nucleus (area of initiation of the urolith growth).
- Stone (body of the urolith).
- Shell (layer of material that surrounds the stone).
- Surface crystals.

It is important to differentiate the layers of the uroliths and determine their composition as prevention of the urolithiasis is better targeted at the mineral composition of the nidus.

It is possible for uroliths to made up exclusively of a single mineral but most often they have more than one mineral and are called mixed. If the nidus of the urolith is composed of different mineral(s) to the outer layer(s) this urolith is called compound. Compound uroliths most frequently occur when:

- Metabolic uroliths (such as calcium oxalate and urate) lead to urinary tract infection with urease-positive bacteria causing deposition of struvite around the initial nidus.
- Suture material or another foreign material leads to deposition of minerals around it.
- Treatment and/or diet administered before urolith removal leads to altered urine pH and solubility of different crystals in the urine.

After uroliths form it is possible for them to pass through the urine tract, continue to grow, dissolve spontaneously or continue to grow potentially leading to clinical signs. Not all uroliths are associated with clinical signs.

Whenever a urolith is detected, the whole urinary tract should be assessed as it is common for uroliths to be present in multiple locations concurrently.

The presence of uroliths can be an inciting cause for an UTI. However, the reverse is also possible, and some urease-producing bacteria can induce the formation of struvite uroliths in dogs and humans although, in cats, the later seems to be a rare cause.

The steps needed for development of an urolith include:

- Favouring of nucleation.
- Promotion of crystal growth and/or aggregation.
- Retention of the urolith in the urinary tract so that more growth can occur.

The importance of each factor on to the development of different types of uroliths will depend on the mineral itself and urine properties.

The formation of some uroliths (struvite, cystine and urate) occurs (although not exclusively) due to higher-than-normal concentration of the solutes in the urine. However, the formation of calcium containing uroliths is a lot more complex and, although increased excretion of calcium or oxalate can play a role in their development, the urine always has a high concentration of the solutes. The lack of factors that reduce growth or aggregation of crystals is also thought to represent an important role in the formation of calcium oxalate uroliths.

Diagnosis

The presence of crystalluria is not necessarily associated with urolithiasis or predisposition to development of uroliths. For example, a small amount of struvite crystals can be normal in healthy cats especially if urine is very concentrated.

Ideally, urinalysis should be performed as soon as possible, and the sample should not have been refrigerated because, as the urine cools down, there is an increased tendency for crystal formation. The best way to assess crystalluria is to perform in house analysis (ideally within 30 minutes of collection), as there is possibility of in vitro formation of crystals with time. The patient should be starved as feeding can lead to postprandial increase in pH.

There is limited usefulness in sending urine to an external laboratory to assess for the presence of crystals as they can form *ex vivo*, especially if the samples are refrigerated. However, the detection of less common crystals such as cystine, xanthine and urate should prompt further investigation.

The presence and type of crystals may be especially useful in some circumstances:

- When pathological crystals are present (e.g. ammonium biurate, cystine and calcium oxalate monohydrate).
- When large amount of struvite or calcium oxalate crystals are seen.
- In patients with urolithiasis assessment of crystals in the urine alongside urine pH, signalment and radiographic density and appearance of urolith can help predict their composition. However, there are studies suggesting that crystalluria is an insensitive and unreliable method of predicting urolith composition as, once uroliths form, crystals associated with that type of stone often decrease or disappear from the urine as it is more favourable for minerals to deposit on the surface of the stone than to form new crystals.

Whenever a urolith is detected, the whole urinary tract should be examined for the potential presence of more uroliths. The detection of uroliths is usually performed by a combination of X-rays and ultrasound (Figure 10). Although most of the uroliths are radiopaque, it is possible for uroliths to be radiolucent and therefore not detectable with radiographs. In addition, some uroliths are too small to be detected by radiography which usually detects uroliths over 2–3 mm.

The most precise **determination of number and location** of uroliths is achieved with a combination of **ultrasound and contrast radiographs** (pneumocystogram and double contrast cystogram) (Figure 11).

It is possible to try to make an educated guess of what type of urolith is present in the lower urinary tract based on signalment, location of calculi, urine pH and presence of crystals, and radiographic opacity.

Calculi that are radiopaque include calcium oxalate and struvite with calcium oxalate being usually more radiopaque. Urate and cystine are variably radiopaque in appearance.

Current data suggests that the most precise determination of number and location of uroliths is done by a

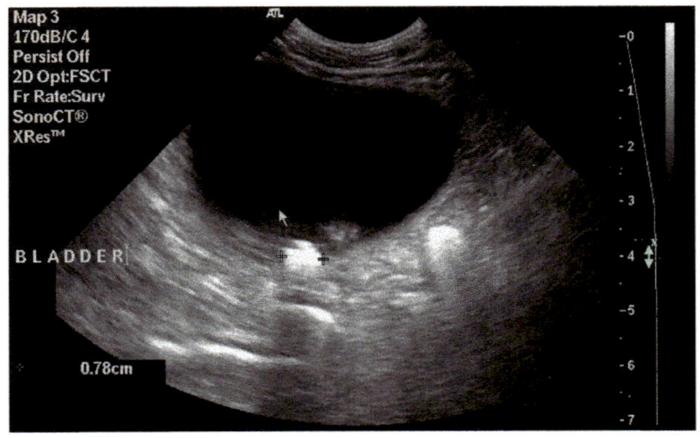

Figure 10. Bladder ultrasound showing an urolith and its acoustic shadowing.

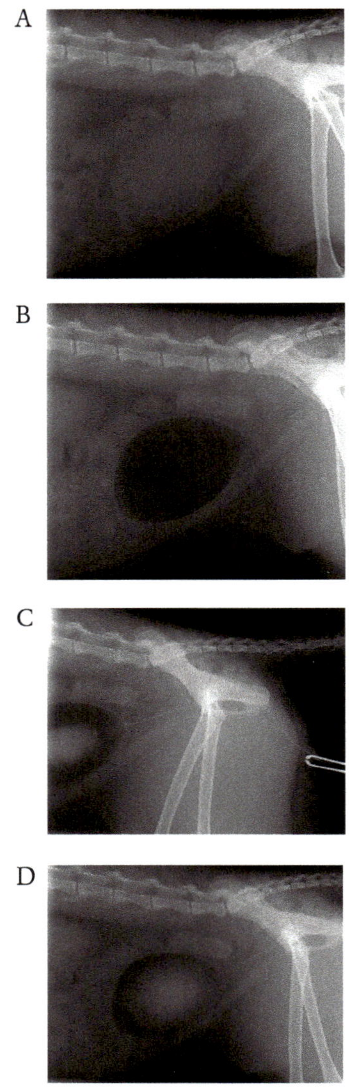

Figure 11. (a) Lateral radiography of the caudal abdomen just before a contrast-enhanced urinary study. (b) Normal pneumocystogram. (c) Retrograde urethrogram after a pneumocystogram. (d) Normal double-contrast cystogram; note the urinary catheter inside the urethra.

combination of ultrasound and contrast radiographs of the urinary tract although advanced imaging can also be used.

Many minerals may form crystals and uroliths in the urinary tract of cats, but the most common types are struvite and calcium oxalate. Purine uroliths (e.g. urate, cystine) are the third most frequent type.

Treatment

The ACVIM (American College of Veterinary Internal Medicine) Small Animal Consensus Recommendations on the Treatment and Prevention of Uroliths in Dogs and Cats has been published in 2016 and is divided into three sections:

1. Treatment of lower urinary tract uroliths (bladder and urethra).
2. Treatment of upper urinary tract uroliths (kidneys and ureters).
3. Urolithiasis prevention.

Although these recommendations are consensus-derived, research and experience supported, the patient-centered recommendations have been formulated as if all management options are available, which might not be the case in some countries. Overall, the main emphasis of the guidelines is to try to dissolve uroliths whenever feasible, to perform urolith removal only whenever essential and, when doing so, using as much as possible minimally invasive techniques.

Uroliths that are amenable to medically dissolution include struvite, urate and cystine. For dissolution to be possible, the urolith must be surrounded by undersaturated urine hence dissolution of nephroliths, ureteroliths and urethroliths is usually not possible. Urethroliths can be flushed by retrograde hydropulsion onto the bladder for medical dissolution or removal.

There are multiple diet manufacturers that have veterinary food specific for urolithiasis (dissolution and/or prevention) and therefore it is recommended that the clinicians contact the manufacturer's literature and local professional representative to help select the best diet for the patient. In patients with multiple health concerns, if there is no available commercially diet that would cater for those conditions simultaneously, it may be preferable to consult with a veterinary nutritionist to create a bespoke diet.

General considerations depending on the location of uroliths

Lower urinary tract urolithiasis

All uroliths causing obstruction should ideally be retrohydropulsed onto the bladder for removal or dissolution.

Dissolution should always be attempted for uroliths that are medically dissolvable. Non-dissolvable urocystoliths associated with clinical signs should ideally be removed by minimally invasive procedures as discussed above, rather than cystotomy.

The ACVIM guidelines suggests that non-dissolvable urocystoliths are unlikely to cause obstruction, that are not leading to clinical signs, do not require removal at that point in time; preventative strategies should be started regardless.

Upper urinary tract urolithiasis

Upper urinary tract uroliths are a lot more frequent in cats than in dogs. Nephroliths are uroliths located in the renal pelvis and/or collecting diverticula of the kidneys. Ureteroliths usually stem from nephroliths that migrated onto the ureter and may lead to ureteric obstruction or pass onto the bladder, subsequently leading to either bladder urolithiasis or they may continue to migrate along the urinary tract and exit the body.

The real prevalence of nephroliths is likely higher than documented in studies as a significant percentage of animals is asymptomatic and the nephroliths are detected incidentally.

Nephroliths can cause distortion of the renal parenchyma, obstruction of the renal pelvis, may migrate onto the ureters (leading to obstruction in some cases) but they can also predispose to pyelonephritis; all the later may cause changes in glomerular filtration rate.

If nephroliths are not causing clinical problems, they are named inactive and when identified the patient should be carefully monitored for disease progression and potential development of complications.

The most frequent clinical signs of nephrolithiasis are haematuria, abdominal pain, recurrent urinary tract infection and progressive renal disease.

The diagnosis of nephroliths is usually made by radiography and/or ultrasound. It is important to differentiate nephrolithiasis from mineralization of the renal pelvis. In recent years, it is also frequent for nephroliths to be detected with advanced imaging as its use is more widespread.

The vast majority of feline upper urinary urolith are not possible to dissolve as calcium oxalate represents around 92% of the nephroliths, solidified blood uroliths around 8% with other types being very uncommon. In the rare situation where the upper urinary tract uroliths are thought to be possible to dissolve (e.g. struvite) dissolution measures should be started.

The therapeutic options for nephroliths include monitoring if they are inactive (with or without dissolution attempt) and surgery or interventional radiology procedures in cases with obstruction or recurrent urinary tract infections. If urolith removal is indicated, the 2016 ACVIM consensus statement recommends, if possible, that minimally invasive techniques are used given that nephrotomy is associated with a significant decrease in GFR.

Unfortunately, extracorporeal shockwave lithotripsy, one of the most common techniques used in dogs cannot be used in cats as there is a high risk of ureteral obstruction with the fragments as they are often larger than the ureteral diameter and, additionally, calcium oxalate uroliths are quite resistant to fragmentation.

Ureterolithiasis has emerged as an important cause of acute and chronic renal disease in cats over the last 15 years, coinciding with a relative increase in the frequency of calcium oxalate urolithiasis in cats.

If only one kidney and/or ureter is affected, the animal may not be azotaemic. However, in around 75% of the cases, studies are suggestive of bilateral renal impairment, or pre-renal azotaemia. In some patients with unilateral upper urinary tract urolithiasis persistently increased SDMA might be the only change detected on biochemistry.

Given the high prevalence of calcium oxalate in the feline upper urinary tract, whenever nephrolithiasis and/or ureterolithiasis is identified the patient should be assessed for hypercalcaemia. Given that in one study 25% of cats with normal total calcium had increased ionised calcium, it is recommended to always measure ionised calcium to maximise detection of hypercalcaemia. Additionally, a thorough history including diet and supplements should be evaluated to target potential supplementation of calcium or feeding of diets high in oxalates.

Identification of ureteroliths with imaging can be challenging and therefore combination of radiography and ultrasound is usually recommended to maximise their detection. Advanced imaging can also be used for the detection of urolithiasis.

At times, on ultrasound, the urolith is not seen and, although identification of a dilated renal pelvis can be seen with multiple conditions, the degree of dilation increases with renal dysfunction, pyelonephritis, and ureteral obstruction. A recent report reported the sensitivity of ultrasound to detect feline ureteroliths associated with obstruction to be 98%.

In cases of ureteral obstruction, the best option will be to use ureteral stents or subcutaneous ureteral bypass (SUBs) as traditional surgery has a high rate of post-operative complications (30–40%) and a high perioperative mortality rate (18–21%). The most common complications with traditional surgery are ureteral oedema, re-obstruction, strictures, incomplete removal of ureteroliths and urine leakage.

If traditional surgical treatment is the only option, medical treatment may be tried for a period of 24–48 hours as there are studies that report a success rate of 8–13% in cats. However, it is important to bear in mind that the risk of recurrence at 1 year is around 40% with either medical treatment or conventional surgery. Additionally, there are studies that document that 33% of cats with nephrolithiasis had concurrent ureteral strictures making stents or SUBs a more sensible approach.

The new interventional techniques lead to quick ureteral decompression, less perioperative complications, lower mortality rate and reduced rate of re-obstruction.

Although stents can be used in cats, nowadays some authors mostly use SUBs for cats given the reported lower rate of post-operative complications in some studies and the fact that they cater for all the different causes of ureteral obstruction (strictures, masses, uroliths).

The most common complications with the newer interventional techniques are dysuria, urinary tract infection, the need to replace the stent due to migration or re-obstruction and the need to change the SUB due to obstruction.

For more information on these techniques please consult the chapter "Medical and Interventional Management of Upper Urinary Tract Uroliths" in the March 2019 volume of Veterinary Clinics of North America.

In the UK, several referral centres are now offering these minimally invasive techniques and one of the centres has recently published a study with data on survival and complications which, in comparison with some of the studies from the USA, may better represent local experience.

As mentioned before, medical management of ureteroliths is not the preferred approach as the rate of success is low (8–13%) and recurrence is common. Additionally, the renal dysfunction and its consequences will continue unaddressed unless the obstruction is released in a swift manner.

Conservative medical management consists of supportive therapy for renal dysfunction and treatments designed to increase the likelihood of relief of ureteral obstruction.

Fluid diuresis alone or in combination with diuretics (frusemide and mannitol) may improve the likelihood of passage of ureteral calculi. Alpha-adrenergic antagonists can be used if there are no specific contraindications; their use is supported by improvement described in anecdotal reports. Analgesia should also be instituted.

In cats treated medically that survived more than one month after diagnosis, the 12-month survival rate is reported at 66%, with a number of cats dying of causes related to chronic renal disease or recurrent ureterolithiasis.

The ACVIM guidelines encourage clinicians to use non-invasive procedures for urolith removal as it is estimated that up to 9% of urolith recurrence is suture-induced. However, the authors of the guidelines recognise that this may not always be feasible due to lack of availability of all options to the clinicians.

If surgical removal is performed, bladder closure should be made using sutures that eliminate the risk of suture exposure to the bladder lumen to avoid suture-induced urolithiasis.

Once uroliths are detected, periodic monitoring (every three to four months) with ultrasound +/− radiographs is essential to detect recurrence. This might allow using voided urohydropulsion in female cats and intensify dissolution techniques for some types of uroliths.

Non-invasive or minimally invasive techniques for urolith removal

Voided urohydropulsion of cystoliths

Voided urohydropulsion can be performed to remove small uroliths in female cats by inducing voiding and encouraging the uroliths to pass through the urethra with the urine. In general, voiding urohydropulsion can be considered for queens with uroliths less than 3 mm in size but some authors report success with uroliths up to 5 mm in diameter. This technique is not usually recommended in males due to the small diameter of the urethra.

The patient must be sedated or anaesthetised for the procedure. The bladder is distended with sterile saline via catheterization, then the urinary catheter is removed, and the patient is positioned vertically so that the long axis of the bladder and the urethra are vertical. The bladder is gently balloted so that the uroliths move to the bladder neck and the bladder is then expressed and emptied relying on gravity and the urine flow for urolith removal. The procedure is repeated until all uroliths are removed as documented by imaging.

The presence of suspected urethral strictures is a potential contra-indication. Voiding urohydropulsion should not be performing within at least a couple of months after surgery as the bladder is unlikely to have regained sufficient integrity to accommodate the significant increase in pressure.

Possible complications include bladder haemorrhage and, although rare, bladder rupture. If the size of the uroliths was miscalculated and they get trapped in the urethra they can be replaced in the bladder by retrograde urohydropulsion.

More information on this procedure is available in the reading/reference list.

Cystoscopic retrieval

Cystoscopic retrieval of small uroliths can only be performed in female cats but this is limited by the size of the endoscopic baskets/snares.

Laser lithotripsy

Laser lithotripsy can be used for urolith fragmentation under cystoscopic assessment in female cats. The fragments can then be removed via cystoscopy or voided urohydropulsion. This procedure is not used in male cats.

Surgery

Surgical removal of uroliths via cystotomy is also possible and complications are uncommon when compared to urethral or ureteral surgery.

The reported percentage of uroliths left in the urinary tract after cystotomy (specialist surgeons) is around 20% in cats. Taking this into consideration, incomplete urolith removal is more frequent than recognised. Not performing radiographs to verify the complete removal of uroliths is usually considered delivering substandard level of care.

What to consider when going ahead for surgical removal of uroliths:

- Inform the client of the risk (legal standpoint).
- Confirm the location and number of uroliths just prior to surgery.
- Reposition all uroliths in the bladder prior to surgery.
- Pre-surgical catheterization to avoid urolith migration to the urethra.
- Flush the bladder.
- Flush the urethra.
- Obtain post-operative radiographs (including contrast) after surgery to look for any remaining uroliths.

Calcium oxalate (CaOx) urolithiasis

Calcium oxalate uroliths tend to occur more commonly in males than in females and are more common in middle-aged to older cats (mean age 7.6 years). Cats of 7–10 years are reported to be 67 times more likely to develop calcium oxalate uroliths than cats of 1–2 years. Male cats were reported to be 1.5 times more likely to develop calcium oxalate calculi than females and males castrated cats were seven times more likely to develop them than intact males.

Some of the reported predisposed breeds are Tonkinese, Burmese, Devon rex, Himalayan, Persian and Siamese.

Calcium oxalate uroliths are moderately to markedly radiopaque and are mostly seen in the lower urinary tract. The most common type of upper urinary tract uroliths is calcium oxalate with other type seen infrequently.

The mechanisms associated with CaOx urolithiasis is incompletely understood but it is thought that urine oversaturation is an important factor and cats with this type of uroliths have increased urinary excretion of calcium (hypercalciuria). As such, controlling factors that promote oversaturation is an important prevention strategy.

The presence of inhibitors in the urine (e.g., citrate and magnesium) cause reduced availability for calcium and oxalate to combine and precipitate and therefore, if they are reduced, the risk of CaOx formation tends to increase.

Hypercalciuria is a risk factor which may be secondary to conditions such as hypercalcaemia, metabolic acidosis, and high sodium consumption.

Marked aciduria (urine pH< 6.2) is thought to represent a significant risk factor for development of CaOx urolithiasis and therefore excessive acidification should be avoided while attempting to dissolve or prevent struvite urolithiasis.

Some studies document that around 33% of cats with CaOx urolithiasis have hypercalcaemia and therefore it is essential to assess both total calcium and ionised calcium in these patients.

Decreased urine volume and concentrated urine are also risk factors for development of CaOx urolithiasis.

It is not possible to dissolve calcium oxalate uroliths and therefore physical removal is the only option.

Ideally, risk factors for CaOx formation, such as hypercalcaemia, should be controlled to help decrease recurrence of CaOx urolithiasis.

The goals of dietary CaOx prevention are:

- Reduction of urine calcium and oxalate concentration.
- Promotion of higher concentration of inhibitors.
- Reducing urine acidity.
- Promoting production of more dilute urine.

Increasing production of urine that is less concentrated (ideally SG< 1.030) allows a decreased urinary concentration of mineral and therefore feeding a canned diet or encouraging increased water consumption with water fountains or flavoured water may help in CaOx prevention.

The recommended target urine pH for CaOx prevention is around 6.5–7.5.

Monitoring of the urine properties and crystal presence in a freshly collected urine is critical for the success of prevention and allows tailoring of treatment as needed.

If urine is consistently with a pH< 6.2, changing to a diet that causes less urinary acidification or the use of urine alkalinizers such as potassium citrate (75 mg/kg PO every 12–24 hours) must be considered.

In patients with recurrent urolithiasis, hydrochlorothiazide (1–2 mg/kg PO BID) can be used but it is contra-indicated in cats with hypercalcaemia.

Given the high risk of recurrence of CaOx urolith and the fact that dissolution is not possible, it is recommended to monitor patients closely to detect very small uroliths which may be amenable to voided urohydropulsion.

A significant percentage of cats will have recurrence within two years of the initial diagnosis if prevention strategies are not implemented.

Struvite urolithiasis

Cats between 2–10 years are at biggest risk of struvite urolithiasis with the bladder and urethra being the almost exclusive location; struvite upper urinary tract urolithiasis is very rare in cats.

For struvite uroliths to form, the urine needs to be oversaturated with magnesium, ammonium, and phosphate.

In cats, struvite uroliths are typically sterile, while in dogs struvite uroliths are mostly infection-induced. However, it is possible, albeit it rare, for cats to have infection induced struvite uroliths.

Sterile struvite urolithiasis

Dietary composition is one of the risk factors for struvite urolithiasis alongside other factors such as alkalinuria, reduced water intake and low urine volume.

Medical dissolution is highly effective, avoids the risk and potential complication of surgical removal and, in many cases, it is significantly cheaper than surgery. There are some concerns about dissolution of uroliths, particularly in male cats due to the very narrow urethra, as urinary obstruction may occur. However, in a few prospective studies, this did not occur, and dissolution was successful in 100% of the cases.

Sterile struvite uroliths can be dissolved by feeding a dissolution diet, which is restricted in magnesium, phosphorus, and protein and that induces aciduria (pH< 6.4). Some studies document dissolution in 6–28 days with a dissolution diet and in 7–52 days with a maintenance diet for prevention of struvite urolithiasis.

During the dissolution phase it is important to assess the urine properties and the presence of struvite crystals in a freshly collected urine sample while, at the same time, monitoring the urolith size with imaging to confirm that it is decreasing over time.

If the urine is not acidic enough the use of methionine or ammonium chloride can be considered.

The dissolution diets should be continued for 2–4 weeks beyond radiographic dissolution as uroliths < 3 mm may not be detected on radiographs.

Prevention of sterile struvite urolithiasis is achieved by feeding a diet restricted in phosphorus and magnesium that induces production of urine with a pH < 6.4. A urine SG < 1.030 is preferrable and the use of canned food, water fountains or flavoured water can help with this.

Monitoring of the urine properties and crystal presence in a freshly collected urine is critical for the success of prevention and allows tailoring of treatment as needed.

Similarly, to the dissolution strategies, methionine or ammonium chloride can be considered for urine acidification if diet is insufficient.

Infection-induced struvite urolithiasis

Infection-induced struvite uroliths occur secondary to an infection with a urease-producing bacteria, which is the driving force for urolith formation.

Infection-induced struvite uroliths can be dissolved by using a struvite dissolution diet alongside appropriate antibiotic treatment with a dissolution time of around 64–92 days. The antibiotic therapy needs to be continued for the whole period of dissolution otherwise bacteria trapped within the urolith may lead to further struvite deposition.

Prevention of this type of urolithiasis is based on prevention of recurrence of the urinary tract infection rather than dietary management. As such, it is important to identify and address potential underlying causes for the urinary tract infection.

Urate urolithiasis

The pathophysiology of **urate stones in cats is not understood and although they can occur with hepatic portovascular anomalies** this is not a frequent cause. To prevent recurrence, a high-moisture protein-restricted diet is recommended; the different diet manufacturers should be consulted for more information.

Solidified blood calculi

Recently, the presence of "dried solidified blood calculi" has been identified in cats; they are firm and stone-like but usually do not contain crystalline material, therefore they are not radiopaque. If they have a significant proportion of incorporate calcium oxalate or calcium phosphate, they can then become radiopaque.

Cystine and silica calculi

Cystine uroliths and silica uroliths are rare in cats.

Mixed composition

Mixed composition uroliths occur in around 13% of cases. The prevention strategies should be implemented for the mineral type found in the core of the calculus.

The Minnesota Urolith Centre website has a lot of extremely useful information on feline (and canine) uroliths and should be consulted for information of management and prevention of urolithiasis.

Matrix-crystalline feline urethral plugs

Feline urethral plugs are a common cause of urinary obstruction in male cats. Plugs may be primary composed of organic material such as blood, protein, or sloughed tissue but some urethral plugs contain aggregates of crystalline minerals. Struvite is the mineral present in over 92% of urethral plugs.

In one study, cats younger than nine years of age represented 82% of the cats identified with urethral plugs.

Urethral plugs should be submitted for mineral analysis to help identify factors that may contribute to obstructive disease (e.g. deposition of struvite in plugs) and therefore best target preventative treatment.

Prevention of urethral plugs should include feeding wet food rather than dry to try to reduce the urine SG and feeding struvite dissolution foods to cats with persistent marked crystalluria.

Controversially, some authors suggest feeding young male cats (until they are 9–10 years) with a struvite dissolution diet, especially if they have persistent struvite crystalluria, with the aim to prevent urethral obstruction this approach.

It is thought that many cats with urethral plugs have underlying idiopathic cystitis which, due to inflammation, is the source of organic components for the urethral plug and therefore treatment for idiopathic cystitis should also be implemented.

Urinary tract infections

Urinary tract infections (UTI's) reportedly account 0.1–2% of feline veterinary visits. Feline bacterial infections are much less common than in dogs and, when present, are more frequent in **older animals (>10 years)**. In general, less than 10% of cats with lower urinary disease signs have bacterial UTI's.

Aetiology

The vast majority of UTIs are caused by **ascending migration of pathogens** from the normal flora of the distal urogenital tract. Should the host's immune defences change, the normal flora may emerge as uropathogens.

For an infection to occur the bacteria have to gain access to the urinary tract, adhere to and colonize the urothelium. The establishment of infection also depends on the **number and virulence of pathogens plus its interaction with the host**.

The urinary tract has several defence mechanisms (see table below).

• Normal micturition
  • Adequate volume
  • Frequent voiding
  • Complete voiding
  • Urinary continence
• Anatomic structures
  • High-pressure zone in the urethra
  • Surface characteristics of the urothelium
  • Urethral peristalsis
  • Length of the urethra (especially in males)
  • Prostatic secretions have antibacterial properties
  • Ureteral vesical flap valves
  • Ureteral peristalsis
  • Extensive renal blood supply and flow
	• Mucosal defence barriers
	  • Antibody production
	  • Surface layer of glycosaminoglycans
	  • Intrinsic mucosal antimicrobial properties
	  • Exfoliation of urothelial cells
	  • Bacterial interference by commensal microbes of distal urogenital tract
	  • Mucosal innate immunity
	• Antimicrobial properties of urine
	  • Urine pH
	  • Hyperosmolality
	  • Organic acids
	  • Tamm-Horsfall mucoproteins
	  • Host defence peptides
	• Systemic immunocompetence
	  • Cell-mediated immunity
	  • Humoral-mediated immunity

In humans and small animals, a **positive urine culture is not the same as having a UTI**. Humans lacking lower urinary tract signs that have persistent bacteriuria are denominated as with **asymptomatic bacteriuria (ASB)**. In those cases, treatment of ASB is not recommended because its eradication does not prevent future bladder re-colonization with bacteria and the presence of ASB may convey a degree of protection against urinary tract colonization with other bacteria.

In veterinary medicine, **recognition of subtle urinary tract signs is challenging** and as such the term subclinical bacteriuria may be more adequate. **Subclinical bacteriuria is defined as the presence of bacteria in the urine (collected by cystocentesis) in the absence of clinical signs of urinary tract infection**. Treatment is not recommended.

Bacterial count (CFU/ml) cannot differentiate subclinical bacteriuria from bacterial cystitis. In the previous guidelines, ISCAID supported the treatment of animals with no clinical signs but with cytological evidence of pyuria (and positive culture) but currently, treatment of animals with active sediment without lower urinary tract signs is not recommended even in the presence of a positive urine culture. Additionally, in these cases culture would not be recommended from the outset.

The reported rate of **subclinical bacteriuria** is 2–12% in healthy dogs and **1–13% in healthy cats**. The frequency of subclinical bacteriuria is reported more frequently in animals with concurrent diseases such as **diabetes mellitus and immunosuppressed animals**. Some studies have looked at the potential effect of subclinical bacteriuria affecting survival when no antibiotics have not been prescribed and no significant effect has been seen either dogs or cats.

Predisposing factors for urinary tract infection and subclinical bacteriuria

- Systemic factors
  - Age
  - Female
  - CKD
  - Diabetes mellitus
  - Hyperthyroidism (recently questioned on a study)
- Local factors
  - Perineal urethrostomy
  - Urinary catheter
  - Urolithiasis
  - Bladder neoplasia
  - Subcutaneous ureteral bypass
  - Ureteral stenting
  - Incontinence

ISCAID recommends **not performing urine culture of animals with no evidence of urinary tract disease when there is no indication to treat based on a positive result**. In animals where there is uncertainty on the presence of clinical signs, a short course (3–5 days) could be considered. The isolation of a multi-resistant organism should not change the decision to not treat subclinical bacteriuria.

Screening may be performed in **difficult to regulate or DKA diabetics** and also in patients in which the ability to demonstrate lower urinary tract signs is questionable (e.g. paralysed patients). Other potential situations where screening may be indicated are:

- Suspected pyelonephritis
- Investigation of the bladder as a potential source of bacteremia/sepsis
- Patients that undergo procedures that will involve entering the urinary tract
- Patients with suspected struvite urolithiasis

ISCAID does not recommend re-testing of subclinical bacteriuric animals as the decision would still be to not treat.

There are some cases in which treatment of subclinical bacteriuria may be considered:

- Isolation of *Corynebacterium urealyticum* and urease-producing bacteria as they can cause encrusting cystitis and struvite-uroliths respectively.
- If there is concern about the risk of ascending infection, systemic infection, or that the bladder maybe a focus of extra-urine infection.
- Patients that are unable to exhibit clinical signs of lower urinary tract disease.

A urinary tract infection should not be diagnosed based exclusively on the presence of lower urinary signs, even if there is concurrent inflammatory sediment. It is essential to perform **culture of urine obtained by cystocentesis**.

The majority of urinary tract infections (>85%) are caused by a single organism. UTI's caused by two different pathogens represent around 13% of the cases and they usually occur in cats with urinary catheters or anomalies of the local defenses.

The pathogens that commonly cause UTIs in dogs and cats are very similar with *E.coli* being the most common and represents 1/3 to 1/2 of the cases. Gram-positive cocci are the second major group (*Staphylococcus spp. Streptococcus spp.* and *Enterococcus spp.*) accounting for 1/3 to 1/4 of the isolates. The remainder of cases are caused by *Proteus, Klebsiella, Pasteurella* and *Pseudomonas*.

Clinical signs

The development of clinical signs of urinary infection depends on the **site and duration of infection**. Signs of lower tract UTI include:

- pollakiuria
- stranguria
- haematuria
- inappropriate urination.

Patients with upper urinary tract can exhibit:

- fever
- pain
- haematuria
- PU/PD
- renal failure
- septicaemia.

Diagnosis

A diagnosis of a UTI should be made based on the results of urinalysis with sediment, urine culture and sensitivity alongside the presence of clinical signs. The presence of **haematuria and proteinuria**, although common with UTI's, is **not specific** and associated with multiple other causes. **Sediment analysis alone is inadequate** for diagnosis of a UTI due to problems with variable quality of interpretation, stain contamination and false-positive bacteriuria.

It is useful to remember the reported sensitivity and specificity for detecting bacteriuria in unstained urine sediment is around 76% and 57% respectively; those figures increase to > 83% and > 98% when stains are used.

In general, in external laboratories, urine sediment is examined unstained therefore it may be sensible to request urine cytology when a UTI is suspected or if there is the need to look at cell morphology (e.g. urothelial neoplasia).

Potential reasons for discrepancy between the cytology and the urine culture results (most common causes in bold)

- Bacteria dead or non-viable
  - **Use of antibiotics**
  - **Transport (time and or conditions)**
  - Extreme pH of urine
- Pseudobacteria (especially if unstained)
  - Cellular debris
  - Lipid droplets
  - **Brownian motion**
  - **Contamination of stains**
  - Anaerobic bacteria
- Bacteria not successfully cultured
  - Fastidious organism
  - Laboratory error

Ideally antibiotic therapy should have been stopped for at least seven days (for short acting antibiotics) before a urine culture is performed; a bare minimum to consider is 72 hours. Cefovecin is a long-acting antibiotic which is slowly eliminated from the body with around 65 days needed to eliminate 97% of the drug from the body.

Even if antibiotics don't kill a specific pathogen *in vivo* they may prevent *in vitro* growth of the pathogens therefore affecting the culture results.

Ideally, urine culture should be performed even in patients with clinical signs for the first time, as it allows identification of the infectious agent and adequate choice of antibiotic therapy.

A **cystocentesis sample** should be used whenever a urine culture is needed and the urine **refrigerated** immediately and submitted for **analysis within 24 hours**. Free-catch samples should be avoided for culture and only used when cystocentesis is contraindicated due to potential for false positive. However, if these are used, culture of cystocentesis collected samples should be used to confirm positive culture from free-catch urine samples.

Lower urinary tract infection

According to the previous ISCAID guidelines, UTIs were classed as uncomplicated or complicated. However, the most recent ISCAID guidelines (2019) reclassified urinary tract infections as **sporadic bacterial cystitis and recurrent bacterial cystitis**. More information on the reason for the change can be found on the guidelines on the ISCAID website.

Sporadic bacterial cystitis

Sporadic bacterial cystitis is very common in dogs but infrequent in cats. In these cases, bacterial infection of the bladder leads to inflammation and lower urinary tract signs (e.g. haematuria, dysuria, pollakiuria, stranguria).

UTI clinical signs are mostly due to inflammation and as such, while awaiting the culture and sensitivity results, non-steroidal anti-inflammatories (provided there is no contra-indication for use) may help with the clinical signs. When the results are available, a UTI can be confirmed and the **antibiotic selection made based on sensitivity**.

In some cases, while awaiting culture results, it may be necessary to start antibiotic therapy and first-line antibiotics to consider are **amoxicillin and trimethoprim sulphonamide** (TMS); amoxicillin-clavulanic may be an acceptable alternative but there is no evidence that the addition of clavulanic acid is needed. The recommended duration of therapy is **three to five days**.

There is potential for concern with **TMS use regarding idiosyncratic and immune-mediated adverse effects** in some patients, particularly if therapy is prolonged. Also, TMS can be bitter when administered in suspension, which can decrease dramatically patient compliance. In cases where treatment over seven days is needed it is recommended to perform a **baseline Shirmer tear test** alongside period re-assessment; TMS should be avoided in patients with KCS, hepatopathy and hypersensitivity.

Fluoroquinolones and **third-generation cephalosporins** should be reserved for cases with proven need based on culture and sensitivity results.

Significant clinical response is expected within 48 hours of appropriate antibiotic therapy, if this is not the case, investigation of complicating factors (e.g. concurrent urolithiasis) should be considered. If there is no clinical response or if it is only partial it is not recommended to change simply antibiotics unless the sensitivity results indicate resistance to the initial choice. In these cases, further investigation is recommended.

If the clinical signs fully resolve there is no indication to repeat the urinalysis or culture after then end of therapy.

Recurrent bacterial cystitis

If the patient has > **3 episodes of bacterial cystitis in a period of 1 year** or > 2 episodes of bacterial cystitis in 6 months it is called **recurrent bacterial cystitis**. This is often associated with underlying causes and therefore **investigation of predisposing factors and comorbidities** is important. If the bacteria isolated is different from previous ones isolated re-infection is likely and there should be a conscious effort to identify and address predisposing factors such as the ones in the table below.

Comorbidities that should be considered in a dog or cat with bacterial cystitis (from ISCAID guidelines 2019)
Endocrinopathy
Kidney disease
Obesity
Abnormal vulvar conformation
Congenital abnormalities (e.g. ectopic ureter)
Prostatic disease
Bladder neoplasia
Polypoid cystitis
Urolithiasis
Immunosupressive therapy
Rectal fistula
Urinary incontinence/ retention

Other considerations to consider in cases of recurrent cystitis are:

- Re-infection
  - If the bacteria isolated is different from previous ones isolated, re-infection is likely and there should be a conscious effort to identify and address predisposing factors.
- Relapse
  - Recurrence of infection with the same strain of bacteria after successful treatment of the initial UTI. This can be due to failure to completely eliminate the pathogen (despite apparent clinical resolution), especially if there is a persistent nidus for infection.
- Persistent infection
  - In some cases, there is persistent positive culture of the same organism despite adequate antibiotic therapy, and this is denominated persistent infection.
- Superinfection
  - The development of infection with a different organism while on antibiotic therapy to address the agent for the initial bacterial cystitis; this is very rare.

For relapsing and persistent infections, it is important to be sure that the drug is achieving adequate concentrations in the bladder and to try to identify a potential nidus for infection to persist.

Previous guidelines suggested a four-week course of antibiotics for recurrent cystitis. The most recent guidelines suggest a short duration of treatment (3–5 days) for re-infection and longer courses (7–14 days) for cases of persistent and potentially relapsing infections. Longer course duration can be considered on a case-by-case approach.

If the treatment prescribed is short there is no recommendation for repeating the urinalysis and culture during the treatment but re-culture by cystocentesis should be considered 5–7 days after the end of the treatment.

In cases where longer treatments are prescribed, it may be reasonable to consider urinalysis and culture 5–7 days into the treatment (to prove that is negative) and repeating urinalysis and culture 5–7 days after then end of the treatment to document resolution.

Due to the lack of evidence-based data on the topic, the ISCAID guidelines don't recommend any preventative strategies such as:

- The use of pulse antibiotic therapy or chronic low-dose antibiotic administration is not recommended.
- Although some compounds in cranberry extract have shown to reduce bacterial attachment to the urothelium there is insufficient clinical data to support its use.
- There is no data on cats on the use of probiotics for prevention of recurrent UTI's; the available data in dogs demonstrated no benefit of oral administration.
- There is no evidence for clinical effect of intravesical instillation of antimicrobials, antiseptics or dimethylsulfoxide (DMSO).
- A small study of intravesical instillation of non-pathogenic *E.coli* in the bladder of dogs with recurrent UTI has shown promising results but a similar study in cats has not been found.

Upper urinary tract infection

The kidneys are reasonably protected against UTIs by virtue of ureteral flaps, ureteral length, and peristalsis and also the relatively hypoxic environment of the renal medulla. **The most common cause of pyelonephritis is ascending UTIs**. Haematogenous infection as a source of pyelonephritis is thought to be rare.

Although a definitive diagnosis of pyelonephritis has to be performed on basis of a positive culture of a pyelocentesis, a **positive culture of a cystocentesis sample** in face of suggestive signs +/− imaging is often used to achieve a diagnosis. In animals that are immunosuppressed or febrile a blood culture is recommended.

Acute presentation can be associated with signs such as anorexia, lethargy, pyrexia, painful kidneys, renomegaly, polyuria, polydipsia and gastrointestinal signs. However, in a study of confirmed pyelonephritis in cats, non-specific signs were the most common finding; pyrexia and renal pain were seen in only a small fraction of cases. Azotemia of varying degrees of severity was seen in all cats, with hyperphosphatemia and non-regenerative anaemia being also very frequent.

Information on chronic feline pyelonephritis is lacking. However, in dogs, chronic pyelonephritis can be associated with minimal clinical signs and can lead to progressive chronic renal disease.

Chronic pyelonephritis should be considered as a differential diagnosis in patients with chronic kidney disease that develop an acute-on chronic episode without another apparent cause.

Diseases that predispose to pyelonephritis include diabetes mellitus, hyperadrenocorticism, chronic renal disease, and urolithiasis of the upper urinary tract. Chronic pyelonephritis should always be considered in patients with chronic kidney disease that develop an acute-on-chronic episode.

In cases of suspected pyelonephritis treatment should start immediately with antibiotics alongside supportive therapy, pending culture and sensitivity results. The ISCAID guidelines recommend a **10–14 day course of treatment for acute bacterial pyelonephritis**.

Marbofloxacin (2.7–5.5 mg/kg PO SID) is considered the first-line drug of choice for pyelonephritis and the ISCAID (International Renal Interest Society) recommendations using the high-end of the dosing range.

Fluoroquinolones, particularly enrofloxacin, have been shown at high doses to cause acute retinal degeneration in cats. Additional risk factors for fluoroquinolone retinal toxicity in cats include old age, renal or hepatic impairment, prolonged administration and intravenous route of administration. **If enrofloxacin administration is required, do not exceed doses of 5 mg/kg** per day and administer it for the shortest duration possible. Owners of cats undergoing treatment with fluoroquinolones should monitor for dilated pupils or signs of vision loss and discontinue use immediately if noted. If a fluoroquinolone is required, some options have a lower risk of ocular toxicity including marbofloxacin or pradofloxacin.

The use of urinary catheters and UTIs

Although the urinary tract has effective defence mechanisms if a large number of iatrogenic pathogenic agents are introduced the development of a UTI is possible.

The most **common cause of iatrogenic UTI is via the introduction of pathogens at the time of placement of a urinary catheter** and during the period of the presence of a urinary catheter with the **ascendant**

migration of bacteria either via the lumen of the catheter or via the external surface of the catheter. The organisms most commonly involved are **enteric bacteria**.

Colonization of the bladder can lead to subclinical bacteriuria and not necessarily bacterial cystitis. Both UTIs and subclinical bacterial colonization of the bladder are common in cats with indwelling urinary catheters and it is important to differentiate one from the other.

Urine culture is not needed if there are no clinical signs of urinary tract disease and routine urine cytology is not recommended for detection of bacteria or active sediment as this other can occur in the absence of bacterial cystitis.

ISCAID guidelines **discourage the culture of the urinary catheter tip** at the time of removal and the routine culture of urine after catheter removal. If after removal of a urinary catheter the patient develops suggestive signs the approach used for sporadic bacterial cystitis (discussed below) should be used.

In catheterized animals, bacterial cystitis should be suspected in those that develop urinary tract signs including fever of unknown origin but it is important to remember that some patients may not demonstrate clinical signs (e.g. paralysed animal). If there is a change in the appearance or smell of urine further investigation is also recommended.

If urine culture is performed in a catheterized animal due to clinical signs of cystitis, the urinary catheter should be removed and a **urine sample collected via cystocentesis**. The need for the continued use of a urinary catheter considered and if possible replacement with a new one should be avoided. If this is not possible or is contraindicated the initial 3–5 ml of urine collected should be discarded before collecting a sample via the existing catheter.

Measures to **avoid iatrogenic UTIs** include:

- avoid indiscriminate use of urinary catheters
- use a closed collection system with indwelling urinary catheters
- avoid indwelling catheters in immunosuppressed animals
- avoid antibiotic usage for patients with a urinary catheter
- appropriate aseptic catheter placement/care with regular inspection for potential issues that can lead to problems
- routine catheter replacement to prevent bacteriuria or cystitis is not recommended (contrary to previous suggestions)
- the use of catheter coated with antibacterial substances (e.g. silver or chlorhexidine) may help reduce the bacterial colonization but currently, there is not sufficient evidence to support this.

Ideally, urine culture should be performed even in patients with clinical signs for the first time, as it allows identification of the infectious agent and adequate choice of antibiotic therapy.

A **cystocentesis sample** should be used whenever a urine culture is needed, and the urine **refrigerated** immediately and submitted for **analysis within 24 hours**. Free-catch samples should be avoided for culture and only used when cystocentesis is contraindicated due to potential for false positive. However, if these are used, culture of cystocentesis collected samples should be used to confirm positive culture from free-catch urine samples.

Feline idiopathic cystitis (FIC)

Feline idiopathic cystitis is thought to be the result of chronic activation of the central threat response system (CTRS), which leads to activation of multiple systems and potential development of a multitude of clinical signs depending on the organ systems affected. Some of the cats with FIC have other comorbidities such as behavioural problems, endocrine disorders, and gastrointestinal disturbances. The complexity of the problem and multisystemic involvement has led to the use of the term "Pandora syndrome" by some authors in an attempt to highlight that FIC is not just a "bladder disease".

Chronic perception of stress leads to chronic activation of CTRS, frequently, very early in life and even *in utero*, resulting in over sensitization of the CTRS to the environment. However, it is possible for it to occur later in life.

The development of lower urinary tract signs results from a complex interaction involving susceptible individuals and provocative environments. Abnormalities that may contribute to the disease include defective bladder lining, neurogenic inflammation, and an abnormal response to stress.

Feline idiopathic cystitis (FIC) is the most common cause of lower urinary tract signs and can only be diagnosed after exclusion of other causes of lower urinary tract disease such as urolithiasis, bacterial UTI, anatomical abnormalities, and neoplasia. At times, it is not possible to completely rule out other causes and FIC is diagnosed presumptively based on signalment, suggestive history, minimal diagnostic tests, and good clinical response to treatment.

The reported **risk factors** for the development of idiopathic cystitis are:

Abnormalities that appear to be common and may contribute to the disease include

Defective bladder lining – The urine contains a high concentration of irritant substances that if it wasn't for a layer of glycosaminoglycans (GAGs) would irritate the bladder wall. In cats with FIC, this layer can be deficient allowing damage to the cells of the bladder wall and leading to ulceration and inflammation.

Neurogenic inflammation – The nerves in the bladder wall can be stimulated by local irritation of the bladder (see above) or also possibly from stimulation of the brain in cases of stress. This stimulation releases neurotransmitters, which can exacerbate pain and inflammation.

Stress – there is evidence that stress plays a very important role in FIC. Exclusively indoors cats and cats in a multicat household are typically more affected; it is important to remember that we (vets) and the owner might not necessarily perceive the presence of stress.

Abnormal response to stress – there is growing evidence that cats with FIC don't handle stress in a "normal" way. Patients with FIC catecholamine concentrations tend to be high and cortisol responses may be subnormal; this is in contrast to "normal" cases.

- neutering (not age of neutering)
- indoor living
- consumption of mostly dry food
- obesity
- sedentary lifestyle.

The pathophysiology of FIC is not fully understood and there is evidence that a large number of body systems such as bladder, nervous system and hypothalamic-pituitary-adrenal axis are involved in the development of disease. Studies of cats with FIC suggest it is multifactorial and the development of clinical signs requires predisposing **intrinsic abnormalities** (bladder, nervous system, adrenal gland) and also **extrinsic factors** (stress factors).

Clinical signs

The clinical signs seen include:

- pollakiuria
- stranguria
- inappropriate urination
- haematuria and/or
- pain on urination.

Clinical signs secondary to urethral obstruction and its consequences (e.g. collapse, acute abdomen) can also occur.

Physical examination reveals a **small painful bladder** and, if there is urinary obstruction, severe signs of systemic disease and an over-distended bladder may be present.

Diagnosis

The diagnosis of FIC is attempted by the **exclusion of other causes** of feline lower urinary tract disease. In chronic cases with multiple relapses, or in cases where there are concerns about potential underlying bladder neoplasia, obtaining bladder biopsies is indicated.

Treatment

Few treatments for FIC have been investigated by well-controlled double-blinded experimental studies. Most treatments are recommended from uncontrolled clinical observations and, as FIC is usually self-limiting, many treatments appear effective.

The goals of treatment are:

- **decrease the severity and duration** of clinical signs during an acute episode.
- **increase the interval** between episodes in patients with recurrent bouts.
- **decrease the severity** of clinical signs in patients with persistent idiopathic cystitis.

The best approach to the management of FIC is to **use multimodal treatment**.

It is important to keep in mind that FIC is **not just a "bladder problem"**. Key points in the treatment of FIC are reducing the output of the sympathetic nervous system, identify and modify suspected predisposing factors such as diet, water intake, indoor living, animal husbandry, stress, and inactivity. **Treatment of pain** is also very important and breaking the cycle of pain-inflammation is crucial; systemic central analgesia seems to be more important than local analgesia.

In the initial stages, in patients with **acute episodes**, the following measures should be considered.

Household cleaning

Ensure all areas where inappropriate urination has occurred are thoroughly cleaned.

Analgesia

FIC is a painful condition and analgesia should be provided. Drugs frequently used are **buprenorphine** or full-agonist opioids (if needed) and **meloxicam**. The use of analgesia alone is insufficient to control FIC.

Diet change

One of the most significant recommendations for management of FIC is diet change, to produce dilute urine

(SG < 1.035) and more frequent urination. Despite some recent controversy, this is still recommended. This is achieved by **switching from dry food to a wet diet (tins or sachets)**. If necessary, water can be added to the food and water fountains provided.

Cats are not usually very compliant with dietary changes. A very gradual introduction of the new diet and warming the food to body temperature might be required while attempting to transition the diet.

Stress reduction

Stress plays a key role in the development of FIC. Potential stress factors include living with another cat from a different social group, abrupt changes in diet or environment, overcrowding, owner stress, and the addition of new pets/people to the household.

At times it might not be possible to remove completely potential stress factors therefore other things such as **environmental enrichment** and provision of synthetic pheromones may play an important role.

- **Synthetic feline pheromones** may help reduce anxiety in cats with FIC in multicat households, however, it should be used in combination with other strategies.
- **Milk protein hydrolysates** may help reduce anxiety in cats and they are found in Zylkene® (MSD), Royal Canin Calm® and Hill's c/d urinary stress®; this diet also contains (L-tryphophan and GAG's).

Environmental enrichment

The indoor environment (www.indoorpet. osu.edu) of some cats is monotonous and predictable which could lead to stress. Also, the presence of other cohabitants (feline or not) might also play a role.

The following measures can be tried to make the environment more stimulating.

- Spending time **playing with the cat** regularly – setting aside time each day and using new and different toys.
- Allowing the cat some **outdoor access**, even in an enclosed run if necessary, can provide interest and stimulation
- Modify the environment so that there is **plenty of interest** for the cat (scratching posts etc) and resting places for the cat. Cats need space and to control their environment, at least to some extent. Also, they require the ability to explore their environment and have hiding places – ideally in elevated locations (e.g., on top of furniture or cupboards).

Modification of urination

Cats with FIC are often stressed and therefore the urination patterns might be altered. Maximising the likelihood that the cat will urinate frequently is very important and the following measures can be implemented and therefore in the household, there should be at least **one litter tray per cat and one spare** if possible. The litter trays should be placed in **different quiet locations** to encourage frequent urination. Most cats are very fussy with litter therefore the choice of litter may also be an important factor to consider.

Other measures

Patients that fail to respond in seven days or that have frequent recurrences should have the same measures instituted and the addition of further drugs should be considered.

Although the use of GAG's may be beneficial, the current published double-blinded, placebo-controlled studies showed no significant difference with their use, either with oral N-acetyl glucosamine (NAG), or with **oral or injectable pentosan polysulphate (PPS)**. However, some individual cats appear to benefit from GAG supplementation. Some of the GAG supplements available in the market such as Cystease® (Ceva Animal Health) contain also hyaluronic acid and L-tryptophan which can help reduce stress.

Tricyclic antidepressants (TCAs) have anticholinergic (increase bladder capacity, relax urethra and ureters), anti-inflammatory, analgesic, and antidepressant properties. However, two studies documented the short-term use of amitriptyline increased the risk of recurrence and in a long-term one-year study, it appeared to reduce clinical signs. TCAs should be reserved for severe chronic cases; liver function should be monitored before and during treatment.

Treatment of cases of obstructive FIC requires the same medical treatment and management as non-obstructive cases; however, relieving the urethral obstruction and dealing with the potentially life-threatening complications is the most important first-line measure.

Although recent literature raised concerns about their efficacy, reducing urethral spasm may reduce the clinical signs of cystitis and reduce the risk of urethral obstruction. The use of anti-spasmodic drugs is rarely associated with side-effects, but it is important to remember that hypotension and hepatotoxicity (amongst others) can occur. Relaxants of both smooth (prazosin, phenoxybenzamine, acepromazine) and skeletal muscle (dantrolene) should be considered.

Prognosis

The prognosis of FIC is vastly dependent on controlling/managing different groups of factors:

- **patient factors**: genetic predisposition, duration of the problem, frequency of episodes, specifics of the inappropriate urination if existing.

- **housing factors**: number of cats in the household, availability of outdoor living, the feasibility of rearranging environment, etc.
- **owner factors**: the ability to identify and modify causes, human bond with affected cat, time dedicated to solving the problem, willingness to follow advise and administer medication.

Treatment is usually considered successful on the basis of the resolution of clinical signs and associated abnormalities such as haematuria, proteinuria, bladder wall thickening and pain.

Patients with chronic FIC are usually more difficult to treat than patients with a single acute episode or infrequent flare-ups. In these two last groups of patients, resolution of clinical signs is often spontaneous and occurs within one week in around 85% of the cases. However, the risk of recurrence is very high within the subsequent six to twelve months. If there is no improvement within seven days, spontaneous resolution is considered unlikely.

Lower urinary tract neoplasia

Neoplasia of the lower urinary tract is very uncommon in cats. However, when encountered, it is more frequent in the bladder than the urethra. The most common neoplasia is urothelial carcinoma or transitional cell carcinoma; other types of tumours are rarer.

Tumours of the bladder are commonly associated with lower urinary tract signs such as haematuria, pollakiuria, inappropriate urination, incontinence, and tenesmus. Urinary obstruction may occur if patients present with a mass in the trigone. Secondary urinary tract infection is common in patients with bladder neoplasia.

Urothelial carcinoma or transitional cell neoplasia is the most common tumour and tends to be an aggressive disease that often has already invaded into the muscular layers of the bladder at the time of initial presentation. Additionally, over 20% of the cats already have metastasis at the time of diagnosis with organs such as liver and lungs more affected than regional lymph nodes.

The location of the neoplasia seems a lot more variable in cats than in dogs with around 27% of cases being in the trigone.

Prostatic neoplasia is extremely rare in cats with most reported cases being prostatic adenocarcinoma in older castrated cats. There is limited information on treatment options, however prostatectomy and chemotherapy might offer longer survival times.

Diagnosis

Imaging is essential in the diagnosis of a bladder mass but a definitive diagnosis of TCC can be difficult to achieve. **FNAs should be avoided** due to the risk of seeding (as per data available in dogs) and therefore catheterization can be used to try to obtain a representative sample of the mass under ultrasound guidance. However, it is frequent for surgical biopsies to be necessary for the diagnosis.

Prognosis

A recent study documented a **median survival time of 46 days without treatment** and 176 days for cats treated without partial cystectomy. The median survival time for cats treated with partial cystectomy +/– other treatments was 294 days and 25% of the cases were alive at 600 days after the diagnosis. In this study, the NSAIDs most frequently used were **meloxicam and piroxicam** with GI signs and worsening of the azotaemia being the most common adverse effects. In some cases, chemotherapy was also used.

Congenital problems of the lower urinary tract

Whenever a congenital problem is detected it is worth considering what other concurrent problems may be present.

Urachal anomalies

The urachus is a foetal connection that allows urine to pass between the foetal bladder and the placenta. Around the time of birth, the urachus should have undergone a complete atrophy and be non-functional as fibrous connective tissue linking the bladder apex to the umbilicus. If there is complete closure and atrophy of the urachus we have then a urachal anomaly.

There are 4 types of urachal anomalies described in small animals: patent urachus, urachal cysts and vesicourachal diverticula are the most common.

If the urachus is patent there is a connection between the bladder and the umbilicus with urine dripping, omphalitis and likely associated urinary infection. If both extremities of the urachal involute and close leaving a focal section unchanged, then we are faced with a urachal cyst which is unlikely to lead to clinical signs.

A vesicourachal diverticulum occurs when a portion of the urachus does not close and remains associated with the bladder apex; if it is a blind diverticulum that protrudes from the bladder apex is called an extramural diverticulum while if it is limited to the thickness of the bladder wall it is called intramural. The diverticulae can be microscopic or macroscopic.

Most of the patients have urachal anomalies diagnosed incidentally with vesicourachal diverticulum being the most frequent urachal anomaly in cats. When clinical signs are present, they are usually signs of lower urinary tract disease such as stranguria and pollakiuria.

Microscopic diverticulae are not usually clinically significant but, in some cases, due to inflammatory conditions or problems that increase intravesical pressure (e.g. cystitis and UTI), they can increase in size and become macroscopic and clinically relevant. It is possible for the macroscopic diverticulum to disappear (usually in 2 to 3 weeks) when the underlying problem is resolved. In some cases, these diverticulae can act as nidus for recurrent UTI's and surgical treatment may be indicated if they don't regress.

Macroscopic diverticula are more likely to be associated with urinary tract infection and clinical signs of lower urinary tract disease.

There are studies that document a high percentage (around 40%) of urachal diverticulae in cats with lower urinary tract problems.

The diagnosis of a urachal diverticulae can be made with radiographic contrast studies, ultrasound, or cystoscopy albeit nowadays they are mostly diagnosed with ultrasound.

Ectopic ureters

Normally, the ureters enter the bladder in the dorsolateral surface of the bladder in the trigonus through an intramural route.

Ectopic ureters enter the bladder in a different location due to congenital problems and it can be uni or bilateral. Ectopic ureters can also be intra or extramural. **Ectopic ureters are very rare in cats.**

Incontinence and urine retention

The urinary tract is mostly designed to store urine and therefore the bladder is in storage phase around 99% of the time and only around 1% in micturition phase.

The coordination of the storage and micturition phases requires complex interactions between the peripheral nervous system and the autonomic nervous system. In addition, the voluntary control of micturition requires the involvement of the cerebral cortex, brainstem and also lumbar and sacral segments of the spinal cord.

Disorders of micturition are broadly divided into those causing urine retention and those causing incontinence. In some animals there is some overlap as urine retention can lead to patients exhibiting signs of incontinence therefore it is important to establish that patients with incontinence can urinate normally at other times. Incontinence is defined as involuntary leakage of urine, which is different from periuria (normal voluntary urination in an inappropriate place).

Bladder storage problems occur due to inadequate tonus of the urethra when the pressure in the bladder is normal or increased. These problems can be secondary to anatomical problems, congenital anomalies or acquired problems of the bladder, urethra, or spinal cord. Bladder storage problems can lead to incontinence.

Lower motor neuron bladder secondary to spinal cord disease is one of the most common causes of storage problems. It occurs due to problems with the spinal segments S1-S3. In these cases, the patient may exhibit overflow incontinence, the bladder is easily expressed, and patients have other associated neurological deficits such as decreased/absent perineal reflex, decreased/absent anal tone. In these patients, it is very important that the bladder is emptied regularly during the day to avoid overdistension, either by manual expression or via catheterization. These patients are at higher risk of developing a UTI.

Although urethral sphincter mechanism incompetence has been reported in cats this is a very rare cause of feline incontinence.

Voiding problems can be the result of functional or mechanical problems that lead to urinary obstruction or problems with contraction of the detrusor muscle. Patients with urinary retention can present with dysuria, stranguria or might not be able to urinate. Most patients have an enlarged bladder and may have urine overflow. Uroabdomen due to bladder rupture is also possible.

Common causes of urinary retention are mechanical in origin (e.g. urolithiasis) or functional (e.g. urethral spasm).

Direct damage to the detrusor muscle due to overdistension can occur secondarily to mechanical or functional urethral obstruction. It is important to assess the primary problem and maintain the bladder small for at least two weeks to allow reversion of the overstretching of the bladder wall and tight junctions. The use of bethanecol may help in these cases and there are some studies that suggest that metoclopramide and cisapride may be of use in some cases.

Dysautonomia has been reported very infrequently in the UK. It has an unknow aetiology but exposure to a neurotoxin has been postulated. Patients with dysautonomia have bladder emptying problems due to bladder atony and they may also have overflow incontinence.

The most common causes of urinary retention are mechanical in origin (e.g. urolithiasis, neoplasia) and, less frequently functional causes, which usually should only be considered after mechanical causes have been ruled out.

True incontinence is extremely rare in cats and therefore it is essential to try to understand if patients with reported incontinence have urinary overflow secondary to bladder overdistension. According to recent studies, congenital and acquired spinal cord disease is the most common cause of feline incontinence. Ectopic ureters in cats are considered very rare and, in the vast majority, are extramural. Bilateral and unilateral ectopic ureters had the same prevalence in this study.

Until recently, there was very little data regarding the cause, treatment, and outcome in cats with clinical signs of urine leakage. In a recent paper, that included both cats with storage phase disorders and emptying phase disorders, documented the frequency of their frequency to be similar. In that study, when problems were classified by anatomic site, spinal cord problems were the most common cause (40% of the cases).

References

Acierno MJ, Brown S, Coleman AE et al. ACVIM consensus statement: Guidelines for the identification, evaluation, and management of systemic hypertension in dogs and cats. Vet Med Intern 2018; 32: 1803–1822.

Bartlett PC, Van Buren JW, Bartlett AD, et al. Case-control study of risk factors associated with feline and canine chronic kidney disease. Vet Med Intern 2010; Article ID 957570.

Berent AC, Weisse CW, Todd K, Bagley DH. Technical and Clinical Outcomes of Ureteral Stenting in Cats with Benign Ureteral Obstruction:69 cases (2006–2010). J Am Vet Med Ass. 2014; 244: 559–576.

Bijsmans ES, Doig M, Jepson RE, et al. Factors influencing the relationship between the dose of amlodipine required for blood pressure control and change in blood pressure in hypertensive cats. J Vet Intern Med 2016; 30: 1939–1676.

Boyd LM, Langston C, Thompson K, Zivin K, Imanishi M. Survival in Cats with Naturally Occurring Chronic Kidney Disease (2000–2002). J Vet Intern Med 2008; 22: 1111–1117.

Braff J, Obare E, Yerramilli M, et al. Relationship between serum symmetric dimethylarginine concentration and glomerular filtration rate in cats. J Vet Intern Med 2014; 28:1699–1701.

Brown CA, Elliott J, Schmiedt CW, Brown SA. Chronic Kidney Disease in Aged Cats: Clinical Features, Morphology, and Proposed Pathogeneses. Vet Pathol 2016; 53: 309–326.

Brown SA (2016) Systemic hypertension (www.iris-kidney.com).

Brown SA (2016) Grading of acute kidney injury (www.iris-kidney.com).

Buffington CA. Idiopathic Cystitis in Domestic Cats- Beyond the Lower Urinary Tract. J Vet Intern Med 2011;25: 784–786.

Buffington CA. Household Resource Checklist. The Indoor Pet Initiative. 2014. www.indoorpet.osu.edu.

Buffington CA, Chew DJ. Management of non-obstructive idiopathic/interstitial cystitis in cats. BSAVA Manual of Canine and Feline Nephrology and Urology 3rd edition. 2017: 317–327.

Buffington CA, Westropp JL, Chew DJ. From FUS to Pandora syndrome. J Fel Med Surg 2014;16:385–394.

Buffington CA, Westropp JL, Chew DJ, Bolus RR. Clinical Evaluation of Multimodal Environmental Modification (MEMO) in the Management of Cats with idiopathic cystitis. J Fel Med Surg 2006; 8:261–268.

Buresova E, Stock E et al. Assessment of symmetric dymethylarginine as a biomarker of renal function in hyperthyroid cats treated with radioiodine. J Vet Intern Med 2019; 33: 516–522.

Carney HC, Sadek TP, Curtis TM et al. AAFP and ISFM Guidelines for Diagnosing and Solving House-soiling Behaviour in cats. J Fel Med Surg 2014;16:579–598.

Chakrabarti S, Syme HM. Elliott J. Clinicopathological variable predicting progression of azotemia in cats with chronic kidney disease. J Vet Intern Med 2012; 26:275–281.

Chalhoub S, Langston CE, Farrely J. The Use of Darbopoetin to Stimulate Erythropoiesis in Anemia of Chronic Kidney Disease in Cats:25 cases. J Vet Intern Med 2012; 26: 363–369.

Cole L, Panagiotis M, Humm K. Ultrasonographic findings in cats with acute kidney injury: a retrospective study. J Fel Med Surg 2019; 21: 475–480.

Coleman AE, Brown SA. Hypertension and the kidney. BSAVA Manual of Small Animal Nephrology and Urology. 2017. 126–223.

Coleman AE, Elliot J (2019) Inhibition of the renin-angiotensin-aldosterone system in dogs and cats: The emerging role of angiotensin receptor blockers.

Connaly HE, Hamar DW and Thrall MA. Inhibition of canine and feline alcohol dehydrogenase activity by fomipezole. Am J Vet Res 200; 61: 450–455.

Cowgill LD, Polzin DJ, Elliott J, et al. Is Progressive Chronic Kidney Disease a Slow Acute Kidney Injury? Vet Clin North Am Small Anim Pract 2016; 46: 995–1013.

Dantas LM, Delgado MM, Johnson I, Buffington T. Food puzzles for cats: feeding for physical and emotional wellbeing. J Fel Med Surg 2016; 18: 723–732.

Dirrig H, Lamb CR, Kulenda N et al. Diagnostic imaging observations in cats treated with the subcutaneous ureteral bypass system. J Small Anim Prac 2020; 61: 24–31.

Ellis SL, Rodan I, Carney HC et al. AAFP and ISFM feline environmental needs guidelines. J Fel Med Surg 2013; 15: 219–230.

Elliot J (2016) Treatment of vomiting, nausea and inappetance in cats with chronic kidney disease (www.iris-kidney.com).

Elliott J, Rawlings JM, Markwell PJ, et al. Survival of cats with naturally occurring chronic renal failure: effect of dietary management. J Small Anim Pract 2000; 41: 235–242.

Elliot J, White J (2019) Overview of the IRIS staging system for CKD (www.iris-kidney.com).

Ferguson LE, McLean MK, Bates JA, Quimby JM. (2016) Mirtazapine toxicity in cats: retrospective study of 84 cases (2006–2011). J Feline Med Surg. 2015 Jul 30. pii: 1098612X15599026.

Finch NC, Geddes RF, Syme HM. Fibroblast growth factor 23 (FGF-23) concentrations in cats with early nonazotemic chronic kidney disease (CKD) and in healthy geriatric cats. J Vet Intern Med 2013; 27: 227–233.

Finch NC, Heiene R, Elliot J, Syme HM, Peters AM. A single sample method of estimating glomerular filtration rate in cats. J Vet Intern Med 2013; 27; 782–790.

Finch NC, Syme HM, Elliott J. Risk Factors for Development of Chronic Kidney Disease in Cats. J Vet Intern Med 2016; 30: 602–610.

Frank D, Beauchamp G, Palestrini C. Systematic review of the use of pheromones for treatment of undesirable behaviour in cats and dogs. J Am Vet Med Assoc 2010; 236: 1308–1316.

Grauer G (2016) Measurement and interpretation of proteinuria and albuminuria (www.iris-kidney.com).

Geddes RF, Biouge V, Chang Y, Syme HM, Elliot J. The Effect of Moderate Dietary Protein and Phosphate Restriction on Calcium-Phosphate Homeostasis in Healthy Older Cats 2016; 30: 1690–1702.

Geddes R, Elliot J (2017) Assessment of calcium and phosphate homeostasis in chronic kidney disease. In BSAVA Manual of Canine and Feline Nephrology and Urology, 2017; 143–150.

Geddes RF, Elliott J, Syme HM. The effects of feeding a renal diet on plasma fibroblast growth factor 23 concentrations in cats with stable azotemic chronic kidney disease. J Vet Intern Med 2013; 27: 1354–1361.

Geddes RF, Finch NC, Syme HM, et al. The role of phosphorus in the pathology of chronic kidney disease. J Vet Emerg Crit Care 2013; 23: 122–133.

Geddes RF, Finch NC, Elliot J, Syme HM. Fibroblast Growth Factor 23 in Feline Chronic Kidney Disease. J Vet Intern Med 2013; 27: 234–241.

Grauer GF (2019) – Reassessment of normal values in dogs and cats with chronic kidney disease (www.iris-kidney.com).

Grauer GF (2019) – Utility of creatinine, UPC and SDMA in the early diagnosis of CKD in dogs and cats.

Greene JP, Lefebvre SL, Wang M, et al. Risk factors associated with the development of chronic kidney disease in cats evaluated at primary care veterinary hospitals. J Am Vet Med Assoc 2014; 244: 320–327.

Griffin MA, Culp WT, Giufridda MA et al. Lower urinary tract transitional cell carcinoma in cats: Clinical findings, treatments and outcomes in 118 cases. J Vet Inter Med 2019; early view article published November 2019.

Hall JE, Yerramilli M, Obare E, et al. Comparison of serum concentrations of symmetric dimethylarginine and creatinine as kidney function biomarkers in cats with chronic kidney disease. J Vet Intern Med 2014; 28: 1676–1683.

Hall JE, Yerramilli, Obare E, et al. Serum concentration of symmetric dimethylarginine in cats with kidney stones. PLos One 2017; 12 (4): e0174854.

Hardy BT, Brito Galvao JF, Green TA, Braudaway SR, DiBartola SP, Lord L, Chew DJ. Treatment of Ionised Hypercalcemia in 12 Cats (2006–2008) Using PO-Administered Alendronate. J Vet Intern Med 2015; 29: 200–206.

Heiene R and Lefebvre HP (2013) Glomerular filtration rate in dogs and cats (www.iris-kidney.com).

Horowitz C, Berent A, Weisse C, Langston C, Bagley D. Predictors of Outcome for Cats with Ureteral Obstructions after Interventional Management Using Ureteral Stents or a Subcutaneous Ureteral Bypass Device. J Fel Med Surg. 2013; 15: 1052–1062.

Hutting A (2016) Urine collection in dogs and cats (www.iris-kidney.com).

Jepson RE. Feline systemic hypertension: Classification and pathogenesis. J Feline Med Surg 2011; 13: 25–34. King JN, Gunn-Moore DA, Tasker S, et al. Tolerability and efficacy of benazepril in cats with chronic kidney disease. J Vet Intern Med 2006; 20: 1054–1064.

Jepson RE. Current Understanding of the Pathogenesis of Progressive Chronic Kidney Disease in Cats. Vet Clin North Am Small Anim Pract 2016; 46: 1015–1048.

Jepson RE, Brodbelt D, Elliott J, et al. Evaluation of the effects of control of systolic blood pressure on survival in cats with systemic hypertension. J Vet Intern Med 2007; 21: 402–409.

Jepson RE, Syme HM, Elliott J. Plasma renin activity and aldosterone concentrations in hypertensive cats with and without azotemia and in response to treatment with amlodipine besylate. J Vet Intern Med 2014; 28: 144–153.

Kopecny L, Palm CA, Drobatz KJ et al. Risk factors for positive urine cultures in cats with subcutaneous ureteral bypass and ureteral stents (2010–2011). J Vet Intern Med 2019; 33: 178–183.

Kruger JM, Lulich JP, MacLeay J et al. Comparison of foods with different nutritional profiles for long-term management of acute non-obstructive idiopathic cystitis in cats. J Am Vet Med Assoc 2015; 247: 508–517.

Kyle AE, Hardie EM, Wooden BG et al. Clinical, clinopathological, radiographic and ultrasonographic abnormalities in cats with ureteral calculi: 163 cases (1984–2002) J Am Vet Med Assoc. 2005; 226: 932–936.

Kyle AE, Hardie EM, Wooden BG et al. Management and outcome of cats with ureteral calculi: 153 cases (1982–2002). 2005 J Am Vet Med Assoc; 226: 937–944.

Lister A, Thompson M, Moss S et al. Feline bacterial urinary tract infections: an update on en evolving clinical problem. Veterinary Journal. 2011; 187: 18–22.

Lonc KM, Kaneene JB et al. Retrospective analysis of diagnoses and outcomes of 45 cats with micturition disorders presenting as urinary incontinence. J Vet Int Med 2019.

Ludovic P, Elliot J. Effects of non-steroidal anti-inflammatory drug treatment on the kidney. BSAVA Manual of Canine and Feline Nephrology and Urology 3rd edition. 2017; 232–245.

Lulich JP, Brent AC, Adams LG, Westropp JL, Bartges JW, Osborne CA. ACVIM Small Animal Consensus Recommendation on the Treatment and Prevention of Uroliths in Dogs and Cats. J Vet Intern Med 2016; 30: 1564–1574.

Maggio F, De Francesco TC, Atkins CE, et al. Ocular lesions associated with systemic hypertension in cats: 69 cases (1985–1998). J Am Vet Med Assoc 2000; 217: 695–702.

Marino CL, Lascelles et al. Prevalence and classification of chronic kidney disease in cats randomly selected from four age groups and in cats recruited for degenerative joint disease studies. J Fel Med Surg 2014; 16: 465–472.

Mason B, Pierce S, Hu T, and Poole M. Open-label pilot efficacy study of recombinant feline erythropoietin in client-owned cats with non-regenerative anemia. Abstract presented at AAFP World Feline Conference 2019 in San Francisco, USA.

Matthews K, Kronen P, et al. Guidelines for recognition, assessment and treatment of pain: WSAVA global pain council. J Small Anim Pract 2014; 55: E10–E68.

Mcloughlin MA. Complications of lower urinary tract surgery in small animals. 2011. Veterinary Clinics of North America: Small Animal Practice; 41: 889–913.

Milligan M, Berent AC. Medical and interventional management of upper urinary tract uroliths. Vet Clin North America 2019; 49: 157–174.

Mizutani H, Koyama H, Watanabe T, et al. Evaluation of the clinical efficacy of benazepril in the treatment of chronic renal insufficiency in cats. J Vet Intern Med 2006; 20: 1074–1079.

Monteiro B, Steagall PVM et al. Long-term use of non-steroidal anti-inflammatory drugs in cats with chronic kidney disease: from controversy to optimism. J Small Anim Pract 2019; 60: 459–462.

Nielsen LK, Bracker K, Price LL. Administration of fenoldopam in critically ill small animal patients with acute kidney injury: 28 dogs and 34 cats (2008–2012). J Vet Emerg Crit Care 2015; 25: 396–404.

Nicoli S, Morello E, Martano M, Pisoni L, Buracco P. Double-J ureteral stenting in nine cats with ureteral obstruction. Veterinary Journal. 2012; 194; 60–65.

Peterson ME, Nichols R and Rishniw. Serum thyroid and thyroid stimulating hormone concentration in hyperthyroid cats that develop azotaemia after radioiodine therapy. J Small Anim Pract 2017; 58: 519–530.

Peterson ME, Varela FV, Rishniw M, Polzin DJ. Evaluation of Serum Symmetric Dimethylarginine Concentration as a Marker for Masked Chronic Kidney Disease in Cats with Hyperthyroidism. J Vet Intern Med 2018; 32: 295–304.

Plantinga EA, Everts H, Kastelein AMC, Beynen AC: Retrospective study of the survival of cats with acquired chronic renal insufficiency offered different commercial diets. Vet Rec 2005; 157: 185–7.

Pollard RE, Phillips KL. Diagnostic imaging of the urinary tract. In BSAVA Manual of Canine and Feline Nephrology and Urology. 2017. 84–115.

Polzin (2016) Diets for cats with chronic kidney disease (www.iris-kidney.com).

Quimby JM, Brock WT, Moses K, Bolotin D, Patricelli K. Chronic use of maropitant for the management of vomiting and inappetance in cats with chronic kidney disease: a blinded, placebo-controlled clinical trial. J Feline Med Surg; 2015; 17: 692–7.

Quimby JM, Gustafson DL, Lunn KF. The pharmacokinetics of mirtazapine in cats with chronic kidney disease and in age-matched control cats. J Vet Intern Med. 2011; 25: 985–9.

Quimby JM, Lunn KF. Mirtazapine as an appetite stimulant and anti-emetic in cats with chronic kidney disease: a masked placebo-controlled crossover clinical trial. Vet J 2013; 197: 651–5.

Ross SJ, Polzin DJ, Osborne CA. Clinical progression of early chronic renal failure and implications for management. In August JR (ed): Consultations in Feline Internal Medicine. St Louis: Elsevier Saunders, 2005, pp. 389–398.

Ross SJ, Osborne CA, Kirk CA, et al. Clinical evaluation of dietary modification for treatment of spontaneous chronic kidney disease in cats. J Am Vet Med Assoc 2006; 229: 949–957.

Ross SJ, Osborne CA, Lekcharoensuk C, et at. A case-control study of the effects of nephrolithiasis in cats with chronic kidney disease. J Am Vet Med Assoc 2007; 230: 1854–1859.

Roudebush P, Polzin DJ, Ross SJ, et al. Therapies for feline chronic kidney disease. What is the evidence? J Fel Med Surg 2009; 11:195–210.

Roura X (2016) Risk factors in dogs and cats for development of chronic kidney disease (www.iris-kidney.com).

Segev G (2018) Biomarkers of kidney disease: potential utilities (www.iris-kidney.com).

Segev G, Kass PH, Cowgill LD. A retrospective Study of Acute Kidney Injury in Cats and Development of a Novel Clinical Scoring System for Predicting Outcome for Cats Managed by Hemodialysis. J Vet Intern Med 2013; 27: 830–839.

Sent U, Gossl R, Elliot J, Syme HM, Zimmering T. Comparison of Efficacy of Long-term Oral Treatment with Telmisartan and Benazepril in Cats with Chronic Kidney Disease. J Vet Intern Med 2015: 29: 1479–1487.

Shropshire S, Quimby J, Cerda R. Comparison of single, averaged and Pooled Urine Protein:creatinine Ratios in Proteinuric Dogs Undergoing Medical Treatment. J Vet Intern Med 2018; 32: 288–294.

Sparkes AH, Caney S, Chalhoub S et al (2016) ISFM Consensus Guidelines on the Diagnosis and Management of Feline Chronic Kidney Disease. J Fel Med Surg 2016; 18: 219–239.

Syme H (2019) CKD early diagnosis (www.iris-kidney.com).

Syme HM, Barber PJ, Markwell PJ, et al. Prevalence of systolic hypertension in cats with chronic renal failure at initial evaluation. J Am Vet Med Assoc 2002; 220: 1799–1804.

Syme HM, Markwell PJ, Pfeiffer D, Elliott J. Survival of cats with naturally occurring chronic renal failure is related to severity of proteinuria. J Vet Intern Med 2006; 20: 528–535.

Takenaka M, Lio A, Sato R, Sakamoto K, Kurumatani H and KT-140 group Clinical Study Group. A Double-Blinded, Placebo-controlled, Multicenter, Prospective, Randomized Study of Beraprost Sodium Treatment for Cats with Chronic Kidney Disease. J Vet Intern Med 2018; 32: 236–248.

Taylor SS, Goodfellow MR, Browne WJ et al. Feline Extranodal Lymphoma: response to chemotherapy and survival in 110 cats. J Small Anim Pract 2009; 50: 584–592.

Taylor SS. Sparkes AH, Briscoe K, Sala SV et al. ISFM Consensus Guidelines on the Diagnosis and Management of Hypertension in Cats. J Fel Med Surg (2017) 19, 288–303.

The IRIS Board. Preventing aminoglycoside-induced AKI (www.iris-kidney.com).

The IRIS Board. IRIS Grading of AKI (www.iris-kidney.com).

The IRIS Board. IRIS Staging of CKD (www.iris-kidney.com).

The IRIS Board. Treatment recommendations for CKD in cats (www.iris-kidney.com).

Vaden SL, Atkins C, Oyama M. Cardiovascular-renal disorders. In BSAVA Manual of Canine and Feline Nephrology and Urology, 2017.196–204.

Vaden SL, Brown C. Renal biopsy. In BSAVA Manual of Canine and Feline Nephrology and Urology. 2017; 161–171.

Van der Broek H, Elliot J (2019) Recent advances in Mineral and Bone disorders in CKD (www.iris-kidney.com).

Van den Broek DHN, Chang YM, Elliot J, Jepson RE. Chronic Kidney Disease in Cats and the Risk of Total Hypercalcemia. J Vet Intern Med 2017; 31: 465–475.

Vaske HH, Schermerhorn T, Grauer GF. Effects of feline hyperthyroidism on kidney function: a review. J Fel Med Surg 2016; 18: 55–59.

Watson ADJ, Lefebvre HP, Elliot J (2015) Using urine specific gravity (www.iris-kidney.com).

Weese JS et al. Brent. International Society for Companion Animal Infectious Diseases (ISCAID) guidelines for the diagnosis and management of bacterial urinary tract infections in dogs and cats. Vet Journal 2019; 247: 8–25.

Westropp JL, Delgao M, Buffington CAT. Chronic lower urinary tract signs in cats: current understanding of pathophysiology and management. Vet Clin North America 2019; 49: 187–209.

White JD, Cave NJ, Grinberg A, Thomas SG, Heuer C. Subclinical Bacteriuria in Older Cats and its Association with Survival. J Vet Intern Med 2016; 30: 1824–1829.

Williams T (2017) Hyperthyroidism and the feline kidney. In BSAVA Manual of Canine and Feline Nephrology and Urology. 2017, 205–215.

Williams TL, Elliot J, Syme HM. Effect on renal function of restoration of euthyroidism in hyperthyroid cats with iatrogenic hypothyroidism. J Vet Intern Med 2014; 28: 1251–1255.

Williams TL, Peak KJ et al. Survival and the development of azotemia after treatment of hyperthyroidism in cats. J Vet Intern Med 2010; 24: 863–869.

Wormser C, Reetz JA, Drobatz KJ, Aronson LR. Diagnostic Utility of Ultrasonography for Detection of the Cause and Location of Ureteral Obstructions in Cats: 71 cases (2010–2016). J Am Med Vet Assoc 2019; 254: 710–715.

Zaid MS, Berent AC, Weisse C, Caceres A. Feline Ureteral Strictures:10 cases (2007–2009). J Vet Intern Med 2011; 25: 222–229.

Further Reading

Buresova E, Stock E, Paepe D, Stammeleer L, Vandermeulen E, Smets P et al. Assessment of symmetric dimethylarginine as a biomarker of renal function in hyperthyroid cats treated with radioiodine. Journal of veterinary internal medicine. 2019 Jan; 33:2, pp- 516–22. doi.org/10.1111/jvim.15407.

DeltaDOT/RVC Iohexol assay. Veterinary diagnostics. http://www.deltadot.com/veterinary-diagnostics/.

Finch N. Measurement of glomerular filtration rate Measurement of glomerular filtration rate in cats: Methods and advantages over routine markers of renal function. Journal of feline medicine and surgery. 2014 Aug. doi.org/10.1177/1098612X14545274.

Finch NC; Geddes RF, Syme HM, Elliott J. Fibroblast Growth Factor 23 (FGF-23) Concentrations in Cats with Early Nonazotemic Chronic Kidney Disease (CKD) and in Healthy Geriatric Cats. Journal of veterinary internal medicine. 2013 march/April; 27:2; pp. 227–33. https://doi.org/10.1111/jvim.12036.

Geddes RF, Finch NC, Elliott J, Syme HM. Fibroblast Growth Factor 23 in Feline Chronic Kidney Disease. Journal of veterinary internal medicine. 2013 Jan; 27:2, pp. 234–41. https://doi.org/10.1111/jvim.12044.

Hall JA, Yerramilli M, Obare E, Jewell DE. Comparison of Serum Concentrations of Symmetric Dimethylarginine and Creatinine as Kidney Function Biomarkers in Cats with Chronic Kidney Disease. Journal of veterinary internal medicine. 2014 Sept; 28:6, pp. 1676–83. doi.org/10.1111/jvim.12445.

Hardcastle MR, Dittmer KE. A new dimension to diseases of calcium-phosphorus metabolism. Veterinary pathology. 2015; vol. 52(5), pp. 770–94. doi/pdf/10.1177/0300985815586222.

Heiene R, Lefebvre HP. Glomerular filtration rate in dogs and cats (2013). International renal interest society. http://www.iris-kidney.com/education/gfr.html.

Heiene R. GFR in practice: assessmen of glomerular filtration rate in dogs (2022). International renal interest society. http://www.iris-kidney.com/education/gfr_in_practice.html.

Hendrik D, van den Broek N, Chang Yu-Mei, Elliott J, Jepson RE. Prognostic importance of plasma total magnesium in a cohort of cats with azotemic chronic kidney disease. Journal of veterinary internal medicine. 2018 April; 32:4, pp. 1359–71. https://doi.org/10.1111/jvim.15141.

Langhorn R, Kieler IN, Koch, J, Christiansen LB, Jessen LR. Symmetric Dimethylarginine in Cats with Hypertrophic Cardiomyopathy and Diabetes Mellitus. Journal of veterinary internal medicine. 2017 dec; 32:1, pp. 57–63. doi.org/10.1111/jvim.14902.mineral_bone_disorders_ckd.html.

Peterson ME, Varela FV, Rishniw M, Polzin DJ. Evaluation of Serum Symmetric Dimethylarginine Concentration as a Marker for Masked Chronic Kidney Disease in Cats With Hyperthyroidism. J Vet Intern Med. 2018 Jan;32(1):295–304. doi: 10.1111/jvim.15036. PMID: 29377360; PMCID: PMC5787157.

Szlosek D, Robertson J, Quimby J, Mack R, Ogeer J, Clements C, et al. A retrospective evaluation of the relationship between symmetric dimethylarginine, creatinine and body weight in hyperthyroid cats. PLoS ONE. 2020. 15(1): e0227964. https://doi.org/10.1371/journal.pone.0227964.

Taylor S, Chan DL, Chalhoub S. 2022 ISFM Consensus Guidelines on Management of the Inappetent Hospitalised Cat. Journal of feline medicine and surgery. 2022 july. doi.org/10.1177/1098612X221106353.

Van den Broek H, Elliott J. Recent advances in mineral and bone disorders in CKD. International Renal Interest Society (IRIS). http://www.iris-kidney.com/education/recent_advances_mineral_bone_disorders_ckd.html.

Van den Broek H. Hypercalcemia in chronic kidney disease (updated 2022). International renal interest society. http://www.iris-kidney.com/education/hypercalcemia_in_ckd.html.

Test

1. **What are the parameters used to stage CKD according to IRIS?**
   A) Creatinine and Urine protein to creatinine ratio (UPC).
   B) Creatinine alone.
   C) Creatinine and systolic blood pressure.
   D) Creatinine and SDMA.
2. **Which of the following parameters is potentially more useful to distinguish chronic kidney disease from acute kidney disease?**
   A) Single creatinine measurement.
   B) Urinary density.
   C) Kidney size.
   D) Serum calcium.
3. **Regarding feline urinary tract tumours, which of the following options is correct?**
   A) Lymphoma is the most common kidney tumour and biopsies are often required to diagnose it.
   B) Transitional cell tumours of the bladder are usually in the region of the ureteral entrance into the bladder, significantly reducing surgical options for treatment.
   C) Transitional cell tumours of the bladder have a very reserved short-term prognosis with medical treatment.
   D) The two main differential diagnoses for a thickened cranial bladder wall are urinary tract infection and neoplasia.
4. **Regarding IRIS guidelines for the classification and management of CKD, which of the following is correct?**
   A) Now that symmetric dimethylarginine (SDMA) is available, it should be used instead of creatinine for classification of chronic kidney disease.
   B) There is no point in testing SDMA in patients who already have elevated creatinine levels.
   C) Stage I is assigned to patients with normal creatinine levels.
   D) The IRIS classification system can be used as soon as the patient is identified as having azotaemia.
5. **Regarding urinary tract infections (UTIs) in cats, which of the following is correct?**
   A) A urine culture is only needed when urine sediment is active.
   B) A cat with stable chronic renal disease and showing signs of UTI for the first time should always have a very long course of antibiotics.
   C) It is assumed that older cats presenting with UTI always have complicated infections and looking for an underlying cause is recommended.
   D) The use of antibiotics is recommended in patients with urinary catheters to avoid a UTI.
6. **What is the lowest lethal dose of ethylene glycol in cats?**
   A) 25 ml/kg.
   B) 0.5 ml/kg.
   C) 1.5 ml/kg.
   D) 5 ml/kg.
7. **Which of the following statements regarding acute kidney injury (AKI) is correct?**
   A) The use of diuretics improves the outcome of AKI.
   B) Dopamine should be used in patients with oliguria or anuria to promote diuresis.
   C) The IRIS classification of AKI assumes that the disease is not stable and therefore the grade of AKI may change several times during an episode of renal failure.
   D) According to the IRIS classification, patients with AKI are assigned one of four grades based on serum creatinine.
8. **Regarding urolithiasis in cats, which of the following is correct?**
   A) In feline nephrolithiasis, it is usually possible to get an educated guess of their composition.
   B) Calcium gluconate reduces serum potassium and therefore can be used to address hyperkalaemia in patients with urethral obstruction.
   C) Surgery is always indicated in patients with nephrolithiasis.
   D) Patients with struvite urolithiasis suffer from infection-induced urolithiasis most frequently.
9. **Regarding the management of chronic kidney disease, which of the following statements is correct?**
   A) Both telmisartan and benazepril are licensed for the treatment of proteinuria in cats.
   B) Dietary phosphate restriction is only needed in stage III and stage IV patients.

C) A diet rich in protein should be chosen for patients with kidney disease with protein loss to avoid the development of hypalbuminaemia.
D) Hypertension is common in patients with CKD and ACE inhibitors are the best option for the treatment of feline hypertension.

10. Which of the following characteristics is not commonly seen in patients with ethylene glycol toxicity?
A) Metabolic acidosis.
B) Hypercalcaemia.
C) Calcium oxalate crystalluria.
D) Hypocalcaemia.

11. Hypertension is commonly seen in patients with kidney disease. The treatment of choice for cats with significant systemic hypertension is:
A) Propranolol.
B) Telmisartan.
C) Enalapril.
D) Amlodipine.

12. Regarding acute kidney injury (AKI), which of the following statements is correct?
A) AKI can be differentiated from CKD based on serum creatinine.
B) There is evidence that mannitol can help feline AKI patients.
C) According to the IRIS system, AKI is classified based on urine output and blood pressure.
D) According to the IRIS system, AKI is classified based on urine production and the need for renal replacement therapy.

13. In patients with chronic kidney disease (CKD), which of the following is correct?
A) Switching a patient to a renal prescription diet should lead to a significant decrease in serum phosphate within two weeks.
B) In patients with late stage III CKD, the renal diet is generally insufficient to control hyperphosphataemia. Therefore, the use of phosphate binders should be considered as an initial measure alongside the diet.
C) Patients with stage I CKD always have normal blood pressure.
D) The combination of phosphate binders from different groups is not recommended.

14. Which of the following is correct regarding biochemical tests for kidney disease?
A) Creatinine and glomerular filtration rate (GFR) have a linear correlation.
B) Serum creatinine is not affected by muscle mass contrary to SDMA.
C) Creatinine does not have a linear correlation with GFR and, as such, significant changes in GFR are possible with normal creatinine levels.
D) If phosphorus is normal in CKD patients, it means that there is no secondary renal hyperparathyroidism.

15. Regarding the treatment of chronic kidney disease (CKD), which of the following is correct?
A) The use of darbepoetin is recommended in all patients with anaemia secondary to CKD.
B) Iron supplementation is necessary in patients receiving darbepoetin.
C) There is clear evidence that calcitriol is beneficial in cats with CKD.
D) Patients with CKD should be started on a renal diet, regardless of their IRIS stage.

Clinical case 1

Neutered 9-year-old short haired female cat, who lives indoors and is allowed outside.

Two-week history of lethargy and reduced appetite.

The owner comments that she has recently had an episode of urinating on the owner's bed who already had had a cat with idiopathic cystitis and brought in a urine sample collected the day before.

Clinical examination

Mild dental disease, but otherwise nothing remarkable. Possible caudal abdominal pain. The bladder is small in size. Systolic blood pressure, 150 mmHg.

Questions

(some answers were left blank to not bias your assessment of the case – take notes of your thoughts as you progress through the case).

1. **What are the problems identified and their respective differential diagnoses? (some answers were left blank to not bias your assessment of the case – take notes of your thoughts as you progress through the case).**
2. **What is the interpretation of the urinalysis below?**
   Urinalysis results:

Parameter	Result	Reference
Colour	Yellow	
Appearance	Clear	
USG (urine specific gravity)	1.035	
pH	7.0	
Protein	++ in the test strip	
Glucose	Negative	
Bilirubin	Negative	
Acetone bodies	Negative	
Blood / Haemoglobin	++ in the test strip	
White blood cells	5–10	<5 / HPF
Red blood cells	100	<5 / HPF
Epithelial cells	Not seen	
Crystals	Struvite ++	
Bacteria	++ (cocco y bacilli)	

3. **At this point, a complete blood count with smear and serum biochemistry were carried out. A new urine sample was collected for culture and urinalysis was repeated. See the results in the text below. What is your interpretation of these results?**
   - Complete blood count and biochemistry showed no abnormalities.
   - Urinalysis is similar to the previous one. No crystals are identified in the fresh sediment.
   - Urine culture was positive for *E. coli*, which was resistant to some antibiotics but sensitive to marbofloxacin.
4. **After analysis of the results of the previous tests, imaging was performed. The following images were obtained. What is your interpretation of the imaging and how would you consider managing the patient?**

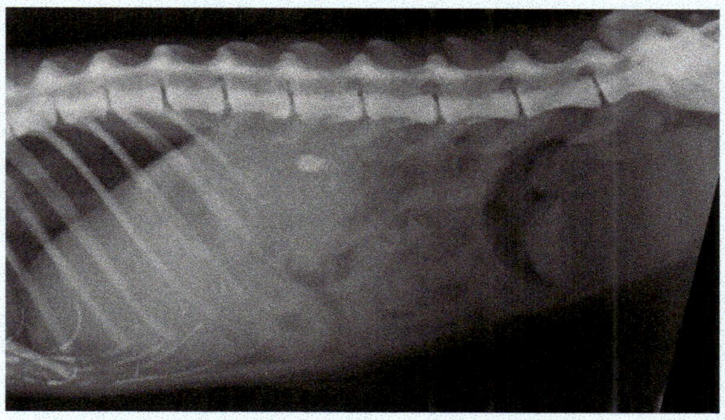

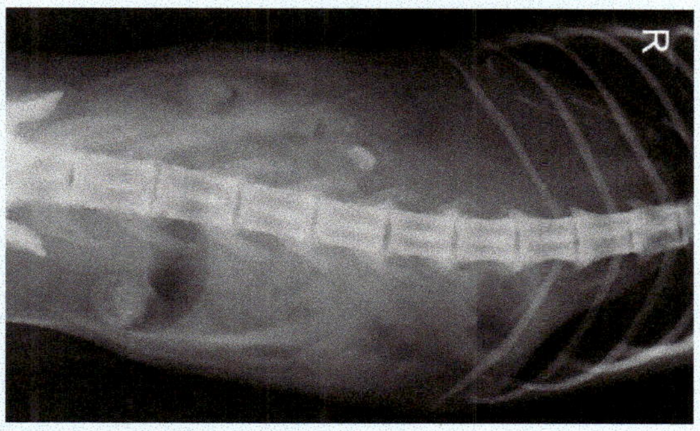

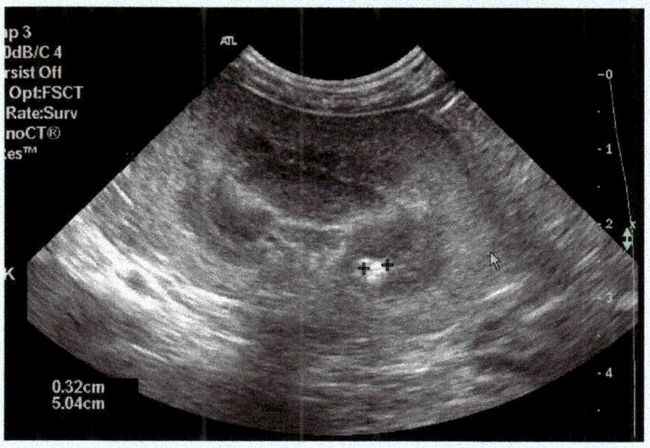

Clinical case 2

12-year-old male neutered domestic shorthair. Brought to the practice to investigate possible polyuria/polydipsia (PU/PD). Up to date with all vaccinations.

Clinical examination

On clinical examination nothing remarkable was noticed except for moderate dental disease. Systolic blood pressure was 160 mmHg with no visible changes to the retina.

Questions

(some answers were left blank to not bias your assessment of the case – take notes of your thoughts as you progress through the case).

1. **What are the problems identified and their respective differential diagnoses? What tests would be sensible to consider at this point? (some answers were left blank to not bias your assessment of the case – take notes of your thoughts as you progress through the case).**

2. **You decide to perform routine haematology, serum biochemistry and urinalysis (see the results below). What is your interpretation of the results?**

 - Complete blood count

Parameter	Result	Units	Reference
Red blood cells	9.96	10^{12}/l	7.12–11.46
Haemoglobin	14.9	g/dl	10.3–16.2
PCV	0.512	l/l	0.281–0.527
MCV (Mean corpuscular volume)	51.4	fl	39.0–56.0
MCH (Mean corpuscular hemoblobin)	15.0	pg	12.6–16.5
MCHC (Mean corpuscular hemoglobin concentration)	29.1	g/dl	28.5–37.8
Reticulocytes	23.9	10^9/l	<50
White blood cells	9.00	10^9/l	3.9–19.0
Neutrophils	6.39	10^9/l	2.62–15.17
Lymphocytes	1.80	10^9/l	0.85–5.85
Monocytes	0.18	10^9/l	0.04–0.53
Eosinophils	0.63	10^9/l	0.09–2.18
Platelets	157	10^9/l	155–641

Platelet aggregates are seen and neither red nor white blood cells show abnormal morphologies.

 - Biochemistry

Parameter	Result	Units	Reference
Total protein	74.5	g/l	60.0–80.0
Albumin	29.6	g/l	25.0–45.0
Globulin	44.9	g/l	25.0–45.0
BUN	9.8	mmol/l	2.5–9.9
Creatinine	130	μmol/l	80.0–203.0
ALT	**125**	**IU/l**	**5.0–60.0**
ALP	26	IU/l	<60
GGT	2.2	IU/l	0.1–9.0
Cholesterol	3.86	mmol/l	2.20–4.00
Sodium	156	mmol/l	145.0–157.0
Potassium	4.01	mmol/l	3.50–5.50
Ratio Na/K	31.14		28.00–40.00
Chloride	124	mmol/l	100.0–124.0
Phosphorus	2.2	mmol/l	0.90–2.20
Calcium	2.43	mmol/l	2.05–2.95
Glucose	6	mmol/l	3.9–8.0

- Urinalysis

Parameter	Result	Reference
Urine specific gravity (USG)	1.020	
Colour/Appearance	Yellow/Clear	
pH	7.5	
Bilirubin	–	
Protein	+	
Blood/Haemoglobin	–	
Glucose	–	
White blood cells	Not found	<5 HPF
Red blood cells	Not found	<5 HPF
Epithelial cells	Not found	
Casts	Not found	
Crystals	Not found	

3. Given that you have not reached a diagnosis, you discuss possible causes and tests that may be indicated with the owner, who elects to have all blood tests done at once to try to avoid another visit to the practice. What additional tests would be appropriate to run in this patient?

4. See below the results of the additional tests that you decided to perform. What is your interpretation of the results?

Test	Result	Reference
SDMA	16 μg/dl	1–14
Total T4	75.0 nmol/l	10.0–60.0
Fasting bile acids	1.0 μmol/l	0.1–5.0
Postpandrial bile acids	5.0 μmol/l	0.5–10.0
Urine P/C Ratio	0.5	<0.4
FeLV	negative	
FIV	negative	

5. How would you manage the patient? (some answers were left blank to not bias your assessment of the case – take notes of your thoughts as you progress through the case).

Answers

Test

1. D	7. C	13. B
2. C	8. A	14. C
3. D	9. A	15. B
4. C	10. B	
5. C	11. D	
6. C	12. D	

Clinical case 1

1. What are the problems identified and their respective differential diagnoses?

Inappropriate urination is usually secondary to lower urinary tract problems and/or behavioural problems.
Abdominal pain points to inflammatory, infectious, or neoplastic disorders of the intra-abdominal structures.
Lethargy and reduced appetite are non-specific problems and likely secondary to the main problem.
Mild dental disease is considered unlikely to be related to the clinical signs identified.

2. What is the interpretation of the urinalysis?
The urine is well concentrated. The urinalysis raises suspicion of inflammation and/or infection and therefore a urine culture is needed. This is the reason why a new urine sample was collected via cystocentesis.

The bacteria seen in the sediment may be real and consistent with a urinary tract infection, but contamination cannot be ruled out especially as the urine was collected by the owner from the litter tray.

3. What is your interpretation of these results?
Considering the clinical signs and the positive urine culture from a cystocentesis sample, bacterial cystitis can be diagnosed.

Bacterial cystitis in cats is rare and, when present, generally they have an underlying cause. The blood tests revealed no concerns. To try to identify the problem, abdominal imaging was performed.

4. What is your interpretation of the imaging and how would you consider managing the patient?
Interpretation of the imaging:

- Radiographs show the presence of a nephrolith in the right kidney.
- On ultrasound, the presence of a nephrolith was confirmed on the right kidney. There was no evidence of renal pelvis dilation or ureteral dilation. No other uroliths were identified in the urinary tract.
- The vast majority of feline nephroliths are calcium oxalate and cannot be dissolved. Urine pH and radiographic opacity would support the presence of a calcium oxalate (CaOx) nephrolith. There is no evidence that the nephroliths are causing clinical disease and they are thought to be an incidental finding when looking for underlying causes for bacterial cystitis.
- Given the clinical signs and positive urine culture from a cystocentesis sample, the patient was diagnosed with bacterial cystitis. According to the ISCAID guidelines, for a sporadic bacterial cystitis, a 3-to-5-day course of an appropriate antibiotic based on culture is recommended. In this case a 5-day course of marbofloxacin was prescribed; there is no clear indication to repeat the urine culture if the clinical signs resolve.
- The upper urinary tract uroliths are suspected to be CaOx and therefore (following the ACVIM guidelines on urolithiasis) underlying causes leading to excessive calcium in the urine should be investigated alongside implementation of preventative measures for CaOx urolithiasis. Serum calcium was normal on the serum biochemistry performed however, up to 25% of the cat with CaOx urolithiasis and normal serum calcium, can have elevated ionised hypercalcemia. In this patient, serum ionised calcium was normal.

Management of the patient:

- The patient should be monitored regularly with urinalysis including sediment to assess for the efficacy of the preventative measures for CaOx urolithiasis. Repeated imaging may also be indicated to assess progression and/or consequences of the upper urinary tract urolithiasis.

Clinical case 2

1. What are the problems identified and their respective differential diagnoses? What tests would be sensible to consider at this point?

Problems and differential diagnoses

a. The patient has PU/PD and the differentials considered are:
   - Primary polydipsia – can be psychogenic or a manifestation of a systemic disease such as hepatic encephalopathy and hyperthyroidism.
   - Primary polyuria occurs either due to osmotic diuresis (e.g. diabetes mellitus) or due to problems with anti-diuretic hormone (ADH). ADH can be reduced or absent (central diabetes insipidus) or response to ADH may be inappropriate (nephrogenic diabetic insipidus).
   - Central diabetes insipidus can occur due to congenital central nervous system defects, trauma, or neoplasia. Inappropriate response to ADH can be seen as a primary problem or it can occur secondarily to several diseases such as chronic kidney disease, hyperthyroidism, hypercalcaemia, liver disease, pyelonephritis, and acromegaly.

b. There is mild hypertension without retinal changes, which will need to be reassessed to see if is persistent. It is possible that this mild increase, represents stress rather than real hypertension.

c. The dental disease is not thought to be linked to the clinical signs reported.

Tests to consider performing at this point

It would be sensible to perform routine haematology, biochemistry with electrolytes and urinalysis to try to identify or rule out some of the differential diagnoses.

2. What is your interpretation of the results?

There is little to note in the routine complete blood count and biochemistry results, except for the elevation of ALT (around twice normal). In cats, even mild increases in ALT are relevant and are consistent with hepatocellular damage, which could be primary or secondary to other disorders.

Urine is not as concentrated as we normal expect in a cat.

The normal renal parameters do not rule out the presence of kidney disease and therefore it would be indicated to measure SDMA as it is a more sensitive to smaller changes in glomerular filtration rate (GFR).

3. What additional tests would be appropriate to run in this patient?

- Serum SDMA to assess for possible early-stage CKD.
- Total T4 in case of hyperthyroidism.
- FeLV antigen and FIV antibody as indicated in all cats that are unwell.
- Bile acid stimulation test to look at liver function.
- Urine protein:creatine ratio (UPC) – as hypertension can lead to proteinuria.

4. What is your interpretation of the results?

- The SDMA is mildly elevated and need to be rechecked as, if persistently elevated, would be consistent with early-stage CKD.
- Total T4 is increased, and the results are consistent with hyperthyroidism.
- The UPC is mildly increased. It is recommended to assess for the persistence of proteinuria. Additionally, hypertension can exacerbate proteinuria and, in this patient, initial assessment of blood pressure revealed a mild increase. Re-assessment of blood pressure and UPC is needed before making decisions.
- Bile acid stimulation test is normal making primary liver disease unlikely.

The patient is diagnosed with hyperthyroidism which can explain the PU/PD and can also be the cause of the mild increase in ALT.

5. How would you manage the patient?

The patient was started on methimazole. The initial dose was low (1.25 mg orally once daily) as there is only PU/PD as a clinical sign and there is uncertainty about the presence of renal disease.

After reassessment of the patient and blood tests, the dose will be increased as appropriate, with the aim of obtaining euthyroidism. Hyperthyroidism can have impact on the GFR therefore we need to reassess the renal parameters when the patient is euthyroid.

Re-evaluation of the blood pressure and urinalysis with UPC is also indicated.

8

Feline cardiology

Domingo Casamián Sorrosal, Dolores María Porteiro Vázquez

Contents

Evaluation of cardiac disease

Be it in first opinion practice or a specialist referral centre, feline cardiovascular diseases are an important part of a clinicians' caseload. Of these **myocardial disease**, both primary and secondary, are the most frequent feline cardiac pathologies. This chapter focuses on those feline heart diseases likely to be encountered in practice, including their clinical presentation, diagnosis, and treatment.

Clinical history

Cats with heart disease may present within **one of the following clinical pictures**:

1. The **asymptomatic** preclinical cat.
2. The cat in **congestive heart failure** presenting with tachypnoea and dyspnoea or, less commonly, ascites.
3. The cat with **arterial thromboembolism** with hindleg or right foreleg paresis or paralysis.
4. The cat with **syncopal episodes**.

In addition **non-specific general signs** may be observed, such as lethargy, hyporexia or anorexia, and/or weight loss.

As part of a complete history aspects such as **age, breed, and diet** should be considered. For example, young cats (under 6 months) are more likely to have congenital diseases, while hyperthyroidism usually occurs in cats over seven or eight years old, and certain breeds have a predisposition to breed-related cardiomyopathies. Finally, it is important to find out about the cat's diet since taurine deficient foods can cause dilated cardiomyopathy.

Physical examination

A thorough physical examination is made up of a general exam that encompasses the cat's overall health, plus a detailed assessment of the cardiovascular system.

General clinical examination

The general physical examination starts by **observing the cat from a distance**. This involves **watching their breathing** and observing the presence or absence of:

- tachypnoea (rapid breathing)
- dyspnoea (respiratory distress)
- asynchronous or paradoxical respiration (where the chest and the abdomen move asynchronously)
- abnormal respiratory sounds (for example, whistles or snoring from the upper airways, which indicate dyspnoea of upper airway respiratory origin).

After observing the cat, a complete physical examination should be performed either before or after the cardiovascular or cardiothoracic exam.

In particular, the following should be evaluated specifically:

- **Mucous membranes**: normal, pale, or cyanotic.
- **Capillary refill time**: normal, decreased, or increased.
- **Jugular veins**: normal, distended, or pulsatile.
- **Abdominal palpation**, for ascites.
- Evaluation of **femoral pulse quality**: reduced, normal, hyperkinetic, or absent.
- When there is a suspicion of arterial aortic. thromboembolism (ATE) the pads, skin and muscles of the hind legs, the **metatarsal pulse**, and their **neurological status** should be assessed (degree and location of paresis or paralysis).
- In patients over seven or eight years of age, **the neck area should be examined** for the possible presence of hyperthyroid goitre.
- When taurine deficiency or systemic hypertension is suspected, **the retina should be evaluated** as part of a complete eye examination.

Physical examination of the cardiorespiratory system

The clinician should systematically assess the cardiorespiratory system. To start with the upper airways should be auscultated, to evaluate abnormal sounds (such as whistling or snoring) over the larynx and cervical trachea. Auscultation should then progress downwards to the thorax and care should be taken when listening to the lungs to assess:

- Are the bronchiovesicular sounds are normal or not?
  - **Increased** sounds may indicate bronchopulmonary disease:
    - **Crepitations** indicate oedema, mucus, pus, haemorrhage, or interstitial disease such as pulmonary fibrosis.
    - **Wheezing** indicates lower airway bronchoconstriction and is typical of feline asthma, but can occur with other lung diseases.
  - **Decreased** sounds may indicate the presence of a pleural effusion, pneumothorax, or lung consolidation.

Cats in heart failure often present with:

- crackles on auscultation due to pulmonary oedema
- attenuated lung and heart sounds due to pleural effusion.

After a thorough examination of the respiratory system, breathing sounds can be "mentally withdrawn"

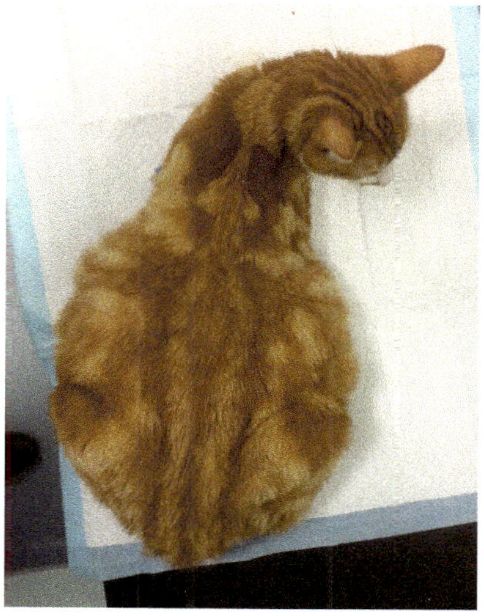

Figure 1. Distended abdomen in a cat with severe abdominal effusion and poor body condition due to ride-sided heart failure (also accompanied by jugular distension). The cat also showed signs of left-sided heart failure with mild to moderate pulmonary oedema and tachypnoea (biventricular heart failure). The underlying disease was an unclassified cardiomyopathy.

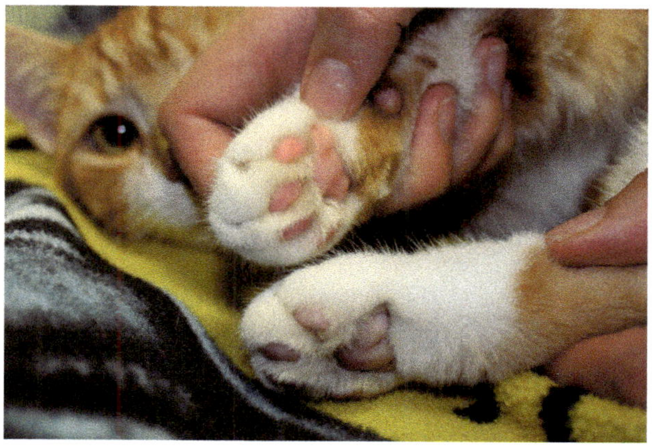

Figure 2. Comparison of a normal pad from the front leg (upper leg) with the pad from the hind leg which has suffered a thromboembolism (cyanotic).

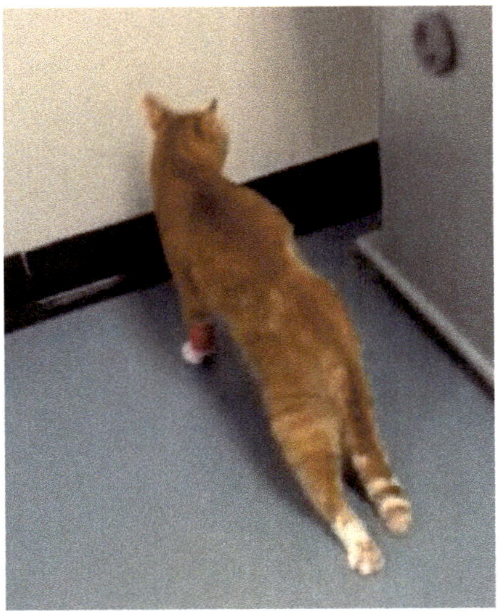

Figure 3. Cat with paralysis of the left hindlimb. Cats with arterial thromboembolism can suffer varying levels of neurological deficits in the affected limbs depending on the grade of neurological and muscular ischaemia.

or subtracted from cardiac auscultation and to avoid confusing breath sounds with heart sounds.

Heart assessment starts by using open palms placed against the chest wall to **palpate the heart's apex**. This enables detection of any concussion of the cardiac tip (the apex) against the thoracic wall, first it should be established if the apex is displaced, and the mitral and tricuspid valves located. Palpation is essential to identify a cardiac thrill (a vibration of the chest wall) and is used to classify murmurs according to their intensity.

Heart auscultation

After palpation, the chest should be auscultated to answer three fundamental questions:

1. Is there a **murmur**?
2. Is there an **arrhythmia**?
3. Is there an **abnormal heart sound**?

If there is a murmur, it should be characterized according to its location, intensity (grade I to IV), and timing.

Murmur location

To establish the murmur's location, **the point of maximum intensity** (**PMI**) should be listened for. To do this the heart's apex should be located by palpation first since this helps orientation and identification of the heart valves. For a strong murmur, the PMI is located where the thrill is palpable. Firstly, it is important to identify if the PMI is in the left or right hemithorax, and at the heart's base or apex.

The feline heart is less upright than in the dog, and the apex area is considered "caudal" with the mitral valves located on the left hand side and the tricuspid valves to the right hand side. The cardiac base is located in a more cranial or cranio-dorsal position, with the parasternal area encompassing the pulmonary and aortic valves, and the outflow tracts of the left and right ventricles.

Murmur intensity

To determine a murmur's intensity, the intensity of the murmur should be compared with that of the heart sounds.

Although this is not a perfect system (since heart sounds vary in intensity) it is an objective way of evaluating murmurs, especially for the inexperienced clinician:

- **Grade I**: murmur only detected after several minutes of auscultation and is very soft.
- **Grade II**: murmur easy to detect, but less intense than heart sounds.
- **Grade III**: murmur of equal intensity to heart sounds.
- **Grade IV**: murmur of greater intensity than the heart sounds, but without cardiac thrill.
- **Grade V and VI**: murmur of higher intensity than the cardiac sounds with cardiac thrill; grade VI murmurs can be auscultated with a stethoscope away from the chest wall.

Murmur timing

The **timing of the murmur** differentiates whether a murmur is **systolic, diastolic or continuous**:

- If the murmur occurs between the "lup" (S1) and "dup" (S2), the murmur is **systolic**.
- If it occurs between the "dup" and the "lup" it is **diastolic**.
- If it can be heard permanently, during systole and diastole, the murmur is **continuous**.

The high feline heart-rate can make it difficult to differentiate the murmur's timing. In addition, murmurs can obliterate or almost obliterate heart sounds (pansystolic or holosystolic), which complicates assessment of their timing. One method that helps is palpation of the pulse while listening: if the murmur occurs during the pulse wave, it is systolic. Also, from a practical point of view, it is important to remember that **most murmurs are systolic**, which are those the ear is most used to. Therefore, if at any time the clinician hears "an unusual murmur," it may be a diastolic murmur and should be auscultated for longer in a quiet location.

Table 1 lists the most common differentials for murmurs according to their location and timing. If the exact location is not identified, but only that the murmur is left or right-sided, this remains useful information. A list of differentials can be made starting from this first left/right location, including cranial (base) or caudal (apex) murmurs on one side or the other.

Pathological and non-pathological heart murmurs

Most of the murmurs are associated with structural cardiac disease and are defined as pathological heart murmurs, but when no structural cardiac disease is present, murmurs are defined as non-pathological heart murmurs and include innocent and physiologic murmurs. Non-pathological heart murmurs are understood to be "benign" murmurs in which turbulent flow occurs in the outflow tract of the ventricle, but without associated structural cardiac disease and clinical consequences. Non-pathological murmurs can occur in puppies (innocent murmurs) or associated with systemic disturbance reducing blood viscosity, such as anaemia (physiologic murmurs). Non-pathological murmurs are soft or quiet (grade 1/6 or 2/6), located on the left heart base and predominantly heard in systole. Another common non-pathological murmur is caused by dynamic right ventricular outflow tract obstruction (DRVOT). This murmur is caused by dynamic systolic narrowing of the proximal outflow region of the right ventricle associated with a hyperdynamic state (stress, hyperthyroidism), decrease cardiac volume (dehydration) or can be iatrogenic. DRVOT can happen in cats during auscultation due to the pressure against the chest with the stethoscope or the ultrasound probe during echocardiography.

For **grade IV murmurs or louder**, or those in a location not suggestive of a physiological murmur, further investigation by a cardiologist is advised since there is a high probability the patient is suffering from heart disease. In most cases **the greater the intensity of the murmur, the more severe the disease causing it**. However, there are exceptions where the opposite occurs, of which the most frequent is a murmur caused by an interventricular septal defect.

Location and type of murmur		Cause
Left base (left hemithorax craniodorsal to the apex/left parasternal)	Systolic	– Physiological murmurs (up to grade III) – HCM (normally with SAM) – Mitral valve dysplasia with SAM – Aortic stenosis – Pulmonary stenosis
	Diastolic	– Aortic regurgitation due to endocarditis
	Continuous	– Persistent ductus arteriosus (normally high in the craniodorsal area, the murmur is often systolic in cats)
Left apex	Systolic	– Mitral regurgitation caused by any of the cardiomyopathies – Regurgitation caused by mitral valve dysplasia or endocarditis
	Diastolic	– Mitral valve dysplasia which causes valvular stenosis
Right base (right hemithorax craniodorsal to the apex/right parasternal)	Systolic	– Physiological murmurs – Right ventricular outflow tract obstruction (benign) murmurs – HCM – Interventricular septal defect
Right apex	Systolic	– Tricuspid dysplasia causing valvular regurgitation – Arrhythmogenic right ventricular cardiomyopathy
	Diastolic	– Tricuspid valve dysplasia causing valvular stenosis

Gallop rhythms

The most common abnormal heart sounds in cats are **diastolic sounds (S3 and S4) that form the "canter" rhythm by the cadence "lup-dup-dup"**. The S3 sound occurs in early diastole and is usually a consequence of diseases that occur with a volume overload such as **chronic anaemia or DCM**. The S4 sound occurs at the end of diastole and is usually associated with cardiomyopathies such as **HCM or RCM**. In practice, considering the usually high heart rates in cats, it is not possible to differentiate between S3 or S4 and the finding is referred to as "evidence of a gallop rhythm" or "there is a diastolic sound".

Contrary to quiet to moderate murmurs (many are physiological and benign); a **patient with a gallop rhythm should be considered to have cardiac disease until proven otherwise** using echocardiography. Sometimes a cat has a gallop rhythm and does not have primary heart disease or obvious heart changes secondary to systemic disease. This may be because there is or has been an unidentified diastolic dysfunction or abrupt change in volume during echocardiography, or the gallop rhythm is not such that the auscultated "extra" sounds are systolic clicks or, is in fact, separation (splitting) of the S1 or S2, sounds, for example.

An exception to the suggested rule of always investigating when a gallop rhythm exists is the cat diagnosed with **hyperthyroidism and no evidence of heart**

failure. A complete echocardiographic examination is always desirable in these cases, but it is also acceptable to **treat hyperthyroidism and monitor the gallop rhythm**, observing if it disappears during the following months, together with the rest of the clinical signs when the euthyroid state stabilizes.

Arrhythmias

If an **arrhythmia** is detected, it should be established whether there are **associated pulse deficits** by palpating the femoral arteries at the same time as auscultation. A complete **electrocardiogram** (ECG) should then be performed. If no abnormalities are observed during the ECG it is advisable, especially for the novice clinician, to auscultate whilst taking the ECG. This helps assess if the arrhythmia is no longer present or the auscultated arrhythmia was an abnormal heart sound, a murmur, or a respiratory sound.

Occasionally, the clinician is confident they heard a severe arrhythmia that was not seen during the ECG. If so, especially if the patient has clinical signs, evaluation of the patient by a cardiologist is recommended, since performing a continuous **ECG (24-hour Holter)** may be necessary.

The asymptomatic cat

These cats are usually examined because they are **breeds predisposed to HCM** as part of a screening programme and belong to breeders. Also included in this group are cats that are examined due to an abnormality (canter, murmur, or arrhythmia) found during a routine examination.

The cat in congestive heart failure (CHF)

Diastolic failure in HCM and RCM eventually leads to high pressure in the atrium and pulmonary veins and, ultimately, to **left-sided heart failure**. In the cat, this manifests as **pulmonary oedema** and/or **pleural effusion**. The most important clinical sign is tachypnoea and acute respiratory distress. The presence of **coughing is rare**, unlike in the dog.

Clinical signs of right-sided heart failure (ascites or peripheral oedema) rarely occur.

Due to a sedentary feline lifestyle, the initial mild clinical signs may go unnoticed by the owner and these cats present in an advanced clinical stage. **Sinus tachycardia** or arrhythmias are often present but, unlike the dog, cats in CHF may have normal sinus rhythms or even sinus bradycardia.

Sometimes an event, such as a stressful situation, triggers fulminant heart failure in a cat that was stable. Sometimes heart failure develops when previously in the hidden phase of the disease, due to the administration of intravenous fluids for another disease.

The cat with arterial systemic thromboembolism

Left atrial dilatation, damage to the endothelium, and exposure of sub-endothelial collagen occur as a result of heart disease and favour slower blood flow. Several studies suggest the third factor of the Virchow triad (**hypercoagulability**) may also play a role in the development of thromboembolism.

The incidence of thromboembolism in cats with HCM is estimated to be 6–17%. Clots form in the left atrium and then enter the systemic circulation. In most cases (90%) the clots become **fixed in the aortic trifurcation** and extend to the iliac arteries, with a saddle appearance. Disruption of flow causes general **unilateral or bilateral signs**, including loss of femoral pulse, cold extremities, pain, paleness or cyanosis, and paresis or paralysis of the hind limbs.

Clinical signs and Doppler flow analysis are usually sufficient to reach a diagnosis. However, it should be remembered that paralysis of the hind limbs may be due to **neurological disease** and that not all thrombi are the result of heart disease. A small percentage of thrombi may be due to other diseases, such as pulmonary neoplasms.

Thrombi may terminate in other arteries such as the brachial, renal, mesenteric, coronary, or cerebral arteries, causing specific signs related to these locations.

Cats with thromboembolism usually present with **tachypnoea**, but it is important to note that only 44% of these cats have heart failure and need furosemide. In many cases, tachypnoea is due to extra-thoracic causes such as **pain or metabolic acidosis**, which must be taken into account since cats with a thromboembolism are usually dehydrated and hypothermic and an unnecessary dose of diuretics could be fatal. If the thromboembolism is intracranial it causes **central neurological signs**, whereas animals with mesenteric thromboembolisms are usually in shock and have **acute abdominal pain**. Cats suffering from renal thromboembolism may have signs of abdominal (peri-renal) pain and signs of acute kidney failure, depending on the functional status of the other kidney.

The cat with syncope

This is the least common presentation and may be due to **haemodynamic** (e.g. severe SAM in OHCM) or **structural** (such as cardiomyopathies or congenital diseases) causes and/or the presence of **arrhythmias**.

Classic syncope follows the pattern of very short episodes with loss of consciousness, flaccid extremities and occurs during exercise or stressful situations. Cardiovascular episodes in cats can be very heterogeneous and it is not abnormal to observe rigid extremities with opisthotonos or symptoms that give the impression of neurological disease.

In addition, **transient thromboembolic episodes** can occur that cause temporary hind leg weakness.

Diagnostic tests

Electrocardiogram

The **electrocardiogram (ECG) is a graphic recording of the electrical potentials generated by the heart muscle during the cardiac cycle.** Electrodes placed on the extremities detect electrical potentials which are represented on the ECG as a trace on paper roll marked in millimetres. On this trace the **X-axis represents time** and the **Y-axis millivolts**. The main function of the ECG is to **detect heart arrhythmias**, although it may sometimes indicate structural changes in the heart.

Obtaining the electrocardiographic trace

The basic ECG evaluates the electrical activity in the frontal axis. For this the following are put in place:

- Red electrode on the right foreleg.
- Yellow electrode on the left foreleg.
- Green electrode on the left hind leg.
- Black electrode on the right hind leg.

An ECG is ideally performed in **right lateral recumbency**. In cats sometimes this not possible and in which case an ECG with the animal in the sternal position is acceptable for the detection of arrhythmias and calculating the duration of the waves. (However, the measurements of wave amplitudes may vary.)

Whenever possible the ECG should be taken **without sedation or anaesthesia** as both can cause variations in heart rate. It is advisable to take the ECG in an area of the clinic or hospital with the least possible electrical/electromagnetic interference from electrical devices, avoiding placing the cat directly on a metal table (to avoid it working as an antenna) and alcohol should be applied to the electrodes (if no patches are used) in previously clipped areas to improve conduction.

The most **common artefacts** are caused by alternating current, breathing, tremors and muscle movements. Ideally, wires should not pass over the chest so that they do not interfere with breathing. Initially the ECG should be attempted without filters and then these applied later. For example, filters can be tested on the ECG if the types of filters and how they affect each artefact are unknown. In cats, a low-pass filter (allows only lower frequencies) at 150 Hz is commonly used.

ECG interpretation

The **paper speed is usually 25 or 50 mm/s**, and the **amplitude 10 mV/cm**. (In cats, an amplitude of 20 mV/cm may aid visualisation of the waves.) A trace is run and the entire log examined to check for artefacts and unusual rhythms. If different rhythms are present, these are analysed separately. Once an artefact-free trace is obtained, the ECG waves, intervals, and segments are measured (Figure 4). The main ones include:

- P wave: represents the depolarization of the atria.
- QRS wave: represents the depolarization of the ventricles.
- T wave: represents the repolarization of the ventricles.
- PR interval: distance from the beginning of the P wave to the beginning of the Q wave.
- ST segment: distance from the end of the QRS wave to the beginning of the T wave.
- QT interval: distance from the beginning of the QRS wave to the end of the T wave.

Table 2 shows measurements considered normal for cats. However, the main function of the electrocardiogram is detecting arrhythmias, which is where the initial emphasis is focussed.

There are four main objectives when assessing an ECG:

1. Calculating the **heart rate**.
2. Establishing whether the rhythm or complex/es is/are **supraventricular or ventricular**.

Table 2. Normal electrocardiographic measurements in the cat.

Electrocardiographic measurement	Value
Heart rate	140–220 beats per minute*
Normal cardiac rhythm	Sinus
Amplitude (P wave)	<0.2 mV
Duration (P wave)	<35 ms
PQ interval	50–90 ms
R wave amplitude	<0.9 mV
Duration (QRS)	<40 ms
Frontal plane electrical axis (QRS)	From 0 to +´60 degrees
Right deviation	From +160 degrees to −80 degrees
Left deviation	From 0 degrees to −60 degrees
ST segment	Isoelectric
QT interval	70–200 ms

*In a minority of cats a wide range (120–240) is normal.

3. Establishing whether the rhythm is **regular or irregular**.
4. Determining the **relationship between the P wave and the QRS complex**. Is there a P wave for each QRS complex? Is there a QRS complex for each P wave?

When these questions are answered, a diagnosis of the rhythm or rhythms present is made and placed in the context of the case for clinical decision making.

Heart rate

The heart rate is calculated by measuring 15 cm (3 seconds at 50 mm/s) or 7.5 cm (3 seconds at 25 mm/s) on the ECG and then multiplying by 20 or, if the rhythm is very short and regular, measuring the distance between two QRS complexes and dividing 3.000 by the measured mm (at 50 mm/s) or 1.500 by the measured mm (at 25 mm/s).

QRS morphology

Supraventricular complexes are narrow and similar in appearance to sinus complexes, since ventricular depolarization occurs normally. **Ventricular complexes are wider than normal or "bizarre."** If there are doubts, they can also be measured (QRS complexes should be less than 40 ms in the cat). On occasion, however, some impulses originating above the atrioventricular node present abnormal conduction due to the presence of a bundle branch block, aberrant conduction, or accessory conduction pathway.

Rhythm

To establish whether the rhythm is regular or irregular, it is advisable to mark several QRS complexes on a piece of paper (at the height of the R or Q wave) or to evaluate their distance with a compass and move along the ECG to do so. "Doing it by eye" is not recommended as this can lead to misunderstandings. The classic irregular rhythms are atrial fibrillation, which in cats is practically always associated with atrial enlargement and sinus arrhythmia, which is less common in cats than in dogs. The presence of frequent supraventricular or ventricular ectopic beats can also lead to a highly irregular overall rhythm.

P-QRS relationship

A P-wave not followed by a corresponding QRS complex suggests the presence of a second- or third-degree atrioventricular block. Atrial activity or P waves may not be visible or not associated with the QRS complex (atrioventricular dissociation). If the QRS complex is wide it is most likely that the ectopic beat is ventricular and if the QRS complex is narrow the origin is supraventricular.

Cardiac rhythms and arrhythmias

The most common heart rhythms or arrhythmias in cats include:

Rhythms originating from the sinus node:

- Sinus rhythm.
- Sinus tachycardia.
- Sinus bradycardia.
- Sinus arrhythmia.

Rhythms of supraventricular origin, (from the atrioventricular node, atria, and pulmonary veins) include:

- Supraventricular ectopic complexes.
- Supraventricular tachycardia.
- Atrial fibrillation.

Rhythms originating from the ventricles include:

- Ventricular ectopic complexes.
- Idioventricular rhythm.
- Ventricular tachycardia.
- Ventricular fibrillation.

Deficits in the formation or conduction of the electrical impulse:

- Pauses, arrests or sinus blocks.
- First, second, or third-degree atrioventricular blocks.
- Left or right bundle branch or left anterior bundle blocks.

Figures 5 to 9 show examples of different rhythms and their main characteristics. The main forms of treatment are set out later in the text.

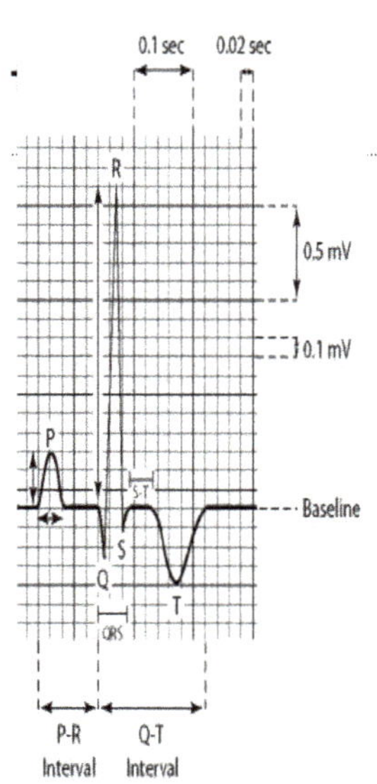

Figure 4. Normal electrocardiographic complexes and measurements with a paper speed of 25mm/second. The P wave represents atrial depolarization. The QRS complex represents ventricular depolarization.

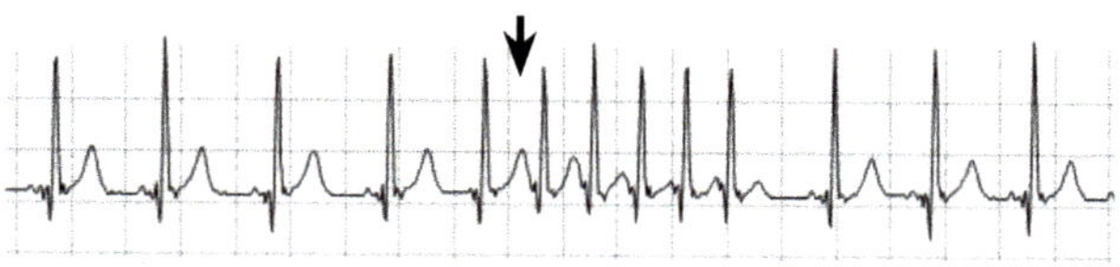

Figure 5. Non-sustained supraventricular tachycardia (for less than 30 seconds, and only a few beats) during the recording of continuous monitoring in a cat with frequent syncope's. After a sinus rhythm the abrupt presence of 5/6 supraventricular ectopic beats (arrow) which cause a supraventricular tachycardia can be seen. The rhythm is mildly irregular (depending on the mechanism, supraventricular tachycardia can be mildly irregular, but they are often regular). The heart rate is 300 beats per minute. The complexes are narrow (supraventricular). It is difficult to assess the presence of P waves (if they are present) as in this derivation they are hidden under the T waves.

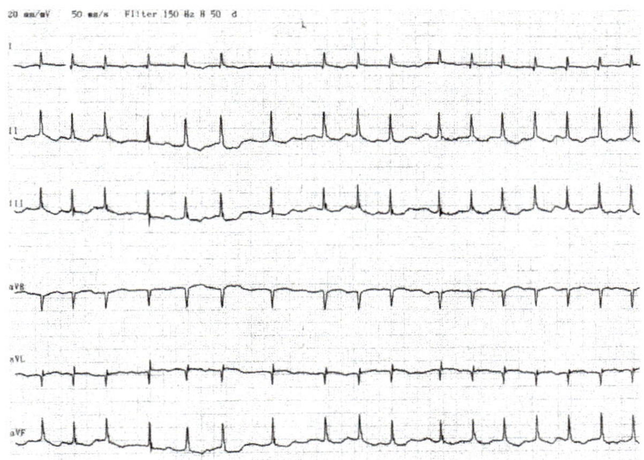

Figure 6. Atrial fibrillation in a cat with underlying RCM. The heart rate is 220 beats per minute, the rhythm is irregular, the complexes are narrow (supraventricular) and there are no evident P waves. It is unusual to see f waves in cats (especially after applying filters) and diagnosis of atrial fibrillation should be based in the existence of an irregular supraventricular rhythm with the absence of P waves.

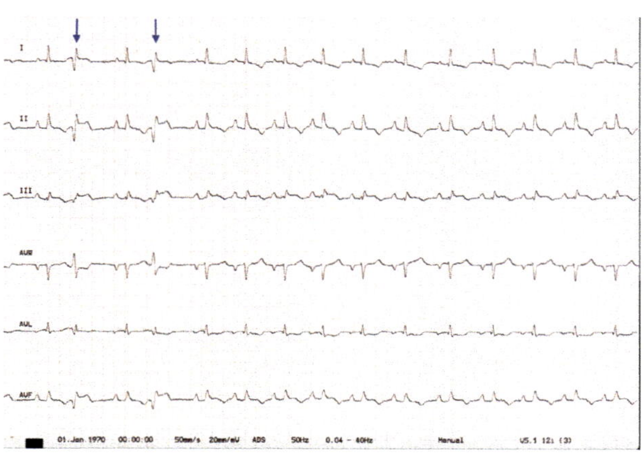

Figure 7. Sinus rhythm (heart rate of 160 beats per minute) interrupted by two simple premature ectopic ventricular complexes in a cat with RCM. These are premature because they occur before the next sinus complex should (which is not occurring as the ventricle is depolarised by the ventricular complex) and are ventricular because they are wide and bizarre.

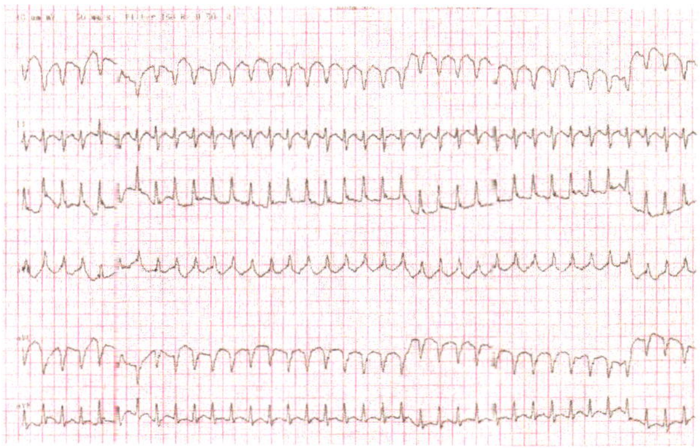

Figure 8. Ventricular tachycardia in a cat with HCM. The tachycardia (increased rhythm) is regular with wide (bizarre) complexes and dissociation (or non-visualisation) of P waves.

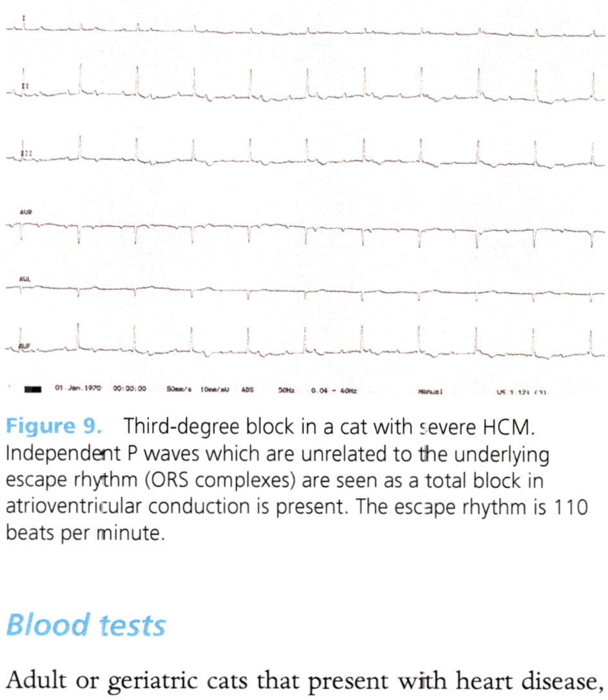

Figure 9. Third-degree block in a cat with severe HCM. Independent P waves which are unrelated to the underlying escape rhythm (QRS complexes) are seen as a total block in atrioventricular conduction is present. The escape rhythm is 110 beats per minute.

Blood tests

Adult or geriatric cats that present with heart disease, especially those in heart failure, may have concurrent diseases. Thus it is advisable to run a **complete blood count and biochemistry including electrolytes**. This establishes if kidney function and electrolyte levels are normal before starting cardiac therapy. In cats older than 7–8 years measurement of **total T4** is recommended, especially if there are concurrent signs of hyperthyroidism such as weight loss, polyphagia, polydipsia, and polyuria, or if a palpable goitre is detected.

NT-proBNP

NT-proBNP natriuretic peptide residue is a functional marker of increased myocardial stress. It can be useful to identify whether cats are in acute respiratory distress secondary to cardiac or respiratory disease. However, results should be interpreted with caution because both false negatives and false positives can occur. A quantitative assessment as well as a semi-quantitative assessment (NT-proBNP SNAP test) are available. SNAP tests are useful to identify the origin of dyspnoea in cats in an emergency (cardiac or non-cardiac). The SNAP tests can be performed with blood or pleural fluid. The SNAP test is a colorimetric test and the result is available in 10 minutes. It is positive with a NTproBNP concentration cut-off greater than 200 pmol/l and equivocal between 150–200 pmol/l. The quantitative blood test results needs to be shipped to the laboratory and provide an exact quantification. Quantitative tests can be used to screen for underlying moderate-severe cardiomyopathy in situations where an echocardiogram is not avaliable.

- Values above 270 pmol/l indicate heart disease as a likely cause of clinical signs and further investigation is warranted.
- Values below 50 pmol/l in asymptomatic cats indicate cardiac disease is unlikely.
- Values above 100 pmol/l indicate heart disease is probable and requires investigation.

Troponin I

Troponin I is a marker of myocardial damage. It is less useful than proBNP for distinguishing between cardiac or respiratory disease. However, levels are an independent risk factor for reduced life expectancy in cats with HCM. Caution is recommended with the use of markers, which are best used as a tool for decision making rather than as a definitive diagnostic test.

Blood pressure measurement

Systemic hypertension can cause structural changes to the heart, aggravate the remodelling of cardiomyopathy, or make it difficult to treat heart failure. In turn, patients with heart disease, especially those with heart failure, may have systemic hypotension.

During the cardiac screening process, **all cats should have their blood pressure measured**. This is recommended especially in adult or geriatric animals, those with kidney disease or CHF, or when changes associated with hypertension are present (e.g. slight symmetrical hypertrophy of the left ventricle.)

The **"white coat" effect** caused by stress complicates the diagnosis of systemic hypertension. If possible at least **five measurements should be taken and the mean calculated** (which should fluctuate by no more than 20%). This should be repeated several times and once the cat has acclimatized to the clinic. The correct diagnosis of hypertension, more than any other condition, depends on having cat-friendly facilities that minimize stress.

Values considered abnormal or potentially dangerous are described in Table 3.

Radiography

Radiography is often undertaken as the first step when determining if dyspnoea is due to cardiac, respiratory or intrathoracic pathology. However, an initial **rapid chest ultrasound** (**FAST scan**) is potentially more useful especially when pleural effusion is suspected.

Dyspnoeic patients must be stabilized before taking radiographs. In an emergency situation, stress should be avoided and a **single dorsoventral radiograph** may be the only view possible. In many cases, this is enough to diagnose cardiomegaly and heart failure. In more stable patients **dorsoventral and lateral views** are required, preferably with both right and left laterals, especially when respiratory disease is suspected.

When sedation is needed in patients with suspected heart disease, the author uses **butorphanol**, and where this is insufficient **butorphanol is combined with intravenous alfaxan** until adequate sedation is achieved. Other recommendations include a combination of **butorphanol, midazolam, and ketamine**.

Radiographic evaluation

The following steps outline the evaluation of thoracic radiographs with an emphasis on the heart (more details on acquiring thoracic radiographs and their evaluation are included in the "Diagnostic Imaging Techniques" chapter of this book):

1. **The quality** of the radiographs should be evaluated and they should be repeated if suboptimal.
2. The **entire chest cavity** should be reviewed and checked for pleural effusion or pneumothorax.
3. The portion of the **abdomen** included in the radiograph should also be examined.
4. The position, course and diameter of the **trachea and main bronchi** should be analysed.

Table 3. Classification of systolic and diastolic arterial pressure measure in mmHg in dogs and cats relative to the risk of damage to target organs (adapted from Brown, 2007).

Risk level	Systolic arterial pressure (mmHg)	Diastolic arterial pressure (mmHg)	Risk of injury in target organs
I	<150	<95	Minimal
II	150–159	95–99	Slight
III	160–179	100–119	Moderate
IV	≥180	≥120	Severe

5. The position of the **cardiac apex and the caudal mediastinum** should be checked.
6. The **margins of the heart** should be evaluated to detect cardiac enlargement (with the analogy of the clock as explained in the "Diagnostic Imaging Techniques" chapter).
7. The size, shape, and course of the main **pulmonary artery and peripheral pulmonary vessels** should be reviewed.
8. The **caudal vena cava** should be observed to detect elevation or enlargement.
9. The **lung field** should be assessed and the presence of hyper/hypoinflation or increased opacity, the pattern (bronchial, interstitial, alveolar) and its distribution assessed.

When evaluating feline radiographs for cardiac disease it is important to be aware that:

- In cats, particularly geriatric cats, the **cardiac axis** (the imaginary line between the carina and cardiac apex) becomes **more horizontal** with increased sternal contact on lateral radiography.
- The "area" where the left atrium is located in the cat is positioned more caudoventral to the carina, rather than caudodorsally as in the dog.
- The maximum **vertebral heart score (VHS) is 8**.
- The **absence of cardiomegaly does not rule out heart disease**, such as the presence of HCM, since the heart thickens but may not show an apparent increase in size.
- In cats with **left heart failure**, cardiomegaly is sometimes seen accompanied by distension of the pulmonary veins. These patients may present with pulmonary oedema or pleural effusion.
- In cats with **pulmonary oedema**, the lung pattern is very heterogeneous and interstitial. Broncho interstitial, interstitial-alveolar or alveolar patterns with a variable or multifocal location can be observed.
- In cats with **pleural effusion**, an increase in "soft tissue" opacity is observed that separates the lung lobules from each other (pleural fissure lines) and the sternum and, depending on the severity, there may be an absence of visualization of the diaphragmatic line.

Figures 10 to 14 illustrate the above.

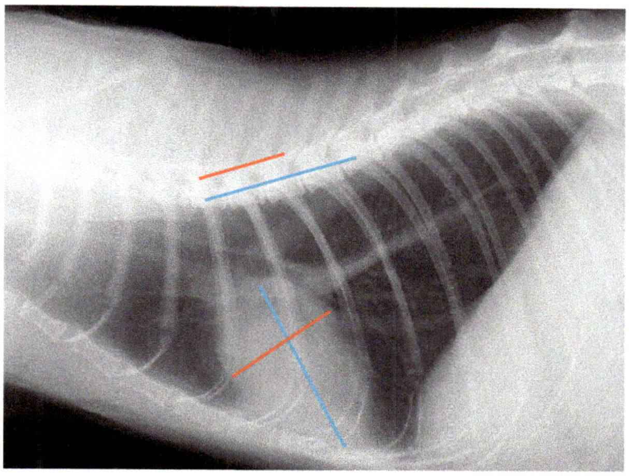

Figure 10. Thoracic radiograph of a normal cat to illustrate the vertebral heart score (VHS). Using a ruler or line on a digital radiograph to trace the longitudinal axis of the heart, which is measured (in blue) from the carina to the apex. This measurement is transferred to the vertebrae from the beginning of T4, counting the number of vertebrae which is covers (3.7 in this case). Later the transverse axis of the heart (in red) is calculated and measured again from T4 (3 vertebrae in this case) Both measurements are added together, and this is the VHS. In normal cats this should be less than 8.

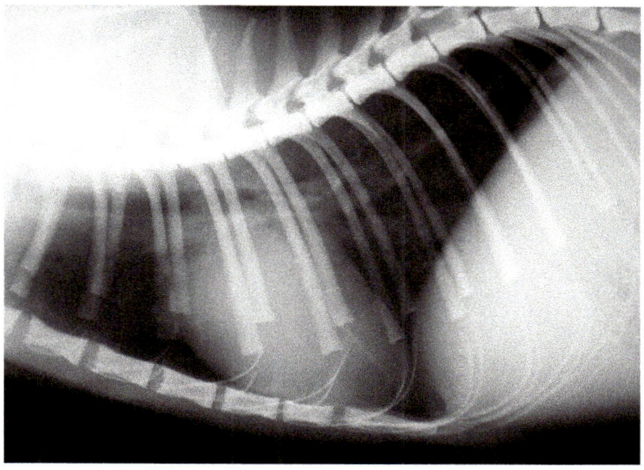

Figure 11. Lateral thoracic radiograph of a cat with HCM where severe cardiomegaly can be seen, with an absence of venous distension, pulmonary oedema or pleural effusion.

Thoracic ultrasound

Thoracic ultrasound (Figure 15) is a useful tool to investigate in cats presenting with dyspnoea. An important use is to **detect pleural effusion**, a common presentation of congestive heart failure.

For basic chest ultrasound, unlike echocardiography, virtually **any type of probe** can be used. The thorax is divided into **four imaginary parts** (ventrocranial, ventrocaudal, dorsocranial, and dorsoventral), which are evaluated one after the other. This examination can be performed with the animal sitting or standing, which is helpful for patients with dyspnoea.

The **normal appearance** of the lung is the visualization of the pleural line followed by **reverberation artefact** (A-lines, which represent the pleural line repeated in the distance) as can be seen in Figure 15A. It is important to remember this artefactual appearance of the normal lung for subsequent detection of abnormalities.

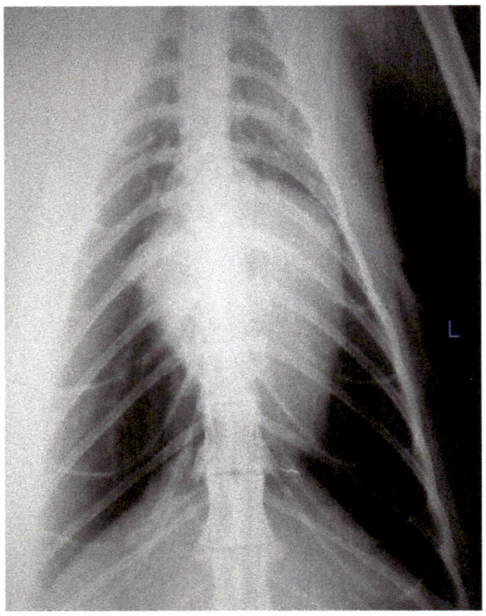

Figure 12. Lateral thoracic radiograph in which cardiomegaly and a broad heart base can be seen (Saint Valentines heart), suggesting atrial enlargement in a cat with HCM. There is no evidence of decompensation, as no venous distension, pulmonary oedema or pleural effusion.

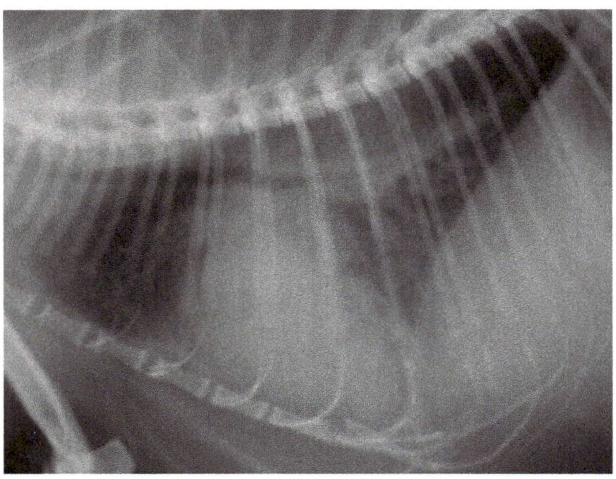

Figure 13. Radiograph of a cat with RCM with severe cardiomegaly and pulmonary oedema.

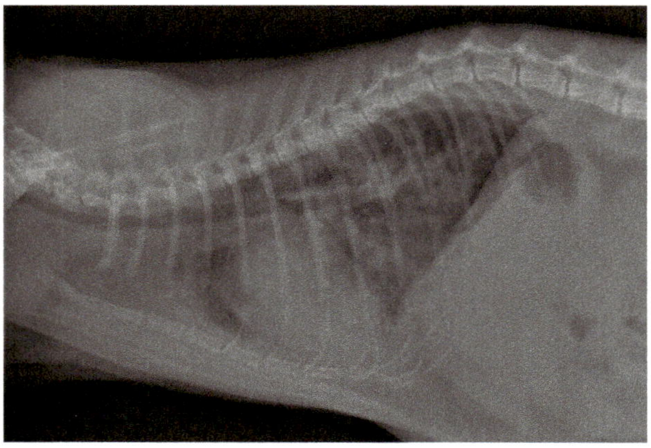

Figure 14. Radiograph of a cat with HCM illustrating cardiomegaly and pulmonary oedema, which in this case is manifested as an interstitial and multifocal alveolar pulmonary pattern with mild to moderate pleural effusion.

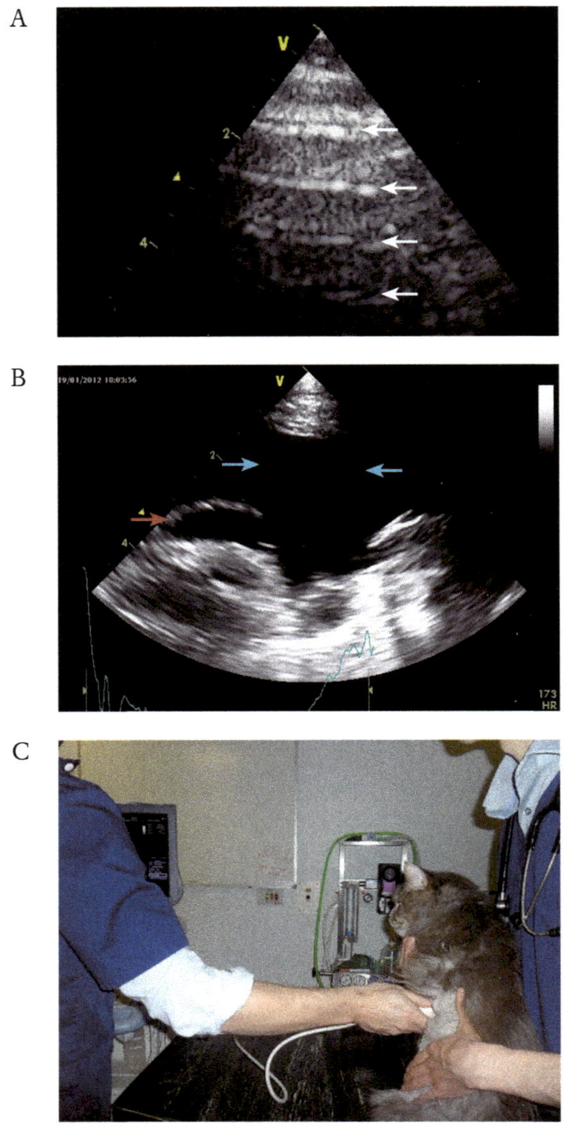

Figure 15. In Figure 15A a normal thoracic ultrasound with a typical image of the normal lung (interphase soft tissue artefact with pulmonary air) can be seen. The pleural line and its repetition in the reverberation time is seen (A lines – white arrows). In Figure 15B a thoracic ultrasound of a cat with pleural effusion. The normal thoracic-pulmonary appearance is substituted with a hypoechogenic space (blue arrows) where the pleural mediastinal leaflets are seen floating (red arrow). In Figure 15C an ultrasound carried out in a cat in a comfortable sternal position can be seen.

If the patient has a **pleural effusion**, the normal appearance of the lung is replaced by a **hypoechoic layer** in which (especially for moderate or severe effusions) the thoracic structures appear to float. Ultrasound can also be used to guide fluid aspiration.

The detection of interstitial disease such as pulmonary oedema is more complex. Operator experience is necessary and corroboration with chest radiography is recommended due to great variability in appearance. **Vertical B lines** are often seen as laser beams starting from the pleural line, obliterating A-lines, and moving with lung movement. However, in the same way that pleural effusion may be of cardiac origin; pulmonary oedema, interstitial or alveolar disease can arise from other aetiologies.

Echocardiography

Echocardiography is the most important tool for diagnosing heart disease in cats. Although echocardiography is best undertaken by cardiologists, a basic understanding of echocardiography and thoracic ultrasound helps the general practitioner make correct decisions at specific times or in an emergency, such as the cat with acute dyspnoea.

Preparation to perform the ultrasound

Echocardiography is carried out in **lateral recumbency (a baseline view in right lateral recumbency)** using a **special table with a hole** so the probe is manipulated under the cat. But in many emergency cases, basic chest and cardiac ultrasound are undertaken in **sternal recumbency** (to reduce patient stress) **to identify pleural effusion and atrial enlargement**.

Probes used for feline echocardiography must be of **high frequency** with a **small footprint**. These are usually small sector phased array or, if this is not available, a micro convex probe can be used. The **frequency varies but is usually 7.5–10 MHz**.

It is important to **clip the patient**, especially when using high frequencies or in obese animals. First, the location of the **cardiac apex should be palpated and a small square clipped** at this point. (It is common to clip too high or too far back given the heart is usually fairly horizontal.) The probe should be held with the thumb on the probe marker, which helps orientate the image. The operator should be comfortable, and while one hand holds the probe, the other adjusts the image settings on the machine's control panel.

Image settings

The feline heart moves rapidly, which makes **temporal resolution especially important**. Temporal resolution is the ability to differentiate heart structures in relation to time, that is, follow the dynamic movements of the heart and place them in the context of the heart's cycle. Optimal temporal resolution is a function of the frame rate and pulse repetition frequency and can be improved by **reducing the sector width and image depth**.

As with abdominal ultrasound, lateral and axial resolution are important in echocardiography and can be improved using higher frequencies, the approach to the structure, and the use of harmonics. The gain should be adjusted appropriately, as in abdominal ultrasound.

Echocardiographic artefacts

The most common echocardiographic artefacts are those caused by **breathing and movement**, the **side lobe** artefact, and the **reverberation/mirror** artefact. They must be taken into account so as not to confuse them with cardiac abnormalities:

- **Movement artefacts** can be minimized by good cat management or sedation (with the aforementioned sedation protocols).
- **Side-lobe artefact**. All probes generate beams lateral to the central sound beam. Reflections of these lateral beams in the different tissues return to the probe and the echocardiograph may erroneously interpret this information comes from the central beam if there is no reflection of the central beam at that level/moment. This artefact is similar to that produced in the urinary bladder, for example, and commonly occurs in the heart in a right longitudinal parasternal view.
- **Mirror artefact**. Reverberation occurs when sound waves collide with tissues that reflect them intensely, return to the probe, and then a second time to the heart, which reflects them again. The result is two sound echoes reflected by the same structure that return to the probe twice within a time interval and the machine interprets the second echo as coming from deeper (twice the distance). The typical mirror artefact is seen on an echocardiogram due to a strong reflex from the pericardium, which causes a mirror image below it (the heart may be seen twice). This artefact is the same one that commonly occurs in the liver and diaphragm (double liver on both sides of the diaphragm).

Sedation during echocardiography

The decision to sedate a patient during echocardiography is made on a case by case basis. It depends on the animal's behaviour, the underlying disease, and the cat's health. Echocardiography without sedation is preferable to minimize the effects of various drugs on the cardiovascular system. It is normally possible in a cat-friendly environment and with adequate training in handling these pets.

Possible protocols are outlined in the radiography section.

Basic echocardiographic views

Right parasternal view

Longitudinal four chamber view (Figure 16).

Position.

- The cat must be in right lateral recumbency.
- The probe should be placed on the right hemithorax.

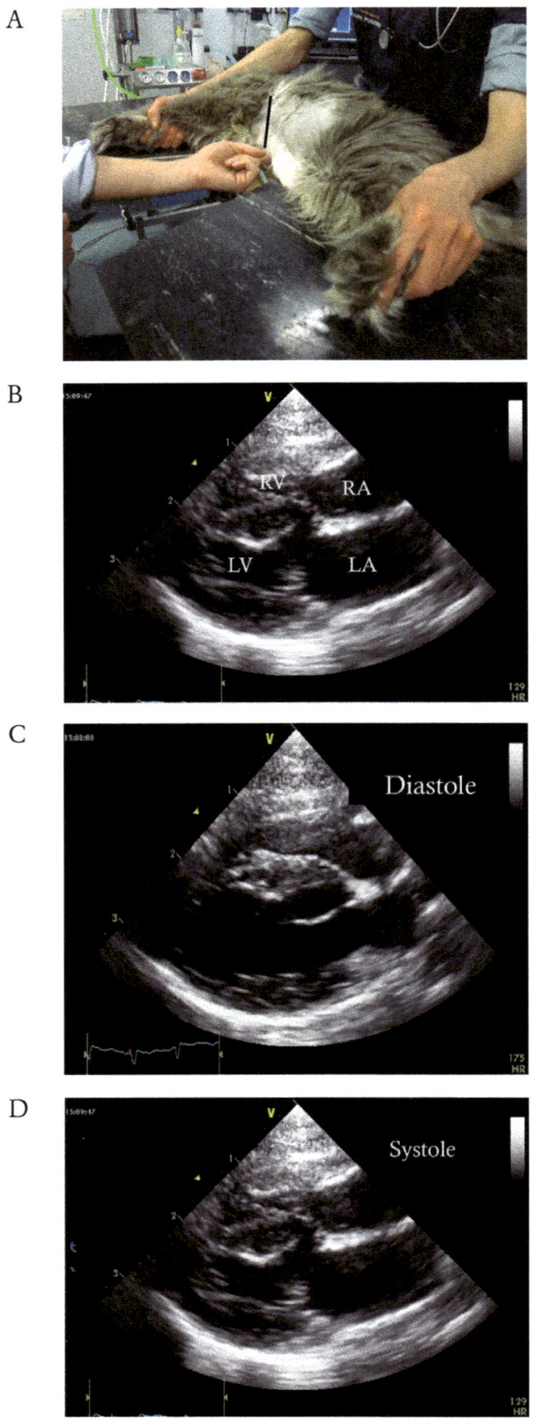

Figure 16. In Figure 16A the position needed to obtain right parasternal views can be seen and the direction from which to take the initial view of the 4 longitudinal chambers. In the frozen images C and D, the images which should be obtained from this angle can be seen, showing the four longitudinal chambers in both diastole and systole.

- The probe should be held with the thumb on the marker line of the probe.
- The cardiac apex is palpated, and the probe is placed there.
- The thumb should be pointing towards the echocardiographer the probe should be directed towards the scapula on the other side.
- Adjustments must be made to obtain a correct image.

This view can be used to:

- Assess of cardiac size: RV 1/3 of LV; IVS similar to LVFW; RVFW half IVSW/LVFW.
- Subjective evaluation of the heart particularly of increases in size and thickening of the heart and systolic function.
- Diagnosis of pericardial effusion.
- Assessment of atrial size (LA should be less than 1.6 cm at the end of systole) and echocardiographic smoke (blood that moves slowly).
- Subjective evaluation of the mitral and tricuspid valves.

Right parasternal view

Right longitudinal view optimized to view the left ventricular outflow tract (Figure 17).

Position:

From the right parasternal view:

- Rotate 10 degrees counter clockwise.
- Optimize the image to view the left ventricular outflow tract, the aortic valve, and, if possible, the ascending aorta.
- In cats this is sometimes the first view to be found and it can be difficult for the inexperienced clinician to "remove the aorta from the screen" and obtain a perfect four-chamber view.

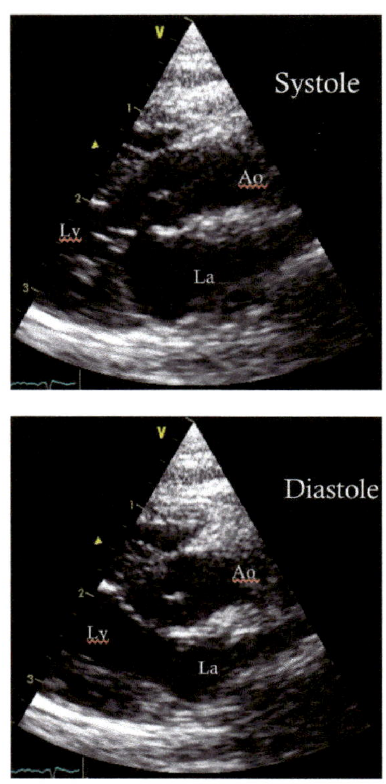

Figure 17. Right longitudinal parasternal view optimised to visualize the left ventricular outflow tract in diastole and systole.

A B C

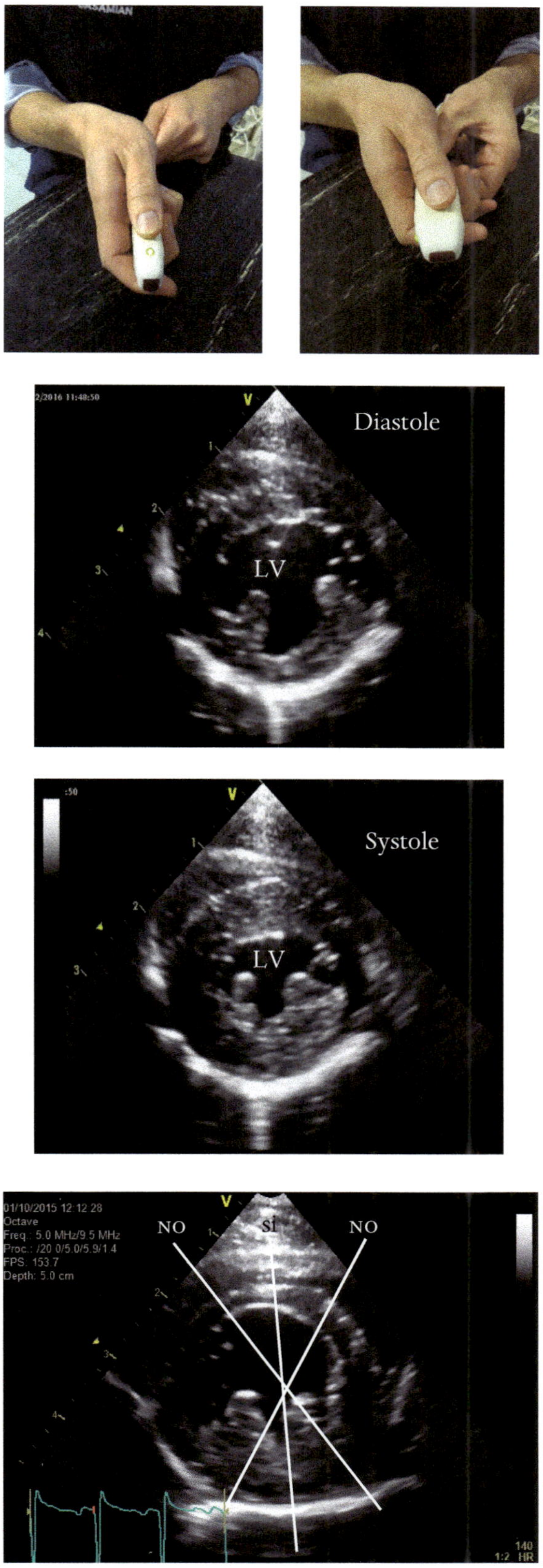

Figure 18. Rotation and positioning to obtain right parasternal transverse views after longitudinal views (A). In B an image of the left ventricle can be seen in systole and diastole. Image C shows how to obtain a section in M mode which should be perpendicular to the left ventricle. However, as explained in the text, measuring the size and ventricular thickening in the two planes is normal and adequate in the cat.

This view is used to:

- Evaluate the aortic valve.
- Evaluate the SAM from the mitral valve.
- Evaluation of ventricular septal defects.

Transverse right parasternal view (short axis)

Left ventricle (Figure 18).

Position:

- From the longitudinal four-chamber view.
- Rotate 90 degrees.
- To improve rotation, the wrist should be kept stable while rotating the probe 90 degrees. This should allow the probe to be manoeuvred more comfortably.
- The probe should be moved up or down or angled until the papillary muscles (below the mitral valve) are clearly visible.
- To achieve an M mode (one-dimensional ultrasound) the image should be optimized so that the line crosses the left ventricle perpendicularly, without touching the papillary muscles (difficult in cats).

This view can be used for the following:

- To measure the ventricular wall (detect hypertrophy) and calculate the ventricular dimensions in systole (when the ventricular dimension is smaller) and diastole (at the beginning of the QRS or if there is no ECG connected when the ventricle is larger). Two-dimensional ultrasound in cats is preferred to avoid inclusion of the papillary muscles.
- For the diagnosis of pericardial effusion.
- To calculate the shortening fraction (assess systolic function).

Transverse right parasternal view (short axis)

Height of cardiac base (Figure 19).

Position:

- From the anterior view, at the level of the left ventricle move (preferable) or angulate dorsally.
- Normally, the probe has to be moved cranially (often skipping an intercostal space) and the view is angled slightly.
- A transverse section of the aorta can be visualised (Mercedes sign) and the left atrium can be seen.

This view can be used to:

- Evaluate the size of the left atrium (normally the aorta/atrial ratio is less than 1.5). Measurement is recommended early in diastole (the frame after the aortic valve is closed).
- Visualize echocardiographic smoke or thrombi.

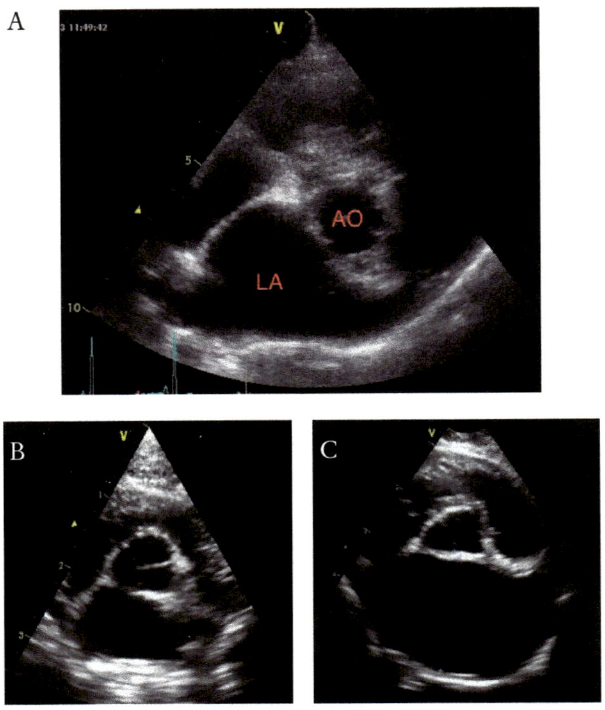

Figure 19. Figure 19A shows the appearance of the right transverse parasternal view at the level of the aortic valve and left atrium. In Figure 19B a normal sized atrium can be seen, while in Figure 19C a markedly enlarged atrium can be seen.

Basic echocardiographic findings in cats with cardiopathies

Basic echocardiography is a valuable tool when investigating the dyspnoeic patient. The presence of an **enlarged left atrium usually indicates the presence of heart disease**. If this is combined with the presence of **pleural effusion** (as long as it is a modified transudate or chylothorax) and/or pulmonary oedema on radiographs, a working diagnosis of congestive heart failure can usually be made.

The **risk of thromboembolism** is assessed by the presence of a **severely enlarged atrium**, the presence of echocardiographic smoke (slow blood movement), and intracardiac thrombi. An initial working diagnosis can be made by subjectively evaluating the possible presence of one of the most common cardiomyopathies (HCM or RCM). However, a cardiologist should make a definitive diagnosis, including evaluating systolic and diastolic function by performing a complete or advanced echocardiogram that includes other echocardiographic views and Doppler techniques.

Hypertrophic cardiomyopathy (HCM)

- Left ventricle wall thicknesses above 6 mm are considered hypertrophic and a grey zone of 5–6 mm may be considered equivocal for left ventricular hypertrophy. Hypertrophy is often asymmetric.
- In cats with obstructive HCM, the anterior movement of the mitral valve (SAM) can be observed on many occasions.
- Enlarged left atrium: the size of the left atrium depends on the severity of the disease and is the most important prognostic factor.
- Sometimes obliteration of the left ventricular cavity is observed (the interventricular and free walls come into contact).
- A heterogeneous myocardium is often seen.
- Areas of myocardial infarction (hypo or akinetic and thin-walled areas) are often seen.

Restrictive cardiomyopathy (RCM)

- Normal ventricular wall thickness.
- The size of the left ventricle is normal.
- In the endomyocardial form, the endocardium is affected and sometimes thickened and hyperechoic, with fibrous bands in the left ventricle.
- Normal systolic function is seen (the shortening fraction and ventricular dimension in systole are usually normal).
- An enlarged atrium is seen and, normally, greatly enlarged (> 2.0 cm) at the time of diagnosis, since practically all cases of RCM present in cardiac failure.
- As patients usually present in heart failure, pleural effusion can be seen.

Dilated cardiomyopathy (DCM)

- Intraluminal enlargement of the left ventricle and atrium and, very commonly, also of the right.
- Left ventricle with a spherical appearance.
- Severe systolic dysfunction: marked increase in ventricular dimensions in systole and a significant decrease in the shortening fraction.
- Possible presence of smoke and clots, as in other cardiomyopathies.
- Cats normally also present in cardiac failure, and pleural effusion can be observed.

Pericardial effusion

- There is a gap without acoustic or hypoechoic echo between the epicardium and the pericardial sac.

Table 4. Cardiac measurements in a normal heart and in those affected by DCM, HCM and RCM.

	Normal	DCM	HCM	RCM
LVDs (mm)	6.7–9.7 (<12)	>11–12	Normal or reduced	Normal or reduced
LVDd (mm)	14–17 (<18)	>18	Normal or reduced	Normal or reduced
LVPWd/ IVSWd (mm)	3.0–4.2 (<6)	Normal or reduced	>6 mm	<6 mm
FS (%)	36–52% (<55)	<30%	Normal or increased	Normal or mildly reduced

- LVDs: left ventricular dimension in systole; LVDd: left ventricular dimension in diastole; LVP Wd: left ventricular posterior wall thickness in diastole; IVS Wd: interventricular septum wall thickness in diastole; FS: shortening fraction.
- The heart appears with an oscillating movement, which "floats in the liquid" when the effusion is significant.
- Cardiac tamponade results in diastolic collapse of the right atrium and right ventricle in severe cases.
- Effusion is not seen behind the aortic base (left and right atria), which helps to differentiate it from the presence of pleural effusion.

Common mistakes on ultrasound

Technique

Echocardiography is more difficult in cats than in dogs, since they are more wriggly, the feline structures are smaller, and the heart beats faster. This is why, beyond the basic use that has been outlined, echocardiography should be performed by a cardiologist to avoid erroneous diagnoses.

Some common mistakes include:

- Measurement of the intraluminal dimensions of the left ventricle or atrium at an inappropriate plane and time.
- Measuring ventricular thickening at the wrong ventricular height (too low in the ventricle), which can lead to a misdiagnosis of HCM.
- Including papillary muscles when measuring the left ventricle, which can also lead to an incorrect diagnosis of hypertrophy (especially in M mode).
- Obtaining views in oblique planes, which will give a subjective appearance and erroneous measurements.
- Confusing fibrous bands from the left ventricle with the ventricular endothelium, which can lead to a diagnosis of hypertrophy in a normal cat.
- Using inadequate gain levels, which can lead to echocardiographic smoke going undetected.

Intrinsic to basic echocardiography

Even though the images and measurements are satisfactory, there are some limitations to keep in mind when diagnosing feline heart disease.

Some of these include:

- The presence of thickening of the ventricular wall does not inexorably mean that the patient has HCM. The thickening may be due to hypovolaemia (pseudohypertrophy), hyperthyroidism, systemic arterial hypertension, aortic stenosis, myocarditis, or idiopathic transient thickening (TMF) of the ventricular wall.
- A diagnosis of HCM is not only based on thickening of the ventricular wall. Other factors such as the appearance of the papillary muscles, the presence of SAM and diastolic function are also taken into account.
- The presence of heart disease does not directly mean that the cat has or will have heart failure. Heart disease and heart failure are different terms.
- Although cardiomyopathies are the most common heart diseases, they are not the only ones: heart disease and heart failure do not inexorably mean cardiomyopathy.
- Echocardiographic smoke and/or thrombi may be "hidden" in the left auricle and left parasternal views may be necessary for their diagnosis. Furthermore, cats with cardiopathies causing large atria may be at risk of thromboembolism in the absence of obvious echocardiographic smoke.
- There may be superimpositions and overlaps. For example, a hyperthyroid cardiomyopathy with early HCM.

Cardiomyopathies

A consensus on the diagnosis of feline cardiomyopathy was recently released by the American College of Veterinary Internal Medicine, which adapted the European Society of Cardiology Cardiomyopathy classification to feline patients. The cardiomyopathies classification is performed based on cardiac structure and function (phenotype). This scheme is based on phenotypic features without assumptions regarding underlying cause. Primary cardiomyopathy is suspected when other underling diseases causing myocardial changes are excluded. The phenotypic categories include hypertrophic cardiomyopathy (HCM), restrictive cardiomyopathy (RCM), dilated cardiomyopathy (DCM), unclassified cardiomyopathy (UCM), and arrhythmogenic right ventricular cardiomyopathy (ARVC). Sometimes it is not possible to include cardiac phenotype in these groups and this is defined as a non specific phenotype.

The consensus includes a staging system. This considers cats predisposed to develop cardiomyopathy as stage A, cats with cardiomyopathy that do not show clinical signs of CHF or ATE belong to stage B, and cats that developed CHF/ATE are classified as stage C. Cats that have been treated for CHF/ATE in the past but develop refractory heart failure are classified as stage D. Stage B is further subclassified as B1 or B2 based on the perceived risk of development of clinical signs: low risk patients are classified as B1, high risk patients are classified as B2.

Primary cardiomyopathies

Hypertrophic cardiomyopathy (HCM)

The most common feline cardiomyopathy is HCM, which represents 60–70% of all cardiomyopathy cases. This section considers the idiopathic or primary forms of HCM. The pathologies that cause secondary ventricular wall thickening (such as high blood pressure, hyperthyroidism, acromegaly, neoplasms such as lymphoma, or FIP) are covered in the section on secondary cardiomyopathies.

Definition

HCM is characterized by **thickening of the ventricular wall and papillary muscles**. A high percentage of cats (25–67%) have **obstruction of the left outflow tract** due to systolic movement of the anterior mitral valve leaflet (SAM), and these cases are subclassified as obstructive hypertrophic cardiomyopathy (OHCM).

Incidence

This varies depending on the breed, geographical location, and the upper limit used for the thickened wall (8–16%). In most studies there is a **male predisposition**, although it has been suggested (for the Maine Coon) males may appear predisposed as they develop the disease earlier.

Aetiology

The specific **cause is unknown**. However, the disease has been shown to run in families and is **hereditary in breeds** such as the Maine Coon, Persian, British Shorthair, Norwegian Forest, Ragdoll, Turkish Van and Scottish Fold. The disease is also very common in the common cat. Breeds such as Siamese, Abyssinian and Burmese have a low incidence of HCM.

In human medicine, many mutations in genes encoding sarcomeric proteins have been discovered, as responsible for causing disease. Similarly, two different mutations have been identified in the gene encoding myosin-binding protein C in the Maine Coon and Ragdoll.

Pathophysiology

HCM causes **diastolic dysfunction** which leads to heart failure in moderate and severe cases. Thickening of the myocardium causes stiffness of the ventricular cavity, and together with ischaemia, cell death, and fibrosis causes decreased ventricular relaxation and compliance.

Other factors associated with the disease that can cause clinical signs include the presence of:

- **arrhythmias** (mainly supra or ventricular but also bradyarrhythmias), which reduce diastolic filling, increase pressure gradients, and reduce cardiac output.
- **SAM**, which increases intraventricular systolic pressure increasing the stress on the ventricular wall and its hypertrophy.
- **mitral regurgitation** (often associated with SAM, but also seen in the non-obstructive subtype), which can increase preload.

Although HCM is primarily a **diastolic disease**, Doppler studies show mild systolic dysfunction may also occur. The presence of severe, regional systolic dysfunction due to heart attacks or, in the advanced, final stage, generalized systolic failure can be observed with conventional echocardiography.

Diagnosis

Electrocardiography

ECG may show ventricular, supraventricular, bradyarrhythmias or findings associated with left ventricular enlargement (R wave greater than 0.9 mV). In many cases, the presence of a left deviation of the electrical axis is compatible with left anterior fascicular block (11–33%). Episodic arrhythmias may cause syncope and **Holter analysis** is necessary for a definitive diagnosis.

Genetic mutation test

Genetic testing is available for two breeds, the Maine Coon and the Ragdoll, but caution is required when interpreting the results. The finding of a **homozygous positive** indicates the individual has a **high risk of developing the disease** and, therefore, breeding from them is not advised. If the individual is heterozygous, the evolution is much less predictable, since many individuals may not develop the disease. A negative test does not rule out HCM either, as the gene mutation is not its only cause.

Blood markers for myocardial disease

Blood biomarkers may indicate the absence or presence of cardiac muscle distress, such as due to HCM, but do not provide a definitive diagnosis of the cause.

Echocardiography

Echocardiography is the main diagnostic tool for detecting myocardial diseases in the cat. With HCM, **hypertrophy (thickening) of the left ventricle** and occasionally of the right ventricle is seen. The ventricular wall **measured at the end of diastole should be less than 6 mm** (some cardiologists use 5.5 mm). The disease is heterogeneous in distribution and severity, with areas of focal thickening possible.

Measurements are taken using **2D mode with the heart in diastole.** This requires a scanner with a good frame rate, preferably with the simultaneous use of an ECG.

Other common findings include:

- enlarged left and right atria
- decreased ventricular luminal dimensions
- hypertrophy of papillary muscles
- mitral regurgitation
- normal or elevated shortening fraction.

SAM can be detected with 2D or M-mode. It is associated with left ventricular outflow tract obstruction and is quantified using spectral Doppler of the left, five-chamber parasternal view. The flow has a characteristic dagger appearance (suggesting a dynamic obstruction). In colour Doppler, this is typified by mitral regurgitation with a bi-lobed jet that begins at the level of the outlet tract obstruction.

The aetiology of SAM is not clear, but may be due to hypertrophied papillary stretching of the mitral apparatus during systole. This obstruction is often labile and present only under stress in periods of

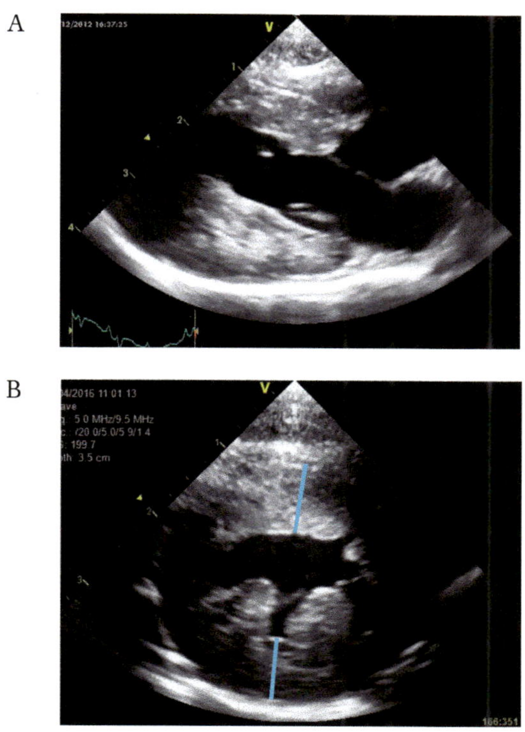

Figure 20. Two-dimensional echocardiography in two hearts from cats with HCM. In Figure 20A a right longitudinal parasternal view shows a severely thickened free wall with heterogeneous intramural echogenicity. In Figure 20B the heart of a cat with hypertrophic cardiomyopathy shows moderate thickening of the interventricular and free walls (blue lines indicate the measurement of the enlarged ventricular walls).

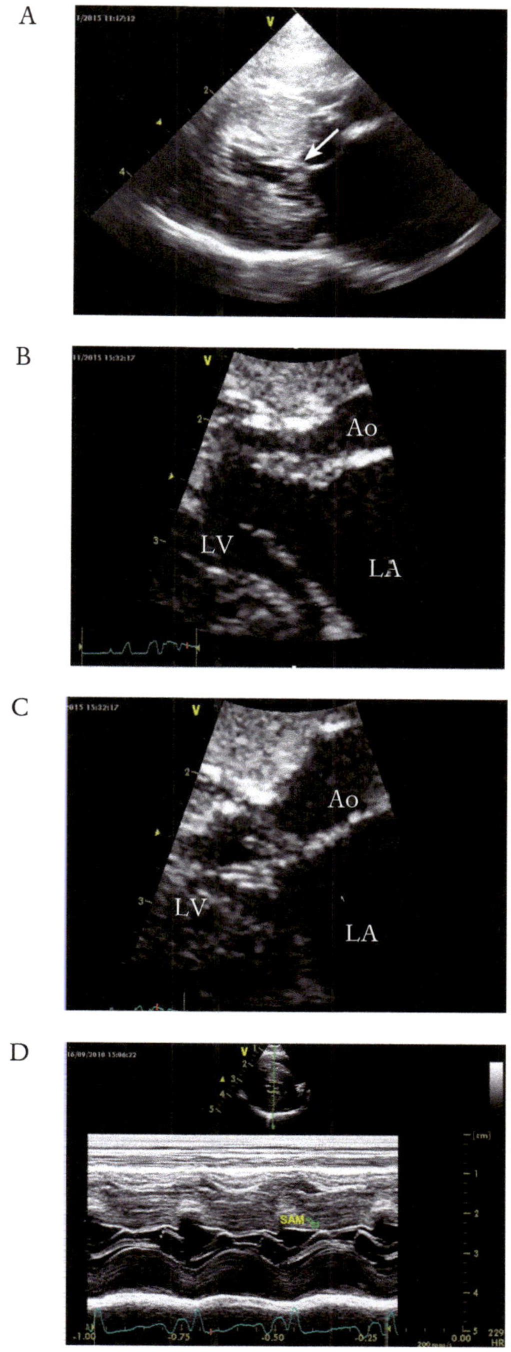

Figure 21. Echocardiographic studies showing systolic movement (motion) of the anterior valve of the mitral valve (SAM) in two cats with hypertrophic cardiomyopathy. In the first image (A) the anterior valve is shown moving towards the septum (arrow) in a right longitudinal parasternal view. In Image B this area has been magnified and can be seen in diastole with the mitral valve open and in systole (C) the presence of the anterior part of the mitral valve in the left ventricular outflow tract can be seen. In Image D SAM can be seen in M mode.

high sympathetic tone. Before diagnosing HCM it is important to **rule out other causes of concentric ventricular hypertrophy** such as aortic stenosis, systemic arterial hypertension, hyperthyroidism, acromegaly, TMF, and infiltrative diseases (lymphoma or FIP). Similarly, some hypovolaemic cats may present with pseudo hypertrophy due to a severe decrease in total plasma volume.

Cats with **HCM have abnormal diastolic function**, which is evaluated clinically by means of transmitral flow, evaluation of the isovolumetric relaxation time of the flow of the pulmonary veins, and by pulsed tissue or longitudinal colour Doppler. Other techniques such as cardiac function analysis by speckle tracking are not used in day to day practice.

Three main patterns are observed depending on the stage of the disease:

- Impaired relaxation
- Pseudo normalisation
- Restrictive filling

In some cats it is not possible to reliably differentiate between normal and mild HCM. These cases are **classified as ambiguous** and the echocardiogram repeated six months later.

Treatment

In **asymptomatic cats**, there is no evidence any treatment (diltiazem, ACE inhibitors, β-blockers) changes disease progression and improves the prognosis. In a recent study, the administration of atenolol during this phase did not improve life expectancy (the vast majority of cases in this study had no significant left outlet obstruction). However, the Feline Consensus statement suggests that atenolol may be considered in cats with stage B1 cardiomyopathy and severe dynamic left ventricle outflow obstruction. Atenolol is not recommended in stage B2, C or D. Animals with **significant arrhythmias that cause symptoms** are treated with drugs appropriate to the arrhythmia.

Finally, an important group that require treatment in the **asymptomatic phase are those at risk of aortic thromboembolism**, as characterized by an enlarged atrium, slow-moving blood visualized as "smoke", reduced appendicular velocities, or visualization of a clot (stage B2). Treatment involves using agents such as **clopidogrel and/or aspirin**.

Congestive heart failure: basic acute therapy

The initial and primary goal of treating these patients (stage C) is thoracocentesis to **drain pleural effusion** if present and **relieve congestion** by reducing preload. In this **acute phase oxygen therapy, furosemide and vasodilators** (such as nitro-glycerine ointment) are used, as well as pimobendan. This improves systolic and diastolic function, especially in the absence of severe left outflow tract obstruction.

Two key aspects of management are to minimize stress and avoid severe dehydration. Response to treatment is monitored through **observation of respiratory rate** and repeat transthoracic ultrasound (to detect pleural effusion), and thoracic radiography. Echocardiography is helpful to evaluate left-filling pressures.

It is important **not to over-treat with diuretics** as this can lead to hypotension, dehydration and hypokalaemia, which can lead to anorexia and a dangerous cycle of further dehydration. Sometimes administering appetite stimulants or water via a naso-oesophageal feeding tube is necessary. It is important to monitor blood pressure, electrolytes, and kidney parameters during treatment.

Basic chronic therapy

Once the respiratory rate is below **40–45 breaths per minute, the furosemide dose should be reduced** to standard levels (2–3 mg/kg BID or TID). An **angiotensin-converting enzyme (ACE) inhibitor** is often added at this time because of its multiple theoretical benefits (such as vasodilation or attenuation of the renin-angiotensin cascade) and its proven benefits in other species for congestive heart failure (people and dogs). However, a clinical study in cats confirms that ACE inhibitors (benazepril) do not delay the onset of a new episode of congestive heart failure.

Pimobendan (a positive ionotrope and vasodilator) may be given at this point. There is evidence cats tolerate the medication well, and the results suggest it may have clinical benefits. However, at the time of writing, there are no robust studies confirming the possible clinical benefits of this product. **Pimobendan usage should be avoided in patients with left ventricular outflow obstruction** (particularly with severe obstructions) because a potential increase in contractibility could potentially aggravate the obstruction.

In this phase, treatment with spironolactone should be considered: an anti-remodelling, ant fibrotic and light diuretic drug. A recent study shows it is a well-tolerated medication, but more studies are needed to determine if there is a clinical benefit to its use.

An important point is monitoring of **the respiratory rate at home at rest**, to achieve the most effective minimum dose. A respiratory rate below 30–40 normally indicates the absence of CHF, although there are individual variations and it is important to know the patient's normal respiratory rate.

After discharging the patient, it is advisable to consult and/or provide updates by phone to find out how the condition evolves: appetite, activity, respiratory rate and weight and adjust the dose until a stable situation is reached and less frequent monitoring is required.

Table 5. Commonly used medications for the treatment of cats with hypertrophic cardiomyopathy (HCM).

Active ingredient	Dose
Enoxaparin (low molecular weight heparin)	0.75–1.0mg/kg SC q 6–12 hours
Rivaroxaban (anti factor Xa)	0.5–1.0 mg/kg PO q 24 hours
Benazepril (ACEI)	0.25–0.5 mg/kg PO q 24 h
Enalapril (ACEI)	0.5 mg/kg PO q 12–24 h
Ramipril (ACEI)	0.125 mg/kg PO q 24 h
Imidapril (ACEI)	0.5 mg/kg PO q 24 h
Propranolol (B1, B2 blocker)	2.5–5 mg/cat PO q 8 h
Atenolol (B1 blocker)	6.25–12.5 mg/cat PO q 12–24 h[1]
Diltiazem (calcium channel blocker)	0.5–2 mg/kg PO q 8h
Aspirin (inhibition of platelet aggregation)	High dose: 75 mg/cat PO every 3 days Low dose: 5 mg/cat PO every 3 days[2]
Clopidogrel (inhibition of platelet aggregation)	18.5–75 mg/cat PO q 24 h[3]
Delteparin (low molecular weight heparin, coagulation inhibitor)	100 IU/kg SC q 12 h
Nitro-glycerine (cream) (vasodilator)	0.5–0.75 cm q 8 h on an area of skin without hair or which is clipped
Furosemide (loop diuretic)	Variable. PO, SC, IM, IV (possible doses are mentioned in the text)
Spironolactone (potassium-sparing diuretic)	2–4 mg/kg PO q 24 h

1: Preferably twice a day.
2: The author uses a quarter of a 75 mg tablet per cat every three days, the lowest possible dose available without reformulating.
3: The author uses 18.75 mg because this dose seems to provide the same benefits as 75 mg.

It is **important to follow-up on the patient**, even if by phone to avoid the stress of going to the vet until a stable situation is achieved. Not to do so risks the patient decompensating and needing hospitalization again, which can lead to euthanasia due to cost and owner frustration.

If the furosemide dose is high (more than 10 mg/kg/day), another diuretic can be added such as thiazide. Some cats require very high doses of furosemide and kidney indicator values and electrolytes should be monitored frequently. A small study showed there was no benefit in β-blocker or diltiazem therapy at this stage. In general, it is best to avoid these medications (particularly β-blockers) in heart failure as they can cause severe decompensation of myocardial function. The only exception is if there are serious arrhythmias, in which case advice should be sought or the case referred to a cardiologist.

Treatment and prevention of arterial thromboembolism

The ideal time to **start prevention with antithrombotic medication** in HCM is unknown Antithrombotic treatment is usually started when:

- The left atrium is moderately large (> 2.0 cm).
- There is "echocardiographic smoke" that indicates slowing of blood movement.
- There are low appendicular velocities on Doppler (below 0.2 m/s).
- In cases in which a thrombus is observed on the heart.
- In cases where a previous episode of thromboembolism is documented.

Clopidogrel is the preferred treatment of choice, rather than aspirin, as it is more effective, or the two may be combined. Where the cost of clopidogrel is a barrier to treatment, then aspirin should be used. Warfarins have fallen out of favour due to their side effects. Dalteparin (low molecular weight heparin) is sometimes used by cardiologists in severe cases, although there are no clinical studies documenting its efficacy and/or superior effect compared to clopidogrel. Some theoretically more potent agents, such as rivaroxaban (factor Xa inhibitor) are used sporadically in refractory patients, but to date there are no clinical studies available.

Treatment of aortic thromboembolism is based on:

- Rest.
- Analgesia.
- Nutritional and fluid support.
- Prevention of further thrombus formation.
- Treatment of heart failure if present (44% of cases).

Dissolution of the thrombus with fibrinolytics (such **as tPA) or removal by surgical techniques is not recommended**, as this does not improve survival, but increases morbidity and the cost of treatment. In many cases, given negative prognostic factors or the absence of improvement within 24–48 hours, owners **choose euthanasia**.

Prognosis

The **prognosis for HCM is very variable**:

- Asymptomatic cats with mild or moderate disease and a normal left atrium have a good prognosis in the short term and many also in the long term.

- In cats with an enlarged left atrium, heart failure is more likely to develop in the future, and if the enlargement is significant, heart failure is more likely in the short term.

The **most important prognostic factors** are:

- Presence of extreme hypertrophy.
- Atrial dysfunction or systolic ventricular dysfunction.
- Enlarged left atrium.
- Heart failure.
- Presence of aortic thromboembolism.

In one study, the life expectancy (as medians) described for asymptomatic cats with a normal atrium was 3,617 days and for asymptomatic cats from 1,129 to 1,830 days. Life expectancy for cats with an enlarged left atrium but not in heart failure was 229 days, while for those in heart failure was 194 days.

However, according to data from the same study, 20% of cats with heart failure lived for many years. In contrast, other studies describe survival rates of between 91 and 561 days. The life expectancy for cats with thromboembolism and HCM is 61 to 184 days, depending on the study. About 35–39% of cats survive an episode of thromboembolism.

Restrictive cardiomyopathy (RCM)

Restrictive cardiomyopathy (RCM) is more common in cats than dilated cardiomyopathy, but less common than hypertrophic cardiomyopathy.

RCM is characterized by normal or slightly reduced systolic function, normal ventricular wall thickness, and severe diastolic dysfunction. Diagnosis depends on the demonstration of a **restrictive pattern during transmitral flow**. There are two main forms: the purely myocardial form and the endomyocardial form.

Unclassified cardiomyopathy does not meet the definition of any of the other cardiomyopathies and, in many cases, has the characteristics of restrictive cardiomyopathy but without the presence of a restrictive pattern, because there is no separation of transmitral E and A waves.

Aetiology and pathophysiology

The aetiology of RCM is unknown. There are four main hypotheses:

1. The presence of **feline panleukopoenia virus in the myocardium** of some RCM cats has been documented, and may result in myocarditis.
2. In human medicine, there is an **eosinophilic form** of RCM. This is described in a single feline case and is unlikely to be common.
3. Results from **genetic mutations** (as occurs in people) of proteins in myocardial cells, such as troponin I or T or actin.
4. **HCM and RCM are grouped as a single disease** with a different phenotypic expression. Some of the genetic mutations (see 3) may evolve into different phenotypes (RCM or HCM). Both diseases are characterized by diastolic function and a recent review article showed the histopathology of the two diseases is similar:
   a. Areas of structural disorganization and myocardial disorganisation.
   b. Alterations to the intramural coronary arteries.
   c. Replacement fibrosis due to ischaemia and cell death.
   d. Severe changes in the left, and often right, ventricle lead to severe diastolic dysfunction and left heart failure with pulmonary oedema and/or pleural or sometimes biventricular effusion.

Clinical presentation and physical examination

Patients are usually adult animals (average age of 7 or 10 years in two different studies).

The clinical presentation is similar to that of cats with HCM, however, cats with RCM most commonly present with **heart failure or an episode of thromboembolism. Cats may have murmurs (33% of cases), gallop sounds, or no auscultation abnormalities.**

Pleural effusion is typified by tachypnoea, with muffled heart and respiratory sounds. The heart rate (unlike in dogs in heart failure) can be normal, high and even low. There may be ventricular or supraventricular arrhythmias. Some cases show clinical signs of arterial thromboembolism.

Diagnostic tests

The findings on physical examination, functional analysis, and radiography are similar to those described for HCM.

Ventricular or supraventricular arrhythmias may be present on the ECG.

Echocardiography shows an **enlarged left or binaural atrium, normal ventricular thickness, and normal or very slightly reduced systolic function.** Some patients have endomyocardial fibrosis, which can obstruct much of the ventricular lumen. In diastolic studies, severe alterations with a classic restrictive transmitral pattern are observed. Although there are no studies regarding this, serious abnormalities in diastolic function can be appreciated when it is evaluated with tissue Doppler or speckle tracking.

Treatment

The treatment of heart failure in RCM is as for HCM.

Prognosis

The **prognosis is relatively poor**. Although some cats live for a few months with a good quality of life, the life expectancy (median) in three different studies is 105, 132 and 273 days respectively.

Arrhythmogenic right ventricular cardiomyopathy (ARVC)

Arrhythmogenic right ventricular cardiomyopathy (ARVC) is a **myocardial disease** characterized by anatomical and functional dysfunction of the right ventricle which results in **replacement of ventricular tissue with fibrous or fatty-fibrous tissue.**

In the cat ARVC is a **rare cardiomyopathy** (1–2% of all cardiomyopathies). It usually occurs in **adult or older** cats, although it is described in cats from 1 to 20 years old. It is suspected that Burmese cats may have a predisposition.

In humans, **ARVC is a disease affecting desmosome proteins** that causes problems with cell adhesion, death of myocytes, and subsequent replacement of myocytes by fat and fibrous tissue. There are more than 800 types of human genetic variants in 12 genes that encode for five desmosomal and some non-desmosomal proteins, but only about 300 cause problems and 35 of them are responsible for 65% of cases.

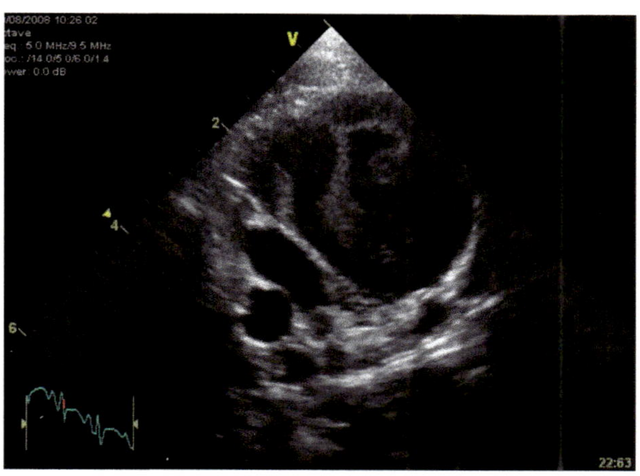

Figure 22. Echocardiographic study in a patient with restrictive cardiomyopathy (left cranial parasternal view not described in this chapter) where echocardiographic 'smoke' is seen (blood which moves slowly and seems like moving hyperechogenic waves) in the left atrium which indicates that the patient is at risk of thromboembolism. This "smoke" can also be seen in right parasternal views.

A B C

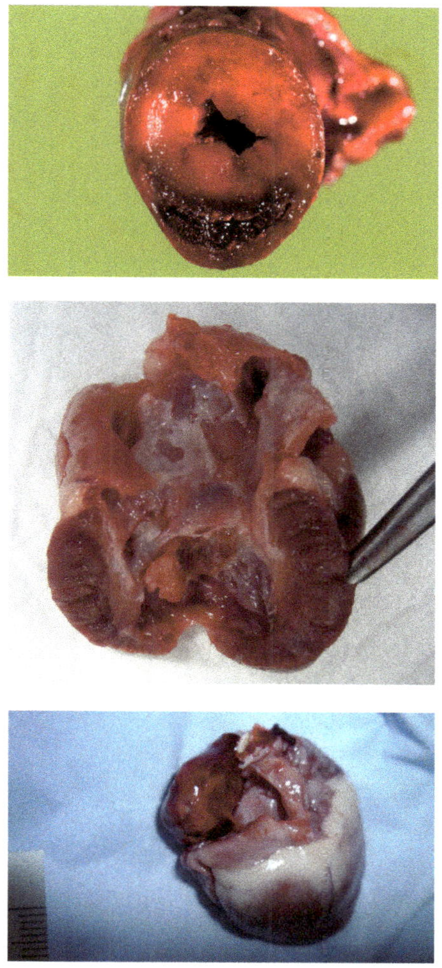

Figure 23. Histopathological analysis in three cats. In Figure 23A the left ventricle from a cat with hypertrophic cardiomyopathy can be seen. In Figure 23B the left ventricle with a mildly thickened, irregular endocardium and a severely enlarged atrium can be seen from a cat with restrictive cardiomyopathy. In Figure 23C a thrombus from a cat with restrictive cardiomyopathy can be seen inside the left atrium which is increased in size.

In the dog, the disease has been associated with a genetic mutation, by deletion of the striatin gene located on chromosome 17. However, subsequent studies have shown this abnormality also occurs in healthy individuals and it is currently thought it may play a role in the development of the disease but is not the direct cause. There **are no studies on the possible association of a genetic mutation with the disease in cats.**

In people and dogs the disease is inherited as autosomal dominant with incomplete penetration; but due to the low number of cases described, its hereditary pattern in cats is unknown. Desmosomal abnormalities lead to impaired function and structure of myocardial cells, which in the dog often lead to arrhythmias and myocardial dysfunction.

Although their pathophysiology and pathology is similar to that of the dog, **feline patients usually present with congestive heart failure and severe right**

heart dysfunction instead of arrhythmias and syncope. Changes in the right ventricle are usually severe, with enlargement and decreased right ventricular movement. There may also be **aneurysms in the right ventricle** (as in the dog.) Left ventricular function may be slightly or moderately altered but is often normal.

A differential diagnosis to rule out is tricuspid valve dysplasia, in which the valve is abnormal. This occurs in younger patients and the prognosis is poor, with most cats euthanized in the first few months after diagnosis.

Dilated cardiomyopathy (DCM)

DCM is characterized by **ventricular enlargement accompanied by systolic dysfunction**, and frequently also diastolic dysfunction. The disease commonly affects the left or both ventricles. Although the disease is often diagnosed as idiopathic (the cause is unknown), it is likely the result of viral, toxic, nutritional, or genetic myocardial insults.

DCM was the most common myocardial disease of cats until 1987. Following the discovery by Dr Paul Pion in 1987 that many of these cats suffered from **taurine deficiency**, this was supplemented in feline diets to the effect that the disease is now very rare. **Plasma taurine should be measured in every cat with DCM.** If the level is low (and arguably if it is not) it should be supplemented with this essential amino acid, alongside treatment for heart failure. Taurine deficiency occurs mainly due to diets with an absence of animal protein.

DCM due to taurine deficiency is reversible, although the cat needs to survive the first 2–3 months whilst taurine supplementation takes effect. The treatment of congestive heart failure is similar to that in dogs with DCM and/or cats with HCM, although when there is severe systolic dysfunction, **the use of pimobendan in the acute and chronic phases and dobutamine in the acute phase are recommended.** However, the majority of cases observed today are not associated with taurine deficiency and **the prognosis is very poor** (with a survival time of 49 days in a recent study with the inclusion of pimobendan in treatment, 15 days without its use).

Secondary cardiomyopathies

Cardiomyopathy can occur secondary to systemic diseases such as hyperthyroidism, hypertension, or acromegaly.

Feline hyperthyroidism

The thyroid glands secrete two biologically active hormones: triiodothyronine (T3) and thyroxine (T4). T3 is the more active form and T4 is largely a reservoir for T3 production outside the thyroid gland.

Thyroid hormones affect a multitude of metabolic, enzymatic, and hormonal processes throughout the body. There are few tissues or organs that escape the influence of thyroid hormones. They affect the heart both directly and indirectly, and their excess or absence can cause cardiac and vascular abnormalities. The most important thyroid disease in cats is feline hyperthyroidism.

Feline hyperthyroidism is caused by overproduction of thyroid hormones, usually due to **benign thyroid tumours** (adenomas or multinodular adenomatous goitre) or, more rarely thyroid carcinoma (2% of cases).

Thyroid effects on the cardiovascular system

Thyroid hormones have multiple effects on the cardiovascular system including:

- Inducing production of a myosin isoform which increases the speed of the interaction between myosin and actin, and thus **increases contractility**.
- Increasing the number of calcium channels and the activity of Ca^{2+} -ATPase in the sarcoplasmic reticulum, which leads to an increase in the contractility and efficacy of diastole.
- Regulation of other ion transporters which in **hyperthyroidism results in an increase in heart rate, contractility and speed of diastolic function**, (with the opposite effect seen in hypothyroidism.)
- Influencing the number of β-adrenergic receptors, which contributes to increased cardiac contractility and hypertrophy.
- The changes caused by thyroid hormones and adrenergic receptors affect the electrical activity of the heart.

Effects on peripheral circulation

Hyperthyroidism increases cellular metabolism causing increased oxygen consumption. This results in release of vasodilatory substances, which together with the direct vasodilator effects of T3, **cause peripheral vasodilation.**

Hyperthyroidism results in increased systolic pressure (due to increased cardiac output) but decreased diastolic pressure (due to peripheral vasodilation). The result is an increase in pulse pressure. The blood volume remains normal or increased, which contributes to the **systolic hypertension** so commonly observed in hyperthyroid cats.

Cardiovascular involvement

When untreated the cardiovascular effects are significant, and were more commonly seen in the 1980s when hyperthyroid disease was new and went undiagnosed. Now, due to widespread recognition of the condition, there are fewer cases of heart failure (less than 3–5%) compared to 20–25% in the 80s.

Some of the clinical signs seen in hyperthyroid cats, such as **tachypnoea, dyspnoea, or weakness**, may be due to heart failure or severe arrhythmias. However, in most cases, these clinical signs are the result of general and metabolic consequences of the disease such as **muscle weakness, increased CO_2 production, or heat intolerance**.

Physical examination commonly reveals cardiovascular findings which include:

- tachycardia (48% of cases).
- murmurs (40%).
- gallop sounds (10%).
- other arrhythmias (8%).
- systolic hypertension.

Hyperthyroidism causes secondary cardiomyopathy due to the action of the thyroid hormone in the heart, an increase in adrenergic receptors, and increased blood volume.

Hyperthyroid cardiomyopathy has various presentations depending on **the duration of thyrotoxicosis, concurrent factors** (such as systemic systolic hypertension), or **underlying heart disease**.

In reality, the majority of cases do not present with heart failure, and with normal or slightly altered echocardiographic values. Only **10% of cases manifest clinically significant abnormal cardiac parameters**. Within this group, once **euthyroidism occurs most parameters return to normal**, although a minority do not. The latter group may be explained by the presence of concurrent cardiomyopathy or that thyrotoxicosis has caused advanced, irreversible structural damage.

Echocardiogram changes

Some hyperthyroid cats do not have echocardiographic changes, while others have diverse abnormalities with changes in several parameters. Some of the changes seen on echocardiography include:

- Unilateral or bilateral **increase in atrial size**.
- **Thickening** of the free wall of the left ventricle and the interventricular septum.
- Increased left ventricular diastolic dimension.
- Decrease (occasionally increase) in the ventricular systolic dimension.
- Increased (occasionally decrease) fractional shortening.
- Dynamic left and right ventricular **outflow tract obstructions**.
- Increased systolic function (occasionally decreased) on Doppler.
- Impaired diastolic function on standard echocardiography or Doppler.

Radiographs may occasionally show cardiomegaly or (more rarely) signs of heart failure such as pleural effusion or pulmonary oedema.

Arrythmias

On **electrocardiographic** analysis, abnormalities are frequent but usually not clinically significant. The most significant or dangerous abnormalities are **marked sinus tachycardias** or the presence of other **supraventricular or ventricular tachycardias**.

The following findings can be seen:

- Sinus tachycardia (42%).
- Increased R wave amplitude (22%).
- Axis deviation to the right (7%).
- Premature atrial contractions (5%).
- Axis deviation to the left (4%).
- Wide QRS complexes (4%).
- Supraventricular tachycardia (2%).
- Ventricular complexes or ventricular tachycardias (1%).

Hypertension

Some hyperthyroid cats have mild or **moderate hypertension** (systolic), however, the proportion affected is lower than in other diseases such as kidney failure. Also, clinical signs of hypertension (such as retinal abnormalities) are unusual in hyperthyroid cats.

The cause of hyperthyroid hypertension is primarily due to an **increase in blood volume and cardiac output**. In many cases the **hypertension does not resolve with attainment of the euthyroid state**. This suggests other factors are involved such as age, kidney disease, or chronic vascular remodelling, and the **hypertension is a concurrent disease** along with hyperthyroidism.

Treatment

There are **four treatment modalities**, each with various associated advantages and disadvantages:

1. Treatment with carbimazole (oral) or methimazole (oral or transdermal).
2. Surgery (thyroidectomy).
3. Radioactive iodine therapy (I131).
4. Special low-iodine diets.

The majority of cats respond to treatment, but a detailed discussion is beyond the scope of this chapter. For cases with mild to moderate cardiac remodelling, both the cardiac and vascular complications do not normally require treatment and are self- correcting once the euthyroid state is reached with treatment. Most of the clinical signs, physical findings, and changes in echocardiography resolve **within the following weeks to months.** But for those cases already in cardiac failure and/or with severe cardiac remodelling, this persists despite a euthyroid state, which significantly worsens the prognosis.

In addition to therapy for hyperthyroidism, other treatments may be required for patients that respond poorly and require stabilisation prior to surgery or ahead of radioactive iodine therapy. β-blockers are sometimes used for patients with **marked tachycardia** (atenolol at 6.25–12.5 mg BID) or **hypertensive patients** (amlodipine at 0.625 mg–1.25 mg SID). The treatment of heart failure or severe arrhythmias is similar to that for any other cardiomyopathy, combined with specific therapy for hyperthyroidism.

Important practical points to consider

1. Hyperthyroidism causes numerous **cardiovascular effects**, although in many cases these are not clinically significant and resolve once a euthyroid state is achieved. In most cases, specific treatment of cardiovascular abnormalities is not necessary.
2. Hyperthyroidism should be considered as a differential diagnosis when murmurs, gallop sounds, arrhythmias, hypertension and certain echocardiographic abnormalities are detected in adult and geriatric cats (over 6 years of age). These **cardiovascular abnormalities may be the first clue to the presence of hyperthyroidism**.
3. In patients requiring anaesthesia, cardiovascular abnormalities should be assessed in cases with uncontrolled hyperthyroidism or those which have only recently achieved a euthyroid state.

Systemic arterial hypertension

In cats, **systemic arterial hypertension is a common cardiovascular disease** and most common in geriatric cats, so diagnosis and treatment are very important.

Hypertension causes **damage to target** organs such as the eyes, kidney, heart, and central nervous system. In cats the disease is mainly associated with **kidney disease** (acute or chronic) or **endocrinopathies** such as hyperaldosteronism, hyperadrenocorticism or pheochromocytomas. Direct association with diabetic and hyperthyroid disease is more variable and controversial. There is a percentage of cases (up to 20% in some studies) in which the disease is **idiopathic**.

Clinical signs

The clinical signs depend on the affected target organ, but the most common ones are associated with eye damage:

- **In the eyes**, systemic hypertension causes arteriolar tortuosity, retinal oedema and haemorrhage, retinal detachment, and hyphaema leading to visual defects and blindness if not treated promptly.
- **In the kidney**, hypertension can contribute to kidney damage and proteinuria.
- In the **central nervous system**, it can cause vascular events such as fainting or cerebellar accidents.
- The **effect on the heart** is based on increased afterload due to increased peripheral vascular resistance. This can cause concentric hypertrophy of the left ventricle, abnormal cardiac auscultation, and potentially arrhythmias. However, it is extremely rare for clinical signs of cardiovascular failure to be associated solely with systemic hypertension. But in cats with pre-existing cardiomyopathies, the presence of systemic hypertension accelerates disease progression.

In cats, the main treatment is amlodipine 0.1–0.5 mg/kg SID. ACE inhibitors such as benazepril may be added, especially when proteinuria is present. The need for other therapeutic agents such as hydralazine, β or α±-blockers or diuretics is rare.

The diagram in Figure 24 can assist in decision-making about when to treat a patient with systemic arterial hypertension.

Acromegaly

Feline acromegaly is caused by an adenoma of the somatotropic cells of the pituitary *pars distalis* producing **excessive secretion of growth hormone**. Clinical and laboratory findings are associated with the **anabolic effects** of this hormone on various tissues (e.g. respiratory rattle due to the thickening of the oropharyngeal tissues) and **secondary diabetes mellitus** (polyuria, polydipsia, or polyphagia). The diagnosis is made by detection of **high IGF-1 (insulin growth factor 1)** levels in the blood.

Cardiovascular effects

The cardiac changes are probably secondary to growth hormone stimulating **increased protein synthesis in the myocardium**, and to **hypertension** where present. Clinical findings include **systolic murmurs, gallop rhythms**, radiographic evidence of cardiomegaly, and (rarely or in advanced cases) heart failure.

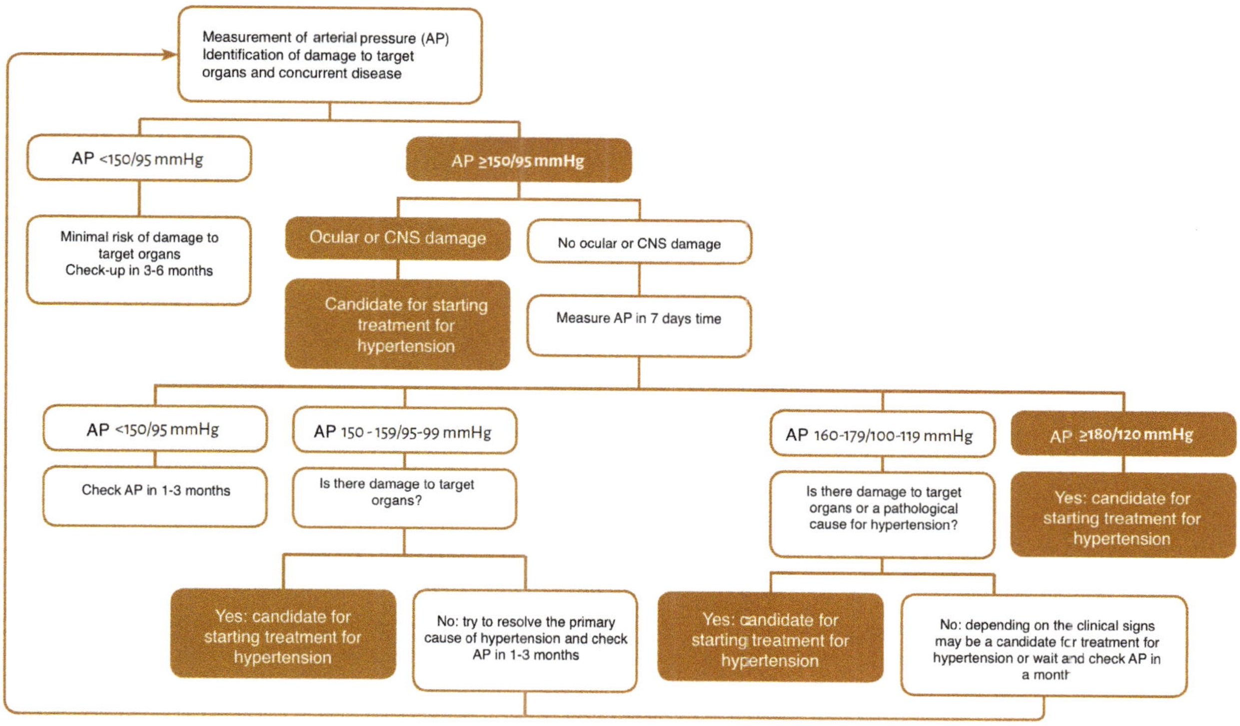

Figure 24. Diagram to show the decision-making process of whether to treat or not in a patient with systemic arterial hypertension. (adapted from Atkins, JVIM, 2007).

The echocardiographic changes include:

- an enlarged left or right atrium
- localized or generalized ventricular hypertrophy
- impaired diastolic function
- anterior systolic movement of the mitral valve
- dynamic obstructions of the right and left ventricular outflow tract.

Hypertension is seen in a small number of cases.

The treatment of choice is **hypophysectomy** and management of diabetes should the condition persist afterwards. In cases where hypophysectomy is not possible, treatment focuses on diabetes management. The use of somatostatin analogues such as pasireotide and radiotherapy have been described.

Myocarditis

Inflammation of the myocardium, or myocarditis is a rare diagnosis, since almost all myocardial diseases are diagnosed within the range of primary myocardial disease. Possible causes of myocarditis include infection (various bacteria, FIP, parvovirus, *Bartonella henselae*, *Toxoplasma gondii*), traumatic, neoplastic, toxic, metabolic, immune-mediated, secondary to generalized inflammation, SIRS, sepsis, or idiopathic. The majority of cases fall into the idiopathic category, although many of these may be of viral or immune-mediated origin.

Diagnosis

Inflammation of the myocardium is diagnosed on histopathology by observing myocyte necrosis, degeneration, or inflammatory infiltrates. However, endomyocardial biopsies are not performed in most cats, and the **diagnosis is almost always presumptive**, based on clinical presentation, ECG (arrhythmia) -Holter or echocardiographic findings, and **significant elevation of cardiac troponin I**.

When the inflammation resolves, the initial clinical signs, arrhythmias, and cardiac dysfunction usually resolve. However, if the damage is intense and prolonged, there may be sequelae in the form of cardiac dysfunction (usually the DCM phenotype) and tachyarrhythmias or bradyarrhythmias.

If the cause is known, this should be addressed specifically. The supportive treatment of arrhythmias and cardiac function, as well as nutritional and supportive care is most important.

Cardiac arrythmias

Cardiac arrhythmias are common in cats, especially those associated with **cardiomyopathies, but rarely require treatment**.

In general, all ventricular arrhythmias and some supraventricular *arrhythmias have an extracardiac cause or* trigger such as electrolyte or acid-base disorders, shock or inflammatory states, neoplasms and all those diseases that may cause changes in vagal or sympathetic tone such as abdominal, thoracic or intracranial diseases.

However, many arrhythmias are caused by any of the aforementioned heart diseases, congenital heart diseases, or are idiopathic.

Supraventricular arrhythmias, particularly atrial fibrillation, are normally a consequence of changes in the structure or size of the atrium, whereas **ventricular ones are often a consequence of myocardial diseases**.

In general, if there is supraventricular or ventricular ectopia, cardiac and systemic causes should be excluded. If there is a treatable cause (e.g. hypovolaemic shock or CHF), this should be treated and the arrhythmia re-evaluated afterwards. If the arrhythmia needs to be treated because it is causing clinical signs or haemodynamic abnormalities or because it is very serious and presupposes a risk for clinical signs or sudden death, the most common antiarrhythmics used include:

- Supraventricular arrhythmias: diltiazem, atenolol or sotalol.
- Ventricular arrhythmias: atenolol or sotalol.

Feline arrhythmias rarely require treatment and conferring with a cardiologist is recommended before starting therapy.

Clinical bradycardia is rare in cats but can be clinically significant. Both sinus node deficits and atrioventricular blocks can result from cardiomyopathy (and are exacerbated by increased vagal tone) but can also be idiopathic.

Many cats with **third-degree blocks** typically have escape rhythms above 100 beats per minute and remain asymptomatic (or only slightly less active than normal). In other cases, especially those with heart rates below 100–110 beats per minute, clinical signs such as fainting, or lethargy are seen and may need treatment.

Medical treatment with terbutaline (β agonist) or theophylline (methylxanthine) can be trialled, although often have no effect. Patients who do not respond to medical treatment need permanent pacemaker treatment, which is usually successful and eliminates clinical signs.

Other secondary myocardial diseases

Diabetic cardiomyopathy is significant in human medicine, and cats with diabetes mellitus have been found to have a higher prevalence of heart failure than cats of the same age without the disease. Systolic dysfunction and myocardial changes have also been demonstrated on histopathology. Many of these patients also have systemic hypertension, which can complicate the condition.

The presence of **sepsis or acute inflammatory response** syndrome causes myocardial inflammation that is typically seen phenotypically as ventricular enlargement and systolic dysfunction and may play a role in the hypotension seen in these patients, along with generalized vasodilation.

The **presence of anaemia** can cause volume overload in cats, leading to cardiac failure. This is mainly seen in cases of chronic anaemia not caused by bleeding (with an increase in total plasma volume).

Ischaemic cardiomyopathy is rare but not non-existent in cats and dogs. Patients often present with severe arrhythmias and/or acute heart failure and may manifest changes on the ECG (ST-segment elevation), echocardiography (regional hypokinesia), or blood markers (extreme elevations of cardiac troponin). Underlying causes should always be sought, although they are often not found. In cats, heart attacks or ischaemic conditions can be observed in the natural course of HCM.

Abbreviations

ATE:	aortic thromboembolism
ARVC:	arrhythmogenic right ventricular cardiomyopathy
DCM:	dilated cardiomyopathy
HCM:	hypertrophic cardiomyopathy
UCM:	unclassified cardiomyopathy
RCM:	restrictive cardiomyopathy
OHCM:	obstructive hypertrophic cardiomyopathy
ECG:	electrocardiogram
CHF:	congestive heart failure
IVS:	interventricular septum
IVSW:	interventricular septum wall
LA:	left atrium
LV:	left ventricle
LVFW:	left ventricular free wall
RV:	right ventricle
PMI:	point of maximum intensity
SAM:	systolic anterior motion of the mitral valve
VSD:	ventricular septum defect

List of feline cardiopathies

The most common cardiomyopathies appear in bold:

- Congenital diseases (such as persistent ductus arteriosus, mitral dysplasia, tricuspid dysplasia, or ventricular septum defects).
- Dilated cardiomyopathy (DCM).

- **Hypertrophic cardiomyopathy** (**HCM**).
- **Restrictive cardiomyopathy** (**RCM**).
- Arrhythmogenic right ventricular cardiomyopathy (ARVC).
- **Unclassified cardiomyopathy** (**UCM**).
- Nutritional cardiomyopathy (due to taurine deficiency).
- Arrhythmia-induced cardiomyopathy.
- **Secondary cardiomyopathies:**
  - **Hyperthyroidism, hypertension**, sepsis, anaemia, acromegaly.
- Specific cardiomyopathies:
  - Myocarditis, infiltrative (lymphoma, FIP).

Bibliography

Atkins, C. E., Gallo, A. M., Kurzman, I. D. & Cowen, P. (1992) *Risk factors, clinical signs, and survival in cats with a clinical diagnosis of idiopathic hypertrophic cardiomyopathy: 74 cases (1985–1989)*. Journal of the American Veterinary Medical Association 201, 613–618.

Boon, J. A. (1998) *Manual of Veterinary Echocardiography*. Williams & Wilkins, Baltimore, MD.

Borgarelli, M., Santilli, R. A., Chiavegato, D., D'agnolo, Sisson, D., O'grady, M. & Calvert, C. A. (1999) *Myocardial disease of dogs. In: Textbook of Canine and Feline Cardiology*. 2nd ed. Eds P. R. Fox, D. Sisson and N. S. Moise. W. B. Saunders, Philadelphia, PA, USA. pp. 581–619.

Cardiology/European Society of Cardiology Clinical Expert Consensus Document on Hypertrophic Cardiomyopathy – a report of the American College of Cardiology Foundation Task Force on Clinical Expert Consensus Documents and the European Society of Cardiology Committee for Practice Guidelines. Journal of the American College of Cardiology 42, 1687–1713.

Ciaramella, P., Basso, C., Di Loria, A., & Piantedosi, D. (2009). *Arrhythmogenic right ventricular cardiomyopathy associated with severe left ventricular involvement in a cat*. Journal of Veterinary Cardiology, 11(1), 41–45. http://doi.org/10.1016/j.jvc.2009.02.007.

Cote, E. et al. 2011. *Restrictive/Unclassified cardiomyopathy. In Feline Cardiology*. Eds John Wiley and sons. 177–181.

Côté, E, Edwards, N. J., Ettinger, S. J., Fuentes, V. L., MacDonald, K. A., Scansen, B. A., Sisson, D. D., Abbott, J. A. (2015)Management of incidentally detected heart murmurs in dogs and cats. *J Vet Cardiol*, 245–61.

Côté, E., Harpster, N. K., Laste, N. J., Macdonald, K. A., Kittleson, M. D., Bond, B. R., Barrett, K. A., Ettinger, S. J. & Atkins, C. E. (2004) *Atrial fibrillation in cats: 50 cases (1979–2002)*. Journal of the American Veterinary Medical Association 225, 256–260.

Ferasin, L. et al., 2003. *Feline idiopathic cardiomyopathy: A retrospective study of 106 cats (1994–2001)*. Journal of Feline Medicine and Surgery, 5(2003), pp. 151–159.

Ferasin, L., Sturgess, C. P., Cannon, M. J., Caney, S. M. A., Gruffydd-Jones, T. J. & Wotton, P. R. (2003) *Feline idiopathic cardiomyopathy: a retrospective study of 106 cats (1994–2001)*. Journal of Feline Medicine & Surgery 5, 151–159.

Fox, P. R., Liu, S. K. & Maron, B. J. (1995) *Echocardiographic assessment of spontaneously occurring feline hypertrophic cardiomyopathy. An animal model of human disease*. Circulation 92, 2645–2651.

Fox, P. R., Maron, B. J., Basso, C., Liu, S. K., & Thiene, G. (2000). *Spontaneously occurring arrhythmogenic right ventricular cardiomyopathy in the domestic cat: A new animal model similar to the human disease*. Circulation, 102(15), 1863–1870. http://doi.org/10.1161/01.CIR.102.15.1863.

Fox, P. R. et al. (2000) *Spontaneously occurring arrhythmogenic right ventricular cardiomyopathy in the domestic cat: a new animal model similar to the human disease*. Circulation 102, 1863–1870.

Fox, P. R. et al., 2014. *Spontaneously occurring restrictive nonhypertrophied cardiomyopathy in domestic cats: A new animal model of human disease*. Cardiovascular Pathology, 23(1), pp. 28–34. Available at: http://dx.doi.org/10.1016/j.carpath.2013.08.001.

Fox, P. R., 2004. *Endomyocardial fibrosis and restrictive cardiomyopathy: pathologic and clinical features*. Journal of Veterinary Cardiology, 6(1), pp. 25–31.

Fuentes, V. L. Jonathan Abbott, J., Chetboul, V., Côté, E., Fox, P. R., Häggström, J., Kittleson, M. D., Schober, K., Stern, J. A. (2020) ACVIM consensus statement guidelines for the classification, diagnosis, and management of cardiomyopathies in cats. *J Vet Intern Med*, 34:1062–1077.

Harvey, A. M., Battersby, I. A., Faena, M., Fews, D., Darke, P. G. G., & Ferasin, L. (2005). *Arrhythmogenic right ventricular cardiomyopathy in two cats*. The Journal of Small Animal Practice, 46(3), 151–156.

Lefbom, B. K., Rosenthal, S. L., Tyrell, W. D. J., Saunders, T. G., Ferguson, M. J., Rush, J. E. & Lesser, M. B. (2001) *Severe hypertrophic cardio- myopathy in 10 young Ragdoll cats*. Journal of Veterinary Internal Medicine 15, 308.

Maron, B. J., Gardin, J. M., Flack, J. M., Gidding, S. S., Kurosaki, T. T. & Bild, D. E. (1995) *Prevalence of hypertrophic cardiomyopathy in a general population of young adults: echocardiographic analysis of 4111 subjects in the CARDIA Study*. Circulation 92, 785–789.

Maron, B. J., Mckenna, W. J., Danielson, G. K., Kappenberger, J. K. B., Kuhn, H. J., Seidman, C. E., Shah, P. M., Spencer, W. H., Spirito, P., Cate, F. J. T. & Wigle, E. D. (2003) *American College of Journal of Small Animal Practice*. Vol 51, October 2010, © 2010 British Small Animal Veterinary Association.

Maron, B. J., Olivotto, I., Spirito, P., Casey, S. A., Bellone, P., Gohman, T. E., Graham, K. J., Burton, D. A. & Cecchi, F. (2000) *Epidemiology of hypertrophic cardiomyopathy-related death – revisited in a large non-referral-based patient population*. Circulation 102, 858–864.

Meurs, K. M., Norgard, M. M., Ederer, M. M., Hendrix, K. P. & Kittleson, M. D. (2007) *A substitution mutation in the myosin binding protein C gene in Ragdoll hypertrophic cardiomyopathy*. Genomics 90, 261–264.

Meurs, K. M. et al. (2002) *Comparison of the effects of four antiarrhythmic treatments for familial ventricular arrhythmias in boxers*. J Am Vet Med Assoc 221, 522–527.

Meurs, K. M. et al., 2000. *Molecular screening by polymerase chain reaction detects panleukopenia virus DNA in formalin-fixed hearts from cats with idiopathic cardiomyopathy and myocarditis*. Cardiovascular pathology: the official journal of the Society for Cardiovascular Pathology, 9(2), pp. 119–26. Available at: http://www.ncbi.nlm.nih.gov/pubmed/10867362.

Ox, P. R. (2003) *Hypertrophic cardiomyopathy. Clinical and pathologic correlates.* Journal of Veterinary Cardiology 5, 39–45.

Paige, C. F., Abbott, J. A., Elvinger, F. & Pyle, R. L. (2009). *Prevalence of cardiomyopathy in apparently healthy cats.* Journal of the American Veterinary Medical Association 234, 1398–1403.

Peterson, E. N., Moise, N. S., Brown, C. A., Erb, H. N. & Slater, M. R. (1993) *Heterogeneity of hypertrophy in feline hypertrophic heart disease.* Journal of Veterinary Internal Medicine 7, 183–189.

Rush, J. E., Freeman, L. M., Fenollosa, N. K. & Brown, D. J. (2002) *Population and survival characteristics of cats with hypertrophic cardiomyopathy: 260 cases (1990–1999).* Journal of the American Veterinary Medical Association 220, 202–207.

Schober, K. & Todd, A. (2010) *Echocardiographic assessment of geometry and the mitral valve apparatus in cats with hypertrophic cardiomyopathy.* Journal of Veterinary Cardiology 12, 1–16.

Spalla, I. et al., 2015. *Survival in cats with primary and secondary cardiomyopathies. Journal of Feline Medicine and Surgery.* Available at: http://jfm.sagepub.com/lookup/doi/10.1177/1098612X15588797.

Tidholm, A. & Jönsson, L. (2005) *Histologic characterization of canine dilated cardiomyopathy.* Veterinary Pathology 42, 1–8.

Test

1. **Which of these statements about heart disease in cats is false?**
   A) Left-sided heart failure can present as a chylothorax.
   B) Left-sided heart failure can present as a thoracic effusion (a modified transudate).
   C) Left-sided heart failure can present as a haemorrhagic effusion.
   D) Left-sided heart failure can present as pulmonary oedema.
2. **Which of these statements about heart disease in cats is false?**
   A) Maine Coon cats are predisposed to hypertrophic cardiomyopathy.
   B) A genetic mutation causing hypertrophic cardiomyopathy has been discovered in the Maine Coon and in the Persian.
   C) It is suspected that a large proportion of cases of HCM in the cat are caused (as in people) by a genetic defect in sarcomeric proteins.
   D) The anterior movement of the mitral valve causes obstruction of the left ventricular outflow tract.
3. **Which of these statements is false?**
   A) Upper respiratory tract diseases usually present with snoring or wheezing from the upper airways.
   B) With pleural effusion, crepitations and wheezing are usually auscultated.
   C) With pleural effusion, the respiratory pattern can be restrictive or paradoxical.
   D) Lung whistles are characteristic of bronchoconstriction in diseases such as feline asthma, for example.
4. **Which of these statements is true?**
   A) The approximate upper limit of a cat's normal heart rate is 220–230 beats per minute.
   B) The approximate lower limit for heart rate in a cat is 80–100 beats per minute.
   C) The approximate lower limit for heart rate in a cat is 160–180 beats per minute.
   D) The approximate upper limit for a normal heart rate in a cat is 160–180 beats per minute.
5. **Which of these statements is true?**
   A) The normal resting respiratory rate for a cat at home is approximately <35 bpm.
   B) The normal resting respiratory rate for a cat at home is approximately <20 bpm.
   C) The normal resting respiratory rate for a cat at home is approximately <50 bpm.
   D) The normal resting respiratory rate for a cat at home is approximately <25 bpm.
6. **Which of these statements is true?**
   A) In hyperthyroidism, the heart always returns to normal once hypothyroidism has been treated, although the left atrium is greatly enlarged, and the patient is in cardiac failure.
   B) In patients with acromegaly, dilation of the left ventricle occurs.
   C) A common treatment used in ventricular arrhythmias is diltiazem.
   D) Cats with systemic arterial hypertension may have associated mild left ventricular hypertrophy.
7. **Which of these statements is false regarding secondary cardiomyopathies in the cat?**
   A) Cardiomyopathy secondary to taurine deficiency is the second most common at present.
   B) Sepsis can cause myocarditis and secondary cardiomyopathy.
   C) Hyperthyroidism can cause thickening of the ventricular wall.
   D) Cats with chronic anaemia may have generalized cardiomegaly.

8. Which of these statements is false regarding cardiomyopathy in cats?
A) Hypertrophic cardiomyopathy is the most common.
B) Arrhythmogenic right ventricular cardiomyopathy is very rare.
C) Cats in heart failure can present with normal or low heart rates.
D) Cats with restrictive cardiomyopathy have moderate or severe systolic dysfunction.

9. Which of these statements is true?
A) The Persian breed and common cat regularly suffer from hypertrophic cardiomyopathy.
B) The Siamese and Burmese breeds commonly suffer from restrictive cardiomyopathy.
C) The Burmese and Birman breeds often suffer from restrictive cardiomyopathy.
D) The Sphynx and Bengali breeds often suffer from dilated cardiomyopathy.

10. Which of these statements is true?
A) In a patient with a heart with a normal vertebral cardiac index, a chest radiograph can rule out cardiomyopathy as long as the heart rate is normal.
B) The presence of a "Valentine's" shaped heart on radiography indicates aortic, ventricular, and left atrial enlargement.
C) The absence of an enlarged pulmonary vein rules out left-sided heart failure.
D) In pulmonary oedema in cats, the increase in opacity is very often multifocal or heterogeneous.

11. Which of these statements is true regarding feline hypertrophic cardiomyopathy?
A) Treatment with pimobendan is indicated only in cases where there is an obstruction of the left ventricular outflow tract.
B) Clopidogrel combined with aspirin has been shown to be more effective in preventing thromboembolism than aspirin.
C) Administration of ACE inhibitors is not indicated in the occult phase but has been shown to be beneficial in cats in heart failure with HCM.
D) Furosemide is the most important drug in the treatment of heart failure.

12. Which of these statements is true?
A) The right transverse parasternal view at the level of the left ventricle is the best to observe the presence of smoke in the atrium.
B) A left ventricle larger than 6 mm at the end of the systole is considered as suffering from ventricular hypertrophy.
C) A left atrium larger than 1.6 cm in systole on a right parasternal longitudinal view is abnormal.
D) Ventricular dimensions and ventricular wall thickness in a right parasternal transverse view are always measured in systole.

13. Which of these drugs is least likely to lower blood pressure in a cat?
A) Amlodipine.
B) Benazepril.
C) Terbutaline.
D) Prazosin.

14. Which of these drugs could be used to decrease left ventricular outflow tract obstruction caused by anterior movement of the mitral valve?
A) Pimobendan.
B) Torsemide.
C) Atenolol.
D) Ramipril.

15. What was the median survival time in cats with hypertrophic cardiomyopathy and heart failure in a recent study?
A) Approximately 550 days.
B) Approximately 100 days.
C) Approximately 200 days.
D) Approximately 350 days.

Clinical case

Bailey is a 9-year-old neutered male cat. He lives indoors, is vaccinated and dewormed and eats a complete, balanced cat food. In the history the owner describes a four-day story of lethargy, poor appetite, and progressively faster and more laboured breathing.

On physical examination, Bailey responds to light stimuli, but is depressed. His temperature is 37.9 °C, he has a weak pulse with a heart rate of 250 bpm and a capillary refill time of 2.5 s. His body condition is 2.5/5.

He has a respiratory rate of 55 breaths per minute with obvious dyspnoea (respiratory distress). There are no obvious upper-airway or lung sounds, and in fact cardiac and respiratory sounds are attenuated on the ventral side. He presents a gallop rhythm on auscultation and there is no murmur. The rhythm is regular with no pulse deficits. There is no goitre upon palpation of the neck.

Questions:

1.

- What is the problem list? (Try to group them together)
- Taking all the findings into consideration, what are the differential diagnoses?
- Describe and reason regarding the importance of the absence of some findings on physical examination.

Progression of the case

At the same time that oxygen is administered through a face mask that Bailey tolerates well, a basic ultrasound of the chest is performed in the sternal position. The following images are seen during the procedure:

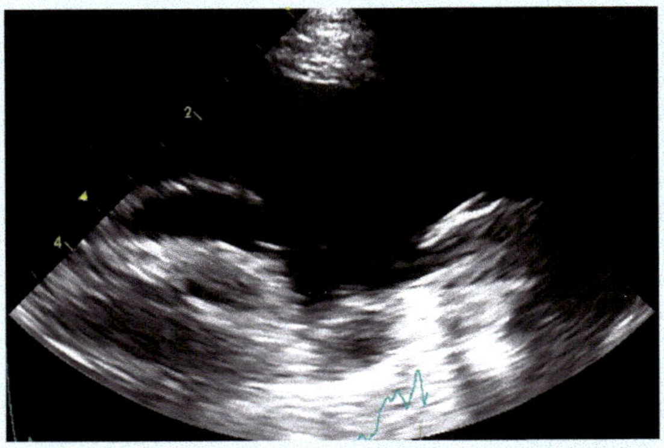

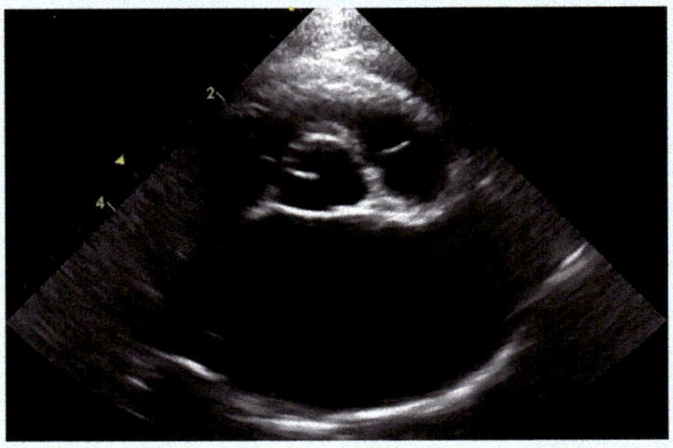

2. **Describe the images, their clinical significance, and the next steps that should be taken with the patient.**

Progression of the case

Thoracentesis is carried out with light sedation (butorphanol at 0.3 mg/kg) and local anaesthesia and 260 ml are drained.

3. What type of fluid is seen in the image and what are the most common causes of its presence in cats? What should the next step(s) be?

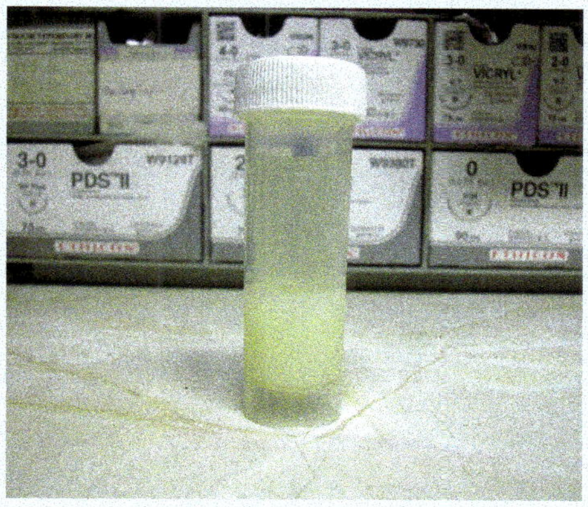

Progression of the case

Following thoracentesis, a 2 mg/kg IV injection of furosemide is administered, and the patient is kept in a special oxygen cage. Breathing returns to normal (26 bpm) and heart rate drops to 190 bpm. A few more tests are done to sequentially characterize the heart disease, avoiding stress. An ECG is performed that shows a sinus rhythm with a frequency of 190 bpm without axis alterations.

A blood test is first performed to determine the presence of concomitant diseases and to assess the possible presence of azotaemia or electrolyte deficits before chronic cardiac treatment, and the results are all within normal limits. T4 is also measured and results are normal, but at the lower end of the range. Blood pressure is also measured to rule out idiopathic systemic hypertension and hypotension due to heart disease. The arterial blood pressure measured with Doppler is 135 mmHg. With Bailey stable, a cardiologist performs a complete echocardiogram (no image) and thoracic radiographs (image below).

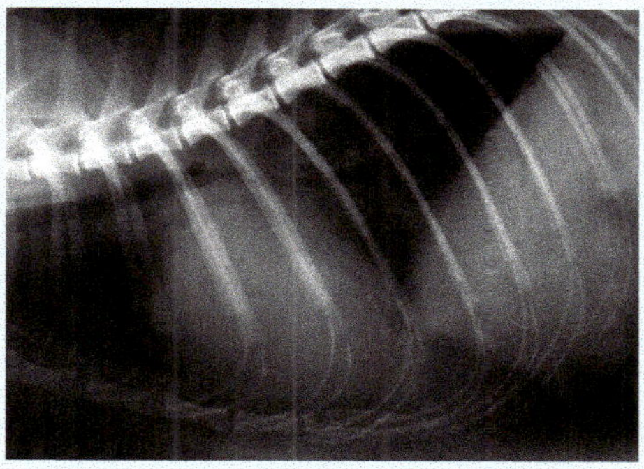

Echocardiography shows a severely enlarged atrium and evidence of light "echocardiographic smoke". A left ventricle of normal to slightly diminished ventricular size is observed with normal-sized ventricular walls. There is no significant regurgitation or valvular abnormalities. Ventricular systolic function appears normal. A restrictive pattern is observed in diastolic studies with an E/A wave ratio greater than 2 and a decreased isovolumic relaxation time.

4. Describe the findings from the echocardiographic description and thoracic radiography and their meaning. How should the treatment be continued?

Progression of the case

Bailey is hospitalized for 24 hours, furosemide at 2 mg/kg is administered every 8 hours. Clopidogrel is also added with a first dose of 75 mg (loading dose) followed by a daily dose of 18.75 mg once a day.

The parameters (respiratory rate, heart rate and blood pressure) remain stable. Bailey eats and drinks well in the hospital, which is very important in cats to prevent dehydration. He is discharged and the owner closely monitors his breathing rate at rest (while sleeping), weight, his appetite, and overall activity at home. The owner is advised to contact the hospital if the respiratory rate is more than 35 bpm.

Bailey is doing well at home, comes back for a check-up after a week, and the owner mentions that the resting breathing rate is 27 bpm, he is eating well, and his weight remains constant. The physical examination shows the previous gallop rhythm, but the rest of parameters are normal. Creatinine, urea, blood pressure, and electrolytes are in normal ranges, although potassium is at the lower limit. Benazepril (0.5 mg/kg once daily) and spironolactone (2 mg/kg once daily) are added and furosemide is decreased to 2 mg/kg twice daily. There is no robust evidence for or against the use of benazepril, spironolactone or pimobendan to improve survival or quality of life in cats with cardiomyopathies and the use of these drugs depends on the case, on how tolerant the cat is of taking pills and the author's preference (in the text the basis of treatments are described in more detail).

The owner is advised to continue monitoring the same parameters, call and provide an update in three weeks and come in for a follow-up consultation in six weeks time.

Answers

Test

1. C
2. B
3. B
4. A
5. A
6. D
7. A
8. D
9. A
10. D
11. D
12. C
13. C
14. C
15. C

Clinical case

1. Questions 1:

- What is the problem list? (Try to group them together)
- Taking all the findings into consideration, what are the differential diagnoses?
- Describe and reason regarding the importance of the absence of some findings on physical examination

The low body temperature and the presence of tachycardia, weak pulse and increased capillary refill time reflect circulatory collapse (or shock). This can be cardiogenic, hypovolaemic, or potentially -although less likely- distributive (caused by sepsis, for example).

The presence of tachypnoea and dyspnoea without upper respiratory sounds and attenuated ventral sounds in the thorax leads to suspicions of pleural effusion as the cause or, at least, a factor in the tachypnoea.

A gallop rhythm is normally associated with primary or secondary cardiac disease although, on some occasions, it may be associated with changes in cardiac volume or the sound heard may not be an abnormal diastolic sound (more information about this in the text).

The absence of a murmur is not unusual in cats with cardiomyopathies, and therefore does not rule out heart disease. The absence of a goitre does not rule out hyperthyroidism, but it makes it less likely.

In general, with suspected heart disease (due to a gallop rhythm), pleural effusion, and circulatory collapse, the presence of heart disease with associated heart failure is most likely.

2. Describe the images, their clinical significance, and the next steps that should be taken with the patient.

In the first image, the presence of a hypoechogenic layer in the thorax below the line of the pleura can be observed, with loss of the normal lung ultrasound pattern and floating mediastinal structures or pleural folds, consistent with severe pleural effusion.

The second image shows a right parasternal transverse view of the heart (short axis) at the level of the left atrium and the aorta with an evident increase in the size of the left atrium (subjective ratio greater than 1.6). Pleural effusion would explain tachypnoea, and the presence of an enlarged left atrium indicates that this pleural effusion is most likely secondary to left-sided congestive heart failure.

3. What type of fluid is seen in the image and what are the most common causes of its presence in cats? What should the next step(s) be?

The fluid looks like chylothorax. Cytologically it is characterized by a cellular increase with the presence of small lymphocytes and a variable protein content. If unsure, triglyceride/cholesterol ratio can be measured or triglycerides in the blood and in the fluid can be compared (there is usually a high concentration of triglycerides, since these are absorbed through the lymphatic system).

The main causes of chylothorax in the cat are secondary to congestive heart failure, secondary to intrathoracic mediastinal masses (usually neoplasia) or due to a traumatic cause. Idiopathic chylothorax is less common than in dogs, but it can also occur. In this case, having evidence of heart disease, the working diagnosis would be that chylothorax is secondary to heart failure.

4. Describe the findings from the echocardiographic description and thoracic radiography and their meaning. How should the treatment be continued?

The lateral radiograph shows severe generalized cardiomegaly. There is no evidence of residual pleural effusion. Nor is there dilation of the pulmonary vein of the cranial lobe or an increase in pulmonary opacities.

Echocardiographic findings are consistent with restrictive cardiomyopathy with normal ventricular size, normal systolic function, normal thickening of the ventricular wall, and severe diastolic dysfunction. There is also a risk of arterial thromboembolism.

9

Infectious diseases

Albert Lloret Roca

Contents

Feline coronavirus infections

Over the past two decades views have changed regarding coronavirus infections and their role in the development of feline infectious peritonitis. It is now clear that it is too simplistic to divide the group into benign enteric coronaviruses and those causing feline infectious peritonitis. Indeed many cats, especially those living in groups are either temporarily or permanently infected with feline coronaviruses (FCoV). However, the majority have no clinical signs and never become sick, with less than 10% of those infected developing the disease known as **feline infectious peritonitis** (**FIP**).

Feline infectious peritonitis (FIP)

Aetiopathogenesis

Feline coronaviruses (FCoV order *Nidovirales*, family *Coronaviridae*, genus *Alphacoronavirus*), are **RNA viruses with an extraordinary mutational capacity and genetic variability**. They are widely distributed in multi-cat groups and the environment where they are extremely resistant (they can remain infectious for up to seven weeks in dry conditions). However, as enveloped viruses, they are **quickly inactivated by disinfectants, steam, and cleaning at high temperatures** (60°).

Many cats acquire infection from contact with either **faeces from carrier cats** or FCoV contaminated environments. FCoV's show a predominant **tropism for enterocytes** and produce a transient or permanent intestinal infection, which may or may not cause **mild clinical signs**. They can also produce a low viral load viraemia and systemic infection, without clinical consequences.

During replication, FCoV suffers continuous mutations and genetic variations due to errors in RNA polymerase producing deletions, insertions, and recombinations. The multiple variants or biotypes of FCoV that may appear during intestinal replication show **variations in cell tropism** and therefore the type of cells they infect.

There are biotypes with an exclusive or mainly **intestinal tropism** and biotypes with a high capacity for entry into the **systemic circulation**. The latter subsequently infect monocytes/macrophages, escape the immune system's defence mechanisms, and cause cats to develop clinical signs of FIP. This model of pathogenesis, known as **the theory of internal mutation**, is widely proven and accepted by the majority of researchers and clinicians.

The genes responsible for the greater virulence of some biotypes have not been precisely identified, but some important **genes which allow the virus to change its cellular tropism** (**spike protein gene and genes 3c and 7b**) have been identified more recently. These spike protein (protein S) facilitate entry of the virus into cells. Recently, amino acid sequences have been identified in the fusion peptides of different S proteins according to the tropism of the FCoV. In short, **lesions and clinical signs of FIP occur when a cat is infected with a biotype or mutated form of FCoV with greater systemic tropism and virulence, which cannot be blocked by the host's immune response.**

In these circumstances, **if the cellular immune response is inadequate, the cat develops the disease known as FIP. FIP lesions are immune-mediated and focused on vascular capillaries**. The virus does not cause direct cytolysis of cells or epithelia but hides in monocytes and tissue macrophages to avoid the cellular immune response. This triggers an exaggerated and ineffective humoral immune response with immune complex deposition and complement activation which causes different forms of the active disease:

- **Wet form**. In the most severe and acute forms, vasculitis occurs in the serosa, especially of the peritoneum and pleura, with extravasation of a protein-rich exudate into cavities.
- **Dry form**. In the most chronic forms, a perivascular pyogranulomatous inflammatory infiltrate in solid organs (lymph nodes, spleen, central nervous system, eyes) occurs.

These two clinical forms are not exclusive but represent the extremes of a dynamic process influenced by the cat's immune response. Both types of lesions can coexist in the same animal suffering from FIP and it is useful to look for the presence of an effusions since the diagnosis is easier to confirm in liquid samples.

The **probability that an FCoV carrier develops FIP is higher in young cats that live in groups** especially if environmental or nutritional conditions are not optimal. Therefore, environmental stress is an important factor in the development of FIP given its impact on the immune response.

In general, **FIP is not a disease that spreads from one sick cat to another**. Mutant viruses do not usually replicate in the intestines, and consequently are not excreted in faeces or spread in the environment. Cats suffering from FIP generally continue to spread FCoV biotypes in their faeces (the virus is not responsible for causing FIP). However, there are exceptions to this model since in some rare cases of outbreaks of FIP have been described in cats in contact with natural infection. This phenomenon has also been described in experimental infections. That is, **there are variants of virus capable of producing FIP and maintaining intestinal replication to contaminate the environment or other cats**.

Epidemiology

FCoV infections are prevalent in cat populations due to the high environmental resistance of these viruses and the large number of cats with transient or permanent intestinal infections. Most cats which come from groups suffer from FCoV infections from an early age, especially if the mother is a carrier. In colonies or groups of cats where FCoV is endemic, seroprevalence is close to 100% in individuals. Intestinal infection with FCoV can be intermittent, permanent, or self-limiting. **The percentage of cats that suffer from FIP is low in relation to the large number of coronavirus carriers**. The main risk factors for the development of FIP are those that prevent the immune system mounting an appropriate response to the mutated pathogenic variants capable of causing systemic infection in monocytes.

- **Age**: less than 2 years old and old cats
- **Poor environmental conditions**: overcrowding, poor nutrition
- **Breed**: there are studies that show a higher prevalence in pedigree cats compared to mixed breed cats. Some breeds (Bengal, Burmese, Ragdoll, Devon Rex, British Shorthair and Abyssinian) may have a higher predisposition
- Stress

- **Immunosuppression**: other diseases, surgery, feline leukaemia virus infection.

Clinical signs

Cats with FCoV intestinal infection do not show clinical signs or at most suffer acute diarrhoea which remises spontaneously after a few days. **Persistent FCoV infections have not been shown to be a cause of chronic diarrhoea** (Figure 1).

Cats with **FIP usually show systemic signs** of illness such as anorexia, apathy, fever, and weight loss.

Cats with the **wet form** of disease may have:

- Abdominal distention (peritoneal effusion) (Figure 2).
- Respiratory distress (pleural effusion) (Figures 3 and 4).
- There are rare cases in which joint, pericardial, and scrotal effusions are present.

When the **dry form predominates** the clinical signs are less specific and depend on which organ is affected. Apart from the systemic signs that develop over months, other symptoms may appear including:

- Kidney disease (Figure 5)
- Palpable or visible **mesenteric lymphadenopathy** on abdominal ultrasound (Figure 6)
- Increases in bilirubin
- **Ocular and/or neurological** lesions (more frequent in the dry or granulomatous form but also appear in cats with effusions)
- **Eye disease**: keratitis, keratic precipitates, exudative uveitis, hyphaema, and is generally bilateral) (Figure 7)

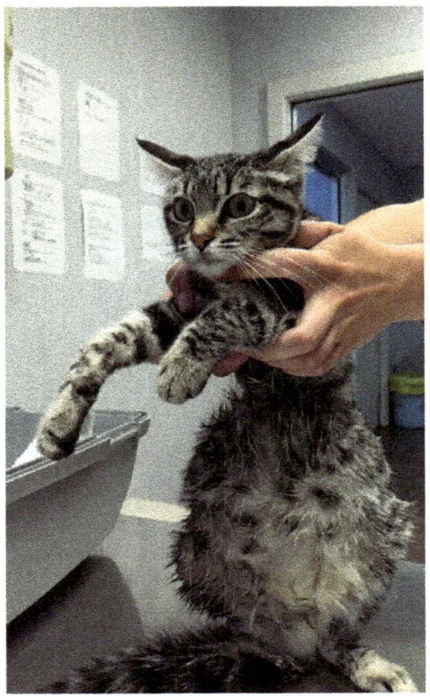

Figure 2. Abdominal effusion in a cat with FIP.

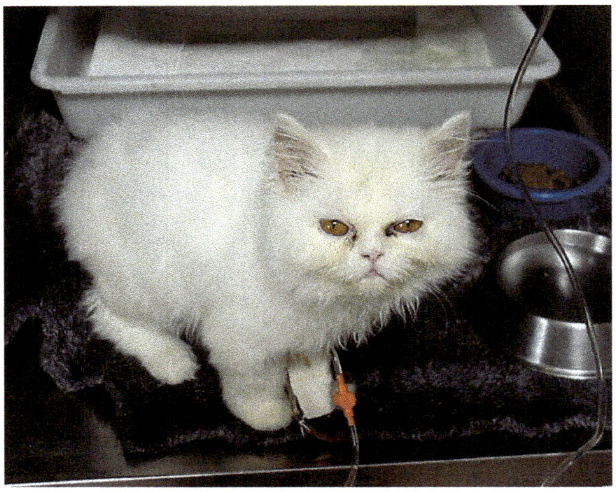

Figure 3. Cat with respiratory distress.

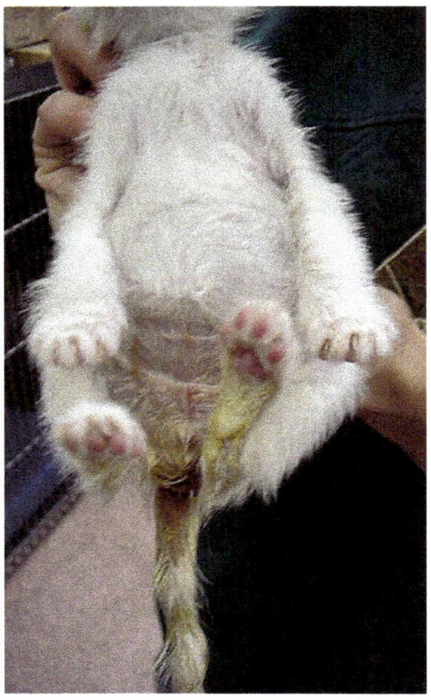

Figure 1. Acute diarrhoea due to coronavirus.

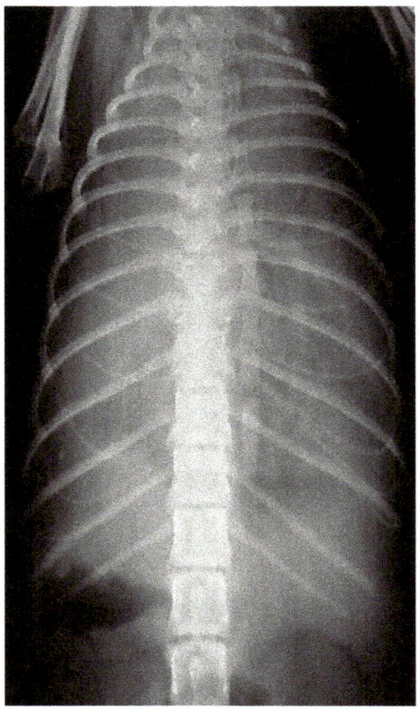

Figure 4. Radiograph showing pleural effusion in a cat with FIP.

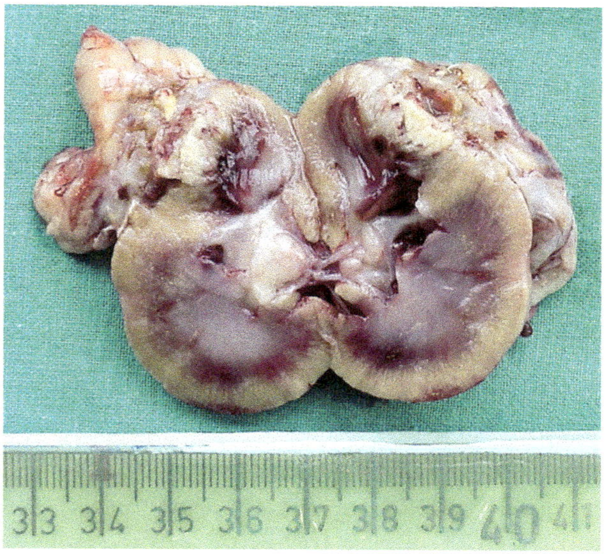

Figure 5. Granulomatous nephritis caused by FIP.

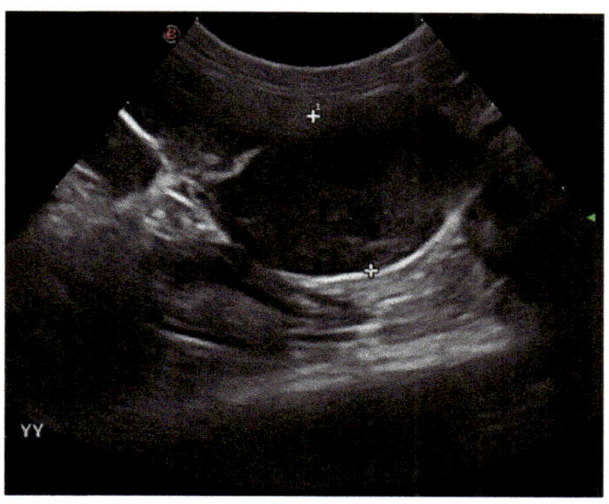

Figure 6. Mesenteric lymphadenopathy in a young cat suffering from FIP.

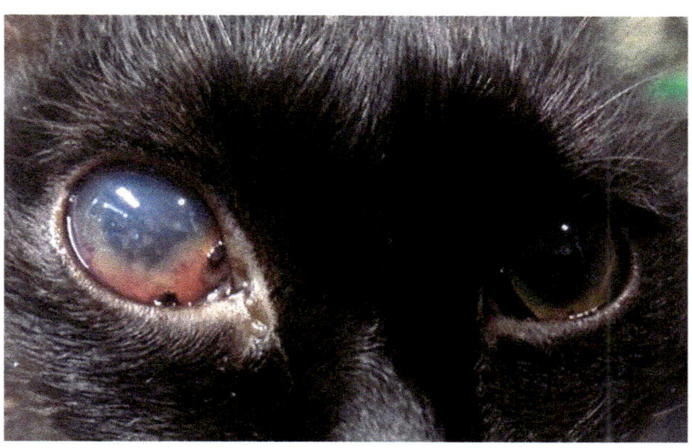

Figure 7. Uveitis, hyphaema and keratic precipitates in a cat with FIP (Photo credit: Juanjo Vega).

- Signs of **CNS disease**: ataxia, depression, seizures, paresis or paralysis compatible with vestibular syndrome or multifocal disease. Many cats only present with CNS signs, but should be checked for abdominal or thoracic effusions (Figure 8)
- Cats with neurological FIP present multifocal intracranial disease, or vestibular syndrome or **myelopathy at T3-L3**.

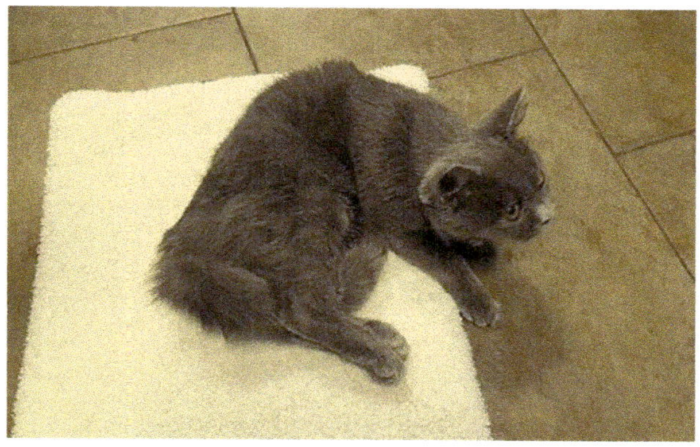

Figure 8. Cat with signs of myelitis from T3-L3 caused by FIP. The presence of abdominal fluid allowed diagnostic confirmation using non-invasive methods.

Atypical forms have also been described with the following symptoms:

- Cutaneous granulomas
- Intestinal granulomas (Figure 9)
- Cutaneous fragility.

Diagnosis

Diagnosis of FIP is difficult, especially in chronic cases with formation of pyogranulomas in different organs.

FCoV antibody titres

Serological techniques that detect **anti-FCoV antibodies do not discriminate between antibodies caused by intestinal or systemic infection**. Diagnosis of FIP solely based on an antibody titre is unreliable. It is also incorrect to think that a healthy anti-FCoV antibody positive cat that does not present signs of FIP will develop the disease sooner or later. **A high percentage of healthy cats are seropositive** and most never develop FIP. To the contrary, there are documented cases of cats with FIP that were seronegative (antibodies are bound in antigen-antibody complexes

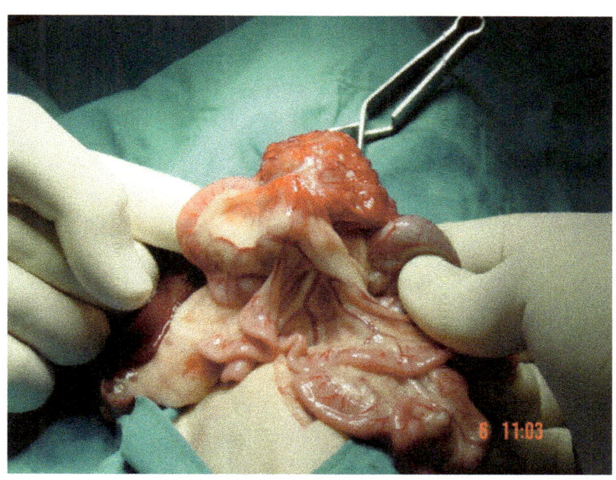

Figure 9. Intestinal granuloma from a cat with FIP.

and not detected by the test). Consequently, **antibody titres against FCoV should always be interpreted alongside the clinical signs**.

The maximum titre from a laboratory together with highly suggestive clinical-analytical signs of FIP and having ruled out other diseases with similar signs leads to a suspicion of FIP, but it never constitutes a definitive diagnostic confirmatory test. On the other hand, **a negative antibody titre makes it less likely, though not impossible, for a diagnosis of FIP**. Also, there is variability between laboratories regarding the serological techniques used for FCoV identification, which implies the results may not be reliable.

PCR

Nor are PCR tests that **detect the FCoV genome** the definitive solution for the diagnosis of FIP, since **conventional PCR does not discriminate between FCoV and the FIP virus**. There are minimal differences in the genome between the two variants (the result of deletions in the genome) which make it difficult to design a PCR that differentiates pathogenic from non-pathogenic forms. However, in recent years it is possible to detect at least two mutations in the spike protein associated with variants with a greater tropism to produce systemic infections using RT-PCR and pyrosequencing techniques.

In general, **RT-PCR techniques on blood samples have low sensitivity** and most cats with FIP have negative results. To the contrary, the sensitivity of **RT-PCR increases considerably in effusion samples, cerebrospinal fluid (CSF) and biopsies** from organs in which there is a granulomatous lesion. Currently, if a good real-time PCR (RT-PCR) on a sample of this type is positive and one of the two mutations associated with systemic infection is detected in pyrosequencing, a diagnosis is confirmed. However, even in samples such as these, RT-PCR can be negative, even if FIP is the final diagnosis. If RT-PCR is positive and mutations are not detected FIP diagnosis is still confirmed, so the utility of this test for the detection of mutations is sometimes controversial.

On the other hand, blood RT-PCR might be positive in certain cats infected with FCoV but not suffering from FIP since, although in small quantities, the virus is not only present and replicating in the intestine but also in circulating monocytes. In these cases, the known mutations associated with FIP may be detected since these variants acquire the capacity to produce systemic infection, but do not necessarily cause FIP if the immune response is adequate.

Diagnostic suspicion

In summary, diagnosis of FIP is complex, clinical and clinical-pathological aspects must always be interpreted together with results of specific tests (molecular or immunohistochemistry).

The **wet form**, characterized by vasculitis in serosal membranes, is **easier to diagnose**. The effusions caused by FIP have specific characteristics which allow a clinical diagnosis to be reached with a reliable prognostic value (Figure 10). These effusions are characterised by:

- Low or moderate cellularity
- Presence of neutrophils and macrophages
- High levels of globulins
- Albumin/globulin ratio <0.8
- Positive Rivalta test.

FCoV can be detected using the following techniques:

- Immunofluorescence.
- RT-PCR.
- Pyrosequencing.

The effusive form is typical, although not exclusive, of **young cats** (under 2 years of age), **pure bred cats**, and those from breeders.

Cases without effusions are harder to confirm and ruling out other diseases and correct interpretation of laboratory tests is very important. The organs that most frequently present with lesions due to FIP are:

- Mesenteric lymph nodes
- Liver
- Kidneys
- Eyes
- CNS.

Most cats with non-effusive FIP have:

- **Fever**
- **Weight loss.**

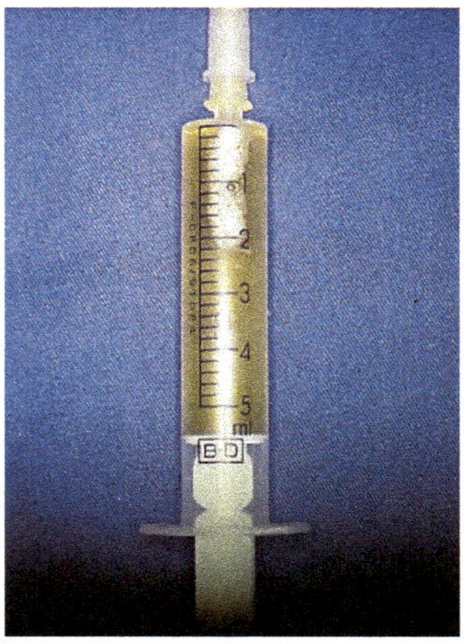

Figure 10. Fluid from an effusion with the characteristic appearance of a case of FIP.

Abnormalities or clinical signs related to the involvement of one or more of these organs.

The most frequent laboratory abnormalities are:

- Lymphopenia
- Non-regenerative anaemia
- Microcytosis
- **Hyperbilirubinaemia**
- **Hyperglobulinaemia** or decreased albumin/globulin ratio. Although it has always been considered a very consistent abnormality in cats with FIP, it currently occurs in approximately no more than 50% of cases
- **High levels of α-1 glycoprotein**. A high value does not confirm the diagnosis, but normal values make the diagnosis of FIP unlikely
- High antibody titres against FCoV.

If a cat has several of these abnormalities and other diseases are ruled out, a diagnosis of FIP is highly probable, although not definitive.

Diagnostic confirmation

The only way to fully confirm the diagnosis is to **demonstrate typical histological lesions** (pyogranulomas) in affected organs and to test for, by means of immunohistochemical techniques (or RT-PCR), the presence of FCoV inside macrophages (Figure 11).

Treatment

FIP is considered a deadly disease with no curative treatment available. Veterinarians who claim to have cured cases of FIP or observed abnormally high survival with different treatments, probably start from **erroneous diagnoses** given the complexity of confirmation and the existence of diseases (lymphoma, lymphocytic cholangitis, pyothorax) with similar clinical presentations. However, there are well-documented cases of FIP with longer survival times than usual, even for several years or with complete recovery, although these are exceptional cases.

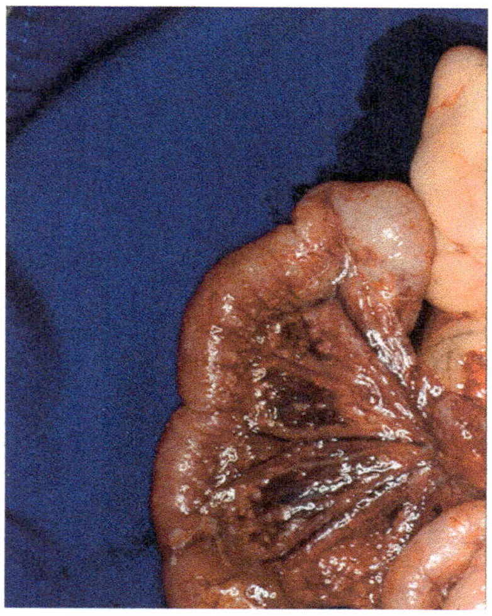

Figure 11. Nodular lesions in the mesentery found post-mortem in a cat suffering from FIP.

Palliative or symptomatic treatment for FIP is based on the suppression of the inflammatory/immune mediated cause of the lesions.

Corticosteroids

The most widely accepted is the use of **high-dose corticosteroids (prednisolone 2–3 mg/kg/day)** through systemic or intracavitary routes (although there are no controlled studies.)

Pentoxifylline, ozagrel, aspirin

Other drugs tested include **pentoxifylline** (vasculitis), **ozagrel** (thromboxane synthesis inhibitor) and **aspirin** (inflammation and vasculitis) although existing studies do not clearly demonstrate clinical benefits and there are no controlled clinical studies.

Feline omega interferon

There are two clinical studies on the treatment of FIP with **feline omega interferon at high doses of 10^6 IU/kg/24 h SC for 7 days and then every 7 days:**

- The first gave promising results, since the survival rate of some cats was high. In some cases, the diagnosis of FIP was not fully confirmed and there was no control group.
- Only cats with confirmed FIP were included in the second, and two groups were compared: those treated with interferon and cortisone and those treated with cortisone and placebo. No statistically significant differences were observed between groups, but one of the cats treated with interferon had a longer than expected survival time.

Studies with a greater number of cats are needed. Although there are no prospective studies, at low doses human alpha interferon, used as an immunostimulant, is contra-indicated, since with FIP **non-specific stimulation of the immune system should be avoided.**

Polyprenil Immunostimulant®

There are also case series of **dry FIP treated with the immune stimulator Polyprenil Immunostimulant®** marketed in the United States:

- In a first series of three cases of confirmed FIP, survival was unexpectedly high, more than two years in two cats and 14 months in another.
- In a second series of 60 cats, the results were not so good: only 4 cats survived more than 200 days and eight cats more than 300 days. However, this drug may be a

good alternative in cats with dry forms of FIP. In this study, cats treated with Polyprenyl Immunostimulant® without corticosteroids had a better survival rate than those who also received corticosteroids.

Protease inhibitor antiviral drugs

Recent studies looked at the use of protease inhibitor antivirals in FIP cats. Studies followed 20 cats with natural infection and experimentally infected cats. In both, remission of clinical signs occurred either temporarily or in the long term. This drug (3c-like protease inhibitor, 15 mg/kg/12 h SC) is not yet commercially available, but is promising as an effective treatment in the future.

Nucleoside analogues

Another promising treatment is the use of **nucleoside analogues which act as an alternative substrate for viral RNA synthesis**. The compound GS-441524 is non-toxic in vitro and effectively inhibited replication of FIP-associated FCoV strains and field isolates in two different cell culture systems. In ten young cats with experimentally induced FIP, GS-441524 (SC q 12 h) caused a rapid reversal of clinical signs and return to a clinically healthy status within two weeks of treatment in all ten cats. Two of the ten treated cats had recurrences of clinical signs at four and six weeks post treatment, respectively. These two cats were treated a second time with GS-441524 for two weeks and responded again, identically to the response seen with the first treatment. All ten cats remained clinically healthy eight months post infection with no signs of toxicity.

GS-441524 treatment was recently evaluated in an un-controlled field study in 31 cats with FIP. The cats started a primary treatment course of GS-441524 at 2 mg/kg SC q 24 h for at least 12 weeks. The dosage was increased to 4 mg/kg SC q 24 h for later treatments in the trial, when cats relapsed or when a treatment course of longer than 12 weeks was deemed necessary. Five of the 31 cats died or were euthanized within 26 days of the first treatment. The remaining 26 cats completed 12 or more weeks of GS-441524 treatment and showed rapid clinical improvement within two weeks. Of these 26 cats, 18 remained healthy, while eight others showed signs of FIP relapses (six cats with non-neurological FIP and two cats with neurological FIP) at a mean of 23 days following treatment. Three of the eight cats with relapses were treated again with GS-441524 at 2 mg/kg SC q 24 h; one of these three cats relapsed with neurological FIP and was euthanized whilst the two remaining cats responded well but relapsed with FIP again and were treated again with GS-441524 but at a higher dosage of 4 mg/kg SC q 24 h. Of the original 31 cats, 25 were classified as long-time survivors after successful treatment. **Neither GC376 nor GS-441524 is currently commercially available.**

Prognosis

The prognosis for cats with FIP is poor, except for rare cases with a longer than normal survival time. Those suffering from the effusive or wet form die within a few weeks of diagnosis, while those affected by dry forms can survive a few months.

In a prospective study of cats with wet forms, the average survival was nine days (50% of cats) and only one cat lived more than six months (200 days).

Prevention

The prevention of FIP is based on the **management of feline communities** to avoid a large number of in-contact cats carrying FCoV, however, this is difficult to put into practice.

An **intranasal vaccine** is available, based on thermo-sensitive variants of the virus which only replicate in the nasal mucosa to induce a local humoral response. It has been shown that **while the vaccine is safe, it does not protect cats that are already seropositive or FCoV carriers from FIP.** However, it can protect cats that are seronegative (not yet exposed to FCoV), and enter an environment where the virus is present. But this situation is unlikely in real life, since many cats have contact with FCoV before the age at which the vaccine can be used (4 months). This is considered a **non-essential vaccine** in committee guides by experts such as those of the AAFP, ABCD and WSAVA.

Retrovirus infections

There are several retroviruses, pathogenic and non-pathogenic, which can infect the cat. The most important are:

- **Feline leukaemia virus** (FeLV)
- **Feline immunodeficiency virus** (FIV).

FeLV and FIV infections have some features in common, for example, both viruses may be present in clinically healthy cats and both can produce an acquired

Table 1. FCoV vaccination programme. Non-essential vaccine, use should be considered in seronegative cats at risk of exposure to FCoV.

Primary vaccination	Revaccination	Adult revaccination
2 doses: 16 and 19 weeks	A year after the last dose	Annual

immunodeficiency syndrome. However, there are many epidemiological, pathogenic and diagnostic differences. In any healthy or sick cat it is essential to know their retrovirus infection status, so diagnostic tests for both viruses are frequently performed.

Retroviruses have a characteristic and unique infection mechanism: they are single-stranded RNA viruses that have a reverse transcriptase enzyme through which they copy their own genome to double-stranded DNA and integrate it into the genome of the cell they infect. In general, retroviruses **infect cells without killing them and produce chronic persistent infections**. During the infection they modify the normal functioning of the cells and produce neoplastic diseases, immunodeficiency syndrome, and immune-mediated diseases.

Depending on the virus and host immunity, the infection can be active or subclinical, but in both cases the viral genome (provirus) becomes integrated into the genome of cells. This may not have clinical consequences, but sometimes it is at the origin of reactivation of the infection or neoplastic transformation of infected cells.

Feline leukaemia virus infection

Aetiopathogenesis

FeLV is an oncogenic gamma retrovirus with the ability to transform the cells it infects into neoplastic ones. It is a fragile RNA virus in the environment, **easily inactivated with common disinfectants**. Indirect infection by fomites is unlikely, unless the transfer is immediate.

FeLV is transmitted horizontally (saliva, urine, faeces, milk) **and vertically** (intrauterine), therefore, any positive cat that eliminates virus in saliva or other secretions is a source of infection for cats in direct contact and their own offspring. The virus is fragile in the environment, but cats that share food and water bowls at close intervals could be a source of indirect infection.

Adults, even if unvaccinated, are naturally more resistant to infection but they may **become infected if the viral load** is high or the animal's immune status is not optimal.

After a cat becomes infected, viraemia occurs which may be:

- **Transitory.** Presence of free and lymphocyte-associated virus. If the cat develops good immunity it is blocked.
- **Persistent.** If immunity is not enough to stop the infection, the virus infects and replicates in the bone marrow progenitor cells. It causes a neutrophilic and platelet associated viraemia. Subsequently, epithelia and glands are infected and the virus spreads throughout the body.

Sometimes the immune response contains the virus before it reaches the bone marrow in high loads, and prevents persistent viraemia from developing. Consequently, **the interaction between the virus and the immune response determines the course of the infection**, as follows:

- **Abortive.** There is **no viraemia** after exposure to the virus.
- **Regressive.** A **transient viraemia** is blocked by the immune response, although some cells may be left with DNA provirus integrated into their genome. These cats do not show signs of disease, but some may suffer from neoplastic or degenerative diseases due to the presence of provirus which is not actively replicating. A small percentage of cats (<10% in one study) suffer reactivation of infection and progressive infection, probably associated with immunosuppression or unknown factors.
- **Progressive. Persistent viraemia** and infection of epithelia and glands. Clinical disease develops within months or years and cats die. In some exceptional cases cats can remain asymptomatic for several years without suffering from a progressive infection.

Epidemiology

Retrovirus infections in cats vary in prevalence depending on the geographical area and animal's lifestyle. In fact, in many countries the prevalence of FeLV infection has decreased considerably thanks to good management programmes and vaccination. There are some countries (for example, Holland) in which the prevalence of infection with FeLV is extremely low or even zero.

At risk cats have continued direct intimate contact with persistently viraemic cats excreting virus in body secretions.

Given the possibility for vertical transmission, cats used for breeding and blood donor cats must always be tested and found negative. **Performing provirus PCR on potential donor cats is advisable.** If they are positive, their blood should be rejected, even if they are not viral (ELISA negative).

Cats which are regressive (positive provirus PCR, negative ELISA) are perfectly healthy and **safe to live with other cats**, although there is a small likelihood of reactivation and viraemia (estimated at below 10%, although the exact percentage and trigger factors are not fully understood).

Clinical signs

Cats with progressive FeLV infection may manifest a wide variety of diseases, however they can also remain healthy for a relatively long time (up to three or four years). In a healthy cat or one with mild signs of illness,

a single positive FeLV test result does not always imply a progressive infection; but could signal a transient viremia or regressive infection. In these cases, **tests should be repeated after six to eight weeks.**

The **most frequent clinical-pathological abnormalities in cats with progressive infections** are:

- Anemia: regenerative or non-regenerative
- Macrocytosis
- Cytopenias: neutropenia, lymphopenia, thrombocytopenia, or pancytopenia
- In cases of neutrophilic leukaemia's, lymphocytosis, or extreme monocytosis with immature neoplastic forms
- Hyperglobulinaemia and gammopathy
- Proteinuria and azotemia in cases of renal involvement.

Cats suffering from **progressive infections** may also manifest the following:

- Neoplasms: lymphoma, leukaemia, others
- Non-neoplastic haematological diseases: myelodysplastic syndromes, bone marrow aplasia
- Immunodeficiency syndrome: opportunistic diseases, chronic or recurrent oral, respiratory, skin or gastrointestinal infections
- Immune mediated diseases: glomerulonephritis, uveitis, polyarthritis, haemolytic anemia
- Peripheral neuropathies: anisocoria, urinary incontinence
- Reproductive disorders: abortions, neonatal mortality
- Lymphoid hyperplasia
- Virus associated dermatosis.

Diagnosis

There are several diagnostic tests for FeLV which should be interpreted together and always taking into consideration whether the cat is sick or healthy.

ELISA or immunochromatographic (IC) tests

These tests **detect a virus circulating antigen, specifically p27, whose presence** in blood or serum (antigenaemia) **means that there is infection and viremia.** The sensitivity and specificity are good (>95%), although not perfect, which is of vital importance when interpreting results in healthy or low-risk cats (Figure 12).

As **sensitivity is high (few false negatives) the predictive value of the negative results is high.** Studies that compared the sensitivity and specificity of rapid diagnostic kits to tests done in commercial laboratories indicate a good correlation.

The specificity is also high (**few false positives**), **although the predictive value of a positive result is not as high as for the negative ones.** These tests are

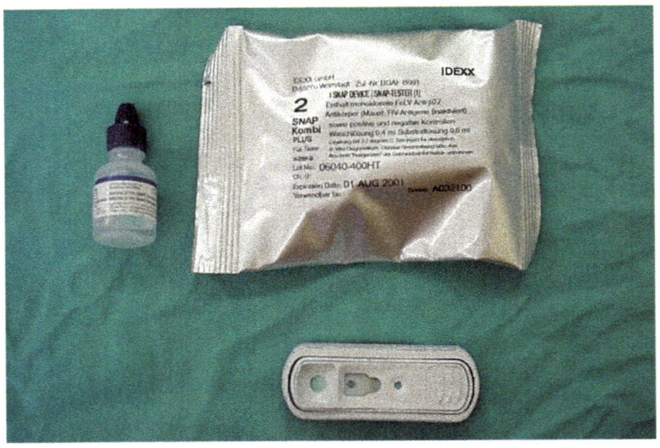

Figure 12. Commercial test for FIV/FeLV detection.

positive both in a transient viremia (regressive infection from which the cat can recover) and in a persistent viremia (progressive infection). Therefore, **in a healthy animal** or one with clinical signs attributable to other diseases, **a single positive result is not definitive** and should never lead to euthanasia.

In addition, in **populations with low prevalence** (2–5%) the probability of finding a positive cat is the same or similar to that of the small percentage of false positives, so the predictive value of a positive may be low or unacceptable. In these situations, **the test must be repeated with other kits or a confirmatory test.**

In a sick cat, especially with abnormalities or diseases typically associated with FeLV (anemia, lymphoma, immunosuppression, myeloproliferative diseases), **a positive ELISA result is enough to establish a diagnosis** since the clinical signs increase the positive predictive value of the test.

In a healthy cat, or one with abnormalities or clinical signs that can be attributed to other causes, **a positive ELISA result must be confirmed by provirus PCR** (to rule out false positives) and by repeated ELISA (or IFA if available) weeks or months later (to differentiate regressive infection from progressive).

Immunofluorescence (IFA)

This test is not widely used in some countries. In the United Kingdom it is used frequently and considered good for **differentiating between transient and persistent viremia** in the face of a positive ELISA result. It is based on the **detection of intracellular p27**, not the soluble or circulating p27, so it confirms **persistent viremias** (progressive infection).

On the other hand, it can give false positives (eosinophils) and false negatives (leucopoenia).

DNA or provirus PCR

In the last decade numerous laboratories have begun to offer DNA or provirus PCR tests. A positive result means that the **virus genome is integrated into some**

Table 2. Joint evaluation of provirus PCR and ELISA/IC.

PCR provirus	ELISA/IC	Interpretation
Positive	Negative	Cats with good immunity where the virus did not reach the bone marrow, but which have cells where the virus genome has become integrated. They do not pose a risk of infection to other cats and the infection rarely reactivates.
Positive	Persistent positive (two positive tests 2–3 months apart)	The cat has a progressive infection.
Negative	Positive or doubtful	The positive ELISA/IC tests are false positives.

of the cat's cells, and confirms FeLV infection (regressive or progressive).

Provirus PCR must always be interpreted in conjunction with the ELISA/IC result and **never used as the sole test**. Its main utility is to confirm the presence of infection in cases of doubtful or inconclusive ELISA results (Table 2). **Provirus PCR is positive in transient and persistent viremia.**

PCR for virus RNA detection

This is a new test not yet performed routinely in diagnostic laboratories. It allows the **detection and quantification of free virus in the absence of cells**: for example, an ELISA negative cat, positive on provirus PCR and negative on RNA PCR is not viraemic.

Another utility of RNA PCR could be to detect virus genome in ELISA-negative cats given its greater sensitivity. The test has been shown to have good sensitivity in whole blood, serum and plasma, saliva and faeces. Its good sensitivity in saliva allows easy, non-invasive diagnosis in domestic cats, but also, in colonies or feral cats to establish the prevalence of the virus in populations. Technically it is a difficult test to perform and a highly specialized laboratory is needed.

Detection of neutralizing antibodies

This is generally not used for diagnosis and the results are difficult to interpret. Many cats develop antibodies against endogenous retroviruses that are integrated into their cells. Few laboratories offer this test routinely. However, a cat positive for neutralizing antibodies is a cat protected against infection and viremia. Therefore, **the test could be used to detect cats resistant to infection and disease.**

Treatment

The first measure is to **isolate cats**, avoid infecting others, and decrease the likelihood of acquiring other infections.

If the cat has an opportunistic disease or chronic infection, these should be treated as normal. If suffering from lymphoma, cats should be treated with chemotherapy in the same way as cats with virus-negative lymphomas, although the prognosis is generally worse (Figure 13 and 14).

Retrovirus infections can be treated with **antiretroviral drugs and/or immunostimulatory or immunomodulatory drugs** such as interferons (amongst others.)

Below is a summary of studies looking at the effects of antiretroviral and immune modulatory or stimulatory drugs in infected cats:

- A controlled clinical study with several treatment groups showed no benefits in the use of **AZT (zidovudine)** in cats with progressive infection.
- Recent experimental and clinical studies with **raltegravir** (integrase inhibitor) demonstrate beneficial effects in FeLV positive cats. Tolerance of raltegravir is

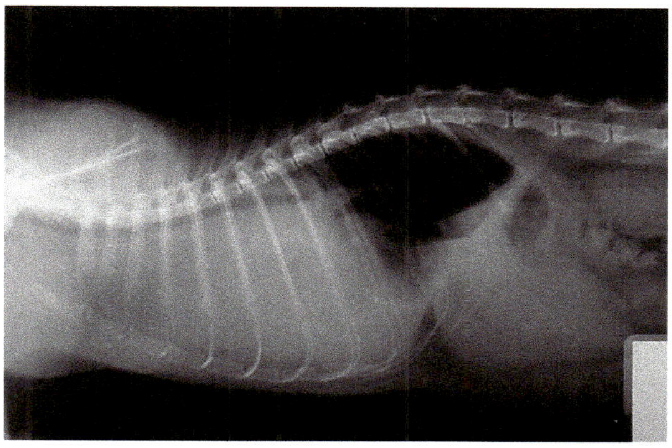

Figure 13. Lateral radiograph of a cat with mediastinal lymphoma.

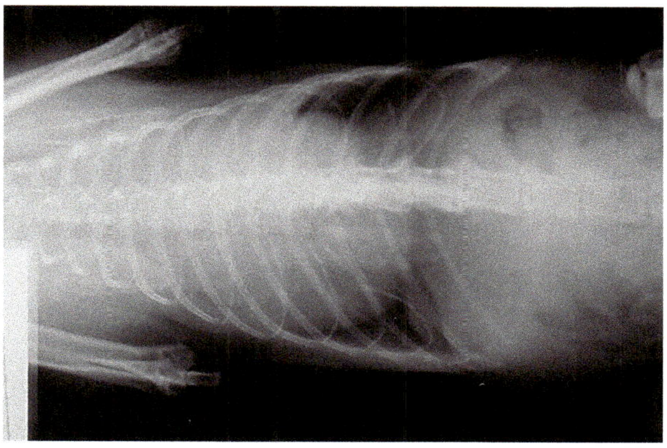

Figure 14. Ventrodorsal radiograph with mediastinal lymphoma.

good at a dose of 20 mg/kg/12 h PO and has shown a beneficial effect both in clinical-pathological aspects and infection parameters as well as viral load. Viremia did not remiss in any cats, therefore, treatment should be continuous.

- A controlled study showed that the use of **feline omega interferon** (10^6 U/kg/day SC for 5 days repeated at two weeks and two months) in positive cats improves clinical status and survival. It was not evaluated whether the positive effect was due to the antiviral action or the immunological effect on infections or opportunistic diseases.
- In a subsequent study, with the same treatment regime, the viral load (RNA PCR) was evaluated and no decreases were observed, so it follows that interferon acts as an immunomodulator rather than as an antiviral.
- There are clinical cases or case series with the use of **other immune stimulants** with diverse results, although in some cases they seem hopeful. However, to validate the benefits of any treatment there should be a controlled clinical study which is compared to a placebo or other treatment.

Prognosis

The prognosis is poor for sick cats with progressive viremia, and should be considered a deadly disease. The life expectancy of FeLV positive cats is variable:

- A healthy cat without any serious associated illness: one to three years. Cases with longer survival times have been documented.
- If the cat has lymphoma: around six months.
- If the cat lives in a group: less than three years, although a small percentage may live longer.

Prevention

Infection prevention is based on **isolation and vaccination**. Since the virus is not transmitted via aerosols and fomites, if a cat lives at home alone or with other negative cats, without contact with unknown cats, the risk of acquiring the infection is zero. Therefore, vaccination recommendations established by some expert committees (AAFP, ABCD, WSAVA) do not consider feline leukaemia vaccination as essential in indoor cats.

To the contrary, vaccination is strongly recommended in cats with the potential to have contact with uncontrolled cats because of their lifestyle. Although the cat is at low risk, it is better to administer the annual vaccination and revaccination since it is not possible to guarantee the cat will not come into contact with uncontrolled cats.

Current vaccines against feline leukaemia are very effective overall. They induce a **good cellular immunity** that does not protect from infection, but from clinical disease and p27 antigenaemia. A vaccinated cat may be provirus PCR positive if it is subsequently infected, but it will be ELISA negative and is not a source of infection for others. **Cats at risk of being in contact with unknown cats should be vaccinated.** Primary vaccination at 9 and 12 weeks is very important given the greater susceptibility in kittens and annual revaccination is also essential, and if the risk of infection persists, annual revaccination is recommended, although with age the risk of infection decreases. A recent study of duration of immunity showed the vaccine is effective for at least two years, consequently the revaccination in cats over three years of age, in which natural immunity is greater, could be every two years.

It is important to **know if the cat is positive or not before vaccinating.** Vaccination of an already positive cat is not dangerous and does not accelerate the infection or disease but will lead to a "vaccine failure" in the opinion of the owner or even thinking that the infection has been caused by the vaccine.

Inactivated feline leukaemia vaccines are epidemiologically associated with the development of sarcomas at injection sites, as they are vaccines with adjuvant and produce an inflammatory reaction that in some predisposed cats is the trigger for the appearance of such sarcomas. The new recombinant vaccines that use a canarypox viral vector do not carry adjuvant and produce less inflammation in the injection area, which should reduce the risk of sarcomas in susceptible cats, although this has not yet been proven.

Feline immunodeficiency virus (FIV) infection

Aetiopathogenesis

FIV is a lentivirus, which causes chronic and persistent infections in cats. It is a fragile virus which does not last long in the environment and distribution

Table 3. Vaccination schedule for FeLV. Vaccination is highly recommended in outdoor cats or those which may be in contact with other cats and is not essential for indoor cats or those which have no contact with other cats.

Primary vaccination	Revaccination	Adult revaccination
2 doses: 9 and 12 weeks	A year after the last dose	Annual until 3 years of age. Cats >3 years, every 2 or 3 years.

varies between countries. There are up to six different variants which have different levels of virulence. The most common route of transmission is natural infection through **bites between a positive and a negative cat, since contact with saliva and/or blood is necessary for effective infection.**

Although transmission from positive mothers to kittens has been demonstrated under experimental conditions, this seems to be ineffective in natural infection unless the cat is infected near or during pregnancy, (since the viral load is higher in the early stages of the infection).

When a cat is infected, FIV **replicates in lymphoid tissue and produces viremia**, initially creating a considerable viral load. At this point humoral and cellular immune responses develop that reduce, but do not eliminate, the viremia. In this first phase of acute infection, the cat may **manifest non-specific signs of** viremia (fever, discomfort, neutropoenia, diarrhoea and lymphadenopathy).

The condition progresses to the **subclinical or asymptomatic phase, which can last for months or years**, without clinical signs although the cat is seropositive. During this phase, FIV progressively destroys CD4+ lymphocytes, which is the main direct action of the virus. When CD4+ levels are very low, serious dysfunction of cellular immunity occurs and an acquired immunodeficiency syndrome appears with chronic infections, opportunistic disease, and certain neoplasms.

Many cats also suffer from **chronic oral and respiratory infections**. Immune mediated diseases associated with the **deposition of immune complexes** (uveitis, glomerulonephritis) may also appear, in fact a significant number of cats who become ill may develop chronic proteinuric kidney disease.

It is common for elderly seropositive cats living in good environmental and nutritional conditions to die of other age-related conditions, without developing immunodeficiency syndrome.

Blood transfusions are another route of infection; therefore, donor cats should be screened and found to be seronegative.

Epidemiology

The **prevalence of FIV largely depends on the cat's lifestyle.**

- Among unneutered outdoor cats, which manifest territorial aggressiveness and fight with other cats, it stands at ≥20% of the population, and may even be higher in some areas of prevalence.
- In indoor cats and in some geographical areas, <5%. A cat which is not in contact with other cats or where contact is not aggressive will never become infected with FIV.

Clinical signs

In the advanced stages of FIV infection a wide variety of diseases may be present.

However, if the cat lives indoors in good environmental conditions and consume a healthy diet, it is unlikely they will develop the disease and, even though they are seropositive the majority die of diseases unrelated to the FIV infection. Therefore, in a healthy cat or one with mild signs of disease a positive FIV result does not imply they are deteriorating or entering the immunodeficiency stage.

Cats that enter an immunodeficient state or are pre-immunodeficiency generally suffer from the following:

- Chronic **inflammatory or infectious diseases** in the oral, gastrointestinal or respiratory tract mucosa (Figure 15).
- **Immunodeficiency syndrome**: opportunistic diseases, and chronic or recurrent oral, respiratory, cutaneous or gastrointestinal infections) (Figure 16).

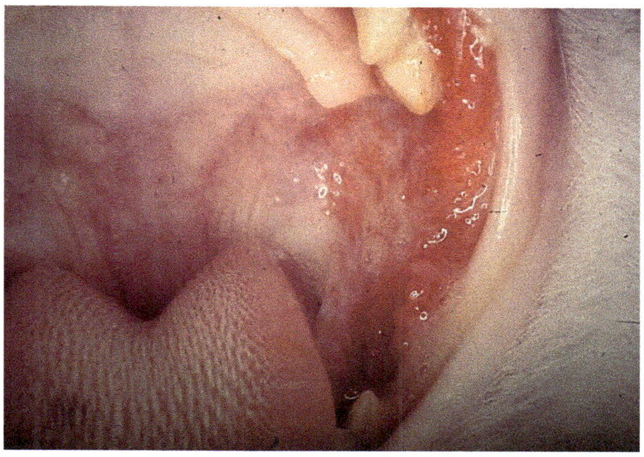

Figure 15. Gingivitis and stomatitis in a cat with immunodeficiency due to FIV.

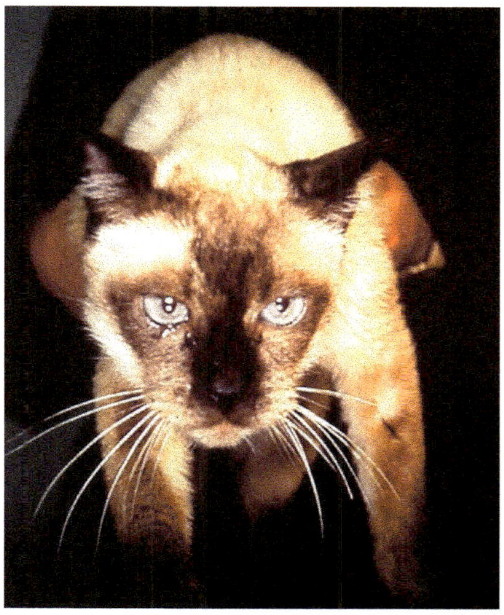

Figure 16. Cat with immunodeficiency due to FIV with fever of unknown origin.

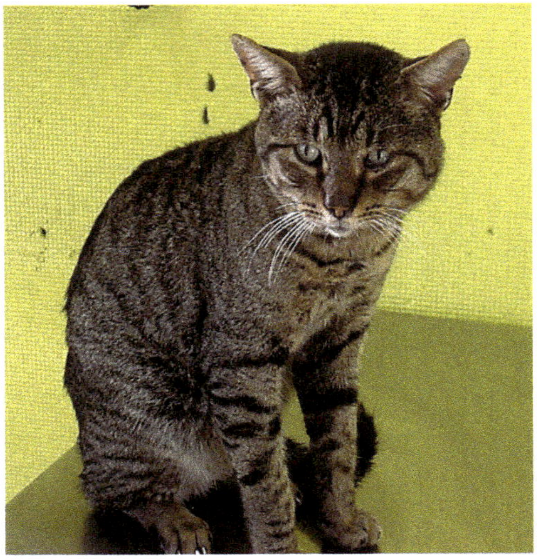

Figure 17. Cat with immunodeficiency due to FIV with chronic kidney disease.

- **Neurological signs of meningoencephalitis** associated with opportunistic diseases or the virus itself).
- **Immune mediated diseases**: e.g. glomerulonephritis, uveitis, especially chronic kidney disease (Figure 17).

The most frequent clinical-pathological abnormalities in cats are:

- Anemia (non-regenerative)
- Different cytopoenias (neutropenia, lymphopenia, thrombocytopenia)
- Hyperglobulinemia
- Polyclonal gammopathy
- Proteinuria
- Azotemia.

Diagnosis

Diagnosis of FIV infection is based on the **detection of antibodies**, which appear within a few weeks of infection and are linked to the permanent presence of the virus.

ELISA or IC

Antibodies are detected by ELISA or IC tests, either using kits in practice or in the laboratory. These tests have **good sensitivity and specificity** (>95%).

However, there may be **some false positives**, which is important when testing healthy or low-risk cats. Another type of false positive is due to detection of maternal antibodies from an infected mother, in a kitten younger than 6 months old. **Intrauterine virus transmission is ineffective** and only occurs if the cat is infected during pregnancy, so a young seropositive kitten is most likely to have antibodies that disappear after 6 months and not be a carrier of the virus. The **positive predictive value of a positive result may not be good in healthy cats** and/or cats in areas with a low prevalence, as previously explained with the diagnosis of FeLV.

False negatives can occur when the test is performed in the early stages of infection prior to seroconversion, for example, in a cat with signs of viremia or in a terminal immunodeficiency stage in which antibody production has been depleted, situations both possible but unlikely in practice. **The negative predictive value of a negative result is very high**.

WBA (Western Blot Assay)

In dubious cases or healthy cats with positive ELISA tests a **WBA (Western Blot Assay) should be performed, which detects several specific antibodies against the virus** instead of just one. **This is considered a confirmatory test**. For years this test has not been widely available, but is now currently offered by some commercial laboratories.

PCR

PCR tests for the detection of FIV DNA provirus are not as well developed as those for FeLV. Their sensitivity and specificity are not well established, and there are **great variabilities and discrepancies in the results**, as demonstrated in some studies. Detection of the A-variant of the virus is good, but for detection of other variants this test does not seem to work as well. Consequently, it is **not considered the test of choice**.

Some commercial laboratories are developing new PCR tests with improved sensitivity and specificity. Recent studies with provirus PCR from a commercial laboratory showed an improvement in sensitivity and specificity. However, there are still discordant results between ELISA and FIV PCR.

- PCR can give false positive results in some cats that are negative for ELISA and viral isolation.
- In some cats ELISA and viral isolation positive cats, it can be negative, probably due to a very low viral load or the virus variant being different to that detected by the primer (initiator) in the test.

The use of PCR in the diagnosis of FIV infection is important in countries where the FIV vaccine is marketed, since in vaccinated cats diagnosis by antibody detection is unreliable. However, in recent years, published studies prove a combination of serological tests that detect different antibodies against different antigens, can discriminate between a cat which is seropositive by vaccination or by natural infection. This is only important in countries where the FIV vaccine exists and is used regularly.

Flow cytometry

Flow cytometry techniques allow **quantification of CD4+ T lymphocytes**, the main targets of FIV. In humans, values below 200 CD4+ lymphocytes are associated with the onset of immunodeficiency syndrome. In cats, different studies have unsuccessfully tried to demonstrate the relationship between the numbers of CD4+ and the clinical signs. Some cats with normal values are very sick and others with low values have no signs of disease. What has been shown to be of interest is the **monitoring of CD4+ values in the same patient: a marked decrease in CD4+ levels are associated with clinical deterioration**, while stable values are not. Currently, some commercial laboratories routinely perform flow cytometry techniques and their use could be of benefit in FIV positive cats, especially if they begin to show signs of disease.

Treatment

The first measure is to **isolate seropositive cats**, to avoid infecting other cats and decrease the likelihood of acquiring other infections. The life expectancy of a healthy positive cat can be many years and may not even develop the disease.

Opportunistic disease or chronic infection must be treated appropriately. A poor response to treatment may indicate that the cat is in an advanced stage of immunodeficiency. Cats which are FIV seropositive and who have chronic gingivostomatitis and caudal stomatitis can benefit from complete exodontics (as for a seronegative cat with the disease). However, a careful decision should be made since it could be the cat is really entering the immunodeficiency phase and is affected by other diseases that could worsen the response or prognosis.

Numerous studies of the treatment of seropositive cats with antiretroviral and/or immunostimulatory or modulatory drugs have been published:

- **AZT (zidovudine)** at a dose of 5 to 10 mg/kg/12 h PO or SC improved chronic stomatitis, increased survival, decreased viral load and increased CD4+ levels. However, as in humans, resistance appears around 6 months and the effect diminishes or disappears.
- With **other antiretrovirals** (PMEA, FPMPA, tenofovir analogue, plerixafor) the clinical and virologic results are good and tolerance is good in cats. They are difficult to obtain and expensive, and therefore not widely used. The studies that exist are experimental in centres where they have been able to access these drugs, but this is not the case for most veterinary clinics.
- For many years, FIV seropositive cats have been treated with **immunomodulatory drugs**, mainly interferons, with the intention of restoring immune function and promoting non-specific antiviral action:
  - High-dose treatments with human interferon alpha (105 IU/kg/24 h SC) have not proven to be very effective. In addition, antibodies are produced within a few months.
  - The use of human interferon alpha at low doses (30 to 50 IU/24 h PO) generally showed clinical improvement and, in some cases, increased survival, but with no effect on viral load or immunological parameters such as CD4+ levels.
- **Feline interferon omega** was marketed in 1992 and studies have been published in seropositive cats using protocols at high doses (106 IU/kg/24 h for 5 days SC, 3 rounds) and at low doses (104 IU/24 h PO for 6 weeks) in both symptomatic and asymptomatic cats:
  - Asymptomatic cats did not show changes in viral load and immunological parameters.
  - In recent studies with low doses 0.1 IU/24 h PO improvements of clinical signs and the quality of life of cats were shown without changes in viral load.
  - In a control study, survival did not improve, compared to the placebo group.
  - Other studies with case series treated with human interferon alpha at low doses showed an improvement in clinical signs and survival time.

Prognosis

The **prognosis is good for healthy, seropositive cats.** At least two studies and numerous clinical experiences show that with good living conditions, life expectancy is relatively long and the disease may not develop, with cats dying from unrelated geriatric pathologies. Moreover, in feline communities seropositive cats do not have a lower life expectancy than the seronegative cats that live with them.

However, the **prognosis is poor for seropositive cats with** diseases associated with immunodeficiency syndrome. In general, inflammatory or opportunistic diseases, or the development of neoplasms such as lymphomas, respond poorly to treatment and can cause death relatively quickly.

Prevention

Prevention is mainly based on the avoidance of fighting between cats through castration or an indoor life. The risk of infection by direct or intimate contact between cats that do not fight is low, but not impossible.

In the U.S.A., Japan and Oceania inactivated vaccine has been marketed since 2002 that has created some division of opinion, since vaccinated cats test positive on diagnostic tests and it is impossible to differentiate an infected cat from a vaccinated cat. On the other hand, this vaccine mainly protects against infections by the A-variant of FIV, so it would probably not be very effective in Europe, where most of the viruses identified are from other variants, mainly B variants.

Haemotropic mycoplasma infections

Haemoplasmosis

Aetiopathogenesis

Haemotropic mycoplasmas (or haemoplasmas) are small **bacteria** that parasitize the periphery of red blood cells and can **trigger immune mediated haemolytic anemia**. Initially they were classified within the rickettsias and denominated *Haemobartonella* spp., but genetic studies showed them to be mycoplasmas.

Routes of infection:

- **Fights** are currently considered the most significant route of infection. It seems contact with blood is a more effective means of transmission than contact with saliva. It is also suspected that direct, non-aggressive contact could be a route of transmission for *Candidatus Mycoplasma haemominutum,* but not *Mycoplasma haemofelis* (Figure 18).
- **Fleas**, *Ctnenocephalides felis*: haemoplasmic DNA in fleas has been isolated. This was considered the most important route of infection, but the most recent studies contradict this hypothesis and it is not currently considered a significant route of transmission.
- **Vertical transmission.**
- **Blood transfusions**: blood donor cats must be PCR negative for the 3 known species of haemoplasm.

Molecular studies confirm the existence of different haemoplasma species with varying pathogenicity:

- ***Mycoplasma haemofelis (Mh).* Acute infection causes severe haemolytic anemia**, but chronic infection does not cause anemia. Prevalence varies depending on whether the cats are healthy or thought to be infected, and the geographical area.
- ***Candidatus Mycoplasma haemominutum (CMh).*** This is a **less pathogenic** variety. Acute infection may trigger a **decrease in erythrocyte numbers** but this is not severe enough to cause clinical anemia in otherwise healthy cats. However, it may cause signs of anemia in immunosuppressed cats or those with concurrent diseases, especially FeLV infections or co-infections with FeLV and FIV. In one study an association was found between the presence of CMh and chronic kidney disease, but this may be coincidental given the age of the cats. According to some studies this is the **most prevalent species**, although there are large differences between studies.
- ***Candidatus Mycoplasma turicensis (CMt).*** This species was described a few years ago. In some cases it can induce mild to severe anemia, especially in immunosuppressed cats. Its presence is frequently associated with coinfection with one or both other haemoplasmas, especially CMh.

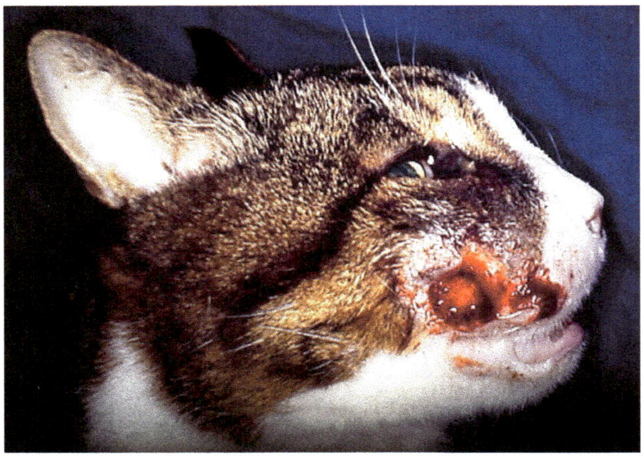

Figure 18. Subcutaneous abscess due to a fight.

Epidemiology

Haemoplasma infections are **most common in male cats**, especially outdoor cats with a history of fighting and subcutaneous abscesses.

There are numerous epidemiological studies on the prevalence of haemoplasmic DNA in the blood of healthy and diseased cats in numerous countries. The prevalence is generally high, with **CMh being the most frequent**, followed by Mh and CMt. The prevalence is high in healthy animals and in those with other diseases, which means **many cats are asymptomatic carriers.**

Feline haemoplasma infection is not considered a zoonotic disease, but haemoplasma infections have been documented very rarely in immunosuppressed humans and in one case the infection apparently originated from contact with a cat. However, it is a single case and could be purely co-incidental.

Clinical signs

After acquiring infection the resulting disease depends on:

- The haemoplasma **species**
- If infection is **acute or chronic**
- The presence of **concurrent diseases** and/or immune status.

The most frequent clinical and pathological clinical signs are:

- Dehydration
- Anorexia

- Depression
- Weight loss
- Intermittent **fever**
- **Anemia**. Typically, this is regenerative hypochromic macrocytic anemia, although marked reticulocytosis may not be present. Increase in osmotic fragility (Mh and CMt)
- **Splenomegaly**. Erythrocyte sequestration in the spleen, which may be obviously enlarged, and decreased haematocrit
- Jaundice. Possible, but not constant
- Leukopoenia, lymphopoenia, eosinopoenia, monocytosis. Changes to leukograms are rare, but possible
- **Hyperglobulinemia and polyclonal gammopathy**. This may occur in chronic cases, although it is not frequent and may be due to concurrent disease.

Haemoplasma infections cause **haemolytic anemia**. Coombs tests may be positive, and sometimes **self-agglutination** is observed, and the presence of anti-erythrocyte antibodies demonstrated. Recently, the importance of these anti-erythrocyte antibodies has been questioned, since it has been observed in some cases they appear once haemolysis has begun and in addition the response to treatment is good with the use of antibiotics without corticosteroids.

Some studies show that retrovirus infection increases the risk of CMh and Mh coinfection, however, the influence of retrovirus infection status on haemoplasmosis is not fully understood. **Performing retrovirus tests on cats with haemoplasmosis is advisable.**

Some cats are **chronic carriers**, especially those infected with CMh. Generally, **chronic carriers are subclinical**, although in some cases the infection can be reactivated.

It has been shown that many cats infected with Mh and CMt completely eliminate the infection after a few months but a general rule is hard to establish because of the wide variability in the course of infection in chronic carriers.

Diagnosis

Peripheral blood smear

Examination of peripheral blood smears has a **very low sensitivity and variable specificity**. Haemoplasmas are visible cyclically, for a short period of time that coincides with the peak of bacteraemia after acute infection. In addition, **smears do not allow differentiation** between species. Haemoplasmas located on the periphery of erythrocytes can also be confused with other basophilic corpuscles, especially staining precipitates or Howell-Joly bodies.

PCR

PCR, performed in a reliable laboratory, is the **test of choice for the diagnosis of haemoplasmosis**. PCR is extremely **sensitive and specific**, allows diagnosis of the infection, and differentiation between the different species, and quantification of the DNA of haemoplasmas, which can be useful for:

- Determining the significance of the infection
- Monitoring the course of the infection
- Monitoring the response to treatment.

However, the interpretation of quantitative PCR can be complicated, given the large fluctuation in the number of haemoplasmas demonstrated in studies on experimental Mh infection. The reason for this large fluctuation is not fully understood, although the possibility of infection sequestered in organs such as the spleen has been investigated, and antigenic variability suggested as another possible cause. Results should be interpreted taking this factor into account and **to classify a cat as having eliminated the infection, a single negative PCR is not enough, several PCRs must be performed over a period of time**. This fluctuation is characteristic of Mh infection and has not been seen in CMh and CMt infections.

Treatment

Administration of any of the following antibiotics resolves the clinical signs, but the infection is not always eliminated completely and permanently:

- **Tetracyclines**, especially doxycycline (10 mg/kg/24 h PO for 1 month), are the medications of choice to treat feline haemoplasmosis. Although only controlled studies of Mh treatment are available, it has been found to be effective in CMh and CMt infections. Doxycycline should be administered preferably in solution, or if it is in tablets, it should be ensured that the cat ingests water or food straight after, to avoid oesophagitis.
- **Quinolones** (enrofloxacin and marbofloxacin) are also clinically effective, although there may be variability in response depending on the haemoplasma species. Pradofloxacin (5 to 10 mg/kg/24 h PO for 1 month) may be more effective at permanently eliminating the infection than traditional quinolones.
- Recent studies show that **sequential treatment** with one month of doxycycline followed by two weeks of a quinolone (marbofloxacin) could be more effective in eradicating haemoplasmas and preventing the chronic carrier state.
- **Imidocarb** (5 mg/kg/14 d IM) is used in resistant cases or those that do not respond to treatment, but controlled efficacy studies are lacking.

In severe cases of haemolytic anemia, especially if the Coombs test is positive or the response to the antibiotic is inadequate, the use of prednisolone is indicated (2 to 4 mg/kg/24 h). There is clinical evidence that the use of cortisone is not necessary in all cases, many respond well to doxycycline without the need for administration of corticosteroids.

Supportive treatment consists of fluid therapy and, in the most severe cases, blood transfusion.

Prognosis

The prognosis is good if the cat does not reach the practice in a critical condition with hypovolaemic shock. Even in these severe cases, if supportive treatment is started and doxycycline is administered quickly, the cat is very likely to survive.

Prevention

Prevention is based on cats living indoors and not fighting with other cats. Although it is currently thought fleas are not the main source of infection, maintaining good control of external parasites (fleas and ticks) is advisable. There are no vaccines or other type of preventive measure available.

Gastrointestinal infections

Diarrhoea of infectious origin is common in cats, especially in kittens and young cats. There are several pathogens that can cause acute and, in some cases, chronic diarrhoea.

For any case of diarrhoea, it is essential to identify whether it is of **small or large intestinal** origin, as the differential diagnosis list for some infectious or parasitic causes will vary. For example, in large intestinal diarrhoea *Tritrichomonas* should be suspected, but not in small intestinal diarrhea.

The **general condition** of the cat is also important. Sometimes, in addition to diarrhoea there are systemic signs or the involvement of other organs, while for others the only clinical sign is diarrhoea. For example, cats with feline panleukopoenia usually have other systemic signs such as fever, anorexia and dehydration, while a cat with giardiasis presents with diarrhoea without systemic signs.

Diagnostic tests

The diagnosis of infectious or parasitic causes of diarrhoea is based on the detection of the pathogen in faeces, either by microscopic observation, serological detection of antigens, or PCR to detect the pathogen's genome.

Table 4. The main causes of infectious/parasitic diarrhoea in cats.

Viral	Feline panleukopoenia virus
	Feline coronaviruses
	Other viruses (Rotavirus, Torovirus)
Bacterial	*Campylobacter*
	Clostridium
	Salmonella
	E. coli
Helminth parasites	*Toxocara*
	Ancylostoma
	Strongyloides
Protozoal parasites	*Giardia*
	Trichomonas
	Isospora
	Cryptosporidium
	Toxoplasma

Microscopic appearance

Microscopic observation is by direct observation in fresh stool samples, rectal cytology, or after zinc sulphate flotation techniques. The **sensitivity** depends on the pathogen, but in some cases is **zero (virus) or low** (bacteria or parasites excreted intermittently or in low numbers). Stools should be **analysed as quickly as possible** after collection to increase the sensitivity of parasite detection.

In general, **zinc sulphate flotation techniques improve sensitivity for the detection of parasites**, especially if several samples are taken on different days. Flotation techniques are sensitive and effective for the diagnosis of **helminth parasites and some protozoa such as *Giardia***. But in other cases this is not very sensitive, e.g. *Cryptosporidium* protozoa are very small and difficult to see, and flotation is not a sensitive technique for diagnosis.

Serological tests

Serological tests to detect pathogen antigens are available for parasites such as ***Giardia* (for which the test is highly sensitive) and *Cryptosporidium***. Diagnostic in-house test kits are sensitive and give rapid results, but do have their limitations.

PCR techniques

PCR techniques are useful for the diagnosis of pathogens and bacteria toxins which are otherwise difficult to detect, therefore, increasing sensitivity in the diagnosis of some infections. It should be remembered that faeces contain DNase enzymes that degrade DNA and may **decrease test sensitivity**; alternatively genetic material may be detected from faecal pathogens which are not the cause of diarrhoea (causing **decreased specificity**). Therefore, the clinical interpretation of the results is important.

Currently some commercial laboratories offer **complete PCR panels** from a single stool sample for detection of the main intestinal pathogens. However, this is not always the test of choice: for example, for the diagnosis of *Giardia* the sensitivity is low, and flotation or antigen detection is preferable. In contrast, for the diagnosis of *Tritrichomonas* PCR is superior to flotation.

Feline parvovirus/panleukopenia virus infection

Aetiopathogenesis

Feline panleukopenia is a disease caused by infection with **feline parvovirus (FPV)**, a single-stranded DNA virus which is **highly resistant in the environment**, where it can persist for months. This virus has been long recognised as infecting cats and other felines. Canine parvovirus appeared in the late 70s from a mutation of FPV. The new variants of canine parvovirus (2b, 2c) can re-infect cats again, but do not usually cause disease.

The virus enters the cat orally resulting in a rapid viremia which provides access to all the organs. FPV has a special **tropism for cells with a high rate of replication**, particularly those in the S phase of cell growth, where it replicates and subsequently destroys them. **Enterocytes and myeloid cells** are particularly affected, resulting in **haemorrhagic enteritis and marked neutropoenia**. Severe panleukopenia infections result in **sepsis due to the bacterial translocation phenomena**. In some cases, it can cause septic shock, disseminated intravascular coagulation and multiorgan failure. **The virus is present in large amounts in blood and faeces.**

Purkinje cells of the cerebellum can also be attacked by the virus in foetuses and neonates. Consequently, infection or application of attenuated vaccines in pregnant cats can lead to the birth of kittens with cerebellar hypoplasia and non-progressive ataxia.

It has not been fully demonstrated whether FPV has a myocardial tropism as can occur with canine parvovirus.

Feline parvovirus infection is an **acute infection** which can be subclinical in the face of a good immune response. The **incubation time is about 7 days**, and a week after the clinical signs have appeared, the animal is cured or dies due to associated complications.

Epidemiology

Oro-faecal transmission is possible by **direct contact** with sick or infected cats or by **indirect infection** in contaminated environments, given the virus's high level of environmental resistance. The disease is very common in **young cats under 1 year of age**, but can occur in older cats, adults or elderly animals, who are not well immunised naturally or by vaccination and then exposed to the virus.

The prevalence of infection is **high, especially in feline communities** where the virus can circulate freely and is present in the environment. The prevalence of infection is low in indoor cats which are not in contact with other cats, although infection is not impossible since the **virus can enter the house through fomites**, especially if the owner has regular contact with other cats or environments where cats live.

Clinical signs

Panleukopenia may present acutely with a wide spectrum of clinical signs. These can be very acute with sudden death without presenting digestive or other clinical signs, especially in kittens living in communities.

Common clinical signs include:

- Anorexia.
- Apathy.
- Fever.
- Vomiting.
- Diarrhoea. Sometimes it is not very profuse and may be undetectable (Figure 19).
- Dehydration (Figure 20).

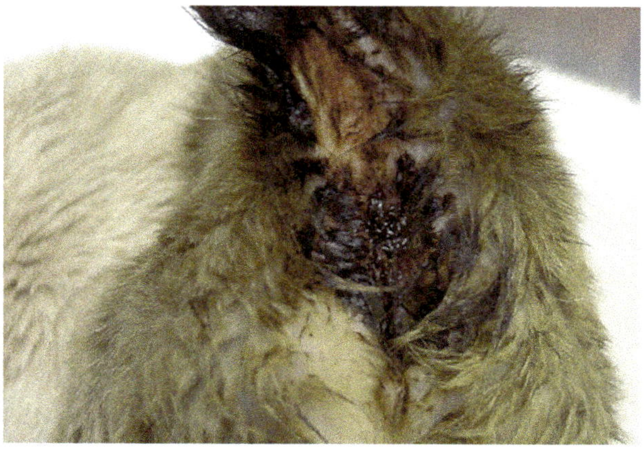

Figure 19. Diarrhoea in a cat with feline panleukopoenia.

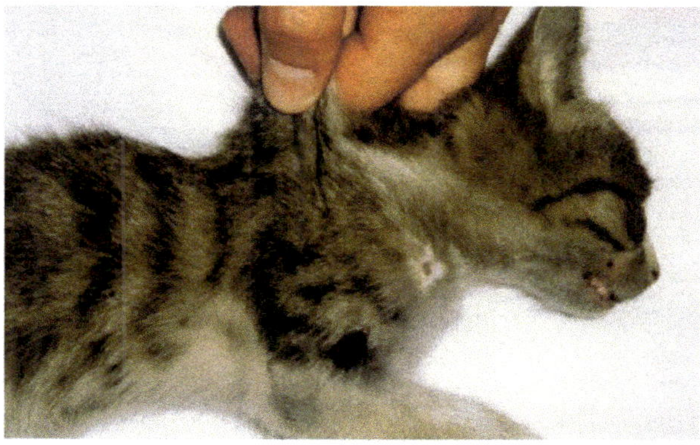

Figure 20. Severe dehydration in a kitten with panleukopoenia. (Image: Diane Addie).

Clinical-pathological abnormalities include:

- Leukopenia due to marked neutropoenia (often less than 1000/µl)
- Thrombocytopenia
- Mild anemia
- Prerenal azotemia
- Electrolyte abnormalities (due to serious dehydration)
- Increase in bilirubin (associated with septicaemia).

Clinical signs in **kittens with cerebellar hypoplasia** include:

- Ataxia. Non-progressive (Video 1).
- Intention tremor.
- Hypermetric gait, without any abnormalities in mental state or other neurological signs.
- Good general body condition.

Diagnosis

Clinical diagnosis is based on the characteristic clinical-pathological appearance. Confirmation is by tests that detect the virus in faeces or blood.

ELISA

ELISA tests have good sensitivity and specificity for the detection of virus antigens in faeces. They can be done in the practice and useful for a quick diagnosis. However, **false negatives can occur**, especially in the initial stages of infection when the antigenic load is below the test's detection limit. But also, and more importantly, during the course of the disease if the viral antigens are blocked by antibodies that have already been formed. In short, a **negative result does not rule out panleukopenia** in a cat where this disease is suspected.

PCR

The use of **feline parvovirus PCR** is widespread. This is a **highly sensitive test in faeces and blood** and not affected by the presence of antibodies. The main problem is **false positives** due to poor quality laboratory technique or detection of virus as a result of vaccination (if the cat has been vaccinated with an attenuated vaccine in the weeks prior to testing.)

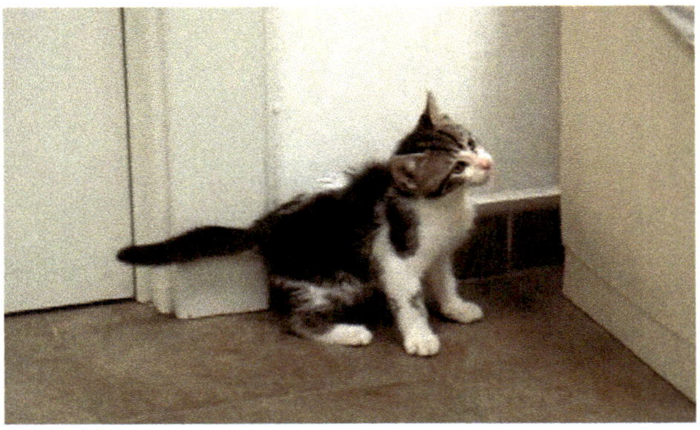

Video 1. Kitten with ataxia due to cerebellar hypoplasia. (Full video available at: http://publication.improveinternational.com).

Electron microscopy

Electron microscopy on faeces has also been used in a research setting, but it is not a test for day to day use in practice.

Antibody detection

Diagnosis by **antibody detection is not useful**, since there are no antibody titres that differentiate between disease, subclinical infection, exposure or previous vaccination. The technique can be used for epidemiological studies or to assess the immune response, but not for disease diagnosis.

Post-mortem

In cases of death in communities, **post-mortem is useful** due to the characteristic histological intestinal lesions, which allow confirmation that death was due to panleukopenia.

Treatment

There are no controlled clinical studies looking at treatment of feline panleukopenia.

Therapy is mainly supportive:

- Adequate **fluid therapy** to correct dehydration and continuous losses due to vomiting and diarrhoea (crystalloids and colloids)
- **Broad spectrum antibiotic** therapy (β-lactams plus quinolones or aminoglycosides)
- Antiemetics (maropitant)
- Analgesics (buprenorphine).

In the most severe cases and in very young or weakened kittens some clinicians administer fresh plasma from vaccinated cats or recovered cats, so as to passively **transfer antibodies (5 ml/kg/d for 2 or 3 days)**. Alternatively, whole blood transfusions can be used to transfer antibodies or if the animal is suspected of having DIC. In some countries there are commercial hyperimmune serums available to administer passive immunity to sick kittens or those in contact with sick cats.

There are no studies on the use of **feline interferon omega** in cats with panleukopenia, but there are in canine parvovirus in dogs. The aim is to try and **enhance a non-specific immune response**, and it may also have some antiviral action. Studies in dogs indicate a shorter hospitalization time, but not necessarily an improved survival rate.

It is essential to **start feeding an enteral or micro enteral diet** as soon as possible, once the most intense vomiting subsides. The necrotised intestine (which is in the process of repairing itself) requires nutrients in order to recover as soon as possible. Enteral nutrition is probably beneficial for the prevention of sepsis due to bacterial translocation, although it has not yet been proven.

Prognosis

Prognosis is reserved and depends on the severity of the condition, age and nutritional status of the cat, and access to supportive treatment. The prognosis is poor in kittens in communities and rehoming centres, with high mortality, close to 80% where there is no access to intensive hospital treatment. To the contrary, if the animal can be treated thoroughly and intensively, depending on the severity of the condition, survival rate is more than 80%.

Prevention

Prevention is based on the control of infections in colonies and thorough **disinfection of the environment with bleach**.

Attenuated vaccines against feline parvovirus have been available for many years. These are **very effective** and produce robust or sterilising immunity. A well immunised cat will not be infected even when exposed to the virus.

However, it is common to see infected cats during the primary vaccination process or shortly thereafter. These cases are because immunization has either not been done correctly or due to interference from maternal antibodies.

Many cats between **8 and 16 weeks still have a sufficient level of maternal antibodies** (especially from well-immunised mothers) to block subclinical infection by the vaccine. In contrast, these antibody levels are not enough to protect against natural infection by a pathogenic virus. Due to this phenomenon, **three doses of vaccine are recommended** for primary vaccination and **one revaccination after a year**. In the latest WSAVA vaccination guides revaccination before a year is proposed, at around 6 months.

Table 5. Feline parvovirus vaccination programme. Core vaccine recommended for all cats.

Primary vaccination	Re-vaccination	Adult re-vaccination
3 doses: 8, 12 and 16 weeks	A year after the last dose	Annual in cats at risk of exposure
		Every 3 years in cats which are at low risk

Giardia infections

Aetiopathogenesis

Giardia (G. duodenalis, G. lamblia, G. intestinalis) is a **flagellated protozoan** which can infect numerous species, including the cat. Several variants have been identified (A, B, C, D, E, F and G):

- **F and G** are the variants that mainly affect the cat
- Recent studies have identified variant A in cats.

The Giardia cycle is **direct, with oro-faecal infection.** It has two different stages:

- Mobile forms or trophozoites
- Oocysts, which are formed by binary division.

Both forms can be identified in faeces. *Giardia* is a parasite with a **tropism for the small intestine**, where it produces lesions in enterocytes, an inflammatory response, and atrophy of the intestinal villi, which results in nutrient malabsorption and **acute or chronic diarrhoea**.

Epidemiology

Oocysts excreted in faeces remain infective in the environment for months, and **infection can be direct or indirect**. The most effective method of transmission between cats is via environmental or indirect contact with oocysts, rather than direct contact with trophozoites which are fragile and only persist for a short time in the environment.

Prevalence is generally high, with a similar incidence in cats with diarrhoea as those without. Most of those with diarrhoea are **kittens or young cats under one year old**. There are numerous studies in different countries with a **variable prevalence of up to 20%**. Co-infections with other parasites are common.

Clinical signs

Although the **diarrhoea is usually due to small intestinal involvement** with malabsorption and weight loss, some cases show large intestinal signs, such as mucus and fresh blood.

Infected cats do not show systemic symptoms, such as fever or anorexia. When a cat with diarrhoea has systemic signs then **other causes should be suspected**, even when coprological tests are positive for *Giardia*.

Diagnosis

Direct observation of faeces

Direct observation of faeces for the detection of trophozoites (Z-type movement) or oocysts is **not very sensitive but is highly specific** and if observation is positive, no further tests are needed.

Flotation with zinc sulphate

Since oocyst excretion is erratic, **several samples from different days are required** to improve the sensitivity of zinc sulphate flotation (making it better than that of direct stool observation).

ELISA

The sensitivity of a single ELISA test is good and similar to that of three flotations on alternate days.

PCR

The *Giardia* PCR has a **moderately high sensitivity** and allows the different variants to be distinguished, which may be important for determining the zoonotic potential but gives a large number of positives where *Giardia* is not the cause of diarrhoea.

Response to treatment

In the initial stages of the diagnostic protocol (even when tests are negative) it is common practice to treat cats with chronic diarrhoea with antiparasitic agents that have an anti-Giardia action

Treatment

The treatment of choice is **fenbendazole at 50 mg/kg/24 h for 5 days**, which has a response rate greater than 90%. If a cat with chronic diarrhoea and *Giardia* does not respond to correct treatment with fenbendazole it is unlikely this is the cause.

Alternative treatments:

- **Metronidazole** (15 to 25 mg/kg/12 h for seven days).
- Combination of febantel, pyrantel pamoate and praziquantel at the standard dose for three days in a row.
- Secnidazole (30 mg/kg single dose). There is an experimental study with good results with a single dose of this drug. It could be the ideal treatment in hard-to-handle cats, but clinical studies and experience in infections in practice are lacking.

Prognosis

Prognosis is good, no treatment-resistant giardiasis has been identified.

Reinfection indicates an ongoing source of environmental infection, although persistent diarrhoea in a treated cat suggests another disease is the cause.

Prevention

There is no vaccine or preventive treatment. Years ago, in the United States, an inactivated vaccine was marketed that was used both as prevention and treatment, but in Europe it was not commercialised and is not currently available.

Hygiene standards are important to avoid infection and reinfection.

Tritrichomonas infection

Aetiopathogenesis

The first description of *Tritrichomonas* diarrhoea in cats dates from 2003. *Tritrichomonas foetus* is a **flagellated protozoan parasite** of cattle, which is increasingly diagnosed in cats. Currently, there is ongoing research into whether the species that causes disease in cats is different from that in cattle and *T. blagburni* has been proposed as a name (pending confirmation).

The parasites cycle is direct from trophozoites excreted in faeces and spread by **oro-faecal contact** to other cats, either directly or by contamination of food or water. Unlike *Giardia*, there are no oocysts in the faeces and trophozoites are fragile in the environment and environmental and **indirect infection is ineffective**.

Tritrichomonas has a **tropism for the colon and the distal ileum**, where the parasite lingers and causes an intense inflammatory response (neutrophilic and lymphoplasmacytic). They may be present in the colon without causing clinical signs, but in some cats the inflammation is intense.

Epidemiology

Since the appearance of the first cases the disease has been **documented globally**. Tritrichomoniasis usually occurs in **pure breed cats, especially in young cats** less than one year old, from a breeder or environment where there are many animals. Adults and the elderly can be subclinical carriers. **Co-infections with other protozoa are frequent**, especially with *Giardia* and *Isospora*.

Clinical signs

Typical clinical signs include chronic large intestinal diarrhoea with:

- Foul smelling stools
- Large amount of mucous (Figure 21)
- Presence of fresh blood.

Sometimes there is a **marked proctitis that occurs with faecal incontinence** and even rectal prolapse. The presence of systemic signs is rare, but in some cases (<25%) there may be anorexia and apathy. Affected cats have no abnormalities on blood tests. Although

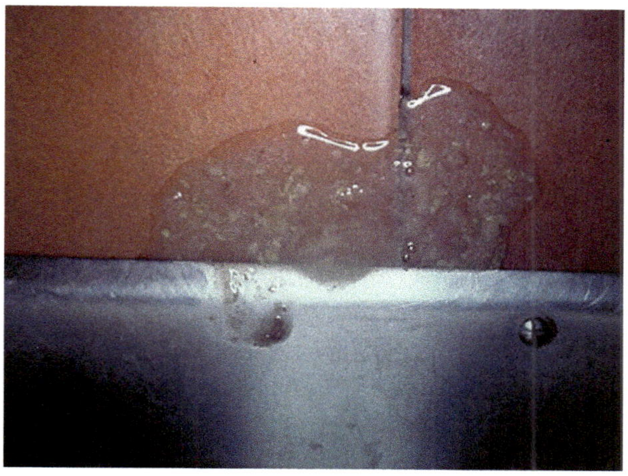

Figure 21. Large amounts of mucus present in the faeces of a cat suffering from tritrichomoniasis.

parasites have been found in the genital tracts of some cats, no associated clinical signs have been observed.

Diagnosis

Diagnostic confirmation of tritrichomoniasis is important, otherwise cats with chronic colitis may be treated with immunosuppressants if erroneously diagnosed as idiopathic or primary lymphoplasmacytic inflammatory colitis.

To obtain samples from the colon area, rectal catheterisation can obtain stool samples with a higher parasite content and thus increase the sensitivity of diagnostic techniques.

Direct observation of faeces

Direct observation of trophozoites in fresh stool samples is easy, immediate and cheap, but **sensitivity is <20%**. Samples should be examined immediately, and mucus samples are helpful. Trophozoites move rectilinearly, unlike *Giardia*. A negative result does not rule out the disease (Video 2).

Specific cultures

Faeces are **incubated for a few days** in a special culture medium (InPouch™ TF) so the parasites proliferate and can be observed under a microscope. The **sensitivity is 60%**.

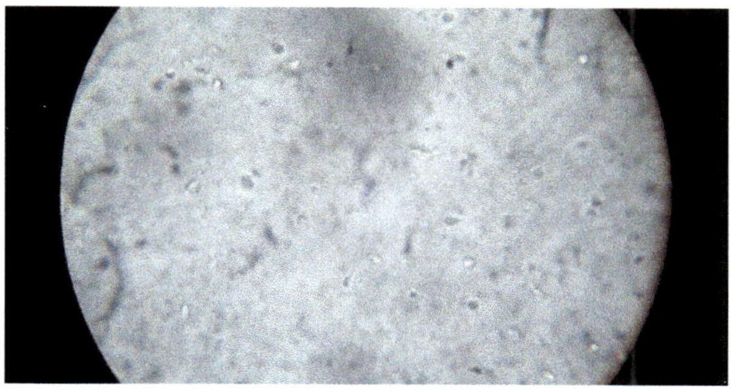

Video 2. Microscopic image of *Giardia* trophozoites. They can be seen moving in a straight line. (Complete video available at: http://publication.improveinternational.com).

PCR

PCR is currently considered the **technique of choice** although it is more expensive and requires a few days to obtain results. Given the low sensitivity of the other tests, it is always preferable to send stool samples to the laboratory for PCR detection if tritrichomoniasis is suspected. PCR does not need the parasites to be alive for detection so fresh samples are not essential.

Other

Sometimes *tritrichomona* can be seen on histology of biopsies of the colon, although the sensitivity is low.

Treatment

Firstly, it is essential to **treat any coinfections**, since another pathogen may be the cause of symptoms. **Tritrichomoniasis heals spontaneously** in most cases, but as it may take time (**from 5 months to 2 years**) the diarrhoea must be treated to improve the animal's quality of life and the inconvenience due to large intestine diarrhoea with faecal incontinence.

There is no effective commercially registered treatment for this disease, but the drug that provides the best results is **ronidazole with approximately 70% efficacy at a dose of 30 mg/kg/24 h for 2 weeks** (at higher doses it frequently causes neurological toxicity [vestibular]). Higher doses improve clinical outcomes, but increase the **risk of neurotoxicity**, so it is preferable to first treat with a conservative dose and decide whether to increase the dose based on the response. Many cats remain infected after treatment, but the diarrhoea disappears or improves.

Recent studies show **treatment with probiotics** (as a sole treatment or accompanying ronidazole) **accelerate the resolution of diarrhoea** and decrease the risk of relapse after the end of treatment with ronidazole.

Cats that recover spontaneously may remain **asymptomatic chronic carriers** and a source of infection for other in-contact cats.

Prognosis

The prognosis is good, although some cats do not respond to safe doses of ronidazole and their diarrhoea persists, or they relapse shortly after being treated.

Prevention

At the time of writing there is no vaccine or preventive treatment for this parasitosis. Implementation of good hygienic and sanitary standards at breeders is essential to reduce the possibility of infection. It is important to treat cats with diarrhoea to reduce the environmental parasitic burden.

Respiratory infections

Upper respiratory tract infections (URTI) are common in cats. URTI signs are general and it is not possible to determine which pathogen is responsible, based solely on presentation.

Symptoms of acute URTI

- Sneezing
- Nasal discharge (serous, mucous or purulent)
- Coughing
- Aphonia
- Oral ulceration
- Gingivitis
- Conjunctivitis
- Keratitis.

In non-serious, acute cases the use of symptomatic and supportive treatment is often initiated on a presumptive diagnosis:

- If the condition is accompanied by **ocular signs** (conjunctivitis, keratitis or corneal ulcers), the most likely diagnosis is **feline herpesvirus infection** (FHV-1)
- If it is accompanied by **superficial ulcers** on the tongue or oral mucosa, the diagnosis is **feline calicivirus** (FCV).

In many cats presenting with URTI, **viral or viral and bacterial coinfections are common**. Commensal bacteria of the upper respiratory tract (*Pasteurella, Streptococcus, Klebsiella*, and others) colonise and infect tissues affected by the primary viral infection (Figure 22). However, apart from the commensals which cause secondary infection, there are bacteria which cause **primary infection of the upper respiratory tract**:

- *Chlamydia felis*
- *Mycoplasma felis*
- *Mycoplasma gateae*
- *Bordetella bronchiseptica*
- *Streptococcus equi subsp. zooepidemicus.*

In an animal predisposed by an underlying anatomical/congenital anomaly or an idiopathic inflammatory disease then recurrent or chronic infection may be common. There are also infectious causes that may become chronic or recurrent, such as feline herpesvirus,

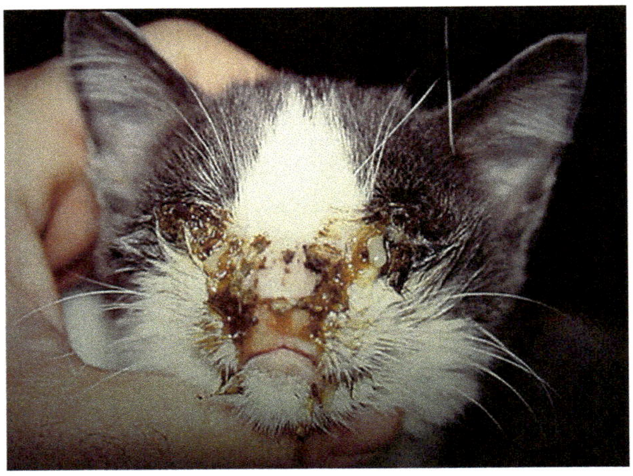

Figure 22. Upper respiratory tract infection.

Table 6. Causes of URTI in cats.

Infectious	Viral (FHV-1, FCV, poxvirus) Bacterial (*Bordetella, Mycoplasma, Chlamydia, Streptococcus*) Fungal (*Cryptococcus, Aspergillus*)
Anatomical/congenital	Nasopharyngeal polyps Brachycephalic syndrome Nasopharyngeal stenosis Soft palate membranes or adhesions
Inflammatory/ immune-mediated	Chronic idiopathic rhinosinusitis Lymphoplasmacytic rhinitis Allergic rhinitis (eosinophilic)?
Neoplasms	Nasal lymphoma Epithelial neoplasms (carcinoma) Sarcoma

Mycoplasma, and fungal infections (cryptococcosis and aspergillosis).

However, especially with atypical or chronic disease all causes of URTI should be included on the list of differential diagnoses. Above all, when there are signs of upper respiratory tract obstruction and/or inspiratory rales or stridor, **an obstructive anatomical abnormality** (e.g. nasopharyngeal polyps, nasopharyngeal stenosis) should be suspected.

Diagnostic tests

In many cases of URTI the diagnosis is based on clinical presentation. Where confirmation of the pathogen is required, this is done using PCR techniques offered by commercial laboratories. However, a pathogen's presence does not mean it is the cause of disease, and **correct interpretation is crucial** with a good understanding of the sensitivity and specificity of each test.

In cases with **chronic URT signs, tests should be run to rule out other diseases or abnormalities**, in addition to tests to detect pathogens.

Diagnostic imaging tests:

- Computerised tomography (CT)
- Flexible endoscopy
- Tests under anaesthesia:
  - Visual examination (Figure 23)
  - Nasal lavage or flushing (Figures 24 and 25).

Feline herpesvirus infections

Aetiopathogenesis

FHV-1 is a DNA virus of the *Herpesviridae* family. It shows little genetic variability and is relatively unstable in the environment, only remaining infective for a few hours at most. It is also **sensitive to most disinfectants** (e.g. sodium hypochlorite).

FHV-1 has a **special tropism for the nasal, oropharyngeal, conjunctival, and corneal mucous membranes. Infection is by direct contact** with an infected cat (indirect contagion is less frequent) and after an **incubation period of two to six days**, the virus produces **necrotic and inflammatory lesions in the nasal and ocular** epithelia with associated acute clinical signs. **Less frequently, FHV-1 can cause ulcerative skin lesions**, and lesions (herpetic dermatitis) with an eosinophilic inflammatory component in the dermis. These occur mainly in the facial area, near the nasal cavity and mouth.

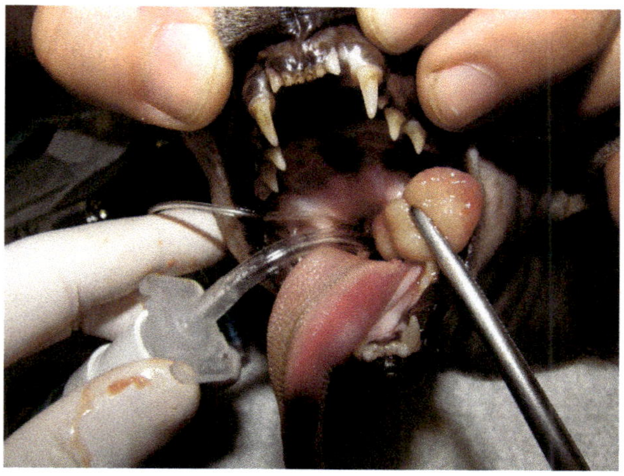

Figure 23. Traction of a nasopharyngeal polyp in a cat.

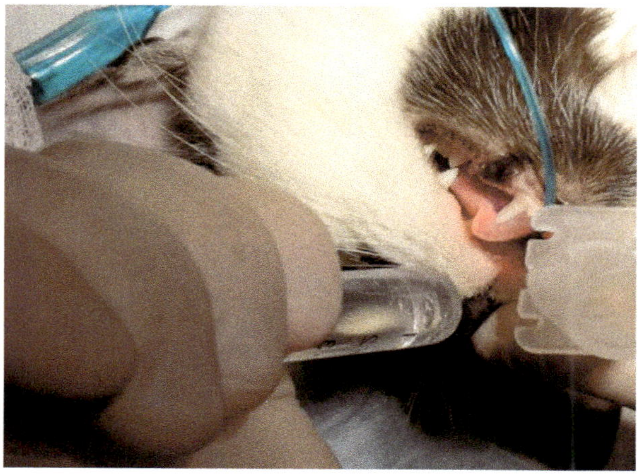

Figure 24. Nasal lavage or flushing under general anaesthesia. (Photo: Diego Esteban).

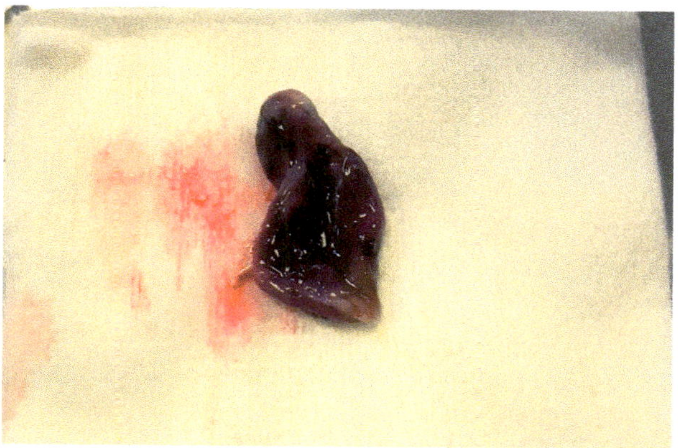

Figure 25. Large nasal polyp extracted via nasal lavage.

In most cats, disease regression is spontaneous without high mortality. But the **virus is excreted in respiratory and ocular secretions for two to three weeks**, during which time it can infect other in-contact cats. **Viremia and pneumonia are rare**, although may occur in weak, malnourished or immunosuppressed cats, where mortality can be high. On some occasions, virus has been isolated in the central nervous system (CNS), but only one documented case of FHV-1 was related to meningoencephalitis. Unlike herpesviruses in the dog, in cats FHV-1 **does not cause abortions** as a result of direct viral replication in the genital organs.

After acute infection and clinical cure, in most cats the virus remains dormant in the trigeminal nerve ganglion without clinical signs or and for long periods virus is not present in secretions. **Stress and other immunosuppressive factors can reactivate viral replication** with or without clinical signs, which can cause a recurrence of virus excretion. This phenomenon of reactivation and new virus outflow maintains a presence in communities, even though the virus is fragile in the environment.

The exact pathogenesis of chronic herpesvirus disease is not well understood. The chronic nasal and ocular disease associated with herpesviruses are mainly immune-mediated inflammatory conditions and the virus is not detectable:

- **Stromal ulcers**. The immune-mediated response causes serious corneal inflammatory lesions leading to blindness.

- **Chronic rhinosinusitis**. A similar mechanism of action is suspected.

Once the virus has ceased replication, the mechanisms of inflammation and destruction persist. **Destruction of the nasal turbinates** is common, with secondary bacterial infections that worsen the inflammation. **Corneal necrosis and eosinophilic keratitis** may also be related to FHV-1, although the mechanism is unclear, and the virus cannot always be identified. Likewise, some cases of uveitis associated with FHV-1, are documented, although the cause-effect association has yet to be demonstrated.

Epidemiology

The prevalence of feline herpesvirus infections in feline communities is high at 20–50%. The presence of virus in communities is perpetuated by latent carrier cats that undergo viral reactivation and excretion and put kittens at risk. In contrast, the herpesvirus prevalence in indoor cats or those living in isolation is less than 5%. However, it should be noted that a cat living alone may undergo herpesvirus reactivation which can result in clinical signs.

Clinical signs

In acute cases the most frequent clinical signs are:

- **Sneezing**
- Nasal discharge
  - Serous: if the condition is only viral.
  - Purulent: due to bacterial coinfection. Very frequent.
- **Coughing**
- May be accompanied by conjunctivitis and ocular secretion
- Superficial **corneal ulcers**: very frequent, especially dendritic ulcers.

Herpetic dermatitis consists of **ulcerative lesions in the nasal septum area** or around the lips in cats which show or have shown respiratory signs, but which have not always been identified. Often, the lesions develop **secondary bacterial infections**, which can be acute or chronic, and histologically an eosinophilic inflammatory component is seen which is sometimes mistakenly diagnosed as being of allergic inflammatory origin (Figures 26 and 27).

The most frequent chronic symptoms are:

- **Chronic rhinosinusitis**: with sneezing and chronic or recurrent purulent nasal discharge in cats showing no signs of systemic disease
- **Keratitis or stromal corneal ulcers**: deep ulcers that are difficult to cure which may cause corneal perforation and loss of vision.

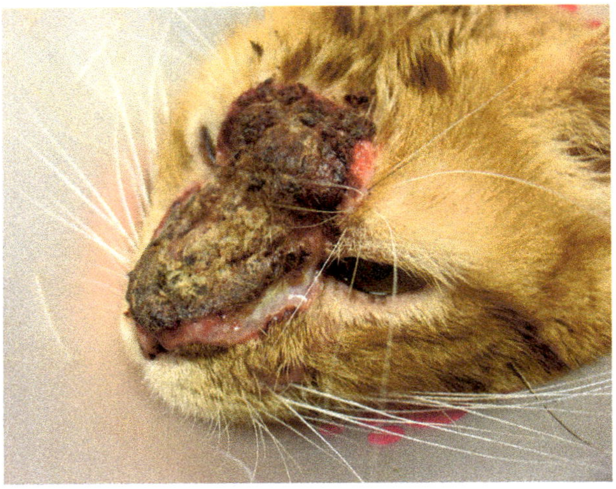

Figure 26. Severe herpetic dermatitis.

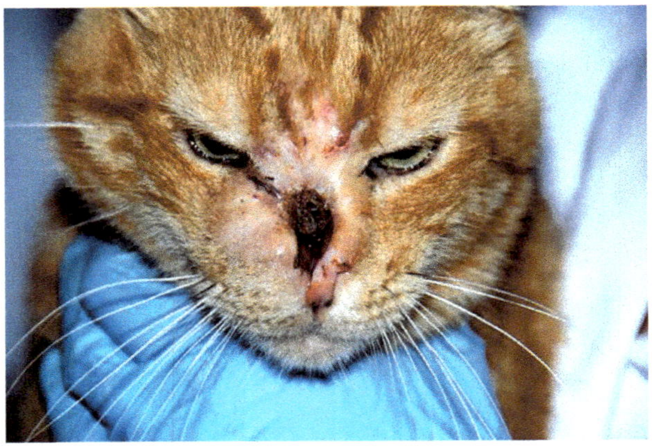

Figure 27. Sequelae of herpetic dermatitis.

Diagnosis

A presumptive diagnosis is often made for the acute condition, based on the typical clinical signs and response to symptomatic or supportive treatment. However, nowadays using **PCR (polymerase chain reaction)** techniques can easily confirm viral presence. This represents significant advances in virus detection in day-to-day practice compared to other less practical techniques such as immunofluorescence or virus isolation. Any veterinarian can confirm the presence of **FHV-1 through nasal, conjunctival, oropharyngeal or corneal swabs** sent to laboratories capable of performing good quality PCR techniques. In cases of herpetic dermatitis, PCR can also be done on biopsies or skin swabs.

There are, however, limitations in the interpretation of PCR for FHV-1:

- The presence of the virus's DNA does not necessarily mean the virus is replicating and therefore the cause of the cat's disease. **PCR can detect DNA from the virus in a sample because there is replication of the virus (latent carrier),** even if the clinical signs are caused by another disease.

- **DNA detection of the vaccine virus.** Herpes virus vaccines are attenuated and produce a subclinical infection, which stimulates the immunological memory response, especially in the weeks following vaccination.

Although there are currently no clinical studies to prove it, quantitative real-time PCR (RT-PCR) techniques could be extremely helpful:

- A **small amount of DNA suggests latency** or low levels of replication and no involvement in the clinical signs.
- **High levels of DNA suggest high levels of replication** and a greater involvement in the clinical signs.

Serological antibody detection techniques are not useful for diagnosis of herpesvirus, since the presence of antibodies has no correlation with the disease and active infection. Given the high prevalence of natural infection and vaccination, many cats are seropositive. Consequently, serology is useful for seroprevalence studies or to assess the humoral immune response against the virus, but not for clinical diagnosis.

Treatment

Herpesvirus treatment is based on:

- **Supportive treatment** (hydration, nutritional, mucolytics)
- **Antibiotics** suitable for respiratory infections (doxycycline, amoxicillin, azithromycin, fluoroquinolones)
- In some cases, **antiviral drugs.**

Numerous antiviral drugs against FHV-1 have been tested, all with good activity in vitro, but this does not always correspond to efficacy in vivo. Most studies are case series or clinical cases; therefore, treatment **recommendations are not based on controlled studies.** There is a wide range of anti-herpetic action (nucleoside analogues).

Topical ocular antiherpetic agents should be administered **every 2–4 hours** as they have a virostatic action and require continuous concentrations to inhibit viral replication. In the past, the most commonly used were trifluridine and idoxuridine (whose efficacy in vivo has not been demonstrated). **Ganciclovir** is currently used more frequently in ophthalmic ointment (two or three times a day, although there are no clinical studies) or **0.5% cidofovir** (there is a clinical study which proves efficacy when applied twice a day). However, cidofovir is a preparation for intravenous use and must be reformulated for ocular use and is expensive.

In recent years, there is widespread use of systemic antiherpetic agents such as **famciclovir** (prodrug of penciclovir). Studies in experimentally and naturally infected cats show tolerance is good and clinical improvement is significant. **The dose for famciclovir is 40 to 90 mg/kg/8 h PO for 3 or 4 weeks** and should never be less than 40 mg/kg/8–12 h or it may not be effective.

Other treatments for herpesvirus include **L-lysine and interferon.** Lysine (amino acid) is widely used at doses of 500 mg/12 h. Its mechanism of action is competition for and displacement of arginine, an essential amino acid for herpesvirus replication. A systematic review of experimental and clinical studies on lysine concluded there were **no clinical benefits**. Even an in vitro study did not observe the inhibition of feline herpesvirus replication against various concentrations of lysine.

There are some publications on the use of interferon, human alpha and feline omega, systemically or topically in FHV-1 infections. The **results are inconclusive**, but in general they reduce the intensity of clinical signs. Recently there is evidence based on some studies that the use of **some probiotics** (*Enterococcus faecium SF 68*) causes stimulation of cellular immunity which may decrease clinical signs and accelerate recovery from FHV-1 infections.

Because stress is an important cause of reactivation of latent FHV-1, infections, environmental enrichment and adequate sanitary, hygienic, and nutritional conditions are helpful in reducing clinical signs in colonies or catteries where the infection is endemic and there are large number of cats that are latent carriers.

Prognosis

The prognosis for herpesvirus is:

- Good, in the vast majority of cases.
- Bad in some weakened or immunosuppressed kittens in which systemic dissemination or pneumonia occurs.
- Reserved in chronic cases, as many do not respond to antiherpetic treatments. These should be treated continuously with a combination of antibiotics and anti-inflammatory drugs (non-steroidals and sometimes, corticosteroids).

Prevention

In group situations latent carriers make prevention of herpesvirus infection difficult, due to reactivation and further shedding of virus. Cats that recover from herpesvirus are not immunised and can manifest the disease again.

Attenuated vaccines against feline herpesvirus prevent the appearance of clinical signs and decrease their intensity. However, they do not produce a robust or sterilising immunity which prevents infection or latency. Consequently, **vaccinated cats can become infected or be latent carriers, but do not show clinical signs**. Although an annual revaccination programme is recommended by vaccine producers, studies on the duration of immunity (DOI) with experimental infection show protection is at least three years. Annual revaccination or vaccination every three years should be a decision based on the individual's risk, such as their lifestyle and likely exposure to infection.

Chlamydia infections

Aetiopathogenesis

Chlamydia felis is a bacterium from the *Chlamydiaceae* family, which is fragile in the environment. Infection is by direct contact between cats. *C. felis'* main tropism is ocular, specifically the conjunctiva, causing **inflammation and ocular secretions** but with no corneal involvement.

C. felis was thought to produce infection and clinical signs in the upper respiratory tract, but current thinking is that it is only a **conjunctival pathogen**. Chronic carriers may exist in a subclinical state.

Epidemiology

There is a high prevalence of *C. felis* in groups of felines, but low prevalence in cats living in isolation. Sick cats or chronic carriers are the main source of infection.

Clinical signs

The signs are those of acute or chronic conjunctivitis. Initially, this is a unilateral, serous conjunctivitis (inflammation and serous secretion), which becomes bilateral and worsens to manifest **blepharospasm, purulent secretions and a marked conjunctival inflammation and chemosis** -the latter being a clinical feature of this infection (Figure 28).

Generally, there are **no systemic or respiratory signs** and if present these are likely due to coinfection with respiratory pathogens. Chronic carrier cats can be asymptomatic or suffer chronic conjunctivitis. Up to **30% of cases of chronic feline conjunctivitis** are due to *C. felis*.

Table 7. *C. felis* vaccination programme. Essential vaccine recommended in all cats.

Primary vaccination	Re-vaccination	Adult re-vaccination
3 doses: 8, 12 and 16 weeks	A year after the last dose	Annual in cats at risk of exposure
		Every 3 years in low-risk cats

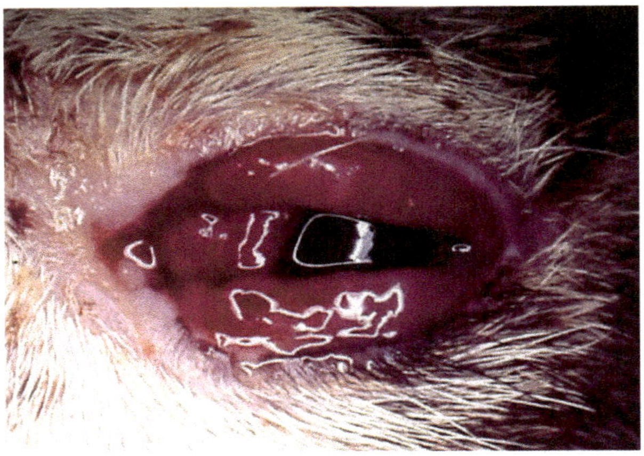

Figure 28. Infectious conjunctivitis with chemosis.

Diagnosis

Clinical suspicion is raised in cats with acute or chronic conjunctivitis, especially with a **marked chemosis**. Diagnosis can be confirmed by observing inclusion bodies in conjunctival cytology (low sensitivity) or PCR of a conjunctival swab (high sensitivity).

PCR is the technique of choice for confirmation of diagnosis and detection of chronic carriers.

Treatment

Tetracyclines are the treatment of choice, as eye drops or ophthalmic ointment. However, it is preferable to administer **doxycycline (10 mg/kg/24 h for 3–4 weeks) orally** to completely eradicate the bacteria from the conjunctiva and prevent the chronic carrier state.

It is important to treat all in contact cats even if they have no clinical signs. Quinolones can also be effective, especially pradofloxacin (5–10 mg/kg every 24 hours).

Prognosis

The prognosis is good. This is not an infection that causes death and if treated properly can be cured. It may be more difficult to eliminate or eradicate *C. felis* in a community where it is endemic, since all cats should be treated, systematic vaccination initiated, and the cat population reduced.

Prevention

Prevention is based on the treatment of affected cats and those which have been in contact. There are vaccines against *C. felis* although they do not prevent infection, but do decrease the appearance or intensity of clinical signs. Vaccination is not considered essential for all cats, but should be considered as part of a broader plan to eradicate *C. felis* from a community (which includes doxycycline treatment, systematic vaccination and improvements to the community's environmental conditions).

Mycoplasma infections

Aetiopathogenesis

Mycoplasma spp. are bacteria without a cell wall which are part of the normal bacterial flora of the respiratory tract in cats and are ubiquitous in the environment. They are difficult to grow in laboratory conditions.

Some *Mycoplasma species* act as primary pathogens in cats, mainly producing signs of **respiratory infection, conjunctivitis and (rarely) polyarthritis**. The *Mycoplasma* species that have been documented as causing disease in cats are *M. felis*, *M. gateae* and *M. feliminutum*.

Epidemiology

The prevalence of respiratory infections due to *Mycoplasma* spp. is unknown, but in recent epidemiological studies in different countries it tends to be high, especially in feline communities.

Groups with an excessive number of cats in poor hygienic and sanitary conditions are likely to be affected.

Clinical signs

Mycoplasma spp. mainly produce **acute upper respiratory infections** (acute rhinitis and tracheitis) and conjunctivitis. There is evidence that a high percentage (16 to 26%) of infectious conjunctivitis are caused primarily by *M. felis*. Cases with corneal involvement and ulcerative keratitis, with *M. gateae* and *M. felis* as the primary pathogens have been described. This is important since corneal disease in cats has traditionally been linked FHV-1 whereas in some cases *Mycoplasma* is responsible

Studies of cats with chronic rhinitis or rhinosinusitis (chronic clinical signs and chronic lesions observed in advanced CT type imaging tests) are documented as caused by *Mycoplasma* as a **primary pathogen and respond well to antibiotics**.

In addition, there are cases of **lower respiratory tract infections and pneumonia** caused by these *Mycoplasma* species. Rarely, cases of polyarthritis (generalized pain, joint pain, joint effusions, fever) due to systemic *Mycoplasma* infections have been documented.

Diagnosis

Clinical suspicion should be high in cats with conjunctivitis, keratitis or upper respiratory infection, mainly with signs of rhinitis. In many cases there will be **viral and bacterial coinfection**.

In **acute cases**, diagnostic tests are rarely performed to establish the aetiology. However, the possible involvement of *Mycoplasma* as a primary pathogen or in coinfection, indicates an **antibiotic should be selected with good efficacy against *Mycoplasma***.

In chronic cases and in cases of pneumonia confirmation of the aetiological diagnosis is important. Although respiratory mycoplasmas can be grown in the laboratory, this is a difficult and slow technique. Therefore, **PCR techniques** using conjunctival, nasal or bronchoalveolar wash samples are generally preferred.

Table 8. *Mycoplasma* vaccination programme. Non-essential vaccine recommended in colonies and groups where there is endemic infection and in cats at risk of exposure.

Primary vaccination	Re-vaccination	Adult re-vaccination
2 doses: 8 and 12 weeks	A year after the last dose	Annual

Treatment

The treatment of choice is **tetracyclines, both topically (ocular) and orally in all cases**. Oral administration of doxycycline (10 mg/kg every 24 hours for 3–4 weeks) is preferable to completely eradicate the bacteria.

Quinolones (enrofloxacin, marbofloxacin, pradofloxacin) are also effective, as are macrolides (azithromycin, clarithromycin).

In general, the most commonly used antibiotics are doxycycline, marbofloxacin and pradofloxacin. Due to the possible involvement of *Mycoplasma* in numerous respiratory infections in cats and the poor response of these bacteria to β-lactam antibiotics (amoxicillin, cephalosporins), the empirical use of these antibiotics as a first choice in an acute or chronic respiratory condition is not advised, even if it is a kitten which is only a few weeks or months old. Doxycycline is considered a safe antibiotic in young kittens (>4 weeks old) provided the risk of oesophagitis is considered, which can be minimized by giving food and water straight after administration.

Prognosis

The prognosis is apparently good, although there are no clinical studies which look at a high number of cases. Cats with chronic conditions may respond well to treatment, but these tend to recur as the pathogenesis of chronic rhinosinusitis is complex and multifactorial.

Prevention

There are **no vaccines** available for the prevention of respiratory mycoplasma infections. Prevention is based on good environmental management and living conditions for cat colonies.

Feline calicivirus (FCV) infections

Aetiopathogenesis

FCV is an RNA virus belonging to the *Caliciviridae* family. *Caliciviridae* are **resistant in the environment**

and remain infectious for up to a month in cold, dry conditions, making indirect transmission possible. There is also great genetic variability within the group, with numerous variants arising in different cat populations.

Different genetic variants show varying virulence, and consequently **clinical signs may vary in severity**. In addition, the evolutionary ability of the virus allows it to adapt its genome to evade the cat's immune response.

FCV has a **special tropism for the nasal, oropharyngeal, and oral mucous membranes**. When a cat is infected, by direct or indirect contact, after a **few days incubation** the virus produces necrotic and inflammatory lesions in the epithelia with associated acute clinical signs (nasal and oral). Less frequently, it **replicates in synovial tissue and causes polyarthritis** (on rare occasions this is an adverse effect of attenuated vaccines). Variants with higher virulence can produce **systemic signs, fever and pneumonia**. FCV spreads in blood producing significant viremia and is **excreted in saliva, respiratory secretions, faeces and urine**.

Most cats **manifest the acute clinical condition, which goes into spontaneous remission** without causing death, whilst the virus continues to be excreted for a month or so and is a source of infection to in-contact animals. Some cats (up to 20%) remain **chronic carriers** of FCV without demonstrating clinical signs, but continuously excrete the virus and contaminate the environment.

Several outbreaks of a severe systemic disease caused by **virulent variants of FCV (virulent systemic calicivirus, VS-FCV)** have been described in the last decade. These outbreaks described in the US, United Kingdom and in other countries in Europe have similar characteristics:

- Systemic inflammation syndrome: vasculitis, involvement of the liver and pancreas, disseminated intravascular coagulation and multiorgan failure.
- Clinical signs are most serious in adult and older cats.
- High mortality, close to 50%.
- It also affects cats vaccinated against FCV.
- Indirect transmission of the virus through fomites is extremely effective.

Epidemiology

There is a **high prevalence of feline FCV infection in colonies (20 to 50%)**, where chronic carriers of FCV infect young kittens and maintain and perpetuate the presence of the virus in the environment. The prevalence of FCV is lower in isolated indoor cats.

Infection is caused by **direct contact with respiratory secretions**, but also by **indirect contact with contaminated environments and fomites**. It has also been shown the virus can be transmitted through **flea faeces in which it remains infective for a few days** and infection has been demonstrated experimentally by contact with fleas and their faeces.

Clinical signs

Most characteristic acute clinical signs:

- Sneezing
- Nasal discharge
- Ocular discharge
- Superficial ulcers on tongue and palate (anorexia, sialorrhoea and odynophagia) (Figure 29).

Some cases present with **fever and apathy** which may be accompanied by joint or generalized pain (polyarthritis) (Figure 30). Recently, corneal ulcers caused by FCV have been described, although this is a poorly documented lesion.

Given the diversity of genomes and genetic variants of FCV, clinical conditions vary from mild to severe, and in some cases, mortality can be high.

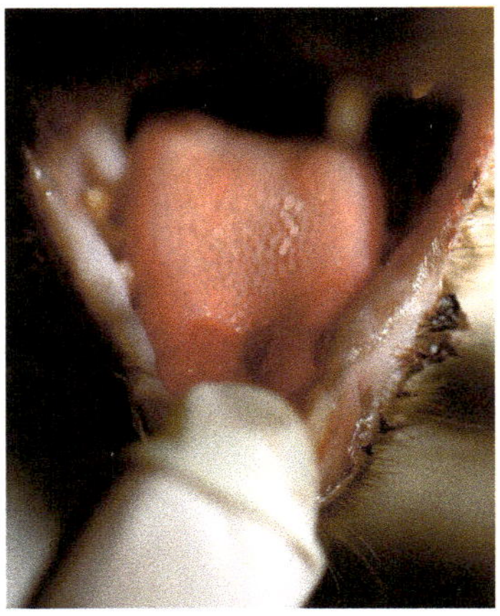

Figure 29. Ulcer on the tongue of a patient suffering from calicivirus.

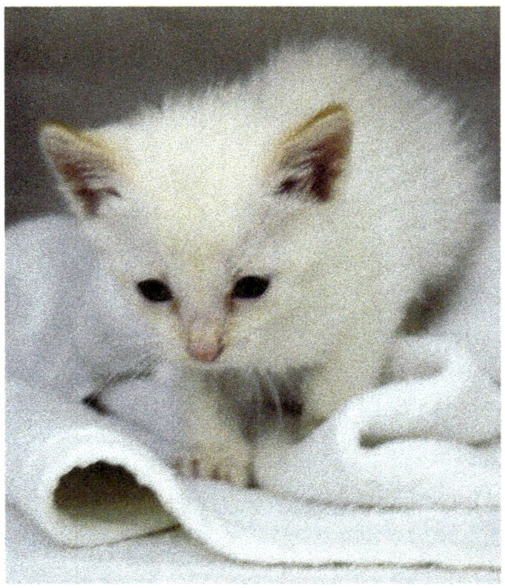

Figure 30. Polyarthritis, as a consequence of calicivirus infection.

The clinical signs associated with **virulent systemic calicivirus** include:

- Oedema of extremities
- Ulcerated pads
- Mouth ulcers
- Fever
- Jaundice
- Vomiting
- Diarrhoea
- Respiratory distress
- Possibility of bleeding, hepatitis, pancreatitis, pneumonia, disseminated intravascular coagulation and multiorgan failure.

Diagnosis

In acute cases a presumptive diagnosis is made based on the clinical signs. Confirmation of the presence of the virus through **PCR techniques** is easy using an **oral, conjunctival, or blood swab** sent to laboratories performing good quality PCR techniques. However, given the variability in the genome of different strains and variants, the **sensitivity of the FCV PCR can be reduced, giving false negatives**. Also, as with **FHV-1, the presence of calicivirus RNA does not necessarily mean it is the cause of the disease**, since many cats carry the virus asymptomatically. There may also be **false positive results** for PCR in the weeks after vaccination with attenuated vaccines.

Diagnosis by detection and titration of **antibodies is not useful**, since antibodies produced by previous infection, active infection, or vaccination cannot be differentiated and discriminated between. In addition, **chronic carrier cats have antibodies present permanently**.

Diagnosis by **immunohistochemistry on biopsies** from oral lesions or internal organs to detect virus antigens inside the cells is also feasible. This diagnostic technique is especially useful for confirmation of cases of VS-FCV and sequencing FCV variants.

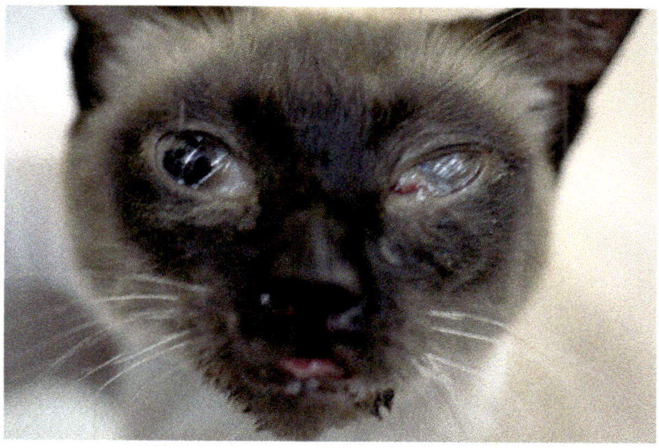

Figure 31. Systemic calicivirus: ocular involvement.

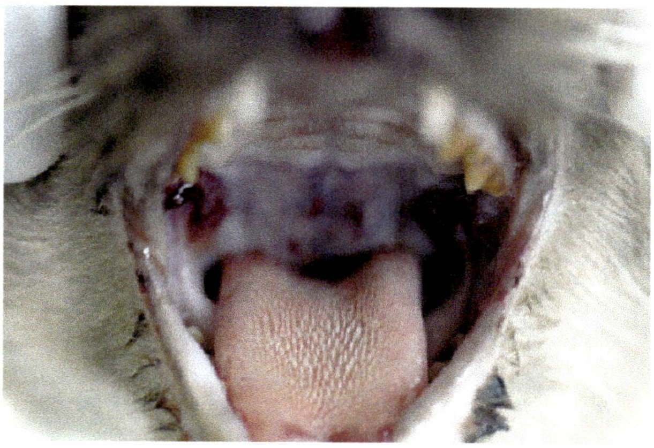

Figure 32. Systemic calicivirus: lesions in the oral cavity.

Treatment

There is **no specific antiviral treatment** against FCV. Many antivirals which are useful against RNA viruses, such as **ribavirin or vidarabine, are toxic in** cats and cannot be used safely. The approach to acute calicivirosis is based on **supportive treatment** (hydration, nutritional, antibiotics and analgesics). In experimental studies**, feline omega interferon can inhibit in vitro replication**, although its efficacy in diseased cats is unknown. However, in the most severe cases, its use is worthwhile to try to increase the chances of cure, given its non-specific antiviral action.

To date there is no specific treatment for virulent systemic calicivirosis, but the use of feline omega interferon is logical. Given the immune mediated component of vasculitis and the lesions caused by this condition, **corticosteroids may be indicated**, even at the risk of immunosuppression, but there are no clinical studies.

Prognosis

With mild and moderate FCV the prognosis is good. With severe disease with systemic signs, the prognosis is poor. With virulent systemic calicivirus, mortality is high.

Prevention

Prevention of FCV infection is difficult in feline colonies or communities due the presence of chronic carriers. Also, **recovered cats are not immune to future infections**. Vaccines are available against FCV, both attenuated and inactivated, which are generally effective either by preventing the appearance of clinical signs or by reducing their intensity. However, these **vaccines do not produce a robust or sterilising immunity** which prevents infection or latency. Consequently, **vaccinated cats may be infected and latent** carriers without any clinical signs. Also, given the diversity of FCV genomic variants and their ability

Table 9. FCV vaccination programme. Essential vaccine recommended in all cats.

Primary vaccination	Re-vaccination	Adult re-vaccination
3 doses: 8, 12 and 16 weeks	A year after the last dose	Annual in cats at risk of exposure
		Every 3 years in low-risk cats

to evolve within cat colonies, vaccines may not be able to fully immunise against all existing FCV variants.

In an attempt to improve the preventative capacity of FCV vaccines, new variants (G1 and 431) have been added to those already included (F9 and 255). If clinical signs of caliciviruses are observed in already vaccinated cats, **it is advisable to vary the type of vaccine administered**.

Although the revaccination schedule recommended in the datasheet is annual, there are studies of duration of immunity (DOI) and experimental infection that show the **DOI is at least 3 years**. However, given the high pressure of infection in some communities and the great genetic variability of FCV, **annual revaccination is highly recommended for cats which are at higher risk**, which live in groups or are in contact with street cats.

Feline chronic gingivostomatitis (FCGS)

Feline chronic gingivostomatitis (FCGS) is a relatively common disease characterised by **diffuse and widespread proliferative and ulcerative inflammation of the gums and oral mucosa** and which appears mainly in adult cats.

FCGS is often associated with a chronic FCV infection; however, it does not fulfil Koch's postulates of infectious disease and it has not been possible to reproduce the disease experimentally. A significant number of cats affected by this disease are positive or carriers of FCV, but in other cats no FCV is detected and the inflammation responds to treatment that does not involve a reduction in viral load.

Consequently, this disease should not be considered as a "chronic calicivirosis" but rather a **chronic inflammatory disease most likely of immune-mediated origin**.

Aetiopathogenesis

Although the exact cause is unknown, the most widely accepted hypothesis is that FCGS is a **multifactorial immune mediated disease due to a loss of immune system tolerance to the antigens frequently present in the oral mucosa** of cats, mainly bacteria from plaque and calicivirus.

Numerous oral and systemic immunological abnormalities have been demonstrated in cats with FCGS. Early studies showed that the **level of immunoglobulins A and G were abnormal in saliva and serum** when compared to healthy cats. More recent studies used cytokine patterns to evaluate the inflammatory response, and found that in the mouth of healthy cats a Th1, pattern predominates, whilst in **cats suffering from CGS there is a mixed pattern of Th1 and Th2.** The immune-mediated basis for disease is supported by histology showing an inflammatory pattern with a predominance of lymphoctyes and plasma cells in the absence of pathogens and the clinical response to anti-inflammatory or immunosuppressive treatments.

A variable percentage (0–70% in various studies) of cats with FCGS are FCV positive with PCR techniques in oral samples. However, the **presence of FCV in oral mucosa does not demonstrate the cause-effect relationship**, since a variable but significant percentage of healthy cats also test positive for FCV in the oral mucosa, and also a significant group of cats with the disease are negative for FCV. It is likely that the **presence of FCV is one of several trigger factors** which contribute to inflammation in cats with this disease, but it is not the direct cause. In addition, in general, treatments with an antiviral mechanism, such as high dose interferons, are not effective. In a recent study, immunohistochemistry (IHC) techniques specific to FCV were performed on biopsies from 26 cats with CGS and all were negative, as well as with the PCR for FCV.

The disease has also been **linked to retrovirus, FeLV and FIV infections**. Coinfections by retrovirus and calicivirus could increase the proinflammatory response and predispose to the appearance of CGS. Cats with **FIV infections have a high prevalence of chronic gingivitis and stomatitis,** although this has not been shown to have a direct relationship with the virus. Rather, they are related to immunodeficiency, chronic bacterial infections, or a pro-inflammatory state related to FIV infection. In a recent study IHC detected FeLV antigens in oral lesions, which suggests that they have a direct influence on inflammation.

Recent studies have evaluated the **type of oral bacteria** in cats with FCGS. These studies detected bacteria by traditional techniques such as bacteriological cultures, with the most recent ones using detection by PCR of bacteria which cannot be cultured. In general, these studies show **important differences in the oral bacterial flora of cats with** FCGS compared to that of healthy cats. Specifically:

- Less bacterial diversity
- Predominance of *Pasteurella multocida*
- Increased presence of *Pseudomonas* spp., *Tannerella forsythia,* and *Porphyromonas circumdentaria.*

Years ago, some studies associated this disease with *Bartonella henselae* infection, but more recently it has been shown that the prevalence of ***B. henselae* is no different** from that observed in healthy cats.

The hypothesis for **bacterial antigenic influence** is reinforced by the clinical improvement with antibiotic administration (especially with effects on *Pasteurella* and anaerobes) and the large percentage of total cure or remission of inflammation after complete dental extraction.

A recent study showed that most cats with CGS also have **inflammatory lesions in the oesophagus** observed by oesophagoscopy. However, no clinical signs associated with oesophagitis were observed and the **significance of this finding is unknown**.

Epidemiology

CGS usually occurs in adult cats, although for some cat's inflammation begins at an early age. Predisposing risk factors include:

- Presence of FCV
- Cats that live in communities
- Elements of environmental stress.

Clinical signs

The main external clinical signs are:

- Odynophagia
- Pseudo anorexia
- Submandibular lymphadenopathy
- Sialorrhoea, sometimes with blood.

There may also be systemic signs such as:

- Weight loss
- Poor hair quality.

And, in advanced cases:

- **Hyperglobulinemia**
- Polyclonal gammopathy
- Proteinuria
- Chronic kidney disease.

Oral examination may show:

- Intense 360° gingivitis around the teeth
- Alveolitis
- **Caudal stomatitis** (glossopalatine angle). Inflammation varies in intensity from erythema to **intense proliferative inflammation with ulcerated areas** (Figure 33). Lesions may be covered with purulent secretion and bleed easily, in some cases they extend to the oropharynx and/or have deep ulcers on the tongue, although this is unusual.

The disease can be mild, moderate or intense depending on:

- Degree of pain
- Proliferation (Figure 34)
- Ulceration
- Chronicity.

Diagnosis

Diagnosis is based on several criteria, but mainly the **type and distribution of the lesions**. The presence of **inflammation in the caudal part of the mouth and caudal stomatitis** is what determines the clinical diagnosis and helps to differentiate from other oral or dental pathologies such as periodontal disease, dental resorption, or juvenile hyperplastic gingivitis. Lesions are **diffuse and symmetrical** which distinguishes them from proliferative lesions which do not have to be symmetrical, such as eosinophilic granulomas or oral neoplasms.

In case of doubt about the diagnosis, or if a histological diagnosis is desired, **biopsies of the lesions**

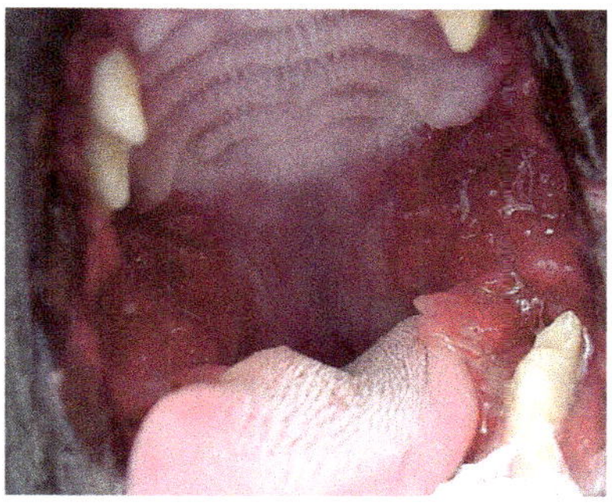

Figure 33. Moderate feline gingivostomatitis.

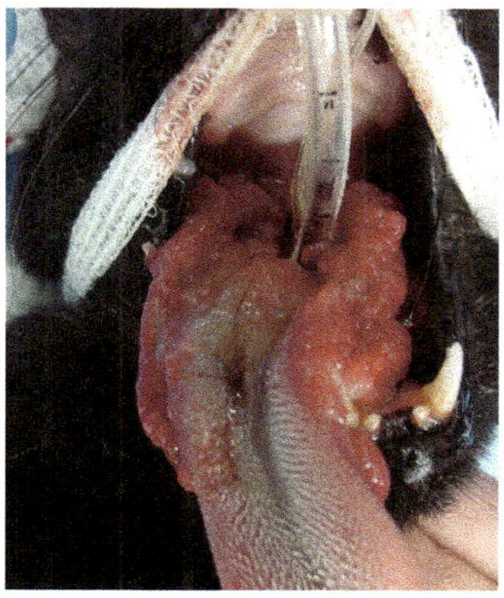

Figure 34. Maximum grade gingivostomatitis.

should be performed. The histological pattern of CGS is a lymphoplasmacytic inflammation although there can be a neutrophilic component especially in ulcerated areas. IHC techniques can be applied to the same samples to detect the presence of pathogens such as FCV or FeLV.

In many cases FCV PCR is performed, even though treatment decisions are not influenced by the result (since there is no effective antiviral treatment for FCV) It is important to **know the retrovirus status**, because the presence of FeLV or FIV can influence the choice of treatment, for example, whether or not to use immunosuppressive treatments. In addition, there may be other diseases associated with retroviruses.

Normally, in first opinion practice, bacterial microbiological cultures of the secretions are not performed, except in cases where antimicrobial resistance is suspected.

To assess if systemic abnormalities are associated with oral disease, the following tests should be performed:

- Complete blood count
- Serum biochemistry
- Proteinogram
- Urinalysis.

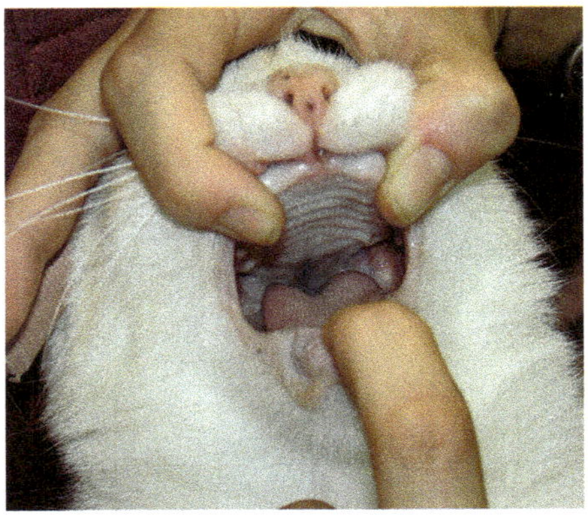

Figure 35. Case of cured stomatitis after complete exodontics.

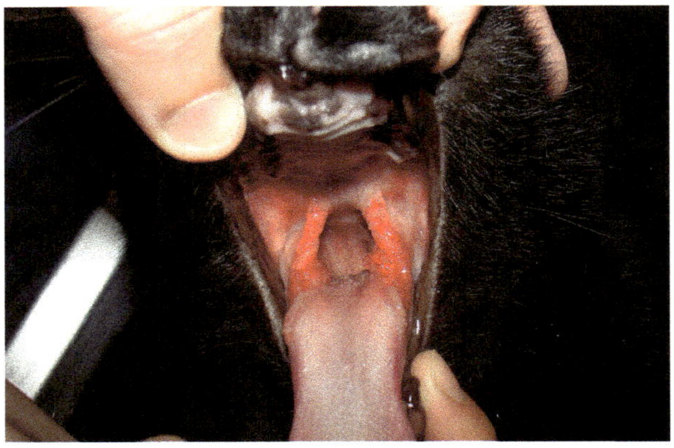

Figure 36. Caudal stomatitis after complete exodontics.

Treatment

There is currently no known treatment with 100% cure for cats with CGS.

- Milder cases usually respond to medical treatment
- Antibiotics (amoxicillin-clavulanic, clindamycin, spiramycin-metronidazole)
- Dental hygiene
- Non-steroidal anti-inflammatories and analgesics.

The response to antibiotics and analgesics usually reduces over time. In moderate states, for the relief of inflammation and pain, corticosteroids are necessary at anti-inflammatory doses, and possibly even immunosuppressants. Occasionally, a temporary remission of the signs and inflammation is achieved, but many cats do not respond or soon stop responding to treatment.

In 1994 a first series of cases was published which demonstrated **complete exodontics** of all the teeth (except, in some cases, the canines) allowed complete **healing in approximately 70% of the cats** (Figure 35). In the remaining 30%, although the disease was not cured, there was a partial improvement with the usual treatments and better control of pain and inflammation.

In the last 20 years, many cats have been treated using exodontics (performed by experienced surgeons and avoiding retained tooth roots) with the same phenomenon observed: a large number of patients slowly improved and were cured 4–6 months after teeth removal, with a smaller group, that although not cured were more easily controlled with corticosteroids, oral feline omega interferon at low doses or cyclosporine (Figure 36). One study showed those that did not fully respond to exodontics were controlled with **oral feline omega interferon at a continuous dose of 0.1 IU/24 h PO**. The response to interferon was similar to that to prednisolone for the control of pain and inflammation.

Other treatments, documented in a small number of cats, are natural or **hypoallergenic diets**, **CO_2 laser** to remove proliferative lesions, and **stem cell treatments**. Two studies using stem cells in cats refractory to the usual treatments have been published. In one study autologous mesenchymal stem cells of adipose tissue origin were used. Of seven cats treated, in five the inflammation subsided completely or partially and only two did not respond. Also a change in the mouth's immune response was noted, using cytokine studies and other parameters. Therefore, the treatment produced a **normalization of the immune response** or pattern and the remission of inflammatory lesions. A second study with allogeneic stem cells did not show the same beneficial results.

Prognosis

The **prognosis for cure is reserved** or poor unless all teeth are removed. Some owners are reluctant to use such an aggressive technique if it does not guarantee total healing. However, the quality of life of cats with moderate and intense CGS is very poor and sometimes they are not able to eat without high, continuous doses of corticosteroids which end up causing serious adverse systemic effects (diabetes mellitus, urine infections, hypercortisolism). In addition, over time, corticosteroids become less effective and, in some cats, the lack of response to treatment leads to euthanasia.

The prognosis after exodontics is good with 70–80% of cats completely cured and 30–20% showing a partial improvement. **Cats without teeth that are not cured are managed more easily** with medical treatments (prednisolone, low dose interferon omega, cyclosporine or autologous stem cells are the best alternatives).

Prevention

There are currently no preventive measures. However, given the association with FCV in a significant percentage of cats, **prevention of FCV infection may be useful.**

Ensuring optimal living conditions, without overcrowding and avoiding environmental stress can also show good results. In any case, some affected animals are indoor cats and no obvious stress factors or environment deficits are identified.

Fading kitten syndrome (neonatal mortality in kittens)

Fading kitten syndrome (FKS) is mortality or morbidity in young kittens occurring from the neonatal period to weaning. The **causes are multiple and diverse** and mainly infectious, although there are also congenital and environmental causes. At this young age, disease manifestation is similar regardless of the cause, so **clinical signs are non-specific**, and it is often difficult to reach an aetiological diagnosis. The age at which the kitten becomes ill or dies is useful in establishing differential aetiological diagnoses. **Post-mortem is of a high diagnostic value** in the event of an outbreak of neonatal mortality.

The causes of morbidity and mortality in litters of kittens are numerous. FKS may be caused by:

- Congenital diseases
- Metabolic diseases
- Infectious and parasitic diseases
- Nutritional problems
- Psychogenic or environmental problems that affect the mother.

Clinical signs are the same or similar regardless of the cause. Typical clinical signs are:

- abnormal excessive vocalization
- the absence of, or ineffective lactation
- weakness and inactivity which leads to hypothermia and hypoglycaemia
- loss of the suckling reflex
- weight loss
- abdominal distention.

Mortality may be due to the primary disease or the secondary consequences of the disease.

Identifying the cause is often difficult given diagnostic limitations in kittens of these ages. It is useful to remember **that non-infectious causes are most frequent during the first two weeks of life** (congenital, trauma, premature birth, nutritional, environmental problems and neonatal isoerythrolysis). **Infectious causes are more prevalent after three to four weeks of age** in kittens.

The prognosis is reserved to poor. Although in some cases, if the cause is reversible and intensive supportive treatment is provided, the outlook can be favourable. The mortality associated with FKS is high.

Congenital diseases

These are infrequent and major ones are:

- **Cleft palate.** Typified by milk coming out of the nostrils.
- **Portosystemic shunts.** The signs usually appear after weaning, special attention should be given to Persian cats with cooper coloured irises.
- **Congenital heart disease** such as the presence of murmurs or signs of congestive heart failure, but can also be asymptomatic.
- **Gastrointestinal disorders** such as megaoesophagus, blind ending intestinal loops, and anal atresia.

Most of these problems produce **rapid mortality and there is no effective treatment.** However, sometimes signs may occur at more advanced ages and surgical (shunt, cleft palate) or medical (megaoesophagus) treatment may be possible.

Metabolic diseases

Neonatal isoerythrolysis

This occurs infrequently in domestic short-haired cats as most are type-A blood groups. **Neonatal**

isoerythrolysis occurs with greater frequency in some purebred cats, since more more than 50% of these cats are type-B, for example: Devon Rex, Sphinx, Scottish Fold, Somali, Persian, Burmese, Abyssinian and some others.

Acute haemolytic anemia occurs in the first two days of life in blood group-A kittens with group-B mothers. Cats with group-B naturally produce anti-A antibodies, even if they have not received transfusions or undergone previous pregnancies. These anti-A antibodies can be passed onto kittens through colostrum. When a kitten is type-A (inherited from the father) and absorbs the anti-A antibodies from the type-B mother, it may suffer **acute signs of haemolytic anemia.**

These may manifest as **sudden death on the first day of life** or as signs of weakness and death may occur over the following days. The presence of **anemia and haemoglobinuria** are characteristic of the condition and confirm the diagnosis. In some cases, necrosis of the tip of the tail is observed.

The prevention of this problem means not mating type A males with type B females. If this is impossible, it is advisable to remove the kittens from the mother during the first two days of life and administer serum from type-A cats or find an adoptive type-A mother. From the third day of life they can be returned to the mother because absorption of antibodies is no longer taking place. In the case of diagnosis of the problem in a kitten, separating it from the mother and if necessary, administering a type-B blood transfusion from which the plasma containing the anti-A antibodies has been separated is recommended.

The disease can be very serious, even causing sudden death without previous clinical signs and, in some cases, it can be mild or moderate manifesting signs of haemolysis (haemoglobinuria), without presenting serious clinical signs of disease and without requiring treatment. Kittens which recover from the acute crisis have no sequelae or other problems.

Hypoglycaemia

This is a **frequent, serious secondary complication** of diseases, such as sepsis, malnutrition, hypothermia, and parasitosis. Clinical signs are usually seen in kittens up to 6 weeks of age, and include weakness, anorexia, ataxia, disorientation, agitation, seizures, blindness, coma and death. In kittens of less than three weeks of age inactivity is the dominant clinical sign, while later ataxia, disorientation and nervousness predominate.

In any case of **FKS glucose levels should be evaluated**: **levels below 60 mg/dl are compatible with hypoglycaemia** that causes clinical signs. The clinical response after administration of **oral or intravenous glucose** is usually rapid and helps confirm the diagnosis. The **presence of other concurrent diseases** as a cause of hypoglycaemia should always be assessed.

Premature kittens

Premature kittens are not common. The condition is characterized by **respiratory failure** due to pulmonary immaturity, absence of hair on the ventral area and legs, poor suckling ability, and average corpuscular volume greater than 90 fl during the first days of life. Treatment is supportive, with forced nutrition and oxygen therapy. The prognosis is poor if dyspnoea persists for more than a few days.

Nutritional diseases

Nutritional problems may arise as a result of **problems with lactation** (agalactia or mastitis), **kitten weakness**, excessive **competition** from litter mates, or due to **congenital abnormalities**. Occasionally, inadequate hand-rearing may be a problem.

Clinical signs seen during the first week of life include weight loss, weakness and ineffective nutrition.

Weaning stress

A delay in physical development may cause problems when the kitten transitions onto solid food, and likewise kittens with locomotor problems may have difficulties in adapting to sucking a bottle. Most kittens (6 to 8 weeks) do not accept solid food but have a good sucking reflex.

Psychogenic diseases

Neglect by the mother

Maternal neglect occurs in **inexperienced mothers** or cats which are sick or suffering from environmental stress and then leads to abandonment of kittens. The mother may even actively reject or attack kittens.

Kittens show weakness, vocalize excessively, are small and show little sucking activity usually during the first week of life.

Physical or environmental diseases

Hypothermia

Hypothermia develops rapidly in neonates deprived of a heat source or secondary to disease. **It produces gastrointestinal stasis, bradycardia, hypoglycaemia and dehydration**. It usually occurs in kittens under three weeks of age but can be as a problem secondary to any other disease occurring until six weeks of age.

The clinical signs are ceasing to suckle, inactivity and kittens which feel cold on palpation. **The normal body**

temperature in kittens is 35°C until 2 weeks of age and 37°C thereafter. In general, primary hypothermia only occurs in case of unfavourable environmental conditions or if the mother abandons the kittens. In most cases, hypothermia is a secondary sequela to any of the causes of disease in kittens, usually along with hypoglycaemia.

Treatment consists of correcting the cause, treating hypoglycaemia and heating using external heat sources. In very severe cases (<32°C) it is preferable to heat by means of fluids or enemas tempered to 37°C first before applying external heat to avoid peripheral vasodilation which the kitten is unable to compensate for. Although empirical, **any hypothermic kitten should be treated as if it were hypoglycaemic**.

It is important to keep in mind that below 32°C intestinal function is paralyzed and any medical and nutritional treatment must be parenteral until the temperature rises (Figure 37).

Infectious diseases

Feline leukaemia virus

FeLV can cause abortions, and foetal and neonatal deaths, as well as in kittens at weaning. But in general it is more common as a **cause of disease after eight weeks of age**. It can affect just one kitten or the entire litter.

The signs in neonatal kittens are not specific and consist of **lack of appetite, weight loss, hypothermia and inactivity**.

Diagnosis is based on performing the **p27 antigen detection test** in the mother and in all kittens. Sometimes false negative results are obtained in infected kittens since there is not enough antigen to be detected by the kit. It is advisable to perform the test in all kittens in the litter and serially in those that come back negative.

Treatment is mainly **supportive and anti retrovirals or interferons** can also be used. However, the prognosis in new-born kittens is poor and they do not usually respond to any treatment.

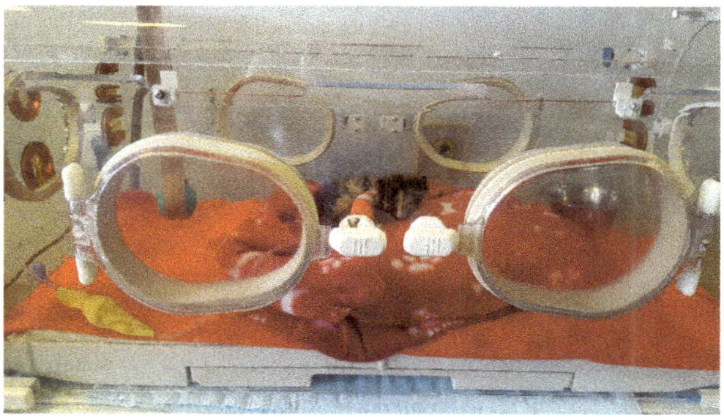

Figure 37. Hypothermic kitten receiving fluids in an incubator.

Feline infectious peritonitis virus

Perinatal infection can cause abortions, foetal and neonatal deaths and deaths of kittens at weaning, but it is more commonly a cause of disease in kittens over eight weeks of age.

The most frequent clinical signs are **weight loss, bloating and/or dyspnoea, and chronic fever with no apparent cause**. FIP usually appears as a sporadic disease that affects one of the kittens in the litter. On rare occasions it can affect whole litters

There are no effective treatments in this situation.

Feline panleukopoenia

Panleukopenia is one of the **most frequent causes of morbidity and mortality** in kittens.

It causes **vomiting, diarrhoea, dehydration and leukopenia**, most frequently in kittens over six weeks of age. It usually affects entire litters, although it is not impossible for some kittens not to be affected if maternal immunity has been adequate. It can also cause sudden-acute death without the typical clinical signs.

Intrauterine infection can cause **cerebellar hypoplasia** (feline ataxia) with classic neurological signs that manifest themselves evidently after four or five weeks of age. This is a **non-progressive condition** and many cats can have a good quality of life.

Diagnosis is based on the **clinical presentation**, the presence of **leukopenia**, and the detection of **parvovirus antigen in faeces by ELISA**. The clinical presentation is similar to that of sepsis, bacterial enteritis and FeLV infection in some cases.

Treatment consists of intensive care, fluid therapy, broad-spectrum antibiotics, antiemetics, blood transfusion, and plasma administration. Mortality in untreated kittens is high, being a common cause of mortality in cat colonies.

Upper respiratory tract infection (herpesvirus and calicivirus)

URTI can cause disease from two weeks of age.

Clinical signs include inactivity, crying, anorexia, weight loss, hypothermia or hyperthermia, sneezing, discharges, oral and corneal ulcers, and conjunctivitis. It is common for the infection to be a mixture of the two viruses and complicated **with secondary bacterial infections**. Neonatal kittens around **two weeks of age can develop severe respiratory infections** and, apart from the typical upper airway signs, manifest severe dyspnoea due to bronchopneumonia that can be viral and/or bacterial.

From six weeks of age the respiratory symptoms are usually less intense. Some FCV-infected kittens may manifest fever and joint pain without presenting the typical respiratory or oral signs.

Treatment consists of supportive measures such as fluid therapy, forced nutrition and antibiotics to treat or prevent secondary bacterial infections (doxycycline, azithromycin or amoxicillin-clavulanic). Topical ocular treatment is important through antibiotics and antivirals.

Bacterial infection/sepsis

This is the most frequent cause of death in kittens from one to six weeks of age. The bacteria usually come from the normal skin and intestinal flora of the mother and the environment.

The clinical signs range from sudden death to clinical signs which can take hours or a few days to develop. Inactivity, weakness, vocalization, inadequate suckling, hypothermia (this is more frequent than fever), gastrointestinal stasis and abdominal distension, presence of subcutaneous or umbilical abscesses and dyspnoea (bronchopneumonia) can be observed. It can affect whole litters causing sickness and death in hours to days. Sometimes clinical signs appear very quickly in kittens that seemed healthy a few hours earlier. The **causes of bacterial sepsis are diverse**: lack of colostrum, poor nutrition, environmental stress and other concurrent diseases that predispose to infection.

In most cases there are no external signs of infection, so the diagnosis is not obvious. The most typical analytical abnormalities are leukocytosis or leukopenia with a left shift and toxicity and hypoglycaemia. Urine, blood or exudate cultures confirm diagnosis, but **antibiotic treatment should be initiated at the slightest suspicion of bacterial infection**, although the results are not yet available. Post-mortem of the kittens that die is of great importance for diagnosis and helps avoid other deaths in the litter.

Treatment consists of fluid therapy and vital support (intravenous, intraosseous, subcutaneous or intraperitoneal access), antibiotics (amoxicillin-clavulanic acid, enrofloxacin plus ampicillin) and nutritional support (forced enteral nutrition or nasogastric tube). In case of a death by sepsis in the litter it is important to treat the rest of the litter with antibiotics, even if they do not show signs of disease.

Parasitism

Intestinal parasites (ascaris, coccidia, Giardia)

Intestinal parasites can be the cause of problems after four weeks of age.

The most frequent signs are diarrhoea, weight loss and bloating. Severe coccidial infestations can occur with dehydration and cachexia. Ascaris infestations are very frequent and cause weight loss, diarrhoea and even intestinal obstruction in kittens of eight weeks of age and older.

Diagnosis is based on faecal analysis and/or response to treatment. All kittens should be **dewormed regularly and routinely** against ascarid parasites.

Fleas

Serious infestations in kittens from two to eight weeks can cause severe anemia. Diagnosis is obvious, although other problems (intestinal parasites, FeLV infection, hyperlipidaemia) should be ruled out. Treatment consists in the use of **insecticides which are safe in kittens** (for example fipronil or imidacloprid).

Vector borne diseases

There are **numerous vector-borne** infections in cats. Some are of great importance and relatively common in some geographical locations, whilst others are less common than in the dog, less well understood, and show different clinical signs to the canine equivalent.

The prevalence of disease and its distribution depends on **geographical area and the cat's lifestyle** (e.g. urban and indoor cats are unlikely to contact ticks if they never leave the homes.) Where specific feline prevalence studies have been done, these indicate that prevalence has been underestimated and may be significantly greater than previously thought.

This section covers the main vector-borne diseases in **Europe**.

Feline leishmaniasis

Aetiopathogenesis

Leishmaniasis is a vector-borne disease transmitted by *Phlebotomus* and caused (in Europe) by *Leishmania infantum*. In respective endemic areas cats become infected with the same *Leishmania* species as dogs and humans: *L. infantum* in the Mediterranean basin (also in Iran and Brazil), *L. mexicana* (Texas, United States), *L. braziliensis* and *L. amazonensis* (Brazil) and *L. venezuelensis* (Venezuela).

Cats are more resistant to infection than dogs, as shown in experimental studies and epidemiological data. The immune response against infection is probably more effective than in most dogs, with a Th1. type cellular response.

In those cats where disease develops the **pathogenesis is similar to in dogs**: mainly a persistent intracellular infection of macrophages in some tissues that produces an **inflammatory granulomatous reaction** and, in some cats (and to a lesser extent compared to dogs) a **non-protective humoral response** which involves a **type III hypersensitivity** reaction in target organs, such as the glomerulus, uvea and synovial membrane.

Epidemiology

The life cycle and transmission of *Leishmania* is the same as in dogs, although there are fewer specific feline studies. ***Phlebotomus* females bite the cat and transmit flagellated promastigotes.** No other transmission routes are documented in cats, although blood transfusion has the potential to do so and therefore donor cats should be tested in endemic regions.

Several epidemiological studies in cats have shown that disease **prevalence is high in endemic areas.** The results vary significantly according to geographical area, cat population or whether DNA or antibodies were detected, in a global range of 0 to 60%. In most studies the **prevalence of antibodies was 15 to 25%** and the presence of DNA was around 5 to 10%. These results underscore not only that the infection rate in cats is important, but also they can act as **potential secondary reservoirs** in endemic areas. However, the efficacy of sand-flies in ingesting amastigotes after biting an infected cat is unknown.

Clinical signs

The clinical signs in cats show significant differences compared to the dog. The most common clinical problem is **skin lesions** mainly in the form of **nodules and/or ulcers** (on the head and neck more frequently than on the trunk and extremities).

Local or generalized lymphadenopathy is common, but not always present. Diffuse **exfoliative seborrhoeic dermatitis is less frequent** in cats than in dogs (Figures 38 and 39).

The **second most frequent manifestation is ocular disease.** Granulomatous lesions with parasites present have been documented in **all layers of the eye**: nodular blepharitis and conjunctivitis, ulcerative keratitis, uveitis and panophthalmitis. Lesions on the eyelids and conjunctiva have sometimes been described as pseudotumoural, due to the nodular and proliferative appearance and considerable size (Figures 40 and 41).

Visceral involvement and associated systemic signs were observed in 30–50% of cats, including:

- non-specific signs: anorexia, weight loss, lethargy
- haematological abnormalities: anemia, pancytopoenia, polyclonal gammopathy
- splenomegaly
- renal involvement: polyuria/polydipsia, proteinuria, chronic kidney disease
- liver involvement: hepatomegaly, jaundice, increased liver enzymes

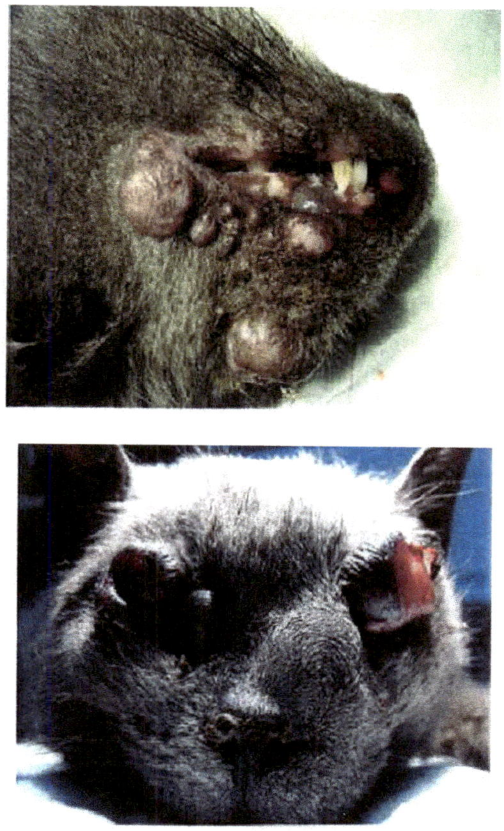

Figure 38. Cutaneous nodules due to leishmaniasis.

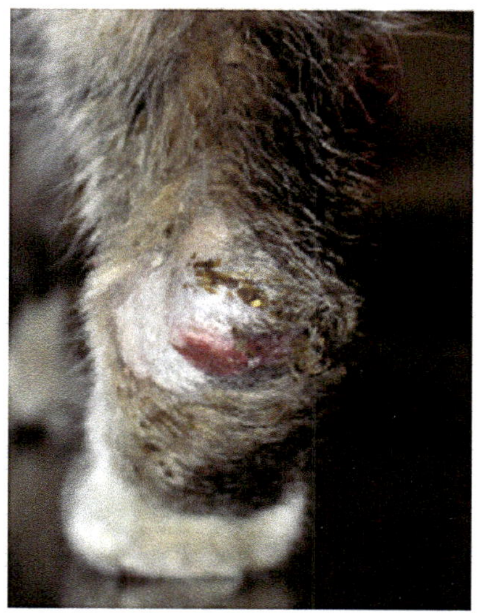

Figure 39. Pressure point sores due to leishmaniasis.

- respiratory problems: chronic nasal discharge and dyspnoea.

It is interesting to note that inflammatory granulomatous stomatitis with the presence of *Leishmania* has been observed in some cats with chronic proliferative-ulcerative gingivostomatitis (Figure 42).

Leishmaniasis is over-represented in cats suffering from concurrent disease, especially those associated

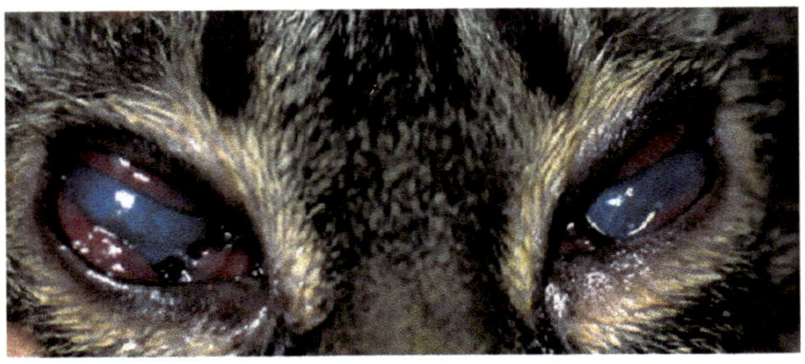

Figure 40. Bilateral uveitis and keratitis due to leishmaniasis.

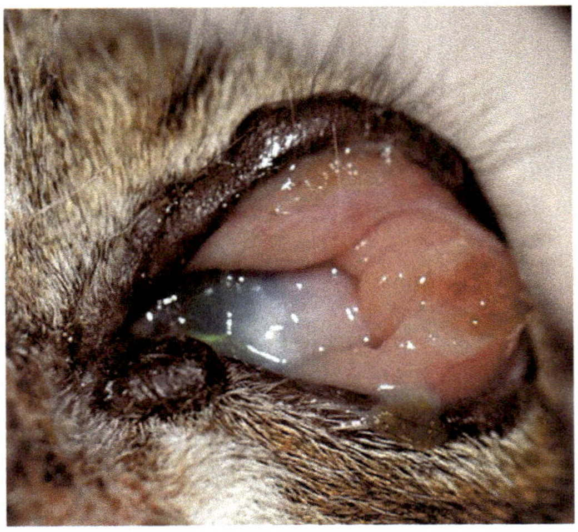

Figure 41. Uveitis and proliferative conjunctivitis due to leishmaniasis.

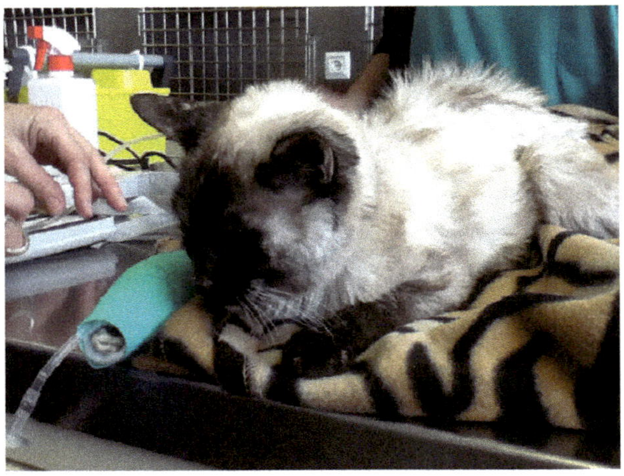

Figure 42. Cat with stage IV renal proteinuria, which is FIV positive and was diagnosed with leishmaniasis.

with immunosuppression such as retroviral infections, cancer or treatment with corticosteroids and/or immunosuppressive drugs. In these cats, immunosuppression could be responsible for a subclinical infection becoming clinical and the prognosis is poor or reserved. However, this is not always the case since leishmaniosis has also been diagnosed in immunocompetent cats that respond well to treatment. Immunosuppressed cats can also respond well to treatment as long as the existing immune disorder is reversible (for example, corticosteroids).

Diagnosis

In most cats the diagnosis is initially suspected by **cytological or histological visualization** of parasites from the skin and/or nodular or ulcerative eye lesions after cytology. The presence of the parasite in these samples is commonly subsequently confirmed by **immunohistochemistry and/or PCR techniques** (Figure 43).

Serology (IFA, ELISA, DAT or WBA) is also useful for diagnosis, since cats with clinical signs may have **high titres of anti-Leishmania antibodies** along with **hypergammaglobulinaemia**. When serum samples are sent to commercial laboratories for serology it is best to check they can perform the test on feline samples. The Th2 humoral immune response may not be as marked as in dogs. However, as with dogs, a **positive titre on its own is not a diagnosis of active disease** and should be interpreted according to the clinical context. A cat suffering from leishmaniasis may have low or medium positive antibody levels or even be negative. Indeed, in cats there is no clear association between high antibody titres and the presence of clinical signs or lesions, as occurs in the dog.

Since many cats with leishmaniasis have **nodular lesions from which samples are obtained for cytology or biopsy**, usually serology or bone marrow aspiration is subsequently performed to confirm any systemic involvement. However, in cats with uveitis, chronic stomatitis and proteinuric renal disease, without lesions to aspirate or biopsy, serology should be performed initially, especially if other diagnostic tests for more common diseases are negative. If **antibody titres are positive**, the diagnosis must be confirmed by detection of the parasite, either in the bone marrow, by lymph node cytology or by PCR. Blood PCR has been positive in sick cats, but to a lesser extent than on bone marrow or lymph node tests. Blood PCR can also be positive in infected cats that are not ill, as is the case in dogs.

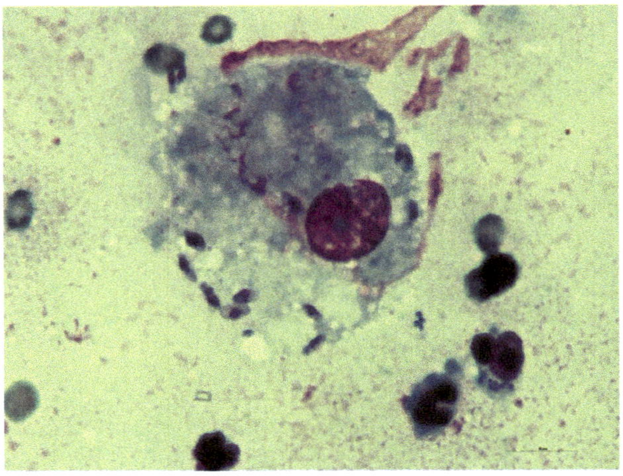

Figure 43. Leishmania amastigotes on cytology of fine needle aspirate of a nodular lesion in a cat.

There is a greater discrepancy between serological and PCR results in the cat compared to the dog.

Retrovirus tests should be performed in suspected or confirmed cases of leishmaniasis in cats.

Treatment

There are no prospective studies of large numbers of cats, so the information on the treatment of feline leishmaniasis and its prognosis are based on clinical cases or retrospective studies of a small number of patients.

The most frequent treatment is with **allopurinol for several months (10 to 20 mg/kg PO every 12–24 h)**. In some cats an excellent response is observed, especially in cats where the immune response is not compromised. Some cats do not relapse once the treatment is withdrawn, although others do. Therefore, allopurinol can be considered the first line of treatment in cats with skin or eye lesions without or with minor systemic involvement. Recently, combined treatment with allopurinol and domperidone has also been documented as stimulating the cellular immune response.

Meglumine antimonate (5 to 50 mg/kg or 375 mg/cat every 24 h SC) has also been used successfully in some cats, but the lack of specific studies on its safety in this species suggests that it should be reserved for patients with serious systemic disease and/or those that are immunosuppressed. The dose of meglumine should be reduced in cats with renal insufficiency to avoid the accumulation of antimonate and intolerance.

There are no clinical data on the use of miltefosine in cats, but some veterinarians have started using it. Surgery has also been used in some cats to remove nodular lesions, but **surgery itself is not curative** and cats should receive systemic treatment afterwards. These recommendations are empirical and based on the results of the few monitored cases that have been published. Because of the lack of specific studies, the prognosis is not sufficiently documented.

Prognosis

From clinical experience and published cases, the prognosis is considered good in cats with external skin and eye lesions without concurrent immunosuppression. Even in these cats, future relapses and/or kidney disease can occur if the parasite has not been completely erradicated. Some cats with skin lesions have survived for long periods without treatment, but the lesions persisted and some of them died of kidney disease.

On the other hand, the prognosis in cats with kidney disease and/or retroviral infection or other causes of severe immunosuppression is poor and most die shortly after being diagnosed.

Prevention

Vaccines available in some countries are only registered for use in dogs. Topical preventive products used in dogs contain pyrethroids that are toxic to cats, so they cannot be used.

A **flumethrin collar** against fleas and ticks registered for cats has shown repellent activity against sand-flies in dogs and recently a study has been published that demonstrates its repellent efficacy against *Phlebotomus*.

Feline anaplasmosis

Feline anaplasmosis is a poorly documented disease, although in recent years cases have been described and some cats infected experimentally.

Disease is caused by ***Anaplasma phagocytophilum* and transmitted by *Ixodes* spp. ticks**, and in geographical areas where this genus of ticks exists cats may become infected. There are epidemiological studies in various European countries and the United States in which antibodies or *Anaplasma* DNA were detected in feline blood. The pathogenesis of the disease is not completely understood.

The most frequent clinical signs are **fever, anorexia, and acute apathy**. In some cases, joint and abdominal pain have been observed. It is not known whether anaplasmosis may be associated with chronic or recurrent signs. Clinical-pathological abnormalities observed are **thrombocytopoenia, lymphopoenia and mild anemia**.

The method of choice for diagnosis is by **detecting blood DNA with PCR techniques**. Antibody detection is also useful, but there are false negatives due to cats developing clinical signs before seroconversion, so **a negative antibody result does not rule out infection**. The Snap 4Dx rapid diagnostic kit for dogs has proven useful for the detection of antibodies against *Anaplasma* in cats. The detection of **morulae in neutrophils** in blood smears is highly specific and diagnostic of the disease, but the sensitivity is low, and the likelihood of seeing them is low. To increase the sensitivity, performing **blood smears from the buffy coat** with microhaematocrit capillaries is preferable.

The treatment of choice is **doxycycline (10 mg/kg/24 h PO for 3–4 weeks)** and the clinical response is fast: clinical signs usually remiss within a few days. It is not known if the treatment completely eradicates the infection or if some cats remain subclinical carriers.

Prevention is based on the application of effective **preventive products against ticks**. There is currently a great variety (collars, pipettes, aerosols, tablets) that adapt to any circumstance.

Feline ehrlichiosis

Feline ehrlichiosis is a **poorly documented disease**, although cases have been described and cats have been infected experimentally. There are also epidemiological studies in which antibodies and DNA from the bacteria have been detected in the blood of cats. *Ehrlichia* morulae have been observed in lymphocytes and monocytes of cats with **fever and lameness** in various countries. In cats the infection is caused by *E. canis*, but another species has been detected (*Ehrlichia canis-like*) that is different from that which infects the dog. Both are transmitted by the **tick *Rhipicephalus sanguineus*** and in all those areas where ehrlichiosis is present in dogs the condition can be diagnosed in cats.

The clinical signs of feline ehrlichiosis are **fever, malaise and joint pain**. In some cases, **splenomegaly** and generalized pain have also been observed. The clinical-pathological abnormalities which have been seen include thrombocytopenia, anemia, pancytopenia and polyclonal gammopathy in chronic cases.

The diagnosis of choice is by **PCR techniques**, since serological tests for the detection of antibodies may not be specific to the species that causes infection in cats. The observation of morulae in monocytes or lymphocytes is diagnostic of the disease, but it is not very sensitive since in most cases they are not seen (Figure 44).

The treatment of choice is **doxycycline (10 mg/kg/24 h PO for 3–4 weeks**) and the clinical response is fast: clinical signs usually remiss within a few days. It is not known if the treatment fully eliminates the infection and, therefore, if some cats remain as subclinical carriers. **Imidocarb dipropionate** has also been used in some patients (5 mg/kg SC, 2 separate doses 14 days apart).

Zoonotic diseases of feline origin

A zoonotic disease is an infectious or parasitic disease that is transferred from animals to people (or vice versa), either **directly or indirectly** through contaminated environments. There are numerous zoonotic disease, some serious and some minor.

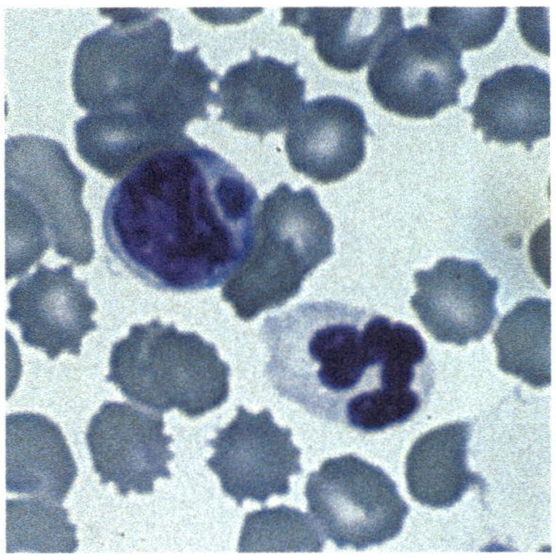

Figure 44. Ehrlichia morula in a monocyte. (Photo courtesy of: Josep Pastor).

This chapter is not intended as an exhaustive compilation of all feline zoonotic diseases, but as a guide to the most important conditions and the advice given to cat owners to avoid infection.

Rabies

Aetiopathogenesis

Rabies is a viral disease, caused by infection with **Lyssavirus**, one of the few viruses that is not species specific.

The bat is the definitive host, which can also be an asymptomatic carrier. All other animals, including humans, suffer from **progressive viral encephalitis** that is fatal once clinical signs develop.

Humans can be **infected through animal bites**, including dogs and cats suffering from signs of the disease, one of which is aggression. Infection is also spread by contact of open wounds with saliva or nerve tissue from affected animals.

People bitten by a dog or cat suspected of having rabies should be treated quickly with prophylactic fluids that prevent the infection from progressing to disease.

Prevention

In endemic areas, prevention of infection in people is based on vaccination of wild animals (bats) and the **mandatory vaccination of domestic pets such as dogs, cats, and ferrets**.

In **rabies-free countries**, the health authorities' guidelines must be followed, and in some cases vaccination is mandatory. Travelling pets must be vaccinated to cross borders and authorities, especially in rabies-free countries, and the entry of unvaccinated animals or those during the incubation period prohibited.

For a few years, to travel to the United Kingdom (as part of the Pet Travel Scheme) and Scandinavian countries, measurement of antibody levels (>0.5 IU/ml) in official laboratories was obligatory, but currently this is no longer necessary.

Veterinarians who suspect an animal may have rabies should notify official health authorities.

Toxocariasis (visceral larval migrans)

Aetiopathogenesis

Nematode parasites or roundworms ***Toxocara canis* (dog) and *Toxocara cati*** (cat) are commonly present in the gastrointestinal tract, especially in puppies.

Humans are accidentally infected by contact with environments contaminated with eggs of these parasites excreted in faeces, which can persist in the environment for weeks to months. Most people who become infected do not develop disease, but in some cases, they can suffer serious consequences due to **erratic migration of larvae in viscera, the eyes, or central nervous system**.

Toxoplasmosis

Aetiopathogenesis

Toxoplasmosis is an infection caused by the *Toxoplasma gondii* protozoan and **cats are the only definitive hosts**. Cats are the only animal in which the parasite can infest the intestine, undergo sexual reproduction and, after a series of changes and transformations, be excreted in the faeces in the form of non-sporulated oocysts. After between one and five days of contact with the air, the non-sporulated oocysts change and **sporulate into infective forms with environmental resistance which lasts for months or years. These sporulated oocysts are the forms that indirectly infect the intermediate hosts** (food production animals or humans) and once the infection and the asexual cycle (tachyzoites) of the parasite have been completed (Figure 45), may become dormant in muscles or CNS as tissue cysts with bradyzoites (forms of low pathogenicity) in a totally subclinical manner.

The most frequent routes of infection in people are:

- The **ingestion of raw meat** carrying tissue cysts
- The consumption of **water or food contaminated** with sporulated oocysts
- Contact with **soil and earth contaminated** with sporulated oocysts (gardening, agriculture).

Infection in humans (and cats) is generally subclinical and of low pathogenicity, however, it can have serious consequences in the first third of pregnancy (abortions or malformations) or in immunosuppressed people (systemic infections with risk of death).

Direct infection with the cat's own faeces is difficult since, normally, the faeces are not handled, and this is even less likely after 24 hours or more. On the other hand, intestinal infection in cats usually occurs once in a lifetime during which they excrete oocysts for a period of 7 to 15 days, and this does not happen again, even if they become infected again. The percentage of people seropositive to antibodies against *T. gondii* is not significantly different between those who have direct contact with cats and those who do not. This fact reinforces the concept that **direct contact with cats is not a frequent or important form of transmission**.

Clinical signs in cats

In general, infected or carrier cats do not become ill, however, some **cases do manifest clinical signs**. Toxoplasmosis in cats can occur with an **acute and severe course** of disease with clinical signs or a more **chronic and insidious** course.

The acute form usually occurs in immunosuppressed cats which produces systemic toxoplasmosis. This form is diagnosed in FIV-positive cats that are in a severely immunodeficient state. Toxoplasma tachyzoites actively replicate and produce necrotic and **inflammatory lesions in various organs**, mainly the lungs (cough, respiratory distress, pleural effusion), heart (arrhythmias, pericardial effusion), liver (jaundice, elevation of liver enzymes) and the central nervous system (CNS, signs of multifocal disease). In these cases, tachyzoites can be observed on cytology of the different organs and even circulating in peripheral blood (Figure 46).

Chronic conditions occur in cats with a normal immune system. They are characterized by persistent or recurrent fever, hyperesthesia and muscle pain, neurological signs and uveitis. This form is associated with the presence of **cystic bradyzoites in muscle or**

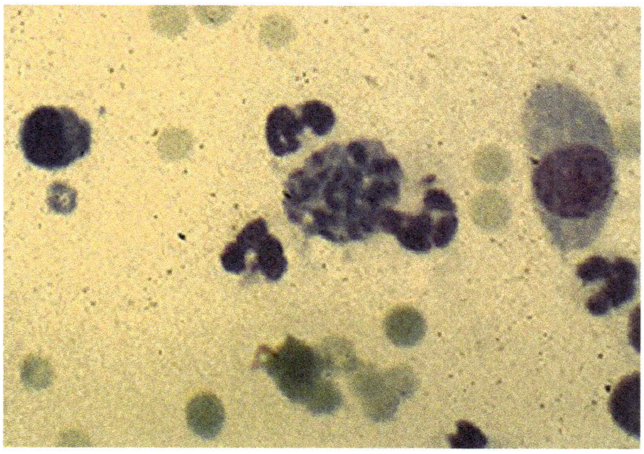

Figure 45. Tachyzoites on cytology of a bronchoalveolar lavage performed on a cat with interstitial pneumonia.

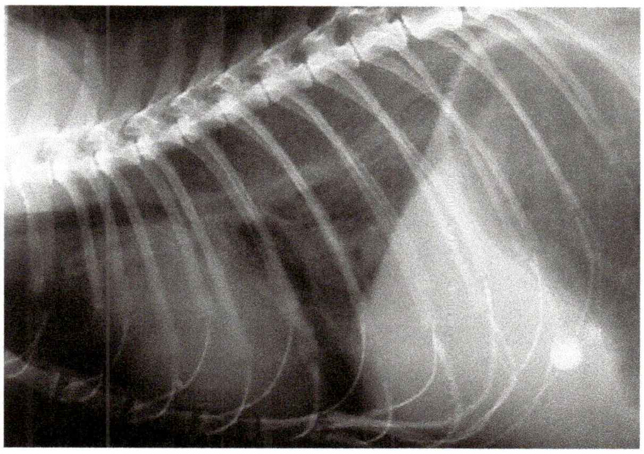

Figure 46. Lateral radiograph of a patient with interstitial pneumonia.

CNS and the inflammatory or immune-mediated reaction that occurs in response. Diagnosis of this form is difficult, since it is based on the detection of elevated antibodies (IgM), the exclusion of other diseases and the response to treatment.

Diagnosis

Diagnosis is based on the **detection of tachyzoites on cytology** or biopsy of the affected organs (muscle, respiratory secretions, cerebrospinal fluid, liver aspirations or lymph nodes). Their presence is diagnostic of toxoplasmosis, but this only occurs in acute systemic toxoplasmosis.

The **PCR for the detection of *Toxoplasma* DNA** is a more sensitive alternative to the observation of tachyzoites, especially in samples where there may be little cellularity such as cerebrospinal fluid, respiratory cytology or aqueous humour.

Therefore, in many cats the diagnosis is based on **serological tests to detect antibody titres** or levels. However, many cats are subclinical carriers of *Toxoplasma* so they have elevated positive levels of IgG against the parasite. A positive IgG result does not confirm the diagnosis. Joint interpretation of IgG and IgM, which are immunoglobulins found with active infection, is preferable. **High levels of IgM suggest a diagnosis of toxoplasmosis**. Even so, there is some overlap and numerous healthy cats that can have positive IgM titres. Therefore, **repeating the titres after a few weeks** is preferable to demonstrate that there is seroconversion or elevation of the titres.

In many cats, especially in the chronic forms, the diagnosis is based on the presence of compatible clinical signs, ruling out other diseases, high IgM titres and a favourable response to treatment.

The detection of oocysts in faeces by flotation is diagnostic that the cat is suffering from the parasite's intestinal cycle, but it is not indicative that the cat is ill with toxoplasmosis. However, the detection of oocysts in a domestic cat's faeces indicates taking preventive measures to avoid infection of the people who live with it, since this is the only moment in which the cat could transmit the parasite to the people in contact with its faeces.

Treatment

The treatment of choice for toxoplasmosis in a cat is **clindamycin, 10 to 12 mg/kg every 12 hours for one month**. The response is usually quick within two to three days and good in cats with fever and muscle pain. Cats with severe systemic conditions (pulmonary, hepatic) may take longer to improve or may not improve, especially if they are severely or irreversibly immunosuppressed. Ocular and/or CNS signs may also take longer to improve. In cases of uveitis, adding topical and systemic corticosteroids to rapidly reduce inflammation and prevent secondary glaucoma and lens dislocation is indicated.

Other drugs that may be effective in the treatment are sulphonamides enhanced with trimethoprim (15 mg/kg PO every 12 hours for 1 month), but most cats do not tolerate sulphonamides by mouth.

Drugs from the triazine family (ponazuril, toltrazuril) have a good anticoccidial action and could be effective in the management of toxoplasma infections. However, there are currently no clinical studies that have proven their effectiveness.

Prevention

The most effective measures to prevent toxoplasmosis in people are:

- Avoid eating raw or undercooked meat
- Wear gloves for gardening and agriculture
- Wash vegetables well
- Remove faeces from litter boxes daily avoiding contact
- Wash hands after coming into contact with earth or meat, or after removing faeces from litter boxes.

The most effective measures to prevent toxoplasmosis in cats are:

- Restrict them to indoors
- Ensure they do not have the chance to hunt and ingest prey
- Do not feed them raw meat.

Bartonellosis

Aetiopathogenesis

Bartonella henselae infection is the main cause of bartonellosis or **cat scratch disease** in humans. Cats can be subclinical carriers of this intraerythrocytic bacteria in the blood (bacteraemia), rarely showing signs of disease or bartonellosis. The route of transmission between cats is through the ingestion of fleas and/or their faeces.

The **spread from cats to people occurs through close direct contact**, playing or sleeping with the cat in bed, by scratches or licking. The transmission of the bacteria to people is associated with the contact with faeces from the bacteria-carrying fleas with erosions or wounds on the skin or mucous membranes. There is not always a history of cat scratches in every human patient with bartonellosis.

Bartonellosis in humans is a generally subclinical infection, but it can sometimes cause **fever and lymphadenitis** in immunocompetent people (cat scratch disease) that heal spontaneously or with antibiotics. However, in immunosuppressed people (AIDS patients, chronic patients, immunosuppressive treatments) it can cause a severe form with fever, endocarditis, sepsis, neuroretinitis, peliosis and bacillary angiomatosis, which can even be fatal in patients with AIDS.

Epidemiology

The prevalence of antibodies in domestic cats is relatively high, especially in the young.

The prevalence of DNA in cat blood samples is generally low, although blood PCR techniques have sensitivity problems.

Clinical signs in cats

Cats infected with Bartonella do not usually present clinical signs, it is mainly a subclinical infection. In experimental infections has been shown to **cause fever, mild anemia and granulomatous lymphadenitis**. There are few well-documented cases of bartonellosis in cats.

Bartonella infection has been associated with numerous chronic inflammatory diseases (gingivostomatitis, rhinosinusitis, cystitis) in cats, but when comparing the prevalence in these cats and in healthy cats, it is the same and therefore the cause-effect relationship cannot be established. However, the presence of Bartonella has been confirmed in a few cases of aortic endocarditis, uveitis, recurrent fever and recurrent polyarthritis and osteomyelitis.

Diagnosis

Diagnosis of bartonellosis is difficult. A significant number of cats, especially under two years old, are or have been bacteraemic and are therefore seropositive. **Antibody titres or levels do not discriminate between previous or active infection**, so the positive predictive value of a positive result is low. However, a negative antibody result has a good predictive value to rule out infection and disease.

Confirmation of the diagnosis is based on the **detection of Bartonella by culture or PCR** or combinations of both. However, there are sensitivity problems with PCR techniques especially in blood. It is preferable to perform PCR on tissues where the presence of the bacteria may indicate that it is the cause of the lesion, for example, in lymph nodes, heart valves and other tissues, cerebrospinal fluid or aqueous humour.

In some laboratories a previous culture is combined with a specific medium plus detection and subsequent sequencing by PCR techniques.

Treatment

Different antibiotics have been used, **mainly doxycycline** (10 mg/kg/24 h PO), but also quinolones (marbofloxacin, enrofloxacin), macrolides (azithromycin) and even amoxicillin-clavulanic acid. Treatments should be long, from six to eight weeks, although there are few well-documented cases in order to give an exact recommendation. As in other species with bartonellosis, it may be better to combine two antibiotics, for example, amoxicillin-clavulanic acid with azithromycin. Some antibiotics could promote the emergence of resistance and it is preferable not to use them as a first choice, azithromycin is probably one of them. Doxycycline is still a good option as a first line treatment, although there is currently some evidence that pradofloxacin (7.5 mg/kg PO every 24 hours) could be more effective and not promote resistance as easily as other antibiotics.

Prevention

The prevention of bartonellosis in cats is based on **the use of effective ectoparasitic** treatments against fleas.

Prevention in people is based on:

- Washing hands after being in contact with cats
- Avoiding aggressive play with cats
- Avoiding close contact (licking, sleeping) with cats, especially in the case of older people or those with immunodeficiencies.

Vaccines and vaccination programmes

Vaccine use in both people and animals has reduced the prevalence of numerous significant infectious diseases and zoonoses, and should be **considered a success story**. However, the emergence of people and movements opposed to vaccination has caused reduced uptake in some places. Opposition to vaccination is a complex topic, with one of the main objections being the risk of adverse effects.

With this in mind, in the past two decades **expert panels** in the United States and Europe, have **developed protocols and guidelines for the vaccination of dogs and cats**. These recommendations are based on the **best available scientific evidence**, without economic pressure from the companies that manufacture and sell vaccines. Thus, veterinarians can offer **independent advice regarding the best vaccination plan for an individual patient** based on environmental challenges and the risk factors for each animal. Whilst there are small differences in criteria between the different panels, this should not be seen as a weakness. There are many aspects of vaccination and the prevention of infectious disease where more knowledge is needed, and the conclusions are those drawn by experts from existing information so discrepancies may well arise.

The general objective (and recommendations) is to **vaccinate as many cats as possible against those diseases for which protection is considered essential.**

One important concept is that of population or **herd immunity**.There are epidemiological studies in human medicine that show where more than **70% of the population are vaccinated** and have good immunity, then the prevalence of that infectious disease decreases and over time it may even be eradicated. (Figure 47).

With robust population or herd immunity, immunised individuals block infection with the consequent reduction in clinical (and subclinical) cases that excrete the pathogen and a decreased possibility of infecting other individuals. Consequently **pathogen circulation may be reduced to the point that even the unvaccinated percentage is protected.**

Unfortunately, **in cats and dogs the average percentage that are vaccinated is around 30–50% and a long way from the desirable 70–80%.** This is a key reason why diseases such as distemper or parvovirus remain prevalent, despite an effective vaccine. Also, as the percentage of vaccinated individuals decreases (vaccine antagonism), the burden of circulating pathogens is potentially higher and the prevalence of infection and disease increases.

In recent years, an important development is the classification of vaccines as those that are **essential (core)** and **non-essential (non-core)** or even not recommended. From the point of view of the vaccine manufacturers all vaccines are necessary, but from the clinicians, owners, and patients' perspective this is debatable. For example, some cats will not encounter certain pathogens due to the lack of prevalence in their region or the animal's lifestyle. In that case the vaccine is considered non-core and advice given as to situations when it may become necessary. Also, there are vaccines whose efficacy is doubtful for the general population and should only be recommended under specific circumstances.

Core vaccines are those whose administration is recommended in all cats whatever their lifestyle and living conditions. They are mainly vaccines against **viral diseases** in which the resulting immunity is good, even sterilizing, and against viruses with a high prevalence and/or environmental resistance, so prevalence is high. The **zoonotic potential of a pathogen** is also important in determining whether a vaccine should be core or even mandatory.

The only vaccine that may be **mandatory** by the authorities of a country or an area is the **rabies vaccine.** In rabies endemic areas it is essential that dogs, cats and ferrets are well immunised, since in most cases it is these species that spread rabies to the people they live with.

Non-core vaccines are those that are recommended depending on the cat's lifestyle or living conditions, and are mainly vaccines against **bacterial diseases.**

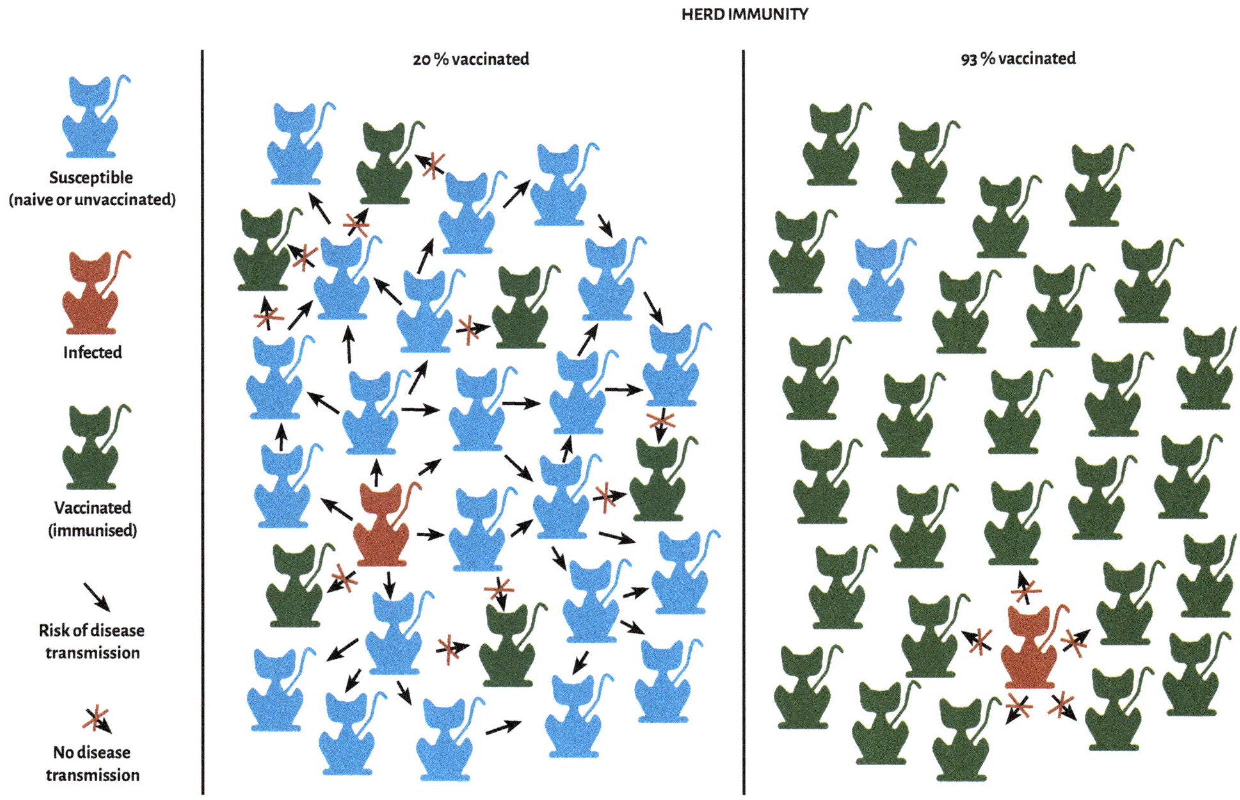

Figure 47. Mechanism of group or herd immunity.

Types of vaccine

There are **different types of vaccines** depending on how the pathogen or antigen is formulated.

Attenuated vaccines

The most frequently used vaccines are **attenuated vaccines**. In these the **pathogen is alive** and produces a subclinical infection in the animal so that it develops an immune and memory response. The pathogens have been attenuated in their virulence or pathogenicity in the laboratory by different techniques. They are safe vaccines when used correctly and, in general, are preferred since they **produce rapid immunity which simulates natural infection.**

Inactivated vaccines

Inactivated vaccines use antigens or **parts of the pathogen** that are not capable of producing subclinical infection, therefore, they are **less immunogenic**. Hence, they must be **accompanied by immunogenic substances** and cause inflammation so that the cells reach the injection site and then recognize the antigen. They are safe vaccines that produce good immunity, although the duration of immunity may be shorter and adjuvants can produce local inflammatory reactions that, in rare cases, evolve into sarcomas, especially in cats.

Recombinant vaccines

In recent years, **recombinant vaccines** have appeared in which viral vectors (non-pathogenic viruses in the vaccinated species) to which a pathogen antigen against which an immune response is desired has been added. They are safe vaccines and **do not require the use of adjuvants**.

Vaccination programmes

Traditional vaccination protocols are usually based on a primary vaccination with two doses (two and three months of age), a revaccination after a year, and annual booster doses throughout life.

The current recommendations propose the following changes to this classic programme:

1. **Primary vaccination**: Administer three (or up to four) doses of the core vaccines in dogs and cats (at two, three, and four months, even a first one at six weeks). This recommendation is based on the results of studies which demonstrate the presence of high levels of maternal immunity up to 12 or more weeks may interfere with the immune response to the vaccine. Consequently, some dogs or cats are not properly immunised after the traditional last dose at 12 weeks.
2. **Revaccination**. Administer when the dog or cat is **one year old**. This recommendation is even being modified to revaccination at six months of age instead of waiting until 12 months. There are no scientific studies on this fact, but it may be better to advance revaccination to give greater immunity to dogs or cats at ages when they are still susceptible to being infected.
3. **Adult vaccinations**. Administer booster doses of core vaccines every three years. This recommendation is based on studies of duration of immunity that demonstrate that for essential vaccines, if the primary vaccination of dogs and cats is correct, it lasts many years (up to seven), but it is preferable to establish a safety margin (three years). This does not include non-core vaccines, of which it is not known whether the duration of immunity lasts more than one year. This recommendation is subject to variation depending on the living conditions and the prevalence or environmental burden of infections or in the case of viruses with frequent genetic modifications (for example, feline calicivirus). In these cases, it is preferable to maintain annual revaccination.

Therefore, the number of vaccinations is increased at the age or stage when cats are most susceptible to infections and decreases at the stage when there is good memory immunity if primary vaccination has been performed correctly (core vaccines). These changes do not affect the herd or population immunity, since these animals are correctly immunised. The real problem is the low percentage of cats that receive a correct vaccination schedule.

Adverse effects

In general, vaccines have few adverse effects. The most frequent are the following:

- **Immediate type I hypersensitivity** reactions with angioedema, hives, vomiting and, very rarely, systemic signs of anaphylaxis or shock.
- Association with **immune mediated or autoimmune diseases** (anemia or thrombocytopenia), although their cause effect relationship has not been demonstrated.
- **Local reactions** with inflammation and pain in the area of application and vasculitis or ischaemia that produces focal or multifocal alopecia.
- **Systemic signs of the disease** which has been vaccinated against (rare, although it may occur by accidental inhalation of the attenuated vaccine during preparation).

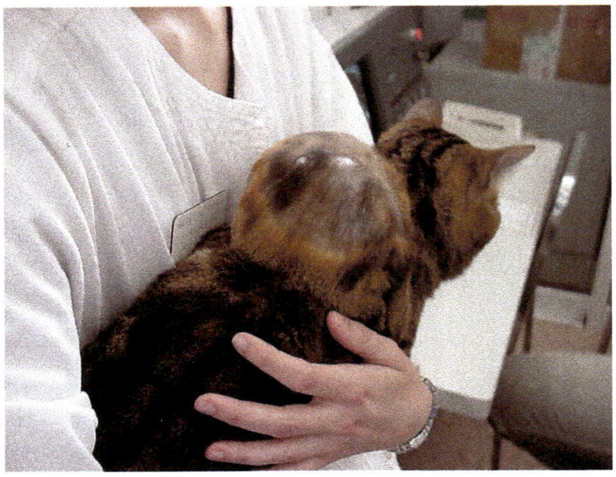

Figure 48. Large sized injection-site associated sarcoma.

- **Vaccine failures** due to poor vaccine preservation, insufficient immunisation or an inadequate vaccination programme.

Injection site sarcomas

A well-known adverse effect in cats is the development of injection-site sarcomas, whose first denomination was sarcomas associated with vaccines or post-vaccination. They appear in a small number of cats associated with chronic or persistent inflammation in places where vaccines were administered, but also other drugs or exogenous materials such as subcutaneous micro-chips.

Therefore, although vaccines are the major risk factor, it is not an adverse effect directly linked to the vaccine product but to a **malignant transformation of an inflammatory reaction in some predisposed cats.**

The type of vaccine most associated with this problem are inactivated vaccines with adjuvants, used to produce a greater inflammatory reaction. Changes in the guidelines (revaccinate every three years) and in the vaccine application sites in cats (avoid inter-scapular area, apply in distal areas of the extremities, lateral wall of the abdomen or tail) were implemented with the objective of reducing prevalence of these sarcomas (Figure 48).

Bibliography

Coronavirus and FIP infections

Addie D, Belák S, Boucraut-Baralon C, Egberink H, Frymus T, Gruffydd-Jones T, et al. *Feline infectious peritonitis: ABCD guidelines on prevention and management.* J Fel Med Surg 2009;11:594–604.

Chang HW, Egberink HF, Halpin R, Spiro DJ, Rottier PJ. *Spike protein fusion peptide and feline coronavirus virulence.* Emerg Infect Dis 2012;18(7):1089–95.

Crawford AH, Stoll AL, Sanchez-Masian D, et al. *Clinicopathologic Features and Magnetic Resonance Imaging Findings in 24 Cats With Histopathologically Confirmed Neurologic Feline Infectious Peritonitis.* J Vet Intern Med. 2017;31(5):1477–1486.

Doenges SJ, Weber K, Dorsch R, Fux R, Fischer A, Matiasek LA, et al. *Detection of feline coronavirus in cerebrospinal fluid for diagnosis of feline infectious peritonitis in cats with and without neurological signs.* J Feline Med Surg 2016;18(2):104–9.

Felten S, Weider K, Doenges S, Gruendl S, Matiasek K, Hermanns W, et al. *Detection of feline coronavirus spike gene mutations as a tool to diagnose feline infectious peritonitis.* J Feline Med Surg 2015. pii: 1098612X15623824.

Gunn-Moore DA, Gruffydd-Jones TJ, Harbour DA. *Detection of feline coronaviruses by culture and RT-PCR of blood samples from healthy cats and cats with clinical feline infectious peritonitis.* Vet Microbiol 1998;8:69–72.

Ishida T, Shibanai A, Tanaka S, Uchida K, Mochizuki MC. *Use of recombinant feline interferon and glucocorticoid in the treatment of feline infectious peritonitis.* J Fel Med Surg 2004;6:107–9.

Legendre AM, Bartges JW. *Effect of Polyprenyl Immunostimulant on the survival times of three cats with the dry form of feline infectious peritonitis.* J Feline Med Surg 2009;11(8):624–6.

Legendre AM, Kuritz T, Galyon G, et al. *Polyprenyl Immunostimulant Treatment of Cats with Presumptive Non-Effusive Feline Infectious Peritonitis In a Field Study.* Front Vet Sci. 2017;14;4:7.

Longstaff L, Porter E, Crossley VJ, Hayhow SE, Helps CR, Tasker S. *Feline coronavirus quantitative reverse transcriptase polymerase chain reaction on effusion samples in cats with and without feline infectious peritonitis.* J Feline Med Surg 2015. pii: 1098612X15606957.

Murphy BG, Perron M, Murakami E, et al. The nucleoside analog GS-441524 strongly inhibits feline infectious peritonitis (FIP) virus in tissue culture and experimental cat infection studies. Vet Microbiol 2018;219, 226–233.

Pedersen NC, Kim Y, Liu H, et al. *Efficacy of a 3C-like protease inhibitor in treating various forms of acquired feline infectious peritonitis.* J Feline Med Surg. 2018;20(4):378–392.

Pedersen NC. *An update on feline infectious peritonitis: diagnostics and therapeutics.* Vet J 2014; 201(2):133–41.

Pedersen NC. *An update on feline infectious peritonitis: virology and immunopathogenesis.* Vet J 2014;201(2):123–32.

Pedersen NC, Perron M, Bannasch M, et al. Efficacy and safety of the nucleoside analog GS-441524 for treatment of cats with naturally occurring feline infectious peritonitis. J Feline Med Surg 2019.

Porter E, Tasker S, Day MJ, Harley R, Kipar A, Siddell SG, et al. *Amino acid changes in the spike protein of feline coronavirus correlate with systemic spread of virus from the intestine and not with feline infectious peritonitis.* Vet Res 2014;45:49.

Riemer F, Kuehner KA, Ritz S, Sauter-Louis C, Hartmann K. *Clinical and laboratory features of cats with feline infectious peritonitis – a retrospective study of 231 confirmed cases (2000–2010).* J Feline Med Surg 2015. pii: 1098612X15586209.

Ritz S, Egberink H, Hartmann K. *Effect of feline interferon-omega on the survival time and quality of life of cats with feline infectious peritonitis.* J Vet Intern Med 2007;21(6):1193–7.

Tasker S. *Diagnosis of feline infectious peritonitis: Update on evidence supporting available tests.* J Feline Med Surg. 2018; 20(3):228–243.

Vennema H, Poland A, Foley J, Pedersen NC. *Feline infectious peritonitis arise by mutation from endemic feline enteric coronaviruses.* Virology 1998;243:150–57.

Retrovirus infections

Bęczkowski PM, Litster A, Lin TL, Mellor DJ, Willett BJ, Hosie MJ. *Contrasting clinical outcomes in two cohorts of cats naturally infected with feline immunodeficiency virus (FIV).* Vet Microbiol 2015;176(1–2):50–60.

Boesch A, Cattori V, Riond B, Willi B, Meli ML, Rentsch KM, et al. *Evaluation of the effect of short-term treatment with the integrase inhibitor raltegravir (Isentress) on the course of progressive feline leukemia virus infection.* Vet Microbiol 2015;175(2–4):167–78.

Crawford PC, Slater MR, Levy JK. *Accuracy of PCR assays for the diagnosis of feline immunodeficiency infection in cats.* J Am Vet Med Assoc 2005;226(9):1503–7.

De Mari K, Maynard L, Sanquer A, Lebreux B, Eun HM. *Therapeutic effects of recombinant feline interferon omega on feline leukemia virus infected cats and felv/fiv coinfected symptomatic cats.* J Vet Int Med 2004;18:477–82.

De Oliveira Medeiros S, Abreu CM, Delvecchio R, Ribeiro AP, Vasconcelos Z, De Moraes Brindeiro R, et al. *Follow-up on long-term antiretroviral therapy for cats infected with feline immunodeficiency virus.* J Feline Med Surg 2015. pii: 1098612X15580144.

Gil S, Leal RO, Mcgahie D, Sepúlveda N, Duarte A, Niza MM, et al. *Oral Recombinant Feline Interferon-Omega as an alternative immune modulation therapy in FIV positive cats: clinical and laboratory evaluation.* Res Vet Sci 2014;96(1):79–85.

Hartmann K. *Efficacy of antiviral chemotherapy for retrovirus-infected cats: What does the current literature tell us?* J Feline Med Surg 2015;17(11):925–39.

Helfer-Hungerbuehler AK, Spiri AM, Riond B, Grest P, Boretti FS, Hofmann-Lehmann R. *No benefit of therapeutic vaccination in clinically healthy cats persistently infected with feline leukemia virus.* Vaccine 2015;33(13):1578–85.

Hosie MJ, Addie D, Belák S, Boucraut-Baralon C, Egberink H, Frymus T, et al. *Feline inmunodeficiecy: ABCD guidelines on prevention and management.* J Fel Med Surg 2009;11:575–584.

Leal RO, Gil S. *The Use of Recombinant Feline Interferon Omega Therapy as an Immune-Modulator in Cats Naturally Infected with Feline Immunodeficiency Virus: New Perspectives.* Vet Sci. 2016; 27;3–4.

Levy JK, Crawford PC, Tucker SJ. *Performance of 4 Point-of-Care Screening Tests for Feline Leukemia Virus and Feline Immunodeficiency Virus.* J Vet Intern Med. 2017; 1(2):521–526.

Lutz H, Addie D, Belák S, Boucraut-Baralon C, Egberink H, Frymus T, et al. *Feline leukemia: ABCD guidelines on prevention and management.* J Fel Med Surg 2009;11:565–74.

Nesina S, Katrin Helfer-Hungerbuehler A, Riond B, Boretti FS, Willi B, Meli ML, et al. *Retroviral DNA–the silent winner: blood transfusion containing latent feline leukemia provirus causes infection and disease in naïve recipient cats.* Retrovirology 2015;12:105.

Pedretti E, Passeri B, Amadori M, Isola P, Di Pede P, Telera A, et al. *Low dose interferon alpha treatment for feline immunodeficiency virus infection.* Vet Immunol Immnupathol 2006;109:245–54.

Stuetzer B, Brunner K, Lutz H, Hartmann K. *A trial with 3'-azido-2',3'-dideoxythymidine and human interferon-α in cats naturally infected with feline leukaemia virus.* J Feline Med Surg 2013;15(8):667–71.

Torres AN, Mathiason CK, Hoover EA. *Re-examination of feline leukemia virus: host relationships using RT-PCR.* Virology 2005; 332:272–83.

Haemoplasmosis

Bergmann M, Englert T, Stuetzer B, et al. *Risk factors of different hemoplasma species infections in cats.* BMC Vet Res. 2017;16;13(1):52.

Novacco M, Sugiarto S, Willi B, et al. *Consecutive antibiotic treatment with doxycycline and marbofloxacin clears bacteremia in Mycoplasma haemofelis-infected cats.* Vet Microbiol. 2018;217:112–120.

Proksch Al, Unterer S, Speck S, Truyen U, Hartmann K. *Influence of clinical and laboratory variables on faecal antigen ELISA results in dogs with canine parvovirus infection.* Vet J. 2015;204(3):304–8.

Reynolds CA, Lappin MR. *"Candidatus Mycoplasma haemominutum" infections in 21 client-owned cats.* J Am Anim Hosp Assoc 2007;43:249–57.

Sykes JE. *Feline hemotropic mycoplasmas.* Vet Clin North Am Small Anim Pract 2010;40(6):1157–70.

Tasker S, Hofmann-Lehmann R, Belák S, et al. *Haemoplasmosis in cats: European guidelines from the ABCD on prevention and management.* J Feline Med Surg. 2018;20(3):256–26.

Tasker S, Peters IR, Papasouliotis K, Cue SM, Willi B, Hofmann-Lehmann R, et al. *Description of outcomes of experimental infection with feline hemoplasmas: copy numbers, haematology, Coombs' testing and blood glucose concentrations.* Vet Microbiol 2009;139:323–32.

Tasker S. *Haemotropic mycoplasmas: what's the real significance in cats?* J Fel Med Surg 2010;12:369–81.

Gastrointestinal infections

Arranz-Solís D, Pedraza-Díaz S, Miró G, et al. *Tritrichomonas foetus infection in cats with diarrhea from densely housed origins.* Vet Parasitol. 2016;15;221:118–22.

Ballweber LR, Xiao L, Bowman DD, Kahn G, Cama VA. *Giardiasis in dogs and cats: update on epidemiology and public health significance.* Trends Parasitol 2010;26:180–9.

Da Silva AS, Castro VS, Tonin AA, et al. *Secnidazole for the treatment of giardiasis in naturally infected cats.* Parasitol Int. 2011; 60(4):429–32.

De Santis-Kerr AC, Raghavan M, Glickman NW, Caldanaro RJ, Moore GE, Lewis HB, Schantz PM, et al. *Prevalence and risk factors for Giardia and coccidia species of pet cats in 2003–2004.* J Feline Med Surg 2006;8:292–301.

Gookin JL, Hanrahan K, Levy MG. *The conundrum of feline Trichomonosis.* J Feline Med Surg. 2017; 19(3):261–27.

Gruffydd-Jones T, Addie D, Belák S, Boucraut-Baralon C, Egberink H, Frymus T, et al. *Giardiasis in cats: ABCD guidelines on prevention and management.* J Feline Med Surg 2013; 15(7):650–2.

Gruffydd-Jones T, Addie D, Belák S, Boucraut-Baralon C, Egberink H, Frymus T, et al. *Tritrichomoniasis in cats: ABCD guidelines on prevention and management.* J Feline Med Surg 2013;15(7):647–9.

Jakel V, Cussler K, Hanschmann KM, Truyen U, König M, Kamphuis E, et al. *Vaccination against Feline Panleukopenia: implications from a field study in kittens.* BMC Vet Res 2012;8:62.

Keith CL, Radecki SV, Lappin MR. *Evaluation of fenbendazole for treatment of Giardia infection in cats concurrently infected with Cryptosporidium parvum.* Am J Vet Res 2003;64:1027–9.

Mcglade TR, Robertson ID, Elliot AD, Thompson RC. *High prevalence of Giardia detected in cats by PCR.* Vet Parasitol 2003;110:197–205.

Miró G, Hernández L, Montoya A, Arranz-Solís D, Dado D, Rojo-Montejo S, et al. *First description of naturally acquired Tritrichomonas foetus infection in a Persian cattery in Spain.* Parasitol Res 2011;109(4):1151–4.

Olson ME, Leonard NJ, Srout J. *Prevalence and diagnosis of Giardia infection in dogs and cats using a fecal antigen test and fecal smear.* Can Vet J 2010;51:640–2.

Paris JK, Wills S, Balzer HJ, Shaw DJ, Gunn-Moore DA. *Enteropathogen co-infection in UK cats with diarrhea.* BMC Vet Res 2014;10:13.

Sotiriadou I, Pantchev N, Gassmann D, Karanis P. *Molecular identification of Giardia and Cryptosporidium from dogs and cats.* Parasite 2013;20:8.

Spada E, Proverbio D, Della Pepa A, Domenichini G, Bagnagatti De Giorgi G, Traldi G, et al. *Prevalence of faecal-borne parasites in colony stray cats in northern Italy.* J Feline Med Surg 2013;15(8):672–7.

Stuetzer B, Hartmann K. *Feline parvovirus infection and associated diseases.* Vet J 2014;201(2):150–5.

Truyen U, Addie D, Belák S, Boucraut-Baralon C, Egberink H, Frymus T, Gruffydd-Jones T, et al. *Feline panleukopenia. ABCD guidelines on prevention and management.* J Feline Med Surg 2009;11(7):538–46.

Truyen U, Parrish CR. *Feline panleukopenia virus: its interesting evolution and current problems in immunoprophylaxis against a serious pathogen.* Vet Microbiol 2013;165(1–2):29–32.

Xenoulis PG, Lopinski DJ, Read SA, Suchodolski JS, Steiner JM. *Intestinal Tritrichomonas foetus infection in cats: a retrospective study of 104 cases.* J Feline Med Surg 2013;15(12):1098–103.

Yao C, Köster LS. *Tritrichomonas foetus infection, a cause of chronic diarrhea in the domestic cat.* Vet Res 2015;46:35.

Respiratory infections

Afonso MM, Pinchbeck GL, Smith SL, et al. *A multi-national European cross-sectional study of feline calicivirus epidemiology, diversity and vaccine cross-reactivity.* Vaccine. 2017;9;35(20):2753–2760.

Ballin AC, Schulz B, Helps C, Sauter-Louis C, Mueller RS, Hartmann K. *Limited efficacy of topical recombinant feline interferon-omega for treatment of cats with acute upper respiratory viral disease.* Vet J 2014;202(3):466–70.

Berger A, Willi B, Meli ML, et al. *Feline calicivirus and other respiratory pathogens in cats with Feline calicivirus-related symptoms and in clinically healthy cats in Switzerland.* BMC Vet Res. 2015; 13;11:282.

Bol S, Bunnik EM. *Lysine supplementation is not effective for the prevention or treatment of feline herpesvirus 1 infection in cats: a systematic review.* BMC Vet Res 2015;11:284.

Fernandez M, Manzanilla EG, Lloret A, León M, Thibault JC. *Prevalence of feline herpesvirus-1, feline calicivirus, Chlamydophila felis and Mycoplasma felis DNA and associated risk factors in cats in Spain with upper respiratory tract disease, conjunctivitis and/or gingivostomatitis.* J Feline Med Surg 2016 Feb 26. pii: 1098612X16634387.

Gruffydd-Jones T, Addie D, Belák S, Boucraut-Baralon C, Egberink H, Frymus T, et al. *Chlamydophila felis infection. ABCD guidelines on prevention and management.* J Feline Med Surg 2009;11(7):605–9.

Hartmann AD, Helps CR, Lappin MR, Werckenthin C, Hartmann K. *Efficacy of pradofloxacin in cats with feline upper respiratory tract disease due to Chlamydophila felis or Mycoplasma infections.* J Vet Intern Med 2008;22(1):44–52.

Hora AS, Tonietti PO, Guerra Jm, Leme MC, Pena HF, Maiorka PC, et al. *Felid herpesvirus 1 as a causative agent of severe nonsuppurative meningoencephalitis in a domestic cat.* J Clin Microbiol 2013, 51(2):676–9.

Jas D, Frances-Duvert V, Vernes D, Guigal PM, Poulet H. *Three-year duration of immunity for feline herpesvirus and calicivirus evaluated in a controlled vaccination-challenge laboratory trial.* Vet Microbiol 2015;177(1–2):123–31.

Le Boedec K. *A systematic review and meta-analysis of the association between Mycoplasma spp and upper and lower respiratory tract disease in cats.* J Am Vet Med Assoc. 2017;15;250(4):397–407.

Lee M, Bosward KL, Norris JM. *Immunohistological evaluation of feline herpesvirus-1 infection in feline eosinophilic dermatoses or stomatitis.* J Fel Med Surg 2010;12:72–9.

Malik R, Lessels NS, Webb S, Meek M, Graham PG, Vitale C, et al. *Treatment of feline herpesvirus-1 associated disease in cats with famciclovir and related drugs.* J Feline Med Surg 2009;11:40–8.

Möstl K, Addie DD, Boucraut-Baralon C, Egberink H, Frymus T, Gruffydd-Jones T, et al. *Something old, something new: Update of the 2009 and 2013 ABCD guidelines on prevention and management of feline infectious diseases.* J Feline Med Surg 2015;17(7):570–82.

Radford AD, Addie D, Belák S, Boucraut-Baralon C, Egberink H, Frymus T, et al. *Feline calicivirus infection: ABCD guidelines on prevention and management.* J Fel Med Surg 2009;11:556–64.

Schulz C, Hartmann K, Mueller Rs, Helps C, Schulz BS. *Sampling sites for detection of feline herpesvirus-1, feline calicivirus and Chlamydia felis in cats with feline upper respiratory tract disease.* J Feline Med Surg 2015;17(12):1012–9.

Stiles J. *Ocular manifestations of feline viral diseases.* Vet J 2014; 201(2):166–73.

Thiry E, Addie D, Belák S, Boucraut-Baralon C, Egberink H, Frymus T, et al. *Feline herpesvirus infection: ABCD guidelines on prevention and management.* J Fel Med Surg 2009;11:547–55.

Thomasy SM, Lim CC, Reilly CM, Kass PH, Lappin MR, Maggs DJ. *Evaluation of orally administered famciclovir in cats experimentally infected with feline herpesvirus type-1.* Am J Vet Res 2011;72(1):85–95.

Thomasy SM, Shull O, Outerbridge CA, et al. *Oral administration of famciclovir for treatment of spontaneous ocular, respiratory, or dermatologic disease attributed to feline herpesvirus type 1: 59 cases (2006–2013).* J Am Vet Med Assoc. 2016; 249(5):526–38.

Chronic gingivostomatitis (FCGS)

Arzi B, Mills-Ko E, Verstraete FJ, Kol A, Walker NJ, Badgley MR, et al. *Therapeutic Efficacy of Fresh, Autologous Mesenchymal Stem Cells for Severe Refractory Gingivostomatitis in Cats.* Stem Cells Transl Med 2016;5(1):75–86.

Belgard S, Truyen U, Thibault JC, et al. *Relevance of feline calicivirus, feline immunodeficiency virus, feline leukemia virus, feline herpesvirus and Bartonella henselae in cats with chronic gingivostomatitis.* Berl Munch Tierarztl Wochenschr 2010;123(9–10):369–76.

Bellei E, Dalla F, Masetti L, Pisoni L, Joechler M. *Surgical therapy in chronic feline gingivostomatitis (FCGS).* Vet Res Commun 2008;32 (Suppl 1): S231–4.

Dolieslager SM, Bennett D, Johnston N, Riggio MP. *Novel bacterial phylotypes associated with the healthy feline oral cavity and feline chronic gingivostomatitis.* Res Vet Sci 2013;94(3):428–32.

Dolieslager SM, Lappin DF, Bennett D, Graham L, Johnston N, Riggio MP. *The influence of oral bacteria on tissue levels of Toll-like receptor and cytokine mRNAs in feline chronic gingivostomatitis and oral health.* Vet Immunol Immunopathol 2013;151(3–4):263–74.

Dolieslager SM, Riggio MP, Lennon A, Lappin DF, Johnston N, Taylor D, et al. *Identification of bacteria associated with feline chronic gingivostomatitis using culture-dependent and culture-independent methods.* Vet Microbiol 2011;24;148(1):93–8.

Dowers KL, Hawley JR, Brewer MM, Morris AK, Radecki SV, Lappin MR. *Association of Bartonella species, feline calicivirus, and feline herpesvirus 1 infection with gingivostomatitis in cats.* J Fel Med Surg 2010;12(4):314–21.

Druet I, Hennet P. *Relationship between Feline calicivirus Load, Oral Lesions, and Outcome in Feline Chronic Gingivostomatitis (Caudal Stomatitis): Retrospective Study in 104 Cats.* Front Vet Sci. 2017; 5;4:209.

Harley R, Gruffydd-Jones TJ, Day MJ. *Immunohistochemical characterization of oral mucosal lesions in cats with chronic gingivostomatitis.* J Comp Pathol 2011;144(4):239–50.

Hennet PR, Camy GA, Mcgahie DM, Albouy MV. *Comparative efficacy of a recombinant feline interferon omega in refractory cases of calicivirus-positive cats with caudal stomatitis: a randomised, multi-centre, controlled, double-blind study in 39 cats.* J Feline Med Surg 2011;13(8):577–87.

Kouki MI, Papadimitriou SA, Psalla D, et al. Chronic Gingivostomatitis with Esophagitis in Cats. J Vet Intern Med. 2017;31(6):1673–1679.

Quimby JM, Elston T, Hawley J, Brewer M, Miller A, Lappin MR. *Evaluation of the association of Bartonella species, feline herpesvirus 1, feline calicivirus, feline leukemia virus and feline immunodeficiency virus with chronic feline gingivostomatitis.* J Feline Med Surg 2008;10(1):66–72.

Rolim VM, Pavarini SP, Campos FS, Pignone V, Faraco C, Muccillo MS, et al. *Clinical, pathological, immunohistochemical and molecular characterization of feline chronic gingivostomatitis.* J Feline Med Surg 2016. pii: 1098612X16628578.

Winer JN, Arzi B, Verstraete FJ. *Therapeutic Management of Feline Chronic Gingivostomatitis: A Systematic Review of the Literature.* Front Vet Sci. 2016;18;3:54.

Fading kitten syndrome

Bücheler J. *Fading kitten syndrome and neonatal isoerythrolysis.* Vet Clin North Am Small Anim Pract. 1999.

Cave TA, Thompson H, Reid SWJ, Hodgson DR, Addie DD. 2002 *Kitten mortality in the United Kingdom: a retrospective analysis of 274 histopathological examinations (1986–2000).* Vet Rec 151: 497–501.

Hoskins JD (ed). *Veterinary Pediatrics: Dogs and Cats from Birth to six months*, 2nd edn. WB Saunders Co, Philadelphia, 1995.

Levy J. *The fading kitten.* En Rand J. Problem-based Feline Medicine. Elsevier-Saunders (eds). 2006;1126–1144.

Vector borne diseases

Fernandez-Gallego A, Feo Bernabe L, Dalmau A, et al. Feline leishmaniosis: diagnosis, treatment and outcome in 16 cats. J Feline Med Surg. 2020;13:1098612X20902865.

Leiva M, Lloret A, Peña T, Roura X. *Therapy of ocular and visceral leishmaniasis in a cat.* Vet Ophthalmol. 2005;8(1):71–5.

Maia C, Campino L. *Can domestic cats be considered reservoir hosts of zoonotic leishmaniasis?* Trends Parasitol. 2011;27(8):341–4.

Pennisi, MG, Hartmann K, Lloret A, et al. *Leismaniosis in cats ABCD guidelines on prevention and management.* J Feline Med Surg 2013;15: 638–642.

Pennisi MG, Cardoso L, Baneth G, et al. *LeishVet update and recommendations on feline leishmaniosis.* Parasit Vectors. 2015;4;8:302.

Pennisi MG, Hofmann-Lehmann R, Radford AD, et al. *Anaplasma, Ehrlichia and Rickettsia species infections in cats: European guidelines from the ABCD on prevention and management.* J Feline Med Surg. 2017; 19(5):542–54.

Main feline zoonoses

Baneth G, Thamsborg SM, Otranto D, Guillot J, Blaga R, Deplazes P, et al. *Major Parasitic Zoonoses Associated with Dogs and Cats in Europe.* J Comp Pathol 2015. pii: S0021–9975(15)00314-X.

European scientific counsel companion animal parasites Guidelines http://www.esccap.org/guidelines/#.VzbX7lTyhdg.

Frymus T, Addie D, Belák S, et al. Feline rabies. *ABCD guidelines on prevention and management.* J Feline Med Surg. 2009;11(7):585–9

Hartmann K, Addie D, Belák S, Boucraut-Baralon C, Egberink H, Frymus T, et al. *Toxoplasma gondii infection in cats: ABCD guidelines on prevention and management.* J Feline Med Surg 2013;15(7):631–7.

Pennisi MG, Marsilio F, Hartmann K, Lloret A, Addie D, BELÁK S, et al. *Bartonella species infection in cats: ABCD guidelines on prevention and management.* J Feline Med Surg 2013;15(7):563–9.

Wang A, Greene CE. *Pet-associated illness.* En Bonagura & Twedt (eds): Kirk's Current Veterinary Therapy XV. St Louis, Missouri: Elsevir Saunders; 2014. p. 1244–9.

Vaccines and vaccination programmes

Day MJ, Horzinek MC, Schultz RD, Squires RA. *WSAVA Guidelines for the vaccination of dogs and cats.* J Small Anim Pract 2016;57(1):E1-E45.

Hartmann K, Day MJ, Thiry E, Lloret A, Frymus T, Addie D, et al. *Feline injection-site sarcoma: ABCD guidelines on prevention and management.* J Feline Med Surg 2015;17(7):606–13.

Horzinek MC, Thiry E. *Vaccines and vaccination: the principles and the polemics.* J Feline Med Surg 2009;11(7):530–7.

Horzinek MC. *Vaccination protocols for companion animals: the veterinarian's perspective.* J Comp Pathol 2010;42(Suppl 1): S129–32.

Hosie MJ, Addie DD, Boucraut-Baralon C, Egberink H, Frymus T, Gruffydd-Jones T, et al. *Matrix vaccination guidelines: 2015 ABCD recommendations for indoor/outdoor cats, rescue shelter cats and breeding catteries.* J Feline Med Surg 2015.17(7):583–7.

Test

1. **Regarding FIP, which of the following statements is correct?**
   A) In a healthy cat, the higher the anti-coronavirus antibody titre, the greater the probability of suffering from FIP.
   B) Corticosteroids improve the clinical signs, but dramatically decrease survival in cats with FIP.
   C) The anti-coronavirus antibody titre has some correlation with the load of coronavirus excreted in faeces in a transient or permanent infection.
   D) Coronavirus PCR on blood is the confirmatory test for FIP, since if the virus is found in blood the cat is ill with FIP.
2. **Regarding rapid diagnostic tests for retroviruses, FeLV and FIV (there is only one correct answer):**
   A) They are tests that detect antibodies, and therefore the results must be confirmed with tests that detect antigen.
   B) It is possible that a 3-month-old kitten positive for FIV may not be infected by the virus.
   C) A 3-month-old kitten which tests positive for FeLV is not considered a reliable result and should be confirmed with a PCR.
   D) A cat recently vaccinated for FeLV may give a false positive in the detection of p27 by ELISA.
3. **A radiograph of a 2-year-old cat with dyspnoea and fever shows pleural effusion, what is the diagnosis?**
   A) If the serum anti-coronavirus antibody titre is high, the diagnosis of FIP is certain.
   B) If the total pleural fluid proteins are high and cytology shows a predominance of neutrophils and lymphocytes, the diagnosis of FIP is certain.
   C) If the coronavirus PCR on the pleural fluid is negative, it is not FIP.
   D) None of the above are correct.
4. **A 14-year-old cat has been diagnosed with diffuse intestinal lymphoma by biopsy ...**
   A) The majority of cases are persistent FeLV viremia's.
   B) Chemotherapy should not be administered, given the risk of immunosuppression and reactivation of a latent FeLV infection.
   C) Although ELISA and provirus PCR on blood and bone marrow are negative, this lymphoma originated from a previous infection with the FeLV virus.
   D) None of the above are correct.
5. **A 6-year-old stray cat which is clinically healthy, with a normal blood count, serum biochemistry and urine tests, tested positive on the FIV ELISA. What conclusion can be drawn from these results?**
   A) It will die before it reaches 3 years of age.
   B) It is advisable to repeat the test in 6–8 weeks to rule out a false positive on the first test.
   C) It is essential to do an FIV PCR, since ELISAs are unreliable. They also detect antibodies and it could be that the cat was not infected.
   D) It would be a very serious mistake to let it live with another cat, since it is a highly contagious infection.
6. **Regarding a cat suffering from confirmed feline chronic gingivostomatitis:**
   A) It is not worth doing the FCV PCR on an oral swab, since 100% of cats are positive. This disease is caused by a chronic FCV infection.
   B) If the FCV PCR of an oral swab is positive, total exodontics are contraindicated.
   C) It is a multifactorial disease with an important immune-mediated component as suggested by the histological pattern, the cytokine pattern and the clinical response to immunosuppressants.
   D) Complete exodontics has good results, with a 40–50% chance of completely healing or significant improvement in the signs of the disease.
7. **Regarding the diagnosis of retroviruses (FeLV and FIV):**
   A) Provirus PCR of FeLV DNA positive in blood means that the cat is infected, is viral and is eliminating the virus through saliva.
   B) The subclinical or asymptomatic phase of FIV infection can last at least 3 years and then the immunodeficiency syndrome develops.
   C) The PCR for provirus DNA from FIV is unreliable because the virus does not integrate into the genome of cat cells in the same way that FeLV does.
   D) IFA on blood smears can be used to discriminate a transient viremia from a permanent viremia in cats with a FeLV positive ELISA.

8. An 8-month-old cat, with obstructive upper respiratory signs (rales, noisy breathing), does not respond to antibiotics, non-steroidal anti-inflammatories or lysine. Over the last few weeks, famciclovir is being given at 80 mg/kg/8 h because the herpesvirus PCR was positive, but it does not improve either. Which option is correct?

A) Most likely, it is chronic herpesvirus that will never be cured.
B) The herpesvirus PCR has been a false positive result, and it may be suffering from another disease, for example, a nasopharyngeal polyp.
C) It probably has a nasopharyngeal polyp, there are studies that have shown that polyps are caused by chronic herpesvirus infections.
D) None of the above are correct.

9. Regarding feline leishmaniasis, which of the following statements is correct?

A) Sick cats are usually only seen if they are severely immunosuppressed.
B) The most frequent skin condition is exfoliative desquamative dermatitis.
C) The species of Leishmania in cats is species specific and is different to that in dogs.
D) The infection rate in endemic areas is not low.

10. A 7-year-old retrovirus-negative cat has bilateral uveitis, polyclonal gammopathy, proteinuria and azotemia:

A) If the coronavirus serology is positive, the most likely diagnosis would be FIP.
B) If there are no effusions in the pleural or peritoneal cavities it is less likely to be FIP.
C) A serology and Leishmania PCR test should be requested.
D) If the anti-toxoplasma IgG titre is high, a safe diagnosis would be toxoplasmosis.

11. In a blood donor cat:

A) While the ELISA is negative for feline leukaemia, it does not matter if the provirus PCR is positive.
B) If haemoplasma are not seen on the blood smear, it can be regarded as negative.
C) A Bartonella PCR should be performed on blood and if it is negative it can be guaranteed that it is not a carrier.
D) None of the above are correct.

12. A cat adopted as a 10 month-old as retrovirus-negative has chronic small intestinal diarrhoea. *Coccidia* and *Giardia* have been observed in coprology, and it has been treated with ponazuril and fenbendazole several times with no response: in the control coprology *Giardia* is still present. The cat's general condition is not very good, and occasionally presents with partial anorexia and does not gain weight.

A) In some cases, *Giardia* infections are persistent and resistant to drugs, it should be treated with metronidazole and secnidazole and the source of reinfection in the environment should be controlled.
B) Trichomoniasis should be suspected and a PCR for *Tritrichomonas* on stools requested.
C) A stool sample should be sent to the laboratory for a complete PCR profile as it is a priority to know what pathogen is causing the diarrhoea.
D) The abdomen should be carefully palpated in search of possible mesenteric lymphadenopathy and an abdominal ultrasound considered since one of the possibilities is that it is a dry form of FIP.

13. Which of the following diseases is not associated with uveitis in cats?

A) Bartonellosis.
B) FIP.
C) Herpesvirus.
D) Mycoplasmosis.

14. A 4-week-old kitten has become acutely ill and is hypothermic, hypoglycaemic and dehydrated, with no other clinical signs:

A) The diagnosis of the cause is complex, but one of the most likely causes would be sepsis/septicaemia or panleukopoenia.
B) Panleukopoenia can be ruled out as it does not have diarrhoea.
C) At that age the most frequent cause of disease is FIP.
D) If the feline leukaemia test is positive, it is not reliable since there may be antibodies from the mother.

15. Regarding vaccination in cats:

A) In general, inactivated vaccines are much less effective than attenuated vaccines.
B) Recombinant vaccines carry adjuvants, so they are immunogenic.
C) Vaccines against feline leukaemia virus are all inactivated.
D) All are incorrect.

16. A gynaecologist, has advised a pregnant owner to get rid of the cat she has at home (an indoor cat that goes out onto a terrace without outdoor access) because she has been positive for toxoplasmosis by antibody detection. What should the veterinarian advise?

A) Although the risk of infection is very low, follow the doctor's advice, to avoid problems.
B) Perform diagnostic tests on the cat, for example, antibody titre in blood: if the cat were positive, the risk is much higher so the owner should follow the doctor's instructions.
C) That there is no risk whatsoever, because it is already seropositive, and that it is precisely because she has a cat at home, and she has already been exposed to the parasite before.
D) None of the above.

Clinical case 1

Signalment: 11 year old, Persian cat weighing 5.2 kg.

Reason for consultation: referred for bilateral uveitis and hyphaema. Undergoing treatment with corticosteroids and clindamycin plus topical ophthalmic treatment.

Clinical history: adopted as a stray a year ago, retrovirus negative, indoor life with 2 other cats, does not show systemic signs of disease.

Physical and eye examination: BC 2/5, hair has poor appearance, alert, hydrated, normal cardiovascular signs, normal abdominal palpation, normal lymph nodes, exudative anterior uveitis, hyphaema in OS, fundus without abnormalities.

- Complete blood count, blood biochemistry and urinalysis: mild mature neutrophilia, monocytosis, moderate azotaemia (creatinine 3.23 mg/dl, urea 167 mg/dl), polyclonal gammopathy (6.04 g/dl), low albumin (2.22 g/dl), urine density 1.020, proteinuria 2+, inactive sediment, UPC ratio 0.8.
- Total T4: normal levels.
- Thoracic radiographs: No abnormalities.
- Abdominal ultrasound: bilateral renomegaly, marked medullary band sign, mild pyelectasis, heterogeneous spleen, mild mesenteric lymphadenopathy, all of the rest is normal.
- FNA and renal cytology: increase in inflammatory cells, neutrophils and macrophages.
- Serologies: cryptococcal latex antigen (–), Ehrlichia antibodies (–), Leishmania antibodies (–), IgG and IgM Toxoplasma (–).

1. Based on these results, what is the most likely cause of this cat's eye disease?

A) FIP.
B) Bartonellosis.
C) Idiopathic.
D) High blood pressure.

2. Which test would be most sensitive to confirm suspicions of FIP?

A) Anti-coronavirus antibody titre.
B) RT-PCR FIP on blood.
C) Biopsy of kidney and/or lymph nodes and immunohistochemistry for coronavirus from the lesion.
D) Kidney FNA and FIP PCR of the sample.

3. What should the initial treatment be until the diagnosis was confirmed?

A) Renal diet, anti-proteinurics and eye treatment according to ophthalmology.
B) Renal diet and eye treatment according to ophthalmology.
C) Renal diet, antiproteinuric drugs, eye treatment according to ophthalmology and prednisolone at 2 mg/kg day.
D) Renal diet, antiproteinuric drugs, eye treatment according to ophthalmology and cyclosporine at 7.5 mg/kg day.

4. How could the diagnosis of bartonellosis be confirmed?

A) If antibody tests are positive, the diagnosis would be confirmed.
B) If antibody tests are negative, it is unlikely to be bartonellosis.
C) If the *Bartonella* PCR on blood is negative, suspicions of bartonellosis could be ruled out.
D) None of the above are correct.

5. If the final diagnosis of the disease was FIP, what would the most appropriate treatment be?

A) Euthanasia, because FIP has a very poor prognosis.

B) Wait and see if the cat responds at least partially to the treatment before making a decision.

C) If polyprenil immunostimulant I was available it should not be added to the treatment, since it only helps in FIP with effusions.

D) None of the above are correct.

Clinical case 2

Signalment: 7-year-old British cat, 4.8 kg.

Reason for consultation: visit for second opinion for chronic rhinitis which has been present for the last year (sneezing and mucopurulent nasal secretion).

History and clinical history: vaccines and de-worming up to date, lives in the city, no history of fleas or ticks. Diagnosed with nasal aspergillosis 6 months ago by culture of positive external nasal secretion to *Aspergillus* spp. and non-significant bacterial culture. Blood tests without abnormalities, negative to retrovirus. Computed tomography (CT) indicated a proliferative lesion in the nasal mucosa in the caudal part of the left nasal cavity, atrophy of the bilateral turbinates, abundant presence of mucus, inflammation and bone remodelling in the right frontal sinus. All these abnormalities are compatible with a fungal type destructive rhinosinusitis compatible with the result of the culture. It was treated for 4 weeks with oral itraconazole and a partial but not complete improvement has been observed. Over the last 3 months it has not received any treatment.

Physical examination: BC 3/5, 4.8 kg, good general condition, 38.5°C, alert, hydrated, normal cardiovascular signs, normal abdominal palpation, normal peripheral lymph nodes, presence of purulent secretion in nostrils, no deformities or asymmetries in nasal and facial septae are observed.

- Complete blood count, serum biochemistry and urinalysis: mild neutrophilic leukocytosis, other results normal.
- Rhinosinusal CT: large tumour in the left nasal cavity with destruction of the frontal bone, rhinitis with atrophy of turbinates in the right nasal cavity, bilateral frontal sinusitis.
- Bacteriological culture (tissue samples obtained from areas with lesions): growth of *Serratia marcescens*, sensitive to quinolones and aminoglycosides.
- Fungal culture (tissue samples obtained from areas with lesion): negative after 2 weeks of incubation.
- Histopathology of the left cavity tumour: squamous cell carcinoma with cytokeratin positive immunohistochemistry.
- Histopathology of the right cavity: intense mixed inflammation with a predominance of neutrophils and macrophages, no infectious agents, Grocott stain for fungi negative.

1. Indicate the most likely differential diagnosis before performing a second CT:

A) Aspergillosis that does not respond to oral itraconazole.

B) Aspergillosis or neoplasia.

C) Aspergillosis, neoplasia or idiopathic chronic rhinosinusitis.

D) Aspergillosis, neoplasia or chronic herpesvirus rhinitis.

2. What tests should have been done in the first round of tests to reach a definitive diagnosis?

A) Rhinoscopy, biopsies, fungal culture and histopathology.

B) *Aspergillus* spp. serology.

C) Nasal flushing, fungal culture and histopathology of the samples recovered in the flushing.

D) A and C are correct.

3. Ideally how should nasal aspergillosis be treated in a cat for better results?

A) Itraconazole for 1 month.

B) Fluconazole for 1 month.

C) Itraconazole for several months and local administration of enilconazole or miconazole under general anaesthesia.

D) Terbinafine for several months.

4. **What treatment would be ideal once the diagnosis of carcinoma of the nasal cavity was confirmed taking the other results into account?**
   A) External radiation therapy, marbofloxacin and meloxicam.
   B) External radiation therapy, marbofloxacin and prednisolone.
   C) Chemotherapy, marbofloxacin and meloxicam.
   D) Marbofloxacin and meloxicam, it makes no sense to treat the carcinoma, they do not respond to any treatment.
5. **How would you interpret the culture of nasal secretions which were positive for *Aspergillus* spp. and the fact that the final diagnosis is different?**
   A) Aspergillosis was present, and the carcinoma developed subsequently.
   B) Cultures of external nasal secretions are not sufficiently sensitive or specific to the causes of rhinitis.
   C) A positive culture to *Aspergillus* spp. in nasal secretions always indicates aspergillosis.
   D) None of the above are correct.

Answers

Test

1. C	7. D	13. D
2. B	8. D	14. A
3. D	9. D	15. D
4. D	10. C	16. D
5. B	11. D	
6. C	12. D	

Clinical case 1

1. A
2. C
3. C
4. B
5. A

Clinical case 2

1. C
2. D
3. C
4. A
5. B

Oncology

10

Pachi Clemente Vicario

Contents

The aetiology of cancer

A study published in 2014 shows **cancer as the leading cause of death in cats** and responsible for 20% of fatalities, as compared with trauma (12%) and kidney disease (12%). In cats, the average age of death due to neoplasia is 14 years old.

Cancer results from a series of genetic changes on a cellular level. After the initial damage, the cell continues to replicate which causes disease, unless cellular control mechanisms are able to repair or destroy altered cells.

The cell cycle is the process during which the cell prepares for division and divides. Normally, a cell needs an **external signal (growth factor)** to activate a receptor and set in motion the cellular replication machinery. During this process **various controls operate which check for alterations and destroy cells that cannot be repaired. This is called apoptosis.**

It is estimated that **at least five or six mutations are necessary** to allow a normal cell to be able to:

1. Be self-sufficient in growth factors.
2. Be insensitive to anti-growth signals.
3. Have the ability to avoid apoptosis.
4. Have unlimited replication potential.
5. Produce angiogenesis.
6. Be able to invade tissues and metastasize.

In general **cancer is a multifactorial disease** and identifying the inciting cause can be difficult. However, in feline oncology there are some well-defined cause-effect relationships, although the mechanism by which these occur is not always clear.

Some of the factors related to tumour development and their involvement in specific feline neoplasms are described in this chapter.

Viral infection and oncogenes

The cat is the domestic animal species which is affected by the greatest number of retroviral infections. In particular, prior to the introduction of an effective vaccine, feline leukaemia virus (FeLV) was associated with a third of deaths. **Natural FeLV infections are associated with proliferative diseases and tumours** such as lymphoma, leukaemia (lymphoid, myeloid, or erythroid), as well as **degenerative diseases such as anaemia.** FeLV does not occur as a single entity, but as a family of closely related viruses.

Different genetic virus variants are associated with different diseases. These varieties are recognized by changes in their genetic material, specifically in the long terminal repeat (LTR), and by the different surface glycoproteins (SG). FeLV is found in nature in four groups (A, B, C and T) differentiated by different sequences in SG and linked to different clinical signs:

- FeLV-A is minimally pathogenic.
- FeLV-B can cause lymphoma, leukaemia, and anaemia.
- FeLV-C pure erythroid aplasia.
- FeLV-T immunosuppression.

On the other hand, different LTRs insert in different sites of the cat genome. When these sites have the same location in different animals, they are called **frequent insertion sites**.

A **proto-oncogene** is a genetic portion in healthy cells, whose functions are important for cell growth and differentiation. A variation of these proto-oncogenes are **oncogenes**, which are genetic portions which alone or in combination with other oncogenes can transform the cell. **Any abnormal expression or mutation of the oncogene can lead to the development of neoplasia.**

Six sites of frequent FeLV insertion have been identified, some of which are oncogenes that are activated producing the neoplasm, including *c-myc*. The highly variable clinical course of FeLV-positive cats probably depends on factors related to both the virus (genetic variations) and the host. **Use of the vaccine has helped to control viral infection** and changed the prevalence of the different clinical forms.

In recent years, information on the role of **protein tyrosine kinase** (and its growth factors) in cancer development has become increasingly abundant. New studies provide data on the potential of molecular drugs targeting these proteins as a treatment option for different tumours, such as vaccine-associated sarcoma. However, much of this data came from *in vitro* trials and must be interpreted with caution until data on their efficacy through phase I and II trials is available.

Physical factors: inflammation

The first data on the FeLV vaccine were published in 1986 and shortly thereafter, in 1991, it was suggested it may cause sarcomas at the injection site, usually around the interscapular area (Figure 1).

Compared to sarcomas at other sites, **injection-site sarcomas tend to grow faster, ulcerate, and necrotize**. They are also **poorly encapsulated**, which makes full surgical resection difficult and recurrence more likely.

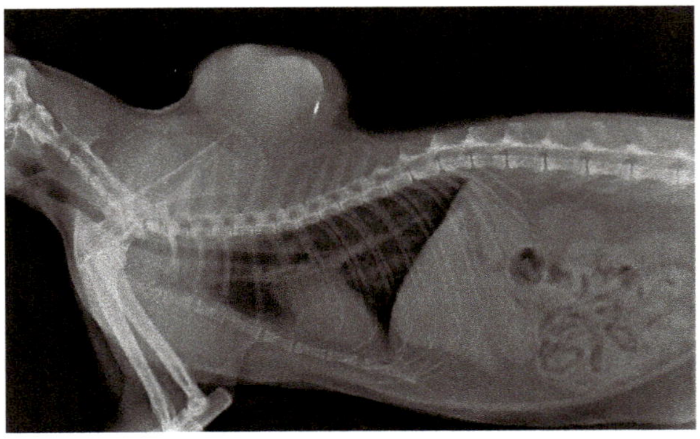

Figure 1. Radiograph of a cat with sarcoma in the interscapular region.

Administering multiple vaccines at the same site increases the risk of sarcoma and also makes it difficult to know the role each vaccine plays. From the start, an association was identified between sarcoma and the FeLV and rabies vaccines, although no specific component (including adjuvants), formulation, or brand has been definitively linked to tumour development. Also, molecular studies have not been able to find viruses in tumours, whilst it has been shown that **inflammation precedes the appearance of the tumour**.

Because cancer is a complex disease with both genetic and environmental factors, a **genetic predisposition** has been suggested as contributing to the development of sarcomas at an injection site. A prospective article published in 2012, with a control group, detected the relationship between various types of vaccines and other injectables with the appearance of sarcomas, and found **no vaccine carried zero risk of producing injection-site sarcoma**. Although local inflammation may be part of the process that ends with tumour development, sarcomas have been documented at the injection sites of corticosteroids (used as anti-inflammatory drugs). In addition, there may be **factors independent of inflammation, such as the aluminium contained in some vaccines**, which aid development of sarcomas. A 2017 study shows how fibroblasts proliferate in concentrations of aluminium that are toxic to other cells.

Tumour suppressor gene: p53

The **p53 tumour suppressor gene plays a key role in the cell cycle; ensuring there are no genetic alterations in the cell and where failures are detected eliminating them through apoptosis**. Cells in which p53 is altered or absent, continue with the cell cycle and divide despite having genetic alterations, which leads to aberrant clones and potentially malignant tumours.

Many of these alterations give rise to abnormal proteins, detectable in tumour tissue by immunohistochemistry. Up to 81% of sarcomas at the injection site present p53 alterations. These present with different clinical symptoms depending on the nuclear or cytoplasmic presentation of the protein, which is associated with alterations in function. **The cytoplasmic expression of p53 is associated with a worse prognosis**, similar to other human tumours.

An interesting finding is the detection **of p53 abnormalities in non-tumour tissues and histologically normal cells as distant as 5 cm** from the initial tumour. This may represent a previous step to these cells becoming malignant under the influence of some carcinogens (which would imply new tumoural foci rather than recurrences) or a genetic predisposition of some cells with defective p53.

The **genetic predisposition** to develop sarcomas at injection sites has been evaluated as it is a tumour that affects young cats, sometimes from the same litter, which may present other additional tumours. The feline genotype has been studied looking for p53 mutations in blood samples, finding that among the eight analysed there is one error present in 42% of cats with sarcoma, compared to 10% of the control population (healthy cats, without sarcoma at the time of the study).

Although injection site sarcoma is likely caused by the presence of **chronic inflammation in a population genetically predisposed to tumours**, a study published in 2012 found no difference in the rate of mutations when comparing 100 healthy cats with 50 cats with sarcoma, so further studies are needed.

Hormonal factors: oestrogens and progestogens

Oestrogens and progesterone play a major role in the development of feline mammary tumours. Early sterilization (before six months old) reduces the risk of future mammary tumours by 91% and when done before 12-months of age this is reduced by 86%. On the other hand, continued treatment with progestogens increases the risk of mammary tumours in cats and felines kept in zoos.

However, there are other factors that influence their appearance and clinical course. The ***Brca2* gene is considered a mammary tumour suppressor gene**, since its mutation (with loss of function) or **absence is associated with an increased risk of mammary tumour** development. Furthermore, after inheriting this condition, the mutation is passed on to the offspring. In women, this explains the risk of some mothers and daughters in developing mammary tumours. **In cats, the Brca2 gene has been described** as in other species. In addition, alteration in the expression of HER-2 (receptor for epithelial growth factor) influences the clinical course of the disease, which is more aggressive in cases that overexpress the HER-2 gene.

Environmental factors: sunlight

Among the possible causes of cancer, **ultraviolet light and sun exposure** are most accepted. The development of tumour lesions in **areas of the skin that do not have protection** against the sun (such as the unpigmented nasal plane, eyelids or tips of the ears in those areas not covered by hair) is frequent in animals with outdoor access in geographical locations with plentiful sunshine (Figure 2).

Long-term accumulated exposure causes **skin tumours through p53 mutations**, with up to 79% of actinic keratitis (precancerous lesion of squamous cell carcinoma) presenting alterations in p53. More recently, different studies have detected the **presence of feline papillomavirus** in squamous cell carcinomas of the skin, nasal plane and oral cavity. A direct relationship in other species has been demonstrated between the development of neoplasms and papillomavirus. If a feline papillomavirus-squamous cell carcinoma relationship is confirmed, it may pave the way for new strategies in the treatment of this common tumour.

Angiogenesis

A growing field of research is the **ability of tumours to generate new blood vessels** which allow them to supply nutrients and oxygen and thus continue growing. Tumours, regardless of their malignancy, cannot grow beyond a few millimetres if they do not receive a blood supply for nourishment. To do this, tumours secrete **vascular endothelial growth factor**, among other substances. Blocking the receptor for this growth factor can be used as anti-angiogenic therapy.

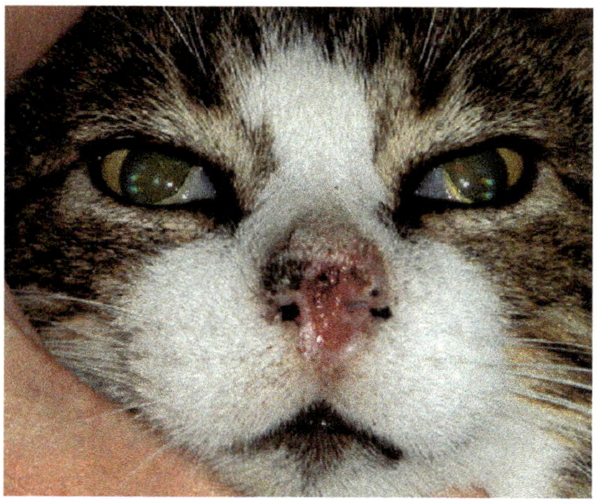

Figure 2. Cat with a tumoural lesion on the unpigmented area of the nasal plane.

Tumour biology is an area under development. New insights have the potential to address many questions about the development of cancer and open the door to new treatment options.

Diagnosis and clinical stage

Cancer represents a large group of diseases with diverse behaviours and response to treatment. Therefore, the first step is always to **reach a specific diagnosis using cytology or histology**.

When managing a patient's neoplasm, the owner must be provided with information about the prognosis and available treatment options. This information depends not just upon the specific type of neoplasm, but on the extent of the neoplastic disease as classified according to accepted **clinical staging**. Knowing the clinical stage prior to treatment allows a more accurate prediction of response to treatment.

Depending on the tumour type, **different approaches are recommended**. For example, many carcinomas and most large cell lymphomas in cats can be diagnosed by cytology (Figure 3).

With other tumours, such as sarcomas or small cell lymphomas, cytology is not helpful and **histopathology** or additional tests are necessary to confirm the diagnosis. **Molecular diagnostic techniques** such as flow cytometry, antigen receptor rearrangements (PARRs), or immunohistochemistry have been proposed as part of the diagnostic work up for small cell lymphomas, because they increase the certainty of the diagnosis when compared with similar clinical signs such as inflammatory bowel disease.

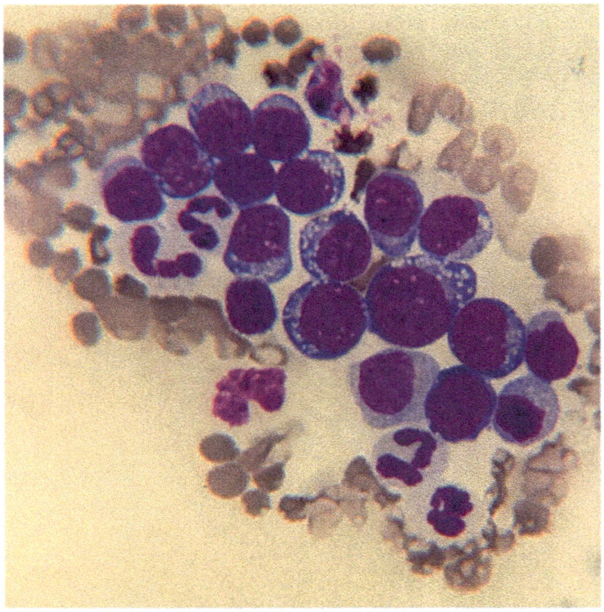

Figure 3. Cytological image of a large cell lymphoma.

The **type of biopsy also varies depending on the type of tumour**. If a vaccine-associated sarcoma is suspected (**Rule of 1-2-3:** mass at the injection site that continues to grow after 1 month, that measures more than 2 cm, or that is present 3 months after the injection) excisional biopsy is not recommended, since the probability of complete excision is very low and complicates definitive surgery. In this case, the biopsy should be incisional.

The basic principles when taking a biopsy include:

- Take several samples.
- That the sample is deep enough to pass through the normal or reactive tissue that covers the tumour.
- That the **biopsy site can subsequently be removed** with the tumour.
- Handle the sample carefully so as not to create artefacts.
- Fix it properly.

If there is a clinical discrepancy or if the diagnosis is unusual, a second opinion on the initial biopsy may be considered before starting treatment. In two studies published in veterinary medicine, there were between 10 and 37% of the cases in which the diagnosis changed significantly, affecting both the prognosis and the tests necessary for the clinical stage.

Although there are specific classifications for each tumour group, **in general the classification is based on data from the primary tumour** (T), **the involvement of the lymph nodes** (N) **and the presence or absence of metastases** (M).

Once diagnosed, by cytology or histopathology, the primary tumour should be **measured**, and its size (using a calliper) and location recorded. **Size is an important prognostic factor** in most tumours: for example, **mammary carcinomas smaller than 2 cm in diameter have a mean survival time greater than 2 years**, while if the diameter exceeds 3 cm, the mean survival time is 4 to 6 months. Furthermore, the histological grade also offers prognostic information, as in the case of feline mammary carcinoma, with a mean survival time of 36 months for grade I, 18 months for grade II, and only 6 months for grade III.

Other prognostic factors that can be obtained from the histopathology report include **lymphovascular embolization** (presence of tumour cells in the lymphatic or venous vessels), which in mammary tumours, for example, is associated with a worse prognosis: the survival rate a year after surgery is 20% in cases with embolization, compared to 67% in cases without embolization.

Equally important is the **clinical evaluation of the lymph nodes** to determine the extent of tumoural disease. Although size assessment is important, it is not definitive in most cases: the fact that the size is normal does not rule out the presence of lymph node metastases. On the other hand, if the size is increased, it does not necessarily mean metastasis is present. For this reason, lymph nodes must be aspirated or biopsied to rule out tumour involvement (Figure 4).

Knowledge of regional lymphatic drainage is essential: for example, two thoracic and one abdominal feline mammary glands can drain both caudally and cranially. However, the first thoracic one always drains cranially (to the axillary lymph node) and last two abdominal ones drain caudally (to the inguinal lymph node). Cases of mammary tumours with lymph node metastasis live on average five months compared to 13 months in animals where the lymph node is not affected.

Finally, the presence of **distant metastases** should be evaluated. Although metastatic spread can affect different organs, **the lungs are affected in a large number of cases**. Thoracic radiology, with right and left lateral and ventrodorsal projections, is a sensitive method for the detection of tumour lesions.

Access to advanced diagnostic techniques, such as computed tomography, allows for more precise studies that allow better clinical decisions to be made.

Once the clinical stage is known, prognostic information appropriate to the specific case is offered and treatment possibilities studied. In addition, data from the initial examination serves as baseline data to evaluate the response to treatment and the evolution of the disease. Boxes 1 and 2 show the clinical stage systems of some tumours.

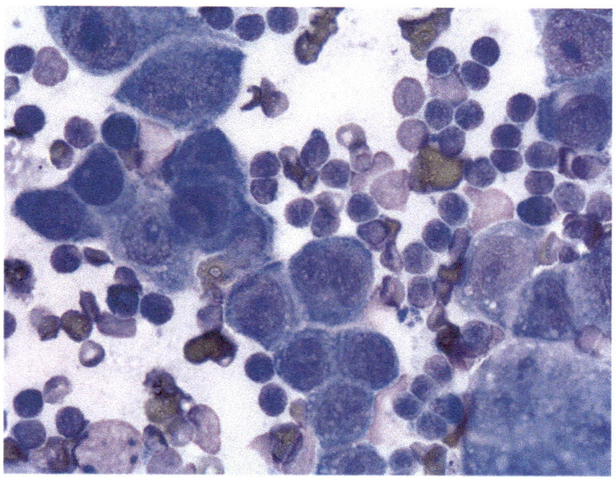

Figure 4. Metastasis from a lymph node carcinoma. There is a population of epithelial cells with marked anisocytosis and anisokaryosis, prominent nucleolus and basophilic cytoplasm. Some small lymphocytes can be seen, with little cytoplasm.

Box 1. Clinical stages of feline mammary tumours.

T – Primary tumour
- T1 <2 cm maximum diameter
- T2 2–3 cm maximum diameter
- T3 >3 cm maximum diameter

N – Regional lymph nodes
- N0 – no metastasis (histology or FNA)
- N1 – with metastasis (histology or FNA)

M – Distant metastasis
- M0 – no evidence of metastasis
- M1 – with distant metastasis

I	T1	N0	M0
II	T2	N0	M0
III	T1, 2	N1	M0
	T3	N0, 1	M0
IV	Any T	Any N	M1

Clinical stages Adapted from: Lana SE, Rutteman GR, Withrow SJ. Tumors of the mammary gland. In: Withrow SJ, Vail DM (eds). Whitrow & MacEwen's Small Animal Clinical Oncology. St. Louis, Saunders, 2007; 619–636.

Box 2. Clinical stages of feline lymphoma.

Stage 1
- Single tumour (extra nodal) or in an anatomical area (ganglionic)
- Includes primary intrathoracic tumours

Stage 2
- Single tumour (extranodal) with regional lymph node involvement.
- Two or more lymph node regions on the same side of the diaphragm.
- Two tumours (extranodal) with or without regional lymph node involvement on the same side of the diaphragm.
- Primary removable gastrointestinal tumour, normally in the ileocaecal region, with or without involvement of mesenteric lymph nodes.

Stage 3
- Two tumours (extranodal) on different sides of the diaphragm.
- Two or more lymph node areas on both sides of the diaphragm.
- Primary intraabdominal disease, unresectable.
- Paraspinal or epidural tumours, independent of tumours in other locations.

Stage 4
- Stages 1,2 and 3 with liver and/or spleen involvement.

Stage 5
- Stages 1,2,3 and 4 with CNS and/or bone marrow involvement.

Adapted from: Vail DM. Feline Lymphoma and Leukemia. In Withrow SJ, Vail DM (eds). Whitrow & MacEwen's Small Animal Clinical Oncology. St. Louis, Saunders, 2007; 733–756.

Prognosis

An awareness of the prognosis for each case provides valuable information when making treatment decisions. However, it should be remembered that prognostic values are **mean values**, and amongst a population the individual survival times may vary greatly and therefore a firm prediction for an individual is difficult and often unreliable.

In feline lymphoma there are different entities, with different prognoses. Therefore, the diagnostic procedure should involve **identifying the specific type of lymphoma** in order to give the most appropriate treatment. Even with gastrointestinal lymphoma (the most common at present) there are up to three histological types with different biological behaviour: small cell lymphoma, large cell lymphoma, and large granular lymphocyte lymphoma (LGL). Well-differentiated, small-cell lymphocytic is low-grade and is sometimes difficult to differentiate from inflammatory intestinal conditions. The lymphoblastic type is high grade and displays more aggressive behaviour. In cats with lymphocytic or lymphoblastic lymphoma, the best prognostic factor is obtaining complete remission. LGL is described as a tumour that is not very sensitive to chemotherapy and has a poor prognosis (57 days median survival).

In some cases, the anatomical location is related to the histological type. This is mainly in the stomach, where up to 100% of the cases are large B-cell lymphomas. In the intestine this association is not so clear, although in the small intestine the majority are from T cells (predominantly small cells) and in the large intestine they are from B cells.

Even the aetiology may be related to the location, since it has been suggested that ***Helicobacter* infection** may be the cause of feline gastric lymphoma, with data suggesting treatment with antibiotics causes remission of the lesions in up to 75% of cases. Thus, interpretation of the tests must be carried out accurately to offer the maximum amount of information to the owners and to choose the treatment that best suits the case.

In extranodal lymphomas, the anatomical location also offers important prognostic information. For example, cases of nasal lymphoma have the best median survival (749 days) and those that affect the CNS the worst (70 days). The majority of extranodal lymphomas (85%) respond to various chemotherapy protocols such as COP (initials of cyclophosphamide, Oncovin®-vincristine and prednisone or prednisolone) or CHOP (cyclophosphamide, hydroxydaunorubicin-doxorubicin, Oncovin®-vincristine and prednisone or prednisolone).

Many of the cases of vaccine-associated sarcomas seen at the author's practice attend after undergoing conservative surgery. In these cases, the most important information for the clinician is the **evaluation of the edges of the excised tissue**. Knowing whether the entire piece was sent for pathology or only a part of the tumour (in this case the edges are always dirty) and how the edges were evaluated is necessary. It is important to investigate cranial, caudal, and both edges as well as the full depth to be able to make a decision on the best treatment.

However, it is important to explain to owners that even **cases with clean borders can recur up to 20% of the time**, a percentage that rises to 70% if tumour cells where found in the margins. A study published in 2011 on almost 100 cats which underwent radical surgery (5 cm margin around the tumour), reported a recurrence rate of 14% although only 3% of the cases showed dirty margins.

Feline mammary carcinomas are associated with high malignancy, with a tendency for frequent recurrences and metastasis. However, groups with different prognoses have been described, so it is important to study the histopathology results in detail when informing the owners. Complex carcinomas (those with tumours in the epithelial and myoepithelial areas) seem to have a low degree of malignancy and are associated with a better prognosis.

Invasive micropapillary carcinoma is associated with more aggressive features such as a large size at the time of presentation, high histological grade of malignancy, deep muscle invasion, and a higher percentage of lymphatic and lymph node invasion than other mammary carcinomas. It is proposed they should be classified in a different subgroup with a worse prognosis.

A rare feline mammary tumour is the **inflammatory mammary carcinoma**. This is characterized by oedema and ulceration of the skin after respective surgery. Histologically, it shows embolization of the superficial lymphatic vessels of the dermis and a strong inflammatory reaction. It is associated with a very poor prognosis.

Treatment

There is no such thing as a single treatment option for any cancer. Each case must be evaluated individually taking into account factors specific to the disease, the patient (presence of other diseases) and the owners (availability of time, money and tolerance to side effects, among other factors).

There are different treatment modalities for each disease:

- surgery
- chemotherapy
- radiotherapy
- immunotherapy
- electrochemotherapy

In addition to weighing up the pros and cons for various conventional treatments, owners often ask about or show interest in alternative therapies. As clinicians, all possibilities should be evaluated so as to identify the best option for a specific patient. Where possible the resulting treatment should have a solid foundation based on evidence. However, in an age of evidence based medicine, it is worth noting that in veterinary medicine, especially feline medicine, data is often limited.

There are **five levels of scientific evidence** on which to base clinical recommendations. In a review of veterinary oncology publications between 1999 and 2007, only 16 of the articles studied aspects of feline oncology (compared to 74% in canine cases): of all published studies (canine, feline and equine oncology) only one 2% were level II (none were level I, the highest evidence level). Most were level IV out of V. Thus, most of decisions are based on the results of small series of clinical cases, sometimes with contradictory results. For example, the two articles published on the use of doxorubicin in feline mammary tumours describe opposite results, so reading them in detail is important in order to draw valid conclusions.

Fortunately, the amount of information available is growing and continually being updated, so consulting sources such as PubMed for recent information on prognostic factors or treatment options is advisable.

Lymphoma

Treatment for lymphoma depends primarily on the grade; for example small cell (low grade) are treated with prednisone and chlorambucil, while large cell (high grade) are treated with multi-drug protocols such as COP or CHOP.

Most small cell lymphomas respond well to treatment, achieve complete remission, and have a good prognosis.

In **high-grade lymphomas**, no big differences are observed between COP and CHOP protocols, either in terms of response rate or in survival. In addition, doxorubicin can cause nephrotoxicity in cats, so the choice of protocol is made taking into account the general health status of the animal.

The **COP-methotrexate protocol is well tolerated by cats** and is used frequently at the authors practice for cats with large cell lymphoma (Box 3, end of chapter). With this protocol it is important to monitor the weight of the cat as the doses of cyclophosphamide and methotrexate cannot be adapted to the weight as they are tablets that cannot be split. If the patient loses weight, the dose (mg/m^2) of these drugs may be too high and treatment may need to be withdrawn.

Once treatment has started, there are factors that indicate the patient's prognosis. In cats with large cell lymphoma, **>5% weight loss one month after initiation of treatment is associated with a lower survival rate** when compared with those that have a stable weight or gain weight during the same period. It is important to check the amount of food eaten and to calculate energy needs.

In general, once they come out of remission, the percentage of animals that achieve remission again is half and the duration of remission, is also half. Using only doxorubicin, the response rate is 22% but if other drugs are added the response is better and longer lasting. Again, survival time is better for cases of small and medium cell lymphoma.

An **important aspect to take into account is that of side effects**, since for the vast majority of owners it is the limiting factor in the author's experience: owners do not want to treat their animals if their quality of life is severely compromised. In this sense, the clinician has to evaluate the side effects and make any necessary treatment adjustments. Side effects are reflected in Table 1.

The CHOP protocol can produce toxicity (neutropoenia) in up to 34% of cases, which leads to a delay in treatment of 5–7 days and a reduction in the dose by 25% for subsequent treatments. At the author's practice, although cats are seen with neutropoenia due to toxicity, they rarely develop infections secondary to neutropoenia or compatible clinical signs (lethargy, anorexia, fever …) so in general treatments are not delayed or reduced if the neutropoenia is grade 1 and the animal is asymptomatic. With more severe neutropoenias, treatment needs to be adjusted.

Table 1. Chemotherapy toxicity (Adapted from: Veterinary and Comparative Oncology, 2004; 2(4):194–213).

Side effect	Grade 1	Grade 2	Grade 3	Grade 4	Grade 5
Haematological toxicity					
Haemoglobin (g/dl)	8.0–LLN1	<8.0–6.5	<6.5–5.0	<5.0	–
Haematocrit	25%–LLN	20–25%	15–20%	<15%	–
Neutrophils (/µl)	1,500–LLN	1,000–1,499	500–999	<500	–
Platelets (/µl)	100,000–LLN	50,000–99,000	25,000–49,000	<25,000	–
Systemic toxicity					
Lethargy-fatigue	Mild	Moderate 2	Compromised 3	Severe4	Death
Fever	1°C above normal	1–2°C above normal	2–3°C above normal	>3°C above normal	Death
Weight loss	5–10%	>10–20%	>20%	–	Death
Gastrointestinal toxicity					
Anorexia	Fussy appetite	Reduced intake over 3 days No weight loss	Reduced intake over 3–5 days Weight loss	Reduced intake for 5 days Severe weight loss	Death
Nausea	Reduced appetite	Salivation over more than 12 h	Salivation between 12 and 24 hours	Salivation lasting more than 24 hours	–
Vomiting	Less than 3 in 24 hours	3–5 in 24 hours Less than 3 per day over 2–4 days	More than 5 in 24 hours One per day over more than 4 days	Severe, shock	Death
Diarrhoea	Defaecates twice more than normal	Defaecates 2–6 times more than normal	Defaecates 6 times more than normal	Severe	Death
Colitis	Asymptomatic	Mucous or blood	Pain, fever	Severe	Death

1: LLN: lower limit of normal; 2: some difficulty leading a normal life (eat, sleep, urinate, defaecate); 3: severe limitations to leading a normal life. Only gets up to eat, defaecate and urinate 4: needs to be force fed and needs help to lead a normal life.

Carcinoma

With regard to **mammary carcinomas**, treatment with doxorubicin (1 mg/kg/IV every three weeks until completion of five treatments) improves survival compared to historical data when treated with surgery only. In any case, the histological grade and the clinical stage strongly influence the evolution and survival time of the animal.

Radical mastectomy followed by adjuvant doxorubicin shows an increase in mean survival, while after conservative surgery, no significant difference was detected compared to the group treated only with surgery. However, the study did not use a sufficient number of cases and its statistical power is low (McNeill, 2009). In the author's practice, treatment of mammary carcinomas with doxorubicin is recommended, except for in those animals in which this drug may be contraindicated (for example, because they are suffering from kidney failure).

Mitoxantrone has also been used in mammary carcinomas, although **studies have not demonstrated benefits from its use**, although the low statistical power means it is unclear whether this is due to lack of efficacy or the design of the studies. Median survival with adjuvant mitoxantrone (about 16 months) is similar to cases treated with only surgery in other studies, and the most common side effects included azotaemia, anorexia, and vomiting.

Nor has adjuvant carboplatin been shown to improve prognosis in queens with stage III mammary carcinoma: median survival is the same in groups treated with surgery alone or with surgery and carboplatin.

Vaccine associated sarcoma

Treatment of vaccine-associated sarcoma requires multimodal treatment.

A **radical initial surgery**, performed by an experienced surgeon, increases the chances of long-term control.

Presurgical or postoperative radiation therapy increases both disease-free period and survival.

Even with aggressive surgeries (a five-centimetre margin), the risk of local recurrence remains around 15% to 20% in cats, which develop distant metastases. Smaller margins of 3 cm are associated with recurrences of around 33% in the first procedure and up to 55% in cases where recurrent tumours were operated on.

Squamous cell carcinoma

Squamous cell carcinoma (SCC) can present in different locations, and treatment varies depending on this factor.

Although aggressive surgery is simple in ear lesions, removing the tumour from the upper or lower eyelids and the nasal plane is more complicated. Surgery for SCC in the oral cavity has not been successful in cats. Photodynamic therapy has achieved very high response rates, but it is not available in all countries. In any case, complete remission can be achieved in 85% of cases with superficial lesions. **Local radiation therapy can achieve complete remission in 88% of cases treated with a single treatment**.

Due to the multiple presentations in many cases and the lack of access to previous therapies, new treatments have been investigated. The response to a new **immunomodulator, imiquimod 5% (Aldara)**, was recently reported in cases of squamous carcinoma in situ, with a response seen in all cases. A response has also been reported in a case of actinic keratitis and SCC on the ear of a cat after 12 weeks of treatment.

Different studies have shown the efficacy of **electrochemotherapy** in the treatment of feline squamous cell carcinoma of the nasal plane and eyelids. This technique consists of the combination of intravenous chemotherapy (bleomycin) with the administration of electrical pulses which increase the permeability of neoplastic cells in such a way that the intracellular concentration of the drug is increased up to several hundred times. Treatment usually consists of a single session and is administered under general anaesthesia. In this way, complete remission is achieved in most cases, which is also durable over time.

The author's experience with this therapy is similar to the published data, obtaining long term complete

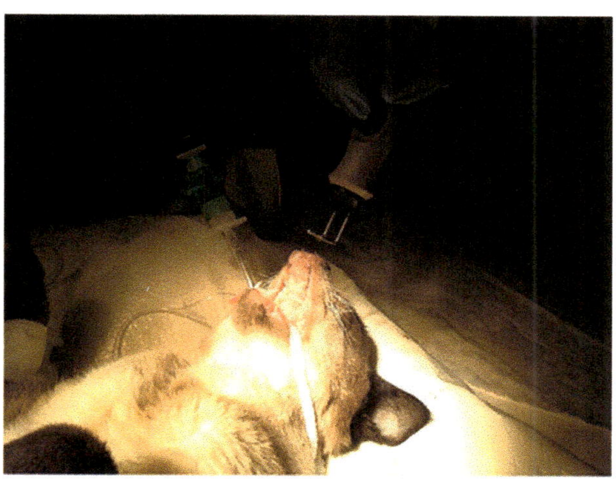

Figure 5. Electrochemotherapy treatment, administered under general anaesthesia.

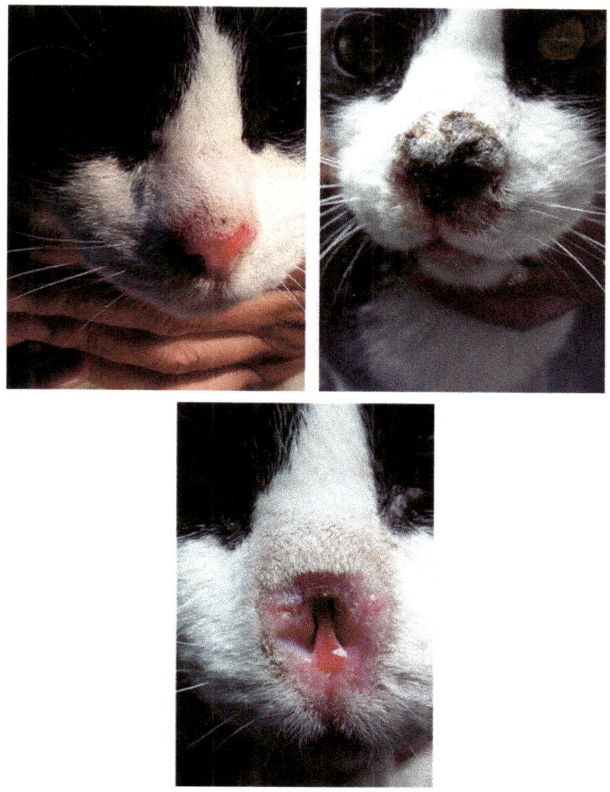

Figure 6. Squamous cell carcinoma on the nasal plane before and after electrochemotherapy treatment. Necrotic tissue can be seen after the initial inflammatory reaction in the second image.

remissions in most cases (Figures 5 and 6). In response to treatment, local inflammation occurs that progresses to necrosis and tissue loss. It is important to communicate these changes to the owners prior to therapy.

In the case of **oral SCC, the prognosis is much worse**, with a one-year survival time in less than 10% of cases. Many of the cases affect the bone locally and although this is not associated with survival, it has been suggested that this group of animals with osteolysis could benefit from zoledronate treatment, both by slowing tumour growth and by controlling lytic changes in the bone, associated with the tumour.

Electrochemotherapy in squamous cell carcinomas of the lips has a high toxicity with extensive necrosis, without achieving good control of the disease, and for this reason the author does not recommend its use, at least with the protocols used so far.

In conclusion, it should be emphasized there have never been so many treatment options for cancer patients as in recent years; with the addition of molecular, metronomic and palliative therapies to the classic options. As clinicians, it is advisable to stop talking about "cancer" and offer owners options tailored to their particular case (histological type, clinical stage, general health status) whilst trying to improve the quality of life for cancer patients.

Safe management of chemotherapy

Cytotoxic drugs should be handled with caution to prevent problems for both the patient and the personnel who administer them, either in the clinic or at home.

The pills and tablets (cyclophosphamide, methotrexate, toceranib, among others) cannot be broken and the capsules (chlorambucil) must not be opened.

Packaging and trade names can be very similar (Figure 7), which can lead to errors. Before administering a drug, checking that it is the drug that has been prescribed along with the weight, dose and total amount to be administered is recommended, ideally by two people to reduce the risk of confusion.

For the administration of **intravenous chemotherapy, closed delivery systems** should be used (Figure 8) to avoid contamination of work surfaces and aerosol formation.

Chemotherapy protocols commonly used in feline oncology are detailed in the following tables.

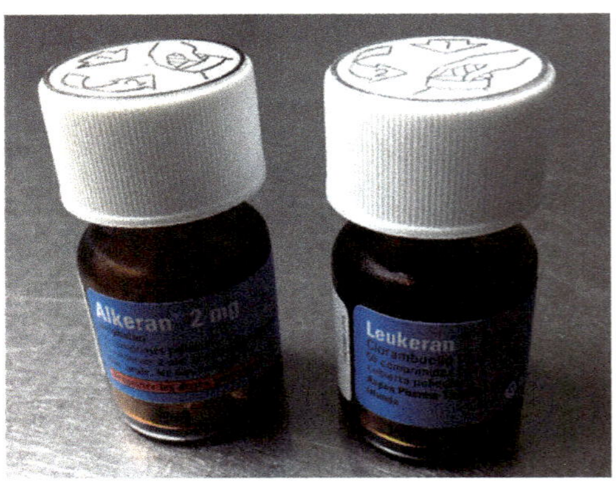

Figure 7. Appearance of melphalan (Alkeran) and chlorambucil (Leukeran) packaging. Both medications come in 2 mg tablets.

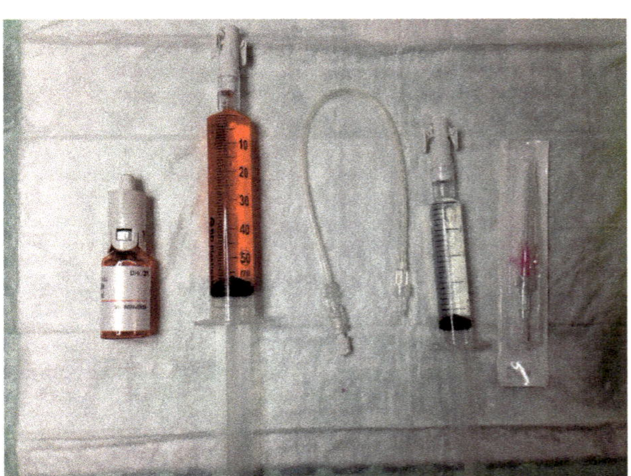

Figure 8. Closed circuit for chemotherapy administration with adaptors for the chemotherapy vial, the syringe with chemotherapy and the injection site. The syringe with saline from flushing the catheter also has an adapter to keep the system closed throughout the whole process.

Box 3. Chemotherapy protocols for sarcomas in cats

5-Fluorouracil is toxic in cats and should not be used in this species

AC protocol (21 days)

- Day 1. Doxorubicin 1 mg/kg IV
- Day 10. Cyclophosphamide: 200–300 mg/m² PO

VAC protocol (28 days)

- Day 1. Doxorubicin 1 mg/kg IV
- Day 8. Vincristine: 0.5 mg/m² IV
- Day 10. Cyclophosphamide: 200–300 mg/m² PO
- Day 15. Vincristine: 0.5 mg/m² IV
- Day 22. Vincristine: 0.5 mg/m² IV

MIC protocol (21 days)

- Day 1. Mitoxantrone 5.5–6.5 mg/m² IV over five minutes
- Day 10. Cyclophosphamide: 200–300 mg/m² PO

Carboplatin: 240 mg/m² IV every 3 weeks

Box 4. Chemotherapy protocols for carcinoma in cats

5-Fluorouracil is toxic in cats and should not be used in this species.

Carboplatin protocol

- Carboplatin. 240 mg/m² IV every 3 weeks

AC protocol (21 days)

- Day 1. Doxorubicin 1 mg/kg IV
- Day 10. Cyclophosphamide: 200–300 mg/m² PO

MIC protocol (21 days)

- Day 1. Mitoxantrone 5.5–6.5 mg/m² IV over five minutes.
- Day 10. Cyclophosphamide: 200–300 mg/m² PO

Box 5. Chemotherapy protocols for high-grade feline lymphoma

COP-Methotrexate protocol

- Week 1. Vincristine 0.5 mg/m² IV
- Week 2. Cyclophosphamide 50 mg/cat PO
- Week 3. Vincristine 0.5 mg/m² IV
- Week 4. Methotrexate 2.5 mg/cat PO

Throughout the protocol, prednisone is maintained at a dose of 1–2 mg/kg/day and the protocol is repeated for the first six months, then every two weeks up to a year of treatment.

COAP

Repeats for six weeks, then maintenance:

- Cyclophosphamide: 200–300 mg/m² PO every 3 weeks
- Vincristine: 0.5 mg/m² IV one day per week
- Cytarabine: 100 mg/m² daily via IV drip over 2 days
- Prednisone: 40–50 mg/m² PO every 24 hours for one week and then 20–25 mg/m² PO every 48 hours

COP

Repeats for six weeks, then maintenance:

- Cyclophosphamide: 300 mg/m² PO every 3 weeks
- Vincristine: 0.5 mg/m² IV one day per week
- Prednisone: 40–50 mg/m² PO every 24 hours for one week and then 20–25 mg/m² PO every 48 hours

Wisconsin-Madison

Does not use maintenance chemotherapy:

- Week 1. Vincristine: 0.5–0.75 mg/m² IV, prednisone: 2 mg/kg PO every 24 hours
- Week 2. Cyclophosphamide: 200–250 mg/m² PO, prednisone: 1.5 mg/kg PO every 24 hours
- Week 3. Vincristine: 0.5–0.75 mg/m² IV, prednisone: 1 mg/kg PO every 24 hours
- Week 4. Doxorubicin: 1 mg/kg IV prednisone: 0.5 mg/kg PO every 24 hours
- Week 5. No treatment
- Week 6. Vincristine: 0.5–0.75 mg/m² IV
- Week 7. Cyclophosphamide: 200–250 mg/m² PO
- Week 8. Vincristine: 0.5–0.75 mg/m² IV
- Week 9. Doxorubicin: 1 mg/kg IV
- Week 10. No treatment
- Week 11. Vincristine: 0.5–0.75 mg/m² IV
- Week 12. Cyclophosphamide: 200–250 mg/m² PO
- Week 13. Vincristine: 0.5–0.75 mg/m² IV
- Week 14: Doxorubicin: 1 mg/kg IV
- Week 15: No treatment
- Week 16: Vincristine: 0.5–0.75 mg/m² IV
- Week 17: Cyclophosphamide: 200–250 mg/m² PO
- Week 18: Vincristine: 0.5–0.75 mg/m² IV
- Week 19: Doxorubicin: 1 mg/kg IV

Bibliography

Cancer aetiology

AbdelMageed MA, Foltopoulou P, McNiel EA. *Feline vaccine-associated sarcomagenesis: Is there an inflammation-independent role for aluminium?* Vet Comp Oncol. 2018 Mar; 16(1):E130–E143.

Argyle AJ, Khanna C. *Tumor Biology and Metastasis.* En: Withrow SJ, Vail DM (eds) Whitrow & MacEwen's Small Animal Clinical Oncology. St. Louis, Saunders, 2007; 31–53.

Banerji N, Kapur V, Kanjilal S. *Association of the Germ-line Polymorphisms in the Feline p53 Gene with Genetic Predisposition to Vaccine-Associated Feline Sarcoma.* Journal of Heredity 2007; 98(5):421–427.

Fujino Y, Ohno K, Tsujimoto H. *Molecular pathogenesis of feline leukemia virus-induced malignancies: insertional mutagenesis.* Vet Immunol Immunopathol. 2008 May 15; 123(1–2): 138–43.

Hendrick MJ, Goldsmith MH. *Do injection site reactions induce fibrosarcomas in cats?* J Am Vet Med Assoc. 1991; 199:968.

Henry CJ. *The epidemiology of Cancer. Chemical, Physical and Hormonal Factors.* En: Withrow SJ, Vail DM (eds) Whitrow & MacEwen's Small Animal Clinical Oncology. St. Louis, Saunders, 2007; 12–19.

Hershey AE, Dubielzig RR, Padilla ML, Helfand SC. *Aberrant p53 Expression in Feline Vaccine-associated Sarcomas and Correlation with Prognosis.* Vet Pathol 2005; 42:805–811.

Lawrence J, Saba C, Gogal Jr R et al. *Masitinib demonstrates anti-proliferative and pro-apoptotic activity in primary and metastatic feline injection-site sarcoma cells.* Vet Comp Oncology. 2011.

Levy LS. *Advances in Understanding Molecular Determinants in FeLV Pathology.* Vet Immunol Immunopathol. 2008 May 15; 123(1–2): 14–22.

Louwerens M, London CA, Pedersen NC, Lyons LA. *Feline lymphoma in the post-feline leukemia virus era.* J Vet Intern Med. 2005 May–Jun; 19(3):329–35.

Macy DW. *The epidemiology of Cancer. Cancer-Causing Viruses.* En: Withrow SJ, Vail DM (eds) Whitrow & MacEwen's Small Animal Clinical Oncology. St. Louis, Saunders, 2007; 19–30.

Millanta F, Calandrella M, Citi S, Della Santa D, Poli A. *Overexpression of HER-2 in Feline Invasive Mammary Carcinomas: An Immunohistochemical Survey and Evaluation of Its Prognosis Potential.* Vet Pathol 2005; 42:30–34.

Modiano JF, Breen M. *The epidemiology of Cancer. Genetic factors.* En: Withrow SJ, Vail DM (eds) Whitrow & MacEwen's Small Animal Clinical Oncology. St. Louis, Saunders, 2007; 3–11.

Morrison WB. *Inflammation and Cancer: A Comparative View.* J Vet Intern Med 2012, 26:18–31.

Mucha D, Laberke S, Meyer S, Hirschberger J. *Lack of association between p53 SNP and FISS in a cat population from Germany.* Vet Comp Oncology 2012.

Munday JS, Dunowska M, De Grey S. *Detection of two different papillomaviruses within a feline cutaneous squamous cell carcinoma: case report and review of the literatura.* N Z Vet J. 2009 Aug; 57(4):248–51.

Munday JS, Howe L, French A, Squires RA, Sugiarto H. *Detection of papillomaviral DNA sequences in a feline oral squamous cell carcinoma.* Res Vet Sci. 2009 Apr; 86(2):359–61.

Munday JS, Kiupel M, French AF, Howe L. *Amplification of papillomaviral DNA sequences from a high proportion of feline cutaneous in situ and invasive squamous cell carcinomas using a nested polymerase chain reaction.* Vet Dermatol. 2008 Oct; 19(5):259–63.

Munson L, Moresco A. *Comparative pathology of mammary gland cancers in domestic and wild animals.* Breast Dis. 2007; 28:7–21.

O'Neill DG, Church DB, McGreevy PD et al. *Longevity and mortality of cats attending primary care veterinary practices in England.* Journal od Feline Medicine and Surgery 2014.

Oonuma T, Morimatsu M, Ochiai K, Syuto B. *Properties of the Tumor Suppresor Gene Brca2 in the Cat*. J. Vet. Med. Sci. 2003; 65(10):1123–1126.

Ordás J, Millán Y, Dios R, Reymundo C, Martín de las Mulas J. *Proto-oncogene HER-2 in normal, dysplastic and tumorous feline mammary glands: an immunohistochemical and chromogenic in situ hybridation study*. BMC Cancer 2007; 7:179–184.

Srivastav A, Kass PH, McGill LD, Farver TB, Kent MS. *Comparative vaccine-specific and other injectable-specific risk of injection-site sarcomas in cats*. J Am Vet Assoc 2012; 241:595–602.

Diagnosis and clinical staging

Biller B et al. 2016 AAHA *Oncology Guidelines for dogs and cats*. J Am Anim Hosp Assoc 2016 Jul–Aug; 52(4):181–204.

Couto CG. *Lymphoma in the Cat and Dog*. En: Nelson RW, Couto CG (eds). Small Animal Internal Medicine. 4th Edition. 2009, St Louis, Mosby Elsevier. 1174–1186.

Forrest LJ. *Computed tomography Imaging in Oncology*. Vet Clin North Am Small Anim Pract 2016 May; 46(3):499–513.

Morris J. *Mammary tumors in the cat: size matters, so early intervention saves lives*. J Feline Med Surg 2013 May; 15(5):391–400.

Novosad CA, Bergman PJ, O'Brien MG, McKnight JA, Charney SC, Selting KA, et al. *Retrospective Evaluation of Adjuntive Doxorubicin for the Treatment of Feline Mammary Gland Adenocarcinoma: 67 Cases*. J Am Anim Hosp Assoc 2006; 42:110–120.

Raharison F, Sautet J. *Lymph drainage of the mammary glands in the female cats*. J Morphol. 2006 Mar; 267(3):292–9.

Regan RC et al. *A prospective evaluation of the impact of second-opinion histopathology on diagnosis testing, cost and treatment in dogs and cats with cancer*. Vet Comp Oncol. 2015 Jun; 13(2):106–16.

Regan RC et al. *Comparison of first-opinion and second-opinion histopathology from dogs and cats with cancer: 430 cases (2001–2008)*. Vet Comp Oncol. 2010 Mar; 8(1):1–10.

Prognosis

Bridgeford EC, Marini RP, Feng Y, Parry NM, Rickman B, Fox JG. *Gastric Helicobacter species as a cause of feline gastric lymphoma: A viable hypothesis*. Vet Immunol Immunopathol. 2008 May 15; 123(1–2):106–113.

Cesari A, Bettini G, Vezzali E. *Feline intestinal T-cell lymphoma: assessment of morphologic and kinetic features in 30 cases*. J Vet Diagn Invest. 2009 Mar; 21(2)277–9.

Guidice C, Stefanello D, Sala M, Cantatore M, Russo F, Romussi S, et al. *Feline injection-site sarcoma: Recurrence, tumor grading and surgical margin status evaluated using the three-dimensional histological technique*. Vet J. 2009 Sep 5. (In press).

Krick EL, Little L, Patel R, Shofer FS, Sorenmo K, Clifford CA, Baez JL. *Description of clinical and pathological findings, treatment and outcome of feline large granular lymphoma (1996–2004)*. Vet Comp Oncol. 2008 Jun; 6(2):102–10.

McNeill CJ, Sorenmo KU, Shofer FS, Gibeo L, Durham AC, Barber LG, et al. *Evaluation of Adjuvant Doxorubicin-Based Chemotherapy for the Treatment of Feline Mammary Carcinoma*. J Vet Intern Med 2009;23:123–129.

Novosad CA, Bergman PJ, O'Brien MG, McKnight JA, Charney SC, Selting KA, et al. *Retrospective Evaluation of Adjuntive Doxorubicin for the Treatment of Feline Mammary Gland Adenocarcinoma: 67 Cases*. J Am Anim Hosp Assoc 2006; 42:110–120.

Pérez-Alenza MD, Jiménez A, Niento A, Peña L. *First description of feline inflammatory mammary carcinoma: clinicopathological and immunohistochemical characteristics of three cases*. Breast Cancer Res 2004, 6:R300–R307.

Phelps HA, Kuntz CA, Milner RJ, Powers BE, Bacon NJ. *Radical excision with five-centimeter margins for treatment of feline injection-site sarcomas: 91 cases (1998–2002)*. JAVMA, 2011, Vol 239, No. 1, July 1.

Pohlman LM, Higginbotham ML, Welles EG, Johnson CM. *Immunophenotypic and histologic classification of 50 cases of feline gastrointestinal lymphoma*. Vet Pathol. 2009 Mar; 46(2):259–68.

Seixas F, Palemira C, Pires MA, Lopes C. *Mammary invasive micropapillary carcinoma in cat: clinicopathologic features and nuclear DNA content*. Vet Pathol. 2007 Nov; 44(6):842–8.

Seixas F, Palmeira C, Pires MA, Lopes C. *Are complex carcinoma of the feline mammary gland and other invasive mammary carcinoma identical tumors? Comparison of clinicopathologic features, DNA ploidy and follow up*. Res Vet Sci. 2008 Jun; 84(3):428–33.

Taylor SS, Goodfellow MR, Browne WJ, Walding B, Murphy S, Tzannes S, et al. *Feline extranodal lymphoma: response to chemotherapy and survival in 110 cats*. J Small Anim Pract. 2009 Nov; 50(11):584–92.

Wilson HM. *Feline alimentary lymphoma: demystifying the enigma*. Top Companion Anim Med. 2008 Nov; 23(4):177–84.

Treatment options

Bexfield NH, Stell AJ, Gear RN, Dobson JM. *Photodynamic therapy of superficial nasal planum squamous cell carcinomas in cats: 55 cases*. J Vet Intern Med. 2008 Nov–Dec; 22(6):1385–9.

Cunha SC et al. *Adjuvant chemotherapy with mitoxantrona for cats with mammary carcinomas treated with radical mastectomy*. J Feline Med Surg 2015 Dec; 17(12):1000–4.

De Campos CB et al. *Use of surgery and carboplatin in feline malignant mammary gland neoplasms with advanced clinical staging*. In Vivo 2014 Sep–Oct; 28(5):863–6.

Gender A, Lewis JR, Reetz JA, Schwarz T. *Computed tomographic features of oral squamous cell carcinoma in cats: 18 cases (2002–2008)*. J Am Vet Med Assoc. 2010 Feb 1; 236(3):319–25.

Gill VL, Bergman PJ, Baer KE, Craft D, Leung C. *Use of imiquimod 5% cream (Aldara) in cats with multicentric squamous cell carcinoma: 12 cases (2002–2005)*. Vet Comp Oncol. 2008 Mar; 6(1)55–64.

Hammond GM, Gordon IK, Theon AP, Kent MS. *Evaluation of strontium Sr 90 for the treatment of superficial aquamous cell carcinoma of the nasal planum in cats: 49 cases (1990–2006)*. J Am Vet Med Assoc. 2007 Sep 1; 231(5):736–41.

Hayes AM, Adams VJ, Scase TJ, Murphy S. *Survival of 54 cats with oral squamous cell carcinoma in United Kingdom general practice*. J Small Anim Pract. 2007 Jul; 48(7):394–9.

Krick EL, Moore RH, Cohen RB, Sorenmo KU. *Prognostic significance of weight changes during treatment of feline lymphoma*. Journal of Feline Medicine and Surgery (2011) 13,976–983.

Mayer MN, Treuil PL, LaRue SM. *Radiotherapy and surgery for feline soft tissue sarcoma*. Vet Radiol Ultrasound. 2009 Nov–Dec; 50(6):669–72.

McNeill CJ, Sorenmo KU, Shofer FS, Gibeo L, Durham AC, Barber LG, et al. *Evaluation of Adjuvant Doxorubicin-Based*

Chemotherapy for the Treatment of Feline Mammary Carcinoma. J Vet Intern Med 2009; 23:123–129.

Milner RJ, Peyton J, Cooke, Fox LE, Gallager A, Gordon P, Hester J. *Response rates and survival times for cats with lymphoma treated with the University of Wisconsin-Madison chemotherapy protocol: 38 cases (1996–2003).* J Am Vet Med Assoc. 2005 Oct 1; 227(7):1118–22.

Müller N, Kessler M. *Curative intent radical en bloc resection using a minimum of a 3 cm margin in feline injection-site sarcomas: a retrospective analysis of 131 cases.* J Feline Med Surg 2017 Jul 1 [Epub ahead of print].

Oberthaler KT, Mauldin E, McManus PM, Shofer FS, Sorenmo KU. *Rescue therapy with doxorubicin-based chemotherapy for relapsing or refreactory feline lymphoma: a retrospective study of 23 cases.* J Fel Med Surg. 2009 Apr; 11(4):259–65.

Ossowska M, Sánchez Requena E, Kravech N, Guizar O, Clemente-Vicario F. *Grade 4/5 local toxicity with treatment with standard electrochemotherapy protocol of labial squamous cell carcinoma in 2 cats.* Proceedings ESVONC 2017.

Peters-Kennedy J, Scott DW, Miller WH Jr. *Apparent clinical resolution of pinnal actinic keratoses and squamous cell carcinoma in a cat using topical imiquimod 5% cream.*

Phelps HA et al. *Radiacl excision with five-centimeter margins for treatment of feline injection-site sarcomas: 91 cases (1998–2002).* J Am Vet Med Assoc. 2011 Jul 1; 239(1):97–106.

Sahora and C. Khanna. *A survey of evidence in the Journal of Veterinary Internal Medicine Oncology Manuscripts from 1999 to 2007.* J Vet Intern Med 2010; 24:51–56.

Spugnini EP et al. *Electroporation enhances bleomycin efficacy in cats with periocular and advanced squamous cell carcinoma of the head.* J Vet Inter Med. 2015 Sep–Oct; 29(5):1368–75.

Taylor SS, Goodfellow MR, Browne WJ, Walding B, Murphy S, Tzannes S, et al. *Feline extranodal lymphoma: response to chemotherapy and survival in 110 cats.* J Small Anim Pract. 2009 Nov; 50(11):584–92.

Tozon N et al. *Electrochemotherapy with intravenous bleomycin injection: an observational study in superficial squamous cell carcinoma in cats.* J Feline Med Surg 2014 Apr; 16(4):291–9.

Wypij JM, Fan TM, Fredrickson RL, Barger AM, de Lorimer LP, Charney SC. *In vivo and in vitro efficacy of zoledronate for treating oral squamous cell carcinoma in cats.* J Vet Intern Med. 2008 Jan–Feb; 22(1)158–63.

Test

1. What is the treatment of choice for feline mammary carcinoma?

A) There is no effective treatment.
B) Conservative surgery and doxorubicin.
C) Aggressive surgery and doxorubicin.
D) Surgery without chemotherapy.

2. What are the side effects of doxorubicin toxicity in cats?

A) Anaphylactic shock.
B) Arrhythmias if administered over less than 30 minutes.
C) All of the above.
D) None of the above.

3. Which of the following factors is of prognostic significance in feline lymphoma?

A) Age.
B) Anatomical location.
C) Serology for detection of FeLV.
D) Pre-treatment with corticosteroids.

4. If the surgery is performed with a 5 cm margin, the recurrence of sarcoma associated with the injection is:

A) 49%.
B) 14%.
C) 20%.
D) 72%.

5. Vaccine associated sarcoma presents distant metastases:

A) In 50% of cases.
B) It depends on the presence of mutation in p.53.
C) The appearance of distant metastases increases after successive surgeries.
D) In 20% of cases.

6. Feline squamous cell carcinoma has been linked to which of the following viruses:

A) Papilloma virus.
B) FeLV.
C) Herpesvirus.
D) FIV.

7. Due to the prevalence of injection site associated sarcoma, clinicians should:

A) Recommend a vaccination plan adapted to each case.
B) Never vaccinate cats that always live indoors.
C) Mix the vaccines and give them in a single injection.
D) All of the above.

8. The clinical stage is determined by:

A) Obtaining prognostic information.
B) Choosing the best treatment option.
C) Assessing the evolution.
D) All of the above are correct.

9. A fellow veterinarian calls you to consult what the prognosis may be for a cat with a 1.5 cm mammary carcinoma. It is the only abnormality on physical examination, and no metastases have been detected on thoracic radiographs. With the limitation of not having examined the animal, you inform them that the average survival time if treated with surgery is:

A) One year.
B) More than two years.
C) Six months.
D) It is impossible to say.

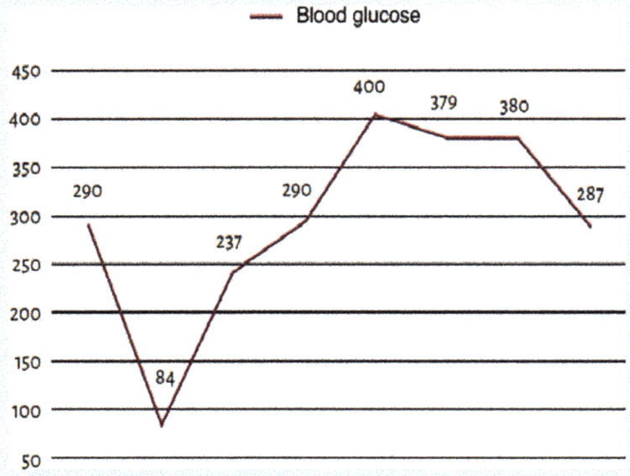

10. The photo shows an enlarged lymph node cytology. What is your diagnosis?

A) Lymphoma.
B) Reactive ganglion.
C) Metastatic ganglion.
D) The sample is not diagnostic.

11. Feline leukaemia virus (FeLV) has different genetic variants that are associated with different pathologies. Which of the following variants is associated with lymphoproliferative diseases such as leukaemia or lymphoma?

A) A.
B) B.
C) C.
D) T.

12. Injection site associated sarcoma was initially associated with adjuvant vaccines. However:

A) No component of the vaccine (including adjuvant), formulation or specific brand, has been definitively related to tumour development.
B) No vaccine has zero risk of producing sarcoma.
C) A and B are incorrect.
D) A and B are correct.

13. Large granular lymphocyte lymphoma (LGL) is a subtype of lymphoma that:

A) Is associated with a slow clinical course.
B) Responds well to chemotherapy.
C) Has a mean survival time of two months.
D) Is diagnosed only by immunophenotype.

14. In cats with lymphoma, it is difficult to provide a prognosis before starting treatment. Once treatment is started, which of the following is associated with longer survival:
A) Minimal weight loss during treatment.
B) Achieve partial remission.
C) Achieve full remission.
D) None of the above.

15. In cats with fibrosarcoma, the primary tumour is the reason for the initial consultation when detected by the owner. When it comes to pulmonary metastases, this tumour:
A) Never presents pulmonary metastases at the time of diagnosis.
B) The risk is low (<10%) initially but increases after successive surgeries.
C) 30% of cases have pulmonary metastasis at the time of diagnosis.
D) The risk is low (<10%) initially and does not increase after successive surgeries.

Answers

1. C	7. A	13. D
2. D	8. D	14. C
3. B	9. B	15. B
4. B	10. C	
5. D	11. B	
6. A	12. D	

11

Endocrinology

Dolores Pérez Alenza

Contents

Feline diabetes mellitus

The **prevalence of diabetes mellitus (DM) in the cat is around 0.4%–1.24%** and rising. It is important to recognize there are different types of feline diabetes because the treatment, progression, and outlook for remission vary depending on type.

- **Type I or insulin-dependent diabetes** occurs due to immune mediated destruction of pancreatic ß cells, is characterized by the inability to produce insulin and the condition is irreversible.
- **Type II diabetes** is characterized by insulin resistance giving rise to hyperglycaemia, although initially there is some capacity for insulin secretion which then becomes exhausted. This is the **most frequent form of diabetes in both humans and felines**, and responsible for 80% of cases in the latter. A sedentary lifestyle and carbohydrate rich diet favours obesity, which is one of the most important factors for its development.
  The aetiology of Type II DM is multifactorial including:
  - **Genetic factors**: the melanocortin receptor gene is implicated, with higher incidence is certain breeds such as the Maine Coon, Russian Blue, Siamese, and Norwegian Forest Cat.
  - Age.
  - Gender: neutered male cats are over-represented.
  - **Obesity**: low adiponectin levels.
  - Lifestyle: such as indoor or inactive cats.
  - **Carbohydrate rich diets**.
  - Amyloid deposits in the pancreatic islets.
  - **Factors causing insulin resistance** such as infection or glucocorticoids.
  - Although Type II DM may or may not be insulin-dependent, treatment with insulin and dietary change is essential. **When diagnosed and treated early, Type II DM may be reversible.**
- **Type III or secondary diabetes** is usually insulin dependent and is the result of triggering factors such as:
  - Diseases such as pancreatitis, acromegaly, or hyperadrenocorticism (HAC).
  - Administration of medications, especially glucocorticoids or progestins.

Removal or correction of the trigger may lead to reversal of Type III diabetes.

In addition, diabetes may be considered uncomplicated or complicated depending on the clinical presentation and severity.

Uncomplicated diabetes is typified by classic clinical signs of:

- polydipsia
- polyuria
- polyphagia
- weight loss
- hyperglycaemia
- glycosuria.

There may be ketones in the blood and urine, but the patient remains compensated and can be treated at home. These cats are eating and drinking freely, are not dehydrated, and do not present with vomiting, diarrhoea, or anorexia.

In **complicated diabetes** the patient is unwell, decompensated, and requires hospitalization for emergency intravenous fluid therapy, electrolyte replacement, and regular insulin administration. On presentation this patient is typically dehydrated, anorexic, vomiting, and ketotic, with moderate to severe ketonuria which is indicative of diabetic ketoacidosis. Mental status is disminished even stupor or comma.

Diagnosis of diabetes

The **clinical signs** of diabetes (polyuria, polydipsia, polyphagia, and weight loss) should raise a **suspicion of diabetes as a differential diagnosis.** This is confirmed by the presence of **persistent hyperglycaemia and glycosuria.**

Fasting blood glucose levels greater than or equal to 180 mg/dl are compatible with diabetes mellitus, although stress hyperglycaemia should always be ruled out. In true cases, **early diagnosis and treatment with insulin and diet adjustment increases the chances of remission**.

In the early stages of type II diabetes, the symptoms may be mild and can go unnoticed.

Diagnosis can then be complicated by stress hyperglycaemia (from concurrent illness). The presence of hyperglycaemia greater 216 mg/dl in a sick cat should be considered as stress hyperglycaemia and if this persists for more than 4–6 hours, treated with low doses of insulin (0.1–0.2 IU/kg/12 h) and progression monitored.

If a cat does not show clinical signs of diabetes but has hyperglycaemia, measurement of **fructosamine levels** and checking for ketonuria/glycosuria helps to differentiate diabetes from stress hyperglycaemia.

A fasting blood glucose level greater than or equal to 180 mg/dl is compatible with DM. However, acute clinical stress such as that experienced during the blood draw elevates blood glucose levels. As a result, a cat with fasting blood glucose levels equal to or greater than 117 mg/dl, should be re-evaluated four hours later and if blood glucose levels remain above 117 mg/dl, re-assessed in 24 hours as the patient is potentially diabetic.

Treatment of diabetes

The goals of treating uncomplicated feline diabetes are:

- **Eliminate clinical signs** (polyuria, polydipsia, polyphagia and weight loss).
- Avoid long-term complications (ketoacidosis, peripheral neuropathy).
- **Control risk factors** that cause insulin resistance and favour the disease (obesity, inactivity, chronic infections, treatment with corticosteroids).
- Avoid the development of hypoglycaemia.

However, the main objective in newly diagnosed type II or type III diabetes (due to pancreatitis or secondary to corticosteroid therapy) is disease **remission (the reversal of the hyperglycaemic cat to a normoglycaemic state without the permanent administration of insulin or glucose-lowering medications**). The main factor to achieve remission is prompt reduction of glucotoxicity, which protects beta cells from further damage so they are able to maintain normal blood glucose levels. This is why it is important to start treatment with insulin as soon as possible.

Key to achieving this goal is **dietary modification, insulin administration, exercise, and treatment of underlying diseases.** To this end good communication and collaboration with the owner is essential.

Exercise

In the type II diabetic cat, **exercise plays a fundamental role** as it helps to reduce insulin resistance. Encourage activity by dividing the daily food allowance into small amounts which are then placed around the home. Owner engagement in play with the cat is also important. Bored, solitary indoor cats are shown to be less active and are predisposed to obesity and diabetes.

Diet

Diet is an important factor in achieving good glycaemic control and remission of disease. The ideal diet aims to achieve and **maintain an ideal body weight** and minimize postprandial hyperglycaemia. The most suitable diet for the diabetic cat is one **low in carbohydrates and high in protein**, since cats are considered obligate carnivores and better adapted to metabolize diets rich in protein. High carbohydrate diets can exacerbate hyperglycaemia and loss of muscle mass, while low carbohydrate and protein rich diets help prevent hyperglycaemia and maintain muscle mass.

The benefits of high protein diets are most evident in cats with incipient diabetes, in which the ability to secrete insulin is conserved. The use of high protein diets increases the probability of remission of diabetes by up to 30–50% in cats. In animals with long-standing diabetes, remission is less likely, but even so, these diets favour the regulation of diabetes. **When switching cats already receiving insulin to this diet, reducing the dose of insulin by 25–50% is recommended** as their insulin needs are expected to decrease.

Diets low in carbohydrates and rich in protein are also recommended in diabetic cats with a normal or low body weight since, depending on the intake, they can promote normalization of body weight.

High fibre, low fat diets (such as indicated for diabetic dogs) have a **limited role** in the management of cats. They are currently only recommended for use in diabetic cats with concurrent fibre-responsive conditions such as constipation, or in those where a high protein diet is contraindicated, such as cats with kidney disease.

Feeding time should coincide with both insulin injections, with the daily ration divided into two doses and given before insulin is administered. For cats accustomed to grazing or ad lib feeding, once at least half the daily ration is consumed then the first dose of insulin is administered, and the remaining food left to be consumed ad libitum. **If the cat fails to eat, the owner must be warned to administer a third or half the dose of insulin,** since a full dose risks hypoglycaemia.

Oral hypoglycaemic agents

Oral hypoglycaemic drugs (e.g. sulphonylureas) stimulate pancreatic insulin secretion. Some cats with uncomplicated type II diabetes mellitus (due to obesity and in the absence of ketone bodies) can be controlled with a low carbohydrate diet and oral hypoglycaemic drugs. However, their **use is not recommended in the long term**, since they can favour the formation of amyloid deposits in the pancreas and depletion of ß cells.

In general, their use is not recommended except in cases where the owner refuses insulin treatment and is considering euthanasia.

The most widely used sulphonyl urea in cats is glipizide and should always be administered with an appropriate diet. Coming soon, a sodium-glucose cotransporter inhibitor 2 (SGLT2) will be available for its use in type II diabetic cats.

Other treatments

Recently, the use of incretins, (gastrointestinal hormones which increase the release of insulin) have been used together with insulin and diet to improve control of DM and cases of remission been described.

Insulin

Although diet is an important factor in achieving remission, insulin administration as soon as possible after diagnosis of diabetes and careful monitoring increases the chances of remission. Also, if **diabetes becomes chronic it becomes insulin dependent and administration is essential.**

There are different types of insulins which vary depending on the duration of action and origin (human, bovine, porcine):

- **Regular insulin** is the fastest acting, shortest and most potent. It is used in complicated patients (ketoacidosis) and can be used intramuscularly or intravenously.
- **Potent, fast-acting insulin analogues** such as lispro, aspart, or glulisine insulins can be used in complicated patients (ketoacidosis).
- **Intermediate-acting insulins (NPH)** have a longer action, although this duration is variable (4–14 hours) and is usually shorter in cats than in dogs.
- **Slow-acting (slow, PZI) insulins** and **long-acting human insulin analogues (glargine, detemir).** are preferable in cats, since the duration after subcutaneous administration is longer. In cats, the duration of action of slow acting insulin is 8–10 h, that of PZI from 13–24 h and that of glargine/detemir 12 up to > 24 h.

The similarity to insulin from the cat depends on the species of origin, with the most similar being bovine, since more amino acids differ in human and porcine insulins. However, both human and porcine insulin analogues are effective in the diabetic cat.

PZI insulin of human origin is highly effective in the management of uncomplicated feline diabetes. In Spain, since 2016, this has been marketed as ProZinc®, Boehringer, and is licensed for use in both cats and dogs. In the UK, slow-acting insulin of porcine origin, Caninsulin® MSD is registered for veterinary use in both cats and dogs.

Recently, various studies showed efficacy of human insulin analogues (especially glargine and to a lesser extent detemir) at achieving prolonged and predictable absorption along with a long duration of action.

For uncomplicated cases of feline diabetes, initial treatment includes switching to a low carbohydrate, high protein diet and starting a low dose insulin. The latter should be prescribed under the cascade, with licensed products chosen in the first instance. The individual veterinarian remains responsible for choosing an appropriate product as licensed in their country. The author uses ProZinc®, Lantus® (glargine).

A conservative dose should be used to start with, which is adjusted gradually as needed to avoid hypoglycaemia.

Dosage regime 1

- 1 IU/cat every 12 hours for cats under 4 kg BW
- 1.5 – 2 IU/cat every 12 hours for cats over 4 kg BW

Or Preferible regimen

- 0.2 – 0.5 IU/kg every 12 hours

In cats with recent onset diabetes, a change of diet may promote diabetes remission and so it is important to monitor treatment well and actively involve the owner. In addition, owners must be taught **how to correctly handle and store insulin**, administer subcutaneous injections, read urine test strips for glycosuria and ketones, and how to recognize and treat hypoglycaemic episodes.

It should be noted that Caninsulin® and ProZinc® insulins are marketed at 40 IU/ml, while human insulins are all 100 IU/ml, so in order to avoid confusion U100 syringes should not be used. Instead, Caninsulin® or ProZinc® U40 units' syringes must be used.

After subcutaneous injection, **glargine insulin (Lantus®)** forms micro precipitates which give rise to a slow, continuous absorption, and so glargine should not be diluted as this alters the absorption rate. In normal cats, its **duration of action is about 23 hours**, however, a better effect is obtained using **0.25 IU/kg/12 hours** rather than using 0.5 IU/kg/24 hours, hence the recommendation for 12-hourly administration.

With respect to the dosage of detemir insulin:

- Cats can need a 30% lower dose of detemir than glargine or other types of insulin.
- 0.5 IU/kg if blood glucose is above 360 mg/dl.
- 0.25 IU/kg if it is lower than <360 mg/dl.

Various studies indicate that the remission percentage is high (60–80%) and similar when either glargine, detemir, PZI or slow-acting insulin are used in combination with a provisional low carbohydrate diet. Ultimately, the most important factor in achieving remission is not the type of insulin but starting insulin treatment promptly and achieving good glycaemic control as soon as possible.

Monitoring the diabetic cat

Newly diagnosed cats on treatment should be **monitored weekly** and then every 1–30 days until remission or stabilization occurs. In these initial check-ups, blood glucose curves should be performed to establish the efficacy, duration of effect and whether or not the insulin dose is adequate.

The owner must monitor the clinical response (changes in thirst, urination, and activity levels) and **check for glucose and ketones in the urine, initially once a day**. The veterinarian should adjust the insulin dose depending on on-going glycosuria and clinical response to treatment. The **agreed dose should be given for at least four to seven days** before it is considered inadequate. If treatment is started with a low dose of insulin 0.2 IU/kg, in most cases this needs increasing by 10–25% of the previous dose. **Adequate control is finally achieved in many cats with a dose of 0.5–1.0 IU/kg insulin.**

When performing blood glucose curves, **portable glucometers specifically designed for veterinary use** should be used (AlphaTrack®, Zoetis; Glucalea®, Wellion). However, the use of continuous blood glucose monitors is becoming more common, among which the Free Style® machine by Abbott stands out due to its ease of use. This machine comes with sensors which are easily applied and last for 12 to 14 days.

It is useful to **measure fructosamine levels at monthly checkups**, since this can help guide treatment adjustments, along with clinical signs and glucosuria.

Poor control of disease is indicated by:

- Persistence of clinical signs e.g., polydipsia, polyuria.
- Blood glucose levels are elevated above 250 mg/dl at any time of the day.
- Above 150 mg/dl between 6–8 h after insulin administration (nadir: the lowest blood glucose level through the curve).
- The levels of fructosamine are elevated (> 450 mmol/l).
- Persistent glycosuria (especially if high doses of insulin are already being administered > 0.7–1 IU/kg).

In the face of poor control of the disease **the patient should be rechecked for concurrent diseases which cause insulin resistance.** Check that the owner is carrying out the treatment properly (e.g., correct diet, timings, insulin and its administration).

Blood glucose curves

Blood glucose curves can be performed at home or at the practice. In the cat, doing them at **home is recommended** as the animal is less stressed, and the results more reliable. Veterinary medicine glucometers, which require a minimal amount of blood, can be used to measure blood glucose. The owner is taught to obtain a **drop of blood** from various areas of the body such as the **ear margin or foot pad.** These glucometers have a margin of measurement error which must be checked and taken into account, for this reason the use of veterinary glucometers (Glucocalea®, Alphatrak®) is preferable.

Continuous glucose monitors are now available, which are placed under the skin and are very useful for performing curves in the practice or at home. **Glucose curve results can be affected by stress and loss of appetite**, therefore, if the cat does not eat its entire ration the results are not valid. Although these problems can be minimized with good management, these glucose curves should be interpreted with caution because there is a high variability in the results of the curves carried out on two consecutive days in the same animal under the same conditions.

A blood glucose curve is performed by **measuring blood glucose every two hours for 12 hours,** whilst maintaining the usual diet and insulin injections. If blood glucose is <90 mg/dl at any time, blood glucose levels should be measured hourly. **Blood glucose levels should remain between 90 and 250 mg/dl for at least 80–90% of the interval between two insulin injections.** The glucose nadir (lowest blood glucose level) indicates whether the insulin dose is adequate and should lie between 90 and 150 mg/dl. If the nadir is below 90 mg/dl there is a risk of rebound hyperglycaemia (Somogyi effect) secondary to hypoglycaemia. The **Somogyi effect subsequently causes severe hyperglycaemia**, which can be confused with a low insulin dose or with insulin resistance, if hypoglycaemia was not seen previously (Figure 1). In this case the insulin dose should be reduced.

A glucose nadir above 150 mg/dl may be due to an insufficient dose or insulin resistance. If the insulin dose is low (<0.5 IU/kg) it should be increased by intervals of 0.5–1 IU. If the dose is high (> 1–1.5 IU/kg per dose),

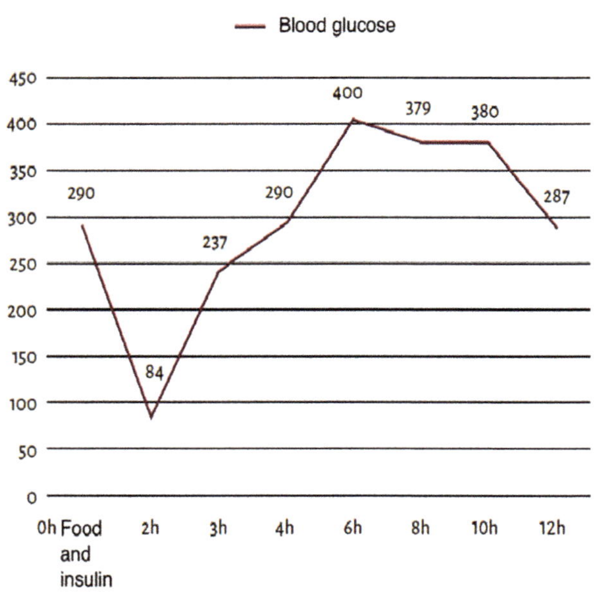

Figure 1. Blood glucose curve showing the Somogyi effect in a Common European neutered female cat being treated with glargine at a dose of 4 IU/12 h.

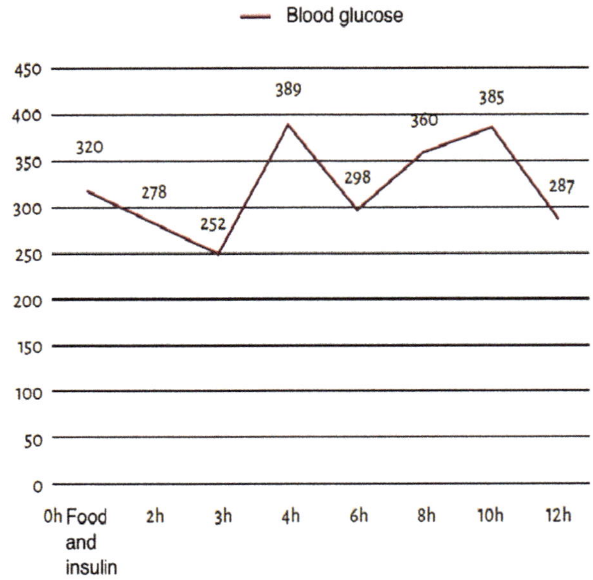

Figure 2. Blood glucose curve showing insulin resistance in a Siamese castrated male cat being treated with glargine at a dose of 7 IU/12 h.

this is generally considered insulin resistance, given the patient receives unusually high doses (Figure 2). This occurs for various reasons such as concurrent diseases/disorders, obesity, infections (oral, urinary), administration of progestins and/or glucocorticoids, hyperadrenocorticism (HAC), kidney disease, pancreatitis, heart disease, liver disease, neoplasia, acromegaly (excess hormone growth), hyperthyroidism and, finally, the existence of anti-insulin antibodies. **HAC is less frequent than in the dog and in most feline cases tends to cause insulin-resistant diabetes mellitus.**

Disease remission

It should be remembered that in **60–80% of cats with recently diagnosed diabetes, remission can be achieved.** That is, insulin administration is no longer necessary, however keeping these cats on a diet low in carbohydrates and avoiding factors that produce insulin resistance (obesity, corticosteroids, infections) is necessary.

For cats receiving an appropriate diet and insulin, remission can occur within one to nine months of the commencement of treatment and is most likely in the first six months but may happen up to two years after diagnosis. Therefore, it is important the check diabetic cats periodically. The sooner treatment is started after diagnosis and adequate glycaemic control achieved, the more likely remission is.

The start of remission is typified by a reduction in polyuria, polydipsia, a slight increase in weight, negative glycosuria for several days, and fructosamine levels below 200–250 mmol/l.

Insulin dose should be progressively reduced (by 0.5–1 IU) and reviewed weekly, until treatment is withdrawn and there is no subsequent hyperglycaemia or glycosuria. Before discontinuing insulin treatment completely, administration can be reduced to every 24 hours and a blood glucose curve performed to identify the nadir and duration of effect of insulin.

Complicated diabetes mellitus: diabetic ketoacidosis and hyperglycaemic hyperosmolar syndrome

Cats with decompensated diabetes (diabetic ketoacidosis DKA or hyperglycaemic- hyperosmolar syndrome) require hospitalization and different management to uncomplicated diabetic cats.

Diagnosis

Complicated diabetes is suspected with a history of anorexia, vomiting, diarrhoea, weakness, and general deterioration; and with physical findings such as dehydration, a prolonged CRT, reduced consciousness, weakness, and hypo or hyperthermia. Such cases are more common in previously undiagnosed cases that are not receiving insulin therapy, although it can occur in poorly controlled diabetics on treatment, especially those with concurrent disease.

In cases of complicated diabetes, the necessary **diagnostic tests include a complete blood count, biochemistry including electrolytes, urinalysis, urine culture, and abdominal ultrasound.** Ketosis can be confirmed indirectly by the use of ketonuria tests strips, which detect acetone. However, **a negative urine result does not rule out ketosis**, since the main ketone body in the bloodstream is β OH butyrate, which is not detected by test strips. The fastest way to detect levels of β OH butyrate in plasma or whole blood is by means of test strips in specialised glucometers.

Hyperglycaemic hyperosmolar syndrome presents with the same clinical and laboratory findings (hyperglycaemia, glycosuria) but without ketosis or ketoacidosis. It is, like DKA, an emergency which requires the same treatment with the exception that acidosis is not as severe. In these cats, insulin administration should be performed at low doses and reduction of blood glucose levels should be even slower than in those with DKA.

Treatment

In the first instance the following should be addressed:

- Restore blood volume and electrolytes.
- Reduce metabolic acidosis.
- Block the production of ketone bodies.
- Achieve stable and close to normal blood glucose levels.

These objectives must be met slowly and progressively, with careful monitoring from the start since fluid therapy, electrolytes, and insulin doses will require modification during the hospitalization period.

Recovery of blood volume

Fluid therapy reduces glucose levels and plasma osmolality and improves perfusion, mainly of the kidney and should be started immediately. The fluid of choice is an isotonic crystalloid such as **sodium chloride (0.9% NaCl), PlasmaLyte 148® or Isofundin®**, or Lactated Ringer's solution, although if liver function is compromised, the former is preferable. Initially, hypotonic solutions are not indicated (for example, 0.45% NaCl), unless hypernatraemia and hyperchloraemia occur after several hours of treatment.

The 24-hour fluid therapy volume is calculated taking into consideration the patient's percentage of dehydration, maintenance needs, and abnormal fluid losses. If the animal is extremely dehydrated (8–12%), approximately half of the dehydration deficit should be administered in the first two to four hours. To calculate these needs, the formula described in Box 1. is used.

Box 1. Calculation of fluid-therapy volume in cats with DKA.

Volume (ml/24 h) =
Percentage of dehydration* × weight (kg) × 10
+
Maintenance (50–70 ml/kg)
+
Additional losses (vomiting, diarrhoea)

* Mild dehydration: 2–5%, moderate: 6–9%, severe ≥10%

Fluid volume is adjusted daily based on monitoring of the cat. Initial fluid therapy should be maintained until blood glucose levels reach 250–300 mg/dl; at which time it should be switched to fluid therapy with 2.5–5% dextrose.

Correct the electrolyte imbalance

Hypokalaemia

The next objective is to correct the electrolyte imbalance, in particular hypokalaemia (K^+ <2 mEq/l). In cats with concurrent diseases such as kidney disease, gastroenteritis with severe diarrhoea, or severe liver disease this can be very important. For this, potassium chloride (KCl) is used, available in vials (2 mEq/ml) (Table 1). Potassium supplements are adjusted daily, depending on plasma levels (6–8 h).

Table 1. Potassium administration in cats with diabetic ketoacidosis.

Serum potassium (mEg/l)	mEg/l KCl to be added per litre of fluid therapy
3.5–5	20
3.0–3.4	30
2.5–2.9	40
2.0–2.4	60
<2.0	80

Hypophosphatemia

Another frequent electrolyte deficit is hypophosphataemia. In the first 24 hours of hospitalization, a serious decrease in phosphorus can occur, which is generally pre-existing but not reflected in serum levels. If **severe muscle weakness, ataxia, tremors, respiratory failure, or haemolytic anaemia are seen**, and whenever phosphorus levels are below 1.5 mg/dl, then levels should be supplemented with potassium phosphate (0.01 to 0.03 mmol phosphate/kg/h), by adding it to fluid therapy (NaCl 0.9%).

In cats with severe hypophosphataemia (<1 mg/dl), potassium phosphate can be administered at higher doses (0.12–0.2 mmol phosphate/kg/h). Two to four administrations of potassium phosphate every six hours should raise serum phosphorus concentrations above 2.5 mg/dl. Phosphorus should not be administered in animals with hypercalcaemia, hyperphosphataemia, or oliguria.

Hypomagnesaemia

Hypomagnesaemia occurs especially when deficits in phosphorus and other electrolytes are not corrected adequately. Mild hypomagnesaemia is treated with replacement magnesium-containing isotonic fluid therapy (e.g., Plasma-Lyte 148® or Isofundin®). If severe (serum magnesium <0.4 mmol/l [1.2 mg/dl]), a magnesium sulphate infusion can be prepared by adding an initial dose of 0.3–0.5 mmol/l/day (0.75–1–1 mEq/kg/day) to a dextrose fluid in water, as a continuous infusion over 24 hours and then reducing this dose to 50% over the following three to five days.

Glycaemic control

Insulin administration should be commenced once the cat is receiving fluid therapy. **The insulin of choice is fast-acting, powerful and short-lived,** that is, crystalline regular type insulin (Actrapid®, Humulin regular®, Humaplus regular®). Other alternatives are lispro insulin (Humalog® 200 IU/ml) and aspart insulin (Novorapid®), which are effective in cats with DKA. Recently, it has been described that in cats treated with insulin within six hours of hospital admission, a better clinical response is achieved than those where insulin administration begins after six hours.

Longer-acting insulins (NPH, slow-acting, PZI, glargine) are not initially indicated in cats with DKA, although they can be used when the animal is compensated, well hydrated, does not vomit, or have diarrhoea, and is eating. However, two retrospective studies indicate that **glargine administration may be effective in cats with DKA**.

Insulin can be administered intramuscularly (IM), intravenously (IV), or subcutaneously (SC). **Initially, IM or IV routes should be used,** and the SC route should only be used after rehydrating the animal. The recommended doses in all the protocols described are low doses, to avoid sudden drops in blood glucose which could cause cerebral oedema.

Glycaemia should initially be checked every hour. The ideal decrease is 50 to 100 mg/dl per hour and, when reaching adequate levels (250–300 mg/dl), administration of insulin should continue, as otherwise lipolysis and the production of ketone bodies will continue. During the first four to six hours, glucose levels must be above 300 mg/dl so that cerebral oedema does not occur. When plasma glucose reaches 250–300 mg/dl, fluid therapy should be modified and a solution containing 2.5–5% dextrose mixed with crystalloid fluids (0.9% or 0.45% NaCl (PlasmaLyte 148® or Isofundin®) should be administered depending on electrolyte levels and insulin administration continued.

If blood glucose falls below 150 mg/dl, insulin should be discontinued and administration of the fluid containing dextrose continued. If blood glucose is less than 100 mg/dl, especially if there are clinical signs of hypoglycaemia, an IV bolus of 50% dextrose solution (0.5–1.0 ml/kg) should be administered, and fluid therapy should be continued thereafter with crystalloid fluids and 2.5% dextrose.

One of the most widely used protocols is the intermittent administration of regular IM insulin, which is started at a low dose (0.1–0.2 IU/kg) and continues with injections of 0.1 IU/kg every hour, monitoring blood glucose every one to two hours, until it reaches 300 mg/dl. Subsequently, insulin is administered SC (every 6–8 h) or IM if the cat is not yet hydrated (every 4–6 h) at a dose of 0.1 to 0.3 IU/kg depending on blood glucose, continuing fluid therapy with a 2.5–5% dextrose solution.

The author and many other authors recommend continuous **low-dose IV insulin infusion** (0.05–0.1 IU/kg/h) as the protocol of choice, especially in cats with severe DKA. This can be prepared by adding 5 IU of regular insulin to 500 ml of crystalloid fluids, to obtain a solution in which 1 ml contains 0.01 IU of insulin. It is administered by a different route to that of fluid therapy and with an infusion pump, to ensure continuous insulin administration. Blood glucose should be checked every hour and when it reaches 250–300 mg/dl the IV insulin infusion should be continued (0.05 IU/kg/h), adding a 2.5–5% dextrose solution to fluid therapy, as described above.

Various studies have been published with two different protocols in cats with DKA: one carried out in 15 patients, in which intermittent IM glargine was administered (with a frequency of between every 2–22 hours) (1–2 IU) combined with SC glargine (1–3 IU), and a good response was obtained in all cases. The other study indicates that administration of glargine SC every 12 hours combined with intermittent regular IM insulin is even more effective than a continuous IV infusion of regular insulin. More studies are needed to confirm these results.

Correct metabolic acidosis

Another **treatment goal is to correct metabolic acidosis**; in most cases fluid therapy and insulin are sufficient to achieve this. In general, **if the plasma bicarbonate concentration is 12 mEq/l or higher, bicarbonate is not recommended** as it can aggravate hypokalaemia, cause sodium overload, and rebound alkalosis. However, if bicarbonate in the blood is ≤11 mEq/l or if the blood pH is less than 7.3, especially if these levels do not improve in the first 8–12 hours, administration of bicarbonate should be undertaken with caution. For this, 1 molar $NaHCO_3$ solutions are used (at 8.4%, 1 mEq/ml) or 1/6 molar (at 1.4%, 1 mEq/6 ml), over one to two hours according to the following formula:

MEq sodium bicarbonate IV = weight (kg) × 0.3 × [15-patient bicarbonate]

Concurrent disease

DKA is often associated with the presence of another disease or concurrent conditions, with the most frequent reasons being infections especially urinary tract, oral cavity, skin and respiratory infections etc. **Broad-spectrum antibiotic therapy** should be used whenever there is a left shift in the leukogram or there are signs of infection, fever, or severe gastrointestinal clinical signs, considering the rational use of antibiotic therapies.

Other **common complications are pancreatitis, triaditis, and hepatic lipidosis**. When pancreatitis is suspected, analgesics (such as butorphanol), antiemetics (maropitant, chlorpromazine, ondansetron), and proton pump inhibitors (omeprazole) should be administered and feeding attempted as soon as possible, to stimulate pancreatic secretion and stop hepatic lipidosis caused by fasting. Therefore, if the cat is not vomiting, force feeding with a low fat and highly digestible diet should be considered and, if this is not possible, a nasoesophageal tube or an oesophagostomy, gastrotomy or enterotomy tube placed.

When **kidney disease is suspected,** the volume of fluids should be increased (without causing volume overload) and urine production (1–2 ml/kg of weight) monitored. If oliguria or anuria persists after the first few hours of treatment, the previously calculated fluid volume should be reviewed and, if everything is correct, mannitol, diuretics and/or dopamine used to force diuresis.

Monitoring

Monitoring is especially important during the first 24 hours, to allow modifications to fluid therapy, electrolyte supplements, and insulin doses. If monitoring is not performed correctly, complications can occur which may cause treatment failure and death. The most frequent complications are hypoglycaemia, hypokalaemia, cerebral oedema due to a rapid decrease in plasma glucose, hypernatraemia and hypochloraemia.

The volume and rate of fluid therapy must be adequate, since if excessive it can cause volume overload (hyperhydration, pulmonary oedema, tachypnoea, tachycardia, etc.) and if insufficient, hypoperfusion (hypoxia, persistent azotaemia, favour pancreatitis, etc.).

Clinical parameters that should be evaluated every two to four hours include mental state, degree of hydration, capillary refill time, pulse, cardiac and pulmonary auscultation, and urine production. Other clinical parameters to be monitored are temperature (every 8–12 h), weight and blood pressure (every 24 h).

The **test parameters that should be monitored** are blood glucose (every one to two hours or with a continuous blood glucose monitor), sodium, potassium, and chlorine levels (every six to eight hours) and every 24 hours blood count, plasma proteins, urea, creatinine, ALT, phosphorus and ketone bodies. Monitoring of ketone bodies should be performed by using **betahydroxy butyrate test strips on plasma**, or, failing that, with test strips that detect acetoacetic acid and acetone, which can be used with plasma or urine samples.

The **most frequent electrolyte abnormality is hypokalaemia**, therefore measuring potassium levels is key to adjusting amounts of potassium chloride supplement. Less frequent complications, but which can occur after several hours of treatment, are hypernatraemia and/or hyperchloraemia, which are corrected by modifying fluid therapy (0.45% saline). If plasma electrolyte levels cannot be monitored frequently, at least one ECG is recommended every six to eight hours.

Venous blood gases are useful for monitoring as they allow the assessment of acid base status, lactate, bicarbonate and electrolyte levels.

The **insulin doses required may vary** from the time of hospitalization until discharge with home treatment (diet and glargine, PZI or slow-acting insulin), meaning monitoring of blood glucose levels are essential, preferably continuously or if not every hour, for at least the first 12 hours, and every two to four hours thereafter until discharge, depending on the route of insulin administration.

In addition to these parameters, all those that are abnormal should be monitored, for example, changes on the complete blood count and azotaemia should be evaluated every 24 hours and elevations of liver enzymes every 24–48 hours.

Food should be introduced orally as soon as possible in a progressive manner. When the cat is hydrated, does not vomit, accepts food (orally or via feeding tube), and ketosis has subsided, it should be **switched to glargine, PZI or slow-acting insulin every 12 hours at an initial dose of 0.2–0.3 IU/kg/12 h**. Four hours before this insulin is administered, regular insulin administration should be discontinued. During the first 12 hours of long-acting insulin administration, performing a blood glucose curve is advisable to adjust the slow-acting insulin dose if necessary. After a recently diagnosed episode of DKA in cats, DM can subside, so animals should be re-assessed weekly, and treatment adjusted.

Feline acromegaly

Acromegaly, or hypersomatotropism, is the syndrome caused by chronic excess growth hormone (GH), and in cats is caused by a pituitary adenoma. The excess of GH causes increased levels of a growth factor similar to insulin-I (IGF-I); chronic excess levels of GH and IGF-I cause the clinical signs of acromegaly.

Although considered a rare disease, current studies indicate it is more common than previously thought. In one study, 32% of diabetic cats had IGF-I levels compatible with acromegaly (> 1,000 ng/ml) and a diagnosis of hypersomatotropism subsequently confirmed in 94%. In other studies, 26% of poorly controlled diabetic cats were found to have IGF-I levels consistent with acromegaly. A subsequent study conducted with a larger number of animals and a four-year follow-up indicates a prevalence of acromegaly in diabetic cats of 26.4%. **Therefore, investigating the possible presence of acromegaly is recommended in all poorly controlled diabetic cats and those that require high doses of insulin.**

Although the main consequence of excess GH is marked insulin resistance, which causes the onset of diabetes, the anabolic effects of excess GH cause tissue overgrowth which causes weight gain, increased body size, and organomegaly. Clinical diagnosis should be confirmed with hormonal and imaging tests to verify the presence of a pituitary tumour.

Clinical diagnosis

Feline acromegaly is more frequent in **males and geriatric adults** (mean age ten years, range 4 to 17 years) but there is no breed predisposition. The symptoms develop slowly, so changes are progressive, and, in some cases, the clinical signs not evident.

The clinical signs are characterized by a slow and progressive increase in the size of organs (abdominal and thoracic), weight gain, an **increase in the size of extremities and face,** mandibular protrusion, increased interdental space, and in the majority of cases diabetes mellitus with marked insulin resistance (> 10 IU per dose) (Figure 2).

In some cases, hypertrophy occurs of the soft tissues of the oropharynx, resulting **in snoring, respiratory stridor, and even dyspnoea.** The most common signs are the presence of polydipsia, polyuria, polyphagia and weight gain in a poorly controlled diabetic cat receiving high doses of insulin. In fact, if a **poorly controlled diabetic cat continues to gain weight despite receiving high doses of insulin, an important differential diagnosis is acromegaly.**

Clinical neurological signs such as depression, lethargy, and although rare, vision disturbances can occur.

In addition, cats with acromegaly may present with signs of diabetic neuropathy and lameness (Figure 3). Other complications that may occur are heart disease (hypertrophic) and glomerulopathy.

Box 2 shows the most frequent clinical signs and physical examination findings in cats with acromegaly.

Box 2. *Clinical signs and findings on physical examination in cats with acromegaly.*

Clinical signs include:

- polydipsia-polyuria
- polyphagia
- **weight gain**
- lameness
- **thickened extremities**
- **increased facial size**
- central neurological signs (lethargy, loss of vision)
- plantigrade posture.

Physical examination findings:

- **organomegaly** (kidney, liver)
- increased facial size

- inferior prognathism
- respiratory stridor
- tachypnoea
- heart murmur.

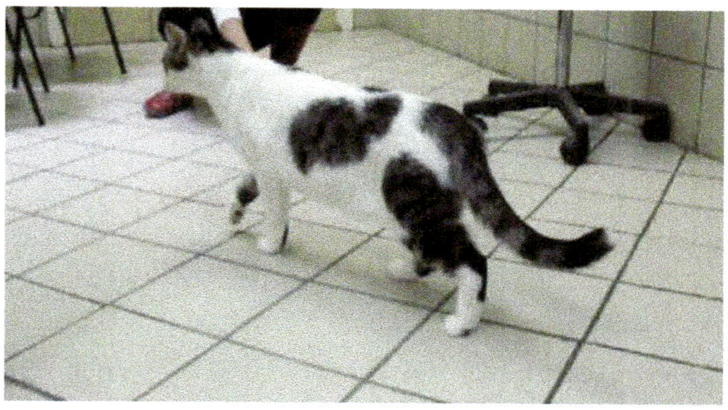

Figure 3. Posture and plantigrade gait in a Common European cat with poor control of diabetes. (Full video available at: http://publication.improveinternational.com).

Diagnosis

In the first instance, clinical signs flag a suspicion of acromegaly. In addition, hypersomatotropism should be suspected in every diabetic cat which remains poorly controlled despite receiving high doses of insulin, and in spite of this gains weight. Cats with acromegaly but without diabetes mellitus have been described, but this is much less common.

Diagnostic tests include blood tests, urinalysis, hormonal tests, and imaging (abdominal ultrasound and MRI or cranial CT). Blood pressure should be measured to assess possible hypertension.

To establish a definitive diagnosis, histological confirmation is required of a pituitary adenoma with proliferation of somatotropic cells, although this is not usually done unless a hypophysectomy is performed or on post-mortem.

The abnormalities found on laboratory tests are similar to those observed in poorly controlled diabetic cats, with the exception of hyperproteinaemia, which is significantly higher in cats with acromegaly. The most notable abnormalities are:

- azotaemia
- hyperglycaemia
- hyperproteinaemia
- hypergammaglobulinaemia
- elevation of hepatic enzymes
- hyperphosphataemia
- glucosuria and proteinuria.

Hormonal tests

The presence of hypersomatotropism can be ascertained by **measuring plasma or serum levels of GH, or serum levels of IGF-I,** where levels are correlated with those of growth hormone.

GH secretion occurs in a pulsatile manner and measurement of feline specific GH (fGH) is not yet commercially available. In a study in which fGH was measured, using an fGH cut-off value of 10 ng/ml, the diagnostic sensitivity and specificity for acromegaly was 84% and 95% respectively. However, IGF-I measurement is available and has a sensitivity of 84% and specificity of 92% so it is used more frequently.

When measuring IGF-I levels in a cat suspected of having acromegaly, the length of time of treatment with insulin must be taken into account, since the synthesis of and therefore, IGF-I levels depend on insulin levels. Therefore, in a cat with acromegaly that has not been treated with insulin, IGF-I levels may be normal, so **repeating the measurement after about six to eight weeks of treatment is recommended.** Likewise, if IGF-I levels are slightly elevated, this may be due to acromegaly or it may be due to insulin treatment, which causes slight increases in levels. In these cases, repeating the IGF-I measurement after one to two months is recommended. If the cat has a clear insulin resistance (it needs more than 1.5–2 IU of insulin/kg/every 8–12 h), carrying out diagnostic imaging tests to evaluate the pituitary is recommended.

Recently, other serum markers have been described which may be useful in diagnosing hypersomatotropism. One of these is **serum procollagen type III propeptide (PIIIP),** which is a peripheral indicator of collagen turnover. PIIIP levels greater than 8 ng/ml have been shown to be diagnostic of hypersomatotropism with a specificity and sensitivity of 100% and 75%. Another potential marker is ghrelin, an endogenous GH secretagogue receptor ligand, however, its measurement does not appear to be useful in differentiating cats with acromegaly from cats which do not suffer from the condition.

Diagnostic imaging

Definitive confirmation of the diagnosis of hypersomatotropism requires imaging techniques to **confirm the presence of a pituitary mass.** Two techniques are used: magnetic resonance imaging (MRI) (Figure 4) or computed tomography (CT); of which CT is more sensitive, but false negatives can occur with either technique. In some cases, the pituitary lesion caused by excess GH is microscopic (hyperplasia or microadenoma) and not visible unless dynamic contrast tests are performed.

Apart from the presence of a pituitary mass, other alterations may appear such as thickening of the frontal bone, the parietal bone and/or accumulation of soft tissue in the nasal cavity, the sinuses and the pharynx.

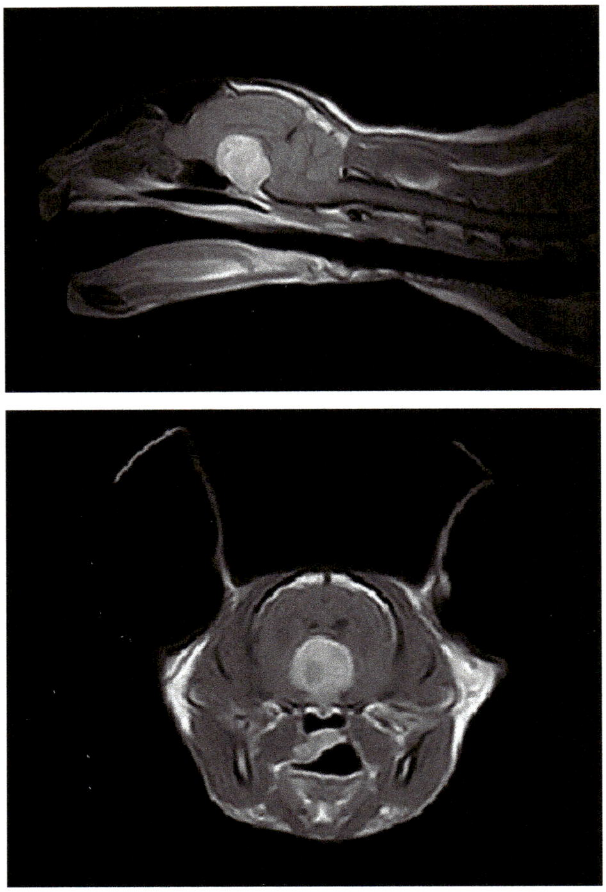

Figure 4. Sagittal (A) and transverse (B) images from MRI, from a cat with acromegaly where a large pituitary neoplasm can be seen. (Published in: Actualizacion en el diagnostico y tratamiento de acromegalia felina, Arenas Bermejo C y Pérez Alenza MD. Canis et Felis, Number 126, February 2014).

False positives may also occur, since a mass in the pituitary seen on CT or MRI may be a pituitary tumour causing pituitary HAC. Therefore, diagnostic imaging should always be performed in cats where there are both clinical and hormonal signs (IGF-I) of acromegaly.

On the other hand, abdominal ultrasound is very useful in cats with acromegaly, since it allows for evaluation of the presence of organomegaly (liver, kidneys, spleen, adrenal glands) and the possible presence of other diseases which produce insulin resistance (pancreatitis, triaditis, HAC, abdominal neoplasms, among others).

Treatment

In cats with acromegaly, **diabetes mellitus must be treated** taking into account insulin resistance caused by excessive levels of GH. These cats need high doses of insulin, a low carbohydrate diet and frequent check-ups to confirm the dose and frequency of insulin are adequate.

On the other hand, the treatment of hypersomatotropism aims to reduce excessive levels of GH (medical treatment) or **eliminate the pituitary tumour** (surgical treatment or radiotherapy). By reducing GH levels, these treatments decrease insulin needs quickly, so insulin doses should be reduced, and the cat checked periodically to adjust the dose and ensure hypoglycaemia does not occur.

Medical treatment

Somatostatin analogues (which inhibit GH synthesis) can be used to reduce GH and IGF-I levels. The most widely used is octreotide (Sandostatin®, Novartis, Switzerland) and more recently pasireotide (Signifor®, Novartis, Switzerland). The efficacy of octreotide is poor: although it has been shown that GH levels drop within 90 minutes of its administration, GH and IGF-I levels subsequently remain high and there is no clinical benefit, especially in the management of diabetes.

However, pasireotide (Signifor®, Novartis, Switzerland), has a high affinity for certain somatostatin receptors (subtypes 1, 2, 3 and 5). It is proven to reduce GH, IGF-I levels and allows better control of diabetes mellitus with lower doses of insulin without side effects. The recommended dose is 0.03 mg/kg SC BID.

Other alternatives to control excess GH are GH receptor antagonists, such as pegvisomant or dopamine agonists, such as bromocriptine or selegiline, but there are no studies in cats with acromegaly that support their efficacy. Cabergolin efficacy remains controversial.

Surgical treatment

Hypophysectomy is the treatment of choice in people with acromegaly. In veterinary medicine, its availability is limited to certain centres in Europe, the United States and Japan, since it requires extensive experience in microsurgery, although more and more centres now offer it.

With adequate experience and postoperative intensive care, results are very good with remission of diabetes described in four out of five cats after hypophysectomy, plus the reduction of GH and IGF-I levels.

The surgical procedure consists of **access through the soft palate**, to expose the sphenoid bone and the pituitary fossa. Postoperatively the procedure requires intensive care (clinical monitoring, blood pressure and tests, including electrolyte levels) and the administration of glucocorticoids (prednisone or hydrocortisone), thyroxine, desmopressin (as a replacement for antidiuretic hormone). The need for administration of thyroxine and prednisone is usually permanent, whereas desmopressin can be withdrawn after a few weeks.

Hypophyseal radiotherapy

As an alternative to hypophysectomy, **pituitary radiotherapy**, is a definitive treatment widely used in cats with acromegaly.

Several pituitary radiotherapy protocols have been described, using total doses between 1,500 and 4,500 cGy, divided over several weeks. In general, pituitary radiotherapy improves neurological symptoms, decreases insulin needs, and in some cases (less frequently than with hypophysectomy), remission of diabetes is achieved in cats with acromegaly.

The drawbacks of radiation therapy are the high cost, the need for frequent anaesthesia, and long-term side effects. **Another type of radiotherapy, the so-called gamma-knife** or radiosurgery, allows administration of the necessary radiotherapy dose in a single administration. It has been available for years in human medicine and more recently at some veterinary centres, and is an alternative to fractionated radiotherapy, with fewer side effects, requiring only one anaesthetic. Recent studies demonstrate that the use of radiosurgery leads to improved survival times and control of diabetes than other treatments.

There are various studies which use **fractionated radiotherapy** in cats with acromegaly, employing protocols which use from 2.7 to 4 Gy/fraction, administering a total of 36–54 Gy. In all of these improvements in neurological signs, better control and even remission of diabetes is described.

Prognosis

Despite insulin resistance and the effects of excess GH and IGF-I, the **quality of life of cats with acromegaly only deteriorates slowly**. Periodic review of these animals is important to verify their quality of life is adequate. Questionnaires can be used for the owner to fill out periodically.

If radiotherapy is available or performing a hypophysectomy is an option, the prognosis is much better, and remission of diabetes can be achieved. Somatostatin analogues used so far do not show good results. However, the use of pasireotide has shown promising results and allows control of the disease, improving prognosis in these cats. Currently the only disadvantage is the high cost.

Feline hyperthyroidism

In recent decades, **feline hyperthyroidism has become the most commonly diagnosed endocrinopathy** in cats and, along with kidney disease, one of the two most important diseases in geriatric felines. The first case was described in 1979, making it a relatively recent disease with a rapid rise in prevalence. The explanations for this increase include:

- A better knowledge of the disease and confirmation of its diagnosis.
- An increase in the life expectancy of cats, due to improved health conditions which have caused the population of geriatric cats to increase.
- A better description of cases.
- A true increase in the prevalence of the disease.

It seems unlikely hyperthyroidism went unnoticed before the 80's, so it is likely the increased incidence today is due to a true increase in prevalence. In the United States, the prevalence of hyperthyroidism in 1978–82 was documented as 0.61 cases per 1,000 patients, while between 1993–1997 it was 29.6 cases per 1,000 patients.

Another surprising fact is the **disparate frequency of disease according to geographical area**. In countries such as the United States, United Kingdom, Netherlands, Germany, and Canada the prevalence is very high (11–25%), while in others such as Spain, Japan, and Scandinavian countries, the prevalence is lower (1.5% in Spain, 8.9% in Japan), albeit rising. However, recent studies in Spain indicate a prevalence of 10% although the feline population is lower in this country than in the first group that has been discussed.

Aetiology and risk factors

The aetiology of this disease is complex and multifactorial. In 98% of cases, it is caused by **functional adenomatous hyperplasia of the thyroid gland**, either bilateral (70%) or unilateral (30%). Only in 2% of cases is hyperthryoidism due to a malignant tumour of the gland. Over time, **feline adenomatous hyperplasia may become malignant,** and the risk increases as the animal ages.

Histologically and clinically the disease is similar to toxic nodular goitre in people. However, involvement of both lobes may indicate a "circulating" aetiological agent is the cause, as with Graves' disease in humans (the most common cause of hyperthyroidism). However, although antibodies (thyroid stimulants) have been found in hyperthyroid cats, their importance and relationship with the disease are not clear. In the cat the disease is not considered to be like Graves' disease, but it is thought that the problem lies in the thyroid gland due to the existence of hyperthyroid cells that function autonomously and cause uncontrolled growth, similar to what happens in human toxic nodular goitre.

A risk factor in toxic nodular goitre in humans is a **mutation in the TSH receptor gene or the G-proteins** (associated with the TSH receptor). There are 11 different mutations in the TSH receptor gene described in feline hyperthyroidism. In one study, 28 out of 50 hyperthyroid cats had at least one mutation of this gene. In addition, altered expression of G proteins and mutations in the G protein encoding gene have been found in hyperthyroid cats.

On the other hand, **various environmental factors** have been associated with the disease, although none of them alone has a dominant role. For example, an increased risk has been associated with:

- advanced age
- indoor cats
- females are at greater risk than males
- living with other cats (in another study this factor is associated with a lower risk)
- chronic periodontal disease
- use of external parasite treatments and pesticides
- use of sand
- consumption of certain varieties of wet food (flavours such as fish, liver and gizzard)
- consumption of canned food in general
- non-purebred cats.

Factors frequently associated with a higher risk in most studies are advanced age and the consumption of a **diet composed of more than 50% of wet canned food**, especially plastic-coated and easy to open (pop-top) cans. A lower risk of the disease is described in the Siamese cat, compared to the common European cat.

Some recent studies indicate a relationship between the iodine content of the diet and the presence of goitrogenic substances (ptalates, diphenyl-polybrominated esters) and the appearance of the disease.

Clinical diagnosis

It is a disease affecting geriatric cats (between 4 and 22 years of age, average age 13 years), 95% of cases are older than nine years of age. There is no clear breed or sex predisposition, although some studies indicate increased risk in cross breed cats.

The clinical signs depend on the stage of the disease at the time of diagnosis. Currently, early diagnosis is common, so the clinical signs are milder than those described years ago.

Weight loss is the most frequent clinical sign of the symptoms observed and appears in approximately 90% of cases (Figure 5). Other common clinical signs, with a frequency of between 25 and 50% are: **polyphagia, polyuria/polydipsia, hyperactivity and vomiting**. The remaining symptoms of thyrotoxicosis are less frequent and include diarrhoea, decreased or loss of appetite, muscle weakness, polypnoea, increased stool volume, lethargy and searching for areas where the temperature is cool.

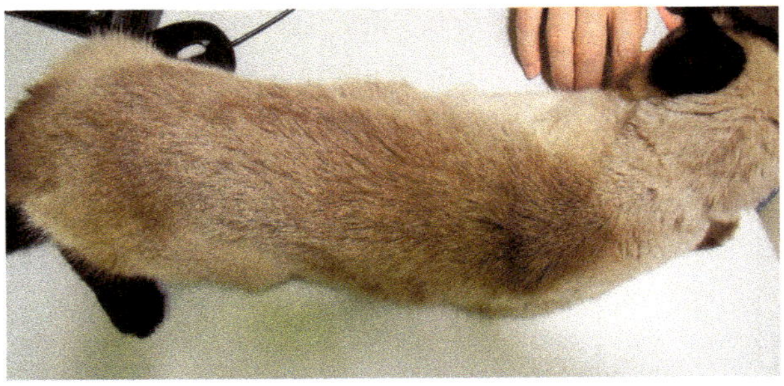

Figure 5. 11-year-old Siamese cross cat with hyperthyroidism. A body condition of 4/9 can be appreciated. Before the onset of the disease the cat weighed 5.2 kg and at the time of the photo it weighed 3.8 kg.

The clinical signs develop progressively, so in the early stages the owner may not be aware a problem exists. But as the disease progresses, the signs become more apparent and complications may develop, such as hypertrophic heart disease. **Some hyperthyroid cats (approximately 10%) present with severe depression**, lethargy, decreased appetite, a condition called "apathetic hyperthyroidism," often caused by severe heart disease.

The most important finding on clinical examination is an **enlarged thyroid gland, bilaterally** (in 70% of cases) or unilaterally (in 30%). In more than 80% of hyperthyroid cats, one or both thyroid glands can be detected (Figure 6). **Palpation of the neck**, together with measurement of plasma thyroxine, are the most useful tools for early detection of the disease. However, sometimes the thyroid nodule is not palpable: for example, because the cat is very tense and does not allow proper palpation, because the nodule is small or because the nodule has moved ventrally and is located at the base of the neck or even intrathoracically.

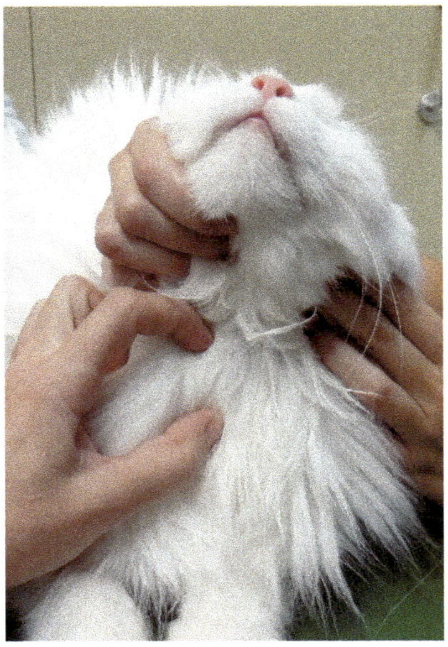

Figure 6. Palpation of a thyroid nodule in a 13-year-old Common European cat with hyperthyroidism.

Other frequent physical findings (between 40 and 65% of cases) are low body condition score, poor coat, heart murmurs and tachycardia. Gallop rhythm, hyperkinesia, aggression, coat disorders, onychogryposis, alopecia, congestive heart failure and ventral neck flexion may also be present (in less than 15% of patients).

Some cats with hyperthyroidism (15–20%) have **systemic arterial hypertension**, considering hypertension as systemic arterial pressure > 150 mmHg, with evidence of retinopathy or > 160 mmHg on two consecutive measurements. This hypertension can cause **ocular abnormalities** (haemorrhages in the anterior, posterior or retinal chambers, retinal oedema, retinal detachment). In most hyperthyroid cats, hypertension is not pronounced unless there is concurrent renal insufficiency. However, 20–25% of initially normotensive hyperthyroid cats develop hypertension after treatment of hyperthyroidism, so it is advisable to measure blood pressure before and during treatment, especially in cats with concurrent renal insufficiency.

Diagnostic tests

Blood tests

In all cases, a **complete blood count, blood biochemistry, and urinalysis** are required. There is usually polycythaemia in 50% and leukocytosis in 20 to 40% of cases. 50–85% of cats with hyperthyroidism have elevated serum alanine aminotransferase, lactate dehydrogenase, alkaline phosphatase, and aspartate aminotransferase levels. **Between 20 and 40% of hyperthyroid cats have concurrent kidney disease.**

Chronic kidney disease is a frequent condition in elderly cats and, although it usually occurs associated with hyperthyroidism, it is not directly caused by the hyperthyroid state. Measurement of urine specific gravity is useful to distinguish prerenal uraemia from primary kidney disease, plus detection of concurrent diseases such as diabetes mellitus or urinary tract infection.

SDMA

Concurrent kidney disease is common in geriatric animals and measuring the serum levels of **SDMA and protein/creatinine ratio** is essential to quantify proteinuria. Urine culture and bile acid measurement are necessary if urinary infection or concurrent liver disease is suspected.

Diagnostic imaging tests

Radiographic evaluation of the thorax is usually necessary in hyperthyroid cats, especially if there are signs of heart disease (murmur, tachycardia). In the most recent studies, cardiomegaly of variable degrees is observed in 30 to 50% of hyperthyroid cats. Radiological findings associated with congestive heart failure (pulmonary oedema, pleural effusion, pericardial effusion) are less frequent (<10%).

Ultrasonographic evaluation of the thyroid is a useful diagnostic tool, although pertechnetate scintigraphy allows better evaluation of the functionality of the gland and is the imaging technique of choice, especially to assess whether it is uni/bilateral or identify ectopic thyroid tissue. Computed tomography is also useful, although it may fail to differentiate between uni/bilateral involvement. Cardiac ultrasound is only necessary in cats with heart failure secondary to hyperthyroidism.

Hormonal tests

Measurement of thyroid hormone levels are necessary to confirm the disease. The first step is to **measure total T4 levels**, which are usually diagnostic in most cases. However, when in a cat with clinical signs of hyperthyroidism and/or thyroid nodule, TT4 levels are normal, other tests must be performed: total T3, free T4 by equilibrium dialysis, TSH levels, suppression or stimulation tests.

Total T4 concentration

A total T4 level above the normal range in a cat with symptoms compatible with hyperthyroidism, confirms the diagnosis. This test is sufficient for diagnosis in over 90% of cases and is very specific (false positive values practically do not occur in sick euthyroid cats).

However, in 10–15% of hyperthyroid cats total T4 values remain within the normal range ("hidden" hyperthyroidism), due to fluctuation of thyroid hormones within and outside the normal range in cats with mild feline hyperthyroidism or due to the decrease in thyroid hormones due to concurrent diseases.

Total T3 concentration

Only between 70 to 75% of hyperthyroid cats have high T3T levels, so the measurement of T3T for the diagnosis of feline hyperthyroidism offers practically no advantage over only the measurement of total T4.

T3 suppression test

The test consists of measuring TT4 levels before and after oral administration of synthetic liothyronine sodium (T3) for three days. After suppression TT4 levels can be used to differentiate between cats with mild hyperthyroidism (elevated TT4) and healthy or diseased cats (TT4 suppressed). In addition, T3T concentrations can be measured by this test to verify the cat has swallowed the medication (correct administration).

The test is effective in diagnosing hidden hyperthyroidism and is not costly, however, it is performed over several days, with several visits to the veterinarian, and its effectiveness depends on the oral administration of the medication, so it is not often used.

Free T4 by the equilibrium dialysis

The most sensitive test for the diagnosis of feline hyperthyroidism is the measurement of free T4 by the dialysis method. The equilibrium dialysis method is considered to be the most valid and is especially useful in hyperthyroid cats with concurrent diseases in which the total T4 concentration remains in the upper-normal limit. However, measurement of free T4 should not be used as the sole diagnostic criterion, since some euthyroid cats with concurrent diseases may have high concentrations of free T4. The presence of elevated free T4 and TT4 levels in the upper half of the normal range is considered compatible with hyperthyroidism.

Free T4 can also be detected by chemiluminescence, although the sensitivity and specificity of this test in the diagnosis of feline hyperthyroidism are lower compared with equilibrium dialysis.

Endogenous TSH

Measurement of plasma TSH levels (using the canine test) has been shown to be useful in confirming hyperthyroidism in the cat, especially in patients with normal or borderline TT4 levels. In hyperthyroid cats, even in subclinical or "hidden" cases, TSH levels are low or undetectable (<0.03 ng/ml, normal TSH values in geriatric cats: 0.03–0.15 ng/ml). Therefore, measurement of levels of TSH together with TT4 are currently recommended to increase the diagnostic efficacy.

Treatment

There are four treatment options for this disease:

- medical treatment (antithyroid drugs)
- surgical thyroidectomy
- radioactive iodine (I131)
- dietary treatment.

Without a doubt, **thyroid ablation with radioactive iodine is the most effective, curative and popular treatment** in many countries.

The **choice of treatment depends on several factors**: the cat's age, the presence of cardiovascular disorders associated with hyperthyroidism, concurrent pathologies (for example, kidney failure), the availability of nuclear medicine, and the owner.

When the clinical signs are very mild or non-existent, or if the cat has advanced concurrent diseases (such as severe kidney disease, IRIS III, IV), the treatment of hyperthyroidism can be temporarily postponed until treatment for kidney disease is established, since decreased thyroxine levels can worsen the condition of a cat with kidney failure (in these cases, relative hyperthyroidism is beneficial, since it increases glomerular filtration).

In patients with renal disease after treatment for CKD has been implemented, medical treatment should be commenced, initially using low doses, which should be progressively adjusted until a euthyroid state is achieved. Medical treatment is preferable in animals which are chronically ill, suffering from severe diseases, or in very old animals as it is reversible as well as in those where the anaesthetic risk is high.

Medical treatment

Antithyroid medications are useful in the short term in preparation for thyroidectomy and in the long term as the only treatment. They decrease the concentrations of thyroid hormones by blocking their synthesis, without destroying the hyper functional thyroid tissue.

Methimazole

Methimazole (Felimazole®, Dechra; Apelka®, Boehringher-Merial) **reversibly reduces the synthesis of thyroid hormones and is the medical treatment of choice.** It is administered orally, although it can be prepared as a gel for topical administration. Topical administration has the advantage of being less toxic, although the efficacy is lower. It is administered by rubbing a PLO gel (organogel) inside the pinna of the ear, at a concentration of 5 mg in 0.5 ml of gel.

The initial dose of methimazole (topical and oral route) is 2.5 mg every 12 hours. Carbimazole can also be used, which is metabolized to methimazole (5 mg of carbimazole is equivalent to 3 mg of methimazole) at an initial dose of 5 mg every 12 hours. An oral carbimazole preparation is also available for once daily administration (Vidalta®, MSD), at an initial dose of 15 mg/24 h.

The goal of treatment is to **keep T4 levels in the middle of the normal range**. After 2 or 3 weeks T4 concentrations should be checked to ensure they are in the desired range, increasing the dose by 2.5–5 mg every 2 or 3 weeks until this is achieved. Some cats require 20 mg of methimazole or 25–30 mg of carbimazole to control hyperthyroidism.

Most side effects occur during the first three months of treatment. Therefore, monitoring that includes a physical examination, measurement of T4 concentration, a blood count, and platelet count are important during this period. In the long term, the minimum effective dose to keep T4 levels in the middle of the normal range should be used. In most cases, this dose is 7.5 to 10 mg/day. Mild and transient side effects such as vomiting, diarrhoea and lethargy are observed in 15% of cases. Other more serious problems include agranulocytosis, thrombocytopaenia, haemorrhage, liver disease, and facial skin reactions which occur in less than 3% of treated cats.

Other medical alternatives indicated in hyperthyroid cats with severe arrhythmias are the ß -adrenergic blockers propranolol (2.5–5 mg/8 h) and atenolol (6.2–12.5 mg/12–24 h).

Dietary treatment

In recent years, it has been shown that administration of a diet containing a very small amount of iodine (0.47 ppm, in dry matter) to hyperthyroid cats, led to the normalization of TT4 levels at 9 weeks in 80% of cases, and by further reducing the iodine content of the diet (0.17 ppm, in dry matter) a euthyroid state was achieved in all cases. These same authors have shown a diet with an iodine content of 0.32 ppm or less is an effective and economical treatment in cats with hyperthyroidism.

It is a safe and effective treatment alternative already available in Europe, which is ideal in cats without concurrent diseases or with mild, compensated disease. Its disadvantages are that it requires **strict adherence to the diet** and periodic check-ups in which, among other parameters, T4 levels and kidney function are evaluated.

It is sold in dry and wet formats, although for some cats the dry version is not very palatable. On the other hand, it is not recommended as a lifelong treatment in a young adult cat, since thyroid hyperplasia can be malignant over time: in these cases, a curative treatment (surgical, iodine) is recommended.

Surgical treatment

Thyroidectomy is an effective treatment for feline hyperthyroidism, even in geriatric cats as long as they are in good clinical condition and with good cardiovascular functionality. **Administration of methimazole for two to three weeks before the procedure** is recommended, as well as propranolol 2.5–5 mg/kg every eight hours, in cats in which antithyroid medication is not sufficient to normalize heart rate.

In patients with only one affected lobe (30%), unilateral thyroidectomy is curative and does not cause a risk of iatrogenic hypoparathyroidism. However, in bilateral hyperthyroidism, thyroidectomy must be bilateral. In order to maintain calcium homeostasis, at least one of the four parathyroid glands must be conserved. Thyroid scintigraphy is useful to determine if one or both thyroid glands are affected, since 15% of hyper functional thyroid glands have a normal macroscopic appearance and failing that, CT may be useful.

There are several surgical techniques:

- The original extracapsular technique, in which the capsule and the thyroid gland are removed, leaving the parathyroid gland and the blood supply intact.
- The modified extracapsular technique, as above, but using electrocautery.
- The original intracapsular technique, in which only the gland but not the capsule is not removed.
- The modified intracapsular technique, in which almost the entire capsule is removed and only the capsular area remains attached to the parathyroid gland.

The original extracapsular technique usually causes postoperative hypocalcaemia, whereas the original intracapsular technique leads to a greater rate of recurrence of hyperthyroidism. Modified intra- or extracapsular techniques are currently recommended.

If a bilateral thyroidectomy is performed, the presence of tremors, involuntary contractions of the limbs and seizures should be monitored for one to four days after the procedure and treatment with vitamin D and calcium should be implemented. **Hypoparathyroidism is usually transient**, and treatment can be discontinued after several weeks or months. Likewise, thyroid hormones (levothyroxine 0.1–0.2 mg) should be administered one or two days after bilateral thyroidectomy, this treatment that can be discontinued several months after the procedure since the thyroid tissue attached to the parathyroid glands is usually enough to maintain euthyroidism. T4 concentration should be measured every 6–12 months to monitor for recurrences of hyperthyroidism.

Radioactive iodine

Radioactive iodine is the treatment of choice, since it has no side effects, is effective, and does not require anaesthesia. A single subcutaneous radioactive iodine treatment is sufficient to achieve a state of euthyroidism in most hyperthyroid cats. The dose used varies between 2 and 6 mCi, depending on the size of the thyroid gland on palpation, the results of scintigraphy, the severity of clinical signs and the concentration of T4.

This treatment reduces T4 concentrations to normal limits and, in some cases, below the reference range in 98% of cats. **Clinical hypothyroidism occurs in approximately 2%** of these patients and 2.5% suffer from a recurrence of hyperthyroidism. The main drawback of this treatment is its limited availability and cost.

Prognosis

The prognosis depends on the state in which the disease is diagnosed, that is, on the presence of hypertrophic heart disease and systemic arterial hypertension.

When cardiovascular function is not affected, the prognosis is good. Another factor associated with poor prognosis is the presence of concurrent kidney disease, although one study indicates that the survival of hyperthyroid cats with and without concurrent kidney disease is similar.

Adrenal neoplasms in cats

Adrenal tumours in the cat are rare, with only an estimated 0.03% of cats developing a primary adrenal tumour. Adrenal metastases from other tumours are also rare. Lymphoma is the tumour that most often metastasizes to these glands.

Feline adrenal neoplasms can **be functional** (producing an excess of one or more adrenal hormones) or **non-functional**. Functional adrenal cortex tumours may secrete glucocorticoids (cortisol), mineralocorticoids (aldosterone), or sex hormones. Tumours of the adrenal medulla (pheochromocytomas) secrete catecholamines.

Hyperadrenocorticism (Cushing's syndrome)

The most common functional adrenal tumour in the cat is a **glucocorticoid-producing adrenal mass.** Feline Cushing's syndrome is rare and in 20% of cases it is due to an adrenal tumour, while the rest are of pituitary origin. The vast majority of pituitary adenomas are benign, whilst approximately one third of adrenal neoplasms are malignant.

Clinical diagnosis

Hyperadrenocorticism (HAC) in cats (both pituitary and adrenal) is a geriatric disease, with a mean age of 12 years. The main clinical characteristics of feline Cushing's disease are **dermal fragility and diabetes mellitus secondary to excess cortisol.**

The **clinical signs are often non-specific, such as lethargy and weakness**, as well as dermatological manifestations including atrophy and dermal fragility, a tendency to suffer from skin lacerations, alopecia, seborrhoea, and a dull coat. Polyuria/polydipsia, bloating, and polyphagia also occur. Polyuria/polydipsia is not usually present in the initial stages of the disease, but appears when the cat develops secondary diabetes, which occurs in 60–90% of cats with HAC.

Diagnostic plan

In cats with HAC, blood counts are varied and non-specific. Only some cats show a stress leukogram (leukocytosis, neutrophilia, lymphopoenia, and eosinopoenia). Most have hyperglycaemia, hypercholesterolaemia, and elevated alanine aminotransferase (ALT) levels. Cats lack the glucocorticoid-induced isoenzyme, so only 20% of HAC patients have a high alkaline phosphatase level. Most cats with this disease have a urine density greater than 1.020 due to glycosuria. Cats with HAC are prone to urine infections, due to the immunosuppressive effect of glucocorticoids and the presence of glucose in the urine. It is advisable to perform a urine culture.

If feline HAC is suspected, blood pressure measurement is advised, as hypertension which requires treatment may be present. Ultrasonographic evaluation of the adrenal glands is useful to confirm enlargement of these glands and differentiate between pituitary and adrenal HAC (Figure 7). The thickness of the adrenal lobes in healthy cats is generally 3.0 to 5.0 mm, while in most cases of feline Cushing's disease the adrenal glands with adrenal hyperplasia or neoplasia have an increased thickness. In cats with adrenal Cushing's disease, the contralateral gland and the possibility of invasion of adjacent structures or metastasis should be evaluated.

Ultrasonography should not be used as the only diagnostic means since other chronic diseases (including feline hyperthyroidism) can lead to a slight increase in the thickness of the adrenal glands (5.3–6.0 mm). However, to differentiate between pituitary and adrenal HAC, abdominal ultrasound or endocrine tests can be used. Abdominal ultrasound is useful since cats with pituitary HAC show bilateral enlargement of the adrenal glands, while in those with adrenal HAC only one gland appears enlarged and the contralateral tends to be atrophied. Furthermore, the enlarged gland may present a loss of its normal morphology.

Adrenal function tests

To confirm HAC, an adrenal function test is necessary. The test of choice is the **low dose dexamethasone suppression test**, since it has a high sensitivity

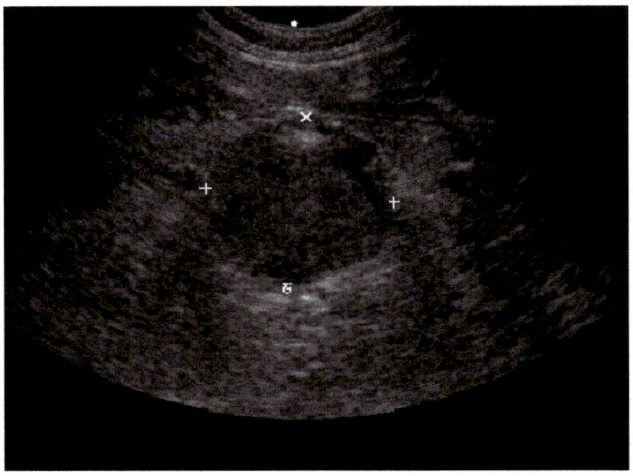

Figure 7. Ultrasonographic image of a mass in the right adrenal gland in a 9-year-old cat with adrenal hyperadrenocorticism.

(90%), compared to the corticotropin stimulation test (ACTH) (40–60%).

Low dose dexamethasone suppression test

In cats, this test is performed with an intravenous dose of dexamethasone of 0.1 mg/kg (ten times higher than that used in dogs: 0.01 mg/kg).

Cortisol levels at four and eight hours should be less than 1.0 µg/dl. If cortisol levels at four or eight hours are higher than 1.4 µg/dl, the result is positive. Results between 1 and 1.4 µg/dl are considered doubtful.

ACTH stimulation test

Maximum cortisol concentration occurs between 60 and 120 minutes after intravenous administration of ACTH, therefore taking two samples to measure cortisol after ACTH administration is recommended: thus, the samples are taken before, at 60 and 90 minutes after intravenous administration of 5 µg/kg or 125 µg ACTH.

In the case of ACTH exclusively for intramuscular use (Nuvacthen depot® 0.125 mg/kg/IM), cortisol should also be measured before, after 60 minutes and at 90 minutes after intramuscular ACTH administration.

In the cat this test is of limited utility for the diagnosis of HAC since its **sensitivity is low** (50%), hence a normal result does not rule out the disease. However, this is still the test of choice if iatrogenic Cushing's disease is suspected. On the other hand, some cats with non-adrenal diseases may respond in an exaggerated manner to ACTH stimulation resulting in false positive results.

ACTH precursors

Due to the limitations of adrenal function tests in the cat, new ways to confirm the diagnosis of HAC are being researched. Measurement of the concentration of an ACTH precursor, POMC (proopiomelanocortin), has been described as useful in the diagnosis of feline Cushing's disease, since its concentration is elevated in patients with pituitary HAC and is maintained at normal concentrations in healthy animals or those with diabetes, both with and without acromegaly.

High dose dexamethasone suppression test

The high-dose dexamethasone suppression test may be necessary if ultrasound does not confirm the origin of the HAC. A dose of 1 mg/kg of dexamethasone is recommended for this test with cortisol samples taken at 0, 4 and 8 hours.

A cortisol level of less than 1.4 µg/dl or a cortisol level of less than 50% of the baseline value at four and/or eight hours is considered suppression. Approximately 50% of cats with pituitary HAC show suppression, while cats with adrenal HAC do not show suppression. Therefore, suppression indicates pituitary origin, but a lack of suppression does not differentiate between both types of HAC.

Plasma ACTH concentration

Measurement of the concentration of ACTH in plasma is useful to differentiate between pituitary and adrenal HAC. In the case of pituitary HAC results will be high or towards the upper end of the normal limit (> 45 pg/ml), while in adrenal HAC it will be low or towards the lower end of the normal limit. The sample must be handled strictly following the laboratory's recommendations, since this is a hormone that breaks down quickly at room temperature.

Some cats with suspected HAC have Cushing's test results within the normal range. If, after repeated tests, the results remain within the reference values, the possibility of an adrenal neoplasm that produces other hormones (sex hormones or precursors of these hormones) should be investigated, which may give rise to symptoms similar to that of Cushing's disease.

Treatment

There are different medical and surgical treatment options. Cats with Cushing's disease often have HAC-related complications (lacerations due to dermal fragility, skin infections and poor healing, diabetes and a predisposition to recurrent bacterial or fungal infections) and concurrent diseases (kidney disease, hyperthyroidism), which must be managed in parallel. 22–47% of cats with HAC suffer from azotaemia at the time of diagnosis.

A large majority of cats with Cushing's have concurrent diabetes mellitus, which should be treated with a low starting dose of insulin (0.2–0.3 IU/kg/12 h PZI, slow-acting or glargine insulin). This initial dose should be gradually increased according to the response. Once treatment for HAC has commenced, insulin needs must be monitored, because the necessary dose may decrease as the animal responds to HAC treatment. Performing periodic urine cultures is recommended.

Medical treatment

Trilostane

Trilostane is the most widely used treatment: it causes a decrease in cortisol levels, the effect is reversible, and it is well tolerated by most cats, although it can cause hypocortisolaemia in 10–15% of feline patients.

In most of the cases described, an initial dose of 2–5 mg/kg/24 hours has been used. The pharmacokinetics of trilostane have not yet been evaluated in cats, but in many patients, who start treatment every 24 hours, the dose ends up being adjusted from 0.5 to 1.5 mg/kg/12 h, which allows better control of the disease. Administering in this way is probably most effective.

Most cats respond well, improving polyuria/polydipsia and lethargy within the first few weeks of treatment. In a study of 15 cats with Cushing's disease treated with trilostane of which nine were diabetic, in six of nine insulin requirements were reduced by 36%. In one of them the needs increased, and diabetes did not remiss in any of them. The median survival time of the treated cats was 617 days and 9 of the 15 animals were euthanized for different reasons such as recurrent urinary infections, kidney disease or pancreatitis.

Mitotane

The efficacy of mitotane (25–50 mg/kg/day) is low and works in approximately 50% of cats with HAC. In addition, signs of intolerance to the drug usually appear, such as anorexia, vomiting and lethargy, so its use is not recommended.

Ketoconazole

The efficacy of ketoconazole (15 mg/kg every 12 hours) is variable. Severe thrombocytopaenia has been described in one cat treated, so this treatment is generally not recommended.

Surgical treatment

Unilateral adrenalectomy is the treatment of choice in cats with adrenal HAC. Before performing surgical treatment, medical treatment is recommended (trilostane) for several weeks to improve clinical signs. The presence of an adrenal tumour causes atrophy of the contralateral gland, so treatment with glucocorticoids is necessary for approximately two months until the contralateral gland recovers. Treatment with mineralocorticoids is not necessary, since the atrophied gland retains the ability to secrete them because their production and release does not depend exclusively on the presence of ACTH.

Bilateral adrenalectomy has been used as treatment for feline pituitary HAC, and the clinical response is satisfactory in most cases. Previous medical treatment with cortisol synthesis inhibitors is also recommended. 20–50% of patients may experience intra or peri-surgical complications such as sepsis, pancreatitis, hypoglycaemia, electrolyte disturbances, or poor wound healing. Cats undergoing bilateral adrenalectomy will need lifetime treatment with glucocorticoids and mineralocorticoids. In cats with diabetes, glucose levels should be monitored because insulin needs may decrease.

Sex-hormone producing adrenal tumours

Adrenal cortex tumours can secrete excessive amounts of progestogens, androgens, or oestrogens. Progestogen-secreting tumours are relatively common in cats and their clinical signs are similar to those seen in cats with cortisol-secreting tumours and include skin atrophy, fragile skin, alopecia, and diabetes.

In most cases, test results for Cushing's diagnosis are normal or low due to suppression of the pituitary-adrenal axis. Diagnosis requires measurement of one or more sex hormones, before and after ACTH administration.

In addition to the hypersecretion of progestogens, different clinical signs have been described which vary depending on the hormone(s) affected, such as aggressiveness (androstenedione and testosterone) or recurring seasons (oestrogens).

Hyperaldosteronism

Primary hyperaldosteronism, also called Conn's syndrome, has been diagnosed more frequently in cats in recent years, although it is still considered as underdiagnosed. It is characterized by an autonomous secretion of mineralocorticoids, usually aldosterone, which gives rise to clinical signs related to high blood pressure and/or hypokalaemia.

This disease is caused by a **benign or malignant unilateral neoplasm of the adrenal cortex**, which comes from the outermost layer of the adrenal cortex (glomerulus zone). Less commonly, feline primary hyperaldosteronism occurs due to nodular hyperplasia or bilateral adenoma of the adrenal cortex.

Clinical diagnosis

High aldosterone concentrations promote sodium retention, potassium elimination and cause hypertension. Most of the clinical signs are non-specific and associated with **hypokalaemia: weakness, lethargy, stiffness, muscle pain, neck ventroflexion, or polyuria/polydipsia**. In addition, hypertensive retinopathy or acute blindness due to intraocular haemorrhage may appear, as well as retinal detachment due to arterial hypertension.

The diagnostic plan in these cases includes a complete blood count and blood biochemistry with electrolytes, urinalysis, abdominal ultrasound and blood pressure measurement. Cats with hyperaldosteronism generally have hypokalaemia and metabolic alkalosis. Sodium concentrations remain within the reference range or only slightly elevated in most of them.

Diagnosis

To diagnose primary hyperaldosteronism and rule out other causes of (renal) hyperaldosteronism, renin activity should be assessed. A high aldosterone concentration together with low renin activity confirm the diagnosis of primary hyperaldosteronism in cats with compatible clinical signs (weakness, hypokalaemia, hypertension, etc.).

Adrenal ultrasound allows identification of the presence of an adrenal mass (aldosteronoma) in most cases. However, in cats with idiopathic primary hyperaldosteronism, the adrenal glands may show an apparently normal ultrasonographic appearance and only mild hyperplasia.

A dynamic test for hyperaldosteronism in cats has recently been described. This oral suppression test with fludrocortisone, consists of measuring the urinary aldosterone: creatinine ratio before and after administration of 0.05 mg/kg/12 h of fludrocortisone for 4 days. In cats with hypertension due to other causes, the administration of fludrocortisone leads to a suppression of more than 50% of the initial measurement, while in most (six of nine, in the study) of cats with hypertension due to hyperaldosteronism, suppression of this ratio is less than 50%.

Treatment

Initially, potassium levels should be stabilised, and hydration and acid-base balance restored. To increase potassium levels, oral potassium gluconate is used at a dose of 2–6 mEq every 12–24 hours and spironolactone at 1–2 mg/kg/12 h. If persistent hypertension exists, amlodipine can be added at 0.1 mg/kg/24 h.

In cases where a unilateral adrenal mass is identified and no metastases detected, adrenalectomy is the treatment of choice. Perioperative complications (abdominal bleeding, sepsis acute kidney disease or thromboembolism) might occur in less than 10% of the cases.

In the presence of distant metastases, bilateral hyperplasia, serious concurrent diseases, or economic limitations, medical treatment is used indefinitely.

Pheochromocytoma

Catecholamine-producing tumours of the adrenal medulla are extremely rare in cats.

Clinical signs are related to excessive secretion of catecholamines (episodic hypertension or tachypnoea), or the space occupied by the adrenal mass. The contralateral gland usually maintains a normal silhouette and size. Measurement of plasma free normetanephrine concentration is useful in the diagnosis of feline pheochromocytoma.

Feline idiopathic hypercalcaemia

Two of the most common causes of hypercalcaemia in cats are **tumour hypercalcaemia** (due to lymphoma, myeloma, carcinomas) and **kidney disease**. In a recent study, of the cats studied with hypercalcaemia, tumoural hypercalcaemia was found in 23% of animals, secondary to kidney disease in 13% and idiopathic in 13%.

However, in recent years, idiopathic hypercalcaemia (of unknown cause after having carried out the appropriate diagnostic tests) has emerged as one of the most frequent types of hypercalcaemia in this species. It has been reported to affect cats between 0.5 and 20 years of age and appears to be more frequent in long-haired animals.

Other causes such as granulomatous diseases (blastomycosis, schistosomiasis, panniculitis, post-injection granulomas), poisonings (plants, rodenticides, creams for psoriasis, xylitol, dried grapes), hypoadrenocorticism, skeletal (non-tumour) lesions and primary hyperparathyroidism are rare in the cat.

Diagnosis

Diagnostic tests to determine the cause should be carried out before treatment starts. This is because the treatment and prognosis of cats with lymphoma or kidney disease is different from that of cats with idiopathic hypercalcaemia. Diagnostic processes include a complete clinical history, detailed physical examination, complete blood count, complete blood biochemistry, urinalysis and diagnostic imaging (thoracic and cervical radiology, abdominal ultrasound).

50% of cats with idiopathic hypercalcaemia are asymptomatic. Those with clinical signs show loss of appetite, lethargy, vomiting, constipation, or even anorexia. Polyuria/polydipsia is less frequent in cats with hypercalcaemia than in dogs: the former maintains the ability to concentrate urine despite having high calcium levels, although dysuria, stranguria or haematuria may occur, secondary to the presence of urinary calculi (usually calcium oxalate). Other less common signs are dehydration, seizures, weakness, and arrhythmias.

Given the finding of a high total calcium level (tCa), hypercalcaemia should be confirmed by repeating a fasting measurement (lipaemia, haemolysis and haemoconcentration interfere) along with albumin levels. The tCa is made up of 3 parts: ionized or free (56%), chelated (phosphate, bicarbonate) (10%) and protein bound (34%). Therefore, if albumin and globulin levels are affected, tCa levels are altered in turn without the biologically active fraction being affected. If tCa is confirmed as being high, ionized calcium (iCa) levels need to be measured, since they reflect the patient's actual calcium levels. Formulas to correct tCa levels in relation to albumin lead to diagnostic errors and are therefore not currently recommended.

Measuring iCa is not difficult or expensive. The sample should be obtained in a vacuum extraction tube (Vacutainer type) without anticoagulant and handled with caution, under the most anaerobic conditions possible. The normal range for ionized calcium is between 1.1 and 1.4 mmol/l.

To establish a diagnosis of idiopathic hypercalcaemia, confirming that PTH levels are normal (in renal disease they are elevated) and those of undetectable parathyroid hormone-like protein (PTHrP) (elevated in tumour hypercalcaemia or due to bone lesions) is recommended, Normal PTH levels in cats are between 2.0 and 13.0 pmol/l. In normal cats, PTHrP levels are almost undetectable (<0.5 pmol/l). The laboratory should be contacted beforehand to send the samples properly (aprotinin EDTA tubes, obtain plasma immediately and freeze).

Treatment

Treatment of hypercalcaemia depends on the cause, the severity of the clinical signs, the degree of hypercalcaemia and serum phosphorus levels. Ideally, an inciting cause should be eliminated. To date, idiopathic treatment is not perfect, as the pathogenesis of the disease is unknown.

When clinical signs are severe, hypercalcaemia appears abruptly (in other causes of hypercalcaemia, for example, rodenticide poisoning) or whenever hypercalcaemia is severe (tCa> 14 mg/dl) especially if hyperphosphataemia is also severe then emergency treatment is necessary. This treatment is focused on increasing renal calcium elimination and consists of:

- **Fluid therapy**: 0.9% NaCl 100–125 ml/kg/day IV, it can also then be administered SC.
- **Furosemide** at a dose of 1–4 mg/kg/8–12 h, IV or in continuous infusion 0.2–1 mg/kg/h initially and, subsequently, at a dose of 1–4 mg/kg/8–12 h SC or PO.
- In severe cases **glucocorticoids** can be administered (once lymphoma has been ruled out): prednisone at a dose of 0.5–2 mg/kg/12 h.
- Another IV drug to reduce hypercalcaemia is zoledronic acid at a dose of 0.2 mg/kg IV as 15 min CRI in 25 ml 0.9% NaCl q 28 d.

In idiopathic hypercalcaemia emergency treatment is not usually necessary since, although iCa levels may be very high, tCa levels are not usually higher than 13 mg/dl and clinical signs are usually mild or moderate. In these cases, the first step is to try to correct hypercalcaemia with a diet rich in fibre, since this reduces intestinal calcium absorption by reducing intestinal transit time. These diets are supplemented with extra calcium, so it is unknown why in some hypercalcaemic cats they reduce calcium levels. However, not all cats with hypercalcaemia respond well to a high fibre diet. Another alternative is administration of renal diets, which contain reduced levels of calcium and phosphorus and are alkalizing (maintenance diets are usually acidifying and increase the availability of ionized calcium, facilitating its intestinal absorption, and may also increase bone resorption).

In cats that do not respond to dietary treatment, oral treatment with prednisone (5–10 mg/cat/day) or prednisolone (20 mg/cat/day) should be trialled for one month, iCa levels should be monitored after 15 days and a month, reducing the initial dose until the minimum effective dose is reached. Animals receiving treatment should be checked every three months. Prednisone has been reported to increase the risk of oxalate stone formation, while prednisolone does not increase this risk.

If hypercalcaemia recurs or if it does not respond to corticosteroids then administration of bisphosphonates should be trialled, which reduce osteoclastic activity and are therefore also useful in tumour hypercalcaemia. Among bisphosphonates, the most useful is alendronate (Fosamax®, MSD), given orally, since pamidronate is for parenteral use and is not usually necessary in idiopathic hypercalcaemia. If required, it is administered at a dose of 1.0–2.0 mg/kg in 40 ml 0.9% NaCl infused IV over 2 hours.

Alendronate (Fosamax®, MSD) is administered at doses of 10 to 30 mg per week per cat. Appearance of oesophagitis and oesophageal stenosis has been described with the use of this medication, so applying butter to the cat's lips and even administering a little water with a syringe after its administration, to ensure that the pill does not stay in the oesophagus is recommended. If alendronate is used, iCa levels should be checked after 15 days, one month and every three months.

Bibliography

C Y Pérez Alenza MD. *Actualización en el diagnóstico y tratamiento de acromegalia felina*. Canis et Felis Número 126 - Febrero 2014.

Ash RA, Harvey AM, Tasker S. *Primary Hyperaldosteronism in the Cat: A Series of 13 Cases* J Feline Med Surg 2005 7:173–182.

Behrend EI, Holford AI, Lathan PI, Rucinsky RI, Schulman RI 2018 AAHA *Diabetes Management Guidelines for Dogs and Cats*. J Am Anim Hosp Assoc. 2018 Jan/Feb;54(1):1–21. doi: 10.5326/JAAHA-MS-6822.

Benchekroun G, De Fornel-Thibaud P, Dubord M, Dossin O, Fracassi F, Rannou B, Garnier F, Maurey-Guenec C, Daminet S, Rosenberg D. *Plasma ACTH precursors in cats with pituitary-dependent hyperadrenocorticism.* J Vet Intern Med 2012 May-Jun;26(3):575–81.

Berg RI, Nelson RW, Feldman EC, et al. *Serum insulin-like growth factor-I concentration in cats with diabetes mellitus and acromegaly.* J Vet Intern Med 2007,21(5):892–8.

Bisignano J, Bruyette DS. *Feline hyperaldosteronism: Recognition and diagnosis.* Veterinary Medicine 2012 Mar 1: 118–125.

Bisignano J, Bruyette DS. *Feline hyperaldosteronism: Treatment and prognosis.* Veterinary Medicine 2012 Mar 1: 126–134.

Bjornvad CR, Rand JS, Tan HY, et al. *Obesity and sex influence insulin resistance and total and multimer adiponectin levels in adult neutered domestic shorthair client-owned cats.* Domest Anim Endocrinol. 2014 Apr;47:55–64.

Bloom CA, Rand J. *Feline Diabetes mellitus: Clinical use of long-acting glargine and detemir.* J Feline Med Surg. 2014 Mar;16(3):205–15.

Boag AK, Neiger R, Church DB. *Trilostane treatment of bilateral adrenal enlargement and excessive sex steroid hormone production in a cat.* J Small Anim Pract 2004 45: 263–266.

Boord M, Griffin C. *Progesterone-secreting adrenal mass in a cat with clinical signs of hyperadrenocorticism.* J Am Vet Med Assoc 1999 214: 666–669.

Briscoe K, Barrs VR, Foster DF, et al. *Hyperaldosteronism and hyperprogesteronism in a cat.* J Fel Med Surg 2009 11: 758–762.

Callegari C, Mercuriali E, Hafner M, et al. *Survival time and prognostic factors in cats with newly diagnosed diabetes mellitus: 114 cases (2000–2009).* J Am Vet Med Assoc. 2013 Jul 1;243(1):91–5.

Calsyn JD, Green RA, Davis GJ, Reilly CM. *Adrenal pheochromocytoma with contralateral adrenocortical adenoma in a cat.* J Am Anim Hosp Assoc 2010,46:36–42.

Caney SM. *Pancreatitis and diabetes in cats.* Vet Clin North Am Small Anim Pract. 2013 Mar;43(2):303–17.

Carney HC, Ward CR, Bailey SJ et al. *2016 AAFP Guidelines for the Management of Feline Hyperthyroidism.* Journal of Feline Medicine and Surgery (2016) 18, 400–416.

Chastain CB, Panciera D, Waters C, et al. *Idiopathic hypercalcemia in cats.* J Vet Intern Med 2000, 14: 619–626.

Claus MA, Silverstein DC, Shofer FS, Mellema MS. *Comparison of regular insulin infusion doses in critically ill diabetic cats: 29 cases (1999–2007).* J Vet Emerg Crit Care (San Antonio). 2010 Oct;20(5):509–17.

Combes A, Pey P, Paepe D, Rosenberg D, Daminet S, Putcuyps I, Bedu AS, Duchateau L, De Fornel-Thibaud P, Benchekroun G, Saunders JH. *Ultrasonographic appearance of adrenal glands in healthy and sick cats.* J Feline Med Surg 2013 Jun;15(6):445–57.

Cook AK. *Monitoring methods for dogs and cats with diabetes mellitus.* J Diabetes Sci Technol. 2012 May 1;6(3):491–5.

Daminet Si, Kooistra HS, Fracassi F, Graham PA, Hibbert A, Lloret A, Mooney CT, Neiger R, Rosenberg D, Syme HM, Villard I, Williams G. *Best practice for the pharmacological management of hyperthyroid cats with antithyroid drugs.* J Small Anim Pract. 2014 Jan;55(1):4–13.

De Brito JF, Chew D, Schenck. *Hipercalcemia: diagnóstico y tratamiento en el perro y en el gato.* Vet Focus 2011, 21: 27–34

DeClue AE, Martin LG, Behrend EN, Cohn LA, Dismukes DI, Lee HP. *Cortisol and aldosterone response to various doses of cosyntropin in healthy cats.* J Am Vet Med Assoc 2011 Jan 15;238(2):176–82.

DiFazio J, and Fletcher DJ. *Retrospective comparison of early-versuslate-insulin therapy regarding effect on time toresolution of diabetic ketosis and ketoacidosisin dogs and cats: 60 cases (2003–2013).* Journal of Veterinary Emergency and Critical Care 26(1) 2016, pp. 108–115 doi: 10.1111/vec.12415.

Djajadiningrat-Laanen S, Galac S, et al. *Evaluation of the Oral Fludrocortisone Suppression Test for Diagnosing Primary Hyperaldosteronism in Cats.* J Vet Intern Med 2013 27:1493–1499.

Djajadiningrat-Laanen S, Galac S, Kooistra H. *Primary hyperaldosteronism: expanding the diagnostic net.* J Feline Med Surg 2011 Sep;13(9):641–50.

Dunning MD, Lowrie CS, Bexfield NH, et al. *Exogenous insulin treatment after hypofractionated radiotherapy in cats with diabetes mellitus and acromegaly.* J Vet Intern Med 2009, 23(2):243–9.

Edinboro CH, Scott-Moncrieff JC, Glickman LT. *Feline hyperthyroidism: potential relationship with iodine supplement requirements of commercial cat foods.* J Feline Med Surg. 2010 Sep;12(9):672–9.

Edinboro CHi, Pearce EN, Pino S, Braverman LE. *Iodine concentration in commercial cat foods from three regions of the USA, 2008–2009.* J Feline Med Surg. 2013 Aug;15(8):717–24.

Fischetti AJ; Gisselman K; Peterson ME. *CT and MRI evaluation of skull bones and soft tissues in six cats with presumed acromegaly versus 12 unaffected cats.* Vet Radiol Ultrasound 2012, 53[5] Sep-Oct: 535–9.

Frénais R, Rosenberg D, Burgaud S, Horspool LJ. *Clinical efficacy and safety of a once-daily formulation of carbimazole in cats with hyperthyroidism.* J Small Anim Pract. 2009. Oct;50(10):510–5.

Gallagher BR, Mahony OM, Rozanski EA, Bujob S, Freeman L. *A pilot study comparing a protocol using intermittent administration of glargine and regular insulin to a continuous rate infusion of regular insulin in cats with naturally occurring diabetic ketoacidosis.* J Vet Emerg Crit Care (San Antonio). 2015 Mar-Apr;25(2):234–9.

Gottlieb S, Rand JS. *Remission in cats: including predictors and risk factors.* Vet Clin North Am Small Anim Pract. 2013 Mar;43(2):245–9.

Hui TY, D.S. Bruyette DS, Moore GE, et al. *Effect of Feeding an Iodine-Restricted Diet in Cats with Spontaneous Hyperthyroidism.* J Vet Intern Med 2015;29:1063–1068.

Lamb CR, Ciasca TC, Mantis P, et al. *Computed tomographic signs of acromegaly in 68 diabetic cats with hypersomatotropism.* J Feline Med Surg. 2014 Feb;16(2):99–108.

Lautenschlaeger IEI, Hartmann A, Sicken J, Mohrs S, Scholz VB, Neiger R, Kramer M. *Comparison between computed tomography and (99m) tc- pertechnetate scintigraphy characteristics of the thyroid gland in cats with hyperthyroidism.* Vet Radiol Ultrasound. 2013 Nov;54(6):666–73.

Marshall RD, Rand JS, Morton JM. *Treatment of newly diagnosed diabetic cats with glargine insulin improves glycaemic control and results in higher probability of remission than protamine zinc and lente insulins.* J Feline Med Surg. 2009 Aug;11(8):683–91.

Marshall RD, Rand JS, Gunew MN, Menrath VH. *Intramuscular glargine with or without concurrent subcutaneous administration for treatment of feline diabetic ketoacidosis.* J Vet Emerg Crit Care (San Antonio). 2013 May-Jun;23(3):286–90.

Meij BP, Auriemma E, Grinwis G, et al. *Successful treatment of acromegaly in a diabetic cat with transsphenoidal hypophysectomy.* J Feline Med Surg 2010, 12:406–10.

MEIJ BP, GALAC S, KOOISTRA H. *Surgical treatment of acromegaly in cats.* In: Voorjaarsdagen Proceedings Committee, editor. Proceedings of the Voorjaarsdagen. Amsterdam (The Netherlands): p. 232–3. 2012.

MELER EN et al. *Cyclic estrous like behavior in a spayed cat associated with excessive sex hormone production from an adrenal carcinoma.* Journal of Feline Medicine and Surgery 2011 13(6):473–8.

MELLETT KEITH AM, BRUYETTE D, STANLEY S. *Trilostane Therapy for Treatment of Spontaneous Hyperadrenocorticism in Cats: 15 Cases (2004–2012).* J Vet Intern Med. 2013.

MICHIELS L, PETRIE G, THOLLOT IG, et al. *Treatment of 46 cats with porcine lente insulin a prospective, multicentre study.* J Fel Med Surg 2008 10:439–451.

Midkiff AM1, Chew DJ, Randolph JF, Center SA, DiBartola SP. *Idiopathic hypercalcemia in cats.* J Vet Intern Med. 2000 Nov-Dec;14(6):619–26.

MILLARD RP, PICKENS EH, WELLS KL. *Excessive production of sex hormones in a cat with an adrenocortical tumour.* J Am Vet Med Assoc 2009 234:505–508.

MILNER RJ, CHANNELL CD, LEVY JK, et al. *Survival times for cats with hyperthyroidism treated with iodine 131, methimazole, or both: 167 cases (1996–2003).* J Am Vet Med Assoc 2006; 228:559–563.

MORETTI S, TSCHUOR F, OSTO M, et al. *Evaluation of a Novel Real-Time Continuous Glucose Monitoring System for use in cats.* J Vet Intern Med 2010 2010: 24: 120–126.

MORROW L, ADMAS VJ, ELLIOT J, et al. *Hypertension in hyperthyroid cats: prevalence, incidence and predictors of its development* J Vet Intern Med 2009; 23: 700 (abstract).

NEIGER R, WITT AL, NOBLE A, AND ALEXANDER J. *Trilostane Therapy for Treatment of Pituitary-Dependent Hyperadrenocorticism in 5 Cats.* J Vet Intern Med 2004 18:160–164.

NELSON RW, HENLEY K, COLE C; *PZIR Clinical Study Group. Field safety and efficacy of protamine zinc recombinant human insulin for treatment of diabetes mellitus in cats.* J Vet Intern Med. 2009 Jul-Aug;23(4):787–93.

NIESSEN SJ, FORCADA Y, CHURCH DB. *Serum type III procollagen propeptide: an alternative measure of growth hormone bioactivity in cats with diabetes mellitus and hypersomatotropism.* J Vet Intern Med 2012, 26(6):1520 TBC.

NIESSEN SJ, PETRIE G, GAUDIANO F, et al. *Feline acromegaly: an underdiagnosed endocrinopathy?* J Vet Intern Med 2007, 21(5):899–905.

NIESSEN SJ. *Feline acromegaly: an essential differential diagnosis for the difficult diabetic.* J Feline Med Surg 2010, 12(1):15–23.

NIESSEN SJM; CHURCH DB; FORCADA Y. *Hypersomatotropism, acromegaly, and hyperadrenocorticism and feline diabetes mellitus.* Vet Clin North Am Small Anim Pract 2013, 43[2] Mar 01: 319–50.

NIESSEN SJM; FORCADA Y; MANTIS P; et al. *Studying Cat (Felis catus) Diabetes: Beware of the Acromegalic Imposter.* PLOS ONE | DOI:10.1371/journal.pone.0127794 May 29, 2015.

NORSWORTHY GD, CARNEY HC, WARD CR.*2016 AAFP Guidelines for the Management of Feline Hyperthyroidism.* J Feline Med Surg. 2016 Sep;18(9):750.

PALM CA, FELDMAN EC. *Oral hypoglycemics in cats with diabetes mellitus.* Vet Clin North Am Small Anim Pract. 2013 Mar;43(2): 407–15.

PETERSON ME, BROOME MR. *Thyroid scintigraphy findings in 2096 cats with hyperthyroidism.* Vet Radiol Ultrasound, Vol. 56, No. 1, 2015, pp 84–95.

PETERSON ME, GUTERL JN, R. NICHOLS R et al. *Evaluation of Serum Thyroid-Stimulating Hormone Concentration as a Diagnostic Test for Hyperthyroidism in Cats.* J Vet Intern Med 2015;29:1327–1334.

PETERSON ME. *Hipertiroidismo.* En: Manual de endocrinología de pequeños animales. Editores: melian C, Pérez Alenza MD. Editorial Multimédica. 2008.

PETERSON ME. *More than just T_4: diagnostic testing for hyperthyroidism in cats.* J Feline Med Surg. 2013 Sep;15(9):765–77.

PINEDA CI, AGUILERA-TEJERO E, RAYA AI, et al. *Feline parathyroid hormone: validation of hormonal assays and dynamics of secretion.* Domest Anim Endocrinol. 2012 May;42(4):256–64.

POSCH B; DOBSON J; HERRTAGE M. *Magnetic resonance imaging findings in 15 acromegalic cats.* Vet Radiol Ultrasound 2011, 52[4] Jul 01: 422–7.

RAMSPOTT S, HARTMANN K, SAUTER-LOUIS C, WEBER K AND WEHNER A. *Adrenal function in cats with Hyperthyroidism.* Journal of Feline Medicine and Surgery 2012 14(4) 262–266.

RAND JS *Diabetic ketoacidosis and hyperosmolar hyperglycemic state in cats.* Vet Clin North Am Small Anim Pract. 2013 Mar;43(2):367–79

RAND JS. *Feline diabetes.*Vet Clin North Am Small Anim Pract. 2013 Mar;43(2).

ROOMP K, RAND J. *Evaluation of detemir in diabetic cats managed with a protocol for intensive blood glucose control.* J Feline Med Surg. 2012 Aug;14(8):566–72.

ROOMP K, RAND JS. *Management of diabetic cats with long-acting insulin.* Vet Clin North Am Small Anim Pract. 2013 Mar;43(2): 251–66.

ROSSMEISL JH, SCOTT-MONCRIEFF JC, SIEMS J, et al. *Hyperadrenocorticism and hyper-progesteronemia in a cat with an adrenocortical adenocarcinoma.* J Am Anim Hosp Assoc 2000, 36: 512–517.

RUCINSKY R, COOK A, HALEY S, NELSON R, ZORAN DL, POUNDSTONE M; *American Animal Hospital Association. AAHA diabetes management guidelines.* J Am Anim Hosp Assoc. 2010 May-Jun;46(3):215–24.

SAVARY KC, PRICE GS, VADEN SL. *Hypercalcemia in cats: a retrospective study of 71 cases (1991–97).* J Vet Intern Med 2000, 14: 184–189.

SCHENCK PA AND CHEW DJ. *Prediction of serum ionized calcium concentration by use of serum total concentration in cats.* Can J Vet Res 2010, 74: 209–13.

SCUDDER CJ, GOSTELOW R, FORCADA Y, et al. *Pasireotide for the Medical Management of Feline Hypersomatotropism.* J Vet Intern Med 2015;29:1074–1080.

SHIEL R, CARMEL M. *Diagnosis and management of primary hyperaldosteronism in cats.* In Practice 2007 29:194–201.

SIEBER-RUCKSTUHL NS, KLEY S, TSCHUOR F, ZINI E, OHLERTH S, BORETTI FS, REUSCH CE. *Remission of diabetes mellitus in cats with diabetic ketoacidosis.* J Vet Intern Med. 2008 Nov-Dec;22(6): 1326–32.

SLINGERLAND LI, VOORHOUT G, RIJNBERK A, et al. *Growth hormone excess and the effect of octreotide in cats with diabetes mellitus.* Domest Anim Endocrinol 2008, 35(4):352–61.

SMITH RR, MAYHEW PD, BERENT AC. *Laparoscopic adrenalectomy for management of a functional adrenal tumour in a cat.* J Am Vet Med Assoc 2012 Aug 1;241(3):368–72.

SPARKES AH. *ISMF Consensus Guidelines on the practical mamagement of feline diabetes mellitus.*

TIMIAN J, LUNN KF. *Evaluation of a long-acting somatostatin receptor ligand for the treatment of feline acromegaly.* J Vet Intern Med 2012, 26:757.

Van der Kooij MI, Becvárová I, Meyer HP, Teske E, Kooistra HS. *Effects of an iodine-restricted food on client-owned cats with hyperthyroidism.* J Feline Med Surg. 2013 Nov 14.

Wakeling J, Elliott J, Syme H. *Evaluation of predictors for the diagnosis of hyperthyroidism in cats.* J Vet Intern Med 2011; 25: 1057–1065.

Watson SG, Radford AD, Kipar A, Ibarrola P, Blackwood L. *Somatic mutations of the thyroid-stimulating hormone receptor gene in feline hyperthyroidism: parallels with human hyperthyroidism.* J Endocrinol. 2005;186(3):523–37.

Wedekind KJ, Blumer ME, Huntington CE, et al. *The feline iodine requirement is lower than the 2006 NRC recommended allowance.* J Anim Physiol and Anim Nutr 2010; 94: 537–539.

Whitney JL, Barrs VRD, Wilkinson MR, et al: *Use of bisphosphonates to treat severe idiopathic hypercalcemia in a young Ragdoll cat.* J Feline Med Surg 2011 Vol 13 (2) pp. 129–34.

Williams TL, Peak KJ, Brodbelt D, et al. *Survival and the development of azotemia after treatment of hyperthyroid cats.* J Vet Intern Med 2010; 24: 863–869.

Wimpole JA, Adagra CF, Billson MF, Pillai DN, Foster DJ. *Plasma free metanephrines in healthy cats, cats with non-adrenal disease and a cat with suspected phaeochromocytoma.* J Feline Med Surg 2010, 12(6):435–40.

Zeugswetter F, Handl S, Iben C, Schwendenwein I. *Efficacy of plasma beta-hydroxybutyrate concentration as a marker for diabetes mellitus in acutely sick cats.* J Feline Med Surg. 2010 Apr;12(4):300–5.

Zeugswetter F, Pagitz M. *Ketone measurements using dipstick methodology in cats with diabetes mellitus.* J Small Anim Pract. 2009 Jan;50(1):4–8.

Test

1. Diabetes mellitus in the cat is:

A) Common and may be transient.
B) Common, usually permanent and causes insulin dependency for life.
C) Is only treated with a diet rich in fibre.
D) Is usually caused by pancreatic neoplasms.

2. Regarding diabetic ketoacidosis in cats:

A) It occurs when there is a slight insulin deficiency and may go unnoticed.
B) It must be confirmed by measuring fructosamine levels.
C) If not treated urgently, it is fatal.
D) Its mortality is low (5%).

3. Regarding feline hyperthyroidism:

A) It is very rare and exclusive to some breeds.
B) It is very common, and its incidence is increasing.
C) It is caused by a malignant lesion in the thyroid gland in most cases.
D) It is one of the most frequent diseases in young cats.

4. Regarding adrenal tumours in feline species:

A) They can produce excessive levels of cortisol.
B) They usually cause hypocortisolism.
C) They are extremely rare.
D) They can cause low blood pressure and severe bradycardia.

5. Regarding feline acromegaly:

A) It is a type of diabetes mellitus.
B) It is caused by growth hormone deficiency.
C) It is caused by excess growth hormone.
D) It is a disease that affects kittens.

6. Regarding diabetes mellitus in the cat:

A) 80% is type II and can be reversible.
B) Type II DM is more common in unneutered females which live outdoors.
C) The diagnosis is simple, with the presence of clinical signs (PD PU PF).
D) In order to achieve remission, treatment should initially be with diet changes and insulin treatment should be delayed.

7. With respect to maintenance treatments for diabetes mellitus and ketoacidosis (DKA), which one is correct?

A) The insulin of choice for maintenance treatment is regular insulin.
B) The diet of choice for maintenance is low in carbohydrates and high in protein.
C) DKA treatment should be given at home, to minimize stress, with slow-release insulin and diet.
D) Cats with acromegaly or diabetic hyperadrenocorticism require low doses of insulin.

8. Which statement is true regarding hyperthyroidism in cats?

A) In Spain and Portugal, the incidence is much lower than in other countries.
B) For clinical detection, the neck should be palpated and TT4 levels should be routinely measured in all geriatric cats.
C) 50% of cases have high levels of TT4 and this should be confirmed with high levels of free T4 in all cases.
D) The most effective treatment is a diet high in sodium and low in iodine.

9. Hyperadrenocorticism (pituitary and adrenal):

A) Causes anorexia, weakness and tremors.
B) It usually occurs with diabetes mellitus, since there is insulin resistance.
C) The treatment of choice is with mitotane.
D) Adrenalectomy is not usually an option, given the high mortality (80%).

10. Regarding hypercalcaemia in the cat:

A) It is very rare and occurs exclusively due to parathyroid adenomas.
B) Requires a comprehensive diagnostic plan, including ionized calcium, serum phosphorus, and diagnostic imaging of the abdomen.
C) Idiopathic hypercalcaemia does not require treatment.
D) Idiopathic hypercalcaemia can be treated with parathyroidectomy.

11. Regarding diabetes mellitus in the cat:

A) Remission happens in between 60–70% of recently diagnosed cats.
B) Treatment with insulin or hypoglycaemics increases the chances of remission regardless of diet.
C) When secondary to pancreatitis, DM never remises.
D) Blood glucose curves should always be performed in the clinic.

12. A cat suffering from diabetic ketoacidosis (DKA):

A) Requires treatment with slow acting insulin or glargine.
B) Can additionally be treated with hypoglycaemic drugs and fluid therapy.
C) Requires treatment with fluid therapy, electrolyte replacement and regular insulin.
D) Insulin should be administered in high doses as soon as possible, to normalize blood glucose as quickly as possible.

13. What is the correct statement regarding cats with hyperthyroidism?

A) Some hyperthyroid cats may have low or normal TT4.
B) In cats with occult hyperthyroidism, TSH is elevated.
C) Treatment of hyperthyroidism does not affect levels of azotaemia.
D) Dietary treatment should be combined with methimazole.

14. Feline acromegaly:

A) Is very rare and over diagnosed.
B) Is diagnosed by checking low IGF-I levels and confirmed by imaging techniques (MRI) to visualize the pituitary.
C) Can be treated with somatostatin analogues.
D) Can be treated with trilostane and low doses of insulin.

15. Adrenal tumours in the cat:

A) Can cause severe hypotension and weakness.
B) Can cause severe hypotension with fatal consequences.
C) Hyperaldosteronism is caused by an injury to the adrenal medulla and causes hyperkalaemia.
D) The low-dose dexamethasone suppression test is the test of choice to confirm hyperadrenocorticism and 0.1 mg/kg is used.

16. Feline hypercalcaemia:

A) The most frequent cause is primary hyperparathyroidism.
B) Is only very rarely caused by a neoplasm.
C) The idiopathic type is treated with a diet rich in fibre, corticosteroids or bisphosphonates.
D) Is usually asymptomatic, even with severe hypercalcaemia.

Clinical case

Rony is a six-and-a-half-year-old male neutered Persian cat. He is brought to the practice because he is depressed and does not play. He has stopped grooming and his coat is in poor condition.

Two days ago, he began to show a lack of appetite. He is fed dry food low in carbohydrates, other foods and canned food. He also shows polydipsia (300 ml/day) and polyuria.

Two months ago, he was diagnosed with diabetes, which is being treated with 2.5 IU glargine/12 h.
He weighs 2.1 kg (1/9 body condition), although he has always been very thin. There is no concurrent illness.

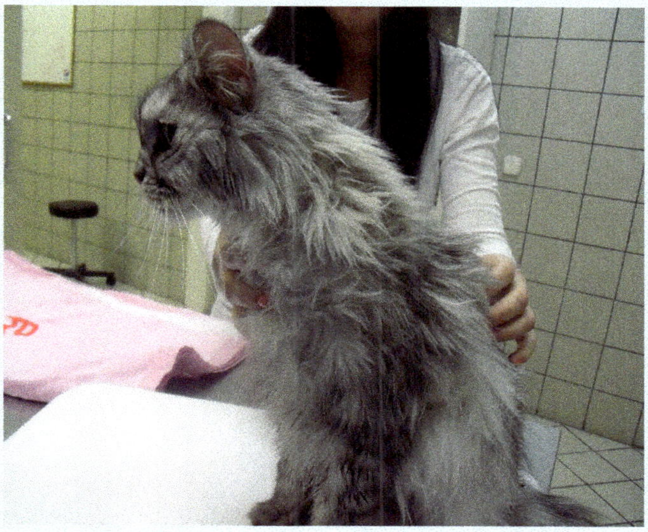

The following information is collected after the history is taken and a first examination is performed:

- Weight 2.1 kg; BCS: 1/9.
- Heart rate: 160 bpm.
- Normal respiratory rate.
- Normal hydration, lymph nodes and mucous membranes.
- Temperature: 38.5°C.
- Poor appearance to the coat.
- Palpation of the neck normal.
- Normal eye examination.
- Systolic blood pressure (Doppler) 140 mmHg.
- Depressed.
- Polyuria/polydipsia.
- Poor control of diabetes (treated with 1 IU/12 h insulin).
- Weight loss.
- Fussy appetite.

1. With this information, what problems would you include in your differential diagnoses?

A diagnostic plan is established in which the following tests will be carried out:

- Complete blood count and blood chemistry.
- TT4 levels.
- Urinalysis and urine culture.
- Ultrasound of the neck and abdomen.

Results of tests are as follows:

Table 1. Complete blood count

Parameter	Result	Reference range
Haematocrit (%)	27	38–58
Haemoglobin (g/dl)	8.8	13–19
Red blood cells (x10^6/µl)	5.64	5.5–8.6
MCV (fl)	54.2	62–74
MCH (pg)	15.6	21–25
MCHC (g/dl)	32.6	31–36
Leukocytes (x10^3/µl)	8.5	6–17
Basophils (%)	4	0–2
Eosinophils (%)	59	2–10
Segmented (%)	35	5–10
Lymphocytes (%)	–	15–43
Monocytes (%)	–	1–7
Platelets	Aggregated	150–500

Table 2. Blood biochemistry

Parameter	Result	Reference range
Glucose (mg/dl)	216	70–120
Urea (mg/dl)	64	20–40
Creatinine (mg/dl)	0.6	0.5–1.4
Total proteins (g/dl)	7.5	5.5–7.5
ALT (U/l)	625	<80
Alkaline phosphatase (U/l)	1,025	<100
Sodium (mEq/l)	144	142–152
Potassium (mEq/l)	3.6	3.5–5.5
Chlorine (mEq/l)	112	110–120
Calcium (mg/dl)	10.7	8–11.6
Phosphorus (mg/dl)	5.1	3.5–6.5

Table 3. Urinalysis and urine culture

Parameter	Result
Protein/creatinine ratio	0.3
UD	1.046
Glucosuria	1,000 mg/dl
Blood	+++
Sediment	–
Leukocytes	1–3/400x
Red blood cells	42–72/400x
Culture	Negative

And with respect to TT4, the result is 1.53 µg/dl (1.5–4.7), while for β OH butyrate it is 0.2 mmol/l.

2. The ultrasound shows the following. Explain what you see in the three images below?

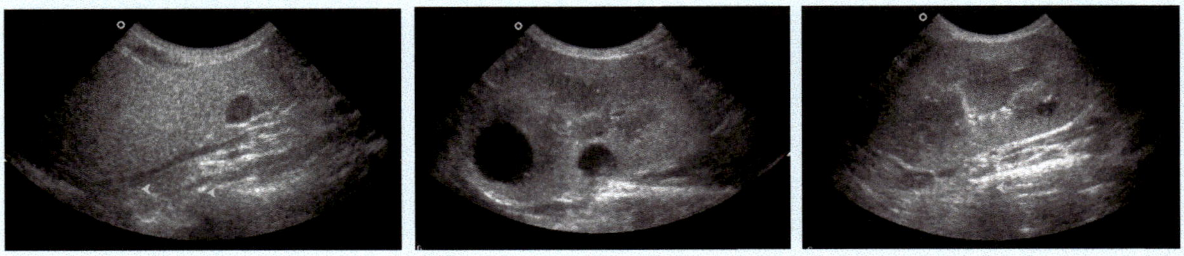

3. What would your diagnosis be?
4. What treatment would you implement?

Answers

Test

1. A	7. B	13. A
2. C	8. B	14. C
3. B	9. B	15. D
4. A	10. B	16. C
5. C	11. A	
6. A	12. C	

Clinical case

1. With this information, what problems would you include in your differential diagnoses?
Kidney disease, urinary tract infection/pyelonephritis, feline hyperthyroidism, liver disease (cholangiohepatitis, lipidosis ...), pancreatitis and triaditis.

2. The ultrasound shows the following. Explain what you see in the three images below?
Ultrasound report: the urine bladder is distended and contains little urinary sediment. In the clinical case in question, cystopuncture was performed.

There are multiple large cystic structures in the left kidney that occupy approximately 30 to 40% of the renal parenchyma. The largest cyst is 1 cm and is located on the cranial pole of the kidney with hyperechogenic content inside.

There are several calculi present in the renal pelvis, the largest measures 6mm. Slightly dilated pelvis (<3 mm), without signs of ureteral calculi or signs compatible with an obstructive condition at the time of the study.

Right kidney with micro-mineralisation in the medullary sinus and presence of two cystic structu-es in the medial zone and caudal pole measuring 5 and 6.6 mm, respectively. Both kidneys have hyperechogenic cortices.

Spleen decreased in size with homogeneous parenchyma and enlarged liver with markedly hyperechogenic parenchyma.

Distended gallbladder with the presence of biliary sludge and dilation of the common bile duct to 4 mm along its entire length.

Image compatible with diffuse liver disease (hepatic lipidosis) and cholecystitis.

Presence of a small amount of free abdominal fluid.

Slight increase in the size of the jejunal lymph nodes, compatible with reactive lymphadenopathy.

Digestive tract shows no ultrasonographic changes.

Adrenal glands of normal ultrasonographic size and morphology.

Rest of the abdomen ultrasonographically normal.

3. What would your diagnosis be?
Diabetes mellitus, hepatic lipidosis and polycystic kidneys.

4. What treatment would you implement?
Diabetes and hepatic lipidosis must be treated:

- Diabetes mellitus:
  - Glargine 3 IU/12 h.
  - Low carbohydrate diet (wet) adjusted for 4 kg (ideal weight).
  - Potassium gluconate (Kaminox®) 1 ml/12 h.
  - Famotidine 2.5 mg/12 h.
  - Maropitant SC for 3 days. Subsequently oral/24 h.
- Hepatic lipidosis:
  - Ursodeoxycholic acid 15 mg/24 h.
  - Amoxicillin clavulanate: 50 mg/12 h.
  - Metronidazole 15 mg/12 h.

Progression

In a week Rony is clinically better. Although she continues to have polyuria/polydipsia, she has a better appetite and has gained weight (500 g more). She does not have vomiting or diarrhoea.

Blood glucose measurement two days before:

- Before insulin, 513 mg/dl.
- 4 hours after insulin administration: 317 mg/dl.
- B-OH butyrate: 0.3 mmol/l.
- ALT: 462 U/l.
- K^+: 4.9 mEq/l.

It was decided to continue administration of glargine 3 IU/12 h and Kaminox and maropitant were withdrawn.

At 15 days, the patient is clinically better, eats well and there is no polyuria/polydipsia. Weight 3 kg.

In addition:

- β-OH butyrate: 0.0 mmol/l.
- ALT: 159 U/l.
- K^+: 4 mEq/l.

The decision was taken to continue with antibiotic treatment.

One month after the start of the treatments, the cat weighs 3.5 kg and the antibiotic and ursodeoxycholic acid treatments are withdrawn.

Due to the blood glucose curve (Table 4), the insulin dose was increased to 4 IU/12 h.

Table 4. **Progress of Rony during the first 2 months of treatment**

Time	Weight	Symptoms	Blood gluose curve (h-mg/dl)	Insuline dose
After one week	2.6 kg	No	13:00–343 15:00–283 17:00–311 19:00–317 21:00–391	5 IU/12 h
After 15 days	3 kg	No	13:00–320 15:00–245 17:00–219 19:00–314 21:00–391	6 IU/12 h
After one month	3.5 kg	No	13:00–394 15:00–343 17:00–362 19:00–375 21:00–421	4 IU/12 h
After two months	4.8 kg	No	13:00–248 15:00–180 17:00–146 19:00–159 21:00–140	6.5 IU/12 h

Clinical neurology

12

Alejandro Luján Feliu-Pascual

Contents

Basic neuroanatomy

For consistency, throughout this chapter the **2012 Nomina Anatomica Veterinaria is used** to concisely define each of the structures found in the nervous system (NS) of domestic animals.

The correct localisation of a neurological lesion and subsequent interpretation of diagnostic tests depends on a good understanding of the "normal" anatomy of the nervous system.

Traditionally the nervous system is divided into the central nervous system (CNS) and the peripheral nervous system (PNS). However, from a functional point of view, these systems do not function independently. For example, the proprioceptive system has components that form part of the PNS (spinal nerve receptors and afferent fibres) and the CNS (ascending tracts, thalamus relay nuclei, connections in the cerebellum, interpretation centres in the cerebral cortex etc.).

The CNS is protected by covering layers, suspended by a series of ligaments and surrounded by **cerebrospinal fluid (CSF), which serves as protection**, in addition to nourishing its parenchyma.

The membranous **CNS coverings, called meninges**, consist of:

- **pia mater**: closely bound to brain tissue and the spinal cord
- **arachnoid mater**: a thin network of connective tissue in the form of a net, which secures the spinal cord and the brain to the dura mater
- **dura mater**: the outermost and hardest layer, formed of fibrous tissue.

CSF mainly forms in the lateral, third and fourth ventricles, and flows caudally from the first to the third ventricle, mesencephalic aqueduct, and fourth ventricle. CSF exits the cranial cavity through the lateral openings to the subarachnoid space, to externally encircle the brain and spinal cord, or the central canal of the spinal cord.

Each anatomical division of the CNS has its own functions which translate into characteristic neurological deficits when these structures are affected; although it is not possible to differentiate the cause simply by identifying the location. However, knowing

Table 1. The most significant components of the CNS.

Encephalon	Telencephalon or cerebrum	Frontal lobe Parietal lobe Temporal lobe Occipital lobe Piriform lobe Hippocampus	
	Brainstem	Diencephalon Mesencephalon	
		Metencephalon	Dorsal: Cerebellum Ventral: Pons
		Myelencephalon or *medulla oblongata*	
Spinal cord	C1-C4		
	C6-T2 or cervical intumescence		
	T3-L3		
	L4-S3 or lumbosacral intumescence		

the characteristic neurological functions and signs that appear as a consequence of focal pathologies of the nervous system is fundamental for clinical examination and choice of the most appropriate diagnostic methods.

It is also important to remember that, as a result of the uneven growth of the spine with respect to nerve structures, in **most dogs (especially large breeds) the lumbar, sacral and caudal spinal segments are displaced cranially** with respect to their respective vertebrae. In cats, however, they are parallel.

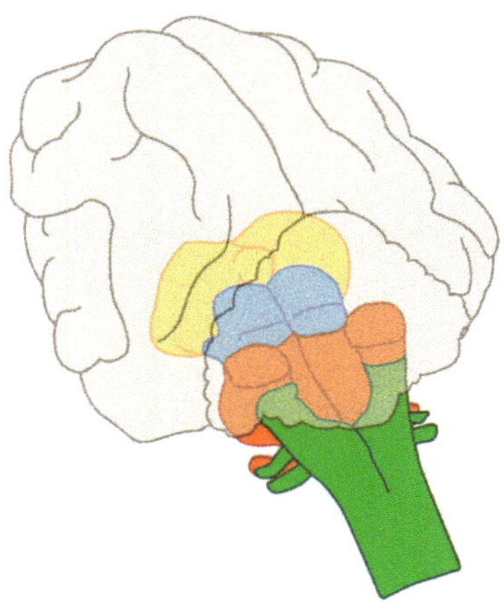

Figure 2. Structures of the feline brainstem: diencephalon (yellow), mesencephalon (blue), pons (brown) and myelencephalon (green).

Functional neuroanatomy

Each part of the nervous system has a specific function and when it suffers an injury, then loss or disorder of that function occurs (Figures 1 and 2).

Telencephalon

- **Frontal lobe**: motor cortex and associative reasoning. Focal lesions cause behavioural changes such as aggression, circling, hyperactivity, compulsive movements, etc.
- **Parietal lobe**: sensory cortex. Focal lesions cause hypoalgesia, anaesthesia and postural delays.
- **Temporal lobe**: memory and hearing.
- **Occipital lobe**: vision: contralateral hemianopia: absence of vision in the contralateral visual field of each eye.
- **Piriform lobe**: smell. Focal lesions cause anosmia.
- **Hippocampus**: behavioural patterns, personality, short-term memory.

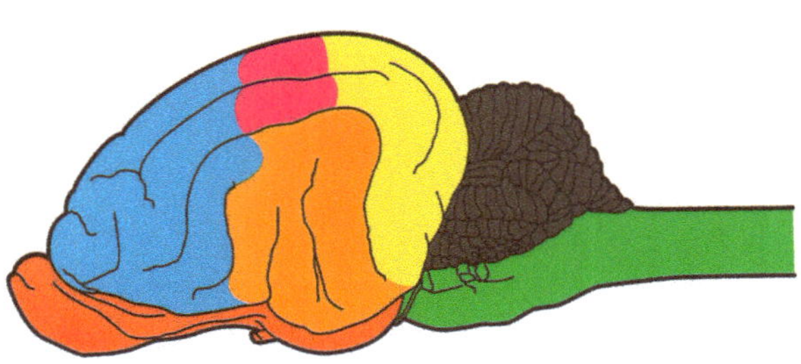

Figure 1. Structures of the feline telencephalon: frontal lobe (blue), parietal lobe (pink), occipital lobe (yellow), piriform lobe and olfactory bulb (brown), brain stem (green), cerebellum (grey) and temporal lobe (orange).

Diencephalon

- **Thalamus**: maintenance of consciousness, centre for ascending and descending connections between the spinal cord and cerebral cortex. All conscious sensations undergo a synapse in the thalamus and project onto the contralateral cortex, except for smell. Similarly, all conscious responses that begin in the cerebral cortex pass through the thalamus to synapse and cross over to the contralateral side of the body.

- **Hypothalamus**: control centre for autonomous functions, regulation of body temperature, hunger and satiety, endocrine function through the pituitary gland. Focal lesions cause, polyuria/polydipsia, anorexia and changes to thermoregulation.
- **Optic chiasm**: cranial nerve II afferent pathway for vision. This is an extension of the CNS where 65% of the fibres on one side decuss contralaterally allowing binocular vision. Injuries to the nerve or chiasm cause ipsilateral blindness if they are located before the decussation.

Mesencephalon

- **Rostral and caudal *colliculi*:** ocular and auditory reflexes, respectively. This reflex allows a quick turn of the head or body to locate sounds or light sources.
- **Cranial nerve motor nuclei**: oculomotor nerve III and trochlear nerve IV. Extraocular movements. Oculomotor involvement causes medial and ventral deviation of the eyeball while trochlear involvement causes a lateral rotation of the dorsal pole of the eyeball.
- **Parasympathetic nucleus of the oculomotor nerve III**: pupillary contraction in response to light stimuli. Injury causes mydriasis that does not respond to light stimuli.
- **Mesencephalic nucleus and tract of trigeminal nerve V**: receives proprioceptive information from face, masticatory muscles and mouth.

Ventral metencephalon (pons)

- **Pontine trigeminal sensory nucleus V**: receives sensitive proprioceptive information from the face, mouth, etc.
- **Trigeminal motor nucleus V**: mandibular movements. Involvement causes masticatory paralysis if it is bilateral in acute lesions and muscular atrophy in chronic lesions.
- **Reticular formation**: diffuse network of interconnected neurons that extends from the diencephalon to the myelencephalon and is responsible for the maintenance of consciousness, the respiratory, vasomotor, protective (cough and vomit) centres.
- **Abducent nerve nucleus VI**: extraocular movements for lateral movement of the eyeball.
- **Facial nerve nucleus VII**: facial musculature movements. Facial paralysis occurs with dropped lips and salivation.
- **Vestibular nuclei**: balance. Involvement causes head tilting, nystagmus, ataxia and weakness.
- **Cochlear nucleus**: hearing. Bilateral involvement causes deafness.

Myelencephalon

- **Area postrema**: chemoreceptor area controlling vomiting.
- **Solitary tract and nucleus**: information relay of visceral reflexes of the pharynx, larynx, oesophagus, trachea and abdominal and thoracic viscera.
- **Parasympathetic nucleus of the glossopharyngeal nerve IX**: innervation to the salivary glands.
- **Parasympathetic nucleus of the vagus nerve X**: motor innervation to the abdominal and thoracic viscera.
- **Hypoglossal nerve nucleus XII**: motor innervation to most lingual muscles. Injury causes unilateral or bilateral atrophy of the tongue.

Cerebellum

The cerebellum's function is **movement coordination through inhibition.** It receives proprioceptive afferent fibres and sends efferent ones to higher motor centres (UMN). There are no direct connections with lower motor nuclei. Involvement in lesions causes increased muscle tone, and an increased range of joint movement and tremors.

Spinal cord

The organization of the spinal cord is somatotopic. The **ascending proprioceptive tracts are located superficially** and the first to be affected by numerous pathologies (Figure 3, areas in blue). Descending motor tracts (Figure 3, red) and the ascending somatic tracts (Figure 3, green) are located more internally. The ascending tracts for deep nociception are located around the grey matter of the spinal cord, which explains why it is the last to be affected and that its involvement means severe injury.

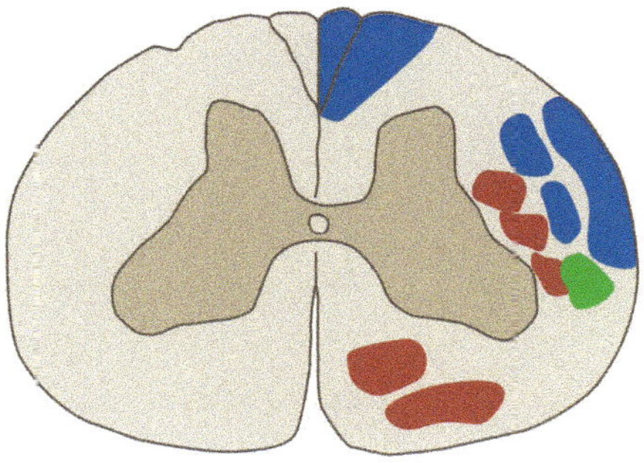

Figure 3. Organisation of the ascending proprioceptive tracts (blue), descending motor pathways (red) and ascending somatic pathways (green) in the spinal cord.

Neurological exam

The first aim of the neurological examination is to identify neurological abnormalities which confirm the presence of a lesion in the nervous system. The second objective is the localisation of the lesion in one of the divisions of the nervous system (central or peripheral nervous system, or neuromuscular junction) or the musculoskeletal system.

In the majority of cases, lesion location requires a basic knowledge of the function of the nervous system and the deficits manifested by lesions in different anatomical divisions. A variety of text books detail the neurological exam and can help with interpretation of results (Garosi, 2009; De Lahunta, 2004; Morales and Montoliu, 2012).

Consultation

An important part of a good neurological examination is taking a complete and exhaustive clinical history. In some cases the underlying cause (e.g. head trauma) can be determined although in some circumstances the owners may not be forthcoming with information. The mention of clinical signs apparently unrelated to the reason for the visit (polyuria, polydipsia etc.) should not be overlooked and may guide the neurological exam and the diagnostic tests required. Special importance should be given to vaccination history, deworming, the cat's environment and behaviour (hunter), exposure to toxins and diet.

The importance of a good physical examination should not be underestimated as it can identify anomalies related to the reason for the visit such as heart murmur in cases of collapse, laryngeal masses in cases of dysphagia, and lack of pulse in aortic thromboembolism.

An orthopaedic examination is equally important, since many **orthopaedic problems can be confused with neurological problems** especially by the inexperienced eye. Special attention should be paid to gait evaluation, palpation and manipulation of the joints and the presence of painful points in bones, muscles and ligaments.

Observation and manipulation

The stages of the neurological examination can be divided into **observation and manipulation**. The reserved nature of many cats means the exam can be tricky, if not impossible. During the observation phase, the cat's mental state, posture and gait are evaluated. During manipulation (if allowed by the patient) postural reactions, spinal myotatic reflexes, cranial nerves, nociception, and presence of painful areas in the head and spine assessed.

Whilst taking the history it is useful to leave the cat loose in the room (first covering any gaps or holes between furniture and walls). While talking to the owner, **the cat's mental state should be observed** and reactions to the environment, along with any evidence of compulsive turning, and postural abnormalities. When assessing mental status, owner reports of any behavioural changes can be more reliable than a one-off neurological examination.

Mental state

There are five mental states:

1. **Normal**: the cat reacts to environmental stimuli in a manner consistent with the intensity of the stimulus.
2. **Obtundation**: due to a neurological cause, obtundation is typified by reduced reactions to environmental stimuli.
3. **Delirium**: the cat reacts inappropriately and often in an exaggerated manner to environmental stimuli.
4. **Stupor**: there is an absence of response to a visual or auditory stimulus but a positive response to painful stimuli.
5. **Coma**: the comatose patient does not respond to any stimulus, even painful ones.

For there to be a **decrease in mental alertness, the ascending activating reticular system must be affected by a focal lesion or the cerebral cortex affected by a diffuse lesion** (for example, hepatic encephalopathy). Focal lesions in the cerebral cortex do not cause a decrease in mental status unless there is an increase in intracranial pressure and secondary compression of the brainstem.

Posture

Evaluation of posture can also occur while taking the clinical history. Evidence of limb abduction, head tilt (Figure 4), scoliosis, kyphosis, lordosis, tremor, myoclonus, pleurothotonus, etc. should be observed.

Gait

In cats, gait assessment can be difficult, so it is helpful to take advantage of their inquisitive nature and do so while they roam the consult room. The patient should be examined from all four angles and particular attention paid to all phases of the walk.

The following steps require direct contact with the patient which, in some cats, can be problematic.

Postural reactions

Postural reactions evaluate both **conscious and unconscious proprioceptive pathways**. The fibres and nerve tracts that carry this information are large and travel

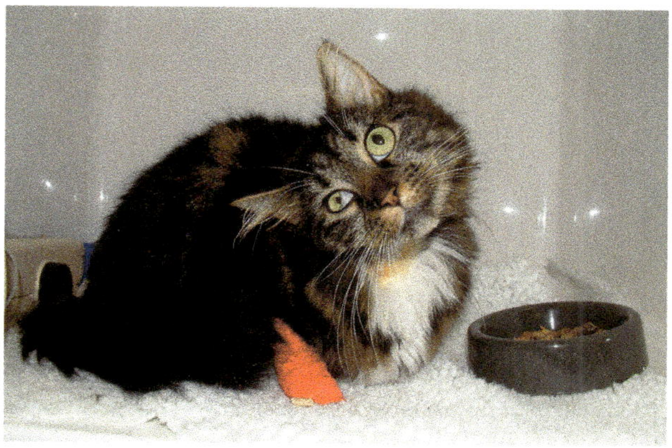

Figure 4. Vestibular syndrome. Horner's syndrome is also present in the right eye.

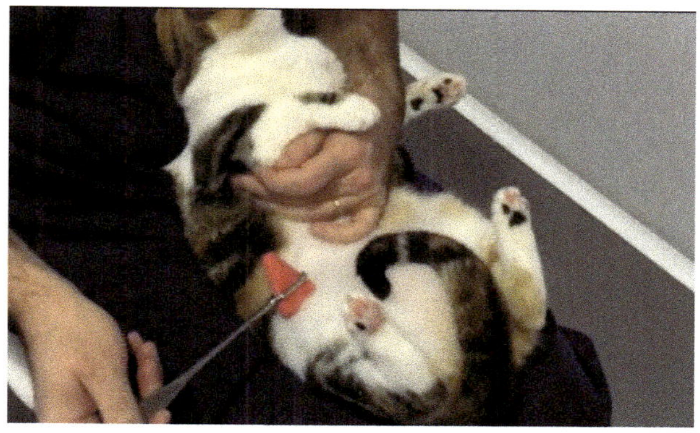

Figure 5. Alternative method of testing spinal reflexes with the cat in dorsal recumbency on a lap.

superficially in the spinal cord (Figure 3, blue). As a result, they are the first to be affected by nerve or spinal injuries.

Information about **joint position and muscle tension** is collected by receptors located in these structures and travels via **ascending pathways to the brain**, where it is subsequently **coordinated by the cerebellum** to initiate a corrective postural action via **descending pathways to the effector muscles**. An injury to peripheral nerves, the spinal cord, or brain can cause delays in these reactions.

The most commonly used tests are the conscious proprioception test, reflex step, hemiwalk, jump, wheelbarrow, extensor postural thrust, balancing, crossed extensor reflex, and visual and tactile postural reactions. All these reactions and reflexes are aimed at **adjusting body position** and, thus, providing the body with a stable position from which to initiate voluntary movements.

The reflex step and the conscious proprioception test preferably use conscious pathways to the cerebral cortex. For the other tests, although the information reaches the sensory cortex, they do not need voluntary initiation of the response.

Spinal reflexes

The evaluation of spinal reflexes plays an important part in the neurological examination since it **provides enough information to locate neurological lesions in the upper motor neuron (UMN) or lower motor neuron (LMN):**

- LMN signs:
  - Muscular atrophy >7 days.
  - Absent or decreased reflexes.
  - Absent or reduced muscle tone.
- UMN signs:
  - Normal or increased muscle tone.
  - Normal or increased reflexes.
  - No muscle atrophy or minimal due to disuse.

Most cats allow examination of their reflexes in lateral recumbency. However, some cats prefer to lie on a lap in dorsal recumbency (Figure 5).

Without a doubt, **the patellar reflex is the most constant** and reliable of all these reflexes. The spinal segments involved are L4-L6 and **it is monosynaptic,** since there is only one direct synapse between the axon of the sensory neuron and the alpha motor neuron responsible for muscle contraction. The reflex may be **absent, diminished, normal, increased, or clonic.** Its absence or decrease may be a consequence of a sensory (polyneuropathy) or motor problem (polyneuropathy, neuromuscular junction such as botulism or myopathy). An increase in the patellar reflex may result from a lesion in the upper motor nuclei that eliminates the inhibitory action of the upper motor neuron or of spinal segments L6-S1 (pseudo hyperreflexia) in which knee extension is not counteracted by the flexor muscles, obtaining an exaggerated extensor contraction. The presence of a clonic reflex indicates a chronic UMN lesion.

The **flexor or withdrawal reflex**, on the other hand, is **polysynaptic** since both excitatory and inhibitory neurons are involved in its function, in the same spinal and adjacent segments. This may be diminished, but not increased.

If there is an extension of the contralateral limb when the flexor reflex is performed, it is called a **cross-extensor reflex**. This is pathological in the adult animal when lying down and indicates chronic damage to the UMN.

In thoracolumbar lesions evaluation of the *cutaneous trunci* reflex (erroneously called the pannicular reflex) is useful. This is tested by stimulation of **thoracolumbar dermatomes from L6 to T3** and is mediated by the *cutaneous trunci* muscle through the **lateral thoracic nerve formed by the ventral roots of the spinal C8 and T1 nerves.** Serious injuries to the spinal cord or spinal nerves can cause bilateral or unilateral absence of this reflex respectively.

More caudally, the **perineal reflex** is evaluated by stimulating the skin around the anal sphincter and observing its contraction. This assesses sensitivity and motor function from **pudendal nerves, S1-S3 nerve roots**, as well as their connections to the lumbar intumescence.

Other myotatic reflexes such as gastrocnemius, cranial tibialis, bicipital and radial carpal extensor are not as reliable or consistent as those mentioned above.

Cranial nerves

Evaluation of the cranial nerves is based on both observation and functional tests.

The patient should be observed for asymmetry of the face, muscular atrophy in the masticatory muscles, deviation of the nose or ears, narrower palpebral fissures, deviation of the eyeball, pupil and tongue, enophthalmos, and exophthalmos.

The **menace response** is examined by moving the hand into the visual field and observing the contraction of the eyelids. The movement must be fast but should not cause air movement since this can stimulate the eyelashes causing a false positive in a blind animal. The menace response **requires the visual system** (retina, optic nerve, chiasma, optic tract, occipital cortex), **cerebellum, mesencephalon and facial nerve to be intact**. Conscious interpretation is necessary, so it is not considered a reflex, but a learned response that manifests for the first time around three months in the cat.

The **palpebral reflex**, on the other hand, does not need interpretation in the cerebral cortex and evaluates facial sensory information collected by the trigeminal nerve V and the motor response of palpebral contraction by the facial nerve VII, as well as its connections in the brainstem.

The **absence of pupillary reflexes** is assessed by shining a bright light into the pupils and observing contraction of the iris constrictor muscle. This reflex involves the retina, optic nerve II, chiasm, optic tract, mesencephalon, and oculomotor nerve III responsible for parasympathetic innervation of the iris.

The **vestibulo-ocular reflex** evaluates the peripheral vestibular system, the vestibular portion of the vestibulocochlear nerve (VIII), the vestibular nuclei in the myelencephalon, the cerebellum and cranial nerves III, IV and VI (which innervate the extraocular muscles and are responsible for eye movements). It is examined by moving the head to the side and observing whether the eyeballs initially remain static but move rapidly in the direction of induced movement as they should do physiologically.

The presence of **spontaneous nystagmus is always pathological** and suggests a lesion in any of the nuclei and projections mentioned for the vestibulo-ocular reflex. This nystagmus can be horizontal, rotatory or vertical and its direction can help locate the lesion in the central or peripheral vestibular system.

Most of the **skin sensory information to the head** is transmitted through the ophthalmic, maxillary and mandibular branches of the trigeminal nerve (V), although the facial nerve has sensory branches that innervate the inner surface of the pinna. Pinching the lips with a haemostat should cause facial contraction and an attempt to move the head away.

To evaluate the **swallowing reflex**, opening the animal's mouth and stimulating the tongue or pharynx is necessary so that weakness or deviation of the tongue muscles can be detected at the same time. Sensory information collected by the facial, glossopharyngeal and vagus nerves, and the motor activity by the glossopharyngeal, vagus, and hypoglossal nerves, as well as their connections in the brainstem can be evaluated. In cats where it is not possible to open the mouth, the pharynx can be stimulated by pressing it through the skin.

Nociception

The last part of the neurological examination is **pain sensation**.

The spine should be palpated by pressing on the spinous process of each vertebra in the thoracic and lumbar spine and paraspinal musculature. In the cervical spine the transverse processes of C1 and C6 can be palpated, and the neck can be manipulated and flexed as long as there is no suspicion of fracture.

Superficial pain is evaluated by pinching the skin with mosquito forceps.

To assess the presence or absence of **deep pain** the metacarpals or metatarsals can be pinched with mosquito forceps or, better still, the distal portion of the tibia with bone forceps. Only the presence of a conscious reaction (meow, turn of the head, attempt to bite or scratch) indicates that nociception is intact.

If superficial pain is present evaluation of deep pain is not necessary.

Special situations

Obviously, in some situations not all reactions and reflexes can be evaluated, for example, in a comatose patient or one suffering from a vertebral fracture. In these cases, the clinician should locate the neurological injury with minimal patient manipulation.

In cases of coma, evaluation of the cranial nerves and especially the vestibulo-ocular and pupillary reflex, while in the case of spinal trauma evaluation of spinal reflexes and the presence of superficial and deep pain is essential.

Neurological lesion localisation

Once a neurological examination is complete the following questions should be answered:

- Does the animal suffer from a neurological condition?
- Where is the neurological lesion located?

To help answer the second question the most common neurological signs associated with the different locations should be listed. The examples illustrated correspond to the locations described, but they do not necessarily show all the signs listed (Table 2).

Table 2. Neurological signs which may be found on neurological examination depending on the location of the lesion.

Lesion location	Clinical signs seen on neurological examination
Telencephalon	Seizures Delayed or absent conscious postural reactions contralateral to the side of the lesion Central blindness with normal pupillary reflexes Pleurothotonus towards the side of the lesion Compulsive turning towards the side of the lesion Head pressing against objects or people No ataxia Facial hypoaesthesia Obtundation to coma with diffuse lesions
Brainstem	Obtundation, stupor or coma Facial paralysis Masticatory muscle atrophy Facial hypoaesthesia Head tilt towards the lesion Pathological nystagmus Reduced pupillary reflexes Strabismus Vestibular ataxia
Cerebellum	Normal mental state Cerebellar ataxia Hypermetria Intention tremor Head tilt contralateral to the lesion Wide based stance Absent menace response Strabismus Pendular nystagmus
C1-C5	Normal mental state Spinal ataxia Hypermetria Delayed postural reactions in all limbs Tetraparesis/tetraplegia Normal or increased spinal reflexes Normal or increased muscle tone
C6-T2	Normal mental state Delayed postural reactions in all limbs Tetraparesis/tetraplegia Reduced spinal reflexes in thoracic limbs Muscle atrophy in thoracic limbs Reduced muscle tone in thoracic limbs Horner's syndrome
T3-L3	Normal mental state Normal thoracic limbs Pelvic limb and trunk ataxia Paraparesis/paraplegia Normal or increased spinal reflexes in pelvic limbs Normal or increased muscle tone in pelvic limbs Reduction or absence of cutaneous trunci reflex Urinary incontinence (full bladder, difficult to empty)

Continued

Table 2. (Continued)

Lesion location	Clinical signs seen on neurological examination
L4-S3	Normal mental state Normal thoracic limbs Pelvic limb ataxia Paraparesis/paraplegia Reduced spinal reflexes in pelvic limbs Reduced muscle tone in pelvic limbs Reduction or absence of cutaneous trunci reflex Muscle atrophy in pelvic limbs Urinary incontinence (full bladder, easy to empty with reduced tone) Reduced anal tone, sensation and perineal reflex
Neuromuscular	Normal mental state Reduced spinal and cranial nerve reflexes Muscular atrophy Reduced muscle tone Weakness/collapse Exercise intolerance Aphonia

The importance of a good neurological examination

A good neurological examination reduces the list of differential diagnoses and the research time required for diagnosis.

The clinician must keep an open mind regarding the **possibility of more than one injury,** which can confuse localisation.

Diagnostic techniques

Correct localisation of an injury to the nervous system allows a differential diagnosis list to be drawn up, and subsequent tests devised according to the location, history, and disease progression.

It is also essential to **investigate systemic diseases** which may secondarily affect the NS, such as diabetes, hypoglycaemia, portosystemic shunt, or renal failure, before subjecting the animal to more expensive tests which require general anaesthesia such as MRI or CT.

Blood tests, serum titres, CSF and PCR analysis

A wide variety of neurological diseases cause changes on blood tests, so the first step in researching any neurological disease is a complete set of tests consisting of complete blood count with smears, electrolytes, hepatic transaminases, glucose, calcium, CK, albumin, total proteins, urea and creatinine. Pre- and post-prandial bile acids and ammonium should be included when tests point towards a metabolic cause as a source. This is to rule out other medical pathologies that may secondarily affect the NS.

The results of **serum titers for infectious diseases should be interpreted with caution** (Nghiem and Schatzberg, 2010). **A positive serum titre only indicates exposure to the pathogen or vaccination**, not necessarily that the neurological disease is caused by this pathogen. This is especially true in diseases such as toxoplasmosis. An increase in serum immunoglobulins requires a competent immune system and a sufficient response period so in early stages of disease or in cases of infectious diseases that cause immunosuppression (FIV) **false negatives** may be obtained. Although a serum titre of IgM has traditionally been associated with recent exposure to the pathogen, in the case of toxoplasmosis the elevation of this immunoglobulin may persist for months or years after exposure (Lappin, 2010).

All positive serum titres should be accompanied by relevant clinical signs and test results compatible with the disease in order to be considered reliable. Therefore, knowledge of the clinical and neurological signs manifested by different infectious diseases, as well as their method of transmission is essential.

In addition, it is important to consider the possibility of cross-reactivity and contamination of the sample as this can produce a false positive (Blevins et al., 1995; Hay and Mackenzie, 1982).

The presence of a positive serum titre for an infectious disease in an animal with neurological involvement without clinical signs or compatible laboratory results is of doubtful reliability (Lappin, 2010; Jaderlund et al.,2007).

Of special importance in neurological investigation is the **analysis of cerebrospinal fluid (CSF), which**

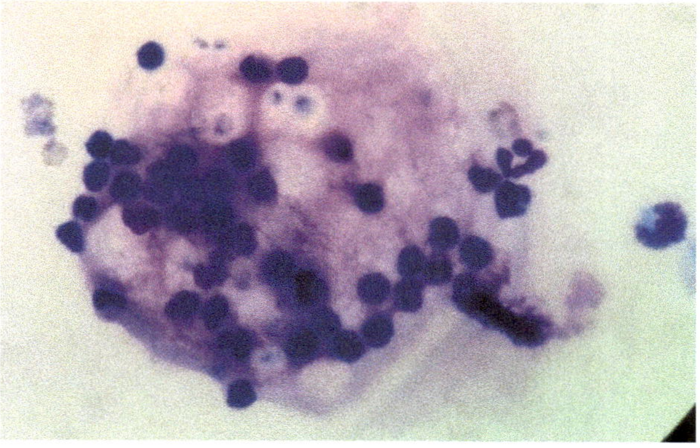

Figure 6. Image of *Cryptococcus spp.*

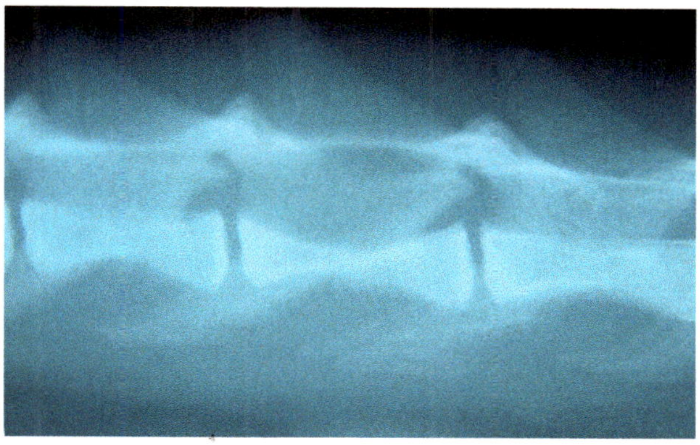

Figure 7. Right lateral radiograph of the lumbar spine of a cat where widening of the spinal canal due to lysis of the body of laminae of L5 can be seen as a consequence of a spinal meningioma.

must be performed within 30 minutes of collection for reliable results (Di Terlizzi and Platt, 2009). An increase in the number of leukocytes in CSF demonstrates inflammation, but not necessarily that the cause is exclusively inflammatory since trauma, seizures, vascular, or tumoral conditions can cause a pathological increase in cell count in cerebrospinal fluid (Di Terlizzi and Platt, 2009). The diagnosis of infectious disease in the central nervous system should be based on demonstrating the presence of the pathogen in CSF or on biopsy. It is possible to detect the pathogen in CSF by cytology as occurs with cryptococcosis (Figure 6) and toxoplasmosis, which provides a definitive diagnosis.

However, the method that has revolutionized the diagnosis of infectious diseases is the **polymerase chain reaction (PCR),** although it also has limitations. PCR uses short segments of single helix nucleotides called primers; whose sequences are complementary to known sequences of pathogen DNA. After an amplification process, the target DNA sequences can be detected by gel electrophoresis. Detection of genetic material from the pathogen in different biological samples is possible in this manner. This method is not completely infallible since **false positives** can occur when there is contamination (therefore obtaining samples under aseptic conditions and choosing a reliable laboratory are essential) and **false negatives** can occur due to the presence of PCR inhibitors. PCR is **not indicated to evaluate the response to treatment** since DNA can persist for a long time after the death of the organism.

Most degenerative and lysosomal diseases are caused by genetic mutations which can be diagnosed by DNA analysis of blood or oral mucosa. Currently, a large number of laboratories offer this service and the range of tests is expanding. However, it is important to understand the limitations of these tests such as breed specificity, the possibility of false positives, and also of concurrent diseases.

Imaging tests

For **brain lesions, CT or MRI are the most appropriate tests**. However, their usefulness is limited in neuromuscular diseases in which studies using **electromyography** and nerve conduction are essential. Both MRI and CT require deep sedation or general anaesthesia, which may be contraindicated in some neurological patients until they are haemodynamically stable.

Plain radiographs allow lesions that affect bony structures or intervertebral discs to be detected. Any lesion that causes bone remodelling either by lysis or proliferation is susceptible to detection by plain radiographs. **Orthogonal projections** under sedation or general anaesthesia are essential for correct interpretation (Figure 7).

Injection of iodised contrast into the subarachnoid space into the cerebellomedullary or lumbar cistern L6-L7 (**myelography**) is particularly useful for demonstrating the absence of spinal compressions that warrant surgical treatment. Myelography allows the complete study of the spinal cord without significantly increasing time or cost.

Both myelography and advanced imaging studies (CT, myelo-CT, MRI) may be useful for this purpose. A recent study, comparing myelography and MRI for thoracolumbar lesions, has shown that there was no difference in terms of treatment outcomes except for a higher cost when MRI was used (Parry et al., 2009). There is no doubt that MRI can show lesions that otherwise, could not be detected, due to its greater sensitivity, especially in vascular diseases of the spinal cord. However, it must be taken into account that the aforementioned imaging techniques (myelography, CT, myelo-CT and MRI) allow for a definitive diagnosis on very few occasions, especially for non-compressive lesions.

Apart from the technique used, the experience of the clinician when interpretating images is essential and, therefore, a good myelography performed and interpreted by an experienced clinician can give more information than an MRI performed by an inexperienced veterinarian. The most important factor is reaching an accurate diagnosis and to apply the appropriate therapeutic measures to that diagnosis.

Several studies show both MRI and CT can show **structural abnormalities that are not clinically significant in clinically normal animals** (Jones and Inzana, 2000; De Decker et al., 2010). Finding vertebral malformations, herniated discs, etc. is common when they are not actually the cause of the current neurological problem. Therefore, it is important to relate findings to the clinical history and neurological examination.

To understand the advantages and limitations of advanced imaging modalities, knowledge of their physical principles is fundamental.

The **CT scan** is based on the emission of X-rays from the periphery of an arch that rotates around the body, crosses the tissues and is detected by a series of receptors on the opposite side of the emitting focus. The main advantage is, like all the modalities that work with this type of radiation, the **good detail for bony structures**, as well as being able to use intrathecal or intravenous contrast, perform 3D reconstructions and quickly obtain images if a helical CT is used (Figure 8).

However, with **CT the resolution obtained from soft tissues is limited**: inflammatory, degenerative lesions and those located next to structures which cause a high degree of attenuation of this radiation (such as caudotentorial structures or those with metal implants) may go unnoticed.

The **principle of MRI** is based on excitation by means of radiofrequency pulses of protons subjected to an electromagnetic field, mainly hydrogen which is present in the largest quantities in the body, and the detection of the emission emitted by said protons when they relax. MRI is especially useful for **visualizing soft tissues such as the brain** (Figure 9) and **spinal cord**, but its main drawback is the cost of the devices, artefacts on images, and the limited resolution of the equipment with low field magnets in small sized animals such as cats.

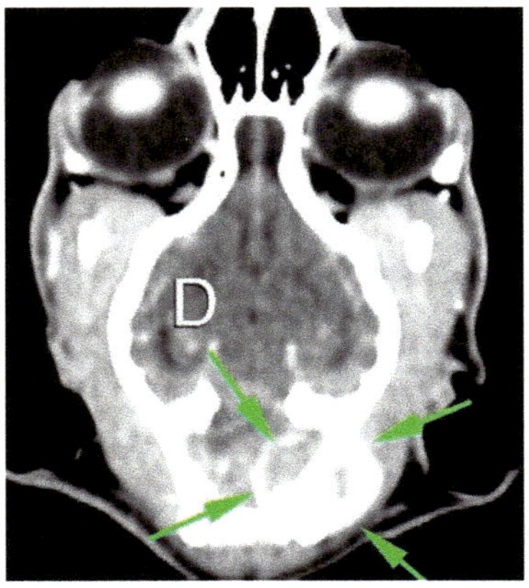

Figure 8. Dorsal reconstruction of a CT post-contrast in a cat which presented with a left cerebellar mass extending into the occipital musculature. The result of cytology was lymphoma.

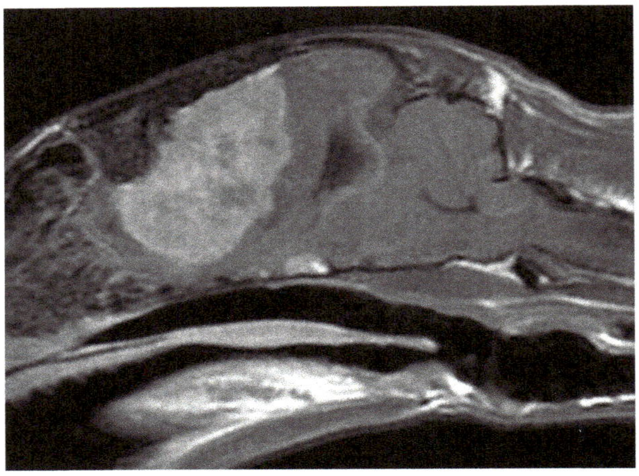

Figure 9. Sagittal image T1-weighted MRI sequence post-contrast where a mass with a well-defined border and intense heterogenous uptake of contrast in the frontal lobe can be seen. Caudal transtentorial herniation through the foramen magnum can be seen. The diagnosis (after surgical removal) was meningioma.

CT or MRI can be used to demonstrate lesions affecting the brain and spinal tissue, thanks to the use of intravenous contrast which highlights lesions where the blood-brain barrier is altered, such as tumours and inflammation.

In cases of **lower motor neuron involvement** (weakness, loss of spinal reflexes, muscular atrophy ...), the most appropriate, and least invasive diagnostic method are **electrodiagnostic tests** (Niederhauser and Holliday, 1989). Electromyography can confirm the presence of spontaneous electrical activity in skeletal musculature suggestive of myopathy or neuropathy. Nerve conduction tests distinguish between muscle or nerve involvement and allow characterization of the type of neuropathy present before confirmation by muscle and/or nerve biopsy. In many cases, the results of electrodiagnostic tests together with the clinical history and the results of the complementary tests allow a diagnosis to be reached without having to resort to biopsy, allowing specific treatments (Figure 10) to be prescribed.

In summary, the diagnostic tests currently available in day to day practice are varied, although they need equipment which is expensive to acquire and maintain and, therefore, the cost of the procedures is high. Thus, for the sake of pets and owners, correct interpretation of findings during the neurological examination is necessary, alongside a list of differential diagnoses adapted to these findings. This allows the clinician to opt for the diagnostic tests most likely to provide a clinical diagnosis and avoid unnecessary procedures for the animal and the associated costs.

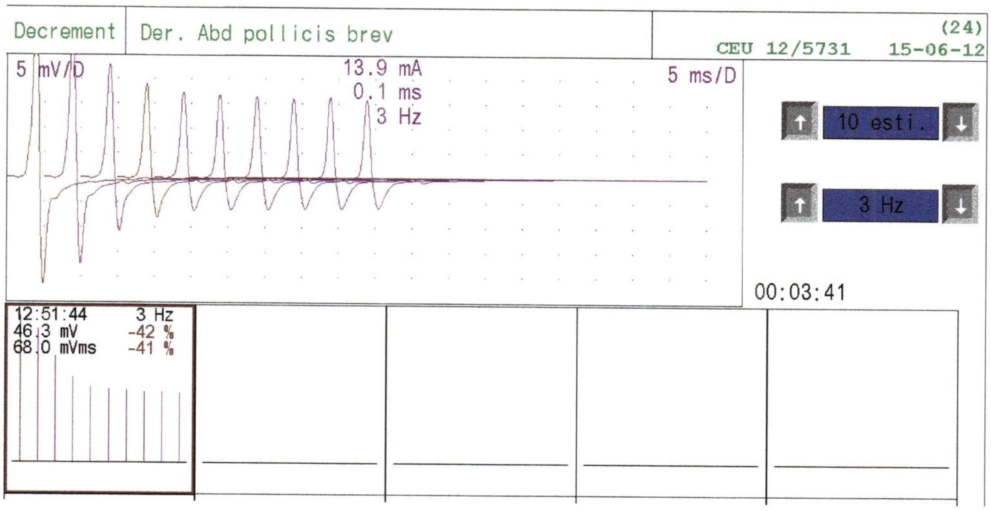

Figure 10. Repetitive stimulation test in a cat with episodic weakness where a reduction can be seen in the amplitude of the waves, which is characteristic of myasthenia gravis.

Common neurological diseases seen in practice

Epilepsy

This section addresses traditional and alternative treatments for epilepsy in cats.

Aetiology and pathogenesis

- **Genetic idiopathic epilepsy** is defined as one in which a **genetic mutation is identified as the cause of seizures.** At the time of writing there are no known genetic epilepsies in cats, since no genetic mutation is associated with seizures in this species.
- **Idiopathic epilepsy of suspected genetic origin** is one where a genetic cause is presupposed, because it appears in a particular family or has a high prevalence in a breed. Most cats with early onset seizures and in which no structural or toxic/metabolic cause is found, fall into this category.
- In **idiopathic epilepsy of unknown cause** there is no evidence of an obvious aetiology despite extensive work-up. A typical example would be a geriatric cat with late onset seizures in which metabolic tests, advanced imaging, cerebrospinal fluid analysis, etc. are performed and no obvious cause found.
- **Structural epilepsy** refers to one in which there is an underlying intracranial structural cause such as tumours, infection, trauma, etc.
- **Reactive seizures** are due to an extracranial cause, whether toxic, endocrine or metabolic. These cases cannot be described as epilepsy since seizures should cease by correcting the imbalance.

Idiopathic epilepsy is a neurological disease whose **diagnosis is presumptive** after the exclusion of other causes of seizures, and its prevalence in cats is approximately 33% (Schriefl et al, 2008; Pakozdy et al., 2010). The most common presentation is in animals between 1–5 years of age with a history of repeated seizures and complete return to neurological normality between episodes. Structural epilepsy has a prevalence of 50% while reactive seizures occurred in 22% in the same study (Schriefl et al,. 2008).

Clinical signs

Epileptic seizures can be classified as focal when the abnormal activity affects only part of the cerebrum. According to the part affected seizures manifest as facial twitches, or rhythmic contractions of limbs in the case of focal motor seizures.

If the autonomic nervous system is involved in the abnormal activity, seizures manifest as excessive salivation, vomiting, defaecation or pupillary dilation and are called focal autonomic. If a behavioural crisis occurs such as episodic aggression, these seizures are called focal behavioural.

Lastly when the whole brain is involved seizures are generalised and invariably affect mental status.

Treatment

Traditionally, the treatment of seizures was based on the administration of anticonvulsants, such as phenobarbital. However, in 60–70% of cases, this medication does not provide effective control. Regardless of the oral dose used, it is essential to measure serum levels regularly, since the success of treatment is fundamentally related to it.

Over the last 15 years the use of anticonvulsants from human medicine, such as levetiracetam or gabapentin, has improved the control of seizures. However, due to their high cost, the use of these medications is often reserved for cases with inadequate seizure control or with serious side effects with traditional anticonvulsants.

When starting anticonvulsant treatment, certain premises should be taken into account: Since in cats most seizures have a structural or reactive cause, it is important to **start treatment as soon as possible**. For idiopathic epilepsy, treatment should start if the frequency of seizures is high (more than one per month), there is an increase in the frequency or duration, and if either partial or generalized status epilepticus occurs.

Phenobarbital

Phenobarbital is the cheapest and most effective anticonvulsant currently available. It comes in 15 mg (human) or 25 mg (dogs) tablet form or slow IV injectable form 200 mg/ml. Its half-life T½ for elimination is 34–50 h and the initial dose 2.5 mg/kg q12 h.

Side effects are minimal in the cat and include sedation, ataxia, polyuria/polydipsia. Hepatoxicities have not been described in cats (as with the dog). Measuring phenobarbital levels in blood 2–3 weeks after starting treatment is important, but, given that it does not cause hepatic induction, regular serum measurement of levels are only necessary every six months or when the dose is changed.

Levetiracetam

Levetiracetam (Keppra) is a second-generation anticonvulsant frequently used as an additional therapy in cases of epilepsy refractory to traditional anticonvulsants or when these are not appropriate, due to liver or kidney disease.

It comes in 100 mg/ml oral syrup and tablet form, but the syrup is more suitable for cats. There is also an intravenous form (100 mg/ml) for the treatment of status epilepticus. Its mechanism of action is not fully understood, although it seems to act on SV2A vesicles in the presynaptic membranes (Lynch et al., 2004). Oral absorption is almost complete, its T½ is about 2–4 hours and elimination is mostly renal. An interesting feature of the pharmacokinetics of this medicine is that despite its short half-life it has a cumulative effect in the brain, so it can be administered every 8 hours. Due to the absence of hepatic metabolism, it is useful in the treatment of seizures due to hepatic encephalopathy or liver damage.

In a recent study, its efficacy for seizure control as an additional therapy has been evaluated (Bailey et al., 2008). The author uses an initial dose of 10–20 mg/kg q8 h and this is gradually increased. On rare occasions, the only side effect observed has been slight sedation. Despite their initial efficacy, some animals may develop a worsening of seizures or even the so-called "honeymoon effect", with their return in the long-term. The introduction of an intravenous format has made its use possible in status epilepticus.

Zonisamide

Zonisamide (Zonegran) is an antiepileptic whose main mechanism of action is the inhibition of presynaptic T-type calcium channels and sodium channels (Hasegawa et al., 2008). Its metabolism is mainly hepatic by microsomal enzymes, although it does not cause liver enzyme induction. The T½ is 15 hours.

Due to its hepatic metabolism, higher doses should be used in patients receiving phenobarbital. The author uses a dose of 5–10 mg/kg q12 h. At a dose of 20 mg/kg, sedation, vomiting and lethargy have been observed in cats (Hasegawa et al., 2008). As with levetiracetam, a "honeymoon" effect has been appreciated. Its main disadvantage is the high cost.

Pregabalin

Pregabalin is another anticonvulsant used occasionally to treat seizures in cats at a dose of 1–2 mg/kg q12 h. However, there are no clinical studies on its effectiveness. The main problem in cats is its capsule format.

Other anticonvulsants from human medicine

Primidone and phenytoin are not used for the treatment of idiopathic epilepsy in domestic animals since they do not provide any advantage over phenobarbital and are associated with a greater probability of liver toxicity.

Valproate has a T½ in the dog (1.7 h), considerably shorter than in humans (9–16 h), so its dosage is difficult. There are no pharmacokinetic studies in cats, but hyperactivity and psychogenic alopecia have been described with continued accidental ingestion (Zoran, Boeckh and Boothe, 2001).

Lamotrigine is metabolized in the dog to a cardiotoxic compound, so it is contraindicated in this species.

Vigabatrin causes blood dyscrasias and is therefore not recommended.

Oral diazepam has a low absorption (<5%) so it is not useful for the control of epilepsy in dogs. In the cat it can cause hepatic necrosis, so if it is used it is important to measure liver transaminases seven days after starting treatment.

Vestibular syndrome

The vestibular system is responsible for maintaining the position of the eyes, trunk and limbs in relation to

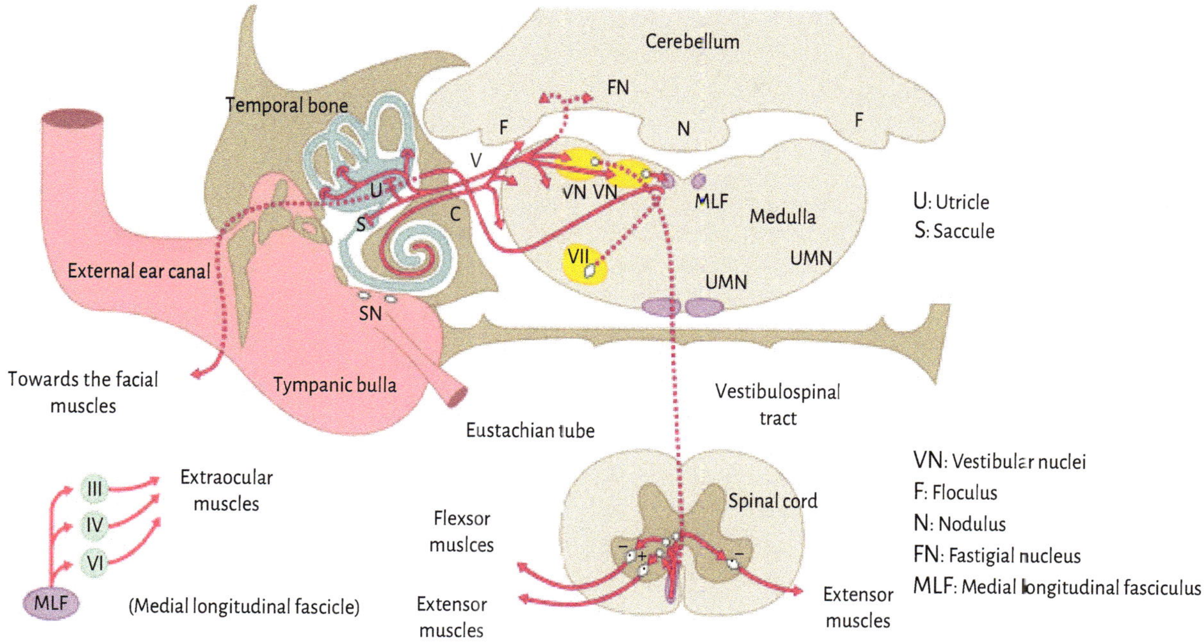

Figure 11. Schematic representation of the vestibular system and its connections with extraocular muscles and UMN tracts. (Illustration adapted from de Lahunta and Glass, Veterinary Neuroanatomy and Clinical Neurology).

the position and movement of the head at any given time. This knowledge helps the brain to obtain a stable position from which to start movements.

It is made up of a **central component** which includes:

- vestibular nuclei of the myelencephalon
- vestibulocerebellum (flocculonodular lobe of the cerebellum)
- associated tracts medial longitudinal fasciculus ascending to nuclei of the extraocular muscles and
- vestibulospinal tract to extensor muscles of the limbs for the maintenance of posture.

A peripheral component which includes:

- the semi-circular canals, utricle, and saccule
- vestibular nerve located in the inner ear (Kent, Platt and Schatzberg, 2010).

The utricle detects movements in the horizontal plane while the saccule in the vertical plane and semi-circular canals detect angular acceleration in the three planes (Figure 11).

Clinical signs

Unilateral vestibular disease

In unilateral peripheral vestibular system disease, the most characteristic neurological sign is **ataxia with preservation of strength**. To the contrary, in central diseases that affect the vestibular nuclei, there is also ipsilateral paresis since the lesion usually also affects the UMN descending tracts (vestibulospinal tract). In addition, mental state can be affected by lesions that affect the ascending reticular formation of the brain stem.

The most common neurological sign in unilateral disease is **the presence of a head tilt towards the side of the lesion.** In extreme cases, the animal may roll over repeatedly. Vision helps compensate for the lack of balance so covering the eyes can exacerbate signs.

In addition, **nystagmus,** involuntary and rhythmic oscillation of the eyeball are common. This is normally from side to side if it is **horizontal**, although it can also be **vertical or rotary** and almost always affects both eyes. Typically, it shows a slow phase in one direction and a fast phase in the opposite direction. Physiological nystagmus occurs when the clinician moves the head to represent normal function. When nystagmus is present in the resting position (horizontal plane) it is called **spontaneous or pathological nystagmus**. The direction of nystagmus is named according to the direction of the rapid phase that is easier to identify. Nystagmus that is seen when the head is placed in an unusual position (for example, raising it) is called **positional nystagmus.**

In cases of unilateral peripheral disease, nystagmus can be horizontal or rotary and **the rapid phase is always towards the opposite side to the lesion.** In cases of CNS disease, nystagmus can be horizontal, rotary or vertical. Thus, a **nystagmus which is vertical or changes direction with changes in head position indicates CNS disease**.

Table 3. Clinical signs of unilateral peripheral vestibular syndrome (PVS), unilateral central vestibular syndrome (CVS), paradoxical vestibular syndrome (PdVS) and bilateral vestibular syndrome.

	Unilateral PVS	Unilateral CVS	Paradoxical PdVS	Bilateral VS
Mental state	Normal	Abnormal	Abnormal	Depends on the cause
Head tilt	Ipsilateral	Ipsilateral	Contralateral	No
Ataxia	Ipsilateral asymmetric	Ipsilateral asymmetric	Ipsilateral asymmetric	Symmetrical
Paresis	No	Ipsilateral	Ipsilateral	Depends on the cause
Nystagmus	Contralateral – horizontal, rotational	Changes direction – horizontal, rotational, vertical	Ipsilateral – horizontal, rotational, vertical	No
Strabismus	Ipsilateral	Ipsilateral	–	No
Postural deficits	No	Ipsilateral	Ipsilateral	Depends on the cause
Vestibulo-ocular reflex	Reduced towards the lesion	Reduced	Reduced	Absent bilaterally
Other cranial nerves	VII, Horner's	V, VII, IX, X, XI, XII	V, VII	Mydriasis, head sway

Vestibular strabismus refers to the ventral or ventrolateral deviation of the eyeball in a non-forced position, which is usually corrected by moving the head to a different position. The deviating eyeball is ipsilateral to the vestibular lesion.

In peripheral disease, the head tilt is ipsilateral to the lesion, the rapid phase of nystagmus is in the opposite direction to the lesion, and strabismus is ipsilateral, which is the case with most CNS diseases. To differentiate between ipsilateral peripheral or central disease, it is important to check for the presence of signs of postural delay, the presence of vertical nystagmus, or a change in direction of the nystagmus.

Paradoxical vestibular disease is always central and occurs with lesions in the caudal cerebellar peduncle, rostral and medial vestibular nuclei, cerebellar flocculonodular lobe or fastigial nucleus. In these cases, the head tilt is contralateral to that of the lesion and the rapid phase of nystagmus is towards the side of the lesion. Only postural reactions are ipsilateral to the lesion, which makes it the most reliable sign for localisation.

Bilateral vestibular disease

Bilateral vestibular disease is characterized by **symmetric ataxia whilst strength is maintained**. The animals show a characteristic movement of the head from side to side (**head sway**) and there is no pathological or physiological nystagmus. In severe cases they remain in a crouched position with a broad based stance.

Table 3 lists the clinical signs of unilateral peripheral vestibular syndrome, unilateral central vestibular syndrome, paradoxical vestibular syndrome and bilateral vestibular syndrome.

Diagnosis

Obtaining a **complete clinical history** from the owner is essential, including the course of the disease, associated clinical signs, history of previous trauma or the administration of ototoxic medications, vaccination history, diet or previous ear disease. The presence of obtundation, paresis, postural deficits, or other neurological signs not characteristic of the vestibular system are indicators of CNS disease.

Diagnostic tests should include **complete blood count and biochemistry, total T4 and urinalysis.**

If peripheral disease is suspected, an otoscopic examination and radiographs of the tympanic bullae should be performed under general anaesthesia (Figure 12). However, the lack of any findings does not rule out otitis media. CT and MRI are the most sensitive methods to demonstrate fluid accumulation or neoplasia in this location, in addition to being able to show contrast uptake of the vestibulocochlear and facial nerves (Figure 13).

Myringotomy to obtain a sample for culture and antibiogram can confirm the diagnosis and indicate which is the most appropriate antibiotic.

When CNS disease is suspected, advanced imaging (CT or MRI) and CSF collection are essential, unless contraindicated due to increased intracranial pressure. Routine analysis (differential count and proteins) in addition to PCR for infectious diseases helps with the diagnosis. The agents commonly involved in vestibular diseases are FIP, toxoplasma, cryptococci and different bacteria due to the spread of otitis media (Figure 14). If results from CSF analysis suggest inflammation in the absence of infectious agents, the most likely cause is immune-mediated encephalitis, which requires immunosuppressive treatment.

Thiamine deficiency (vitamin B1) can cause progressive encephalopathy in cats (Davidson, 1992;

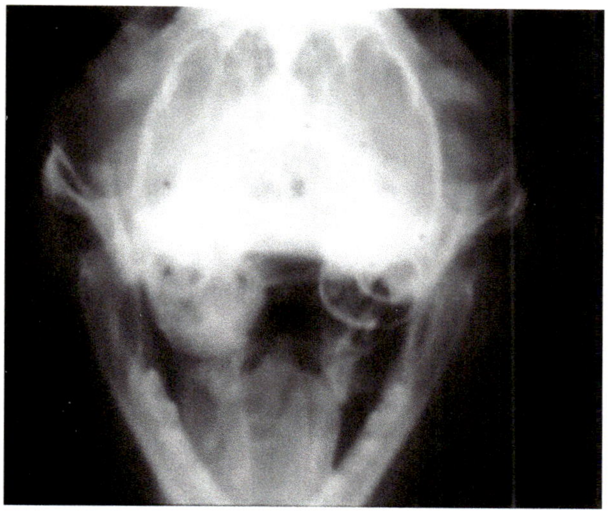

Figure 12. Rostro-caudal radiograph with the mouth open in a cat with right-sided otitis media where an increase in the opacity of the tympanic bulla and its silhouette can be seen.

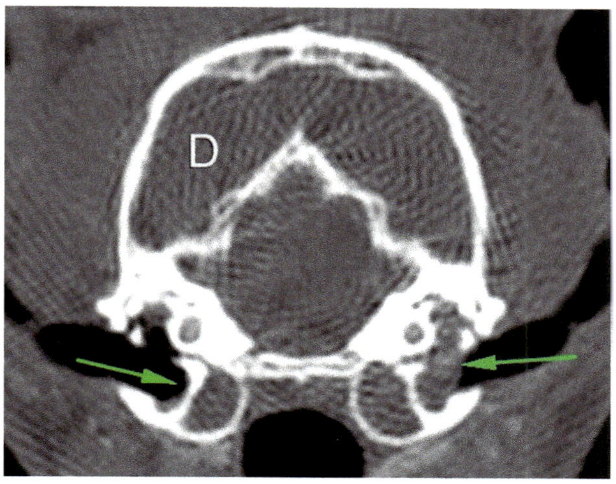

Figure 13. Transverse CT window section of a cat where increased attenuation was seen in both tympanic bullae compatible with otitis media.

Marks et al., 2011; Palus et al., 2010; Penderis, McConnell and Calvin, 2007). The initial signs of anorexia and lethargy precede the signs of bilateral vestibular disease, pupil dilation and seizures. A diagnosis is suspected due to history and blood thiamine levels. MRI images show areas of haemorrhage and symmetric malacia that affect the caudal *colliculus*, vestibular nuclei and cerebellar nuclei. Early treatment with parenteral thiamine 100 mg IM for 7–10 days produces complete recovery.

Idiopathic vestibular disease is common in cats. The key to its diagnosis is the absence of structural, metabolic or inflammatory diseases without signs of central disease. Geriatric animals are the most commonly affected. Treatment is supportive and recurrence is possible.

In recent years vascular diseases, such as cerebellar infarctions, are being diagnosed more frequently.

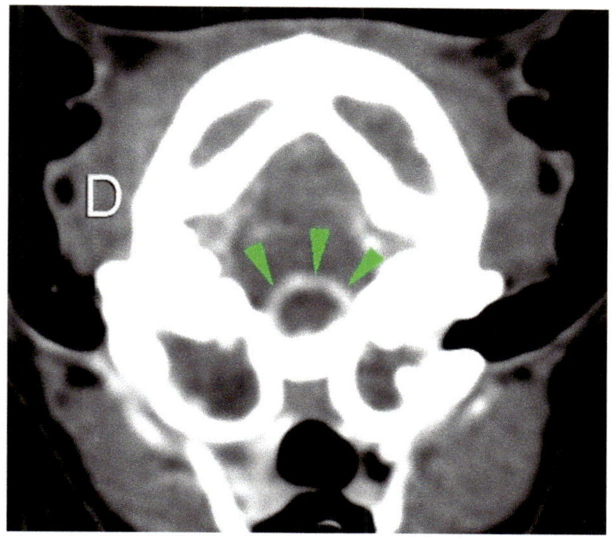

Figure 14. Transverse CT section post-contrast of a cat with central vestibular signs where bilateral filling of the tympanic bullae and ring enhancement of a lesion in the myelencephalon are seen which are compatible with bilateral otitis media and secondary bacterial encephalitis.

The characteristic images obtained on MRI make them easily recognizable to the expert eye, always in conjunction with the clinical history, although other pathologies such as tumours and inflammation may show similar characteristics. In any cat with suspected cerebellar infarction, underlying diseases such as endocrine (hyperthyroidism) or coagulation disorders should be ruled out, however, in more than 50% of cases the primary cause is not found.

Lysosomal diseases or congenital vestibular syndrome in young animals without findings on previous tests including MRI are less common. In some lysosomal diseases, checking for excretion of abnormal organic acids, amino acids or oligosaccharides can give positive results.

Neurological manifestations of systemic diseases

The **central and peripheral nervous system (NS) has a high energy demand,** so any decrease in the supply or use (due to systemic causes) can cause varied and serious neurological effects.

The types of systemic diseases that secondarily affect the nervous system can be divided into:

1. **Haematological or vascular abnormalities** which cause a decrease in the energy supply to the nervous system:
   - hypoxaemia due to cardiopulmonary disease, anaesthetic accidents, coagulopathies, cerebral ischaemia, etc.

   - hypoglycaemia as a result of sepsis, hyperinsulinism or severe liver disease
   - nutritional deficiency, such as thiamine deficiency.
   - arterial hypertension.
2. **Electrolyte abnormalities** which disrupt neuronal or muscular functionality (Na^+, Ca^{2+}, K^+).
3. **Metabolic abnormalities** which produce endogenous neurotoxins, which disrupt the brain's neurochemical balance:
   - hepatic encephalopathy consistent with portosystemic shunt, liver cirrhosis, microvascular dysplasia or hepatitis.
   - uraemic encephalopathy due to renal failure or urinary obstruction.
4. **Endocrine abnormalities** which result in a myriad of systemic effects and secondarily affect the NS:
   - hyperthyroidism.

Clinical signs

The objective of the neurological examination is to establish if the signs observed are caused by nervous system disease and establish the location of the lesion.

Taking a thorough history and physical examination can be sufficient to raise suspicions of the presence of systemic diseases as the causes of neurological signs. Cyanosis, weak pulse, bradycardia, the presence of haemorrhages, abnormal heart or lung sounds are examples of haematological or cardiovascular abnormalities that can affect oxygenation and perfusion of the nervous system.

Neurological signs vary with the location of the lesion. Thus, changes in energy intake, electrolyte imbalances and endocrine and metabolic diseases usually cause diffuse and symmetrical neurological signs, while those caused by haematological changes, infectious diseases, or which are immune mediated are usually more localized.

Diagnostic protocol

The appropriate diagnostic tests depend on the physical and neurological findings during examination.

A complete blood count, including a blood smear along with coagulation tests (PT, PTT, ATT, D-dimer and antithrombin III) may show anaemia, polycythaemia, thrombocytopaenia and coagulopathies that affect oxygenation or perfusion of the NS.

A complete blood biochemistry with electrolytes may show specific abnormalities in other organs such as the kidney and liver, which are responsible for the neurological signs, or electrolyte abnormalities that interfere with NS or muscle function.

Thoracic radiographs and abdominal ultrasound can identify pathologies such as pulmonary or aortic thromboembolism, adrenal masses, renal atrophy, neoplasms, etc.

However, these findings may not be specific and may require another series of functional tests such as the bile acid stimulation test or total T4 to prove suspicions.

Advanced imaging (MRI or CT) is rarely useful for the diagnosis of these systemic diseases and its high cost and the need for general anaesthesia mean its use is not advisable. Examples where they may be useful include pituitary macroadenomas, cerebrovascular accidents, myelinolysis and thiamine deficiency.

In cases where neurological examination suggests generalised LMN involvement, electrodiagnostic techniques allow corroboration of the location and help with choice of the most appropriate laboratory tests.

Hyperthyroidism

Feline hyperthyroidism has been associated with weakness, fatigue and muscle tremors in 12–25% of cats suffering from the condition. Other systemic signs include weight loss, polyphagia, hyperactivity, tachycardia, polyuria/polydipsia, vomiting and diarrhea (Mooney, 2005). A diagnosis is reached by demonstrating high levels of baseline T4 along with clinical signs.

Curative treatment consists of surgical removal of the tumour responsible or ablation with radioactive iodine. Medical treatment is not curative.

Hepatic encephalopathy

The most common cause of hepatic encephalopathy is portosystemic shunt followed by liver cirrhosis, fulminant liver failure and, rarely, congenital defects in the urea cycle (Battersby, Giger and Hall, 2005).

The clinical signs are mainly neurological. The first one to appear is a change in behaviour that suggests bilateral cortical involvement. Subsequently, stupor, blindness, collapse, seizures, deafness and coma can be observed. Growth failure, anorexia, fever, vomiting, polyuria, polydipsia, or struvite urolithiasis are other associated clinical signs. Neurological signs can be episodic and precipitated by a meal, intestinal bleeding, constipation, azotaemia or recent anaesthesia, among others.

Diagnosis is possible by demonstrating high levels of blood ammonia (Gerritzen-Bruning et al., 2006). In cases of vascular anomalies there is an alteration in the enterohepatic cycle, so the measurement of pre and postprandial bile acids can also be diagnostic (Berent and Tobias, 2009). Since the causes can be varied, a complete range of tests, abdominal radiography and ultrasound, urine analysis and serum cobalamin measurement are necessary to identify the aetiology (Battersby, Giger and Hall, 2005; Gerritzen-Bruning et al., 2006; Lamb, 1998; Ruland, Fischer and Hartmann, 2009).

Treatment can be medical or surgical depending on the aetiology and economic resources of the owner. Medical treatment is necessary before surgery to stabilize the patient and consists mainly of a hypoproteic diet, antibiotic therapy and lactulose. When the animal presents with seizures, they should be controlled with levetiracetam 20 mg/kg IV or orally. Surgical treatment is associated with a longer survival period (Greenhalgh et al., 2010).

Hypoglycaemia

Insulin overdose in diabetic animals may produce a drastic reduction in serum glucose levels with severe neurological signs. Glucose is the main energy substrate for the nervous system and is necessary for use by neurons, so any disease that reduces its availability in general circulation has a great impact on this system.

In chronic cases axonal polyneuropathy has been described that causes progressive weakness and hyporeflexia (Braund et al., 1987; Kraje, 2003; Shahar, Rousseaux and Steiss, 1985; Van Hamm et al., 1997; Schrauwen, 1991).

Treatment is based on the restoration of normoglycaemia and support measures. Most neurological signs resolve once normal blood glucose is restored, although residual signs such as blindness or seizures may remain.

Thiamine deficiency

Thiamine deficiency is a rare cause of metabolic encephalopathy that has been described in cats as a result of poor diets and ingestion of thiaminase from fish-exclusive diets (Davidson, 1992; Marks et al., 2011; Palus et al., 2010; Penderis, McConnell and Calvin, 2007). Thiamine (vitamin B1) is an essential vitamin for carbohydrate metabolism in the Krebs cycle.

Clinical and neurological signs in cats include vestibular signs, nystagmus, mydriasis, seizures, absent menace response, stupor and death.

Typical MRI findings reinforce suspicions (Figure 15), but the definitive diagnosis is reached by measuring thiamine in blood in specialized laboratories (Dewey, 2003).

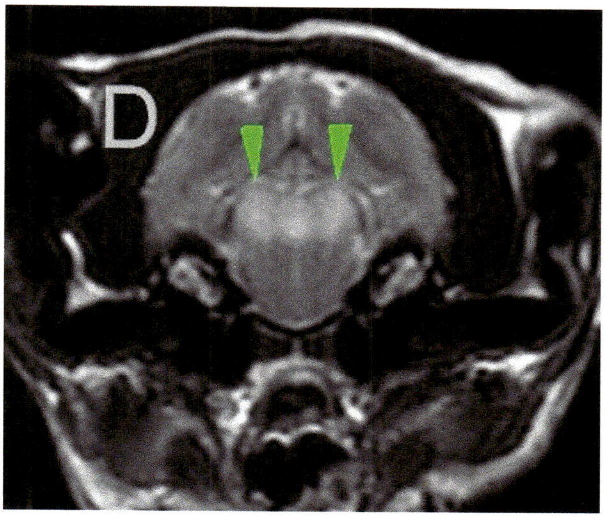

Figure 15. Transverse T2 weighted MRI section of the mesencephalon where hyperintense symmetrical lesions of the mesencephalon can be seen in the caudal colliculi, characteristic of thiamine deficiency.

Treatment should be established early and be aggressive with intramuscular thiamine administration for several days resulting in a full recovery.

Uraemic encephalopathy

Urinary diseases that occur with decreased metabolite excretion and electrolyte imbalances can cause clinical and neurological signs.

Neurological signs include obtundation or stupor, generalized seizures, facial fasciculations, myoclonus and weakness (Dewey, 2003). Seizures are more frequent in cases of acute renal failure, while obtundation usually appears in chronic cases. In cats, when there is hypokalaemia associated with chronic renal failure, it usually manifests as severe neuromuscular weakness with pain and decreased spinal reflexes (Jones, 2009).

Treatment should be directed at the underlying cause and correct electrolyte imbalances and seizures associated with their specific treatment. The prognosis depends on the cause.

Systemic hypertension

Hypertensive encephalopathy is an acute neurological syndrome caused by a sudden increase in systemic blood pressure. The principal cause is kidney disease, but it has also been described with hyperthyroidism (Brown et al., 2005; Littman, 1994).

Associated signs include retinal detachment or blindness due to retinal haemorrhage, polyuria/polydipsia, seizures, ataxia, nystagmus, collapse, paraparesis, and epistaxis. Systemic blood pressure is invariably high with values between 150–300 mmHg. Laboratory findings include elevated creatinine, BUN and phosphorus. Retinal haemorrhages and cerebral oedema with herniation are the causes of neurological signs in these cats.

Management is based on the treatment of arterial hypertension, as well as the underlying cause, so it is very important that it is identified (Littman et al, 2006).

The average survival time is 18 months and does not appear to be influenced by the response to treatment (Littman, 1994).

Bibliography

GAROSI L: *Neurological examination of the cat. How to get started.* J Feline Med Surg. 2009; 11(5): 340–348.

DE LAHUNTA A: *Neurological examination.* In Braund KG (ed): Clinical neurology in small animals: Localisation, diagnosis and treatment, IVIS, 2004;

MORALES C Y MONTOLIU P. *Neurología canina y felina.* Barcelona, Multimédica Ediciones Veterinarias, 2012.

NGHIEM PP Y SCHATZBERG SJ: *Conventional and molecular diagnostic testing for the acute neurologic patient.* J Vet Emerg Crit Care (San. Antonio.) 2010; 20(1): 46–61.

LAPPIN MR: *Update on the diagnosis and management of toxoplasma gondii infection in cats.* Topics in Companion Animal Medicine 2010; 25(3): 136–141.

BLEVINS LB, FENN J, SEGAL H, NEWCOMB-GAYMAN P Y CARROLL KC: *False-positive cryptococcal antigen latex agglutination caused by disinfectants and soaps.* Journal of Clinical Microbiology 1995; 33(6): 1674–1675.

HAY RJ Y MACKENZIE DW: *False positive latex tests for cryptococcal antigen in cerebrospinal fluid.* J Clin Pathol 1982; 35(2): 244–245.

JADERLUND KH, EGENVALL A, BERGSTROM K Y HEDHAMMAR A: *Seroprevalence of borrelia burgdorferi sensu lato and anaplasma phagocytophilum in dogs with neurological signs.* The Veterinary Record 2007; 160(24): 825–831.

DI TERLIZZI R Y PLATT SR: *The function, composition and analysis of cerebrospinal fluid in companion animals: Part ii - analysis.* Vet J 2009; 180(1): 15–32.

PARRY AT, HARRIS A, UPJOHN MM, CHANDLER K Y LAMB CR: *Does choice of imaging modality affect outcome in dogs with thoracolumbar spinal conditions?* J Small Anim Pract 2010; 51(6): 312–317.

JONES JC Y INZANA KD: *Subclinical ct abnormalities in the lumbosacral spine of older large-breed dogs.* Vet Radiol Ultrasound 2000; 41(1): 19–26.

DE DECKER S, GIELEN IM, DUCHATEAU L et al.: *Low-field magnetic resonance imaging findings of the caudal portion of the cervical region in clinically normal doberman pinschers and foxhounds.* Am.J.Vet Res 2010; 71(4): 428–434.

NIEDERHAUSER UB Y HOLLIDAY TA: *Electrodiagnostic studies in diseases of muscles and neuromuscular junctions.* Semin.Vet Med Surg. (SmallAnim) 1989; 4(2): 116–125.

SCHRIEFL S, STEINBERG TA, MATIASEK K, OSSIG A, FENSKE N Y FISCHER A: *Etiologic classification of seizures, signalment, clinical signs, and outcome in cats with seizure disorders: 91 cases* (2000,äì2004). J Am Vet Med Assoc 2008; 233(10): 1591–1597.

PAKOZDY A, LESCHNIK M, SARCHAHI AA, TICHY AG Y THALHAMMER JG: *Clinical comparison of primary versus secondary epilepsy in 125 cats.* J Feline Med Surg 2010; 12(12): 910–916.

LYNCH BA, LAMBENG N, NOCKA K et al.: *The synaptic vesicle protein sv2a is the binding site for the antiepileptic drug levetiracetam.* Proc. Natl.Acad.Sci.U.S.A 2004; 101(26): 9861–9866.

BAILEY KS, DEWEY CW, BOOTHE DM, BARONE G Y KORTZ GD: *Levetiracetam as an adjunct to phenobarbital treatment in cats with suspected idiopathic epilepsy.* J Am Vet Med Assoc 2008; 232(6): 867–872.

HASEGAWA D, KOBAYASHI M, KUWABARA T, OHMURA T, FUJITA M Y ORIMA H: *Pharmacokinetics and toxicity of zonisamide in cats.* J Feline Med Surg 2008; 10(4): 418–421.

ZORAN DL, BOECKH A Y BOOTHE DM: *Hyperactivity and alopecia associated with ingestion of valproic acid in a cat.* J Am Vet Med Assoc 2001; 218(10): 1587–1589.

KENT M, PLATT SR Y SCHATZBERG SJ: *The neurology of balance: Function and dysfunction of the vestibular system in dogs and cats.* Vet J 2010; 185(3): 247–258.

DAVIDSON MG: *Thiamin deficiency in a colony of cats.* Vet.Rec. 1992; 130(5): 94–97.

MARKS SL, LIPSITZ D, VERNAU KM et al.: *Reversible encephalopathy secondary to thiamine deficiency in 3 cats ingesting commercial diets.* J Vet Intern Med 2011; 25(4): 949–953.

PALUS V, PENDERIS J, JAKOVLJEVIC S Y CHERUBINI GB: *Thiamine deficiency in a cat: Resolution of mri abnormalities following thiamine supplementation.* J Feline Med Surg 2010; 12(10): 807–810.

PENDERIS J, MCCONNELL JF Y CALVIN J: *Magnetic resonance imaging features of thiamine deficiency in a cat.* The Veterinary Record 2007; 160(8): 270–272.

MOONEY CT: HYPERTHYROIDISM. EN ETTINGER SJ Y FELDMAN EC (ed): Textbook of veterinary internal medicine, St. Louis, Elsevier Saunders, 2005; 1544–1563.

BATTERSBY IA, GIGER U Y HALL EJ: *Hyperammonaemic encephalopathy secondary to selective cobalamin deficiency in a juvenile border collie.* J.Small Anim Pract. 2005; 46(7): 339–344.

GERRITZEN-BRUNING MJ, VAN DEN INGH TS Y ROTHUIZEN J: *Diagnostic value of fasting plasma ammonia and bile acid concentrations in the identification of portosystemic shunting in dogs.* J Vet Intern Med 2006; 20(1): 13–19.

BERENT AC Y TOBIAS KM: *Portosystemic vascular anomalies.* Vet Clin NA: Small Anim Pract 2009; 39(3): 513–541.

LAMB CR: *Ultrasonography of portosystemic shunts in dogs and cats.* Vet Clin NA: Small Anim Pract 1998; 28(4): 725–753.

RULAND K, FISCHER A Y HARTMANN K: *Sensitivity and specificity of fasting ammonia and serum bile acids in the diagnosis of portosystemic shunts in dogs and cats.* Vet Clin Pathol 2009;

GREENHALGH SN, DUNNING MD, MCKINLEY TJ et al.: *Comparison of survival after surgical or medical treatment in dogs with a congenital portosystemic shunt.* J Am Vet Med Assoc 2010; 236(11): 1215–1220.

BRAUND KG, MCGUIRE JA, AMLING KA Y HENDERSON RA: *Peripheral neuropathy associated with malignant neoplasms in dogs.* Veterinary Pathology 1987; 24(1): 16–21.

KRAJE AC: *Hypoglycemia and irreversible neurologic complications in a cat with insulinoma.* J Am Vet Med Assoc 2003; 223(6): 812–4, 810.

SHAHAR R, ROUSSEAUX C Y STEISS J: *Peripheral polyneuropathy in a dog with functional islet b-cell tumor and widespread metastasis.* J Am Vet Med Assoc 1985; 187(2): 175–177.

VAN HAM L, BRAUND KG, ROELS S Y PUTCUYPS I: *Treatment of a dog with an insulinoma-related peripheral polyneuropathy with corticosteroids.* The Veterinary Record 1997; 141(4): 98–100.

SCHRAUWEN E: *Clinical peripheral polyneuropathy associated with canine insulinoma.* The Veterinary Record 1991; 128(9): 211–212.

DEWEY CW: *Encephalopathies: Disorders of the brain.* En Dewey CW (ed): A practical guide to canine and feline neurology, Iowa, Iowa State Press, 2003; 99–178.

JONES BR: *Hypokalemic myopathy in cats.* En Bonagura JD y Twedt DC (ed): Kirk's current veterinary therapy xiv, St. Louis, Saunders Elsevier, 2009; 1136–1138.

Brown CA, Munday JS, Mathur S y Brown SA: *Hypertensive encephalopathy in cats with reduced renal function.* Veterinary Pathology 2005; 42(5): 642–649.

Littman MP: *Spontaneous systemic hypertension in 24 cats.* J Vet Intern Med 1994; 8(2): 79–86.

Littman MP, Goldstein RE, Labato MA, Lappin MR y Moore GE: *Acvim small animal consensus statement on lyme disease in dogs: Diagnosis, treatment, and prevention.* J Vet Intern Med 2006; 20(2): 422–434.

Test

1. **The frontal lobe of the brain is involved in:**
   A) Conscious visual interpretation of retinal images.
   B) Memory and hearing.
   C) Initiation of conscious movements and associative reasoning.
   D) Smell.
2. **Indicate which of the following statements is true.**
   A) The cerebellum is responsible for initiating movements and therefore movements are hesitant when affected.
   B) Severe spinal compressions only affect nociception.
   C) The pontine nucleus of the trigeminal is the origin of the efferent fibres to the masticatory muscles.
   D) The dorsal metencephalon is responsible for coordinating movements throughout the body.
3. **The objectives of the neurological examination are:**
   A) Identify if the animal has a neurological problem and its location.
   B) Estimate the need for an MRI.
   C) Develop a list of diagnostic tests necessary for the work-up.
   D) All of the above answers are incorrect.
4. **Regarding the neurological examination, indicate which statement is true:**
   A) Postural reactions are only diminished in cases of spinal cord involvement.
   B) Mental status is usually affected even with small focal chronic lesions of the telencephalon.
   C) The patellar reflex is the most reliable for assessing LMN lesions in the pelvic limbs.
   D) All of the above are true.
5. **Indicate which of the following statements is true.**
   A) CSF is mainly produced in the subarachnoid space.
   B) Under physiological conditions, the production of CSF is dependent on intracranial pressure.
   C) The spinal proprioceptive tracts are immediately adjacent to grey matter.
   D) The ventral metencephalon is responsible for coordinating movements throughout the body.
6. **Regarding cerebrospinal fluid, indicate which statement is incorrect:**
   A) Pleocytosis can be observed in all inflammatory and infectious diseases.
   B) Analysis of the sample in less than 30 minutes is essential to avoid cellular changes.
   C) Cytology allows identification of the pathogen that causes myelitis in some cases.
   D) A positive on PCR indicates the presence of genetic material from the pathogen in the CNS provided there has been no contamination of the sample.
7. **It is possible to demonstrate spinal compression by:**
   A) Myelography.
   B) Myelo-CT.
   C) MRI.
   D) All of the above.
8. **Regarding imaging tests in neurological diseases, indicate which statement is false:**
   A) Myelography can show spinal compressions that require surgical decompression.
   B) CT is especially useful in diseases that affect bony structures.
   C) MRI makes it possible to reach a definitive diagnosis for a large number of neurological diseases.
   D) With spinal diseases, the success of the treatment is not influenced by the diagnostic method used (MRI vs. myelography).

9. **Regarding idiopathic epilepsy of unknown cause, indicate which is the true answer:**
   A) It is caused by pathogens of unknown origin.
   B) It is probably due to a structural cause even though extensive research has not been conducted.
   C) No abnormalities are found during exhaustive investigations nor does it have a genetic origin.
   D) Its origin is related to lunar phases.
10. **Regarding veterinary antiepileptic medications, indicate which statement is true:**
   A) Phenytoin is an excellent anticonvulsant because of its prolonged effect and low toxicity.
   B) Diazepam is ideal for chronic seizure control in cats.
   C) Levetiracetam is recommended as an anticonvulsant in hepatic encephalopathy.
   D) Gabapentin is a third-line antiepileptic after phenobarbital, since there is no liver metabolism.
11. **Regarding seizures in cats, indicate which statement is true:**
   A) They do not need treatment, as they resolve spontaneously.
   B) Cluster seizures are neurological emergencies that must be treated promptly.
   C) Serum phenobarbital levels should be monitored at most every 6 months.
   D) The administration of phenobarbital does not influence levetiracetam metabolism.
12. **Regarding unilateral peripheral vestibular syndrome, indicate which statement is true:**
   A) Nystagmus presents with the rapid phase towards the lesion.
   B) Vestibular strabismus is ipsilateral.
   C) The head tilt is contralateral to the side of the lesion.
   D) Delays in postural reactions are ipsilateral to the head tilt.
13. **A 9 year-old entire male cat, presents with a hyperacute onset of obtundation, non-ambulatory tetra paresis, postural reaction delays in the limbs on the left side, circling to the left, left pleurosthotonus, spontaneous horizontal right-sided nystagmus, with no head tilt, left reflexive mydriasis, and left ventrolateral strabismus. Locate the neurological lesion:**
   A) Diffuse lesion in the left myelencephalon.
   B) Focal lesion in the right cerebellum.
   C) Left mesencephalon.
   D) Focal lesion in the right telencephalon.
14. **A 12-month-old female cat with an acute, progressive history over the last two days of hindlimb weakness with diminished spinal reflexes, which has evolved into a partial status epilepticus, consisting of facial tics, and as of two hours ago an obtunded state is brought to the practice. What should the first step be?**
   A) Blood tests with complete blood count and biochemistry including ammonium, electrolytes, glucose, urea, creatinine, T4 and a neurological antibody profile.
   B) General anaesthesia to perform CT/MRI of the thoracolumbar spine, CSF analysis and PCR for infectious diseases.
   C) Head and spine radiographs, electromyography and a nerve conduction study prior to muscle and nerve biopsy samples.
   D) Venous access to administer IV diazepam or, failing that, rectal administration prior to investigation.
15. **A 7-month-old male cat with an acute, progressive history of multifocal syndrome with behavioural disturbance, ataxia, vertical nystagmus, pelvic limb weakness, decreased myotatic reflexes and thoracolumbar pain is brought to the practice. In tests prior to the visit moderate hyperglobulinaemia, elevated ALT, ALP, CK and light neutrophilia are observed. Make a list of differential diagnoses:**
   A) Vertebral metastasis, cerebellar arachnoid cyst.
   B) FIP, toxoplasmosis, multifocal lymphoma.
   C) Non-compressive traumatic disc herniation with associated spinal shock, mucopolysaccharidosis, multiple infarcts.
   D) Portosystemic shunt, thiamine deficiency, abnormalities in the urea cycle, multifocal discospondylitis.
16. **Regarding systemic diseases that cause neurological signs, indicate which is the correct answer:**
   A) Excess T4 in cats is directly responsible for neurological signs due to its neurotoxic effects on neurons.
   B) Thiamine deficiency is only likely with exclusive fish-based diets and is impossible with commercial diets.
   C) In cases of chronic renal failure, the most frequent neurological sign is the presence of seizures.
   D) Hepatic encephalopathy can be triggered in subclinical cases by recent anaesthesia.

Clinical case

A 7-month-old male common European cat with an acute history of vomiting over the last seven days, which has progressed and has been unable to walk for 24 hours, is brought into the practice. Maropitant and omeprazole have been administered with no clinical response.

In the neurological examination there appears to be a normal mental state, slight postural delay in the four limbs, a broad-based stance and the presence of positional vertical nystagmus when raising the head.

1. **Based on the clinical history, what is the location of the neurological lesion?**
   A) C1-C5 spinal segments.
   B) Right telencephalon.
   C) Cerebellum.
   D) Mesencephalon.
2. **Make a list of 5 differential diagnoses based on clinical history and progression:**
   A) Toxoplasmosis.
   B) Immune-mediated encephalitis.
   C) Lymphoma.
   D) FIP.
   E) Cerebellar cyst.
   F) Otitis media/interna.
   G) Thiamine deficiency.
3. **List all the tests that would be necessary to try to cover all the possible differential diagnoses:**
   A) Complete set of blood tests.
   B) Complete blood count and blood smear.
   C) Thoracic radiographs.
   D) Abdominal ultrasound.
   E) CT or MRI of the brain.
   F) Collection and analysis of cerebrospinal fluid.
   G) PCR for infectious diseases.
   H) Measurement of thiamine in blood.
4. **On the blood test, thoracic radiographs, and abdominal ultrasound no abnormalities are observed, however, when performing a CT scan of the brain, this image is observed after the administration of intravenous iodinated contrast (Figure 1, soft tissue CT, and Figure 2, bone CT). Describe the CT findings and a make a list of differential diagnoses.**

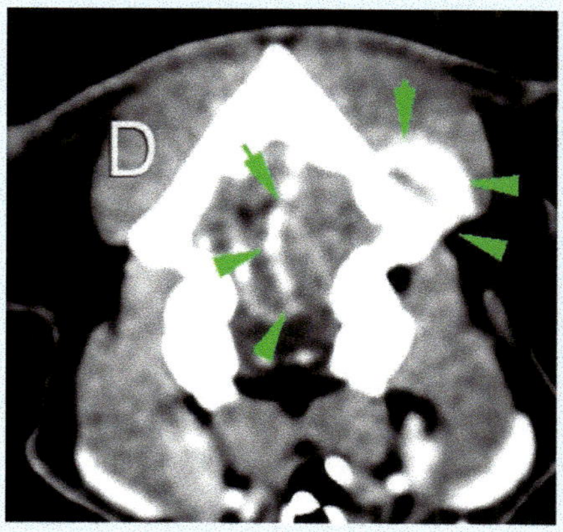

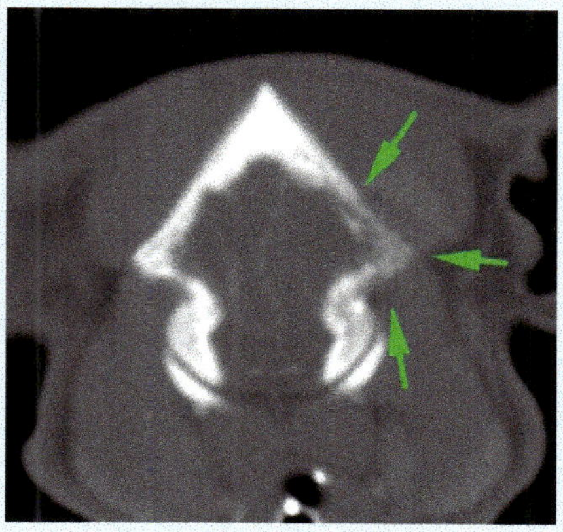

5. **What test should be performed next to make a diagnosis of the nature of the mass? Indicate which is the most appropriate.**
   A) Fine needle aspiration.
   B) Collection and analysis of cerebrospinal fluid.
   C) MRI of the brain.
   D) Measurement of thiamine in blood.
   E) Rule out the possibility of a bacterial infection by PCR.

6. **On fine needle aspiration the cell type in the image below is seen. Describe the findings and the definitive diagnosis.**

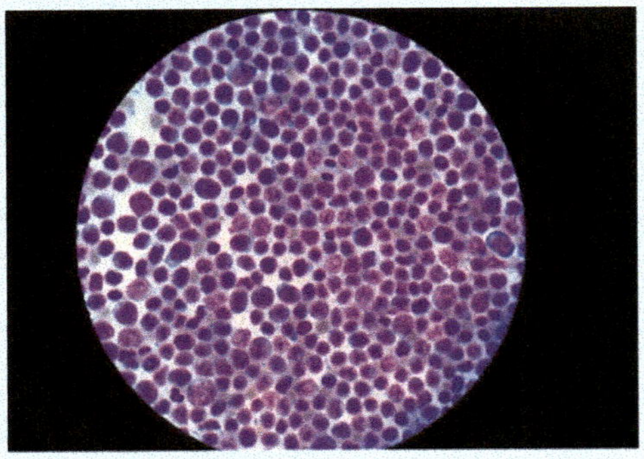

Answers

Test

1. C	7. D	13. C
2. D	8. C	14. D
3. A	9. C	15. B
4. C	10. C	16. D
5. A	11. B	
6. A	12. B	

Clinical case

1. **Based on the clinical history, is the location of the neurological lesion?**
   C) Cerebellum.
2. **Make a list of 5 differential diagnoses based on clinical history and progression:**
   All are valid.
3. **List all the tests that would be necessary to try to cover all the possible differential diagnoses:**
   All are necessary to cover the list.
4. **On the blood test, thoracic radiographs, and abdominal ultrasound no abnormalities are observed, however, when performing a CT scan of the brain, this image is observed after the administration of intravenous iodinated contrast (Figure 1, soft tissue CT, and Figure 2, bone CT). Describe the CT findings and a make a list of differential diagnoses.**
   Post-contrast CT scan of the caudal fossa where a displacement of the cerebellar vermis to the right side is observed due to a mass originating on the left side that has caused osteolysis of the occipital bone and extends extracranially to the left temporal musculature, where it appears ring like. Differential diagnoses for this mass would include abscess, osteosarcoma, fibrosarcoma and lymphoma.
5. **What test should be performed to make a diagnosis of the nature of the mass? Indicate which is the most appropriate.**
   A) Fine needle aspiration.
6. **On fine needle aspiration the cell type in the image below is seen. Describe the findings and the definitive diagnosis.**
   A mononuclear cell population with a variable cytoplasm and prominent nucleolus and the presence of moderate amounts of mitosis is observed. Some of the cells have a larger cytoplasm and double nucleoli. Lymphoma.

Behavioural medicine

13

Jaume Fatjó y Patricia Darder

Contents

In clinical practice, consultations concerning feline behavioural problems are common (Golden and Hanlon, 2018).

Furthermore, the veterinarian is often responsible for identifying behavioural issues owners are not aware of, but which could compromise the cat's welfare and ultimately the family's quality of life too. The veterinarian plays a fundamental role in educating clients on how to improve the behaviour and welfare of their cats (Rodan and Heath, 2016).

This chapter on feline behavioural medicine looks at normal feline behaviour, with a focus on communication and social behaviour, and then examines the **principal signs of stress in the cat** and considers strategies for prevention and treatment. The last section covers inappropriate elimination and aggression.

Social behaviour and communication

Most of the domestic cat's behaviour problems, such as aggression, fear or urine marking, are related to either physical or social stressors (Bradshaw, 2018; Amat et al., 2016; Barcelos et al., 2018). A survey addressed to Spanish first opinion veterinarians suggests the main reasons for feline behaviour consultations are **inappropriate elimination, marking, aggression, scratching, and excessive vocalization** (Fatjó et al., 2006).

Domestication of the cat took place at least 9,500 years ago, probably in the region between the Nile delta and Mesopotamia, known as the Fertile Crescent (Vigne et al., 2004; Discroll et al., 2007). The wild ancestor of the domestic cat is the African/Arabian wild cat, *Felis silvestris lybica*. It is a solitary, small feline, with a tendency to be territorial, adapted to an arid and semi-arid climate.

According to the most widely accepted scientific theory, the most socially tolerant specimens approached human settlements to exploit a new ecological niche which offered an abundant and localized food source. Over time this subpopulation gave rise to the appearance of a new species: the domestic cat. Nevertheless, some authors believe that humans played a more active role in the process by purposefully capturing and keeping wild cats as pets (Serpell, 2013).

The social behaviour of today's cat is the product of inherited tendencies from their wild ancestor and changes introduced through domestication. Most cats show a more or less marked tolerance for living with people or with other cats (Ramos et al., 2013; Vitale et al., 2019).

A good strategy to better understand the social nature of the domestic cat is to observe the behaviour and structure of feline colonies (Bradshaw, 2016), which spontaneously form in places where resources are abundant (Macdonald, 2000).

The typical structure of a **feline colony is matriarchal**, made up of a nucleus of females and their young, with males occupying a more peripheral position (Macdonald, 2000). The size of a medium-sized colony is between 7 and 11 cats, while those of a larger size are formed from around 16–25 individuals. The maximum limit of 25 individuals has been used to set the maximum number of cats that could live in a single facility, for example in a rehoming centre, although ideally the ratio of 10–12 animals/group should not be exceeded (Newbury et al., 2010).

Understanding the dynamics and composition of feline colonies is important, since they account for a significant number of the cats that live in cities. For example, the city of Barcelona, in collaboration with various animal protection entities, manages more than 600 feline colonies (www.barcelona.cat, 2021).

Successful social behaviour requires the regulation of interactions between individuals within the same species, for which frequent and effective exchange of information (in other words **communication**) is essential. Therefore, from a clinical perspective, understanding the natural language of cats is important for the diagnosis, treatment, and prevention of behavioural problems.

Communication and the diagnosis of behavioural problems

Fundamental to the diagnostic protocol in feline behavioural medicine is a **detailed description of the cat's behaviour**, which includes different forms of communication. The **signals given by the animal are the most reliable indicator of their emotional and motivational state** at that moment (Heath, 2016). For example, body posture is a major element used to categorize different forms of aggression (DePorter, 2013). Also, with regards to inappropriate urination, a knowledge of the typical pattern of urine marking allows it to be differentiated from other problems with a similar presentation but different aetiology, and therefore change the therapeutic approach.

Communication, treatment and prevention of behavioural problems

Regarding prevention and treatment, it is important to highlight problems such as fear or aggression can arise or be aggravated by an incorrect interpretation of the cat's language by their owner.

Animals in general, and cats in particular have **four basic communication channels: visual, tactile, olfactory, and auditory**.

Visual communication

In the context of encounters between two cats or a cat with a person, the animal's body language conveys two fundamental messages:

- The desire or not to establish contact.
- The underlying emotional state, that is, whether they are friendly or not.

Visual communication is the most accessible for people and, therefore, is the main source of information about the motivational status of the cat, for their owners, veterinarians, and behaviourists. Investing time in **educating clients to recognise the main patterns of feline visual communication is therefore important**.

Friendly approach posture

The cat approaches another cat or a person and indicates a **friendly mood with a tail perpendicular to the ground** (Fatjó and Heiblum, 2013). This visual signal, the tail raised as a friendly signal, is only observed among felines in the domestic cat and the lion (*Panthera leo*). Interestingly two of the only three species of this carnivore family that show a gregarious tendency (Cafazzo and Natoli, 2009) (Figure 1).

Offensive approach posture

The indicative signs of aggression are varied and appear in varying degrees of intensity (Figures 2 and 3) (Bowen and Heath, 2005). In its clearest presentation, the cat approaches the person or another cat with its body

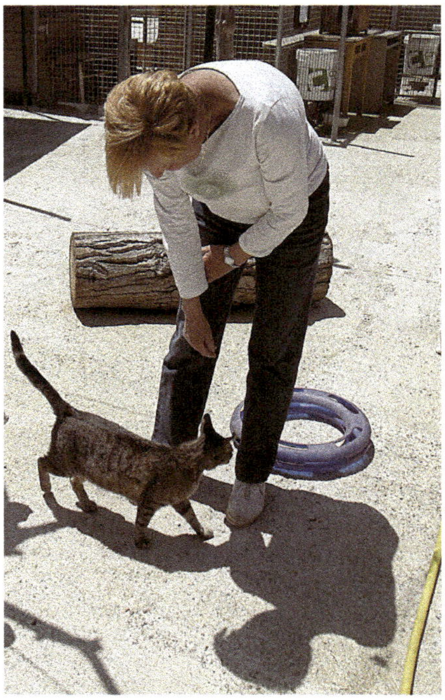

Figure 1. Friendly approach posture: the cat approaches with a relaxed body position and the tail up high, like a flag.

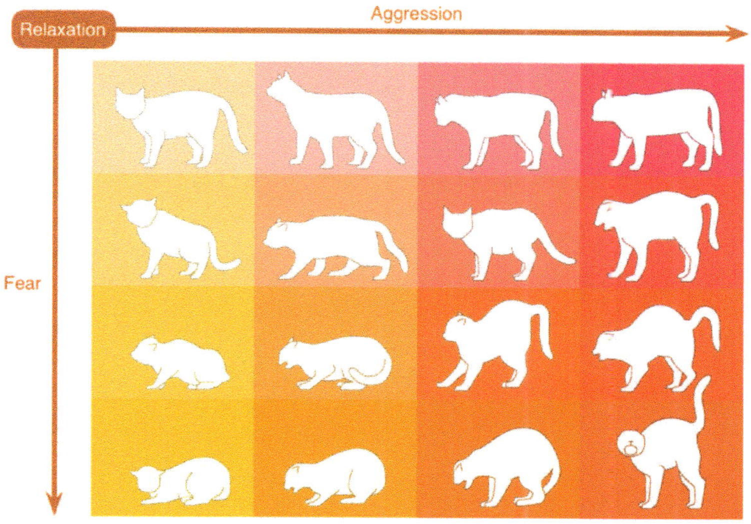

Figure 2. Feline body postures: aggression and fear. In a direct interaction between two cats, body language comes into play in the first instance, before facial expression, as a sign of the animal's motivation. The image shows the main body postures which the cat adopts showing relaxation, and after this growing levels of aggression (from left to right) or fear (from top to bottom). (Modified from: Bowen J, Heath S (2005) An overview of feline social behaviour and communication. In: Bowen, J & Heath, S (eds.) Behaviour Problems in Small Animals: Practical Advice for the Veterinary Team. Elsevier-Saunders, pp. 29–36).

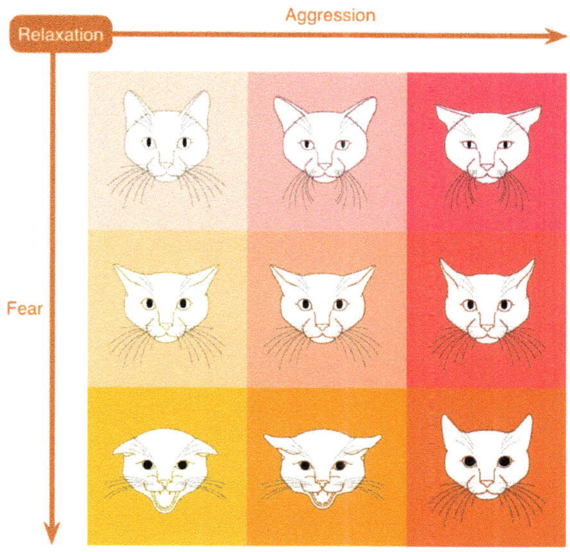

Figure 3. Feline facial expressions: aggression and fear. Once contact is established the facial expression signals the motivational state of the cat more precisely than body posture. From a relaxed expression, aggression increases from left to right and fear from top to bottom. One of the clearest signs of fear is the dilation of the pupils, which is often noted and described by the owner as a "change in the gaze". (Modified from: Bowen J, Heath S (2005) An overview of feline social behaviour and communication. In: Bowen, J & Heath, S (eds.) Behaviour Problems in Small Animals: Practical Advice for the Veterinary Team. Elsevier-Saunders, pp. 29–36).

erect, its gaze directed forward, its pupils contracted, its ears raised and the tail, especially its tip, moving from side to side. On many occasions piloerection is observed on the rump. The **offensive attitude is typical of territorial aggression**, although defence of a cats own territory from intruders may also involve fear and anxiety (DePorter, 2013).

Defensive posture

The warning signs of fear are diverse (Figures 2 and 3) (Bowen and Heath, 2005). In its most distinct presentation, the **fearful cat arches its back and positions itself sideways**, perpendicular to the person or cat with whom it wants to avoid contact. The ears remain lowered in a caudal direction, the lips retracted, and the pupils dilated. The defensive posture expresses the cat's desire to avoid social contact (Beaver, 2004). Therefore, interaction with a cat that shows defensive cues should never be forced. Over-approaching a cat that shows a defensive attitude, especially if the animal has the perception that it cannot escape, can easily trigger an attack.

Appeasing posture

An appeasing posture is defined as one that when displayed by an animal, has the ability to relax or lower the aggression of the individual in front of them and is considered calming. When in contact with another cat, some individuals stretch and roll on the ground, similar to how females behave when in season. This behaviour is frequently accompanied by purring (Figure 4). In groups or colonies of cats it is usually displayed by immature males towards mature ones, to obtain a tolerant attitude from the latter and appease them. Another possible function of rolling-over is scent-marking (Vitale, 2018). Some authors have proposed the position has just been described as indicative of submission (Vitale, 2022; Feldman, 1994). However, most behavioural medicine specialists agree about ruling out stable dominance-submission relationships in the domestic cat.

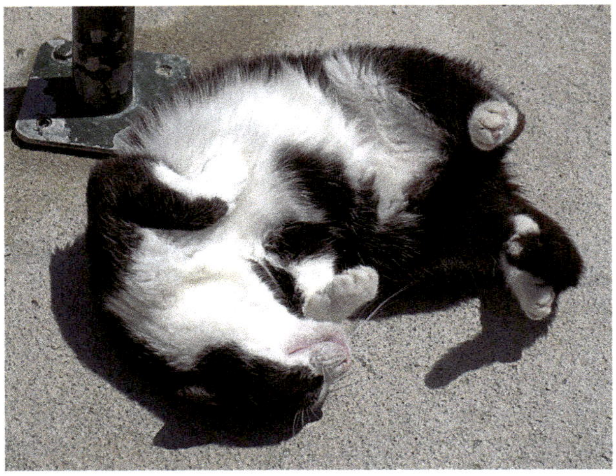

Figure 4. Submissive or appeasing posture.

Tactile communication

From a practical perspective, **feline tactile communication is divided into three fundamental patterns**.

Allorubbing

(From the Greek *allo* = other and from the English rub). In a friendly encounter the cat rubs their head and body against another cat or a person. Often the animal intertwines tails with the other cat (Crowell-Davis, 2003) or, if it is a person, it tries to do the same around their leg (Crowell-Davis et al., 2004). Among cats, allorubbing is more common between females and between males and females, but not between males. This form of mutual tactile stimulation helps to strengthen affectionate bonds between the animals that display it (Fatjó and Heiblum, 2013).

In various species it is proven mutual contact favours the release of various neurotransmitters and neurohormones (such as dopamine, endorphins and oxytocin) involved in the formation and maintenance of social ties (Crockford et al., 2013; Romero et al., 2014).

Furthermore, this behaviour helps mix odours to build a **group odour** (Ley, 2016) which could reduce tensions between individuals sharing the same territory. In small cat species, no allorubbing behaviour is observed in the wild. In the African lion it does occur when two individuals meet after a separation or conflict (Gilfillan et al., 2016), perhaps as a reconciliation behaviour. In short, allorubbing behaviour is interpreted as a way for the cat to indicate acceptance and recognition (Crowell-Davis et al., 2004) of the cat or the person to whom it is directed and, according to some authors, it could be interpreted as a sign of recognition of social status.

Allogrooming

(From the Greek *allo* = other and from the English groom).

This refers to the licking behaviour a cat directs towards the body (especially around the neck and head) of another during an encounter. Although allogrooming is normally understood as a way of reinforcing the bonds between two cats (Curtis et al., 2003; Fatjó and Heiblum, 2013), it could be suggestive of the opposite, that is, of conflict. According to various observations in groups of cats, an individual may attack another shortly after licking it. **Allogrooming behaviour is interpreted here as an expression or redirection of the tension existing between both animals** (van den Bos, 1998).

It is clear more research is needed to clarify the function of a behaviour that must be interpreted with caution in the cat.

Sleeping or resting in contact with another cat

In groups or colonies of cats, individuals often sleep or rest in physical contact with another. This attitude is considered an indicator of tolerance and a good social relationship between both animals (Crowell-Davis et al., 2004).

Visual, tactile communication and social tolerance

Social conflict between two cats often goes unnoticed by their owners. When two cats interact, observing body postures and other visual cues is helpful to assess mutual social tolerance. Systematic, objective, analysis of both positive and negative visual and tactile indicators of social tolerance provide the clinician with essential information to establish a diagnosis.

Whilst problems such as aggression directly confirm the presence of conflict, other behavioural problems (e.g. inappropriate elimination or urine marking) are frequently related to underlying social tensions or conflict (Ramos, 2019).

The presence of positive indicators suggest good social tolerance, whilst their absence suggests the opposite. Likewise, negative indicators point to the appearance of conflict, whilst their absence suggests good tolerance, especially in the presence of positive indicators (Figure 5).

Auditory communication

Vocal messages convey generic information about the emotional or motivational state of the cat in four main contexts (Fatjó and Heiblum, 2013):

- Social conflicts.
- Sexual behaviour.
- Mother-kitten relations.
- Interactions with people.

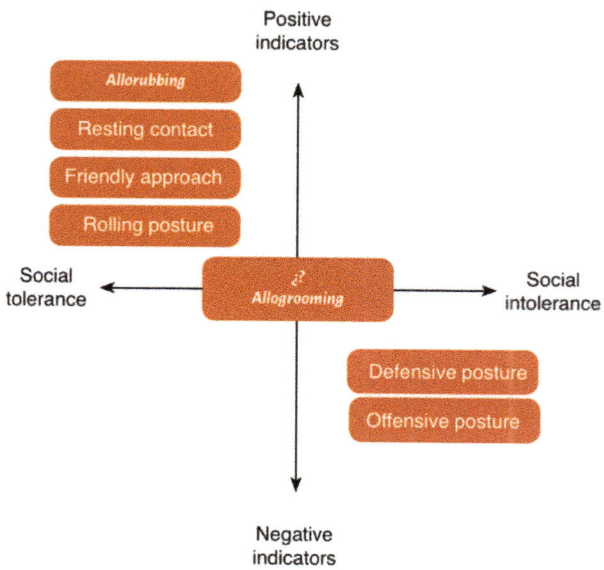

Figure 5. Positive and negative indicators of social tolerance.

Excessive vocalization problems, especially meowing typically occur when animals are in season but are not unique to this context. Many cats present with excessive vocalization after moving to a new territory and in scenarios of frustration, for example, when the possibility of accessing the outdoor area of the home is reduced or eliminated (Fatjó and Heiblum, 2013).

Although spectrogram research has described 21 different vocalization patterns in the cat, in practice four main ones should be highlighted: the meow, the growl, the snort and the purr (Fatjó and Heiblum, 2013).

The meow

This is without a doubt the most characteristic feline vocalization. It is usually seen in social interactions of a **friendly nature**, either in contexts of greeting, contact seeking, territorial marking or for mate attraction (Tavernier et al., 2020). Meow has its most probable evolutionary origin in the vocalizations emitted by the kitten demanding attention from its mother. It is a sound rarely produced between adult cats, but commonly used by pet cats in cat-human interactions (Yeon et al., 2011).

Cats often meow when isolated from their owners or to demand their attention. For this reason, meowing often becomes an annoying behaviour resulting from involuntary reinforcement. Through trial-and-error associative learning, many cats discover meowing enables them to get what they want, whether it's food, play, petting by their owners, or access to a particular place in the home.

The purr

Purring is a form of vocalization produced by the modulating effect of the larynx on the respiratory flow. At just a few days old, kittens already purr while suckling. Some specialists believe it could be a sign from the kitten to the mother that everything is working correctly, comparable to a baby's smile, and could help to strengthen the mother-kitten bond (Fatjó and Heiblum, 2013).

Adult animals retain the ability to purr in the context of social and reproductive interactions. Purring produced by adult individuals is interpreted **as a sign of appeasement and also a demand for attention** (Fatjó and Heiblum, 2013). In this sense, a study indicated there are two purring patterns in the domestic cat, one of a more harmonic nature than the other. The less harmonious purr shares certain acoustic characteristics with children crying and is produced by the cat to get the attention of its owners in general and, in particular, to request food (McComb et al., 2009). Cats may also purr when are involved in stressful situations or are in pain.

The growl

A powerful, long-lasting vocalization, with a harsh timbre and usually a low frequency, associated with **aggressive interactions**.

The hiss

Interpreted as an aggressive vocalization, performed with an open mouth and exposed teeth. **It indicates a defensive motivation** (Tavernier et al., 2020; Schötz, 2015) and its observation is very **useful to differentiate offensive aggression from that caused by fear.**

From a practical point of view, the low or high tone of the vocalizations is an effective way to differentiate the motivation of a cat in an aggressive interaction with another cat or a person. Thus, **high pitched vocalizations suggest defensive aggressiveness, while low pitched ones are more typical of offensive reactions.**

Olfactory communication

Olfactory language allows two or more animals to exchange information without the need to coincide at a certain time, in the same place. Thus, olfactory markings are of great value in regulating the social interactions of a species such as the domestic cat, descendant from a solitary, territorial feline.

Olfactory signals provide information on the identity and physiological state of the cat emitting them and are decisively involved in management of the territory and regulation of reproduction (Ley, 2016).

Cats deposit marks in the environment in three principal ways: facial and body marking, scratching with the claws, and urine marking.

Faecal marking may also happen in cats (middening), although its frequency, communicative relevance and exact function are not clear yet (Feldman, 1994; Pageat and Gaultier, 2003).

Face and body marking

In addition to allorubbing behaviour, cats usually **rub parts of their bodies with high concentrations of sebaceous glands**, either against a person or a cat, or against various objects in their territory. The density of pheromone-producing sebaceous glands is particularly high around the head, especially from the corner of the lips to the base of the ear, in the perineal area and at the base of the tail.

Facial marking against objects, especially furniture, is interpreted by some authors as a way for the cat to increase its degree of familiarity with the territory (Figure 6) (Pageat and Gaultier, 2003). Therefore, many owners mention how their cat rubs its head against objects which have been newly introduced into the home, such as bags or suitcases. This is the main scientific foundation of the synthetic facial pheromone F3 prescribed in the prevention and treatment of problems related to stress (Gaultier et al., 1998; Griffith et al., 1999).

Synthetic analogues of pheromones are a perfect example of the value of basic research in the field of clinical ethology, as a preliminary step in the development of therapeutic strategies.

Scratching with claws

Of the four biological functions attributed to scratching behaviour (Bowen and Heath, 2005), two are related to communication:

- To deposit pheromones on the object being scratched from the interdigital sweat glands.
- To leave a visual mark on the scratched object.

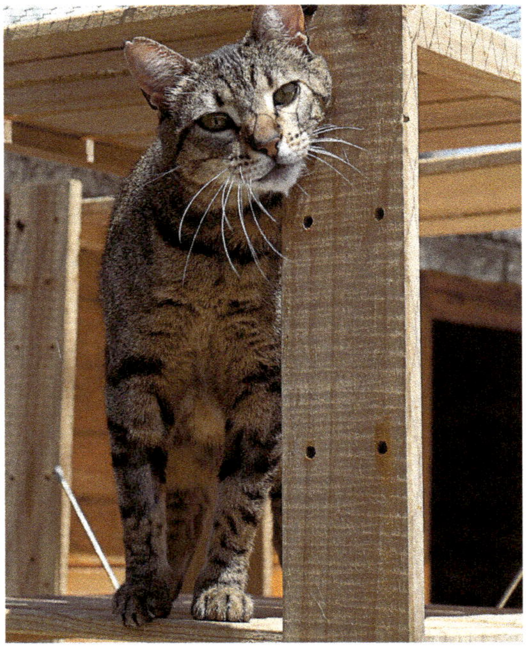

Figure 6. Facial marking.

- To condition the claws.
- To stretch and tone the muscles. In fact, cats often scratch objects after a period of rest.

Scratching does not seem to form a part in delimitation of territory, since the marks deposited by a cat are not usually investigated by other cats. It has been suggested that **these signals could be a way for a cat to assert itself in a certain territory** (Overall et al., 2005) (Figure 7). Cats often mark objects close to their home or resting places. This trend explains the preference of many cats for marking furniture in central areas of their territory and should be taken into account when deciding on placement of a scratching post.

A synthetic pheromone based on the cat scratching pheromone (FeliScratch®; Ceva Animal Health) is commercially available to treat scratching-related problems. Applying the synthetic pheromone to an object increases the likelihood that the cat will use it as an object for its scratching behaviour, and therefore could be used both to treat and prevent inappropriate scratching problems (Vitale, 2018).

Scratching should be considered a behavioural need (Ellis et al., 2013), that is, a behaviour that the cat must be able to express in order to be properly adapted to its environment. Therefore, cat owners must understand that this is a behaviour with which they must learn to live with, although it can be redirected to acceptable objects, such as scratching posts.

Urine marking

Urine marking is a normal behaviour related to territory management and reproduction, which is more frequent in males than in females. In the wild cats often mark the outer limits and pathways of their home range with urine (Feldman, 1994), that is, the area through which they usually move.

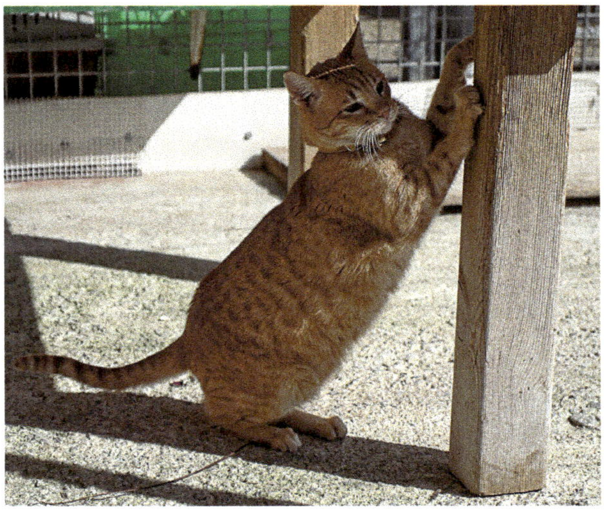

Figure 7. Scratching behaviour.

Urine marks are usually deposited using the typical **spraying posture**. The cat stands with its back to the object it wants to mark, lifts its tail and releases a small stream of urine, which contains secretions from the anal glands and from the prepuce. Some cats assume the squatting posture and mark horizontal surfaces (Landsberg et al., 2013). Thus, although observation of spraying confirms marking behaviour, the deposition of urine in a horizontal position does not rule out a communicative function.

The message contained in a urine mark is different depending not only on the identity of the sender, but also on the receiver. Thus, the urine of a female in season could constitute a warning for another female loitering in the area, while for a male it would be a sexual call (Bowen and Heath, 2005). A urine mark may contain information not only about the identity of its sender, but also about its reproductive and emotional state.

In addition to sexual motivation, **urine marking can itself be a sign of stress** (Landsberg et al., 2013; Amat et al., 2016). Both forms of marking are different in aetiology and neurophysiological mechanisms, and therefore their treatment differs. It has been suggested that **urine marking occurs in situations where there are high levels of emotions**, either positively, as in reproductive behaviour, or negatively, as in a stressful situation. In summary, sexual and social status, arousal, territorial disputes and anxiety can all influence the expression of marking (Neilson, 2003).

Urination problems due to marking have a different clinical presentation than those related to litter tray aversion. In cases of marking the cat usually deposits **urine marks in places in the house somehow related to the triggering stimulus**. For example, the deposition of marks at access points to the house suggests an external stimulus by which the cat feels threatened, such as the presence of another cat. In a marking problem the frequency of urine deposition is high and often the cat continues to use the litter tray for defaecation or urination when there is no communicative purpose (Landsberg et al., 2013).

Well-being and stress

Well-being and quality of life

In recent years the concept of animal welfare has evolved. In the past the existence of well-being used to be equated only with the absence of fear or stress. Indeed, avoiding stress, anxiety, and negative emotional states is a first step to improve the well-being of a cat, but in itself is not enough. **Well-being also means being able to experience positive emotions** or, in other words, being able to express behaviours important to the animal and that make it feel good. In this sense, many specialists prefer the term **quality of life** (Mellor, 2016).

Veterinarians are responsible for promoting attitudes that result in an improvement in the quality of life of their clients' cats, fundamentally through the application of comprehensive environmental enrichment protocols.

Feline stress

Aetiology, diagnosis and treatment

Stress, especially when chronic or non-adaptive, suggests the cat does not cope with its environment.

The appearance of signs of stress depends on the nature of the environmental stimulus and the predisposition of each individual animal to experience stress (Karagiannis, 2016).

Among the various environmental factors responsible for a stress reaction in a cat, the following can be highlighted:

- Related to the **physical environment**:
  - Absence of architectural elements, such as elevated platforms, which allow a **"three-dimensional" use of space**.
  - Absence of a space where the cat can isolate itself and **avoid contact** with people and/or other cats.
  - Inadequate arrangement or **insufficient number of litter trays**.
  - Inadequate provision or **insufficient number of food and water containers, scratching posts, playing areas and resting areas**.
  - Changes in the physical environment (moving to a new home) or introduction of modifications, such as replacing furniture or relocating important resources for the cat (food, water, litter tray, rest area, etc.).
- Related to the **social environment**:
  - **Existence of a conflict** with one or more of the cats that are in the same house or neighbourhood.
  - Inappropriate handling by the owners:
    - Excess handling.
    - Use of punishment, especially physical.
  - Arrival of a new person, another cat or a new dog to the family.

In addition to the characteristics of the environment, there are **individual differences in relation to sensitivity to stress** (Karagiannis, 2016) and its manifestation. These individual differences may be due to genetic factors, but also the environment and in particular

management during the first weeks of life and previous experience of the animal.

Studies carried out in other altricial mammals indicate that the environmental and **tactile stimulation of the offspring during the first weeks of life promotes the maturation of a nervous system which is more resistant to stress** in the adult phase of life (Levine et al., 2016). In this sense, a recent study suggests that early separation from the maternal environment is a risk factor for aggression and stereotypes in adulthood (Ahola et al., 2017).

Previous experiences can influence the animal's response when facing a new environment. Cats coming from a domestic environment are more prone to show acute stress when entering a shelter, often involving hyporexia/anorexia.

Signs of feline stress

Although stress is a response to the environment, it manifests in different ways in different animals. These reactions are broadly described as changes of behaviour and physiological changes which affect the cat's health.

Behavioural changes

Modifications in a cat's behaviour when under stress can be of two types.

Positive (productive) clinical signs of stress

These include all those behaviours that increase in frequency and/or intensity, or that occur for the first time as a result of the state of stress:

- **Aggression and increased alertness**: the cat appears more irritable and reactive to environmental stimuli.
- **Urine marking**: a cat can manifest its stress through urine marking (Landsberg, et al., 2013; Amat et al., 2016). In this sense, many stress urination signs are incorrectly interpreted as sexual behaviour.
- **Excessive grooming**: with the appearance of lesions on the skin and coat. Excessive grooming can manifest itself with sufficient frequency and intensity to be considered a stereotypy, also called obsessive-compulsive disorder or, simply, compulsive disorder by some authors.
- **Increased vocalisation**.
- **Appearance of feline hyperaesthesia syndrome**: which include spasmodic contractions of the dorsal trunk musculature, vocalizations, and self-mutilation of the hair and skin.

Negative (non-productive) clinical signs of stress

These include all behaviours that decrease in their frequency and/or intensity as a result of stress:

- Inhibition of exploratory behaviour.
- Inhibition of playful behaviour.
- Inhibition of grooming behaviour.
- Decrease in facial marking.
- Inhibition of elimination.
- **Hyporexia/anorexia**: the appearance of anorexia is perhaps the clinical sign of stress that requires the fastest and most forceful intervention, due to the associated risk of hepatic lipidosis.
- **Increased rest periods**, especially in areas of the house where the cat can avoid contact with other cats or with people.

The **inhibitory indicators of stress are important** in the feline species, in particular the reduction of exploratory behaviour and prolonged stays in an isolated area. This inhibition of one or more behavioural facets may result from a passive response to an environment which is perceived as threatening or from a gradual reduction in interest in an environment lacking stimuli.

Postural indicators of stress

The body posture of a cat helps assess the presence or absence of a state of stress. For example, dilated pupils, a tail pinned to the body, or a head lowered below the height of the withers could be signs of fear or stress.

Medical conditions

The relationship between stress and medical conditions is bidirectional. On the one hand, chronic stress in animals is associated with a greater tendency to suffer from numerous pathological conditions (Lambert, 2009; Tanaka, 2012), such as gastric and duodenal ulcers, metabolic imbalances, and those related to a reduced immune response, such as infections and neoplasms. On the other hand, the existence of a medical condition, especially if its presentation is painful, in itself constitutes an element of stress for the cat (Karagiannis, 2016).

Feline stress management

This includes three main strategies:

- Techniques for modifying behaviour and adapting the environment.
- Application of synthetic pheromones in the environment.
- The use of anti-anxiety drugs.

Techniques for behaviour modification and environmental adaptation

It is important to act on these two aspects at the same time:

1. Identify and correct (if possible) the specific cause of stress.
2. Address environmental needs.

Identification and correction of the specific cause of stress

A detailed clinical history often allows identification of the main cause of environmental stress, such as a social conflict with another cat or with a person. If such identification is possible, treatment should focus on eliminating or at least reducing the impact of that cause or causes of environmental stress.

Addressing environmental needs

The aim is to improve the welfare of the animal, **by providing an environment rich in stimuli**, which allows expression of natural behavioural patterns. For instance, an impoverished environment, which exceeds the adaptability margin of the animal, could cause the appearance of a chronic stress reaction and, therefore, a loss of well-being. Addressing environmental needs is a non-specific strategy that can be recommended in any case of feline stress, whether or not the cause has been identified.

Some feline behaviour specialists believe the urban environment in which many cats live today strays too far from the conditions of the natural ecosystem typical of their wild ancestor, but also that of their already domestic ancestors, which until the mid-nineteenth century developed in conditions of semi-freedom. In other words, it could be said that in most cases cats have their physical needs covered, although they cannot adequately express some behaviours necessary for their well-being.

Below, the practical recommendations are outlined for a standard environmental needs (Ellis et al., 2013) programme:

1. Provide a **three-dimensional physical space**. Cats like to rest and move around elevated areas within their territory. Therefore, it is advisable to have obstacles and platforms in the house on which the cat is allowed to climb (Figure 8).
2. Promote **food searching behaviour**. Part of their food, if possible wet food, can be hidden around the house, to stimulate tracking behaviour. The places where these food portions are placed should be alternated. Interactive feeders are also useful, where the cat must make an effort to get food (Figure 9).
3. **Provide fresh water in more than one area of the house**, in wide containers. So-called "active drinkers or water fountains" are becoming increasingly popular. These are electronic devices that generate a small stream of water, which seems to be very attractive to cats (Figure 10).

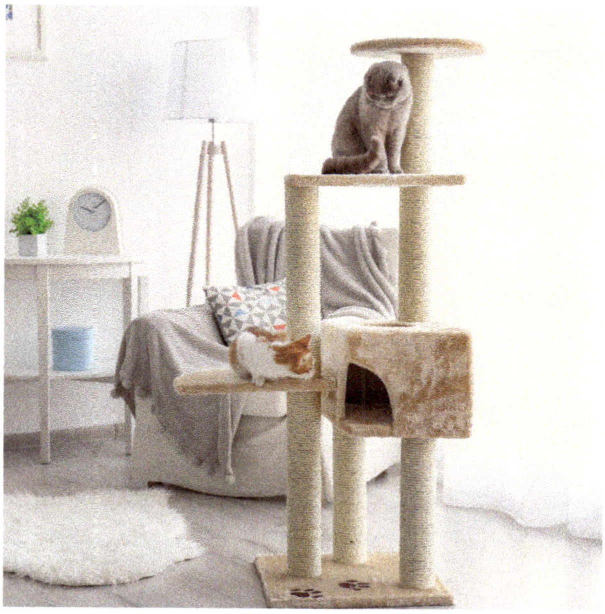

Figure 8. Example of an elevated platform for cats.

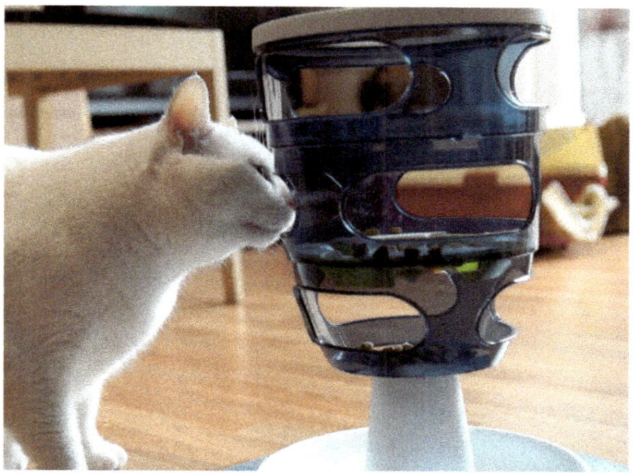

Figure 9. Example of an active feeder.

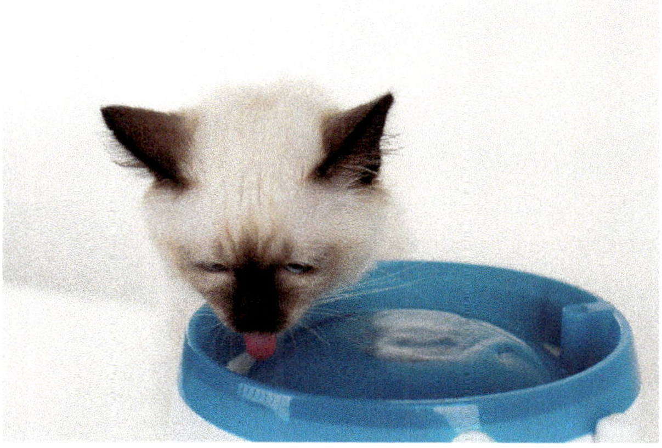

Figure 10. Example of an electronic drinker for cats.

4. One or two **scratching posts** should be placed near the areas most frequented by the cat.
5. Place **more than one litter tray with sand**, in different parts of the house, which are easily accessible and

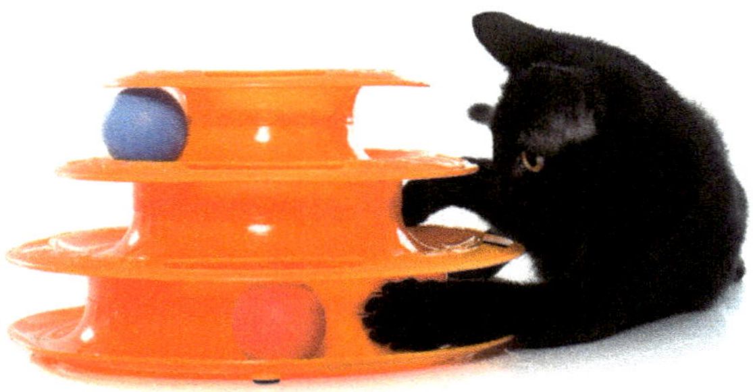

Figure 11. Example of an interactive toy for cats.

away from food and water. Wide, low-edged trays appear to be preferred (Carney et al., 2014).
6. Use **clumping cat litter**.
7. Maintain a **strict daily litter cleaning routine**. Dirty litter is one of the main risk factors for the appearance of inappropriate elimination problems in cats (Ellis et al., 2017).
8. Provide toys and, most importantly, **actively stimulate play behaviour**. Today, there are many toy options on the market designed to stimulate play behaviour (Figure 11).
9. **Avoid excessive handling of the cat**. In general, the animal should be allowed to decide the degree of contact it wants to have with its owners.

Application of synthetic pheromones in the environment

Various clinical trials confirm the efficacy of the **feline synthetic pheromone F3** in the treatment and prevention of feline stress, whatever the aetiology (described in the section on communication).

A new feline pheromone complex (Feliway Optimum®, Ceva Santé Animale) has recently been introduced to prevent and to treat different behavioural problems related to stress in cats (De Jaeger et al., 2021).

Use of anxiolytic medications

These are used in a limited way in feline ethology for two practical reasons:

Firstly, establishing an **environmental management program and the use of synthetic pheromones** offer satisfactory results in most cases.

Secondly, the administration of drugs orally for prolonged periods of time is complicated in the cat, especially in stressed patients. In fact, the administration of the drug can become a stressor in itself, which could further worsen the clinical situation.

The use of anxiolytic drugs from the benzodiazepine family, such as alprazolam, may be useful in acute stress reactions that occur with marked anorexia or hyporexia, where a rapid response with treatment is necessary. An **interesting alternative is mirtazapine** (Vorontsova, 2019), which also offers a quick anxiolytic action and stimulates appetite.

In cases that include self-mutilation behaviour, the combination of anxiolytics with drugs such as **gabapentin or pregabalin** can be useful (Amengual et al., 2019).

Inappropriate elimination

Inappropriate elimination of urine and faeces in the cat is one of the main behavioural problems presented to the first opinion veterinarian (Fatjó et al., 2006).

Until recently, disease-related behavioural changes were clearly differentiated from those seen in healthy patients. However, an increasingly better understanding of behavioural control mechanisms means this boundary is increasingly blurred.

An example that illustrates this new relationship between clinical ethology and internal medicine is idiopathic FLUTD (Feline Lower Urinary Tract Disease) (Cameron et al., 2004).

Ethology

Inappropriate urination problems are attributed to three major causes.

- The existence of a pathology.
- Marking behaviour.
- A problem related to litter tray use.

Inappropriate elimination due to disease

The possibility of illness justifies a comprehensive clinical examination, including at least one physical examination and complete urinalysis. A study carried out in the United States is of interest, which indicates the existence of a history of FLUTD in 60% of cats which were attended for inappropriate elimination behaviour problems (Horwitz, 1997).

According to the classic perspective in clinical ethology, **a behavioural problem can only be suspected after the presence of a pathology has been ruled out.**

Urine marking

Urine marking is a natural form of communication for the cat. The classic marking pattern includes the deposition of small urine marks in various places in the house, usually on vertical surfaces. Although the above suggests urination for marking purposes, sometimes the deposition of larger amounts of urine on horizontal surfaces may also have a communicative purpose.

Urine marking is a behavioural problem controlled by two different motivational systems: **one related to sex hormones and the other to the physiological mechanism of stress**. The first explains the high frequency of marking in uncastrated males, starting at puberty. The second justifies the appearance of inappropriate urination problems in stressful situations. For this reason, aside from castration, the treatment of urine marking includes different measures to reduce stress, from adaptation of the environment, to the administration of synthetic pheromones or anxiolytic drugs, such as fluoxetine.

Inappropriate elimination due to problems using the litter tray

Problems related to the use of the litter tray usually involve both inappropriate urination and defaecation and can be linked to both social and environmental factors (Heath, 2019). Thus, a full assessment of the social and physical background of the cat should be performed.

The modification of the cat's environment constitutes the main treatment strategy, especially the characteristics and location of the tray and the litter.

The internal medicine perspective

FLUTD describes a variable range of clinical signs related to urination, including haematuria, urinary frequency, and periuria (urine deposition in unusual locations). In a significant proportion of cases (54–64%) it is of idiopathic origin resulting from various factors, and is called "feline idiopathic cystitis" by many authors. However, in recent years the hypothesis that stress could be the main reason for the appearance of the problem has gained support. This idea could be the result of three different factors:

- The lesions seen in feline idiopathic cystitis are also seen in female interstitial cystitis; a pathology whose relationship with stress is well established.
- Secondly, the response of many patients to treatment measures to reduce stress empirically demonstrates the relationship between the two phenomena.
- Finally, the use of drugs such as amitriptyline, with analgesic but fundamentally anxiolytic properties, is especially effective in the treatment of some refractory cases of feline idiopathic cystitis.

When considered together, this evidence has led some internal medicine specialists to focus on stress management through environmental enrichment to initially treat cases of feline idiopathic cystitis.

Aggression

Feline aggression can be divided into problems directed towards people and those occurring between cats sharing the same territory.

Clinical characterisation

The clinical characterisation of problems relating to feline aggression is based on four elements:

- The target of attacks.
- The context in which they occur.
- The motivation and underlying emotions involved.
- The cat's body language during the aggressive episode.

Categorization of feline aggression can be done according to different criteria, and may vary depending on the author.

Fear-related aggression

This type of aggression is shown when the cat perceives people or other stimuli as a threat, usually as a defensive strategy when the animal is not able to avoid or escape from the situation. The body posture is typically defensive, although may evolve to be more offensive over time through learning (Casey, 2016).

Territorial-related aggression

Cats may engage in aggression when other conspecifics that do not belong to their same social group invade or spend time in their territory. They can display territorial aggression toward other cats or new pets in the house, and less commonly toward people and children. Although the typical features are offensive (bold attitudes and active approach to the intruder), in some cases fear or anxiety may be also involved (DePorter, 2013).

Play-related aggression

The cat's play is based on predatory behaviour. Owners sometimes stimulate kitten play with their hands or feet, and the kitten literally learns to hunt its owner (Casey, 2016). Over time, this form of play can become a major problem for people. **It is important not to stimulate predatory behaviour in the cat with the hands or feet**, but only by means of toys.

Aggression related to petting intolerance

Aggression appears shortly after a friendly interaction with a person has begun. Suddenly, the cat scratches and/or bites for no apparent reason. Aggression due to intolerance to petting usually appears in cats that show positive social behaviour towards people. In fact, quite often the cat asks to initiate the interaction and it is only later that it shows an aggressive reaction (DePorter, 2013).

There is some debate among ethology specialists about the causes of this form of aggression (Bowen and Heath, 2005).

Redirected aggression

This is characterized by an attack directed at a subject other than that responsible for the aggression, such as sudden noise. According to some authors, redirected aggression can be understood as the product of a high **state of arousal related to frustration or pain**. In fact, cats that show redirected aggression remain agitated long after the initial aggressive episode occurred.

Prevention and risk factors

From a treatment and prevention point of view, it is important to recognize the main risk factors that occur in cases of feline aggression and the main management measures to reduce their impact.

Socialisation deficits

The cat's socialization period runs from approximately the second to the eighth week of life. Lack of contact with people or other cats during this phase of development can result in a rejection attitude in the future, which is difficult to correct.

Therefore, it is important that kittens have contact with people and other cats, to encourage good social tolerance in the future (DePorter, 2013).

Traumatic experiences

A negative experience resulting from an interaction with a person or with another cat can induce fear and a subsequent attitude of avoidance. Sometimes, people maintain interactions of a duration and intensity beyond the natural tolerance levels of the cat, which may generate aversion in the future. In this sense, it is important to let the cat determine the time and duration of its contact with people (Ellis et al., 2013).

Punishment, both physical and verbal, is a negative experience which can cause a defensive aggression problem towards people (Overall et al., 2005). Therefore, **punishment as a means to modify behaviour is totally contraindicated in feline behaviour medicine**.

One of the factors most likely to predispose owners to use punishment is the attribution of intent. In other words, the person mistakenly thinks the cat displayed the behaviour with the conscious intention of upsetting them or causing harm. Therefore, it is important for the vet to spend time explaining the real reasons for the cat's inappropriate behaviour and to ensure the owner does not perceive a component of revenge or spite in their pet.

One of the forms of punishment of greatest concern to behavioural medicine specialists is derived from the placement of electronic devices designed to administer electric shocks when the cat, for example, enters an unwanted place. The use of **this type of device is completely contraindicated** and can seriously harm the welfare of the animal (de Castro et al., 2020).

Communication problems

Many people do not know how to recognise body language related to aggression and the cat's desire not to maintain a particular social interaction. An example of this is found in the aforementioned aggression due to intolerance to petting section (Bowen and Heath, 2005).

A detailed analysis of aggressive episodes often reveals suggestive signs of tension, such as a moving tail or jerking of the skin of the hindquarters. Again, the veterinarian plays a fundamental role in the education of clients as to the best strategy to prevent the appearance of behavioural problems.

Territorial conflicts and limited opportunity for dispersal

Conflicts between cats that share the same territory are frequent and, in some cases, can lead to a serious problem with aggression (Crowell-Davis, 2004).

Under conditions of freedom, most territorial conflicts are resolved through the dispersal of one or more of the animals involved. However, in the domestic environment this possibility is often limited and explains the escalation of aggression.

Management measures to limit tension within the territory include the availability of safety zones and the multiplication of access points to basic resources, such as food, water or the litter tray.

Some cases of intraspecific feline aggressiveness require the initial separation and progressive reintroduction of cats.

The environmental management protocol must sometimes be reinforced with the application of biological treatments, such as synthetic pheromones or drugs such as fluoxetine.

Regarding synthetic pheromones, a synthetic analogue based on the feline appeasing pheromone is available for the treatment of social conflicts between coexisting cats (Feliway-Friends®; CEVA Animal Health) (Pageat and Gaultier, 2003).

Disease associated with pain

There are diverse mechanisms that link pain to aggression. On the one hand, pain can trigger aggression as a strategy to avoid handling. On the other hand, pain causes stress and increases irritability which ultimately lowers the threshold for stimulating aggression.

Behaviour modification protocols

Different protocols are required depending on the type of aggression.

Aggression between cats sharing the same territory

The initial treatment protocol is **based on avoiding aggressive episodes** which result in physical harm. In many cases, this requires the temporary separation of the cats and their subsequent reintroduction through a progressive exposure procedure.

In any case, it is important to apply a general protocol for environmental enrichment that improves the use of the territory and reduces social tension between the different cats that occupy it.

Aggression towards people

This treatment protocol is based on avoiding excessive handling and avoiding any form of physical or verbal punishment. In addition, counterconditioning exercises can be performed to modify the cat's perception of people.

Offensive aggression towards human beings presents a special challenge for the clinician, since response to treatment is modest and the cat's proactive nature increases the risk they pose to people.

Medical treatment

The treatment of aggression can be completed with the application of **synthetic pheromones** and the administration of **psychotropic drugs**.

Either the synthetic analogue based on the F3 fraction of the feline facial pheromone or the synthetic feline pheromone complex (Feliway Optimum®, Ceva Santé Animale) can be applied wherever the existence of a stress element is suspected.

Fluoxetine stands out among the drugs indicated for the treatment of feline aggression, as long as the nature of the problem does not prevent its administration.

Bibliography

Ahola, MK, Vapalahti, K & Lohi, H (2017) Early weaning increases aggression and stereotypic behaviour in cats. Sci Rep 7, 10412. https://doi.org/10.1038/s41598-017-11173-5.

Amat, M, Camps, T, & Manteca, X (2016) Stress in owned cats: behavioural changes and welfare implications. Journal of Feline Medicine and Surgery, 18(8), 577–586.

Amengual Batle, P et al (2019) Feline hyperaesthesia syndrome with self-trauma to the tail: retrospective study of seven cases and proposal for an integrated multidisciplinary diagnostic approach. Journal of feline medicine and surgery, 21(2), 178–185.

Barcelos AM, McPeake K, Affenzeller N et al. (2018) Common Risk Factors for Urinary House Soiling (Periuria) in Cats and Its Differentiation: The Sensitivity and Specificity of Common Diagnostic Signs. Front. Vet. Sci 5:108. doi: 10.3389/fvets.2018.00108.

Beaver, B. (2003) *Feline Behaviour: A Guide for veterinarians.* Philadelphia, WB Saunders.

Beaver, B. (2004) Fractious cats and feline aggression. Journal of Feline Medicine and Surgery 6:13–18.

Bowen J, Heath S (2005) An overview of feline social behaviour and communication. In: Bowen, J & Heath, S (eds.) Behaviour Problems in Small Animals: Practical Advice for the Veterinary Team. Elsevier-Saunders, pp. 29–36.

Bowen J, Heath S (2005) Feline aggression problems. In: Bowen, J & Heath, S (eds.) Behaviour Problems in Small Animals: Practical Advice for the Veterinary Team. Elsevier-Saunders, pp. 205–227.

Bradshaw, J (2016) Sociality in cats: a comparative review. Journal of Veterinary Behavior 11: 113–124.

Bradshaw, J (2018) Normal feline behaviour and why problem behaviours develop. Journal of Feline Medicine and Surgery, 20: 411–21.

Cafazzo, S., Natoli, E. (2009) The social function of tail up in the domestic cat (Felis silvestris catus). Behav Processes, 80:60–66.

Cameron, ME et al (2004) A study of environmental and behavioural factors that may be associated with feline idiopathic cystitis. Journal of Small Animal Practice, 45(3), 144–147.

Carney, HC et al (2014) AAFP and ISFM guidelines for diagnosing and solving house-soiling behavior in cats. Journal of feline medicine and surgery, 16(7), 579–598.

Casey, R (2016) Human-directed aggression in cats. In: Feline Behavioral Health and Welfare. Elsevier, St Louis, pp. 374–80.

Crockford, RM et al (2013) Urinary oxytocin and social bonding in related and unrelated wild chimpanzees. Proc. R. Soc. B., 280: 20122765. https://doi.org/10.1098/rspb.2012.2765.

Crowell-Davis, SL (2003) Social behaviour, communication and development of behaviour in the cat, in: Horwitz, D, Mills, D, Heath, S (Eds.), BSAVA Manual of Canine and Feline Behavioural Medicine. Gloucester, UK. British Small Animal Veterinary Association, pp. 21–29.

Crowell-Davis, SL, Curtis, TM, Knowles, RJ. (2004) Social organization in the cat: a modern understanding J Feline Med Surg, 6:19–28.

Curtis TM, Knowles RJ, Crowell-Davis SL (2003) Influence of familiarity and relatedness on proximity and allogrooming in domestic cats (Felis catus). Am J Vet Res; 64 (9): 1151–1154.

de Castro, ACV et al (2020) Does training method matter? Evidence for the negative impact of aversive-based methods on companion dog welfare. PloS one, 15(12), e0225023.

De Jaeger, X et al (2021) An initial open-label study of a novel pheromone complex for use in cats. Open Journal of Veterinary Medicine, 11(3), 105–116.

De Keuster T, Fatjó J, Heath S. *Understanding and Treating Emotional Disorders in Companion Animals.* Veterinary Masterclass.

British Small Animal Veterinary Association Annual Congress, Birmingham, 12–15 Abril de 2007.

DeFauw, PA et al (2011) Risk factors and clinical presentation of cats with feline idiopathic cystitis. Journal of Feline Medicine & Surgery, 13(12), 967–975.

DePorter, T (2013) Feline aggression. In: Landsberg, G., Hunthausen, W. and Ackerman, L., Behavior Problems of the dog and cat (3rd edition). Saunders Elsevier, pp. 327–343.

Discroll, CA et al. (2007) The Near Eastern origin of cat domestication. Science 317: 519–523.

Ellis, J., McGowan, RTS, & Martin, F (2017) Does previous use affect litter box appeal in multi-cat households? Behavioural processes, 141, 284–290.

Ellis, SL et al (2013) AAFP and ISFM feline environmental needs guidelines. Journal of feline medicine and surgery, 15(3), 219–230.

Fatjó J, Ruiz-de-La-Torre JL, Manteca X (2006) The epidemiology of behavioural problems in dogs and cats: a survey of veterinary practitioners. Animal Welfare 15(2):179–85.

Fatjó, J, Heiblum, M (2013) Developmental, social and communicative behavior. In: Landsberg, G., Hunthausen, W. and Ackerman, L., Behavior Problems of the dog and cat (3rd edition). Saunders Elsevier, pp. 13–28.

Feldman, HN (1994) Domestic cats and passive submission. Animal Behaviour 47, 457–459.

Feldman, HN (1994) Methods of scent marking in the domestic cat. Canadian Journal of Zoology 72, 1093–1099.

Forrester, SD, & Towell, TL (2015) Feline idiopathic cystitis. Veterinary Clinics: Small Animal Practice, 45(4), 783–806.

Gaultier E, Pageat P, Tessier Y (1998) Effect of a feline appeasing pheromone analogue on manifestations of stress in cats during transport. In: Veissier I, Boissey A, editors. Proceedings of the 32nd Congress of the International Society for Applied Ethology, Clermont-Ferrand. INRA; 1998. p. 198.

Gilfillan G, Vitale J, McNutt JW et al. (2016) Cross-modal individual recognition in wild African lions. Biol. Lett. 12: 20160323. http://dx.doi.org/10.1098/rsbl.2016.0323.

Golden, O, Hanlon, AJ (2018) Towards the development of day one competences in veterinary behaviour medicine: survey of veterinary professionals experience in companion animal practice in Ireland. Ir Vet J 71, 12 (2018). https://doi.org/10.1186/s13620-018-0123-3.

Griffith C, Steigerwals E, Buffington CAT (1999) Effects of a synthetic facial pheromone on behavior and food intake of caged cats. In: Proceedings of the 3rd ESVCN Congress, Lyon.

Guidelines for Standards of Care in Animal Shelters (2010) Association of Shelter Veterinarians. Newbury S, Blinn MK, Bushby PA, Barker Cox C, Dinnage JD, Griffin B, Hurley KF, Isaza N, Jones W, Miller L, O'Quin J, Patronek GJ, Smith-Blackmore M and Spindel M. http://www.sheltervet.org/assets/docs/shelter-standards-oct2011-wforward.pdf.

Heath, S (2016) Intercat conflict. In: Rodan I and Heath S. Feline behavioral health and welfare. St Louis, MO: Elsevier, pp. 357–371.

Heath, S (2019) Common feline problem behaviours: unacceptable indoor elimination. Journal of feline medicine and surgery, 21(3), 199–208.

Horwitz, DF (1997) Behavioral and environmental factors associated with elimination behavior problems in cats: a retrospective study. Applied Animal Behaviour Science, 52(1–2), 129–137.

Horwitz DF, Mills DS (2009) BSAVA *Manual of Canine and Feline Behavioural Medicine* (2nd ed.) British Small Animal Veterinary Association.

Karagiannis, C (2016) Stress as a risk factor for disease. In: Feline Behavioral Health and Welfare. Elsevier, St Louis, pp. 138–47.

Lambert GP (2009) Stress-induced gastrointestinal barrier dysfunction and its inflammatory effects. J Anim Sci 87: 101–108.

Landsberg, G, Hunthausen, W and Ackerman, L (2013) Feline housesoiling. In: Landsberg, G, Hunthausen, W and Ackerman, L, Behavior Problems of the dog and cat (3rd edition). Saunders Elsevier, pp. 281–95.

Levine, S et al (1967) Physiological and behavioral effects of infantile stimulation. Physiology & Behavior, 2(1), 55–59.

Ley, JM (2016) Normal but unwanted behavior in cats. In: Feline Behavioral Health and Welfare. Elsevier, St Louis, pp. 320–30.

Ley, JM. (2016) Normal social behavior. In: Feline Behavioral Health and Welfare. Elsevier, St Louis, pp. 34–40.

Macdonald, DW, Yamaguchi, N, Kerby, G (2000) Group-living in the domestic cat: its sociobiology and epidemiology. In: Turner, D. C., Bateson, P. (Ed.) The Domestic Cat: the Biology of its Behaviour, 2nd Edition. Cambridge University Press, Cambridge, pp. 95–118.

McComb, K et al (2009) The cry embedded within the purr. Current Biology, 19(13), R507-R508.

Mellor, DJ (2016) Updating animal welfare thinking: Moving beyond the "Five Freedoms" towards "a Life Worth Living". Animals, 6(3), 21.

Naarden, B, & Corbee, RJ (2020) The effect of a therapeutic urinary stress diet on the short-term recurrence of feline idiopathic cystitis. Veterinary medicine and science, 6(1), 32–38.

Neilson, JC (2003) Feline house soiling: elimination and marking behaviors. Veterinary Clinics: Small Animal Practice, 33(2), 287–301.

Overall KL et al (2005) Panel on Feline Behavior Guidelines; American Association of Feline Practitioners. Feline behavior guidelines from the American Association of Feline Practitioners. J Am Vet Med Assoc Jul 1;227(1):70–84. doi: 10.2460/javma.2005.227.70. PMID: 16013540.

Pageat, P, & Gaultier, E (2003) Current research in canine and feline pheromones. Veterinary Clinics: Small Animal Practice, 33(2), 187–211.

Pryor PA, Hart BL, Bain MJ, et al. (2001) *Causes of urine marking in cats and the effects of environmental management on the frequency of marking*. Journal of the American Veterinary Medical Association 219, 1709–1713.

Ramos, D (2019) Common feline problem behaviors: aggression in multi-cat households. Journal of Feline Medicine and Surgery 21, 221–233.

Ramos, D, Reche-Junior, A, Fragoso, PL et al. (2013) Are Cats (Felis catus) from Multi-Cat Households More Stressed? Evidence from Assessment of Fecal Glucocorticoid Metabolite Analysis. Physiol. Behav. 122, 72–75.

Rodan, I & Heath, S (2016) Importance of Feline Behavior in Veterinary Practice. In: Feline Behavioral Health and Welfare. Elsevier, St Louis, pp. 2–11.

Romero T, Nagasawa M, Mogi K, et al. (2014) Oxytocin promotes social bonding in dogs. Proceedings of the National Academy of Sciences. 2014 Jun 24; 111(25): 9085–90.

Schötz, S (2015) Agonistic vocalisations in domestic cats: a case study. In Fonetik 2015 (pp. 85–90). Lund University.

Serpell, J (2013) Domestication and history of the cat. In D. Turner & P. Bateson (Eds.), The Domestic Cat: The Biology of its Behaviour (pp. 83–100). Cambridge: Cambridge University Press. doi:10.1017/CBO9781139177177.011.

Tanaka A, et al (2012) Associations among weight loss, stress, and upper respiratory tract infection in shelter cats. J Am Vet Med Assoc 240: 570–576.

Tavernier, C, Ahmed, S, Houpt, K A, et al. (2020) Feline vocal communication. Journal of veterinary science, 21(1).

Turner DC & Bateson P (eds.) (2000) *The Domestic Cat: The biology of its behaviour* (2nd ed.) Cambridge University Press, Cambridge.

van den Bos, R. (1998) The function of allogrooming in domestic cats (Felis silvestris catus); a study in a group of cats living in confinement. Journal of Ethology, 16(1), 1–13.

Vigne, J D, Guilaine, J, Debue, K et al. (2004) Early taming of the cat in Cyprus. Science 304:259.

Vitale, KR (2018) Tools for Managing Feline Problem Behaviors: Pheromone therapy. J Feline Med Surg. 2018 Nov; 20(11): 1024–1032. doi: 10.1177/1098612X18806759. PMID: 30375946.

Vitale, KR (2022) The Social Lives of Free-Ranging Cats. Animals 12, 126. https://doi.org/10.3390/ani12010126.

Vitale, KR, Udell, MAR (2019) The Quality of Being Sociable: The Influence of Human Attentional State, Population, and Human Familiarity on Domestic Cat Sociability. Behav. Processes 158, 11–17.

Vorontsova, OA et al (2019) The experience of using drug Mirtazapine in comprehensive therapy of idiopathic cystitis in cats. Pharmacophore, 10(6), 31–6.

Westrop JL, Buffington T, Chew D (2005) *Feline Lower Urinary Tract Diseases.* In: Ettinger & Feldman (Ed) Textbook of Veterinary Internal Medicine (6th ed.)WB Saunders, Philadelphia, pp. 1828–1850.

www.barcelona.cat (2021) Benestar Animal. Descobreix la feina de les entitats gestores de les colònies de gats i el seu paper indispensable a la ciutat de Barcelona. Ajuntament de Barcelona. In: https://ajuntament.barcelona.cat/benestaranimal/ca/noticia/descobreix-les-entitats-gestores-de-les-colonies-de-gats_1049959.

Yeon, SC et al (2011) Differences between vocalization evoked by social stimuli in feral cats and house cats. Behavioural processes, 87(2), 183–189.

Test

1. Which of these psychotropic drugs is considered the first choice for the treatment of a urine marking problem?

A) Diazepam.
B) Alprazolam.
C) Fluoxetine.
D) Trazodone.

2. Regarding the Feliway Classic synthetic pheromone:

A) It is a synthetic analogue of the natural calming pheromone.
B) It should not be applied in the same environment for more than 6 months.
C) The first few days may cause mild sedation.
D) None of the above are correct.

3. The occurrence of feline idiopathic cystitis is linked to:

A) The Siamese breed.
B) Situations of environmental stress.
C) High water intake.
D) None of the above are correct.

4. Regarding redirected aggression:

A) The prognosis is good.
B) It may occur in response to high intensity noise.
C) It is extremely rare.
D) It is usually directed towards other cats, but almost never towards people.

5. Which of the following drugs has been associated with the occurrence of hepatic lipidosis?

A) Fluoxetine.
B) Clomipramine.
C) Diazepam.
D) None of the above are correct.

6. Regarding defensive aggression:
A) It usually includes high pitch vocalizations.
B) It usually includes low pitch vocalizations.
C) It is usually silent.
D) None of the above are correct.

7. Regarding offensive aggression towards people:
A) It typically appears before 6 months of age.
B) It has a poor prognosis.
C) It responds very well to castration.
D) None of the above are correct.

8. Regarding scratching behaviour:
A) Castration is not considered a good strategy to fix the problem.
B) When it occurs near the rest area, it suggests a stress problem.
C) It is usually demonstrated in peripheral areas of the territory.
D) None of the above are correct.

9. Regarding domestication of the cat:
A) The domestic cat comes from the African wild cat.
B) Domestication took place 6,000 years ago.
C) The oldest known fossil comes from a site in northern Europe.
D) None of the above are correct.

10. Which of the following behaviours responds best to castration in the male?
A) Marking with the claws.
B) Urine marking.
C) Excessive grooming.
D) None of the above are correct.

11. Regarding the pharmacological treatment of urine marking:
A) Fluoxetine offers faster results than clomipramine.
B) Clomipramine offers better overall results than fluoxetine.
C) Fluoxetine and clomipramine have similar efficacy.
D) None of the above are correct.

12. Free-living cat colonies are made up of:
A) A central nucleus of males.
B) A central nucleus of females.
C) A mixed central nucleus made up of males and females.
D) Unrelated females and males that associate only temporarily.

13. Regarding the behaviour allorubbing:
A) It does not occur between same sex individuals.
B) It only occurs between females.
C) It occurs between females and also between males and females.
D) It occurs between males and also between males and females.

14. Regarding play aggression:
A) It is typical of cats poorly socialized with people.
B) Its prognosis is good, and it usually disappears spontaneously.
C) It does not respond to castration.
D) None of the above are correct.

Clinical cases

Case 1

A one and half year-old male neutered Common European cat, is brought to the practice for an aggression problem towards the owner.

The problem appeared immediately after the owner adopted him from a rescue centre at a year old. In a typical episode, the cat hides behind furniture or doors and crouches waiting for the owner to pass by. When they do, the cat lunges at the owner's ankles, bites them, and runs away.

Efforts have been made to reduce aggression by punishing the cat with a water spray.

After performing a complete clinical examination, with results within normal limits, a diagnosis of play related aggression is established.

What would your recommendations be to the owners to control the problem?

Case 2

A 2-year-old, female neutered, Siamese cat is brought into the practice due to inappropriate elimination problems with urine and faeces.

The cat was purchased from a pet store at two months of age. Until a few weeks ago, the cat had used the litter tray without problems, which is located in a lit courtyard that is accessed through a cat flap. The clinical history indicates that the cat does not access the patio, even when accompanied by its owners. Urine and faeces appear on the bathmat and on the bed in the guest room. Clinical examination and laboratory tests do not provide evidence of disease.

1. **What would your diagnosis be?**
2. **What treatment would you prescribe to the owners?**

Answers

Test

1. C	6. A	11. C
2. D	7. B	12. B
3. B	8. A	13. C
4. B	9. A	14. C
5. C	10. B	

Clinical case 1

What would your recommendations be to the owners to control the problem?

In this clinical case, the following recommendations were made to the patient's owners:

1. Do not play with the cat using your hands.
2. Stop using punishment.
3. Provide interactive toys and generally increase play sessions with the cat.
4. Apply a general protocol for environmental enrichment.

Progression of the case

Three months after implementing these recommendations, the attacks have subsided.

After a year, the owner again requests help for a slight reccurrence of the attacks. The clinical history indicates that the environmental enrichment and play stimulation protocol has been relaxed. Enrichment intensity is increased, and this is enough to completely suppress attacks.

Conclusion

The present case shows the importance of providing adequate stimulation to indoor cats, not only as a treatment measure, but as a long-term strategy to guarantee good adaptation to the environment.

Clinical case 2

1. What is your diagnosis?

A diagnosis of litter tray aversion is established due to a possible traumatic experience in the patio and secondary development of an alternative preference directed to the bathmat.

2. What treatment would you prescribe to the owners?

Treatment includes placement of two new litter trays, one near the bathmat and one in the guest room. The mat is removed from the bathroom and the guest bed is covered with plastic.

Progress

After a month the cat urinates and defaecates normally in the new trays. By mutual agreement with the owners, it was decided to keep the litter tray in the bathroom and the one in the guest room gradually moved to a storage room.

After four months, the problem remains under control.

Feline critical care and emergency case management

14

Nicki Grint

Contents

The **learning objectives** for this chapter are to enable the reader to:

- perform triage, assess patients, and prioritise cases
- understand the effects, clinical signs, and treatment for common toxicities including insecticides, molluscicides, rodenticides, herbicides, household preparations, and plants
- undertake emergency monitoring and stabilisation
- become familiar with critical therapeutics including fluid and electrolyte therapy, transfusion medicine, cardiovascular and respiratory support, analgesia, and CPR.

Triage, clinical examination, and prioritisation

Cats are masters of disguise and often hide or **conceal critical illness**, with subtle clinical signs being the only clue to a severe clinical condition. Veterinary assessment of feline cases, even those simply described as 'not doing well' by their owners is recommended to identify any life-threatening conditions.

The **three phases** which allow assessment and prioritisation of an emergency case are shown in Figure 1.

Triage is defined by the Oxford English Dictionary as: *The assignment of degrees of urgency to wounds or illnesses to decide the order of treatment of a large number of patients or casualties.*

In a veterinary setting it is **the process of sorting sick or injured animals based on their need for or**

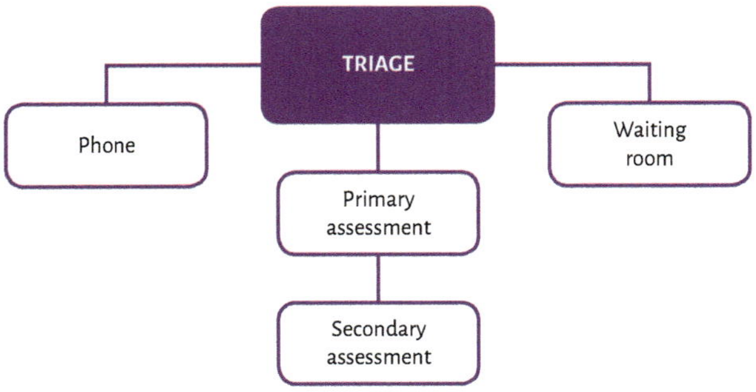

Figure 1. The three phases of triage.

likely benefit from immediate medical treatment (Drobatz and Costello, 2010).

Phone triage

An owner's first point of contact with the practice is usually via a phone call. The staff manning reception should be trained in what information to obtain from owners to facilitate the initial triage of the case.

This involves:

- assessing if the cat needs to be seen and with what urgency
- advice to the owner regarding first aid treatment
- a heads-up for the clinic staff as to what equipment to set up
- calming the owner.

A **checklist of the information** the call handler should ask about is shown in Figure 2.

Phone triage check list

- nature of injury or problem
- wounds
- bleeding
- respiratory status
- colour of mucous membranes
- level of consciousness
- ability to ambulate
- obvious fractures
- vomiting / diarrhoea
- ability to urinate
- abdominal distension
- coughing
- ingestion of toxins
- seizures / altered mentation
- presence of pain

Figure 2. A phone triage check list can be used by the call handler.

The types of cases requiring immediate attention include:

- respiratory distress / dyspnoea
- dysuria / stranguria
- severe haemorrhage
- seizures or altered mentation
- toxin ingestion
- severe coughing
- protracted or severe vomiting or diarrhoea
- pain
- anorexia or marked lethargy.

If in doubt, a consultation should always be offered. If the problem is clear, first aid advice may be given over the phone but a consultation should always be suggested. The owner should be warned that a distressed cat in pain may become aggressive. An injured cat can be transported supported on blankets, towels, or boards to minimise movement of fractures, but the use of home-made splints is not recommended.

Waiting room triage

The next step is waiting room triage which should ideally be performed in a closed consult room by a veterinary surgeon, but if this is not possible, it can be undertaken in the waiting room by trained colleagues. Information to collect during this phase of triage includes **a short history, the nature of the problem, previous medical history, and any medications the cat has received.**

It is important the clinical assessment (Figure 3) is succinct and does not stress the patient.

If at this stage it becomes apparent the cat requires emergency intervention, they should be moved straight to a treatment room where oxygen supplementation, intravenous access, and analgesia can be provided as appropriate. (Further details later in the chapter.)

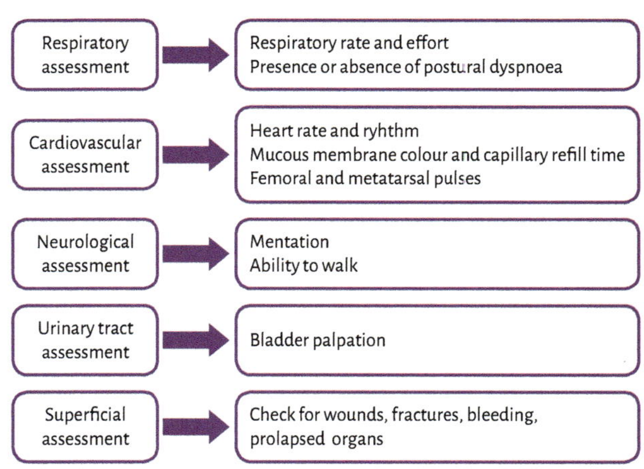

Figure 3. The brief clinical assessment of the different body systems in the 'waiting room triage' phase.

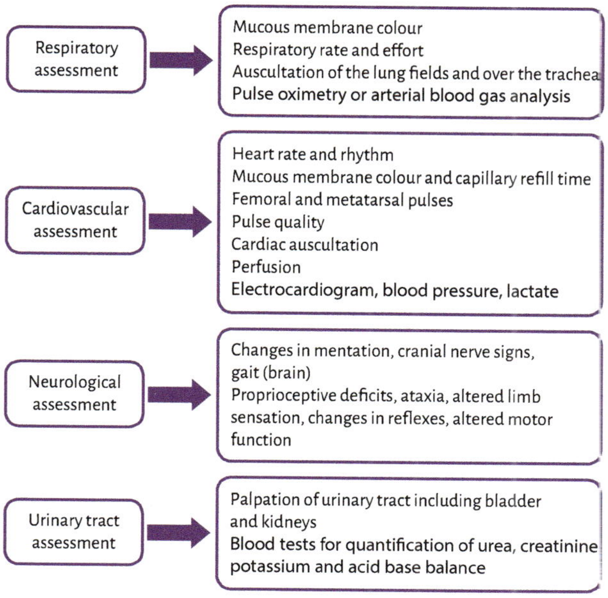

Figure 4. The primary assessment contains both subjective and objective evaluations. Further tests which may be warranted are highlighted in italics.

Primary assessment

The primary assessment is the next stage of examination and should be undertaken by the veterinary surgeon responsible for the case. It gives a more detailed evaluation of the cat than triage and concentrates on **four major body systems**, evaluated both subjectively and objectively.

Secondary assessment

A secondary assessment is carried out **after the initial stabilisation of life threatening injuries**. The secondary assessment includes:

- a thorough clinical examination
- a detailed medical history
- any imaging required
- laboratory tests.

After a secondary assessment, a detailed diagnostic and therapeutic plan is drawn up. In addition, the prognosis and likely costs should be communicated to the owner.

Emergency database

An emergency data base is **run in-house to quickly provide information** on the patient's condition. The emergency data base includes:

- packed cell volume (PCV)
- total protein (TP)
- glucose
- urea
- blood smear.

The cat's PCV and TP should be evaluated together (Figure 5).

Blood glucose must be tested for immediately after sampling, with point-of-care glucose analysers being most accurate when using serum or plasma samples (Tauk et al., 2015).

Figures 6 and 7 include reasons for increased and decreased blood glucose and urea respectively in cats.

Interpretation of a blood smear relies on a good quality smear, this needs:

- a **feathered edge** where abnormal cell types, platelet clumps, and microfilariae are found
- a **monolayer** where white blood cells and red blood cell abnormalities are identified.

PCV normal range 31–48%	TP normal range 6.4–8.6 g/dl	
Increased	Increased	Dehydration
Increased	Normal	Polycythaemia
Increased	Normal	Dehydration with protein loss
Normal	Increased	Dehydration
Normal	Increased	Dehydration with concurrent anaemia
Normal	Increased	Increased globulins, lipaemic sample
Decreased	Decreased	Blood loss
Decreased	Decreased	Non regenerative anaemia plus protein loss
Decreased	Decreased	Non regenerative anaemia plus liver dysfunction
Decreased	Decreased	Red blood cell destruction plus protein loss

Figure 5. The emergency feline patient: possible reasons for increased or decreased packed cell volume or total protein.

Glucose normal range 4.3 – 6.6 mmol/l	Cause
Increased	Stress Diabetes mellitus Iatrogenic overdose of glucose
Decreased	Insulin overdose Liver failure Sepsis Neonate

Figure 6. Causes of increased and decreased blood glucose in emergency feline patients.

Urea normal range 3.5 – 8 mmol/l	
Increased	Pre-renal; dehydration, GI bleeding
	Renal
	Post renal
Decreased	Diuresis
	Liver failure or dysfunction

Figure 7. Causes of increased or decreased blood urea in emergency feline patients.

For emergency purposes; **assessment is required of the three major cell lines** (white blood cells, red blood cells and platelets).

Clinical plan

After collating all the information from the triage and assessments, **a problem list should be created** for each symptom (most life threatening down to least) and a plan formulated which includes **diagnostics, therapeutics and monitoring**. Aspects these plans must cover include:

- fluid therapy: type, route, and rate
- medications: type, route, dose, and frequency
- diagnostic tests
- monitoring: repeated physical exam, clinical pathology, and electronic monitoring of parameters.
- nursing care: pain assessment, toileting, turning the patient, maintaining tissues clean and dry/moist, nutrition.

If you are unable to stay with the patient, a '**Call clinician if**' sheet can be used, where you can include parameters outside of which the staff monitoring the patient should call you. An example of this can be seen in Figure 8.

Patient Label

CALL CLINICIAN IF...

Heart rate:	<	bpm	or	>	bpm
Respiratory rate	<	bpm	or	>	bpm
Temperature	<	°C	or	>	°C
Blood glucose	<	mmol/l	or	>	mmol/l
Lactate	<	mmol/l	or	>	mmol/l
Chest drain output	<	mL	or	>	mL
Urine output	<	mL/h			
Pain score	>				
Systolic arterial blood pressure	<	mmHg		>	mmHg
Mean arterial blood pressure	<	mmHg		>	mmHg
Diastolic arterial blood pressure	<	mmHg		>	mmHg
Central venous pressure	<	cmH_2O		>	cmH_2O

Other:

Figure 8. An example of a 'Call clinician if' sheet.

Toxicities in cats

When compared to dogs, toxicities in cats are less frequent. Out of the calls to the Veterinary Poisons Information Service (VPIS), approximately 10–14% of the total calls are regarding feline patients. This may be due to their more selective eating, but also that clinical signs may go unnoticed, and unfortunately many cats are found dead without toxicities being reported.

Toxicities most frequently reported in cats to the VPIS are included in Figure 9.

An overview of the literature published in 2015, suggested that **drugs intended for human use are commonly involved in poisoning of cats** (although less frequently than dogs). Major drug groups included NSAIDs, antihistamines, cardiovascular drugs, gastrointestinal protectants, drugs for the central nervous system, nutritional supplements, and respiratory drugs (Cortinovis et al. 2015).

Agent name
Non steroidal anti-inflammatory drugs
Quarternary ammonium compounds
Lilium species
Paracetamol
Praziquantel
Benzalkonium chloride
Grapes, raisins etc
Imidacloprid
Permethrin
Moxidectin
Ethylene glycol

Figure 9. Commonly reported toxicities in cats reported to the Veterinary Poisons Information Service.

History taking

During the initial phone call or consultation, the following pieces of information should be obtained:

- identity of toxin
- time of ingestion
- quantity of toxin ingested
- what signs the patient is currently showing
- any treatment the owner administered.

First aid advice includes **washing off topical toxic agents** (including removing collars). However, asking owners to induce emesis is very difficult in feline species and therefore an **immediate consultation should always be offered.**

Prevention of further toxin absorption and aiding elimination

For ingested toxins, either emesis or gastric lavage helps reduce gastrointestinal absorption.

Emesis may be effective if produced within two hours of toxin ingestion, but **contraindicated** in the following cases:

- animal unable to protect airway
- dyspnoeic
- raised intracranial pressure, seizures, altered mentation
- petroleum or caustic substances.

Cats are notoriously difficult to chemically induce to vomit. **Alpha 2 adrenergic agonists** are likely to be the most useful drugs to use. A retrospective study showed that xylazine was effective in producing emesis in 60% of the cats it was administered to, but produced sedation in 30% of cases (Thies et al. (2017).

After emesis, if possible **activated charcoal should be administered**, ensuring the cat can protect its own airway (they are often still sedated). Activated charcoal works to absorb organic compounds, but is not useful against caustic alkalis, ferrous sulphates, mineral acids, or petroleum compounds. **The dose rate is 1–2 g/kg per os.**

Gastric lavage is used if efforts to induce emesis are unsuccessful. The cat should be anaesthetised, with an endotracheal tube in place and the airway further protected with a pharyngeal pack. Warm saline is allowed to passively flow in and out of the stomach via a tube (passed to the level of the 9th rib) and a dose of activated charcoal instilled into the stomach after the final lavage.

Intravenous fluids are useful in toxicity cases to replace gastro-intestinal losses and aid flushing of toxins through the kidneys. Support of renal blood flow helps protect the kidneys where renal failure is a known effect of the toxin. Haemo- and peritoneal- dialysis are two methods of extracorporeal elimination of toxins but not widely available outside of large referral institutions.

Lipid emulsions (such as intralipid) can be used as a lipid sink to bind lipophilic drugs, such as local anaesthetics, macrocylic lactones, and pyrethrins. The reported dose in the cat is **1.5 ml/kg given IV over 30 minutes**. Corneal lipidosis and marked hypertriglyceridaemia has been reported in one cat (Yuh & Keir 2018) but resolved without treatment after 72 hours.

If the toxin is topical, clipping of the fur, application of a buster collar, or washing the coat reduce further absorption either topically or orally through grooming.

Various toxicites

Rodenticides

These toxins all interfere with vitamin K1 activation which is required for hepatic carboxylation of vitamin K dependent coagulation factors. Clinical bleeding is seen within 72-hours of ingestion, and may manifest as bleeding into a body cavity, epistaxis, or pulmonary haemorrhage.

Clinical signs observed in the cat have included signs of **haemorrhaghic shock, bruising, dyspnoea, and lameness.** Minimum tests usually reveal anaemia and low platelet count on the blood smear. Prothrombin time (PT) is prolonged at 48 hours and occurs before activated prothrombin time (APTT) prolongation as factor VII (measured by PT) has a shorter half-life. Clinical signs of bleeding are observed at approximately 72 hours. Emesis or gastric lavage should be attempted in addition to activated charcoal. If PT is not prolonged at 48 hours, no further therapy is required. If it is prolonged, vitamin K supplementation is required. Clinical bleeding may also require whole blood transfusions.

Metaldehyde

This toxin works by decreasing GABA concentrations in the brain and therefore central nervous system (CNS) signs account for many of the clinical signs:

- CNS signs
- seizures
- muscle tremors
- hyperthermia
- salivation
- tachycardia
- nystagmus and dilated pupils
- liver damage (2–3 days later).

Emesis and activated charcoal administration should be attempted. Fluid therapy is suggested as the myoglobinuria, which results from muscle tremors causing muscle damage, can cause renal damage. Anticonvulsants and cooling therapies may also be required. **Dexmedetomidine (2 μg/kg then 0.5 μg/kg/h)** has been used to control similar signs in a cat with a different toxicity (Norkus et al., 2017).

Pyrethrins and pyrethroids

This toxicity is usually secondary to the use of flea spot-on preparations. Clinical signs are mainly neurological:

- hypersalivation
- depression
- muscle tremors
- ataxia
- seizures.

The flea spot-on product should be washed off with mild detergent and water. Anticonvulsants may be required to reduce stimulation and prevent twitchiness. Lipid therapy has been reported with good results in cats (DeGroot, 2014). Fluid therapy should also be used.

Paracetomol

There is **no safe dose of paracetamol in cats**; even very low doses produce toxicity. This is due to the cat's lack of a glucuronidation pathway which is required to metabolise the drug. Instead, N-acetyl-p-benzoquinone is produced and this metabolite is likely (although some evidence also points to paraaminophenol) which produces liver and red blood cell damage. In the cat, hepatic necrosis, methaemoglobinaemia, and Heinz body anaemia may all be seen.

Clinical signs include the following:

- depression
- weakness
- anorexia
- vomiting
- tachypnoea / dyspnoea
- tachycardia
- hypersalivation
- facial oedema
- brown discoloration of mucous membranes.

Treatment includes **emesis or gastric lavage** plus administration of activated charcoal. The **antidote to paracetamol toxicity is N-acetyl cysteine** (140–280 mg/kg orally or 140 mg/kg IV as a loading dose and then maintenance dose of 70 mg/kg orally q 6 hours for 2–3 days).

Non steroidal anti-inflammatory drugs

These include those licensed for use in the cat and also human preparations such as ibuprofen. Due to prostaglandin inhibition, clinical signs are related to **gastro-intestinal and renal dysfunction.** After emesis/gastric lavage and activated charcoal administration, fluid therapy should be used in addition to gastro-protectants.

Onions and garlic

These cause blood dyscrazias in cats due to the presence of sulphides. In addition, gastrointestinal irritation can be caused. Clinical signs include:

- anaemia
- haemoglobinuria
- heinz body anaemia
- vomiting
- diarrhoea.

After gastric lavage or emesis, supportive therapy should be instigated if clinical signs are detected.

Ethylene glycol

The active ingredient of anti-freeze is not toxic per-se, however its two main metabolites, glycolic acid and oxalic acid are. Glycolic acid causes metabolic acidosis, and oxalic acid combines with calcium to produce calcium oxalate crystals, which lodge in the small blood vessels in the kidneys and renal tubules **producing renal failure**. Clinical signs include:

- ataxia
- tachycardia
- tachypnoea
- seizures
- acute renal failure
- polyuria (PU) / polydipsia (PD).

There are three stages of ethylene glycol toxicity described in Figure 10.

Emesis or gastric lavage is rarely useful given the rapid absorption of ethylene glycol from the stomach. Instead, fluid therapy in combination with ethanol or fomepizole (4-methylpyrazole) as an antidote is attempted as therapy. **Ethanol or fomepizole inhibit the metabolism of ethylene glycol.**

- Ethanol dose is 5 ml/kg slow IV q 6 hours (5 doses) then q 8 hours (4 doses).

Phase	Time frame post ingestion	Signs
Phase 1	1–4 hours	Ataxia, tachycardia, tachypnoea, dehydration due to polyuria
Phase 2	4–6 hours	Anorexia, depression, vomiting, miosis, coma and hypothermia
Phase 3	2–7 days	Renal failure

Figure 10. The three stages of ethylene glycol toxicity in the cat.

- Fomepizole dose is 125 mg/kg IV at 1,2 and 3 hours post ingestion and then 31.25 mg/kg IV at 12, 24 and 36 hours.

Lilies

Ingestion of any part of a lily plant can cause **acute renal failure** in the cat although the toxic substance which they contain causing this is not known. Emesis, activated charcoal and decontamination of the coat is recommended, along with fluid therapy. Prognosis is poor if animals are presented later in the development of symptoms with fulminant clinical signs including PU/PD, vomiting, anuria or oliguria.

Disinfectants

There are several toxic substances which can be found in disinfectants, however **phenols are a major problem,** causing chemical burns to the skin and gastrointestinal tract, and renal/hepatic damage.

If the skin has been affected, copious lavage of the area is required, and if ingested, gastroprotectants should be used. Acetylcysteine can help reduce renal/hepatic damage.

White spirit

White spirit can cause toxicity by local contamination, ingestion, or inhalation. **Gastrointestinal signs** after ingestion include vomiting, diarrhoea and nausea. **Renal signs** can include haematuria, albuminuria and oliguria. Hyperexcitability, ataxia and seizures have been observed at high doses, and if inhalation has occurred, dyspneoa and coughing. Depending on the route of contamination, supportive treatment should be used (e.g. oxygen therapy, fluid therapy, anti-convulsants). Emesis or gastric lavage are not recommended due to the irritant nature of the substance.

Locating therapies used to treat toxicities

In collaboration with the Veterinary Poisons Information Service (VPIS) in the UK, several practices hold a variety of medications that can be used to treat various toxicities or prevent further contamination (www.vpisglobal.com/toxbox/). These medications can be purchased 24 hours a day. The **VPIS website** also has a downloadable checklist (www.vpisglobal.com/wp-content/uploads/2019/10/checklist-image-for-website.png) which may be useful for recording details of any toxicities in emergency feline cases.

Cardiovascular and respiratory monitoring and support

Intravenous access

This should be **established as soon as practicable** for emergency cases. Intravenous access facilitates the following:

- emergency drug administration
- fluid therapy
- analgesia administration and anaesthetic induction
- blood sampling
- Central venous pressure measurement (if a jugular catheter or long saphenous catheter is used)
- euthanasia.

Cephalic catheterisation is usually the first peripheral site used in the cat. Restraint and attempts at catheterisation in fractious, stressed, and painful cats may cause decompensation. If appropriate, the cat should be allowed time to acclimatise, and intramuscular opioid pain relief should be administered, along with stress free oxygen supplementation (e.g. in an oxygen tent), local anaesthetic cream over any venepuncture and catheterisation site, as well as gentle handling before catheterisation is attempted.

If hypovolaemia and poor perfusion is suspected, a **cut-down approach** over the site with a scalpel blade can aid visualisation of the vessel. An alternative peripheral site is the **medial saphenous vein** in the cat. If the circulation is so poor that neither of these peripheral sites can be catheterised, two further options are intraosseous catheterisation (see Figure 11 for a step by step guide) or jugular catheterisation.

Jugular catheterisation

Jugular catheters can be placed by a variety of techniques, including over-the-needle catheters, through-the-needle catheters, peel-away catheters, or the over-the-guidewire technique (also known as the Seldinger technique). The **Seldinger technique** allows entry into a vein with minimal trauma to surrounding tissues. The threading of the catheter over a guidewire allows the use of catheters which are too soft, too long, or too flexible for a usual percutaneous technique. A step by step guide on placement of a jugular catheter by Seldinger technique is found in Figure 12.

Jugular catheterisation should not be attempted in cats with raised intra-cranial or intra-ocular pressure, coagulopathies, or that are immunocompromised. The use of jugular catheters is not without complication, for example extravasation (leakage) of fluids or drugs, catheter infection, thrombus/

Intra-osseous catheterisation

The proximal femur, humerus or tibia have been described for intra-osseous catheterisation in the cat:

- intact bone needed
- after strict aseptic preparation, lidocaine (up to 4 mg/kg) can be infiltrated down onto the periosteum
- scalpel blade stab incision
- the catheter should be placed with downward pressure and rotation
- placement should be checked with injection of saline
- flow should be limited to 11 ml/min with gravity flow and 24 ml/min with fluid pump
- the catheter can be left in place for 72 hours or removed once the patient is volume resuscitated and peripheral intravenous catheterisation is achieved.

Figure 11. A step by step guide to intra-osseus catheterisation in the cat.

thrombophlebitis, air embolism, catheter embolism, or exsanguination.

Measurement of blood pressure

Blood pressure measurement is used to **assess the impact of cardiovascular disease or hypovolaemia**, and repeated measurement helps assess response to treatment.

Central venous pressure (CVP)

Central venous pressure represents the pressure in the intra-thoracic vena cava. Central venous pressure is a measure of the relative ability of the heart to pump the blood returning to it, and is a **useful tool if a degree of heart failure is suspected**. Central venous pressure is also an estimate of the relationship between blood volume and blood volume capacity, and is used to monitor and tailor fluid therapy in hypovolaemic animals. **Normal CVP in small animals is between 0–10 cm$H_2$0**. Generally, low value ranges indicate relative hypovolaemia, and if the value is increased, it indicates relative hypervolaemia, and the heart's inability to cope with the venous return.

First, a catheter should be placed in the jugular vein in the direction of the heart. Its tip must lie within the thorax (usually in the anterior vena cava) although if overlong it can contact the endocardium of the right atrium or ventricle and stimulate arrhythmias. This catheter is then attached to either an electrical transducer (as used in arterial blood pressure monitoring) or to a U-manometer. An electrical transducer displays CVP in mmHg, and a U-manometer reading reads as cm$H_2$0. The following conversion should be used; mmHg $\times$ 1.36 = cm$H_2$0

U-manometers are available in commercial sets, but can be easily made in-practice with a bag of normal saline, a drip set, a three way tap, an extension set, a drip stand, and a cut down length of drip tube.

Once flushed through with saline, the three way tap should be turned to connect the jugular catheter and

Step by step guide to jugular catheter placement using the Seldinger technique:

1. Gather prep solution, sterile gloves and drape, dressing materials, suture material, sterile swabs, heparinised saline, and jugular catheter kit.
2. Anaesthetise or sedate (+local anaesthetic) the patient. Clip, prep and drape the area over the jugular vein. Monitoring of the ECG is also advisable.
3. Raise the jugular vein and introduce either a needle or catheter towards the heart.
4. Pull back the J shaped end of the wire into the coil, then insert the end of the coil into the hub of the catheter or needle. Advance the wire into the catheter by pushing the wire with your thumb.
5. Once the wire has been advanced into the vein, remove the needle or catheter, leaving the wire in the vessel.
6. Thread the dilator over the wire and create a tunnel in the skin.
7. Remove the dilator and advance the catheter over the guide wire.
8. Thread the catheter over the wire into the vein up to the hub and then remove the guide wire. Bung the end of the catheter, aspirate any air, and then flush with heparinised saline.
9. Suture the catheter securely in place.
10. Dress the catheter site with a transparent permeable polyurethane layer and then soft dressing material and a cohesive bandage.

Figure 12. A step by step guide to jugular catheter placement via the Seldinger technique.

the column of fluid open to the air. A zero level on the ruler should be drawn at the level of the animals heart and measurements taken in relation to this.

Arterial blood pressure measurement

Direct arterial blood pressure measurement requires the placement of an intra-arterial catheter. **Arterial cannulation is painful**, and so this should be performed when the animal is anaesthetised or the skin above the site desensitised by application of a local anaesthetic cream. The catheter and its attachments must be placed aseptically and secured well, as dislodgement of any part will result in a large haematoma formation, air embolism, or severe blood loss.

The catheter is connected via a saline filled extension tubing to a pressure transducer device which converts the pulsatile pressure signal into a numerical value. Pressures are measured against a reference level (level of the heart), and devices to record pressure need to be "zeroed". Electronic transducers can convert the numerical values into wave forms.

Non-invasive blood pressure

These techniques utilise a cuff to occlude blood flow to an appendage by increasing the inflation pressure to greater than systolic blood pressure. As the cuff is gradually deflated, the resumption of the arterial blood flow is detected by a variety of methods. **The width of a cuff should be 40% of the circumference of the appendage** (limb or tail) it fits around.

Doppler blood pressure monitors (Figure 13) use sound waves emitted from the Doppler probe. When sound waves reflect back from a moving structure (e.g. arterial wall or blood cells) then an audible signal (a whoosh) is heard. Doppler blood pressure correlates with direct blood pressure and is likely to be more reliable in the cat than oscillometric, especially at lower blood pressures. Different studies have produced different correction factors but in general, the blood pressure measured using a Doppler represents a blood pressure between systolic and mean blood pressure values.

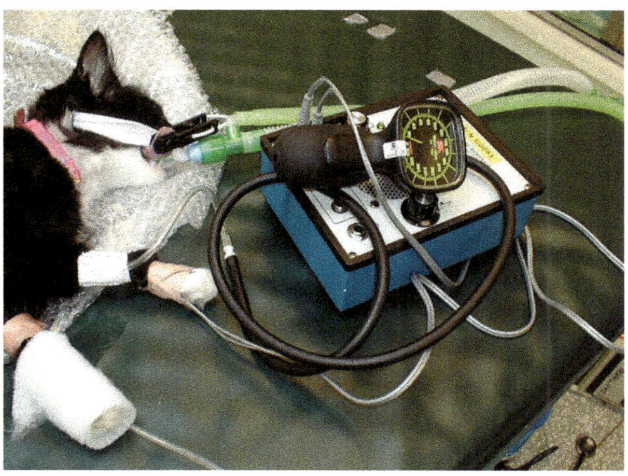

Figure 13. The Doppler technique can be used to measure arterial blood pressure in anaesthetised or conscious cats.

Oscillometric blood pressure monitors are automated and can be programmed to measure blood pressure at set intervals and display the results digitally, alongside a pulse rate. The cuff usually has an arrow indicating which part of the cuff to place over the pulse. After the cuff is in place, the machine cyclically inflates and deflates the cuff, and sensors detect pressure changes in the cuff during its deflation, as pulsatile flow returns to the appendage.

Systolic blood pressure can be predicted well using pulse palpation. Absent metatarsal pulses in cats are associated with a Doppler blood pressure less than 75 mmHg, strong metatarsal pulses are associated with a Doppler blood pressure of 135 mmHg (Reineke et al. (2015)).

Electrocardiogram (ECG)

ECG is a useful tool in the monitoring of critical cases, especially if cardiac or respiratory pathology, trauma, or electrolyte imbalances are suspected. The ECG indicates the electrical activity of the heart, but gives no information on whether the heart is beating satisfactorily.

Electrodes should be placed so they triangulate over the heart. In small animals this is usually achieved by placing leads on the two front limbs and the left hind limb. These are attached to the patient using crocodile clips or sticky pads, the latter are better tolerated in conscious cats. The most useful ECG monitors are those which provide a continuous display, as opposed to paper trace monitors.

Pulse oximetry

Pulse oximetry is a non-invasive, continuous monitor of arterial haemoglobin oxygen saturation. Oxygen can be carried in the blood either dissolved in the blood or bound to haemoglobin, with the vast majority (98%) bound. The percentage saturation of haemoglobin bound with oxygen is known as SpO_2.

Pulse oximetry is based on the absorption of light transmitted through a pulsatile vascular tissue bed. The probe on a pulse oximeter, which can be of several types has a light emitting diode on one side, and a photodetector (which detects light) on the other side. Haemoglobin that is fully saturated with oxygen (oxyhaemoglobin) and haemoglobin with no oxygen bound to it (de-oxyhaemoglobin) absorb light differently, and so the amount of light transmitted through the tissue bed (e.g. the tongue) and reaching the photodetector on the other side depends on the proportions of oxyhaemoglobin and de-oxyhaemoglobin present.

A pulse oximeter measures two things; the haemoglobin oxygen saturation (SpO_2) as a percentage, and the pulse rate in beats per minute. Some pulse oximeters also produce a pulse wave form although some models expand this wave form to fit the screen, which can be misleading. **Pulse oximetry is not an indicator of whether an animal is breathing or ventilating adequately,** (for this assessment capnography is required to measure end-tidal carbon dioxide in intubated patients, or a pCO_2 from a blood gas sample). A pulse oximeter can, however, indicate if there is sufficient peripheral perfusion for the machine to detect a pulse.

All animals should have an oxygen haemoglobin saturation of at least 95%. A value of below 95% is considered moderate hypoxaemia, a value of below 90% is considered profound hypoxaemia, and corrective action should be taken in both circumstances.

Pulse oximetry is a useful tool in monitoring the haemoglobin oxygen saturation of a patient; however, there are several limitations to the technique in the critical care setting.

- May fail in cases where there is poor peripheral perfusion.
- Some models utilise probes with tight springs, this may cause local ischaemia of the tissue bed if the probe is clamped too tightly.
- Pulse oximetry readings may not be accurate in conscious animals which are moving.
- The presence of other haemoglobin species causes inaccurate readings, e.g. carboxyhaemoglobin or methaemoglobin.

Other indicators of perfusion include peripheral pulse palpation, urine output (a minimum of at least 1–2 ml/kg/h), venous lactate (normal 0.37 – 2.81 mmol/l), and rectal temperature.

Oxygen supplementation

There are several techniques appropriate for use in cats to increase the fraction of inspired oxygen concentration (FiO_2) (above that of 21% (or 0.21) in normal atmospheric air), in order to try to improve or prevent hypoxaemia (an abnormally low oxygen content in the blood). These techniques may be appropriate for cats suffering from respiratory, cardiac or neurological pathology as well as post-trauma.

Ideally, techniques should:

- increase FiO_2
- not be stressful to the cat
- not cause accumulation of CO_2 or humidity.

Flow-by oxygen

This is performed by ducting oxygen through tubing to near the animal's nose and mouth. This is a useful initial technique if the cat resents a face mask over its nose or mouth and the ensuing struggle further compromises its clinical condition. Oxygen flow rates of > 5 l/min are commonly used and can increase the inspired oxygen percentage to around 50%. However, this technique is wasteful and requires a member of staff to be present.

Face mask

This technique involves delivering oxygen through tubing or breathing system to a face-mask, snugly applied over the cat's nose and mouth. **The oxygen flow rate normally employed is 5L/min** and this can increase the animal's inspired oxygen percentage greatly, depending on the snugness of fit of the mask.

Oxygen hood

Oxygen hoods may be home-made or purchased from equipment manufacturers. The home-made version is made using an Elizabethan collar by placing the collar over the cat's head, and oxygen is delivered, from a cylinder, into the hood via tubing or a breathing system. Cling film is usually placed over the 'open mouth' of the Elizabethan collar to make a kind of oxygen tent over the animal's head, but can be omitted in an emergency, as high oxygen flow rates delivered near the cat's nose and mouth increase inspired oxygen levels above that of room air.

Oxygen cage

Incubators are usually capable of providing an oxygen enriched environment, although many only deliver an inspired oxygen percentage up to a maximum of 40%. Many practices now use collapsible oxygen tents. These have a variety of venturi devices which deliver different FiO_2 depending on the oxygen flow and the aperture of the device.

An alternative 'makeshift' oxygen cage can be created by placing a cat carrier inside a plastic bag into which a high flow of oxygen is delivered. Black plastic bags are most robust and easily available, but are opaque, therefore a window must be cut into them and a clear plastic piece sellotaped in place to observe the patient. Two holes should be present in the bag/tent – one for the oxygen entry and one for escape of excess gases.

Plastic sheeting can similarly be taped over larger kennel doors to try to make the kennel airspace into an area of oxygen enriched atmosphere. Specially made kennel doors are available which are relatively airtight in order to control the kennel's environment, and provide oxygen enrichment as required. The build-up of carbon dioxide can be prevented by using a 'scubber' pack or tray (containing carbon dioxide absorber such as soda lime), but animal access to this must be prevented as the absorber is caustic (cat litter trays with a fine mesh placed well above the level of granules can help should commercially available 'packs' of CO_2 absorbent not be available); and humidity monitored by utilising an in-cage hygrometer.

Nasopharyngeal catheter

These can be inserted (see Figure 14) to allow nasopharyngeal insufflation of oxygen. **At flow rates of 200 ml/kg/min, FiO_2 can be increased to almost 50%** by this means, and even up to 80% with flow rates of 500 ml/kg/min, although the exact inspired oxygen concentration depends upon the size of tube used, the oxygen flow rate achieved, the position of the tube tip within the nasopharynx, and the breathing pattern of the animal. Soft feeding (naso-oesophageal) tubes are preferred, and placed, with the aid of local anaesthetic, into the ventral nasal meatus, so the tip lies in the nasopharynx.

Placement of a nasopharyngeal oxygen tube

The necessary kit should be collected:

- Soft feeding tube or nasopharyngeal tube
- Tape
- Superglue
- Suture
- Local anaesthetic
- Lubricant
- Elizabethan collar
- Adaptors (for connection to oxygen source)

This is often easier to perform while the cat is still anaesthetised or under sedation, otherwise there will be a large amount of sneezing which often hinders the process.

- One nostril should be desensitised, usually by dribbling lidocaine (up to 4 mg/kg) down it.
- The feeding tube should be pre-measured so the tip lies next to the lateral canthus of the eye.
- Butterfly tape should be attached to the point of the tube which indicates how far it can be advanced.
- The cat's nose should be 'snubbed' – so that it looks 'snooty nosed' and the tube fed (with lubricated tip) through in short sharp motions, holding the tube like a dart.
- Once the tube has been advanced to the point of the tape, superglue should be applied to the tape and used to stick it on to the nasal planum.
- More butterfly tapes should be attached to the rest of the tube and stitched or glued onto the skin, running up the middle of the nose and down the back of the head.
- An Elizabethan collar should be placed on the cat.
- The end of the tube should be connected the oxygen supply and oxygen flow gradually turned up to the desired level.

Figure 14. A step by step guide to placing a nasopharyngeal oxygen catheter.

Trans-tracheal oxygen

This emergency technique is used to buy time if the cat has severe upper respiratory tract obstruction. It involves placement of a needle or catheter between two tracheal rings to insufflate oxygen through into the tracheal lumen. The needle or catheter is attached to a 2 ml syringe barrel, which can then be attached to an Ayre's T-piece via a 7 mm endotracheal tube connector to deliver oxygen (see Figure 15). The bore of the needle or catheter often limits the **oxygen flow possible, so 200 ml/kg/min should be aimed for,** but, through narrow tubes, it is often only possible to achieve a flow of 2 l/min. Oxygen inflow may also be limited by the availability of escape routes for the extra gas volume administered, e.g. if the trachea is blocked above the site of needle entry, then care must be taken not to over-inflate the lungs. A second needle may need to be inserted to allow escape of gases so as to prevent such an over-pressure situation.

Tracheostomy tube

If **severe upper respiratory obstruction** cannot be resolved, then a longer term solution than transtracheal oxygen supplementation is the use of a tracheostomy

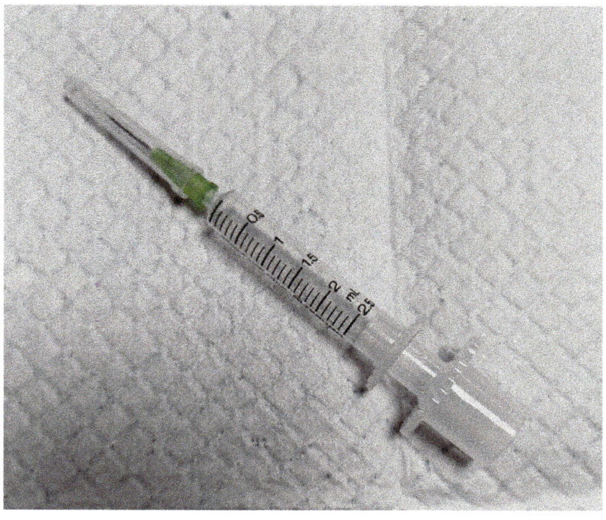

Figure 15. Trans-tracheal oxygen; a needle or catheter is attached via the barrel of a 2 ml syringe to a 7 mm endotracheal tube connector.

Placement of a tracheostomy tube

- The surgical site (ventral neck) should be clipped and prepared aseptically.
- A longitudinal incision should be made along the ventral midline from the caudal border of the cricoid cartilage extending caudally some 2–3 cm (depends upon patient size).
- The paired sternohyoideus muscles should be separated and retracted.
- The trachea should be identified, and an incision made through the annular ligament between two of the tracheal rings – usually in the region of the third or fourth rings.
- The incision should be extended circumferentially but not further than 40% of circumference of the trachea.
- Stay sutures should be placed around the rings on either side of the incision to facilitate placing the tube and changing it for cleaning.
- A suitably sized tube should be chosen and gently inserted.
- If using a cuffed tube, care should be taken not to overinflate the cuff.
- The tube should be secured in place with neck ties or sutures.
- Initially, regular suctioning (after pre-oxygenation) should be employed to ensure tube patency. A small volume of sterile saline may be instilled through the tube lumen prior to suctioning and cleaning.
- Tubes should be replaced for cleaning twice daily.

Figure 16. A step-by-step guide to placement of a tracheostomy tube.

tube. This is easier to perform if the animal is under general anaesthesia. Figure 16 includes a step-by-step guide to placement. Once in place, the cat must be constantly monitored, even when recovered from anaesthesia.

Oxygen humidification

When oxygen from a cylinder, which is cold and dry is breathed for prolonged periods of time via a route which bypasses the nasal passages (which normally warms and moistens inspired gases), then the **oxygen should be humidified**. This is easily achieved by bubbling the oxygen through a chamber containing sterile water.

Oxygen toxicity

When the fraction of inspired oxygen >60% is breathed for prolonged periods, lung damage can occur because of free radical generation with subsequent "attack" of the alveolar membrane. Also, when a high percentage of oxygen is present in alveoli, this can be absorbed and leaves the alveoli "empty" and thus "collapsed" – described as absorption atelectasis.

Thus, oxygen therapy with an FiO_2 >60% is only provided when absolutely necessary, and the FiO_2 reduced as soon as possible to a level sufficient to prevent hypoxaemia.

Ventilation

Whilst oxygen supplementation may improve hypoxaemia, this depends on adequate lung ventilation. Persistently elevated carbon dioxide levels (>60 mmHg) can be treated by mechanical ventilation of the cat's lungs. This is an arduous undertaking, both for the practice and the owner, as it requires constant monitoring and specialist equipment. The cat is either heavily sedated or anaesthetised so as to tolerate an endotracheal tube, and either a volatile agent anaesthesia or a constant rate infusion of a drug such as alfaxalone employed. If prolonged ventilation is necessary, to avoid oxygen toxicity a means to decrease FiO_2 to under 60% must be used.

Initial ventilator settings are suggested below (Figure 17) but altered depending on the patient's carbon dioxide and oxygen tensions.

During ventilation, full anaesthetic monitoring techniques must be employed. Additional nursing requirements include turning the cat, lubricating the eyes and oral cavity, and repositioning the endotracheal tube cuff (if inflated) every 2–4 hours.

Needle thoracocentesis

This technique has both a therapeutic and diagnostic use if pleural space disease is suspected. Ordinary syringe needles or butterfly needles are preferred to catheters, because catheters tend to collapse. If pleural space disease is suspected from the observations of the cat's breathing pattern or from auscultation, needle thoracocentesis (Figure 18) should be performed before attempting other investigations (e.g. radiography) or general anaesthesia.

Parameter	Initial setting
Respiratory rate	20 bpm
Tidal volume	8–10 ml/kg
Maximum peak inspiratory pressure	12 cmH_2O
Inspiratory: expiratory	1:2 or 1:3

Figure 17. Initial ventilator settings for use in cats undergoing ICU ventilation.

A step-by-step guide to needle thoracocentesis

- After clipping and aseptic preparation, insert the needle at 7th or 8th intercostal space (mid to caudal intercostal space), halfway up chest wall.
- The procedure should be attempted with the cat in sternal recumbency.
- Local anaesthesia, either with an intercostal nerve block or a wheal of lidocaine over the needle insertion point should be used.
- A bleb of sterile saline should be put in needle hub before insertion. When entering the pleural space, this fluid bleb will either: be sucked in, because of negative pressure in the space (intrapleural pressure is normally negative) or squirt out, because of positive pressure in the space (from abnormal "filling" of the space i.e. pneumothorax, haemothorax etc.).
- Once in the pleural space, the needle should be advanced parallel to the ribs to cause the least possible laceration to the lungs during breathing movements.
- The needle should be attached to a one-way valve system or 3-way tap.
- The pleural space should be drained.
- This procedure can be repeated on the contra-lateral side of the cat's thorax.
- Any fluid samples should be sent for laboratory assessments.

Figure 18. A step-by-step guide to needle thoracocentesis.

Electrolyte and acid base abnormalities

Electrolytes

A recent multivariable analysis (Goggs et al., 2018) showed that **sodium, potassium, chloride, and calcium are independently and proportionally associated with mortality in cats** and are an important component of assessment of critical care or emergency feline patients.

Potassium

Normal range: 3.5–5.5 mmol/l.

Hyperkalaemia

Potential causes of hyperkalaemia in the cat are listed in Figure 19. If serum potassium increases above 7 mmol/l then arrythmias may develop and ideally this electrolyte abnormality should be corrected.

- increased intake (e.g., iatrogenic infusion)
- decreased excretion (e.g., urinary tract obstruction, acute renal failure)
- severe dehydration
- secondary to acidosis
- secondary to cell lysis
- hypothermia
- blood transfusions
- some drugs e.g. potassium penicillin, ACE inhibitors, heparin.

Figure 19. Potential causes of hyperkalaemia in the cat.

Correction of hyperkalaemia is by:

- Removing excessive potassium from the body by diuresis, using intravenous fluid therapy and aiding the voiding of urine.
- Shifting potassium into the intracellular compartment (where it does not produce negative effects). This can be done by correcting acidosis, as hydrogen moving out of cells will encourage potassium to move into cells. Alternatively, glucose 0.5–1 g/kg intravenously +/− soluble insulin 0.2–0.5 IU per g of glucose can be administered. Glucose (50%) is a hypertonic solution and therefore should be diluted with a crystalloid fluid before administration through a peripheral venous catheter to avoid causing thrombosis.
- The administration of calcium salts will not decrease serum potassium concentrations but does counteract the effects of potassium on cardiac membrane potential and therefore stabilise the cardiomyocyte membrane. Calcium chloride (10%) 0.2 ml/kg IV over 5–10 minutes or calcium gluconate (10%) 0.6 ml/kg IV administered slowly over 5–10 minutes. The effects are transient, lasting approximately 20 minutes before being sequestered into cells.

Hypokalaemia

The potential causes of hypokalaemia in the cat are listed in Figure 20. Treatment for hypokalaemia is intravenous fluid therapy with added potassium (Figure 21). The maximum potassium supplementation rate should not exceed 0.5 m Eq/kg/h.

- gastro-intestinal losses
- inadequate dietary intake
- excessive intravenous fluid therapy
- polyuria / diuresis
- drugs e.g. digitalis, loop diuretics
- hyperinsulinaemia.

Figure 20. Potential causes of hypokalaemia in the cat.

Potassium supplementation

Serum potassium / mmol/l	Amount to add to 500 ml crystalloid
<2	40 mmol
2 – 2.5	30 mmol
2.5 – 3	20 mmol
3 – 3.5	14 mmol
3.5 – 5.5	10 mmol

It is important to ensure that rate of supplementation does not exceed 0.5 mEq/kg/h

Figure 21. Rates of potassium supplementation.

Sodium

Normal range: 135–155 mmol/l.

Hypernatraemia

Causes of hypernatremia in the cat:

- primary hyperaldosteronism
- over infusion of saline
- renal failure
- congestive heart failure
- hypoalbuminaemia
- increased insensible loss of sodium free fluid
- water deprivation.

Treatment: includes free access to oral water or the administration of low sodium fluid, but the aim should always be to change the sodium level slowly, no faster than 1 mmol/h. This is to avoid the formation of cerebral oedema.

Hyponatraemia

Causes of hyponatraemia in the cat:

- Addison's disease
- diabetes mellitus
- excessive diuresis
- sodium rich fluid los
- over administration of free water
- psychogenic polydipsia
- inestinal obstruction
- duodenal vomiting.

Treatment: infusion of 0.9% saline, with the aim to change sodium levels slowly and no faster than 1 mmol/h. **Too rapid an increase in sodium serum concentration leads to demyelination of the central nervous system.**

Calcium

Normal range (total): 2.0–2.7 mmol/l.

Hypocalcaemia

Causes of hypocalcemia in the cat include:

- eclampsia
- burns
- hypoalbuminemia
- chronic renal failure
- acute pancreatitis
- post bilateral thyroidectomy.

Treatment: 5–15 mg/kg of 10% calcium gluconate slowly IV over 15 minutes, or a continuous rate infusion of 10 mg/kg/h.

Hypercalcaemia

Causes of hypercalcaemia in the cat:

- hyperparathyroidism
- neoplasia (less common)
- idiopathic.

Treatment includes diuresis with fluids which do not contain calcium, with or without furosemide.

Chloride

Normal range: 117–123 mmol/l.

Chloride should be corrected for changes in sodium to take into account changes in plasma osmolarity:

$$[\text{Cl}]\ (\text{corrected}) = \frac{[\text{Cl}]\ (\text{measured}) \times [\text{Na}]\ (\text{normal})}{[\text{Na}]\ (\text{measured})}$$

Hypochloraemia

Causes include:

- vomiting
- excessive renal losses (including loop and thiazide diuretics and glucocorticoids)
- over infusion of low chloride fluid therapy
- acute tumour lysis syndrome
- anaemia
- metabolic alkalosis
- urethral obstruction
- hyperadrenocorticism and hyperaldosteronism
- refeeding syndrome
- syndrome of inappropriate ADH release.

Hyperchloraemia

Causes of hyperchloremia in cats include:

- pure water or hypotonic fluid loss
- overcorrected hypochloraemia
- renal failure
- diabetes mellitus
- chronic respiratory alkalosis
- spironolactone administration.

Other than treating the primary cause, fluid therapy with either lower chloride fluids such as Hartmann's solution (to treat hyperchloraemia) or higher chloride fluids (such as 0.9% saline) to treat hypochloraemia help address chloride abnormalities.

Acid-base abnormalities

Blood gas analysis

Blood gas analysis is **useful in the diagnosis, prognosis, and monitoring of several conditions** in small animal clinical practice. It gives information on the respiratory system, perfusion, and acid base balance of the patient. The normal ranges given below are approximate but validated normal ranges for each individual blood gas machine should be used whenever available.

pH

This is an indication as to how acidic or alkaline a solution is and thus the **overall state of acid – base balance.** The pH is inversely related to the number of acidic H^+ ions in a solution. The pH scale is logarithmic, and therefore small decreases in pH represent a large increase in H^+ ion concentration.

The normal pH is 7.35–7.45. If the pH is outside this range there is "acidaemia" (<7.35) or "alkalaemia" (>7.45) present. If the pH goes out of range then the body will try and correct the pH again; chemical buffers in extracellular fluid and intracellular fluid act immediately. If there is a metabolic underlying reason to the pH abnormality then the respiratory system is able to alter CO_2 in the blood as CO_2 is an acidic gas. This is a coarse control that acts in the medium term. The kidneys can excrete excess acids/reabsorb bases as a longer term fine control to compensate for metabolic or respiratory abnormalities.

Base excess

The base excess (BE) is the number of millimoles of acid or alkali that must be added to one litre of blood in order to restore its pH to normal, once the $PaCO_2$ is adjusted to "normal". In theory [BE] should more accurately assess metabolic acid-base disturbances than (HCO_3^-), because it represents all the buffer base, not just bicarbonate. Normal is +5 to –5 (mmol/l); an excessively positive BE indicates metabolic alkalosis and an excessive negative BE indicates metabolic acidosis (a negative BE is also known as base deficit).

Bicarbonate

Normal range is 21–28 mmol/l.

Bicarbonate is an indicator of the metabolic component of blood gas results. A low and high bicarbonate indicates metabolic acidosis and alkalosis, respectively.

Carbon dioxide

The partial pressure or $PaCO_2$ is the dissolved carbon dioxide in the blood, and represents a balance between the amount of CO_2 produced by the body and alveolar ventilation. Usually if there is an abnormality in carbon dioxide tensions this is due to a change in alveolar ventilation, with hypoventilation causing an increase in CO_2, and hyperventilation causing a decrease in CO_2. **Normocapnia is 35–45 mmHg.**

Acid base abnormalities

There are **four basic types of acid base abnormality:**

1. metabolic acidosis
2. metabolic alkalosis
3. respiratory acidosis
4. respiratory alkalosis.

Usually the other body systems compensate (i.e. the respiratory system compensates for metabolic abnormalities, and the metabolic system compensates for respiratory abnormalities).

Figure 22 shows the expected changes for these acid base abnormalities with the expected compensations.

Mixed acid base disorders can also occur; e.g. a respiratory acidosis and metabolic acidosis together.

Correction of acid base abnormalities

Once the primary acid base abnormality is identified, there are ways to assist the animal in correcting their pH back to the normal range.

- **Respiratory acidosis**: accumulation of CO_2, usually through decreased ventilation, and therefore increasing

Primary problem	pH	PCO_2	HCO_3
Metabolic acidosis	↓	↓	↓
Metabolic alkalosis	↑	↑	
Respiratory acidosis	↓	↑	↑
Respiratory alkalosis	↑	↓	↓

Figure 22. Primary acid base abnormalities with compensations.

ventilation (e.g. by provision of intermittent positive pressure ventilation) will help. Rebreathing (inhalation of inspiratory gas laden with CO_2) should also be eliminated (if present) by increasing fresh gas flow (in non-rebreathing systems) and changing the soda-lime (in rebreathing systems).

- **Respiratory alkalosis:** usually from over-ventilation driving down $PaCO_2$. If the cat's lungs are being artificially ventilated, respiratory rate or tidal volume could be decreased to reduce minute ventilation. If the cat is hyperventilating due to pain, analgesia should be administered.
- **Metabolic acidosis**: often due to accumulation of acidic hydrogen ions in the cat's body. If the cat is unable to void urine (containing hydrogen ions) then removal of urine will help. Dilution of the H^+ ions with fluid therapy, especially with an alkalinising fluid such as Hartmann's solution helps. If this is insufficient or the metabolic acidosis is severe (for example base excess >–10 mmol/l), then sodium bicarbonate should be considered. This fluid should not be mixed with calcium containing fluids such as Hartmann's solution. The total dose calculated is (in mmol) = base excess × 0.3 × bodyweight (kg). Usually half of this total dose is infused slowly over 10–20 minutes and then a further blood sample is taken to check acid-base status a further 20 minutes later. Sodium bicarbonate is not an innocuous fluid and should be reserved for use only after other treatment options have been attempted.
- **Metabolic alkalosis**: usually secondary to a loss in hydrogen ions (e.g. pre-pyloric vomiting). Use of an acidifying fluid, such as 0.9% saline assists in correction of the acid base status.

Using blood gas analysis to assess oxygenation

An arterial blood sample will yield information on the patient's oxygenation. The most **commonly used site for arterial blood gas sampling is the dorsal pedal artery**. Sampling can be a noxious stimulus to the cat and therefore local anaesthetic cream should be applied in conscious patients. A 24g needle and pre-heparinised syringe should be used, to facilitate sampling the needle should be bent slightly at the point where it connects to the hub. Once an arterial blood sample is obtained, any air bubbles should be knocked out of the syringe, and the syringe capped. **The blood sample should be analysed immediately**.

Both oxygen bound to haemoglobin and oxygen dissolved in the blood are measured by blood gas analysers; 98% of oxygen is carried bound to haemoglobin (SaO_2) and 2% is carried dissolved in the blood (PaO_2).

- SaO_2 of 95–100% is clinically desirable and suggests good oxygen carriage by haemoglobin
- SaO_2 <95% (but above 90%) indicates moderate hypoxaemia
- SaO_2 <90% indicates severe hypoxaemia
- PaO_2 >90 mmHg = adequate pressure of dissolved oxygen in arterial blood
- PaO_2 80–90 mmHg = mild hypoxaemia
- PaO_2 60–80 mmHg = moderate hypoxaemia
- PaO_2 <60 mmHg = severe hypoxaemia.

The PaO_2 of arterial blood should be approximately five times the fraction of inspired oxygen (FiO_2) (%) e.g. if taking a sample of arterial blood from a patient breathing room air (FiO_2 of 21%); 5 × 21% = 105 mmHg.

So a patient breathing room air with good diffusion of oxygen between alveoli and arterial blood should have a PaO_2 of about 105mmHg. If a patient is having oxygen supplementation it may be difficult to estimate their FiO_2. If the patient's clinical status will allow, oxygen should be discontinued for five minutes before sampling so that accurate estimation of FiO_2 can be made.

Fluid therapy

There are two main types of fluids used in fluid therapy; **crystalloids and colloids**.

Crystalloids

Crystalloids are any solution of crystalline solids that are dissolved in water e.g. sodium based or dextrose based. If the electrolyte composition of the solution is similar to extra cellular fluid (ECF), then the fluid is known as a balanced electrolyte solution.

Extracellular fluid volume replacers

Extracellular fluid volume replacers have a concentration of sodium similar to the ECF, which means these fluids stay in the extracellular compartment and are good at replacing extracellular fluid loss.

These fluids can be infused rapidly as they will not induce changes in electrolyte composition. After IV administration the fluid redistributes between the intravascular and interstitial (outside the blood vessels) fluid compartments; thus for every 1 litre of fluid administered IV, only about 250–300 ml remains in the intravascular space after 1–2 hours.

The two most commonly used extracellular fluid volume replacers in the UK are **Hartmann's solution** (also known as lactated Ringer's solution) and **normal (0.9%) saline.** Outside of the UK, acetated Ringer's solution is also popular. Both Hartmann's and acetated

Electrolytes	Hartmann's solution	Acetated Ringer's solution	Normal (0.9%) saline
Sodium (mmol/l)	131	130	150
Chloride (mmol/l)	111	112	150
Potassium (mmol/l)	5	5	–
Calcium (mmol/l)	1.5	1	–
Magnesium (mmol/l)	0	1	–
Lactate/acetate (mmol/l)	29 (lactate)	28 (acetate)	–

Figure 23. Composition of commonly used extra-cellular volume.

Ringer's solution are similar, they have a different alkalinising component (lactate and acetate respectively), but their electrolyte concentrations are similar (see Figure 23). Normal saline conversely, is an acidifying solution.

In an emergency and critical care setting, the choice between Hartmann's solution/acetated Ringer's and normal saline is dependent on the cat's acid base and electrolyte abnormalities. For example; if a cat has a metabolic acidosis, then choosing an alkalinising fluid (such as Hartmann's solution or acetated Ringer's) is beneficial in trying to restore the pH back to normal. In the past Hartmann's was avoided in clinical situations such as the cat with urethral obstruction because of concerns about administering a small amount of potassium (within the fluids) into an already hyperkalaemic animal. Drobatz et al. (2003) found that when compared to normal saline, a balanced polyionic fluid (similar to Hartmann's solution) did not increase serum potassium in cats with urethral obstruction. The use of the balanced polyionic fluid actually corrected the cats' metabolic acidosis significantly more quickly than fluid therapy with normal saline.

There are some clinical situations where normal saline is the fluid of choice, e.g. pre-pyloric vomiting, where the patient often presents with hypochloraemic metabolic alkalosis (due to loss of HCl in stomach acid) and would benefit from the acidifying nature and higher chloride content of normal saline. This fluid should be used in situations where the calcium content of Hartmann's precludes its use, for example when administering with citrate containing blood products or sodium bicarbonate.

Maintenance solutions

There are other **crystalloids which are appropriate as maintenance solutions or water replacers.** These are used in patients suffering from dehydration after a primary water loss, or if the patient is being hospitalised over several days but needs fluid therapy during this time. These fluids tend to have lower sodium concentrations but are made isotonic by inclusion of glucose based solutes. Once this glucose is metabolised, these fluids can become physiologically hypotonic. Potassium is often added to these fluids, especially if they are used as maintenance fluids when a patient has been anorexic for several days, as these cats are often hypokalaemic (see Table 21). A more suitable alternative in this situation would be placement of a feeding tube if the cat has been anorexic for more than three days.

The amount of dextrose present in the solutions described provides negligible energy at the concentrations used and therefore cannot meet the cat's caloric requirements. Because the sodium concentration is much lower than that in the extra-cellular fluid, these fluids should not be given at fast rates, but infused slowly over 24 hours.

Recommendations from the American Animal Hospital Association include **calculating maintenance requirements on an individual basis** as the smaller the animal, the higher the maintenance rate.

To calculate a cat's maintenance fluid therapy rate, the following formula should be used:

$$\text{Maintenance fluid therapy rate} = 80 \times \text{body weight(kg)}^{0.75}.$$

This calculation provides a total volume over 24 hours, which usually equates to 2–3 ml/kg/h.

Hypertonic Saline

Hypertonic saline can be used in cases of shock. There are several strengths available but a typical concentration is 7.2%. Administration of hypertonic saline causes an increase in blood pressure by several mechanisms, the main action being that it draws water from the interstitial space. Any effect that hypertonic saline has is transient (lasting 30–120 mins). **The suggested dose is 4 ml/kg over 10 mins.**

The use of hypertonic saline must be followed by the administration of isotonic crystalloids to replace "borrowed" water from the interstitial space and provide a long-term increase in circulating volume.

The use of hypertonic saline also carries with it potential side effects; these can include hypernatraemia and hypokalaemia, haemolysis, and ventricular arrhythmias. If the reason for shock is blood loss, there is a possibility of re-haemorrhage after administration of hypertonic saline. This is because the transient increase in blood pressure may dislodge blood clots which are trying to form.

Colloids

Colloid fluids contain large molecular weight particles which cannot pass through the vascular

endothelium. They increase the colloid osmotic pressure of the plasma and in addition to staying in the intravascular compartment, they also "pull" water from the interstitial space into the intravascular space. To avoid dehydrating the interstitium, crystalloids should be used concurrently or just after colloids, to pay back the fluid drawn from the interstitial space.

Colloids should be used in any case where rapid improvement of circulating volume is necessary. As a general rule no more than one quarter of an animal's circulating volume should be administered in a 24-hour period. In a cat this equates to approximately 15 ml/kg, otherwise the haemodilution will dilute clotting factors etc. Colloids can be used intra-operatively to help maintain blood pressure, or if an animal has a total protein of less than 35 g/l in order to prevent extravasation of fluid.

Colloids can be further subdivided into **natural colloids** (including whole blood, packed red cells and plasma), and **artificial colloids** (including starches, gelofusin and dextrans). Some disadvantages of colloids include volume overload, anaphylactic reactions, and clotting problems. Large scale studies in the human field identified potential side effects especially with starches. These results prompted a downturn in starch production for the human medicine field and in turn this has affected supplies to the veterinary sector.

Intravenous fluid therapy calculations

Intravenous fluid therapy infusion volumes and rates must be calculated accurately especially in feline patients so as not to produce overhydration or insufficient restoration of fluid deficits. With the increased popularity of drip pumps in practice, the administration of fluid therapy is more accurate, however it is still necessary to perform calculations and set up fluid therapy plans.

Dehydration

If a cat is admitted with pre-existing dehydration, e.g. persistent vomiting, then this deficit needs to be factored in and compensated for in the fluid therapy plan. First of all, an estimation should be made of how dehydrated the animal is by a combination of **clinical exam and clinical pathology tests**. Moistness of mucous membranes, skin turgor, and sunkenness of eyes should be checked (see Figure 24). This is only a rough guide and there are many factors, not just hydration which affect these signs e.g. fat and paediatric animals have normal skin turgor even when dehydrated, and anecdotally oriental cat breeds often have skin that tents even when well hydrated. So more objective tests e.g. PCV, TP, urea, urine specific gravity, and sodium levels give a more accurate picture of the dehydration.

The signs of dehydration (where water is lost from all fluid compartments) should not be confused with signs of hypoperfusion due to inadequate circulating volume i.e. alterations in heart rate, pulse quality, mucous membrane colour, capillary refill time. Severe dehydration ultimately decreases the intravascular volume and therefore, signs of hypoperfusion are often seen alongside those of dehydration.

Correcting dehydration

The % dehydration value from Figure 24 indicates the amount of water lost as a % of body weight. So if this % is multiplied by the animal's body weight, the fluid deficit can be calculated. For example, if a 3 kg cat is assessed as 10% dehydrated then $10/100 \times 3$ kg $= 0.3$ kg which is the equivalent of 0.3 l or 300 ml fluid deficit.

This fluid deficit, depending on the severity of the animal's dehydration, is given over 12–24 hours. In more acute situations, deficits may need to be addressed in a shorter time frame, e.g. 1–4 hours.

Ongoing losses

Often when animals are hospitalised with dehydration, losses from vomiting and diarrhoea are ongoing. Additional boluses of fluids for each episode of vomiting or diarrhoea should be included, some authors suggest 4 ml/kg per episode of vomiting or diarrhoea.

Assessing response to fluid therapy

The patient must be regularly re-assessed and the plan changed as necessary. In addition, it is good practice

% dehydration	Clinical signs
4%	No clinical signs
5%	Semi dry oral mucous membranes Skin turgor normal Eyes moist
6–7%	Dry oral mucous membranes Eyes moist Mild loss of skin turgor
8–10%	Dry oral mucous membranes Eyes retracted Considerable loss of skin turgor Signs of hypoperfusion
10%	Very dry mucous membranes Severe eyeball retraction Eyes dull Complete loss of skin turgor Altered consciousness Greater signs of hypoperfusion
12%	As 10%, moribund
12–15%	As 10% but dying

Figure 24. Signs of dehydration.

to administer fluid therapy until certain "end-points" i.e. parameters such as heart rate, mentation, mucous membranes, skin turgor etc. return to normal.

Blood loss

All of the information above concerns crystalloid fluid therapy and dehydrated animals. However, as mentioned previously there are other types of fluid losses including haemorrhage which require compensation. If haemorrhage occurs, to decide what type of fluid is needed and how much fluid is required, an **estimation of the amount of blood lost** needs to be made. The latter is difficult if the trauma has occurred before the cat was admitted to the hospital, however there are surgical patients which may be cared for in the ICU where an estimation of surgical blood loss is more accurate. Estimation is by counting and weighing swabs soaked with blood (1 g of weight is approximately 1 ml of blood), looking at how much is in the suction bottle, on the floor and the drapes. The volume of blood lost should then be used to calculate the percentage of blood volume lost. Usually blood loss over 20% of blood volume requires blood product administration. Total blood volume for cats is approximately 56–60 ml/kg.

Blood transfusions

At the time of writing, there are no facilities in the United Kingdom for the production and storage of feline blood products, although there are facilities in Europe from where blood products (including packed red cells and fresh frozen plasma) can be ordered. More often, a whole blood donation is obtained from a local feline donor.

Attributes to look for when choosing a local donor include a friendly, normal large cat ideally over 5 kg lean weight, aged between 1–8 years. The cat should have a high PCV (>30%). Pregnant queens should not be used, but previous pregnancy does not exclude a queen from donating blood. Cats should ideally be indoor cats, tested routinely for FELV, FIV and FIP. Cats should also be free from *Haemobartonella felis*, and *Bartonella*, *Dirofilaria* and *Babesia*. The ACVIM suggest a questionnaire to check the risk profile of donor cats and the Pet Blood Bank (UK) suggests an echocardiogram to rule out occult heart disease.

Feline Blood Groups

- Type A is most common.
- Type B is thought to be common in some breeds, e.g. Persian, British Shorthair.
- Type AB is rarely seen.

There is no universal donor in cats, so cross matching must always be performed – even if checks for compatible blood types between donor and recipient have been performed. A more recently identified red blood cell antigen (Mik) is a potential cause for such non-AB incompatibilities (McClosky et al., 2018).

- A typical "unit" of cat blood is 45 ml; and a "unit" of packed red cells around 20 ml.

To calculate how much blood is required by a recipient, the following equation can be used:

- Ml donor blood required = recipient blood volume × (desired PCV – current PCV)/donor PCV

A retrospective review (Doolin et al., 2017) demonstrated donations can be harvested from unsedated

- A typical "unit" of cat blood is 45 ml; but no more than 12 ml/kg per donation is taken.
- A ratio of 1 ml of anticoagulant (acid citrate dextrose or citrate phophate dextrose adenosine) drawn in a sterile manner from the bag of anti-coagulant, to 7 ml of whole blood should be prepared.
- The area over the jugular vein should be clipped and prepared aseptically.
- Sterile gloves should be worn.
- The butterfly catheter and three way tap should be attached to the 60 ml syringe (containing anti-coagulant amount described above) and some anticoagulant injected through the three way tap into the butterfly needle.
- The jugular vein should be raised and the butterfly catheter inserted into the vessel, bevel uppermost and blood gently aspirated into the syringe. The blood should be withdrawn at a rate of 5 ml/min or greater.
- Once the desired volume has been collected into the syringe, the three way tap should be turned off to the butterfly needle and the needle removed from the vessel.
- Pressure should be applied to the venepuncture site.
- Demeanour, heart rate, mucous membrane colour and pulse quality should be checked. If the donor is showing any signs of hypovolaemia, such as tachycardia or pale mucous membrane colour, then crystalloid fluid therapy (at three times the volume removed) can be administered intravenously.

Figure 25. Step-by-step guide to feline whole blood donation.

cats and that blood volume collection was not affected, however most feline donors do require some sedation. The sedation protocol is selected based on the temperament and health status of the cat. The author has previously used alfaxalone intramuscularly (although this is off-licence), or sevoflurane by mask. Others suggest alpha 2 adrenergic agonist based protocols although this class of drugs prevents compensatory tachycardia as a response to a loss of blood volume. Flow-by oxygen by mask and anaesthetic monitoring should be used for all sedated cats. Their eyes should also be lubricated.

See Figure 25 for a step by step guide on how to take a feline whole blood donation.

Blood administration

A blood donation can never be collected through a 'closed' system so strict asepsis is required. Usually blood is administered straight after harvesting, but if the whole blood has been stored in the fridge, it should be warmed up slowly in a water bath. The blood must be administered via an in-line filter to ensure micro-thrombi and debris are not transfused.

The recipient's baseline temperature, pulse, and respiratory rate should be recorded before the transfusion starts, and repeated observations made during the transfusion to identify transfusion reactions.

Blood products should not be administered through drip lines with Hartmann's or other calcium-containing solutions in them, or else clotting of the blood in the line can occur. The initial administration rate is 0.5 ml/kg/h for the first 15 minutes to check for acute reactions. If necessary the rate can be increased up to 5–20 ml/kg/h. The transfusion should be completed within a four hour time frame.

Transfusion reactions can be immunologic (acute or delayed), and non-immunologic.

Signs of immunological reactions include:

- agitation/restlessness/change in attitude
- nausea, vomiting, salivation
- urticaria with or without pruritus
- anaphylaxis
- pyrexia
- tachypnoea/dyspnoea
- tachycardia
- hypotension
- seizures
- haemolysis, jaundice, haemoglobinuria.

Non-immunological transfusion reactions include hypocalcaemia through citrate toxicity, circulatory and volume overload, hypothermia if the blood is not warmed prior to the transfusion, and transmission of infectious diseases.

Anaesthesia and analgesia for emergency feline cases

Anaesthesia of emergency cases inherently carries an increased risk compared to elective cases. In the Confidential Enquiry into Perioperative Small Animal Fatalities (CEPFSAF) (Brodbelt, 2006), data collected from just under 80,000 cat anaesthetics and sedations showed increased odds ratios of risk of death due to anaesthesia of sick cats compared with American Society of Anesthesiologists (ASA) classification 1 cats (see Figure 26) and elective cases (Figure 27).

This increased risk should be communicated to owners, and then every effort made to stabilise animals before anaesthesia or sedation. **Stabilisation may include analgesia, fluid therapy, oxygen supplementation, and administration of drug therapy.** The anaesthetist's job is to monitor and support the cat's body systems and to minimise the potential adverse effects of anaesthesia.

1. Fit healthy animal with no systemic disease
2. Animal with systemic disease, which is fully compensated for.
3. Animal with systemic disease which is not fully compensated for.
4. Animal with systemic disease which is incapacitating.
5. Animal which is not expected to survive the next 24 hours, whether anaesthetised or not.

Figure 26. American Society of Anesthesiologist's classification system.

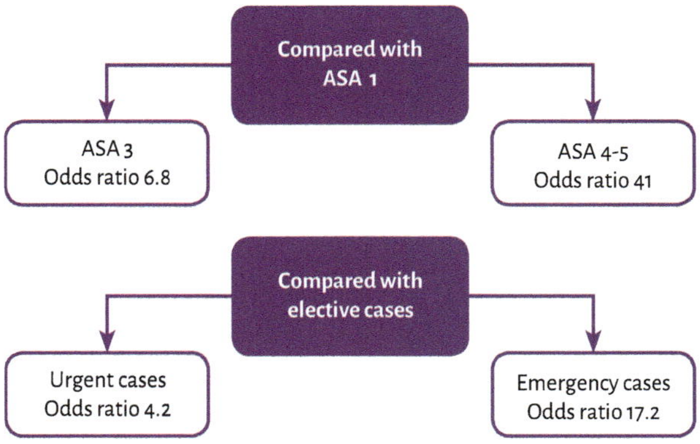

Figure 27. Odds ratios of increased ASA classification and increased case urgency compared with ASA 1 cats and elective cases (Brodbelt et al., 2007).

Analgesia for emergency and critical cases

Analgesia should be one of the first therapeutics provided in an emergency situation, as pain is associated with many presentations. Reasons for the provision of analgesia include:

- welfare considerations
- to facilitate stress-free handling
- to improve ventilation in cats with thoracic wall pain or cranial abdominal pain
- decreases catecholamine release.

Opioids

Opioids are usually the first line analgesics in emergency and critical care cases. Most opioids decrease heart rate, this is of little clinical relevance with methadone, buprenorphine etc. and pethidine tends to increase heart rate somewhat. At normal clinical doses, opioids cause little respiratory depression. Some opioids are emetic (especially morphine) and vomiting may be contra-indicated in certain clinical scenarios, including airway problems, increased intra-ocular pressure, and intra-cranial pressure.

Non-steroidal anti-inflammatory drugs

Non-steroidal anti-inflammatory drugs (NSAIDs) are not recommended as a first line analgesic in feline emergency cases. The rationale is that NSAIDs block the production of prostaglandins, which not only play a role in inflammation, but they are also part of the kidneys' and gut's homeostatic mechanisms. In times of poor perfusion to these organs (e.g. in hypotensive or hypovolaemic patients), these prostaglandins help maintain function and blocking them can lead to serious consequences including intestinal ulceration and kidney dysfunction. Non-steroidal anti-inflammatory drugs also can have an effect on clotting as they block the production of thromboxane-A2, a pro-aggregatory eicosanoid.

Therefore NSAIDs are contraindicated in the following clinical situations:

- when a steroid has been used
- in renal failure
- in cases of hypovolaemia or dehydration
- when an animal is hypotensive
- evidence of gastro-intestinal ulceration
- animals with a clotting dysfunction.

Alpha 2 adrenergic agonists and ketamine

Other drugs to consider which have analgesic properties include alpha 2 adrenergic agonists, ketamine, and local anaesthetics.

Alpha 2 adrenergic agonists are usually used for sedation and rarely as primary analgesics, although at appropriate doses they provide good analgesia. Alpha 2 adrenergic agonists are associated with marked physiological effects including hypertension and bradycardia, and therefore the cardiovascular fitness of the cat must be assured before these drugs are used.

Although ketamine is a widely used anaesthetic induction agent, at **sub-anaesthetic doses, it is a very effective analgesic.** Because these doses are much smaller than those required to induce anaesthesia, the side effects of this drug are also limited. Ketamine works well in animals with chronic pain based on its action as an antagonist at NMDA (N-methyl D-aspartate) receptors which are involved in the development of central sensitisation. Ketamine is also a useful analgesic for somatic pain, i.e. that associated with superficial tissues, skin etc. Ketamine can be administered as bolus doses or in a continuous infusion (between 5 and 20 µg/kg/min).

Local anaesthetics

These drugs are the only ones which can produce a total absence of pain. To stop the transmission of the electrical impulses along nerves, the drugs block sodium channels in the nerve fibres. Both sensory and motor nerves may be affected, so areas of the body can be desensitised, but the animal may also temporarily loose function and movement of that part of the body if the motor nerves are affected.

In an emergency situation, the potential applications for local anaesthesia are limited. However, when the cat is in a stable state for anaesthesia for e.g. surgical repair of its injuries, then local blocks should be used where feasible.

Local anaesthetic can be applied topically, e.g. in creams to desensitise the skin, or dropped on eyes to prevent corneal sensation. They can be injected subcutaneously to create a wheal, through which an instrument or catheter is placed without the animal feeling it. This could be used for drainage of the peritoneal or pleural space. They can be injected into joints (intra-articular). Infiltration of local anaesthetic around specific nerves (perineural analgesia) supplying certain areas of the body can also be performed e.g. intercostal nerve blocks before thoracocentesis. Local anaesthetics can also be injected into the pleural cavity in the chest, usually to aid with pain relief post thoracotomy. In addition, they can be injected into the epidural space to desensitise hind limbs, abdomens, tails etc. although this would usually be performed at a later date when the cat is stable enough for surgical repair of any fractures or soft tissue injuries.

Sedation versus anaesthesia

Once a patient is as stable as possible, the choice must be made as to whether diagnostic tests and procedures are carried out with the animal conscious, sedated, or anaesthetised, with or without local anaesthesia. Sedation often involves the use of drugs with more profound cardiovascular and respiratory effects than general anaesthesia, and without the same level of "support" (e.g. airway protection) and monitoring that is conferred when a general anaesthetic is used. Therefore general anaesthesia is often the more advisable approach.

Pre-oxygenation

Unless it causes the animal to struggle, pre-oxygenation (preferably by mask) is advocated, especially if the cat has cardiovascular or respiratory disease. This can delay the onset of hypoxaemia if the anaesthetist cannot place the endotracheal tube immediately after anaesthetic induction.

Pre-oxygenation is recommended if a difficult endotracheal intubation is expected, e.g. a brachycephalic cat, facial trauma etc. In addition, a range of endotracheal tube sizes, a stylet, a laryngoscope, local anaesthetic spray and suction should be available. Alternative means of providing oxygen (transtracheal) or indeed an airway (tracheostomy tube) can also be considered if endotracheal intubation is not possible.

Head up inductions

This is where the nurse restraining the patient holds the patient's head up and keeps it elevated above the level of the thorax until the trachea is intubated. This position uses gravity to prevent regurgitation of stomach contents, and should be used in patients which have not been starved, or have a history of regurgitation (e.g. megaoesophagus) or delayed gastric emptying.

Head flat inductions

These are useful in cases of animals with neck pain, as it avoids potential wrenching of the neck when animals are held for intubation. It is important to use this position for any suspected cases of cervical vertebral fractures. With this technique, the head is held flat on the table whilst the patient's trachea is intubated. It is technically a little more difficult due to the more awkward angle, and so it may be beneficial to preoxygenate the patient using a mask, and use a laryngoscope to aid visualisation

Cardiopulmonary resuscitation

Unfortunately, respiratory and or/cardiac arrest are a more likely in emergency and critical care cases compared with healthy cats being treated at the practice. **Overall survival rates post cardiac arrest are low,** at between 4 and 9.6% (Hofmeister et al., 2008; Kass & Haskins, 1992; Wingfiled & Pelt (1992)) in small animals. Cardiopulmonary arrests may happen whilst the cat undergoing emergency care is conscious and being stabilised, or during an anaesthetic or sedation.

The likelihood of survival is increased if a cat is under anaesthesia at the time of arrest (Gilroy et al., 1994) compared with a case being cared for in the ICU, but this may be because in this data the cohort of anaesthetised animals likely included healthy animals that became too deeply anaesthetised and suffered from respiratory arrest that was not swiftly recognised, and/or that vascular access and endotracheal intubation had already been secured and animals were likely being monitored so that arrests were recognised early and resuscitation attempts could be instituted without delay and monitored from a very early stage.

Furthermore the state of the interior milieu (the physiological capacity of the body's extracellular fluid to ensure protective stability for the tissues and organs) in healthy animals is optimal before an arrest, which makes post-crash survival more likely. Cats presented for emergency or critical care will often have a sub-optimal interior milieu and therefore this is a likely reason that return of spontaneous circulation (ROSC) in these cats is lower.

Owners of cats admitted in an emergency or critical care situation should be asked for their wishes on the extent of life saving measures in advance if at all possible, especially if a crash situation is anticipated due to the cat's clinical status.

Evidence based recommendations on cardiopulmonary resuscitation in dogs and cats were released in the **RECOVER guidelines** in 2012 (Fletcher et al., 2012) and the reader is directed to these or any updated guidelines for further information.

Signs of respiratory arrest

- no breathing effort seen either with the thorax or the reservoir bag (if under anaesthesia).
- no trace on capnography (if under anaesthesia)
- may have cyanotic mucous membranes.

Signs of cardiac arrest

- either no respiratory effort, or "agonal gasping"
- no heartbeat or pulse palpable

- no haemorrhage at surgical site if surgery is being undertaken.
- grey, cyanosed or pale mucous membranes
- central eye with unresponsive dilated pupils
- no lacrimation or salivation
- no palpebral or corneal reflexes
- flaccid limbs, no reflexes (if cat was conscious).

Respiratory arrest usually precedes cardiac arrest, and on its own, is relatively easily remedied by endotracheal intubation and intermittent positive pressure ventilation whilst the underlying cause is investigated and resolved if possible. Infrequent checks on patients however may mean that respiratory arrest is missed, and the animal is discovered in full cardio-respiratory arrest.

Resuscitation

Airway, breathing and circulation are basic life support which mimics the body's own ventilation and circulation, whilst trying to rectify the underlying cause.

Airway

An endotracheal tube should be placed, or if one is already in place, its position and patency checked.

Breathing

The endotracheal tube should be attached to a suitable breathing system for IPPV (Ayre's T-piece, Mapelson D T-piece or Bain for feline patients) or Ambu-bag, and the patient's lungs ventilatedat a rate of approximately **10 breaths per minute.** Faster rates than this have detrimental effects on the cat's haemodynamic status. The aim should be for just above normal size chest excursions. Sufficient time should be allowed in between ventilations for the chest to deflate. If the cat is under anaesthesia, only oxygen should be supplied and the volatile agent and nitrous oxide discontinued.

Circulation

Compressions are only used if there is no palpable pulse. The "Airway" and "Breathing" parts of basic life support are suitable for respiratory arrests.

External cardiac compression of the heart to pump blood around the body can be done in one of two ways depending on the size of patient.

The patient should be placed in right lateral recumbency if possible. A compression rate of 120 bpm should be aimed for with compressions made to a depth of a third to half of the width of the chest, whilst allowing for full elastic recoil of the chest in between compressions. After every two minute cycle of compressions and ventilation, the person performing the compressions should be rotated to prevent fatigue, aiming for minimal disruption of compressions.

- Fingers and thumbs (circumferential compressions) over the heart can be used for kittens, and small cats.
- Cardiac compressions compressing directly over the heart should be used in larger cats. See Figure 28.

If two people are available for CPR, the compressions and ventilation should be performed simultaneously at the rates indicated above. If only one person is present, then 30 compressions to 2 ventilations should be delivered cyclically.

Another alternative is to perform an emergency thoracotomy and do internal cardiac compressions. This should only be attempted if the practice is able to offer post-thoracotomy care. If the cat's abdominal cavity is open for surgery, an incision can be made in the diaphragm to gain access for internal cardiac compressions.

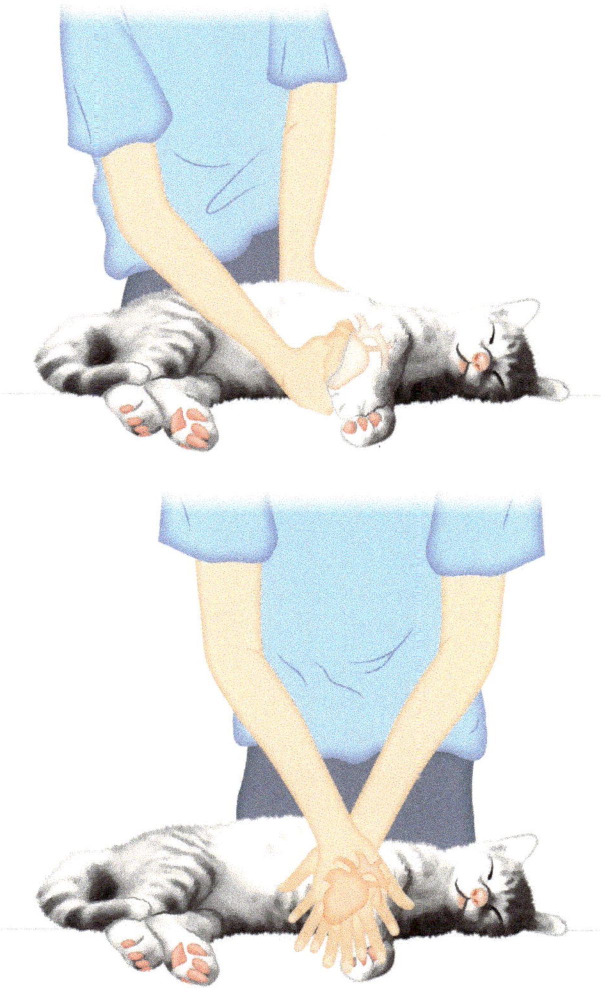

Figure 28. Circumferential compressions (A) and cardiac compressions (B) performed on the cat.

Drug	Dosage	Volume for 2.5 kg cat	Volume for 5 kg cat
Adrenaline (low dose) 1 mg/ml	0.01 mg/kg	0.03 ml	0.05 ml
Atropine (0.6 mg/ml)	0.04 mg/kg	0.17 ml	0.33 ml
Lidocaine (20 mg/ml)	2 mg/kg	0.25 ml	0.5 ml
Naloxone (0.4 mg/ml)	0.04 mg/kg	0.25 ml	0.5 ml
Flumazenil (0.1 mg/ml)	0.01 mg/kg	0.25 ml	0.5 ml
Atipamezole (5 mg/ml)	100 µg/kg	0.06 ml	0.1 ml

Figure 29. CPR drug dosing chart for small and larger cats (adapted from RECOVER guidelines (Fletcher et al., 2012).

After the first two minute cycle of ventilation and compressions, the patient should be evaluated for ROSC including:

- palpable peripheral pulse
- audible heart sounds
- mucous membrane colour improving
- return of spontaneous ventilatory efforts.

An electrocardiogram should be attached to the patient, and the rhythm analysed during this brief pause as the compressors are rotated. This guides the administration of resuscitation drugs.

Drugs

If ventricular fibrillation or ventricular tachycardia (pulseless) is present, then lidocaine and adrenaline (every other two minute cycle) can be used.

If pulseless electrical activity or asystole is observed then atropine and adrenaline (every other two minute cycle) should be used.

Up to a maximum of three doses of adrenaline can be administered.

The drug dosages and volumes for 2.5 kg and 5 kg cats are listed in Figure 29.

If arrest occurred in association with administration of opioids, alpha 2 adrenergic agonists or benzodiazepines, then the antagonist should be administered (naloxone, atipamezole, flumazenil respectively) to antagonize the effects of the drugs. Doses are included in Figure 29.

Electrical defibrillation

Electrical defibrillation (Figure 30) is appropriate if ventricular fibrillation is identified on the electrocardiogram. Immediate defibrillation is recommended if ventricular fibrillation has been present for less than four minutes or if identified in the ECG check between compression cycles. If the patient is believed to have been in ventricular fibrillation for more than four minutes, then one cycle of cardiac compressions should be completed before defibrillation. If one defibrillation shock is unsuccessful, then another two minute cycle of compressions should be completed before re-evaluating the ECG and defibrillating again.

- 4–6 Joules/kg if external paddles (monophasic)
- 2–4 Joules/kg if external paddles (biphasic)
- 0.5–1 Joules/kg if internal paddles (monophasic)
- 0.2–0.4 Joules/kg if internal paddles (biphasic)

Figure 30. Defibrillator settings for internal and external defibrillation.

Fluids

If hypovolaemia is partly responsible for arrest, then intravenous fluid administration is beneficial. However, **if the patient was euvolaemic before**

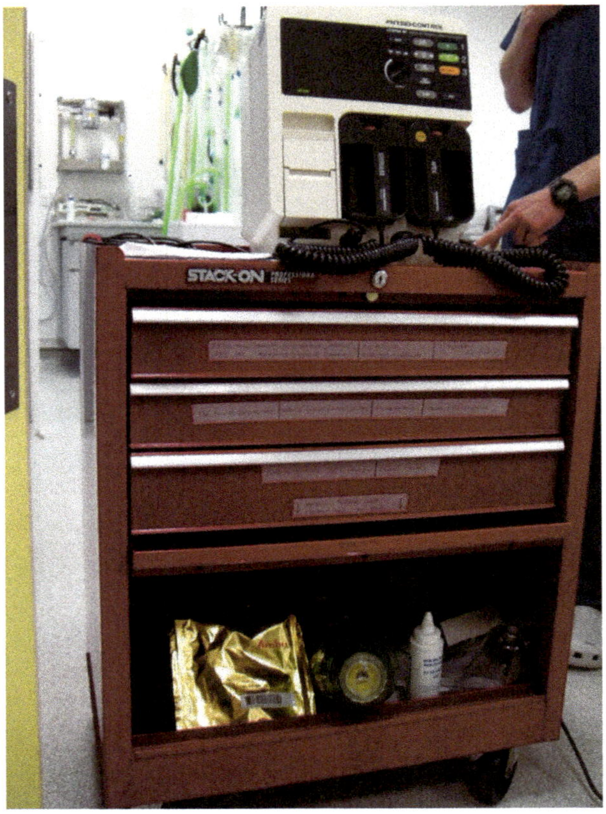

Figure 31. A fully stocked crash trolley with defibrillator.

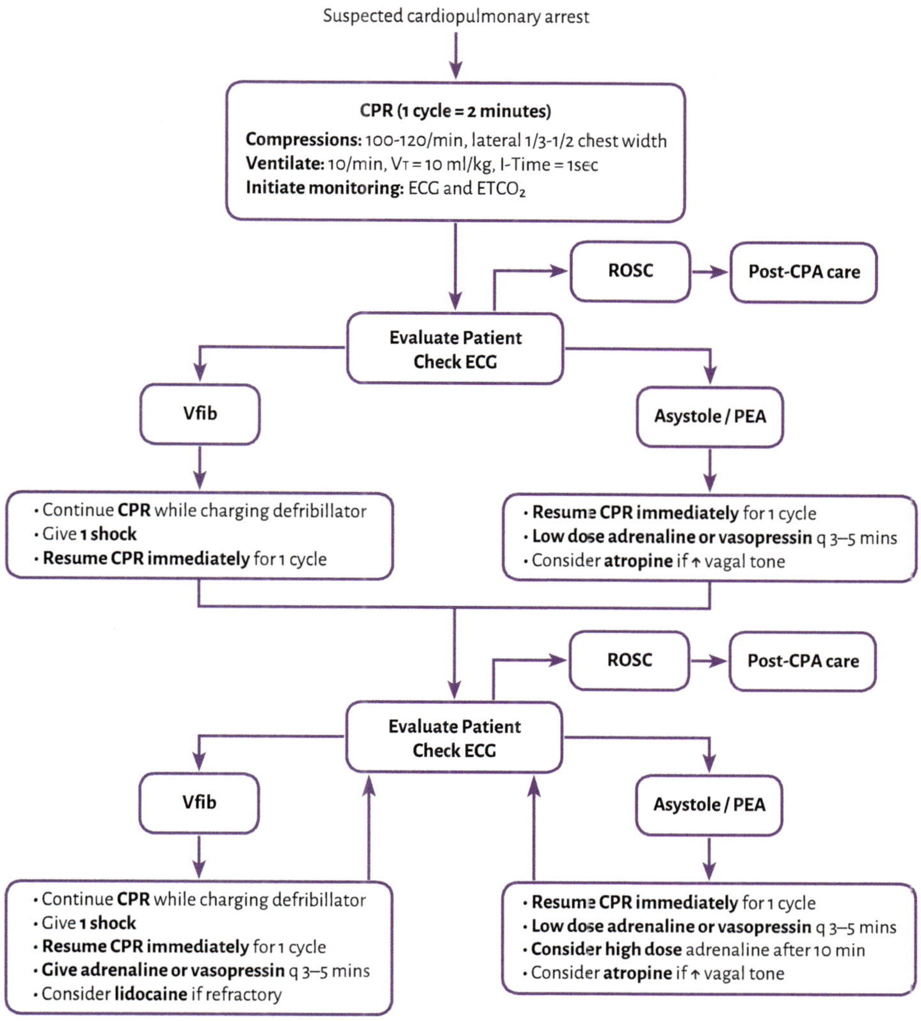

Figure 32. CPR algorithm adapted from RECOVER guidelines (Fletcher et al., 2012).

arrest, the administration of additional fluids is not recommended.

Team work and training

In all resuscitation attempts it is preferable to have **a team of at least four people**, practiced in their roles, with one individual acting as leader of the resuscitation efforts. This leader assigns tasks to other team members; a closed-loop communication style is recommended, i.e. the recipient of the order repeats the order back to the team leader. All clinical staff should undergo regular training (at least every six months) in CPR to refresh their skills. This training should include both didactic and simulator based learning.

Preparedness

Whilst some crash situations occur unexpectedly, there are some patients and surgeries where critical incidents can be anticipated and prepared for. Simple modifications to routine anaesthetic protocols or case management should include early intravenous access, close monitoring, and calculation of "emergency drugs" doses for that animal's weight. Each practice should also have a designated area which is easily accessible from all parts of the building, with the facilities to hand including oxygen, breathing systems, endo-tracheal tubes, fluids, monitoring equipment and emergency drugs (Figure 31). Cognitive aids, such as check-lists, CPR algorithms (Figure 32) and dosing charts (Figure 29) should be easily visible in this area.

References

Brodbelt et al. (2007) Br J Anaesth 99, 617–23.
Cortinovis et al. (2015) Vet J 203, 52–8.
DeGroot (2014) Can Vet J 55, 1253–43.
Doolin et al. (2017) JVECCS 27, 555–560.
Drobatz & Cole (2008) JVECCs 355–361.
Drobatz & Costello (2010) Feline emergency and critical care medicine. Blackwell publishing.
Fletcher et al. (2012) JVECCS 22, S102–S131.
Goggs et al. (2018) JFMS 20, 1072–1081.
Hofmeister et al (2008) JVECCS 18, 142–152.
Kass & Haskins (1992) JVECCS 2, 57–65.

McClosky, ME et al. (2018) *J Vet Intern Med*. 2018; 32: 1934–1942.
Norkus et al. (2017) Can Vet J 58, 261–264.
Reineke et al. (2015) JVECCS.
Tauk et al. (2015) JAVMA 246, 1327–33.
Thies et al. (2017) JVECCS 27, 658–661.
Wingfield & Pelt (1992) JAVMA 200, 1993.
Yuh & Keir 2018.

Clinical cases

Case 1

A 7-year old, 6 kg male cat with urethral obstruction has the following results on a venous blood gas analysis.

- pH 7.112
- pCO_2 28 mmHg
- pO_2 36 mmHg
- BE −12 mmol/l
- K^+ 6.5 mmol/l
- Na^+ 155 mmol/l

1. What is the overall acid base picture?

2. What could another reason be for the cat to be hypocapnic?

3. Which electrolyte abnormalities are present?

4. How should the metabolic acidosis be treated?

5. The cat is now stable enough to anaesthetise for urethral catheterisation. Which pieces of monitoring equipment are most relevant in this case?

6. What analgesia could be used to keep the cat comfortable for the placement of an indwelling urethral catheter?

7. The patient is being assessed the day after urethral catheterisation has taken place, and even though the cat has received fluid therapy at 2 ml/kg/h overnight, the following is found when assessing hydration semi-dry oral mucous membranes, with moist eyes and normal skin turgor. What % dehydration should be estimated and what fluid deficit does this represent?

Case 2

An 11-year-old 3 kg cat is admitted with a history of lethargy. On clinical examination it is noted that the patient has tachycardia, tachypnoea, and very pale mucous membranes.

1. It is decided that initial stabilisation should include oxygen supplementation. Briefly compare and contrast the different methods available and which is most appropriate for this case.

2. Whilst waiting for full haematological and biochemical analysis of the blood, a blood smear is examined. What areas of the blood smear would provide information on the i) the red cells and ii) platelets?

3. Haematological analysis of the blood confirms severe anaemia with a PCV of 10%. A whole blood transfusion from a local donor cat that is the correct blood type, weighs 5 kg and has a PCV of 35% is planned. Ideally enough blood should be transfused to achieve an increase in PCV to 21%. How much donor blood will be required?

4. Is is "safe" to obtain this volume of blood from the donor cat?

5. How much anticoagulant should be drawn from the blood donation bag into the syringe when anticipating this volume of donation?

Test

1. **The last phase of triage is termed:**
   A) Primary assessment.
   B) Secondary assessment.
   C) Waiting room triage.
   D) Phone triage.
2. **When running an emergency data base, the combination of a decreased packed cell volume and a decreased total protein in the blood of a cat could suggest which of the following?**
   A) Dehydration with concurrent anaemia.
   B) Polycythaemia.
   C) Blood loss.
   D) Dehydration with concurrent protein loss.
3. **Metaldehyde toxicity causes clinical signs by decreasing the brain concentrations of which substance?**
   A) GABA.
   B) Adrenaline.
   C) N-methyl D-aspartate.
   D) Endogenous opioids.
4. **When placing a jugular catheter via the Seldinger technique, what is the correct order in which to use the different parts of the catheter kit?**
   A) Jugular catheter, dilator, guidewire, catheter introducer.
   B) Guidewire, catheter introducer, jugular catheter, dilator.
   C) Dilator, catheter introducer, jugular catheter, guidewire.
   D) Catheter introducer, guidewire, dilator, jugular catheter.
5. **In non-invasive blood pressure measurement techniques; the width of the cuff should be approximately what percentage of the circumference of the limb?**
   A) 20%.
   B) 40%.
   C) 60%.
   D) 80%.
6. **The venturi devices that can be added to tubing delivering oxygen to oxygen tents and cages are present for what reason?**
   A) They humidify the inspired oxygen.
   B) They "scrub" the exhaled gases of carbon dioxide.
   C) They influence the fraction of inspired oxygen.
   D) They warm the inspired oxygen.
7. **Chloride should be corrected for changes in which electrolyte to take into account changes in plasma osmolarity?**
   A) Magnesium.
   B) Potassium.
   C) Calcium.
   D) Sodium.
8. **What is the formula for calculating the volume of maintenance fluid therapy for 24 hours in the cat?**
   A) $62 \times \text{bodyweight(kg)}^{0.75}$
   B) $80 \times \text{bodyweight(kg)}^{0.75}$
   C) $132 \times \text{bodyweight(kg)}^{0.75}$
   D) $160 \times \text{bodyweight(kg)}^{0.75}$
9. **Which of the following groups of analgesics can provide a total absence of pain sensation?**
   A) Opioids.
   B) NMDA antagonists.
   C) Alpha 2 adrenergic agonists.
   D) Local anaesthetics.

10. If only one person is available to provide cerebro-pulmonary resuscitation in a cat, the recommended number of compressions to ventilations in every cycle is:

A) 100:10.
B) 30:2.
C) 2:5.
D) 6:1.

Answers

Test

1. B	5. B	9. D
2. C	6. C	10. B
3. A	7. D	
4. D	8. B	

Clinical cases

Case 1

1. Overall the cat is acidaemic (pH<7.35). There is a metabolic acidosis (BE is more negative than –5 mmol/l) with respiratory compensation (pCO_2 <35 mmHg).
2. The cat could be hyperventilating from the pain caused by a distended bladder.
3. The cat is hyperkalaemic, but with normal sodium levels.
4. Fluid therapy with an alkalinising fluid such as Hartmann's solution will help to correct the pH somewhat. However, at levels of BE more negative than –10 mmol/l sodium bicarbonate can be considered.
5. Blood pressure: as the cat may be hypovolaemic, and maintenance of renal perfusion is important.

   ECG: in case the electrolyte abnormalities cause any dysrhythmias.
   Capnograph: in case the distended bladder causes a reduction in tidal volume and resultant hypercapnia.
   Temperature: as cats usually have a high surface area to volume ratio, and are prone to developing hypothermia during anaesthesia.

6. Initially an opioid is most appropriate, probably methadone or buprenorphine. Renal perfusion is initially affected because of back pressure on the kidney from the distended bladder and therefore in the first 24–48 hours, NSAIDs should be avoided, but may be introduced later once renal parameters and volume status are normal.
7. This represents 5% dehydration. In a 6 kg cat this would be 5/100 × 6 = 0.3 kg = 300 g = 300 ml.

Case 2

1. A technique that increases FiO_2, is not stressful to the cat and does not cause accumulation of CO_2 or humidity, should be chosen. Flow by oxygen could be used initially as it can increase FiO_2 to up to 50% but high rates are needed, as well as a member of staff to be present. A face-mask would increase the FiO_2 but may cause stress to the cat. An oxygen cage, whether manufactured or "homemade" could be used as a stress-free way of supplementing oxygen without needing constant supervision by a member of staff. Any interventions would lose FiO_2, however. Oxygen insufflation through a naso-pharyngeal catheter can produce one of the highest FiO_2 of oxygen. If this cat was very depressed, placement of a nasopharyngeal catheter under local anaesthesia is possible, however, in more alert cats, the author often combines nasopharyngeal tube placement with tests or treatments that require sedation or general anaesthesia.
2. The feathered edge is where abnormal cell types, platelet clumps and microfilariae are found and the monolayer is where white blood cells and red blood cell abnormalities are identified.
3. ml donor blood required = recipient blood volume × (desired PCV – current PCV)/donor PCV

   - recipient blood volume = 56 ml/kg × 3 kg = 168 ml

- ml donor blood required = 168 × (21–10)/35
- ml donor blood required = 53 ml

NB. The cat's blood volume used in this calculation is 56 ml/kg. If a different blood volume figure has been used this may generate a slightly different answer.

4. Yes, the maximum a cat should donate is 12 ml/kg, which would be 60 ml.
5. 1 ml citrate-based anticoagulant per 7 ml whole blood should be drawn into the bag, therefore approximately 7.5 ml anticoagulant should be drawn up.

15

Feline Orthopaedics

Fernando Reina

Contents

Introduction

The diagnosis of musculoskeletal disease in cats is often challenging due to the particular demeanour of this species. Despite these difficulties, orthopaedic diseases such as **osteoarthritis (OA) are frequently recognised** and diagnosed in veterinary practice (Lascelles et al., 2010; Hardie, Roe and Martin, 2002).

The most common orthopaedic disorders diagnosed in cats are directly related to trauma (Voss and Steffen, 2009), and as such easy to identify by the clinician. However, those of non- traumatic origin are more challenging to recognise. Cats may develop undetected or subtle gait abnormalities, or they may present to the consult with unspecific clinical signs. In addition, the clinician may experience difficulties performing a full orthopaedic examination compared to dogs. These contributing factors complicate the identification of orthopaedic pathologies in this species.

Proper identification of the cause of lameness requires awareness of specific orthopaedic disorders in this species, a good clinical history, and a thorough orthopaedic and neurological examination (Voss and Steffen, 2009).

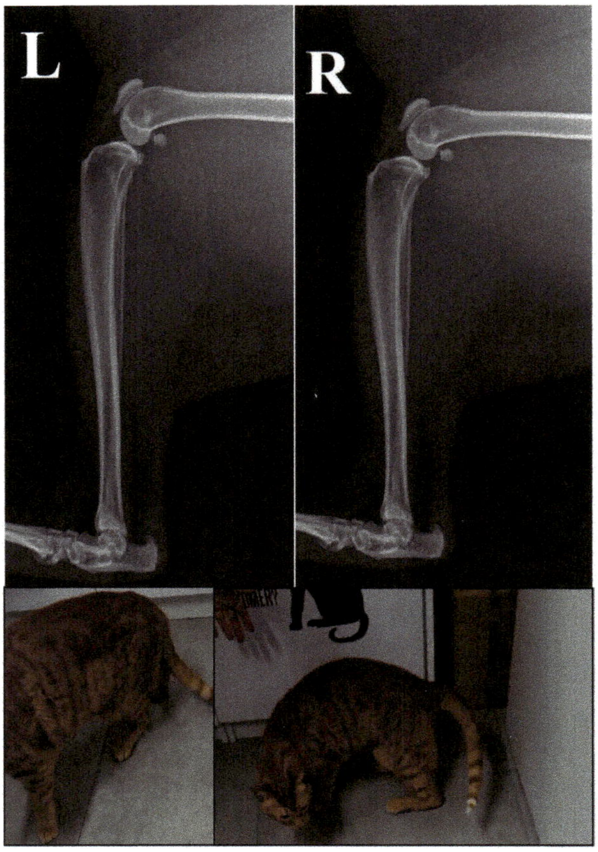

Figure 1. Adult cat with bilateral plantigrade stance due to uncontrolled diabetes mellitus. Taking an inadequate clinical history contributed to erroneous suspicion of an orthopaedic disease.

Orthopaedic examination

Orthopaedic examination requires a rigorous **clinical history, consideration of patient signalment, and**

Signalment
- Age, breed, sex (neutered, entire?)

Environment
- Indoor, outdoor, both
- Any cohabitants?

Immune status
- Vaccinated, unvaccinated, tested for feline viruses

Presenting complaint
- Owner's perception
- Referring vet's perception
- Our impression (not final)

Other clinical signs?
- Gastrointestinal (vomiting, diarrhoea, anorexia, none)
- Respiratory (cough, sneezing, respiratory noises)
- Others?

Medical treament
- Ongoing medication?
- Treatment for lameness (type, duration, response)

Specific questions
- Timing for appearance of presenting complaint
- Changes observed in daily habits (e.g. grooming, activity)
- Previous similar episodes in the past?
- Changes in the condition over time (frequency, severity)

Box 1. Specific questions which should be directed at the cat's owner during initial consultation (adapted from Voss and Steffen, 2009).

a general physical examination. It is important that these steps are completed prior to looking for the cause of lameness. For example, cats with uncontrolled diabetes may develop pelvic limb weakness and a plantigrade stance (Kramek el al., 1984). A poor clinical history can drive the clinician to look for primary orthopaedic or neurological disorders in these cases.

Cats with orthopaedic disorders do not tend to exhibit the same clinical signs as dogs, and often owners do not react to these non-specific signs in the same way. Therefore, **the clinician must ask specific questions** to get useful information. Box 1 details the questions cat owners should ideally be asked when taking a clinical history.

Clinical approach to feline orthopaedic conditions

Once a full clinical history has been obtained an orthopaedic examination should be performed. This examination must be systematic. Therefore, it can be divided into three stages: 1) observation and gait analysis, 2) palpation, and 3) specific orthopaedic manoeuvres.

Observation and gait analysis

Unlike dogs, cats with orthopaedic disease (especially when there is no history of trauma) **may not be overtly lame.** In fact, only 33% of feline patients demonstrate clinical signs during the initial evaluation (Godfrey, 2005). Instead of showing stiffness or lameness, some patients suffer from loss of jumping ability, are unable to jump as high as before, or show decreased activity levels. Others present with decreased appetite, or develop behavioural changes, such as altered grooming or abnormal toilet habits (e.g. urinating out of the litter box) (Kerwin, 2012; Clarke and Bennett, 2006; Bennet and Morton, 2009; Lascelles et al., 2007).

In addition to these non-specific presentations, it is important to remember cats display orthopaedic pathology differently to dogs which means that observation and analysis of their gait requires a different approach.

Cats should be left to walk freely around the examination room, rather than forced into controlled walks (Figure 2). The clinician must observe the cat´s locomotion, posture, and its interaction with different obstacles in the consultation room, such as chairs and tables. Encouraging the cat to jump is helpful in identifying whether the lifting or landing phase of the jump is abnormal (Figure 3).

Some cats need a few minutes to acclimatise before they start walking around the consulting room, while others need stimulation with games or toys commonly used at home. During observation, there may be a clear lameness, abnormal gait, weight shifting, mechanical anomaly (plantigrade stance) or ataxia. However, changes may be subtle (e.g. asymmetry in a stance, sitting or lying position), and therefore **video recording is advised** so that such abnormalities can be evaluated in slow motion afterwards (Figures 4 and 5).

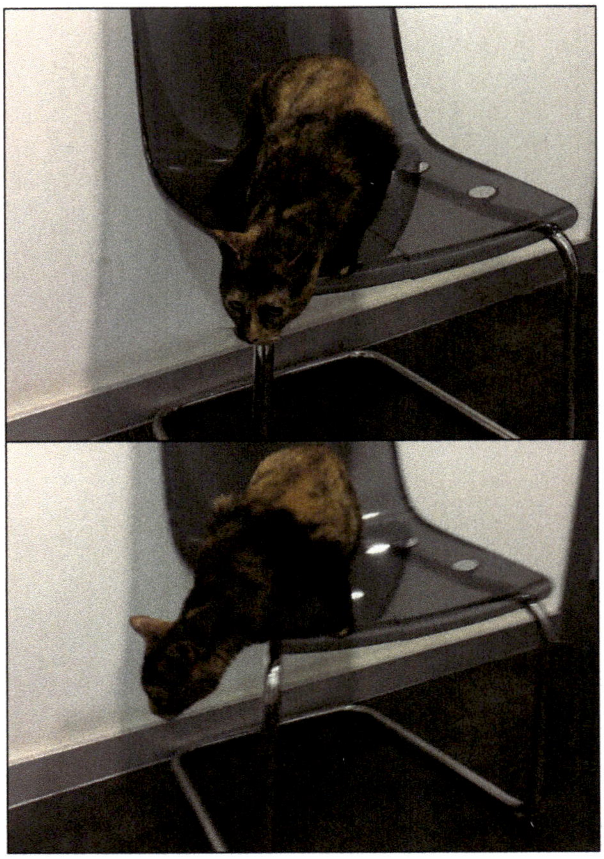

Figure 3. A feline patient who climbed onto a chair. As part of the gait evaluation, the clinician must observe whether the landing phase of the jump is normal (symmetrical) or abnormal (asymmetric).

Palpation

Palpation **is best done with the cat standing** rather than lying down, since many cats do not tolerate lateral recumbency without sedation. Also, cats tend to be more comfortable on the floor, so a standing exam undertaken by a single person is least likely to cause further stress to the patient.

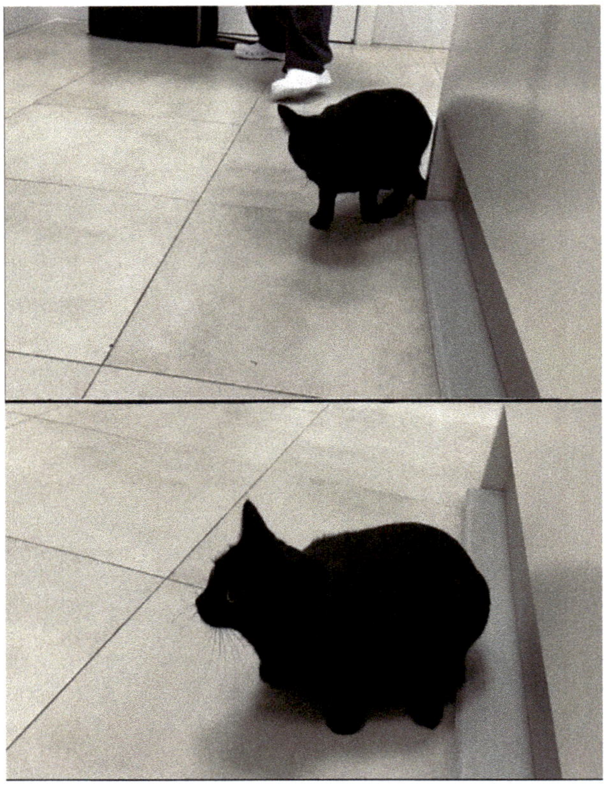

Figure 2. Gait analysis in cats is challenging. Some patients need a few minutes to acclimatise before they start walking around the consulting room.

The key to an adequate orthopaedic palpation is being **systematic**, so as not to miss anything. It is helpful to start the examination with the non-affected limbs, to give the cat time to acclimatise. However, some cats only tolerate handling and palpation for short periods and therefore the exam needs to start with the affected limb, whilst the rest are explored under sedation.

Palpation should follow a distal to proximal direction, whilst looking out for muscle asymmetry, atrophy, masses, and/or swelling which may indicate the origin of the lameness (Lascelles et al., 2010). Palpation should be gentle but firm, spreading finger pressure over the bone edges seeking trigger points for pain. When **examining a joint, any effusion, pain, or crepitus**, should be checked for, since these may be present in cats with arthropathies (Lascelles et al., 2012). However, feline joints are small compared to the dog, and joint effusion may not be as evident. Therefore, **the affected limb should be compared with the contralateral side** to remove any doubt. During joint palpation, the range of motion should be evaluated. Normal joint

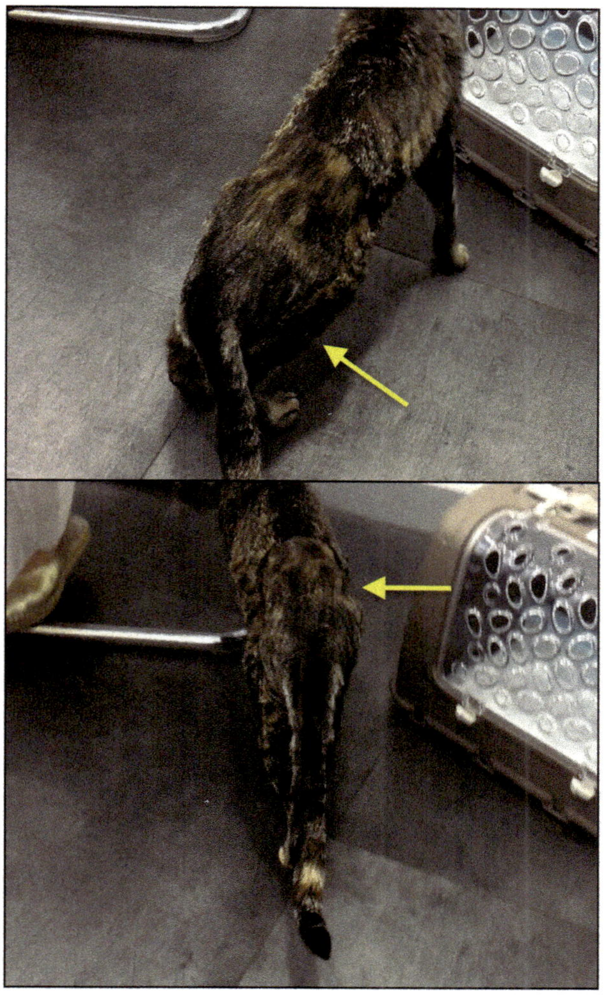

Figure 4. Follow-up orthopaedic examination in an adult cat diagnosed with multiple pelvic fractures, who underwent surgery six weeks before. Although the short-term outcome is so far good, abnormal (asymmetric) gait is still observed in her pelvic limbs (yellow arrows).

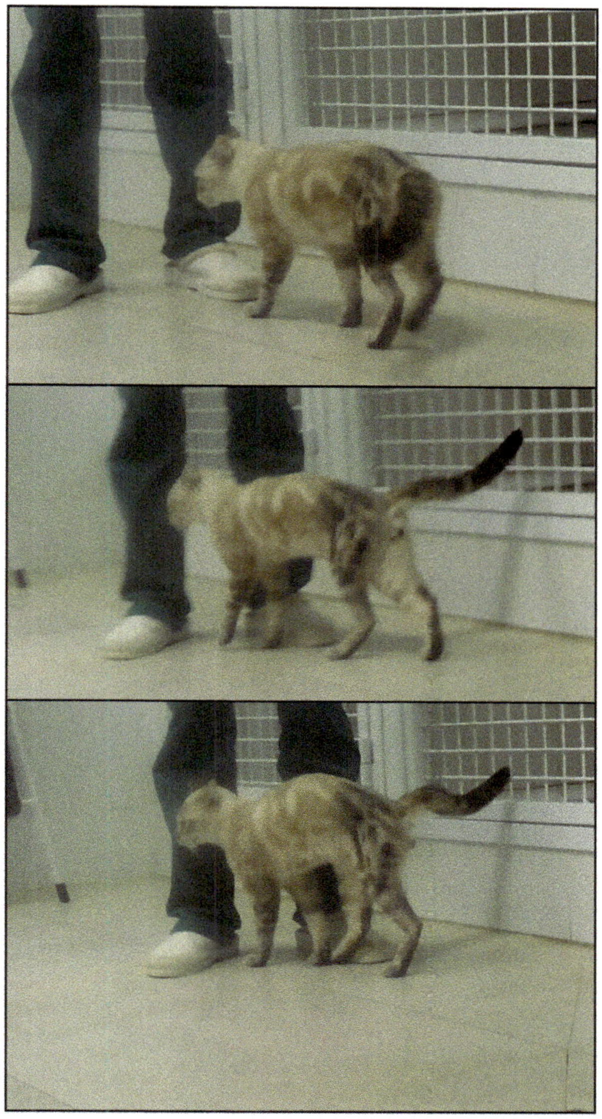

Figure 5. Gait analysis in a young cat 24 hours after left femoral fracture repair. The patient demonstrates an asymmetric gait and a subtle lameness of the left pelvic limb.

Thoracic limb

- Unilateral – head nodding (similar to dogs)
- Bilateral – weight shifting towards the pelvic limbs, short strides
- Changes may be observed during landing after jumping from a low height (table, chair)

Pelvic limb

- Unilateral – elevation of the hip when the affected limb touches the ground, asymmetry of the tail towards the "normal" side when cat is in motion
- Bilateral – weight shifting towards the thoracic limbs, short strides
- Changes may be observed immediately before jumping to a low height (table, chair)

Box 2. Clinical presentations of cats with common orthopaedic disorders (adapted from Voss and Steffen, 2009 and Kerwin, 2012).

Table 1. Anatomical landmarks for joint location, range of motion and normal angles in cats (pelvic limbs). Adapted from Jaeger, 2007 and Gordon-Evans, 2021.

Joint	Anatomical landmarks	ROM†	Normal angles (median values)¶
Carpus	Between the styloid process of radius and ulna (minor depression felt with the joint in flexion)	**Flexion** – paw pads touch antebrachium **Extension** – standing position slightly >180° **Minor valgus and varus** (internal and external rotation of the manus)	**Extension** – 22° **Flexion** – 198° **Valgus** – 10° **Varus** – 6°
Elbow	Distal to lateral and medial humeral epicondyles and cranial to olecranon	**Flexion** – carpus touches the shoulder **Extension** – straight limb from shoulder to carpus	**Flexion** – 22° **Extension** – 164°
Shoulder	Immediately distal to acromion and caudal to greater tubercle of humerus	**Flexion** – elbow travels caudally and lateral to the ribs **Extension** – elbow travels cranially and towards the head **Adduction** – humerus moves towards the thoracic wall **Abduction** – humerus moves away from the thoracic wall	**Flexion** – 32° **Extension** – 168°
Hock	Immediately distal to lateral and medial malleolus of the fibula and tibia, respectively, and slightly cranial to the cranial aspect of the calcaneus	**Flexion** – metatarsal bones touch the tibia if the stifle is in flexion; flexion is minimal with stifle in extension **Extension** – straight limb from tibia to metatarsal bones	**Flexion** – 22° **Extension** – 168° **Valgus** – 7° **Varus** – 11°
Stifle	Lateral and medial aspect of the patella tendon (midpoint of kneecap and tibial tuberosity)	**Flexion** – tuber calcaneus touches the ischium **Extension** – limb straight from femur to tibia seen from lateral side	**Flexion** – 24° **Extension** – 164°
Hip	Immediately cranial to greater trochanter and slightly ventral to it	**Flexion** – stifle touches the ilium ventrally **Extension** – femur extends caudally almost parallel with the spine	**Flexion** – 33° **Extension** – 166°

†Range of motion; ¶minor variations may occur when angles are measured in the conscious or sedated patient.

angles have been described for cats based on orthopaedic (Jaeger et al., 2007) and radiographic (Jaeger et al., 2007; Dantas et al., 2016; Swanson et al., 2012) measurements (Table 1).

In addition to joint and muscle palpation, **spinal palpation** should be performed. Some spinal disorders may cause gait abnormalities which mimic other orthopaedic conditions, whilst also causing spinal pain (Kerwin, 2012). When performing spinal palpation, the tail should also be palpated and manipulated and the lordosis test performed (dorsal displacement of the tail and ventroflexion of the lumbosacral spine). Some cats with lumbosacral disease, particularly, those with a history of difficulty jumping, may exhibit pain when the lordosis test is performed (Harris and Dhupa, 2008).

If insufficient information is obtained during standing palpation, then a full orthopaedic examination should be completed with the cat in lateral recumbency, if necessary under sedation.

Gait evaluation and palpation are important steps in the diagnosis of orthopaedic and neurological disorders, but they are not purely objective. To facilitate further patient reassessments, it is good practice for **findings to be quantified**. Scoring systems for orthopaedic findings can be descriptive (light/mild/moderate/severe lameness) or numerical, either using pre-existing scales (Morton et al., 2011) or one's own system, as long as it is consistently applied by all other staff members.

Specific orthopaedic manoeuvres

Carpus and tarsus

Carpal and tarsal injuries are relatively common in cats, possibly as a result of normal daily activity.

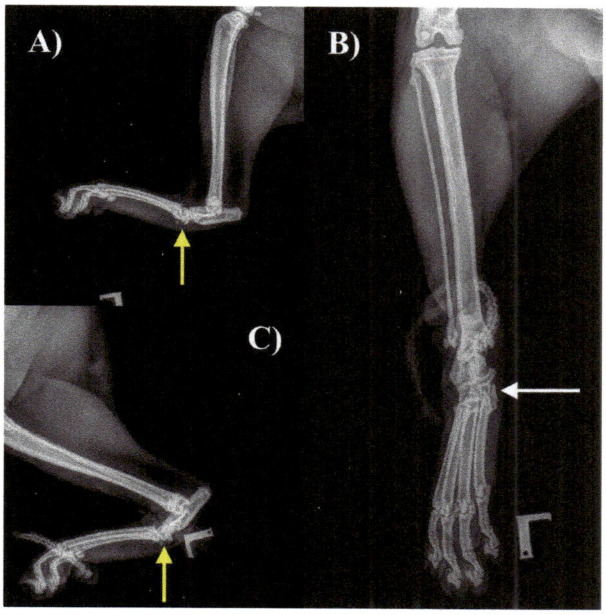

Figure 6. A) Mediolateral, B) caudocranial, and C) mediolateral stress radiographic projections of the left tarsus of an adult Domestic Shorthair presented for left pelvic limb lameness after being attacked by a dog. The patient was diagnosed with a traumatic tarsometatarsal luxation. Observe the abnormal position of the tarsometatarsal joint (yellow arrows) and the rotation of the metatarsal bones (white arrow).

Falls from heights, road traffic accidents, or penetrating wounds such as dog bites may result in **hyperextension injuries, joint luxation, or subluxation** (Basa and Johnson, 2019; Kulendra and Arthurs, 2014) (Figure 6). In some cases, particularly for road traffic accidents, the orthopaedic problem is associated with degloving injuries (Earley and Dee, 1980). **Such cases require appropriate wound management** in addition to the treatment of the orthopaedic condition (Figure 7).

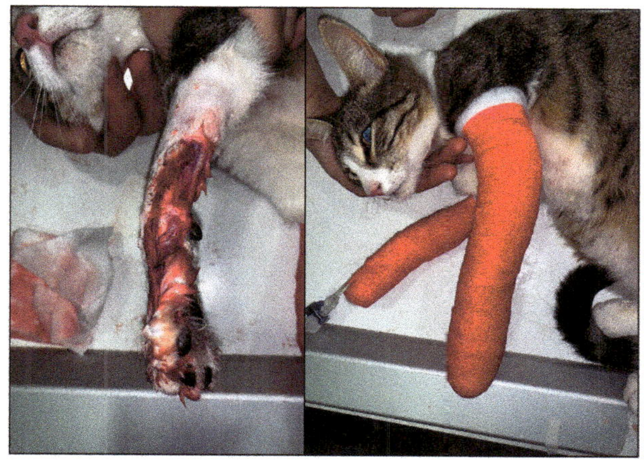

Figure 7. Carpal instability associated with degloving injury in a Domestic Shorthair. Adequate wound management is required prior to addressing the orthopaedic condition.

Due to the nature of trauma involving cats, **multiple injuries are more common than isolated fractures or ligament damage** (Basa and Johnson, 2019). Additionally, the lack of a thick, soft tissue envelope over the carpus and tarsus predisposes them to open fracture-luxations (Own, 2000). Assessment of the normal range of motion of these joints, including flexion-extension and varus-valgus, is crucial to identify suspected injuries. In most cases sedation is required, particularly when open wounds are present. If there is doubt about ligamentous injury, it is best practice to compare the affected limb with the non-affected limb to check for joint instability.

Stifle

Stifle instability occurs less frequently in cats compared to dogs (Umphlet, 1993). While injuries such as a rupture of the cranial cruciate ligament in dogs are extremely common (Hayashi, Manley and Muir, 2004), they are less common in cats, and when reported, frequently related to a traumatic event (Boge et al., 2019) (Figures 8 and 9).

As a result of severe trauma with multiple ligament injuries, the stifle becomes unstable and painful. **In more than 50% of cases, there are also secondary meniscal injuries** (Connery and Rackard, 2000) (Figure 9). Isolated rupture of the cranial cruciate ligament without trauma may occur in cats; however, it is not as frequent as in dogs. When an isolated rupture occurs, it tends to be identified in old overweight male cats and it is often associated with secondary meniscal injuries (Harasen, 2005).

Medial patella luxation also occurs in cats, although it occurs less frequently compared to in dogs (Johnson, 1986). These can be unilateral or bilateral, and may be associated with congenital malformations or be secondary to trauma (Johnson, 1986; Smith et al., 1999). When checking for patella luxation in cats, it is important to acknowledge that **healthy cats may show a degree of laxity** and subluxation of the patella (Smith et al., 1999). A history of intermittent locking of the knee following stifle extension (Johnson, 1986) or a crouching gait increases the suspicion of a luxated patella (Houlton and Meynink, 1989). However, some cats with patella luxation are asymptomatic or display intermittent lameness (Johnson, 1986). Medial patella luxation should be tested with the knee in extension. The severity of the luxation is graded using the same classification scheme used for dogs (Roush, 1993). Medial and lateral stress of the knee and detection of an abnormal varus/valgus signal the need for further testing to check for potential damage to the collateral ligaments (Figure 10). Evaluation of cranial cruciate ligament integrity should be performed in a similar manner to in dogs, using the tibial compression and cranial drawer tests (Figure 11).

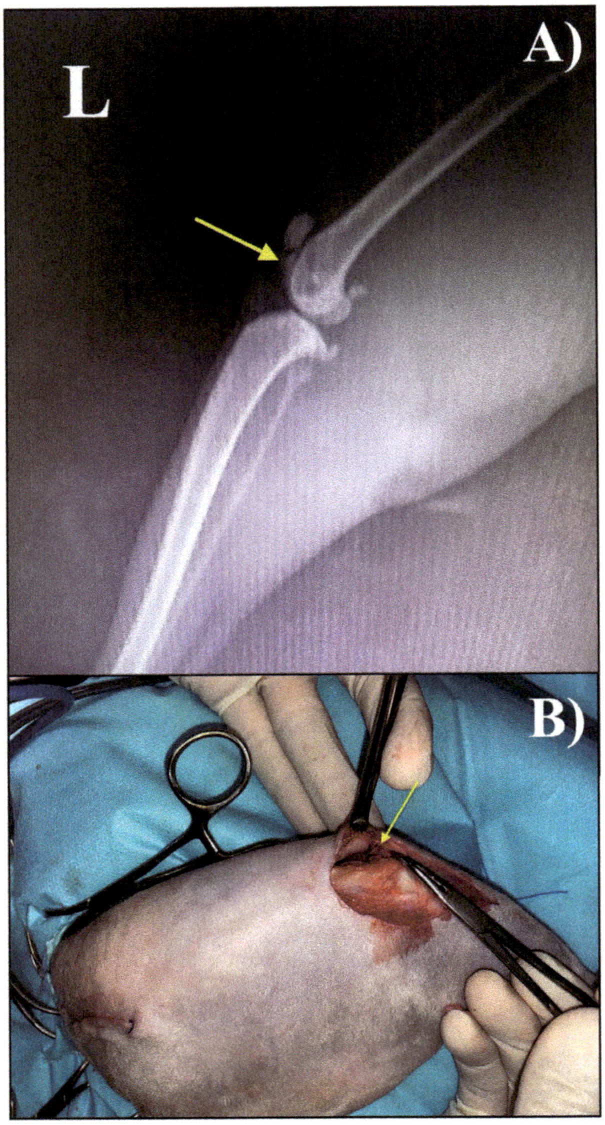

Figure 8. A) Mediolateral radiograph of the left stifle in a female cat with pelvic limb lameness and an unstable knee. X-rays revealed a distal fracture of the patella (yellow arrow). B) Intraoperative image of the same patient. The yellow arrow indicates the location of the patella fracture.

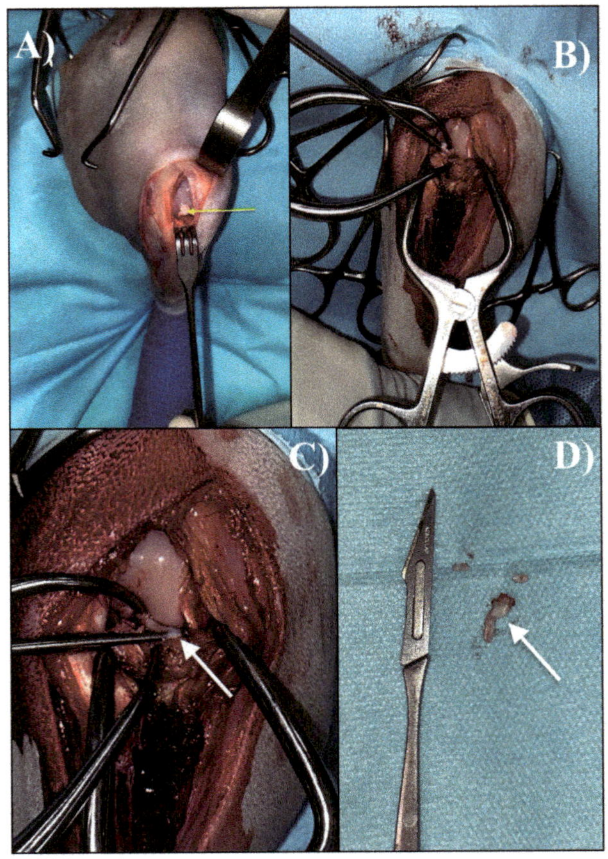

Figure 9. A) and B) The patient shown in Figure 8 was also diagnosed with a complete traumatic rupture of the cranial cruciate ligament (yellow arrow), and C) a secondary meniscal injury (white arrow). The ligament rupture was repaired using a fabello-tibial suture and the meniscal injury with a subtotal meniscectomy D).

Hips

When examining the hip joint, the full range of motion, including flexion, extension, rotation, and abduction should be evaluated. These manoeuvres can be done in a standing position or in lateral recumbency, the latter providing a more objective evaluation due to the inability of the cat to move away from the examiner. Most cats without hip pathology tolerate 90° of pain-free abduction (Kerwin, 2012), whilst lower levels of tolerance may indicate an underlying hip pathology (Kerwin, 2012) (Figure 12).

The Ortolani test can be used for cats, as in dogs, and this test evaluates joint laxity, which can sometimes be detected in young patients (Kerwin, 2012). The test is performed similarly for both cats and dogs (Smith et al., 2017). One hand should be placed over the dorsal

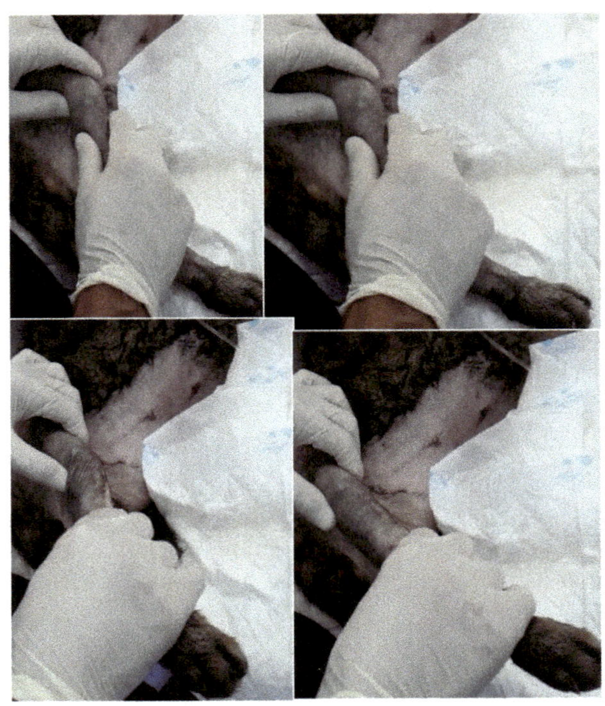

Figure 10. Multiple ligament injury (including collateral ligaments) in an elderly Domestic Shorthair.

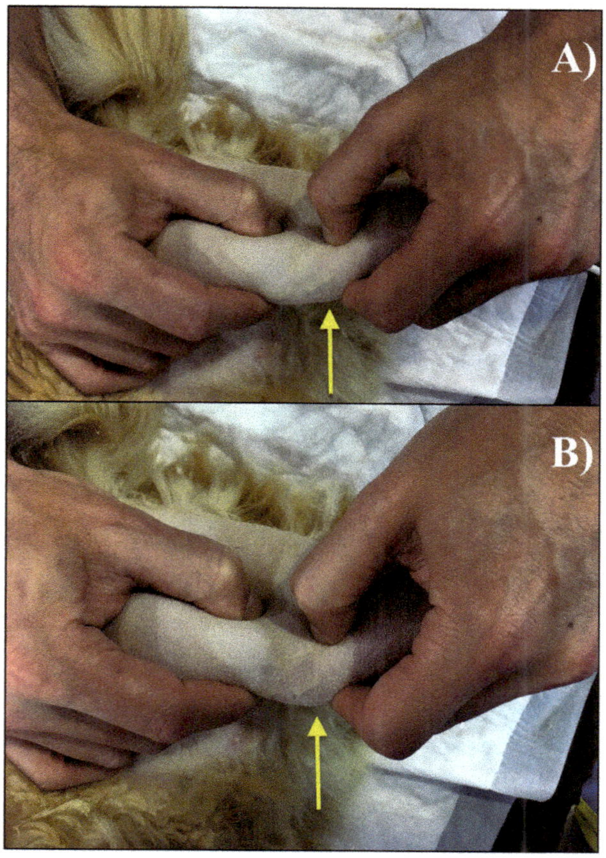

Figure 11. Cranial drawer test in an adult cat with traumatic rupture of the cranial cruciate ligament. The yellow arrow shows the point of insertion of the patella tendon at the tibial tuberosity. A) The right hand holds the distal femur and left hand the proximal tibia. B) A positive test is obtained when the left hand can be moved forward (cranial displacement of the tibia).

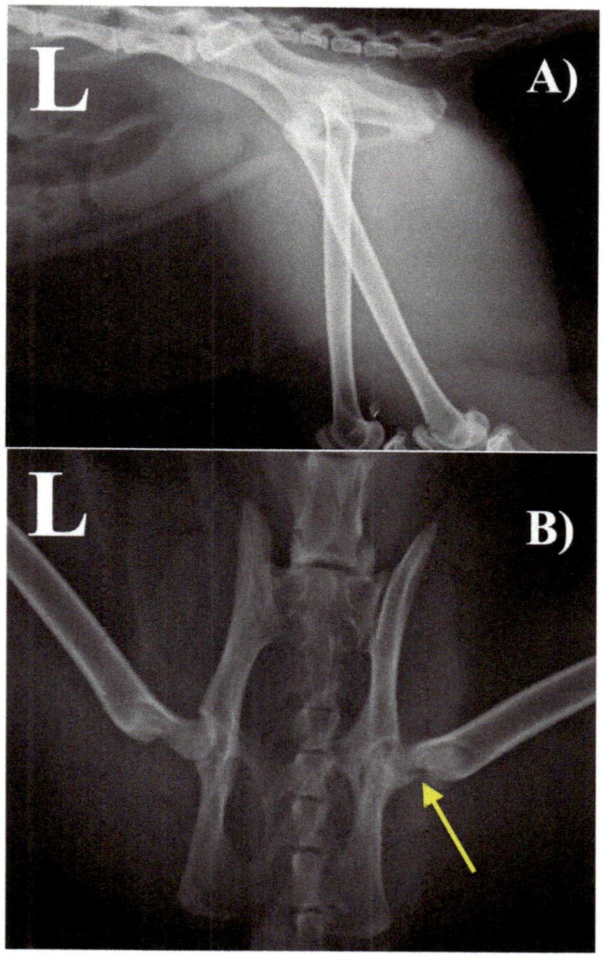

Figure 12. A) Lateral and B) ventrodorsal ('frog-legged') hip radiographs in a 2-year old male Maine Coon with acute lameness in the right pelvic limb. Pain was detected on manipulation of the right hip. Although no abnormalities were detected in the lateral projection, the silhouette of the right femoral head looks slightly abnormal (yellow arrow).

aspect of the pelvis and spine to provide stabilisation, whilst the other is placed at the level of the stifle. First, the hip is adducted while a force is applied in a proximal direction, then the stifle, and therefore the femur are pushed, causing dorsal subluxation of the hip. Once this is achieved, the hip is abducted to relocate the femoral head in the acetabulum, which is consistent with a positive Ortolani sign (Perry, 2016). This test can be performed without sedation; however, in patients with hip subluxation the pain caused by the manipulation may trigger muscle contraction which prevents manipulation, giving a false-negative result (Smith et al., 2017). In the absence of a positive Ortolani sign, pain on hip manipulation in cats may be secondary to OA (Smith et al., 2017) or capital fractures. This pathology can occur after trauma in skeletally immature animals or in mature cats with delayed physeal closure (Rubinos and Meeson, 2021). It has also been reported to spontaneously occur without any history of trauma, secondary to osteopathy at the femoral neck, particularly in heavier, male, adult cats (McNicholas et al., 2002; Queen, 1998) (Figure 13).

Elbow

In the absence of a traumatic condition, cats can still suffer from non-traumatic elbow pathology. **Osteoarthritis is relatively common in cats.** However, unlike in dogs, the underlying cause remains unclear (Lascelles et al., 2010). The most severe form of degenerative joint disease in the feline elbow affects the medial compartment, including the medial coronoid process. However, it is unknown if the mechanisms leading to this pathology are similar to those in the dog (Freire, Meuten and Lascelles, 2014).

The clinical signs of elbow OA in cats are often non-specific, and lameness is not commonly observed (Voss and Steffen, 2009). Examination should check for thickening of the periarticular tissues, joint effusion, reduced range of motion, crepitus, or pain: these may be particularly evident during pronation or supination (Perry, 2016).

A condition with a similar presentation to OA is **medial humeral epicondylitis**. The latter causes pain

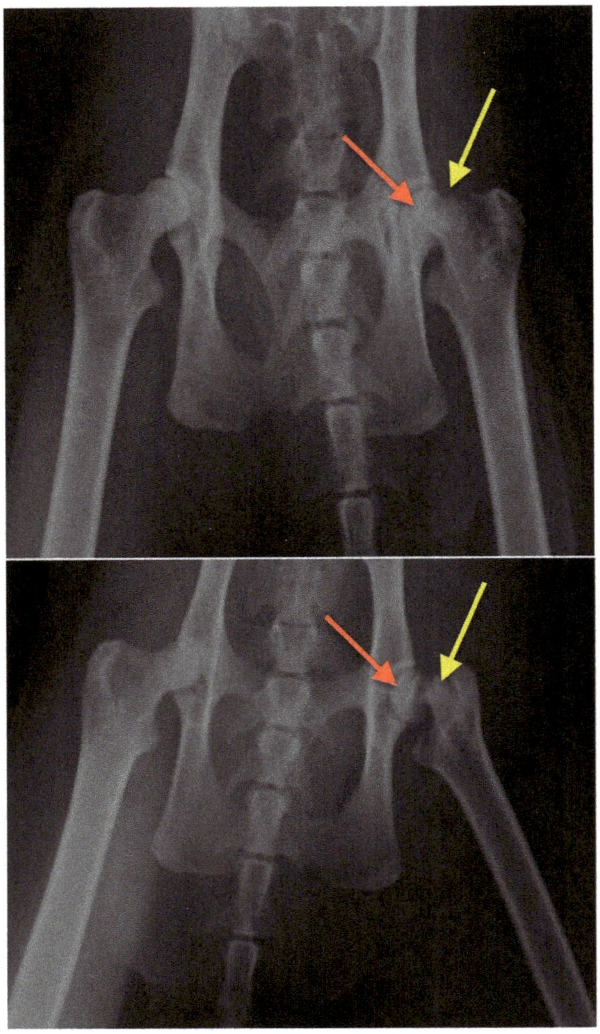

Figure 13. Ventrodorsal (extended legs) hip radiographs in the same patient show in Figure 12. A femoral neck fracture is observed (yellow arrows). It caused separation of the femoral head from the femoral neck (red arrows). The cat was diagnosed with unilateral osteopathy of the femoral neck.

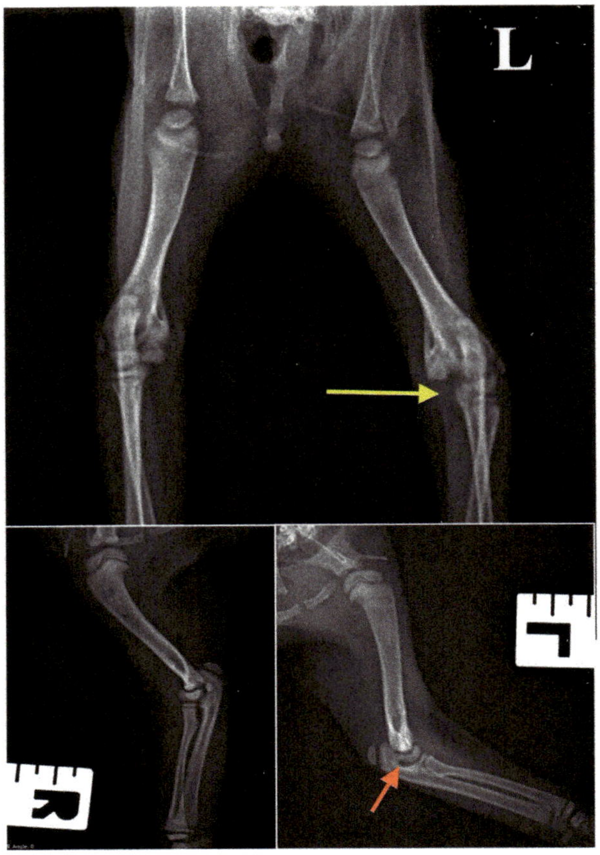

Figure 14. Orthogonal radiographs of the forelimbs in a 4-month-old female Persian with acute left forelimb lameness. A type 1 (radiohumeral) congenital elbow luxation was diagnosed. Lateral deviation of the radial head from the humerus (yellow arrow) and the joint incongruence (red arrow) of the left elbow compared to the right elbow can be observed.

on direct palpation of the medial humeral epicondyle and on flexion of the carpus. However, in some cats this pathology is asymptomatic (Streubel, Geyer and Montavon, 2012). Lifestyle plays an important role in the development of this condition, with active outdoor cats exposed to repetitive pronation and supination motions that cause chronic inflammation of the flexor tendons and development of bony spurs at the origin of the flexor muscles (Streubel et al., 2015).

Congenital elbow luxation/subluxation is rare in cats, and more commonly reported in dogs (Bingel and Riser, 1977). However, it has been described in young cats (Valastro, Di Bello and Crovace, 2005) (Figure 14). Depending on the severity, signs include pain on manipulation, reduced pronation/supination, and mild to moderate lameness (type 1: radiohumeral luxation, Figure 15), decreased flexion-extension and moderate to severe lameness (type 2: humeroulnar luxation), or loss of the normal range of motion of the joint due to lack of contact between the articular surfaces of the radius, ulnar, and humerus (type 3: combination of type 1 + type 2) (Kene, Lee and Bennett, 1982).

Shoulder

Traumatic and non-traumatic shoulder disease is rarely diagnosed in the cat. The most **common pathologies affecting the cat shoulder are traumatic in origin** (Voss and Langley-Hobbs, 2009), whilst congenital conditions such as glenoid dysplasia and osteochondritis dissecans have been reported in young patients (Schwarze, Tano and Carroll, 2015).

Indications of shoulder pathology include moderate to severe non-weight bearing lameness, with the shoulder held in a flexed position, and pain on manipulation of the joint (Voss and Langley-Hobbs, 2009), as well as muscle atrophy, periarticular fibrosis, and joint effusion. The orthopaedic manoeuvres used to assess the shoulder are similar to those used for dogs. For example, the bicipital test, used to assess for bicipital tendinopathy, is performed placing a finger over the greater tubercle of the humerus with the shoulder flexed whilst the elbow is extended.

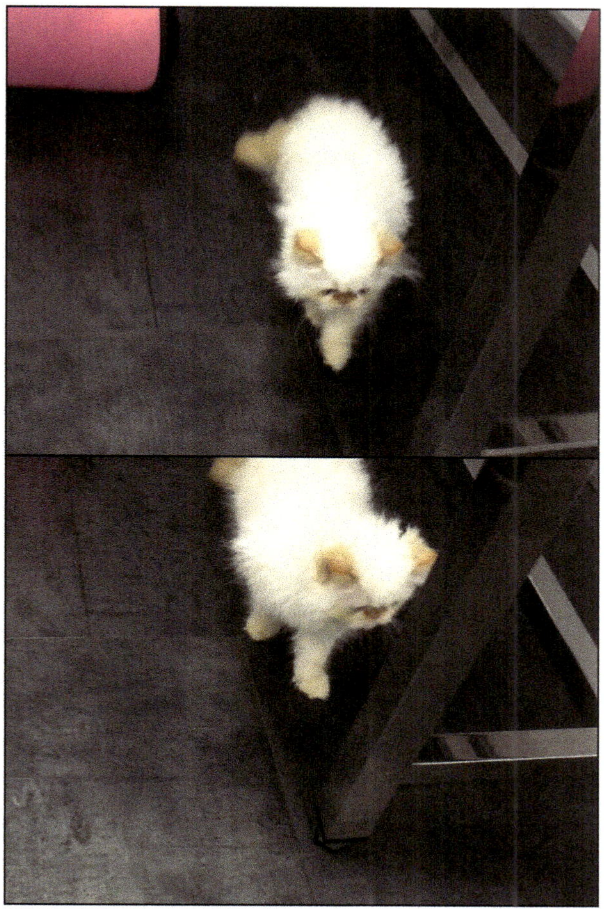

Figure 15. Gait evaluation in the kitten shown in the radiographs in Figure 14. Despite the congenital joint luxation, the cat was not lame. She only demonstrated mild discomfort on manipulation of the left elbow and decreased pronation and supination.

An alternative is the craniocaudal and mediolateral drawer test, which is similar to the stifle cranial drawer test and evaluates mediolateral instability (Voss and Lanley-Hobbs, 2009).

Neurological examination

When a neurological exam is required palpation should be performed first, before the orthopaedic examination. **Neurological disease can also cause lameness and gait abnormalities, which need to be differentiated from orthopaedic problems.** Common presentations of neurological disease include (Voss and Steffen, 2009):

- dragging of one or more limbs
- swaying gait
- scuffing
- arched back
- low head carriage
- abnormal tail position.

Likewise, **some orthopaedic problems can mimic a neurological condition**. For example, hindlimb pathologies such as bilateral cranial cruciate rupture, hip dysplasia, or tarsal luxation may present with an abnormal gait suggestive of thoracolumbar neuropathies. Another example is severe elbow OA or polyarthritis, with presenting signs compatible with pathology affecting the cervical spine or a central neurological disease (Berry, 2014). Hence why **neurological and orthopaedic exams are complementary** and should be performed for every case.

A clinical history is crucial, even when a purely neurological disorder is suspected. This is because occasionally the feline nervous system is affected by metabolic diseases, drug administration, or generalised disease (e.g. toxoplasmosis) (Voss and Steffen, 2009).

As for the orthopaedic exam, the first steps involve **observation and gait analysis, and recording the cat's state of consciousness and awareness** (alterations in these can affect the neurological exam leading to inaccurate findings) (Garosi, 2009). For this reason assessment without sedation, even in fractious patients, is required. The **level of consciousness is classified as:**

- normal
- lethargic
- stuporous
- comatose.

The latter is a total absence of consciousness, which can be associated with complete disruption between the brainstem and the cerebral hemispheres (Voss and Steffen, 2009).

Normal gait requires adequate function of the brainstem, cerebellum, spinal cord, peripheral nerves, muscles, and neuromuscular junctions (Garosi, 2009). When this is not the case and an abnormal gait is present, this may involve:

- all four limbs: ambulatory **tetraparesis**
- generalised, uncoordinated gait: **ataxia**
- pelvic limbs only: **paraparesis**
- just one limb: **monoparesia.**

If the patient drags one or more limbs during ambulation, a differentiation between paresis (weakness with the presence of voluntary muscle movements) and paralysis/plegia (absence of voluntary muscle movements) should be made as the prognosis differs. Despite this, gait abnormalities cannot be used as the sole criteria to identify and localise neurological disorders (Voss and Steffen, 2009).

In some cats performing a full neurological exam is a challenge. Therefore, tests that require minimal restraint should be evaluated first, such as evaluation of the cranial nerves and postural reactions, including the conscious propioception. In a healthy, conscious, alert, and responsive cat, any deficit in the cranial nerves may indicate the injury is outside the forebrain (Voss and Steffen, 2009). Cranial nerve deficits associated with an abnormal level of consciousness, indicate problem is likely centrally located (Voss and Steffen, 2009). See Table 2 for tests for evaluation of the cranial nerves.

Proprioceptive tests are highly sensitive at detecting neurological disorders, but are non-specific with regards to lesion localization. Therefore the results must be combined with other neurological findings. Tests include the proprioceptive positioning reaction (knuckling test) and other postural tests, such as the wheelbarrow, hopping, hemiwalk, placing reaction, extensor postural thrust, and tonic neck reaction tests (Voss and Steffen, 2009).

Evaluation of conscious proprioception is the proprioceptive test best tolerated by cats, particularly in non-cooperative patients. During this test, the foot is placed in a flexed position, and the dorsal surface is forced to contact the floor. The normal response is an immediate reposition of the foot into an extended position (Figure 16).

Spinal reflexes should then be evaluated, which assess the components (sensory and motor) of the reflex arc (Voss and Steffen, 2009). Spinal reflexes may be normal, absent, or depressed (found in lower motor neuron disease), or exaggerated (associated with upper motor neuron disease or deficit of the opposing group muscles) (Voss and Steffen, 2009). A repetitive contraction and relaxation of a muscle, or group of muscles, in response to the stimulus (clonus) may occur when there is an anomaly of the descending inhibitory pathways for the reflex being tested. This may be observed in chronic lesions (Voss and Steffen, 2009). See Table 3 for tests for evaluation of spinal reflexes.

Other peripheral reflexes include the perineal and panniculus. The perineal reflex test allows evaluation of the pudendal and sacral nerve function. The panniculus reflex tests the contraction of the cutaneous trunci muscle. The perineal reflex should be evaluated in cats with a history of sacrocaudal injuries (Tatton, Jeffery and Holmes, 2009) (Figure 17) and pelvic fractures (Messon and Corr, 2011), as some patients may

Table 2. Evaluation of the cranial nerves (adapted from Voss and Steffen, 2009).

Test	Description	Cranial nerve/s tested
Menace response	Slow hand movement towards the eye without touching the face or pushing air onto the cornea	Optic (II) Abducens (VI) Facial (VII)
Visual assessment	Cotton ball dropped in front of the eye	Optic (II) Abducens (VI) Facial (VII)
Palpebral reflex	Gentle finger pressure applied at the medial canthus of the eye to check blinking	Trigeminal (V) Facial (VII)
Vibrissae response	Gentle pressure applied to the upper lip to check for lip movement and head turning	Trigeminal (V) Facial (VII)
Mandibular touch	Similar to vibrissae response but pressure applied to the lower jaw	Trigeminal (V) Facial (VII)
Auricular reflex	Inner pinna touched with a cotton bud. Observe for twitching of the ear, blinking, or head shaking	Facial (VII)
Corneal reflex	Cornea touched slighly with a moistened cotton bud. Observe for retraction of the eyeball	Trigeminal (V) Abducens (VI)
Pupillary light reflex	In a dark room, bright light pointed at the pupil. Check for pupillary contraction (direct pupillary reflex) and slight dilation (indirect pupillary reflex) of the non-illuminated eye This test helps to check for anisocoria (different pupil sizes in the same environment)	Optic (II) Oculomotor (III)
Oculocephalic reflex	Steady, controlled movement of the head performed and head then turned in the opposite direction. Check the eye position. More than a few beats are pathological	Vestibulocochlear (VIII) Oculomotor (III) Trochlear (IV) Abducens (VI)
Gag reflex	Larynx touched with a finger to induce gagging	Glossopharyngeal (IX) Vagus (X)
Tongue movement and symmetry	Visual assessment of the tongue. Check for asymmetry or muscle atrophy	Hypoglossal (XII)
Palpation of the head for symmetry	Check for muscle atrophy, asymmetry, or droopy lips	Trigeminal (V) Facial (VII)
Palpation of the neck	Assess for muscle atrophy	Accessory (XI)

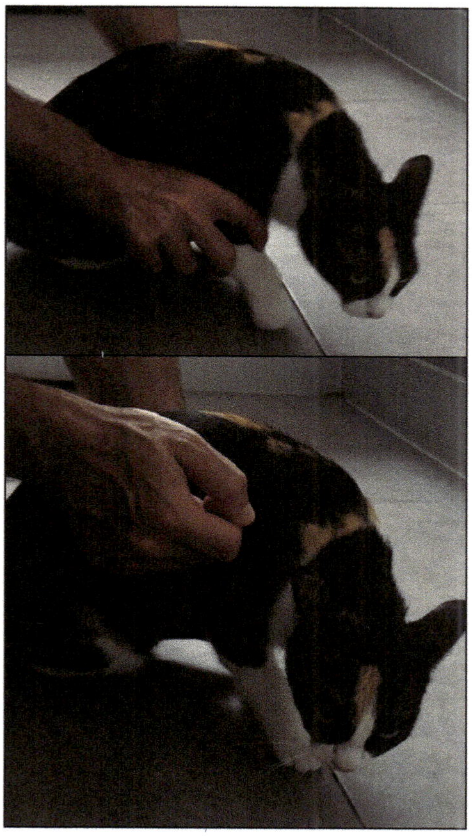

Figure 16. Evaluation of conscious proprioception in the right forelimb in an adult female cat.

experience temporary or permanent urinary and/or faecal incontinence due to neurological damage (Tatton, Jeffery and Holmes, 2009; Messon and Corr, 2011). The panniculus reflex has clinical relevance as a predictive indicator for the recovery of patients with acute thoracolumbar myelopathy (Muguet-Chanoit et al., 2012).

Another important part of the neurological examination, particularly in trauma cases, is evaluation of the dermatomes. **A dermatome is an area of skin innervated by one or several nerves** (Voss and Steffen, 2009). To do this the area of skin to be tested should be pinched; a painful response indicates a positive result (Table 4).

The final part of the neurological exam is evaluation of muscle tone, muscle atrophy, nociception, and the presence/absence of back or neck pain. Testing of back/neck pain and nociception should be done at the end of the exam so as to not affect the remainder of the evaluation. Manoeuvres to test for neck pain include lateral rotation, extension, ventroflexion, and lateral palpation. Tests for back pain should include ventroflexion of the spine (placing one hand under the belly to provide support), extension of the hips with ventroflexion of the lumbosacral area, examination of the tail, and the lordosis test.

Table 3. Evaluation of the spinal reflex (adapted from Voss and Steffen, 2009).

Test	Description	Spinal segment tested
Withdrawal (forelimb)	With the limb extended, area between toes pinched with hands or forceps without causing pain. Normal test causes flexion of the forelimb	C6-T2
Extensor carporradialis	Hammer used at the craneolateral aspect of the proximal antebrachium. A positive response causes extension of the carpus and toes	C7-T2
Tricep contraction	Finger placed on the olecranon (insertion of the triceps) and hammer used. A positive test causes contraction of the muscle bellies	C7-T2
Withdrawal (hindlimbs)	Similar to the forelimb test. A positive response causes retraction of the limb with flexion of the knee	L6-Sacrum
Patella	With the knee in a normal standing angle and the limb relaxed, patella tendon should be hammered. A positive test causes extension of the knee	Femoral nerve (L4-L6)
Cranial tibial	With the hock extended, a finger should be placed at the craniolateral aspect of the proximal tibia to feel Gerdy's tubercule†. The finger should be hammered. A positive response causes flexion of the hock	Peroneal nerve (L6-Sacrum)
Gastrocnemius	A finger should be placed on the calcaneus and hammered. A positive response causes contraction of the gastrocnemius muscles	Tibial nerve (L6-Sacrum)
Sciatic	With the limb relaxed and in a normal standing angle, the area between the greater trochanter of the femur and the ischiatic tuberosity should be hammered. A normal response causes extension of the hock	Sciatic nerve (L6-Sacrum)

†Gerdy's tubercle is used in humans to define the lateral tibial condyle (small bony protuberance at the proximolateral aspect of the tibia). In small animals, Gerdy's tubercle is cranial to the long digital extensor fossa.

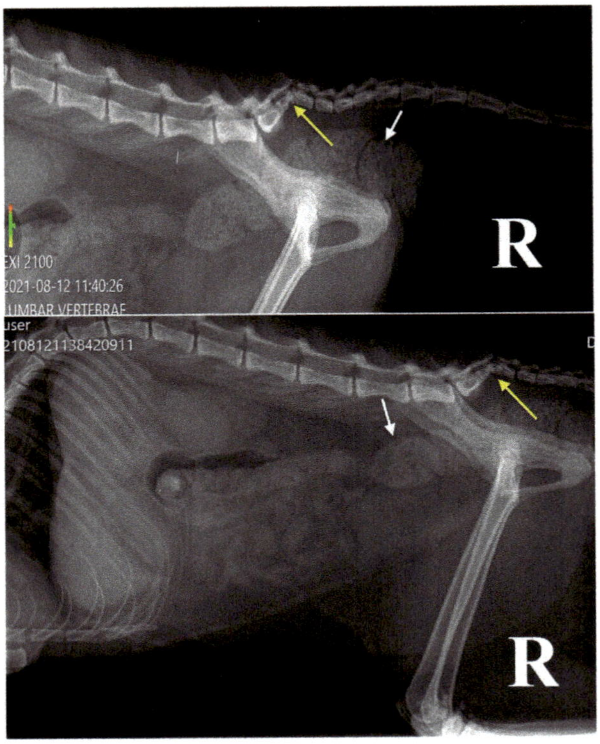

Figure 17. Lateral radiographs of the caudal spine and caudal abdomen in a cat with trauma of unknown origin. The patient was referred for investigation of faecal and urinary incontinence. Radiographs revealed a sacro-coccygeal fracture/luxation (yellow arrow) and faecal accumulation in the colon and rectum. A traumatic injury of the pudendal nerve was diagnosed.

Nociception (conscious perception of a painful stimulus) should only be assessed if paralysis/plegia is suspected. If voluntary movements are present, then nociception should also be present (Voss and Steffen, 2009).

This test should be performed by pinching the digits with a haemostat to check for a painful response. In a positive test, the cat demonstrates a clear painful reaction such as dilation of the pupils, tachycardia/tachypnoea, vocalisation, or an aggressive response. The test should also be performed at the tail, particularly in cases where pelvic trauma is suspected (Tatton, Jeffery and Holmes, 2009; Messon and Corr, 2011). It is important to distinguish between nociception and a positive withdrawal test, as the second only indicates the reflex arch is intact but does not evaluate the integrity of the nociceptive pathways.

With the neurological exam complete, findings should be combined to localise the lesion and select the most appropriate diagnostics test(s).

A broad classification localises neurological lesions into those affecting the spinal cord (C1-C5, C6-T2, T3-L3, L4-Sacrum), forebrain, brainstem or cerebellum, vestibular system (central or peripheral), or peripheral nerves (Voss and Steffen, 2009). Occasionally, some diseases cause multifocal lesions where more than one area is affected.

Table 4. Evaluation of the dermatomes (adapted from Voss and Steffen, 2009).

Dermatome/ nerve tested	Anatomical area
Radial	Digits I to IV Mannus (dorsomedial) Carpus (dorsomedial) Antebrachium (cranial aspect to the level of the elbow)
Ulnar	From the caudolateral aspect of the antebrachium (level of the elbow) towards the lateral aspect of the carpus and digit V It extends in a palmar direction to include the metacarpal pad and digits II to V
Median	From the mediodistal aspect of the brachium towards the mediodistal aspect of the antebrachium. The region includes a small area of the carpus located palmomedially
Peroneal	From the craneolateral aspect of the mid-thigh towards the dorsomedial aspect of the tarsus, including digits II to IV
Saphenous	From the caudal aspect of the mid-thigh towards the tarsus and the plantar aspect of the foot

Ancillary tests

Radiographs

Radiography is a fundamental tool for the investigation of lameness and/or trauma in cats. Depending on the orthopaedic and neurological examination findings, this diagnostic modality will confirm or refute a clinically suspected lesion, show the nature and extent of a suspected lesion, reveal additional non-detected lesions, discard other diagnoses, and provide valuable information for the selection of which diagnostic tests are needed to complement the radiographs. Additionally, radiographs help to monitor the progression of disease or healing and aid in establishing a prognosis for the patient.

The quality of the radiographs depends on the settings selected to obtain the images (Ohlerth, Voss and Steffen, 2009). Although it is out of the scope of this chapter, adequate radiographic quality is achieved when proper settings (kVp, mAs) are used. Moreover, patient positioning directly affects the quality of the images and radiographic interpretation. Many cats do not cooperate during radiograph positioning, even if restraining methods such as ropes and sandbags are used; therefore sedation or general anaesthesia is generally required. Orthogonal views are mandatory for diagnosis and preoperative planning, as some lesions can be missed due to the superimposition of bony structures (Ohlerth, Voss and Steffen, 2009). If needed, orthogonal radiographs of the contralateral limb are taken for comparison. The requirement for additional views, such as horizontal beam projections (Beck, 1991), oblique, or stress radiographs, is indicated depending on the suspected pathology (Basa and Johnson, 2019; Kulendra and Arthurs, 2014; Earley and Dee, 1980; Owen, 2000; Ohlerth, Voss and Steffen, 2009).

Radiographic interpretation should focus on the evaluation of the bones, joints, and surrounding soft tissues. A good example of this is seen in open fractures, as loss of the soft tissue envelope can be detected in conventional radiographs (Figure 18). Having that information before the initial consultation is important for these cases, as the complication rate for open fractures differs significantly compared to closed fractures (Agnello, 2016).

In addition to the diagnosis of bone fractures (Basa and Johnson, 2019; Kulendra and Arthurs, 2014; Earley and Dee, 1980; Connery and Rackard, 2000; Rubinos and Meeson, 2021; McNicholas et al., 2002) radiographs are useful in the diagnosis of degenerative joint disease (Lascelles, 2010; Hardie, Roe and Martin, 2002; Godfrey, 2005; Clarke and Bennett, 2006; Lascelles et al., 2012), evaluation of angular limb deformities (Jaeger et al., 2007; Dantas et al., 2016; Swanson et al., 2012) (Figure 19), and diagnosis of congenital (Johnson, 1986; Valastro, 2005) or developmental diseases (Smith et al., 2017; Queen et al., 1998; Freire, Meuten and Lascelles, 2014).

Radiographic assessment must include evaluation of the soft tissues, presence/absence of periosteal and/or endosteal reaction, and cortical changes (Ohlerth, Voss and Steffen, 2009). For radiographic evaluation of fractures, the anatomical location of the fracture and type of fracture should be described. Additionally, details of the fracture biology should be provided, as prognosis and treatment differ if the fracture has occurred secondary to a neoplastic process or infection or is secondary to trauma. The direction in which the fracture fragments are displaced should also be included in the radiographic description. This description is based on the position of the distal main fragment with regard to the proximal main fragment, as seen in the orthogonal views (Figure 20).

After the fracture has been repaired, proper evaluation of the follow-up radiographs is required to assess bone healing. For postoperative radiograph evaluation, the rule of the 4 A's (Langley-Hobbs, 2003) should be followed:

1. **Apposition**: the amount of end-to-end contact of the fracture fragments.
2. **Alignment**: rotational or angular position of the fracture fragment.

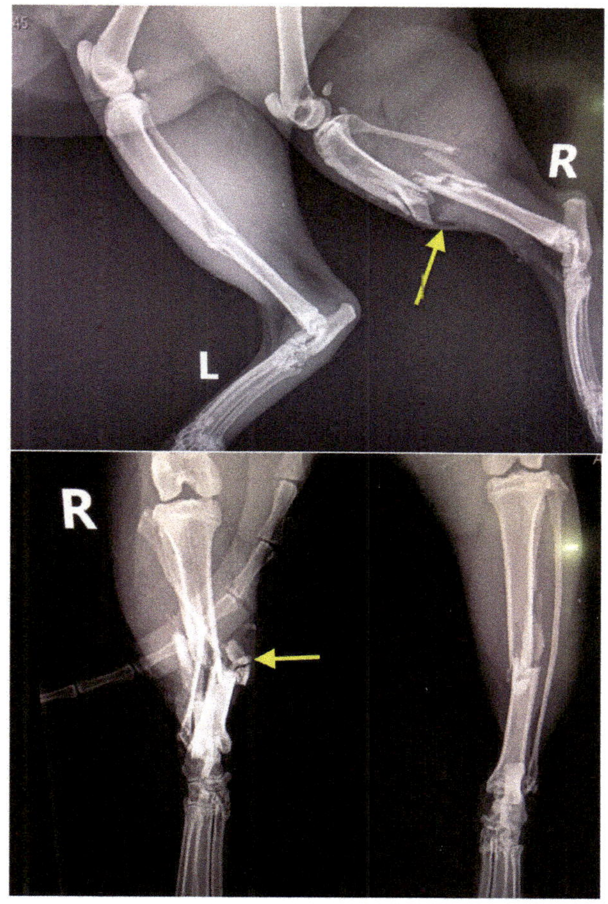

Figure 18. Mediolateral and craniocaudal pelvic limb radiographs in an adult Domestic Shorthair after falling from a height. He was diagnosed with bilateral comminuted diaphyseal fractures of the tibias. Gas opacity is observed under the skin in association with the tibial fracture. This finding is consistent with an open fracture (loss of soft tissue envelope)

3. **Apparatus**: description of the adequate/inadequate position of the orthopaedic implants or issues associated with them (e.g. loosening, breakage).
4. **Activity**: radiographic evidence of bone activity at the fracture site and surrounding structures (periosteal reaction, cortical bridging, bone reabsorption, etc.). Note: activity cannot be assessed in immediate postoperative radiographs.

Radiographic evaluation of bone healing is similar in cats and dogs, provided there are no complications (Ohlerth, Voss and Steffen, 2009). In the early stages of bone healing (approximately two weeks after surgery), the fracture gap appears radiographically wider compared to immediate postoperative radiographs (Ohlerth, Voss and Steffen, 2009) (Figure 21). However, if no complications occur, callus formation is generally visible between 4 – 8 weeks after surgery (earlier in young patients) (Ohlerth, Voss and Steffen, 2009). Once bone bridging occurs at the fracture gap (continuation of the cortical bone), bone healing is

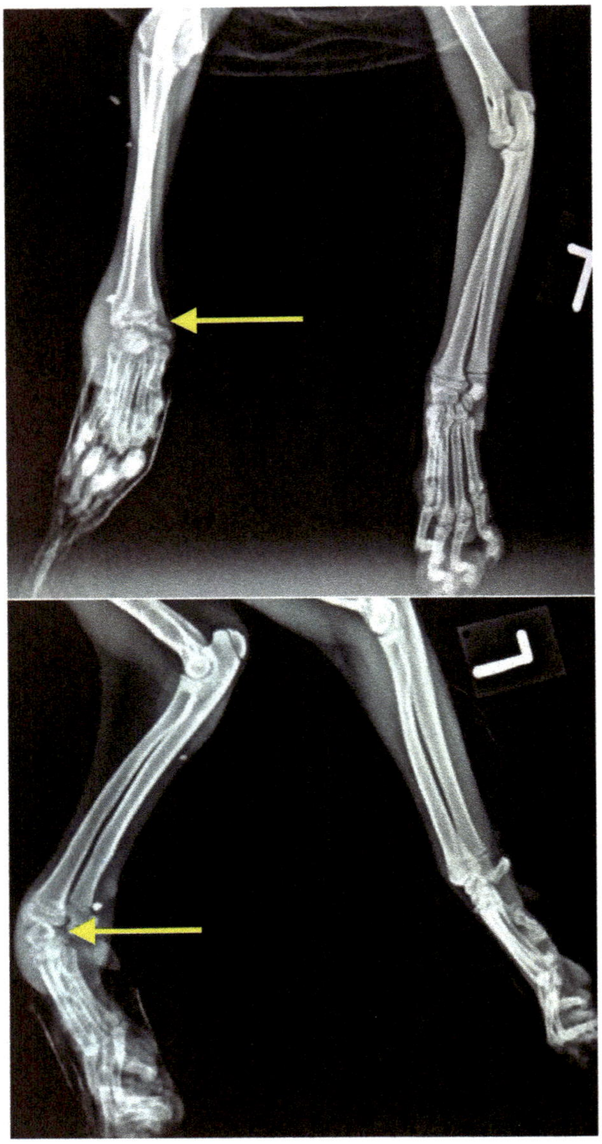

Figure 19. Orthogonal radiographs of the forelimbs in a 8-month old male cat with an angular limb deformity of the right antebrachium. The patient was diagnosed with a radius curvus, which caused significant rotation of the manus (yellow arrows).

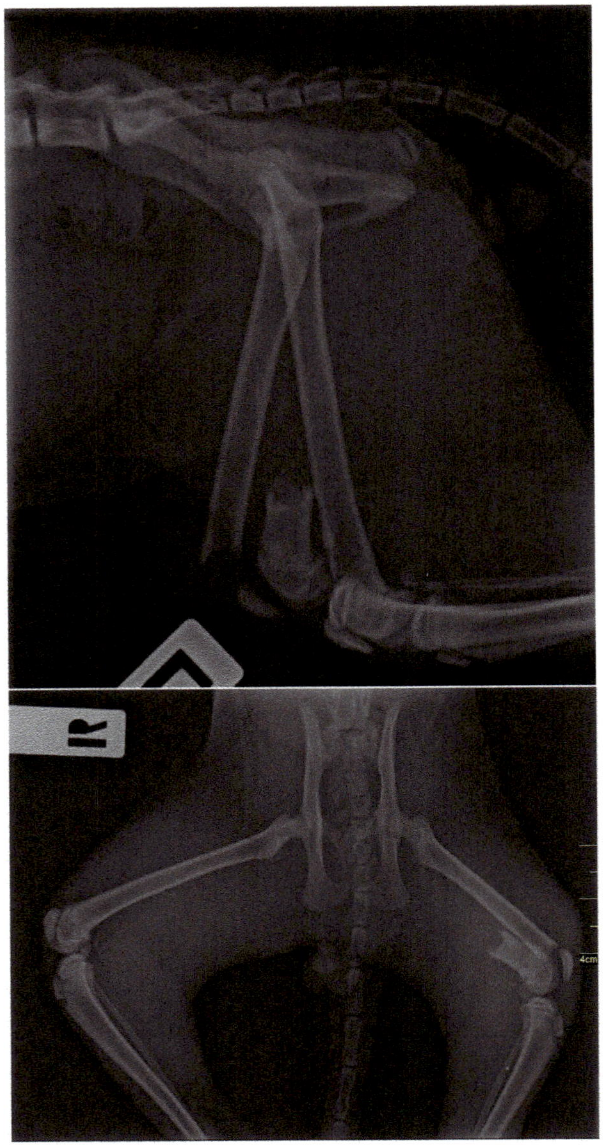

Figure 20. Orthogonal views of a femoral fracture in a male cat. An adequate radiographic description of the fracture would include the following information: *"distal diaphyseal (or supracondylar), transverse fracture of the left femur with caudomedial displacement"*. Additional information to include would be the cause *(traumatic)*, the nature *(close fracture)* and the estimated age of the patient *(young cat, as some of the growth plates are radiographically open)*.

generally completed with no complications. At the latest stages (> 12 weeks after surgery), bone remodelling continues to make the callus smaller and smoother, and corticomedullary continuity can be seen (Ohlerth, Voss and Steffen, 2009) (Figure 22). Complications of fracture healing in cats are similar to those seen in dogs (Griffon, 2016; Johson, 2016). These may be related to the apparatus (implant loosening, failure, infection) (Griffon, 2016) affecting fracture alignment (malunion), precluded bone healing (non-union) (Johson, 2016) or postponed bone healing (delayed union) (Johson, 2016).

Apart from fractures, other pathologies that can be detected with radiographs are those affecting the soft tissues, such as bite wounds. Bite wounds may cause radiographic soft tissue changes, such as disruption of the normal pattern of the subcutaneous fat and fascial planes, showing areas of gas mixed with soft tissue opacity (Ohlerth, Voss and Steffen, 2009). While the diagnosis may be challenging during the early stages, changes such as pain on palpation of the limb, manipulation reluctance, cellulitis, or cutaneous erythema in conjunction with the aforementioned radiographic changes may indicate a bite wound (Leonard and Tillson, 2001). Cat bites involving a joint may cause septic arthritis. Although a final diagnosis cannot be made by radiographs, the presence of intra-articular and/or extra-articular soft tissue swelling, together with the clinical history and examination findings, may increase suspicion (Ohlerth, Voss and Steffen, 2009).

Fracture location	• Diaphysis: proximal, mid, distal • Physeal (growing animals): Salter Harris classification (Salter and Harris, 1963) • Metaphyseal: proximal, distal • Articular
Fracture type	• Transverse • Oblique (short, long) • Spiral • Segmental • Greenstick • Linear • Comminuted • Impacted • Avulsion
Fracture biology	• Traumatic • Pathological • Closed/open • Stress (implant related)

Box 3. Description of fractures based on radiographic assessment.

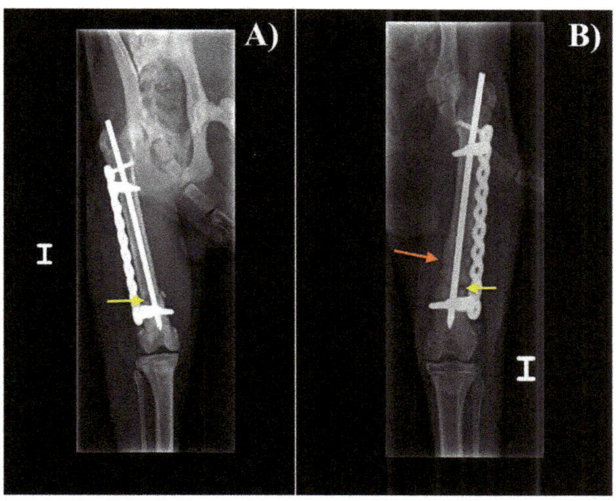

Figure 21. A) Immediate postoperative radiograph of the patient shown in Figure 20 after fracture repair. B) The fracture gap looks wider in the two week postoperative follow-up radiographs (yellow arrow). There is periosteal reaction near the fracture gap, indicating bone activity (red arrow). (Courtesy of Ivan Serra).

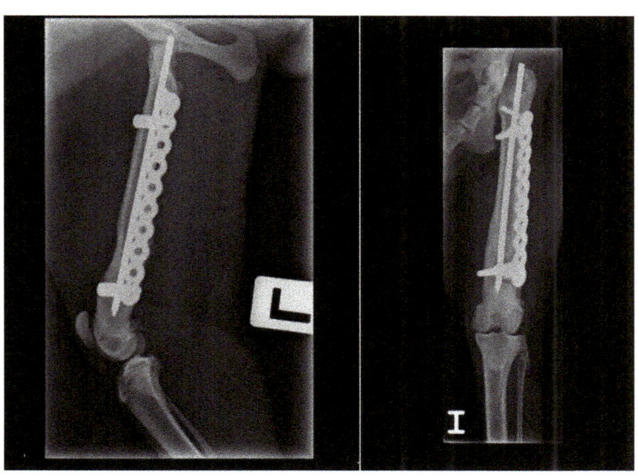

Figure 22. 3-month postoperative follow-up radiographs of the patient shown in Figures 20 and 21. The corticomedullary continuation and the absence of fracture gap can be observed. The fracture line is no longer visible. (Courtesy of Ivan Serra).

Degenerative joint disease (OA) can also be detected in radiographs. Some common findings include subchondral sclerosis, moderate to severe intra-articular soft tissue swelling, irregular articular surfaces with new bone formation (osteophytosis), and mineralisation at the origin or insertion of tendons and/or ligaments (entheseophytes) (Ohlerth, Voss and Steffen, 2009) (Figure 23). However, the absence of these radiographic findings do not exclude this pathology, as occasionally such findings are not visible during the early stages of the disease. Moreover, the presence of new bone formation in articular surfaces is not always associated with clinical lameness. An example of this is the detection of meniscal mineralisation, which is relatively common in domestic cats. Although it appears in association with stifle OA (Figure 23), patients with meniscal mineralisation are not always lame, and therefore this finding is only clinically relevant when gait abnormalities are also detected (Freire-Gonzalez et al., 2010).

Ultrasound

Ultrasonography of the musculoskeletal system in cats is challenging due to the small size of the anatomical structures to be evaluated. Additionally, the changes observed may be subtle, increasing the difficulty to make a diagnosis. In general, a **7.5 MHz linear transducer is used** for its power resolution and to ensure the probe remains in flat contact with the skin, which provides a better view of the structures (Kramer et al., 1997). While evaluation of bone is limited with ultrasonography, articular surfaces and surrounding soft tissues (e.g. muscles and tendons) can be explored

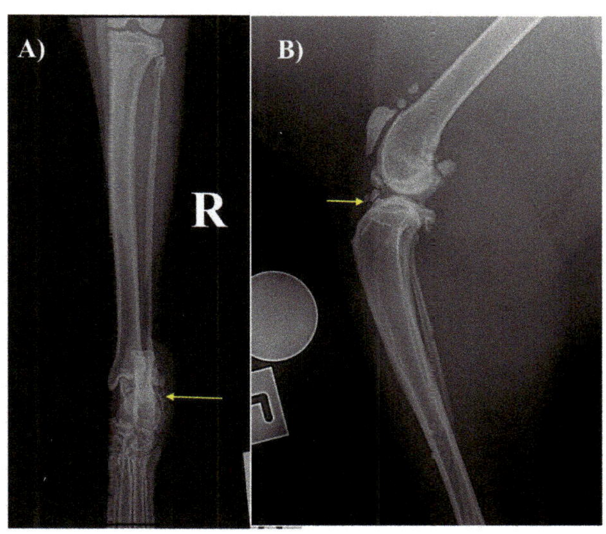

Figure 23. A) Radiographic *new bone formation* at the tarsal joint in a 10-year old Domestic Shorthair. Joint tap and cytology of the lesion confirmed the diagnosis of degenerative joint disease (osteoarthritis). B) Osteophytes and meniscal mineralization (yellow arrow) in an elderly cat with chronic rupture of the cranial cruciate ligament.

dynamically, which can be useful if joint instability is suspected (Kramer et al., 1997).

Despite the technical limitations of ultrasonography, this diagnostic modality can be useful in detecting pathologies such as bite wounds, foreign bodies, and/or soft tissue masses, particularly if combined with ultrasound-guided needle aspiration and cytological examination (Kramer et al., 1997). Ultrasonography is a complementary tool when combined with other diagnostic modalities.

Advance imaging (CT scan, MRI)

CT scan provides higher contrast and resolution, compared to conventional radiography, which allows better visualisation of anatomical structures such as bone and articular surfaces (Ohlerth, Voss and Steffen, 2009). This is of particular interest for small size patients, like cats. CT is also more sensitive at detecting bone lysis (Hoskinson and Tucker, 2001), which is of diagnostic value in cases of suspected neoplastic or infectious disease (Ohlerth, Voss and Steffen, 2009), detecting new bone formation (Hoskinson and Tucker, 2001), and soft tissue mineralisation (Streubel et al., 2015). Other advantages of CT scan include the ability to eliminate opacities caused by superimposed tissues, visualise structures in 3D, and enhance depth perception for observers (Hoskinson and Tucker, 2001). Furthermore, CT scan images can be displayed in different, pre-adjusted settings (window and level), enhancing the visualisation of soft tissues or osseous structures (Hoskinson and Tucker, 2001). Lastly, a CT scan enables the creation of reconstruction images from the original acquisition data, making it possible to create a tri-dimensional image simulation for preoperative planning and enhance understanding of the extent of the pathology (Hoskinson and Tucker, 2001) (Figure 24).

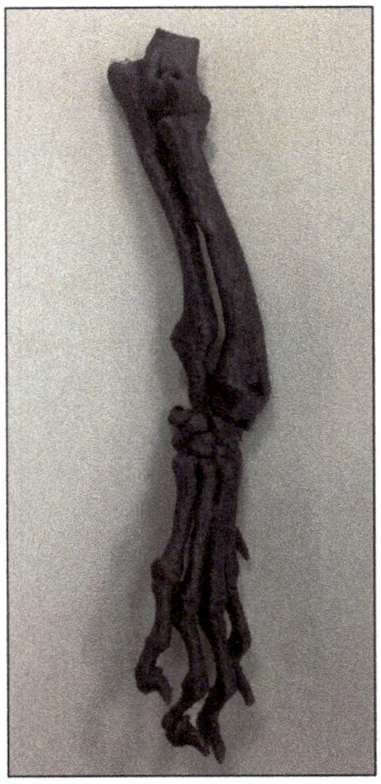

Figure 24. 3D model of the right forelimb in a young cat diagnosed with an angular limb deformity. The model was created using CT scan images and a 3D printer.

Despite these advantages, soft tissue contrast resolution is not as good as alternative imaging modalities, such as MRI. Additionally, metal devices, such as orthopaedic implants cause artefacts which affect image interpretation (Hoskinson and Tucker, 2001).

MRI provides better soft tissue resolution compared to CT, which is useful for evaluating neurological disorders and pathologies affecting muscles, tendons, synovial linings, or ligaments. MRI also enables the acquisition of images in any desired anatomic plane (Hoskinson and Tucker, 2001). In small animal orthopaedics, this diagnostic tool enables early detection of articular cartilage destruction (Hoskinson and Tucker, 2001). However, high-resolution MRI machines (1.5 – 3 Tesla) are needed for small size joints, like those of cats (Hoskinson and Tucker, 2001).

The advantages of MRI for the diagnosis of spinal diseases is well established in humans. MRI is the ideal technique in small animals for investigation of suspected spinal cord, brain, or peripheral nerve pathologies (Hoskinson and Tucker, 2001). However, MRI provides less bone details compared to a CT scan (Ohlerth, Voss and Steffen, 2009). This limitation, along with the small size of feline bones and joints, make this imaging modality less suitable for the evaluation of primary bone disorders in cats (Ohlerth, Voss and Steffen, 2009).

The main limitations of advanced imaging techniques like CT and MRI are cost-related, such as the costs associated with equipment, facilities, and maintenance. Another limitation is the need to obtain the images under general anaesthesia. Furthermore, there is a need to have skilled technical support in order to run the machines and for the interpretation of the images (Hoskinson and Tucker, 2001). Despite these limitations, advanced imaging techniques are essential tools for the diagnosis of musculoskeletal disorders in small animals.

Myelography

The main clinical indication for myelography is the identification of focal spinal cord lesions, when inflammatory/infectious conditions have been excluded during the evaluation of the cerebrospinal fluid (CSF) analysis (Ohlerth, Voss and Steffen, 2009). The information provided by this diagnostic modality helps to identify potential compressive spinal cord lesions as the cause of lameness or abnormal gait. It also helps the clinician to infer whether the patient requires decompressive surgery. Myelography is recommended when other, less invasive diagnostic tests have not identified the cause of the pathology. This is due to the **potential complications which can arise** during the test, such as spinal cord trauma, iatrogenic haemorrhage, blood contamination during needle insertion (which affects CSF analysis), or post-contrast administration seizures (Gaitero, 2017). Fortunately, the incidence of these complications is low when the test is performed by an experienced clinician.

Before performing the spinal tap, plain orthogonal radiographs of the entire spinal vertebrae should be obtained. This helps detect potential anatomic variations (e.g. an abnormal number of vertebrae, abnormal vertebrae, bone lesions) and indicate the ideal patient position.

Thereafter, the side of the spine for the tap should be selected. Lumbar tap is technically more challenging than cerebellomedullary cistern puncture, due to the smaller space for needle insertion, particularly in cats (Figure 25). However, it carries a lower risk of complication during the puncture (Lowrie and Anderson, 2011). Regardless of the site of needle penetration, aseptic techniques should always be used.

The patient should be properly positioned, as oblicuity during the procedure affects needle insertion and it can lead to complications. (Gaitero, 2017; Lowrie and Anderson, 2011). Once the needle is in place, a CSF sample should be collected prior to contrast injection. Cytological examination of the CSF significantly changes with storage due to the low-protein environment which causes rapid lysis of cells (Lowrie and Anderson, 2011). Therefore, CSF samples should be analysed within 30 minutes of collection to avoid misinterpretation of the results (Lowrie and Anderson, 2011). For samples not containing a high enough number of cells, centrifugation, or alternative methods, to remove the supernatant are recommended to improve the interpretation (Lowrie and Anderson,

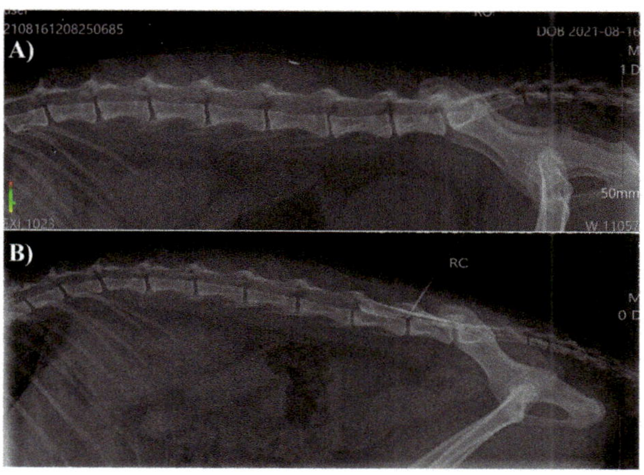

Figure 25. A) Lateral radiographs of the caudal spine (lumbar, sacral and coccygeal vertebrae) in an adult cat with acute onset paraparesia. B) A lumbar puncture has been performed to slowly inject the contrast medium.

2011). Basic analysis of the CSF includes general appearance, cell count, protein quantification, and presence of infectious diseases such as toxoplasmosis, neosporosis, and feline infectious peritonitis (FIP) (Lowrie and Anderson, 2011).

Once CSF analysis has excluded inflammatory or infectious disease, the contrast agent should be injected through the needle at the selected puncture site. Contrast should be injected slowly in conjunction with careful anaesthetic monitoring.

A potential complication is post-contrast administration seizures, which can occur up to 24-hours from contrast administration (Roberts and Selcer, 1993). Although the incidence is low, and newer contrast agents are now used in place of older, more neurotoxic agents, it is recommended that small volumes of contrast are used. Additionally, anticonvulsive drugs should be readily available (diazepam, pentobarbital, and phenobarbital) in case they are required (Roberts and Selcer, 1993).

Immediately after contrast administration, lateral, ventrodorsal, and oblique radiographs should be taken to highlight how the contrast travels cranially (lumbar puncture) or caudally (cisterna magna injection) (Ohlerth, Voss and Steffen, 2009). To facilitate pooling of the contrast in the area of interest, the pelvic limbs or the head can be elevated, respectively (Ohlerth, Voss and Steffen, 2009) (Figure 26). If dynamic compression of the spinal cord is suspected, flexion, extension, compression, or distraction images of the spine should be added to the study (Ohlerth, Voss and Steffen, 2009). In cases of suspected disc herniation, when myelography is combined with a CT scan (CT myelography), an initial, plain CT scan is recommended prior to myelography (Figure 27). In some instances, "normal" CT images may reveal a compressive lesion without the need for contrast administration (Robertson and Thrall, 2011). High field MRI avoids the need for myelography, and is considered the optimal diagnostic modality for myelopathy in small animals (Robertson and Thrall, 2011). In the absence of MRI, CT myelography is the next best option, as it enables CSF evaluation (Robertson and Thrall, 2011).

Arthrocentesis

Arthrocentesis, or joint tap, is the aspiration of synovial fluid from a joint for diagnostic purposes. It is an essential diagnostic tool when joint pathology is suspected. The procedure causes minimal morbidity and, when combined with other diagnostic procedures, such as radiography and CT scan, assists in the diagnosis of joint pathology. Arthrocentesis can be performed in most peripheral appendicular joints. However, because of the small size of feline joints, it is more technically

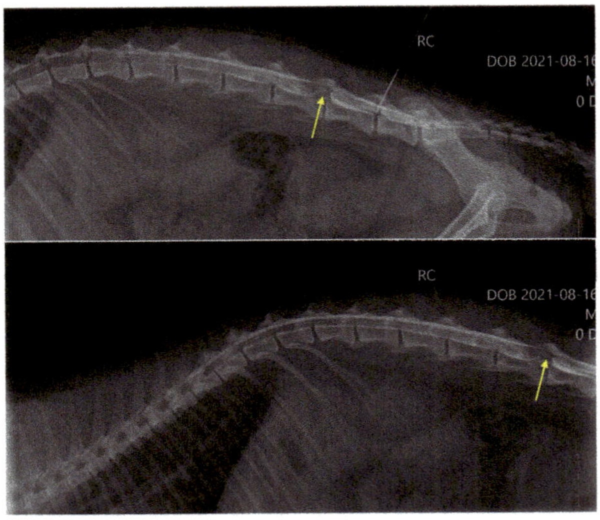

Figure 26. Cranial pooling of contrast medium. The defect in the ventral contrast column at the L5-L6 intervertebral disc space can be observed.

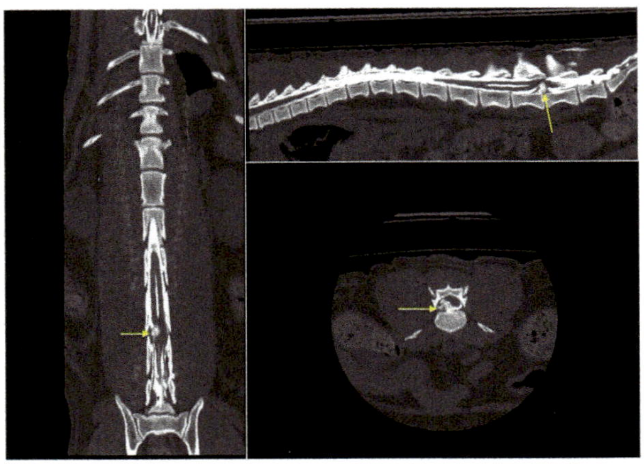

Figure 27. CT myelogram in the same patient shown in Figure 26 (frontal, sagittal and transverse plane images). There is a hyperattenuating structure at the L5-L6 intervertebral disc space causing ventrolateral compression of the spinal cord. The patient was diagnosed with an intervertebral disc herniation (Hansen type 1).

challenging compared to in dogs (Ohlerth, Voss and Steffen, 2009).

The main indications for arthrocentesis are:

- to confirm suspected joint pathology
- to eliminate other causes of lameness or systemic symptoms, such as pyrexia of unknown origin
- to evaluate the response to medical treatment, e.g. in cases of immune-mediated polyarthritis (Clements, 2006).

Analysis of synovial fluid is not helpful for diagnosing joint neoplasia, as this type of tumours do not tend to exfoliate cells into the joint fluid (Clements, 2006).

Arthrocentesis requires the patient to be sedated or under general anaesthesia. Anatomical landmarks for needle insertion on each joint are described in Table 1 (see some examples in Figures 28 and 29). The patient should be placed in lateral recumbency with the affected limb uppermost. The area of interest should be clipped and prepared aseptically, and the needle should also be inserted in a sterile manner.

If the pathology is mono-articular (only one joint affected), a single joint tap is required. If the pathology affects more than one joint, arthrocentesis of at least three joints is recommended (Bennett and Nash, 1988). One of the main causes of monoarthropathy in cats is an infected joint (Bennett and Nash, 1988). Larger joints, like the stifle, are commonly affected. However, as the main cause of septic arthritis in cats is bite wounds, distal joints can also be affected via the inoculation of microorganisms through a penetrating wound (Bennett and Nash, 1988).

Several joints may be affected in diseases such as immune-mediated polyarthritis. Compared to dogs, primary immune-mediated polyarthritis is less common in cats. When it does occur, it tends to appear as a consequence of systemic diseases, such as feline

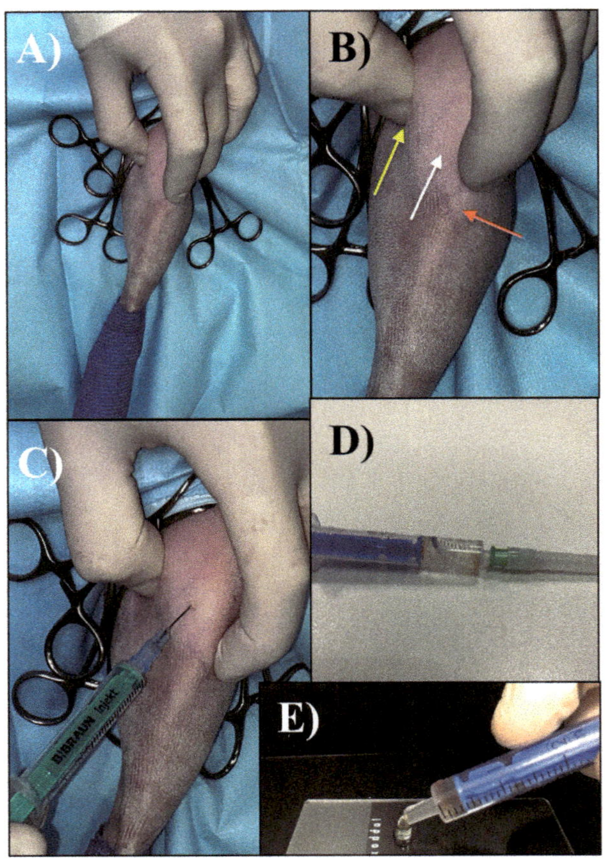

Figure 28. A) Stifle arthrocentesis in an adult cat. B) Anatomical landmarks for stifle arthrocentesis include the medial aspect of the femoral condyle (yellow arrow), the patella tendon and its insertion at the tibial tuberosity (red arrow). The needle is introduced medial (white arrow) or lateral to the patella tendon in a caudoproximal direction (C). Approximately 1 ml (D) of light yellow/clear (E) joint fluid is obtained in healthy joints.

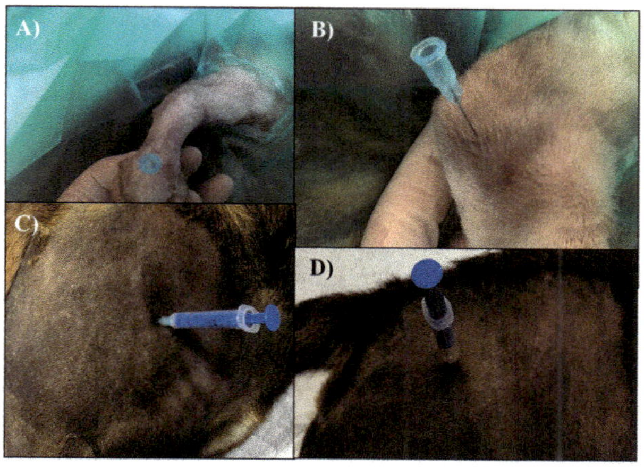

Figure 29. Arthrocentesis of the right carpus (A), elbow (B), shoulder (C) and hip (D) in cadavers to show the site of needle penetration.

immunodeficiency virus (FIV) or feline leukaemia virus (FeLV) (Lemetayer and Taylor, 2014). Immune-mediated arthritis tends to be more pronounced in small distal joints (hock, carpus). However, larger joints can also be affected, so several joint taps are required to make a diagnosis (Bennett and Nash, 1988).

A small needle of normal length (25G, 22G, 5/8 inches) is sufficient to tap most feline joints (Lemetayer and Taylor, 2014). For deeper joints, such as the hip and shoulder, larger needles may be used (Lemetayer and Taylor, 2014). As feline joints are small, negative pressure, using a 3 mL syringe, obtains a small amount of joint fluid (2 – 3 drops) (Lemetayer and Taylor, 2014). Immediately after extraction, the fluid should be evaluated for macroscopic changes in volume, colour, viscosity, and turbidity (Clements, 2006) (Figure 30). Increased volume, abnormal colour, reduced viscosity, or increased turbidity are some of the changes observed with joint pathology (Clements, 2006). Samples should be evaluated under a microscope and then submitted for bacterial culture. If a larger amount of fluid is obtained and cytology cannot be performed in-house, the fluid can be placed in an EDTA tube for submission to an external lab.

Cytology of synovial fluid aims to identify the predominant cells and differentiate inflammatory from non-inflammatory conditions (Clements, 2006). For joint neoplasia, cytology has no diagnostic value (Clements, 2006). When performing cytology of joint fluid, it is important not only to identify the main cell population but also to estimate the cell count. This can be done using automated cell counters or pre-existing formulas (see Table 5).

Abnormal cellularity with the presence of intra/extracellular microorganisms is typical of septic arthritis (Ohlerth, Voss and Steffen, 2009), however, the joint fluid should also be submitted for bacterial culture. As

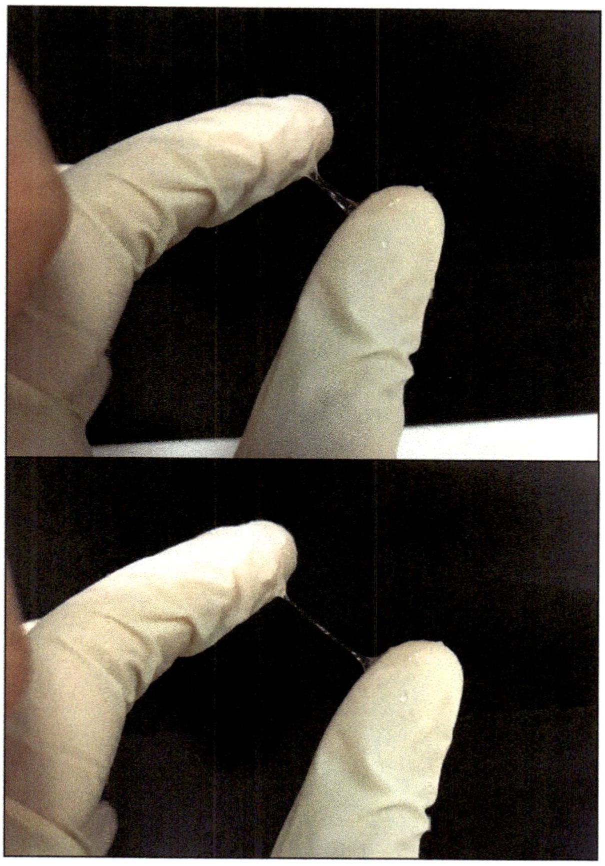

Figure 30. Viscosity of the joint fluid can be checked by observing the length of the string formed between the fingers as they are moved away. Strings of > 1 cm are considered normal.

previously mentioned, bite wounds are the primary cause of septic joints in cats (Bennett and Nash, 1988). In contrast to dog bites, cat bites cause deep puncture wounds which create an ideal environment for anaerobic microorganism growth (Abrahamian and Goldstein, 2011). Therefore, samples should be tested to identify aerobic and anaerobic microorganisms. Although not commonly reported, *Mycoplasma spp.* can cause joint infections. Therefore, samples should be tested for this microorganism (Liehmann et al., 2006). The majority of septic arthritis affect a single joint. Polyarthritic bacterial infections are rare and suggest haematogenous bacterial spreading (Lemetayer and Taylor, 2014). In these cases, when the microorganism is not identified in the joint fluid, an attempt should be made to identify the origin of the infection by running urinalysis, blood analysis, or CSF culture (e.g. for bacterial meningoencephalitis) (Lemetayer and Taylor, 2014). Bacterial culture of joint fluid is not perfectly sensitive, therefore, a negative result does not exclude a septic joint (Montgomery et al., 1989). To decrease the number of false-negative results, samples should be submitted in blood culture bottles (Figure 31B) or other enrichment media rather than in standard bacterial swabs (Montgomery et al., 1989; Taylor and Scott-Moncrieff, 2013).

Table 5. Macroscopic and microscopic changes in the synovial fluid of cats (adapted from Clements, 2006; Bennett and Nash, 1988; Lemetayer and Taylor, 2014).

Diagnosis	Volume	Macroscopic appearance	Viscosity	Cell count[†] (%)	
Normal	0.1 ml (small joints) 0.25 ml (larger joints)	Colourless Light yellow Clear	High (strand of fluid between fingers of > 1 cm)	*Monocytes/ macrophages* > 95%	*PMN cells (neutrophils)* < 10%
DJD (osteoarthritis)	Reduced Normal Increased	Colourless Light yellow Clear	High or slightly reduced	> 95%	< 10%
Traumatic arthropathy[¶]	Normal Increased	Yellow Blood-tinged	Reduced	> 90%	< 10%
Septic arthropathy[‡]	Increased	Yellow Serosanguineous Turbid	Reduced	< 75%	> 25%
Immune-mediated polyarthritis (IMPA)[§]	Normal Increased	Yellow Serosanguineous Turbid	Reduced	< 80%	> 20%

[†]Total cell count can be estimated by calculating the number of cells in a high power (× 400) field. This value corresponds to approximately 1000 cells/μl (Clements, 2006).
[¶]Red blood cells can be identified in non-contaminated samples.
[‡]Intracellular and extracellular bacteria can be identified in non-contaminated samples.
[§]Diagnosis of IMPA is based on clinical signs and abnormal cytological findings in a minimum of 3 joints.

Other synovial fluid tests include the mucin clot test (rarely used in small animals), glucose concentration test (used in humans and horses), and tests to determine protein and lactate levels (Clements, 2006; Proot, De Vicente and Sheahan, 2015). Protein concentration in synovial fluid changes with pathology (Ohlerth, Voss and Steffen, 2009). The protein concentration can be measured with a refractometer and tends to increase with inflammation. However, the test cannot differentiate if the increased concentration is caused by inflammation or by infectious conditions (Clements, 2006). Determination of lactate levels in synovial fluid cannot differentiate between changes that are immune-mediated and changes that are caused by degenerative joint disease. However, it is a quick and cost-effective way to exclude infection, as lactate concentration significantly increases in septic arthritis (Proot, De Vicente and Sheahan, 2015).

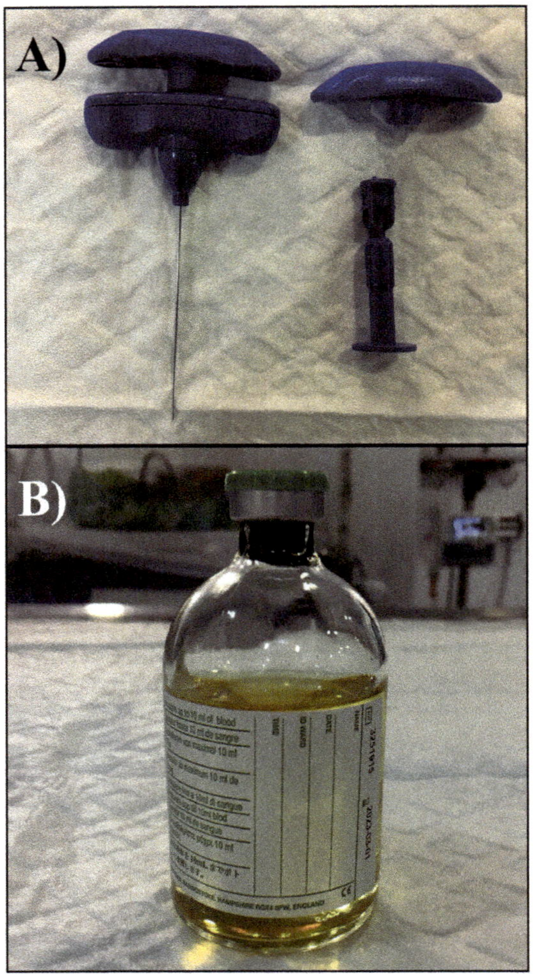

Figure 31. A) Jamshidi biopsy needle; B) Enrichment media (blood culture bottle).

Biopsy (bone, synovium, muscle and nerves)

Bone biopsy is indicated to investigate osteolytic or osteoproliferative lesions and to differentiate between inflammatory, infectious, or neoplastic processes (Ohlerth, Voss and Steffen, 2009). In cases of neoplasia, biopsy also helps identify the tumour type.

Prior to performing a bone biopsy, the viability of other less invasive techniques should be considered (such as fine needle aspirate or cytology) especially for osteolytic lesions.

When correctly performed, FNA and bone cytology is diagnostic in up to 80% of cases (Sabattini et al., 2017). However, the results largely depend on sampling technique and the ability to collect tumour cells. Moreover, cytology may not identify the tumour type, which plays a significant role in determining the prognosis and treatment plan (Ohlerth, Voss and Steffen, 2009). For such cases, bone biopsy should be considered.

Once the area from which the sample will be taken is identified (via radiographs, ultrasound, or CT scan) the patient is anaesthetised, and the biopsy site clipped and prepared in an aseptic manner. Jamshidi biopsy needles are ideal for cats due to their smaller core diameter, which reduces the risk of post-biopsy fracture (Ohlerth, Voss and Steffen, 2009) (Figure 31A). For bone biopsy, the sample should be taken from the centre of the lesion, which is why radiographs are used to identify the target sample site. For some cases a small skin incision, with minimal dissection of soft tissue is required. Samples should be submitted for histopathology and bacterial culture, particularly if the bone lesion is associated with infection. Prior to fixing the sample in formalin, impression smears of the biopsy should be done for microscopic evaluation.

There are few indicators for synovium biopsy as tumours of the joint capsule are rare in cats. When they do occur, they mainly arise from the periarticular soft tissues rather than the joint itself (Liptak and Forrest, 2007). Excluding neoplasia, another indication of biopsy of the joint capsule is to investigate septic arthritis, as cultures of tissue samples may identify microorganisms not identified in the joint fluid (Montgomery et al., 1989). Additionally, joint capsule biopsy may identify rare inflammatory joint conditions (Ohlerth, Voss and Steffen, 2009). Synovial biopsies are obtained from the same locations as arthrocentesis. However, due to the small sizes of feline joints, the procedure requires a minor surgical approach to acquire diagnostic samples (Ohlerth, Voss and Steffen, 2009). Incisional biopsies via direct visualisation by arthrotomy or arthroscopic-assisted procedures are often diagnostic, and therefore the techniques of choice for cats (Ohlerth, Voss and Steffen, 2009).

Muscle and nerve biopsies are used for the diagnosis of neuromuscular diseases in cats. Although less invasive techniques, such as neurological examination and electromyography, can provide valuable information, only nerve and muscle biopsies provide specific information regarding the nature of pathologies affecting the motor unit, sensory or autonomic nerves (Dickinson and LeCouteur, 2002). Clinical indications for this technique are the investigation of generalised or focal muscle conditions (weakness, stiffness, contracture, atrophy, and hypertrophy), underlying motor unit disease (myotonia), biochemical abnormalities in muscle metabolism (lactic acidaemia, elevated creatine kinase, or myoglobinuria), or degenerative processes (demyelination, axonal loss) (Dickinson and LeCouteur, 2002).

Prior to considering the procedure, it is important to rule out systemic pathologies that can cause muscle wastage and weakness, such as neuropathic diabetes mellitus (Godfrey, 2005), or hyperadrenocorticism (Boland and Barrs, 2017). A suitable biopsy site needs to be identified and the sample should be representative of the pathology. For muscular biopsy, criteria to select the biopsy site are described in Table 6.

Some of the common muscles used for biopsy purposes are the *triceps braquii, tibial cranialis* (Figure 32), and masticatory muscles such as the maseter and temporalis (Dickinson and LeCouteur, 2002). Although the procedure can be performed by percutaneous needle biopsy insertion, a minor surgical approach is advantageous, as the clinician can visualise the orientation of the muscle fibres, which is important for laboratory interpretation (Dickinson and LeCouteur, 2002). Criteria for the selection of the nerve biopsy site are similar to those described for muscle biopsy sites. Additionally, a nerve that innervates a muscle where biopsies are routinely taken should be selected (Dickinson and LeCouteur, 2002). The common peroneal (Figure 32) and tibial nerves are commonly selected for the pelvic limbs, while the ulnar nerve is commonly selected for the thoracic limbs (Dickinson and LeCouteur, 2002). If pathology of the ventral nerve roots of the spinal cord is suspected, a more invasive surgical approach (laminectomy) is required (Dickinson and LeCouteur, 2002). Adequate storage and preparation of the biopsies is essential to ensure accurate interpretation of the samples, particularly if they are submitted to external labs or require more complex laboratory tests (Dickinson and LeCouteur, 2002) (Figure 32).

Table 6. Criteria for selection of muscle biopsy sites (adapted from (Dickinson and LeCouteur, 2002).

Criteria	Comments
Clinical examination (acute presentation)	Select the muscle/s which are clinically abnormal (atrophy, hypertrophy, weakness, pain)
Clinical examination (chronic presentation)	Select the muscle/s which are least affected†
Electromyography (EMG)	Select the muscle/s with abnormal EMG data
Surgeon criteria	Muscle/s easily identified Minor surgical approach Low patient morbidity

†Chronic degenerative changes may affect interpretation of the biopsy.

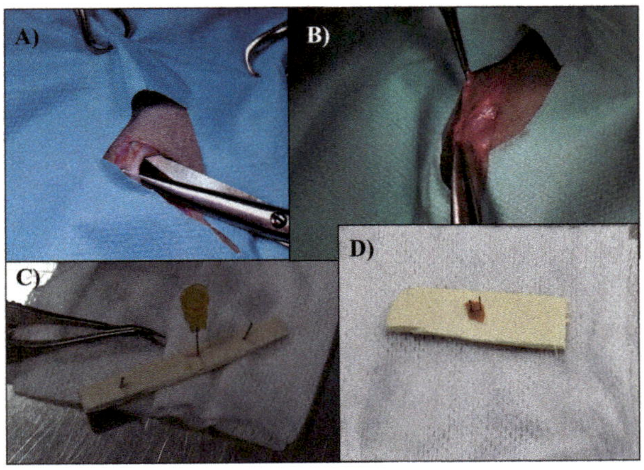

Figure 32. Biopsies of the common peroneal nerve (A) and tibial cranialis muscle (B). Preparation of the nerve (C) and muscle (D) biopsy before submission. (Image courtesy of Alejandro Luján).

The feline trauma patient

General management

When presented with a feline trauma patient, especially one with bone fractures, it is essential to recognise and treat non-orthopaedic injuries which could be potentially life-threatening. High energy traumas (road traffic accident, fall from a height) require that special attention is paid to the ABCs (airway, breathing, circulation) (Hernon, Gurney and Gibson, 2018). It is recommended that a full general physical exam, basic laboratory investigations, thoracic radiographs, and FAST abdominal ultrasound are done to exclude life-threatening conditions. Adequate emergency treatment, including intravenous fluid therapy (IVFT), multimodal analgesia, and/or oxygen therapy, may be required in some cases (Hernon, Gurney and Gibson, 2018). Once the clinician has confirmed the patient does not have life-threatening conditions or those has been adequately treated, the focus can shift to the orthopaedic condition. However, it is important to perform a neurological exam first, as the presence of neurological deficits may affect decision-making.

Emergency orthopaedic treatment is generally not required for trauma patients, with the exception of open and articular fractures. The priority is stabilisation of conditions affecting the ABCs or treatment of soft tissue injuries such as splenic rupture, bladder rupture or traumatic diaphragmatic herniation.

Open fractures commonly occur in anatomical locations with little soft tissue coverage, such as the distal part of the extremities (Figure 33). Primary treatment focuses on open wound management (Zalabras et al., 2007). The wound should be covered with a sterile dressing to prevent contamination. Once the patient is stable, further wound evaluation under sedation or general anaesthesia can be done.

An important part of wound assessment is **checking for adequate blood perfusion to the area**. Indicators of poor tissue viability include:

- lack of an arterial pulse
- low temperature
- severe congestion
- cyanosis.

When in doubt, the wound should be reassessed 12–24 hours after the initial assessment, as further changes may be more obvious.

Good open fracture management involves adequate clipping of the area, aseptic wound manipulation, and cleaning (Millard and Towle, 2012), with the debridement of nonviable tissue considered the most important factor in preventing infection and facilitating wound healing with no complications (Millard and Towle, 2012). Removing unviable tissues brings benefits such as increases in oxygen tension, improvements in blood perfusion, increases the number of local inflammatory cells, and elimination of detritus that acts as a culture for bacterial growth. During wound debridement, a careful manipulation of the bony fragments attached to muscles or tendons is required; however, fragments that are completely loose should be removed to avoid the development of a sequestrum (Millard and Towle, 2012). Following debridement, the area should be covered with a dressing and systemic antibiotics administered immediately for a minimum of 5 – 6 days (Zalabras et al., 2007).

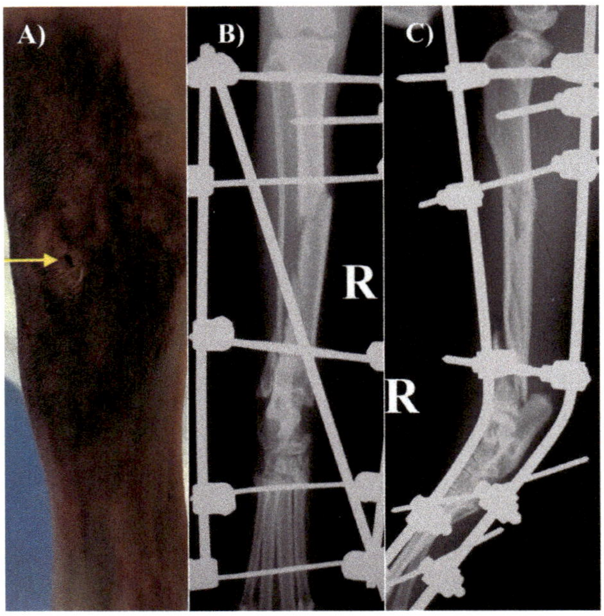

Figure 33. A) Open (yellow arrow) comminuted right tibial fracture in an adult cat. The fracture was repaired with a linear external fixator (B and C). (Courtesy of Carlos Macías.)

For articular fractures (Figure 34), delays in the surgical repair should be avoided because with prolonged joint immobilisation the articular cartilage rapidly degenerates. Considering the basic principles of articular fracture repair as outlined in the following paragraphs, proper surgical planning is mandatory. This occasionally involves the use of advanced imaging techniques, namely a CT scan (Macias and McKee, 2003).

The traumatised cat should always be provided with multimodal analgesia. Drugs available for such cases are well described in previous literature.

Bandages and dressings

In feline orthopaedics, bandages are used to:

- apply or relieve pressure on inflamed soft tissues associated with a fracture
- modulate pain
- restrict or allow safe movements
- provide stabilisation, immobilisation, or support to underlying structures (Campbell, 2006)
- protect wounds associated with areas of bone damage from contamination and mechanical forces from the environment
- if the orthopaedic condition is associated with soft tissue injuries (e.g. open fractures), the bandage provides the wound with additional protection from contamination and mechanical forces exerted by the environment, further aiding wound management (Campbell, 2006).

In rare cases, bandages and dressings are the primary treatment for fracture repair, except for greenstick fractures in young patients. They also provide additional support after a stronger primary treatment, such as in cases of joint luxation or subluxation (Kulendra and Arthurs, 2014; Earley and Dee, 1980).

Splints or casts are appropriate when additional stability is required. Commercial splints are available for cats, with thermomoldable materials such as fibreglass enable the splint to adapt to the shape of the patient's limb (Campbell, 2006). To minimise dressing-associated complications (Figure 35), the patient's hair should be clipped, the skin should be clean and adequate padding should be in place before applying the splint or cast. The dressing should be changed regularly (Campbell, 2006). If the dressing is also used for wound management, an adequate primary layer should be selected to be in direct contact with the wound, and the frequency of dressing changes selected based on the healing phase of the wound (Campbell, 2006).

Keeping a bandage in feline patients is always challenging due to their demeanour. Limb bandages tend to slip distally when the patient ambulates. Furthermore, cats tend to shake the limb causing the bandage to loosen and displace distally. To minimise this, strips of adhesive tape should be applied to healthy skin to act as anchor points. However, this is only possible if the toes do not need to be included in the dressing. The strips should be placed in a proximal to distal direction. The dressing should be applied and once nearly finished, the free ends of the strips rotated 180 degrees in a proximal direction and secured to the outer layers of the dressing.

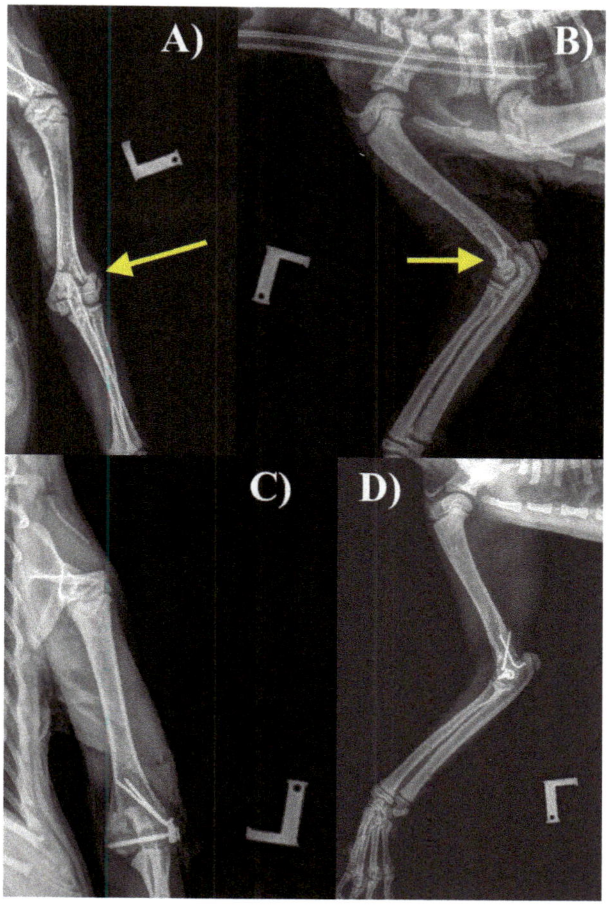

Figure 34. Orthogonal radiographs (A and B) of a 3-month-old Persian cat with a lateral condylar fracture (yellow arrow). The articular fracture was repaired (C and D) with a transcondylar screw and two anti- rotational Kirschner wires.

Another strategy to avoid dressing loosening is placement of adhesive tape or sticky dressing material between the end of the outer layer of the bandage and healthy skin, which acts as an additional anchor point.

Dressing changes often require sedation, especially when the dressing is used for open wound management.

Principles of fracture repair in cats: overview

The principles of fracture repair and joint surgery are similar in both dogs and cats; however, there are some

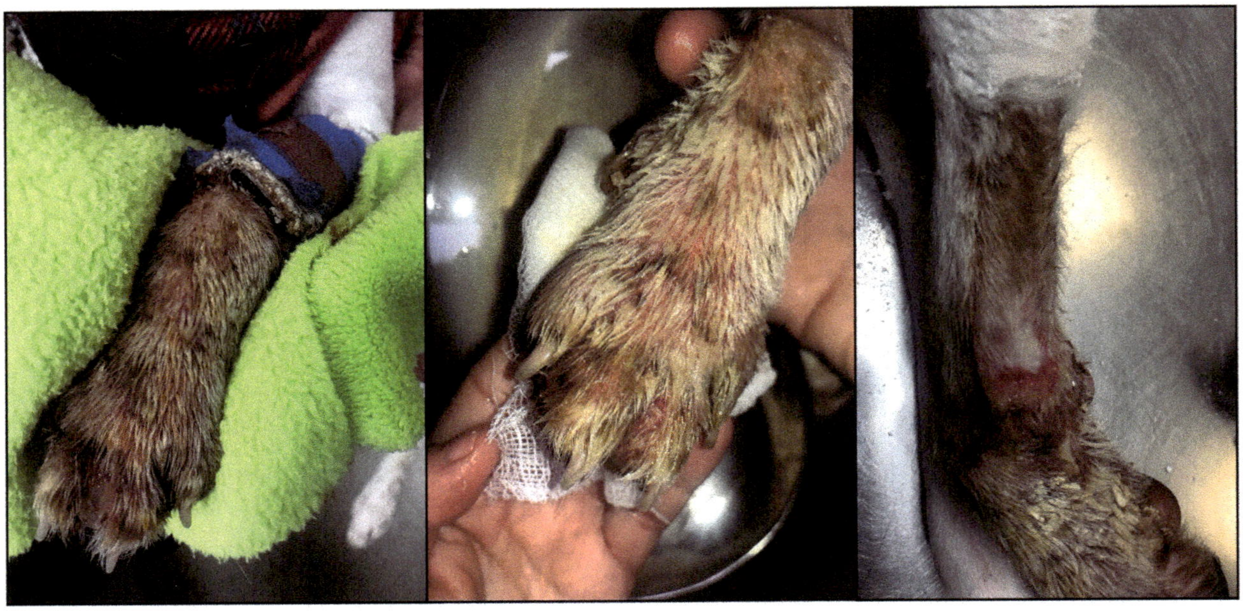

Figure 35. Inappropriate application of a splinted bandage caused severe dressing associated complications in this patient. (Images courtesy of J. José Vilches García).

important differences to note. Compared to dogs, cat bones are straighter, and there is less size variation between breeds (Voss and Montavon, 2009). Despite the lighter bodyweight of cats, complications following fracture repair can still occur, and therefore, the selection of an adequate fixation method that considers both fracture biomechanics and biology is essential for a good outcome.

Decision making regarding the method of fracture repairs **requires consideration of whether a biological or anatomical approach is most appropriate**.

Before selecting a method of fracture repair, one should decide whether an anatomical or a biological approach for fracture resolution should be selected. For some types of fractures (e.g. articular fractures), an **anatomical approach** is typically selected (Figure 34). This means the surgeon tries to put all the pieces of the puzzle together in a near-perfect manner in an attempt to achieve primary bone healing (Voss and Montavon, 2009). For other types of fractures (e.g. highly comminuted diaphyseal fractures or open fractures) a biological approach is typically chosen, so that secondary bone healing occurs. For the latter, the surgeon lines up the main fracture fragments, without disturbing the fracture callus (or with minimal disturbance), so as not to interfere with the biological environment (Figure 36). The surgical approach and the orthopaedic implants selected for fracture fixation vary between these two types of osteosynthesis (Voss and Montavon, 2009).

Another consideration is **fracture biomechanics and the method of fixation**. The surgeon must be aware of the forces acting on the fracture and select a fixation system that neutralises them all.

The main forces acting on bone are **torsion, bending, axial compression, and tension** (Voss and Montavon, 2009). Implants that are considered primary methods of fracture fixation, such as plates, interlocking nails, intramedullary pins and external fixators, can neutralise these forces when applied properly (Johnston et al., 2012). Secondary or supplementary methods of fracture fixation are those that reinforce primary methods of repair or hold bony fragments in place before a primary method is applied (Johnston et al., 2012). Examples of these methods include interfragmentary screws, cerclage and Kirschner wires, and Steinmann pins (Johnston et al., 2012).

Another factor to consider in fracture repair is the patient's age. In mature animals, a more rigid stabilisation is typically used. In immature animals, the abundant extra-osseous blood supply from the periosteum enables faster bone healing (Voss and Montavon, 2009). Moreover, the soft quality of cortical bone in younger animals means that orthopaedic implants are not held in a similar way to adults which impacts on implant selection; the latter typically have increased plasticity and the fixation is less rigid (Voss and Montavon, 2009) (Figures 37 and 38).

Particular considerations are required for specific types of fractures, such as **articular and open fractures**. Articular and periarticular fractures may occur in immature and mature animals. However, they occur more frequently in growing (immature) patients due to relatively weak growth plates at the extremities of the long bones (Macias and McKee, 2003). They also can occur at the insertion sites of tendons and ligaments (avulsion fractures) as the growth plate is weaker than the tendon or ligament attachment to the bone

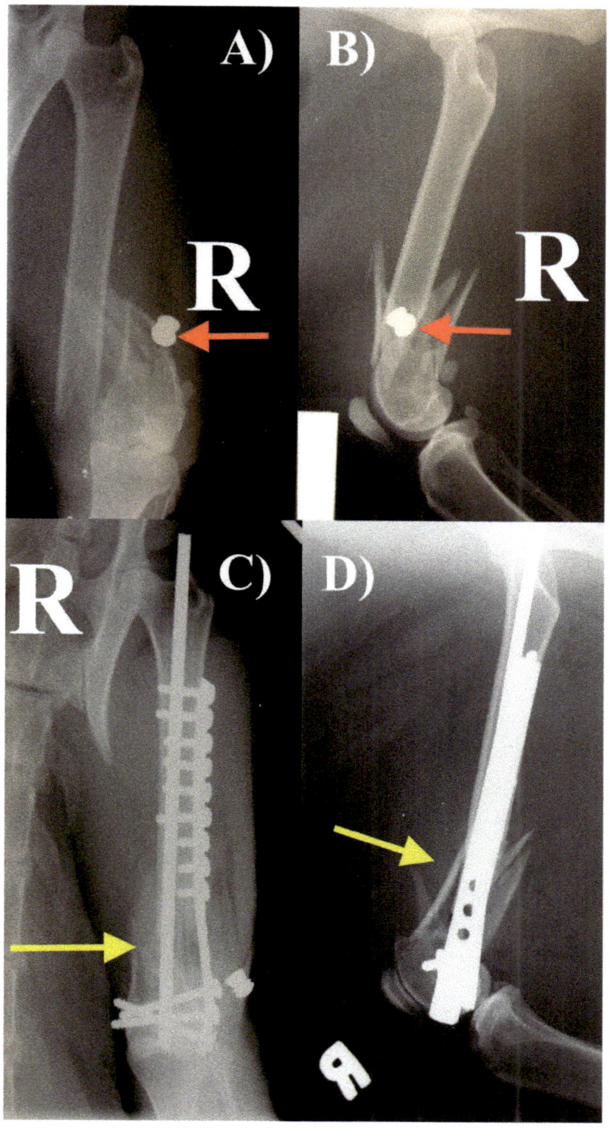

Figure 36. A) and B) Highly comminuted fracture of the distal diaphysis of the right femur in an adult Domestic Shorthair after being shot with a pellet gun (red arrows). C) and D) The fracture was repaired using a more biological approach, with a combination of an intramedullary pin and a bridging plate (plate-rod configuration). No attempts were made to reduce all the small fragments (yellow arrows). Instead, the main fragments were aligned to look for secondary bone healing. (Courtesy of Carlos Macías).

(Macias and McKee, 2003). In mature animals, these types of fractures can occur, but tend to be associated with considerable trauma and present with a degree of comminution. Conversely, in immature patients, they tend to be two-fragment fractures (Macias and McKee, 2003).

The **basic principles of articular fracture repair** in the cat are to achieve a:

- near-perfect anatomical reconstruction
- use rigid fixation
- achieve a rapid return to joint function (Macias and McKee, 2003).

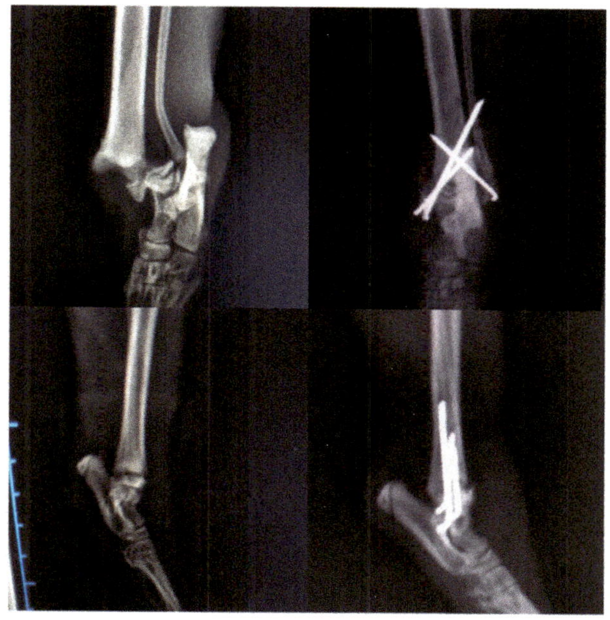

Figure 37. Distal tibial physeal fracture (Sa ter Harris type 1) in a young cat. The fracture was repaired with c-oss-pins. (Images courtesy of Pablo Corpas Laguna).

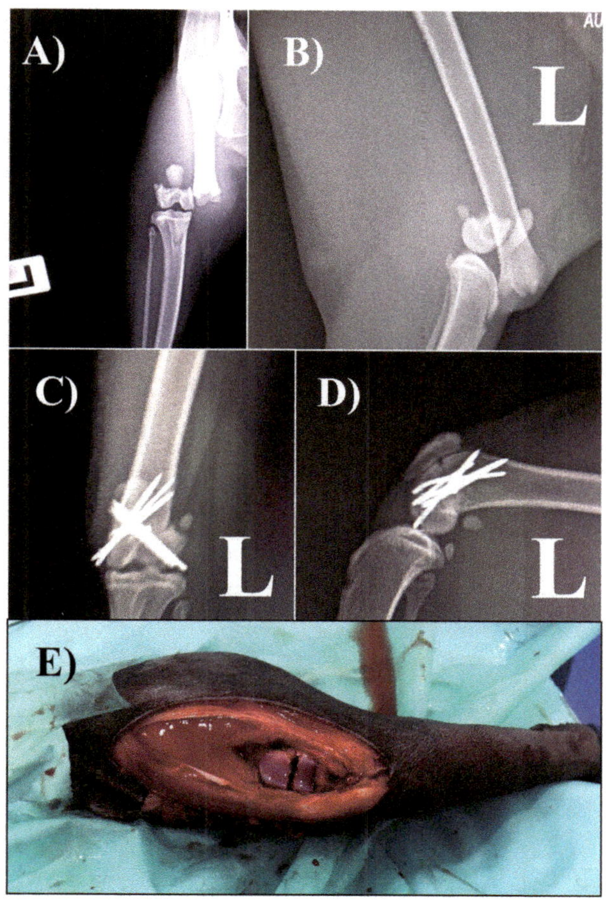

Figure 38. A) and B) Distal femoral physeal fracture (Salter Harris type 1) in an 8-month old male cat. C) and D) The fracture was repaired with cross-pins. E) Intraoperative image before fracture reduction.

In mature animals, this is achieved using primary and/or secondary orthopaedic implants such as plates, screws, and pins. However, in immature animals, implant selection differs, as some implants may interfere with the normal development of the physeal plate, particularly if the patient still has growth potential (Macias and MacKee, 2003; Voss and Montavon, 2009). In such cases, secondary orthopaedic implants (e.g. Kirschner wires or intramedullary pins) are typically selected using different configurations (Macias and MacKee, 2003; Voss and Montavon, 2009). Occasionally, when the fracture has healed, a second surgical procedure for implant removal is necessary in order to avoid interference with the growth plate.

For open fractures, alongside adequate wound management, the clinician must select a method of fixation that provides:

- adequate stability
- preserves the integrity of the remaining viable tissues
- allows for wound assessment (Gustilo and Merkow, 1990).

Linear or circular external fixators are commonly used to treat open fractures as they allow a biological approach as they preserve the local soft tissue, avoid vascular compromise, provide easy access to the wound bed for evaluation of soft tissue healing, and allow easy removal once fracture healing is completed (Gustilo and Merkow, 1990).

When properly applied and configured, they neutralise the forces acting upon the fracture. They are versatile and can be used for temporary immobilization of a joint if necessary (Griffiths and Bellenger, 1979) (Figure 39). Despite the clear advantages of external fixation, some fractures, such as highly comminuted or articular fractures, may require stronger methods of internal fixation.

Complications of fracture repair in the cat are similar to those in dogs. These include fracture union disorders (delayed union, non-union, mal-union), implant-related complications (breakage, migration), and infection (osteomyelitis, implant-associated infection). Union disorder complications may be related to biological factors (age of the patient, blood supply to the affected bone, type of fracture, type of trauma) or mechanical factors (inadequate method of fixation, excessively strong repair method) (Voss and Montavon, 2009).

Once a diagnosis of a union disorder complication is made, the clinician should **analyse which factor led to the complication** and adopt the appropriate strategies to resolve it. If the union disorder complication is related to a biological factor, bone grafting may be required to stimulate bone healing. If a mechanical factor is the cause, the clinician should consider making changes to the method of fixation, such as making it stronger or less rigid. Primary bone infection (post-traumatic osteomyelitis) is not as frequent in cats compared to dogs (Voss and Montavon, 2009). However, when infection occurs, it is mainly by extension from adjacent soft tissues or in association with open fractures (Griffiths and Bellenger, 1979). Although the infection may not arise from the orthopaedic implants, some of the microorganisms commonly isolated have the ability to colonise and survive on the implants, even if appropriate antibiotics are used (Voss and Montavon, 2009). Therefore, implant removal is commonly required once complete fracture healing has occurred to effectively eliminate the infection (Voss and Montavon, 2009) (Figure 40).

Physeal fractures in immature animals may cause premature closure of the growth plates, potentially leading

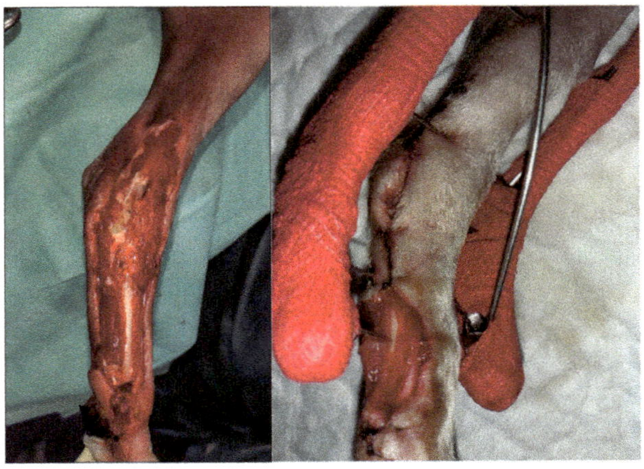

Figure 39. Open tarsal fracture/luxation stabilised with a trans-articular linear external fixator.

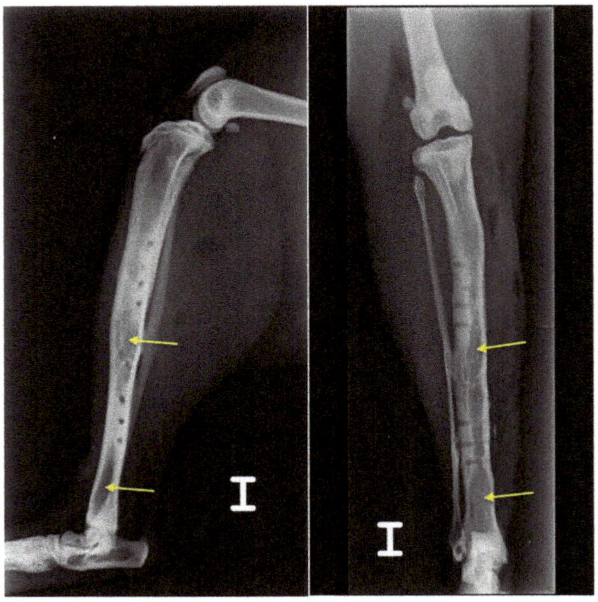

Figure 40. Postoperative radiographs after implant removal in an adult cat diagnosed with osteomyelitis. Observe the abnormal intramedullary pattern (yellow arrows), which suggests the infection is still active. (Image courtesy of Ivan Serra).

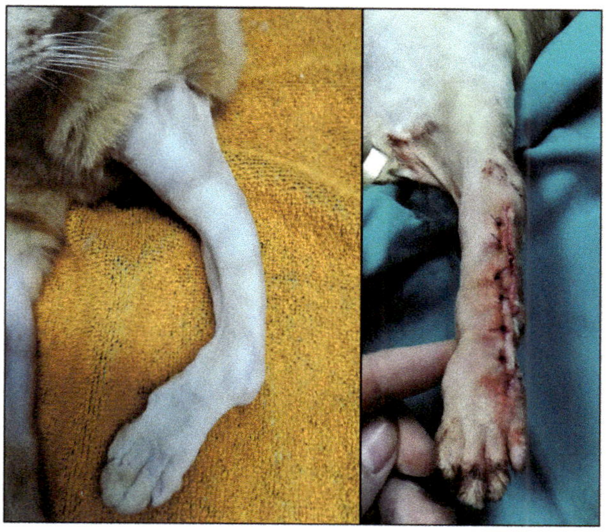

Figure 41. A) 2 year old rescued cat with an angular limb deformity due to premature closure of the distal physis of the left antebrachium. B) Immediate postoperative image after surgical resolution of the limb deformity. (Image courtesy of Pablo Corpas Laguna).

to angular limb deformities (Voss and Montavon, 2009). Although the clinical relevance in cats is not as severe as in dogs (due to the smaller growth potential of domestic cats), regular check-ups and follow-up radiographs are required in suspected cases (Voss and Montavon, 2009). As previously mentioned, removal of the orthopaedic implants used to treat physeal fractures in cats is occasionally required if the patient has growth potential, as the implants may cause premature physeal closure and lead to angular deformities (Figure 41).

References

Abrahamian FM., Goldstein EJC. Microbiology of animal bite wound infections. *Clin Microbiol. Rev.*, 2011; 24: 231–246

Agnello K. Surgical management of open fractures. In: *Small Animal Surgical Emergencies*. Aronson LR., 2016. 1st ed. Wiley-Blackwell, Ames, Iowa; pp. 533–542

Basa RM., Johnson KA. Management of feline carpal injuries. What are the options and when is arthrodesis indicated?. *J Fel Med and Surg.*, 2019; 21: 809–823

Beck KA. Caudocranial horizontal beam radiographic projection for evaluation of femoral fracture and osteotomy repair in dogs and cats. *J Am Vet Med Assoc.*, 1991; 198: 1751–1754

Bennet D., Morton CA. A study of owner observed behavioural and lifestyle changes in cats with musculoskeletal disease before and after analgesic therapy. *J Fel Med Surg.*, 2009; 11: 997–1004

Bennett D., Nash AS. Feline immune-based polyarthritis: a study of thirty-one cases. *J Small Anim Pract.*, 1988; 29: 501–523

Berry W. Is It neurological or orthopaedic?. *World Small Animal Veterinary Association World Congress*. Proceedings, 2014

Bingel SA., Riser WH. Congenital elbow luxation in the dog. *J Small Anim Pract.*, 1977; 18: 445–456

Boge GS., Engdahl K., Moldal ER., Bergström A. Cranial cruciate ligament disease in cats: an epidemiological retrospective study of 50 cats (2011–2016). *J Fel Med Surg.*, 2019; 22: 277–284

Boland LA., Barrs VR. Peculiarities of feline hyperadrenocorticism. Update on diagnosis and treatment. *J Fel Med Surg.*, 2017; 19: 933–947

Campbell BG. Dressings, bandages, and splints for wound management in dogs and cats. *Vet Clin North Am: Small Anim Pract.*, 2006; 36: 759–791

Clements D. Arthrocentesis and synovial fluid analysis in dogs and cats. *In Practice.*, 2006; 28: 256–262

Clarke S., Bennett D. Feline osteoarthritis: a prospective study of 28 cases. *J Small Anim Pract.*, 2006; 47: 439–445

Connery NA., Rackard S. The surgical treatment of traumatic stifle disruption in a cat. *Vet Comp Orthop Traumatol.*, 2000; 13: 208–211

Dantas BD., Durand A., Parkin T. Broome C. Establishment of normal anatomical radial angles in cats. *Vet Comp Orthop Traumatol.*, 2016; 29: 320–324

Dickinson PJ., LeCouteur RA. Muscle and nerve biopsy. *Vet Clin North Am: Small Anim Pract.*, 2002; 32: 62–102

Earley TD., Dee JF. Trauma to the carpus, tarsus, and phalanges of dogs and cats. *Vet Clin North Am: Small Anim Pract.*, 1980; 10: 717–747

Freire M., Meuten D., Lascelles D. Pathology of articular cartilage and synovial membrane from elbow joints with and without degenerative joint disease in domestic cats. *Vet Pathol.*, 2014; 51: 968–978

Freire-Gonzalez M., Brown J., Robertson ID., Pease AP., *et al.* Meniscal mineralization in domestic cats. *Vet Surg.*, 2010; 39: 545–552

Gaitero L. In: Current Techniques in Canine and Feline Neurosurgery. Shores A., and Brisson BA. 2017. 1st ed. Wilet and Sons; New Jersey, USA; pp. 85–91

Garosi L. Neurological examination of the cat. How to get started. *J Fel Med Surg.*, 2009; 11: 340–348

Godfrey D. Osteoarthritis in cats: a retrospective radiological study. *J Small Anim Pract.*, 2005; 46: 425–429

Gordon-Evans WJ. Feline orthopaedic examination. *Clinician's brief 2021*; April / May

Griffiths GL., Bellenger CR. A retrospective study of osteomyelitis in dogs and cats. *Aust Vet J.*, 1979; 55: 587–591

Griffon D. Osteomyelitis. In: *Complications in Small Animal Surgery*. Griffon D, Hamaide A., 2016. 1st ed. Wiley-Blackwell, Hoboken, New Jersey; pp. 28–33

Gustilo RB, Merkow RL, Templeman D. The management of open fractures. *J Bone Joint Surg Am.* 1990; 72: 299–304

Hayashi K., Manley PA., Muir P. Cranial cruciate ligament pathophysiology in dogs with cruciate disease: A review. *J Am Anim Hosp Assoc.*, 2004; 40: 385–390

Harasen GLG. Feline cranial cruciate rupture: 17 cases and a review of the literature. *Vet Comp Orthop Traumatol.*, 2005; 18: 254–257

Harris JE., Dhupa S. Lumbosacral intervertebral disk disease in six cats. *J Am Anim Hosp Assoc.*, 2008; 44: 109–115

Hardie E., Roe S., Martin F. Radiographic evidence of degenerative joint disease in geriatric cats: 100 cases (1994–1997). *J Am Vet Med Assoc.*, 2002; 220: 638–632

Hernon T., Gurney M., Gibson S. A retrospective study of feline trauma patients admitted to a referral centre. *J Small Anim Pract.*, 2018; 59: 243–247

Houlton JEF., Meynink SE. Medial patellar luxation in the cat. *J Small Anim Pract.*, 1989; 30: 349–352

Hoskinson JJ., Tucker RL. Diagnostic imaging of lameness in small animals. *Vet Clin North Am: Small Anim Pract.*, 2001; 31: 165–180

Jaeger GH., Marcellin-Little DJ., PePuy V., Lascelles BDX. Validity of goniometric joint measurements in cats. Am *J Vet Res.*, 2007; 68: 822–826

Johnston SA., von Pfeil DJF., Déjardin LM., Roe SC., *et al.* Internal Fracture Fixation. In: Tobias KM., Johnson SA. *Veterinary Surgery Small Animal.* 2012. 1st ed. Elsevier Saunders, St Louis, MO, USA; pp. 5226–5461

Johnson ME. Feline patellar luxation: a retrospective case study. *J Am Anim. Hosp. Assoc.*, 1986; 22: 835–838

Johson A. Non-Union. In: *Complications in Small Animal Surgery.* Griffon D, Hamaide A., 2016. 1st ed. Wiley-Blackwell, Hoboken, New Jersey; pp. 669–672

Johson A. Delayed Union. In: *Complications in Small Animal Surgery.* Griffon D, Hamaide A., 2016. 1st ed. Wiley-Blackwell, Hoboken, New Jersey; pp. 665–668

Kramek BA., Moise NS., Cooper B., Raffe MR. Neuropathy associated with diabetes mellitus in the cat. *J Am Vet Med Assoc.*, 1984; 184: 42–45

Kramer M., Gerwing M., Hach V., Schimke E. Sonography of the musculoskeletal system in dogs and cats. *Vet Radiol Ultrasound.*, 1997; 38: 139–149

Kerwin S. Orthopaedic examination in the cat. *J Fel Med Surg.*, 2012; 14: 6–12

Kene ROC., Lee R., Bennett D. The radiological features of congenital elbow luxation/subluxation in the dog. *J Small Anim Pract.*, 1982; 23: 621–630

Kulendra E., Arthurs G. Management and treatment of feline tarsal injuries. *In Practice* 2014; 36: 119–132

Lascelles BDX., Henry JB., Brown J., Robertson I., *et al.* Croos-sectional study evaluating the prevalence of radiographic degenerative joint disease in domesticated cats. *Vet Surg.*, 2010; 39: 535–544

Lascelles BDX. Bernie HD., Roe S., DePuy V., *et al.* Evaluation of client-specific outcome measures and activity monitoring to measure pain relief in cats with osteoarthritis. *J Vet Intern Med.*, 2007; 21: 410–416

Lascelles BDX., Dong YH., Marcellin-Little DJ., Thomson A., *et al.* Relationship of orthopaedic examination, goniometric measurements, and radiographic signs of degenerative joint disease in cats. *BMC Vet Research.*, 2012; 8:10

Langley-Hobbs SJ. Biology and radiological assessment of fracture healing. *In Practice*, 2003; 1: 26–35

Leonard CA., Tillson M. Feline Lameness. *Vet Clin North Am: Small Anim Pract.*, 2001; 31: 143–163

Lowrie M., Anderson J. Cerebrospinal fluid: analysis and interpretation in small animals. *In Practice*, 2011; 33: 78–85

Lemetayer J., Taylor S. Inflammatory joint disease in cats. Diagnostic approach and treatment. *J Fel Med. Surg.*, 2014; 16: 547–562

Liehmann L., Degasperi B., Spergser J., Niebauer GW. Mycoplasma felis arthritis in two cats. *J Small Anim Pract.*, 2006; 47: 476–479

Liptak JM., Forrest LJ. Soft tissue sarcomas. In: *Small Animal Clinical Oncology.* Withrow SJ and MacEwen EG., 2007. 4th ed. Saunder WB., Philadelphia, USA., pp. 425–454

Macias C., McKee M. Articular and periarticular fracutures in the dog and cat. *In Practice*, 2003; 25: 446–465

McNicholas WT., Wilkens BE., Blevins WE., Snyder PW., *et al.* Spontaneous femoral capital physeal fractures in adult cats: 26 cases (1996–2001). *J Am Vet Med Assoc.*, 2002; 221: 1731–1736

Messon R., Corr S. Management of pelvic trauma: neurological damage, urinary tract disruption and pelvic fractures. *J Fel Med Surg.*, 2011; 13: 347–361

Millard RP., Towle HA. Open fractures. In: Tobias KM., Johnson SA. *Veterinary Surgery Small Animal.* 2012. 1st ed. Elsevier Saunders, St Louis, MO, USA; pp. 572–575

Morton CM., Grant D., Johnston L., Letellier IM., et al. Clinical evaluation of meloxicam versus ketoprofen in cats suffering from painful acute locomotor disorders. *J Feline Med Surg.*, 2011; 13: 237–243

Montgomery RD., Long IR., Milton JL., DiPinto MN., *et al.* Comparison of aerobic culturette, synovial membrane biopsy, and blood culture medium in detection of canine bacterial arthritis. *Vet Surg.*, 1989: 18: 300–302

Muguet-Chanoit AC., Olby N., Lim JH., Gallagher R. The cutaneous trunci muscle reflex: A predictor of recovery in dogs with acute thoracolumbar myelopathis caused by intervertebral disc extrusions. *Vet Surg.*, 2012; 41: 200–206

Ohlerth S., Voss K., Steffen F. Further diagnostic procedures. In: *Feline Orthopaedic Surgery and Muskuloskeletal Disease.* Montavon PM., Voss K. and Langley-Hobss SJ., 2009. 1st ed. Saunders Elsevier, Philadelphia, USA., pp. 21–38

Owen MA. Use of contoured bar transhock external fixators in 17 cats. *J Small Anim Pract.*, 2000; 41: 440–446

Perry K. Feline hip dysplasia. A challenge to recognise and treat. *J Fel Med Surg.*, 2016; 18: 203–218

Perry KL. Elbow disease in cats. *ESVOT 2016*, London

Proot JLJ., De Vicente F., Sheahan DE. Analysis of lactate concentrations in canine synovial fluid. *Vet Comp Orthop Traumatol.*, 2015; 28: 301–305

Queen J., Bennett D., Carmichael S., Gibson N., *et al.* Femoral neck metaphyseal osteopathy in the cat. *Vet Rec.*, 1998; 142: 159–162

Roberts RE., Selcer BA. Myelography and epidurography. *Vet Clin North Am: Small Anim Pract.*, 1993; 23: 307–329

Robertson I., Thrall DE. Imaging dogs with suspected disc herniation: pros and cons of myelography, computed tomography, and magnetic resonance. *Vet Radiol.* Ultrasound., 2011; 52: S81–84

Rubinos C., Meeson RL. Traumatic physeal fractures in cats: a review of 36 cases (2010–2020). *J Fel Med Surg.*, 2021. doi: 10.1177/1098612X211005886

Roush J.K. Canine patellar luxation. *Vet Clin North Am: Small Anim Pract.*, 1993; 23: 855–858

Salter RB., Harris WR. Injuries involving the epiphyseal plate. *J Bone Joint Surg. Am.*, 1963; 45: 587–622

Sabattini S., Renzi A., Buracco P., Defourny S., *et al.* Comparative assessment of the accurary of cytological and histologic biopsies in the diagnosis of canine bone lesions. *J Vet Intern Med.*, 2017; 31: 864–871

Schwarze RA., Tano CA., Carroll VW. Glenoid displasia and osteochondritis dissecans in a cat. *Can Vet J.*, 2015; 56: 749–752

Smith GK., Langenbach A., Green PA., Rhodes WH., *et al.* Evaluation of the association between medial patellar luxation and hip dysplasia in cats. *J Am Vet Med Assoc.* 1999; 215: 40–45

Smith GK., Leighton EA., Karbe GT., McDonald-Lynch MB. Pathogenesis, diagnosis and control of canine hip dysplasia. In: *Veterinary Surgery Small Animal.* Johnston SA. and Tobias K., 2017. 2nd ed. Saunders Elsevier, Philadelphia, USA., pp. 7289–7504

Swanson EA., Tomlinson JL., Dismukes DI., Fox DB. Measurement of femoral and tibial joint reference angles and pelvic limb alignment in cats. *Vet Surg.*, 2012; 41: 696–704

Streubel R., Bilzer T., Grest P., Damur D. *et al.* Medial humeral epicondylitis in clinically affected cats. *Vet Surg.*, 2015; 44: 905–913

Streubel R., Geyer H., Montavon PM. Medial humeral epicondylitis in cats. *Vet Surg.*, 2012; 41: 795–802

Tatton B., Jeffery N., Holmes N. Predicting recovery of urinary control in cats after sacrocaudal injury: a prospective study. *J Small Anim Pract.*, 2009; 50: 593–596

Taylor SM., Scott-Moncrieff JC. Clinical manifestations of and diagnostic tests for joint disorders. In: Nelson RW., Couto CG. *Small Animal Internal Medicine.*, 2013. 5th ed., St Louis, MO, USA: Elsevier; pp. 1111–1125

Umphlet RC. Feline stifle disease. *Vet Clin North Am: Small Anim Pract.*, 1993; 23: 897–913

Valastro C., Di Bello A., Crovace A. Congenital elbow subluxation in a cat. *Vet Radiol. Ultrasound.*, 2005; 46: 63–64

Voss K., Steffen F. Patient assessment. In: *Feline Orthopaedic Surgery and Musculoskeletal Disease.* Montavon PM., Voss K., and Langley-Hobss SJ., 2009. 1st ed. Saunders Elsevier, Philadelphia, USA., pp. 3–19

Voss K., Langley-Hobbs SJ. Shoulder joint. In: Feline Orthopaedic Surgery and Muskuloskeletal Disease. Montavon PM., Voss K. and Langley-Hobss SJ., 2009. 1st ed. Saunders Elsevier, Philadelphia, USA., pp. 337–358

Voss K., Montavon PM. Fractures. In: *Feline Orthopaedic Surgery and Muskuloskeletal Disease.* Montavon PM., Voss K. and Langley-Hobss SJ., 2009. 1st ed. Saunders Elsevier, Philadelphia, USA., pp. 129–152

Yardimci C., Özak A., Önyay T., Inal KS. Management of traumatic tarsal luxations with transarticular external fixation in cats. *Vet Comp Orthop Traumatol.*, 2016; 29: 232–238

Zalabras CG., Marcus RE., Levin S., Patzakis MJ. Management of open fractures and subsequent complications. *J Bone Joint Surg.*, 2007; 89: 883–895

Clinical cases

Case 1

A 2-year old female neutered Domestic Shorthair was referred with a recent history of trauma of unknown origin. According to information from the owners, the cat was found lying in the garden. She was unable to get up and appeared really uncomfortable. Her general physical examination was unremarkable. Rectal temperature could not be taken and rectal palpation could not be performed because the cat was uncooperative during the examination.

1. Considering the cat's demeanour, which of the following tests should be performed first?

A) Full orthopaedic examination if possible. Otherwise, a target orthopaedic examination.
B) Full neurological examination if possible. Otherwise, a "target" neurological examination.
C) A combined full neurological and orthopaedic examination if possible. Otherwise, a target neurological examination first. Thereafter a full orthopaedic exam under sedation/general anaesthesia.
D) Evaluation of the cranial nerves.

Gait analysis revealed the cat had right pelvic limb monoparesia. Conscious proprioception was absent in her right hind limb and normal in her left hind limb and forelimbs. Evaluation of the cranial nerves was normal. Spinal reflexes were normal in her left pelvic limb and forelimbs. The right patella reflex was normal. However, the withdrawal and sciatic reflexes were markedly reduced (almost absent) in her right pelvic limb. Panniculus and perineal reflexes were normal. There was marked pain on palpation of the caudal lumbar spine. Full orthopaedic examination without sedation could not be performed due to the cat's demeanour.

2. Where is the problem likely to be located?

A) Thoracolumbar spine, as the cat demonstrated pain on palpation of the caudal lumbar spine.
B) Brainstem, cerebellum or forebrain.
C) Sacro-coccygeal spine.
D) Lumbo-sacral spine (cauda equina) and/or nerves of the pelvic plexus (e.g. sciatic nerve).

Thoracic radiographs (Figure 1) revealed a mild pneumothorax (yellow arrow) which was resolved by thoracocentesis. Abdominal radiographs (Figure 2) were unremarkable. Thoracic and abdominal FAST scans were normal. A blood sample

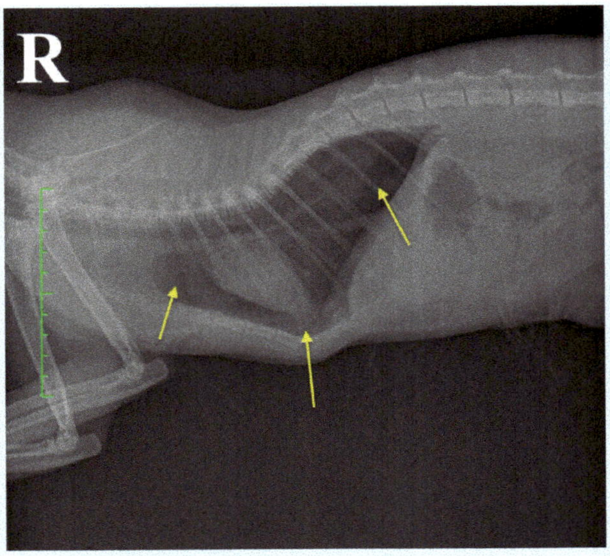

Figure 1. Thoracic radiograph (lateral view) revealed a mild pneumothorax (yellow arrows).

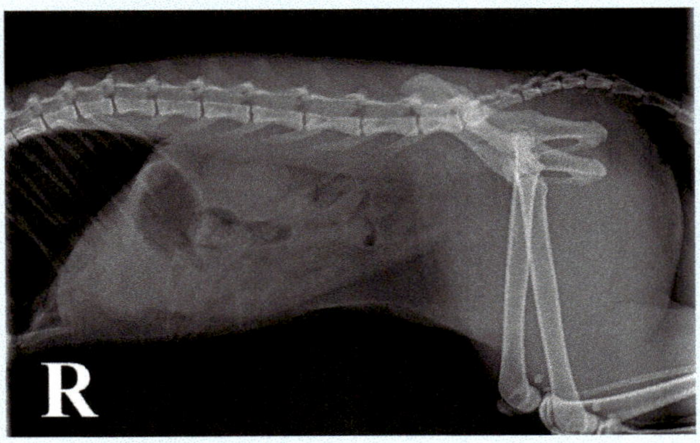

Figure 2. Abdominal radiographs were unremarkable.

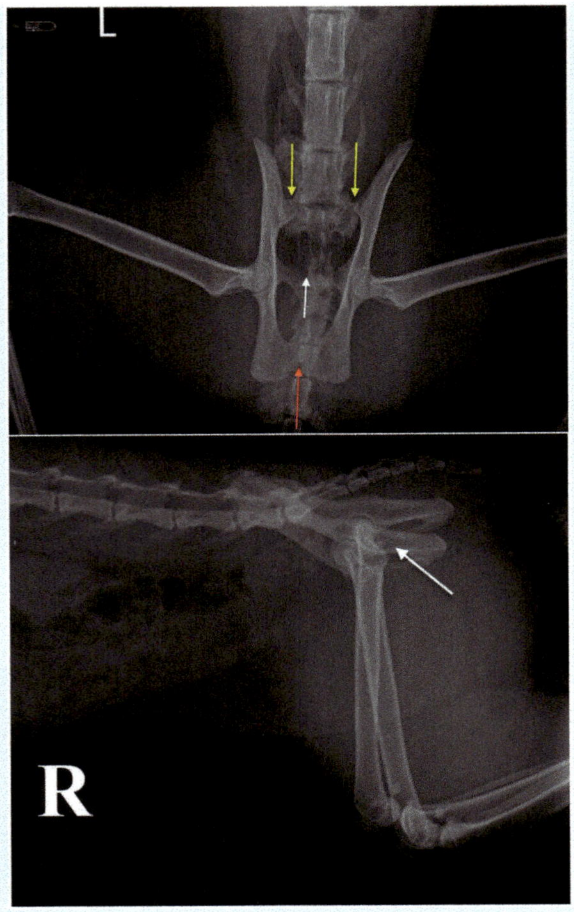

Figure 3. Radiographs of the pelvis revealed fractures of the pubis (white arrow), ischium (red arrow) and bilateral sacroiliac luxations (SI) (yellow arrow).

was taken from an IV catheter placed in the right cephalic vein. No significant abnormalities were detected on the complete blood count, biochemistry and electrolytes. The cat received opioids and IVFT. The ECG was connected and cardiac function was monitored.

Once pain was controlled, the cat was sedated to complete the orthopaedic examination. No abnormalities were detected in the forelimbs, hocks or stifles. There was crepitus and pain on manipulation of the hips. Rectal palpation suggested fractures at the pelvic floor and marked stenosis of the pelvic canal was detected. Hip radiographs were obtained (Figure 3). There were fractures of the pubis (white arrow), ischium (red arrow) and bilateral sacroiliac fracture/luxations (yellow arrows).

3. Which of the following fractures is the likely cause of the neurological signs?

A) Fracture of the pubis.
B) Bilateral sacroiliac luxation.
C) Fracture of the ischium.
D) All of the above.

Following the diagnosis of multiple pelvic fractures, surgical repair versus conservative treatment of the fractures was discussed with the owners. Based on diagnostic findings, surgery was recommended. The patient underwent fracture repair the following day.

4. Why was surgery recommended for this patient?

A) Because the bilateral sacroiliac/fracture luxation had caused a neurological deficit and marked stenosis of the pelvic canal. Moreover, the sacroliliac fracture/luxations were markedly displaced, so conservative treatment was not the best option for this patient.

B) To speed up the recovery.
C) Surgery should have not been recommended because the prognosis is poor in these cases.
D) Because conservative treatment was not an option considering the cat's demeanour.

A bilateral dorsal approach to the sacroiliac joint was performed. The fracture/luxations were repaired using a trans-sacral pin, a transiliac pin and cerclage wires to avoid rotation of the pins. A fluoroscopic assisted technique was used to improve the accuracy of implant positioning (Figure 4).

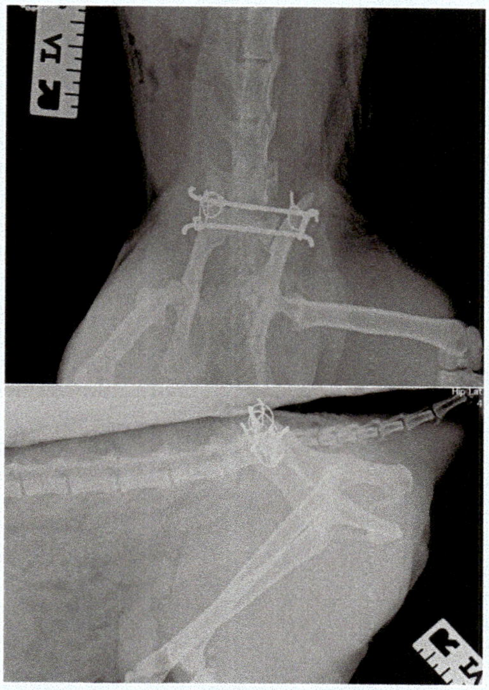

Figure 4. Postoperative hip radiographs. SI luxation was repaired using a trans-sacral pin, a trans-ilial pin, and cerclage wires to avoid pin rotation.

5. Which of the orthopaedic implants used are considered primary methods of fracture fixation?

A) Pins.
B) Cerclage wire.
C) Trans-sacral pin.
D) None of the above. The combination of all these secondary methods of fixation effectively neutralised all the forces acting at the fracture/luxation.

48 hours after surgery, the patient was discharged from the hospital. She was able to use her left hind limb without problems. However, she was intermittently knuckling the right hind foot. Neurological examination was repeated. It was unremarkable in her left hind limb and forelimbs. There was positive but delayed withdrawal and sciatic reflexes in her right hind limb.

Six weeks after surgery, the neurological examination was repeated. Normal conscious proprioception was detected in her right and left hind limbs. Spinal reflexes in her hind limbs were normal. The cat was able to ambulate without assistance and no proprioceptive deficits were observed. However, an asymmetric hind limb gait was still observed. Follow-up radiographs (Figure 5) were normal.

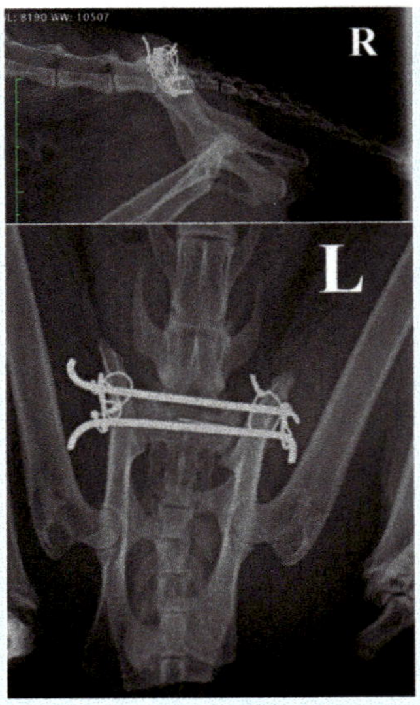

Figure 5. 6-week postoperative radiographs.

6. What was likely the cause of the neurological deficit observed before and immediately after surgery?

A) Spinal cord injury due to pelvic trauma.
B) Pudendal nerve injury due to pelvic trauma.
C) Vascular lesion at the cauda equina.
D) Sacral nerve injury due to pelvic trauma.

A second postoperative check-up was performed 12 weeks after surgery. Orthopaedic and neurological examinations were both normal. Follow up radiographs were normal (Figure 6). The patient was discharged and no further follow-ups were required.

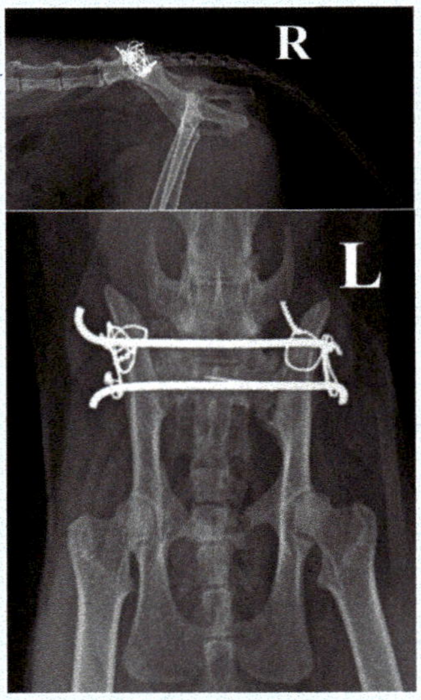

Figure 6. 12-week postoperative radiographs.

7. Which of the following statements is true in relation to this case?

A) Neurological deficits are relatively common in cats diagnosed with multiple pelvic fractures.
B) The presence of neurological deficits and marked stenosis of the pelvic canal are indications for surgical repair of the fracture.
C) The neurological issues were trauma related, including local inflammation at the sciatic nerve and/or contact of the bone fragments with the sciatic nerve.
D) All of the above are correct.

Case 2

A 4-year-old male entire Domestic Shorthair was referred for evaluation of a chronic right hind limb lameness. According to his owner, the cat became lame approximately a month before referral. A short course of the NSAID meloxicam was initiated. However, no response was observed and the treatment was stopped. The referring veterinarian suspected a cranial cruciate ligament rupture. However, he was unsure of the diagnosis during a sedated orthopaedic examination and referred the patient for further investigations. The referring veterinarian radiographs and basic blood work (complete blood count and biochemistry) were normal. According to the owner, the cat lived with other cats; some of which were diagnosed with FeLV (Feline leukaemia virus) in the past. However, recent blood tests done in this patient were negative for feline viral diseases.

The general physical examination was unremarkable. No abnormalities were detected in the neurological exam. On gait analysis, no lameness was observed. However, in a video recorded by his owner, a mild to moderate weight bearing lameness of the right hind limb was observed. Palpation of the right hind limb revealed a very mild muscle atrophy at the thigh. No abnormalities were detected in the forelimbs or left hind limb. No abnormalities were detected during manipulation of the right hock. Pain was detected on manipulation of the right hip and stifle. Additionally, there was a very mild joint effusion in the right stifle.

8. What would the next steps be?

A) Repeat the orthopaedic examination under sedation.
B) Take radiographs of the right hip and stifle as they may show changes that were not observed in the previous radiographs taken by the referring veterinarian.
C) Consider a joint tap, as the clinical history may indicate the lameness could be associated with a penetrating injury (bite wound).
D) All of the above are correct.

Hip radiographs were unremarkable. Radiographs of the right stifle revealed a very mild joint effusion (Figure 1). Orthopaedic examination under sedation only revealed a very subtle cranial drawer test in flexion and slight movement of the patella at the femoral groove. However, the knee felt stable and the patella could not be medially luxated. The remainder of the orthopaedic examination was unremarkable. Stifle arthrocentesis revealed the following findings:

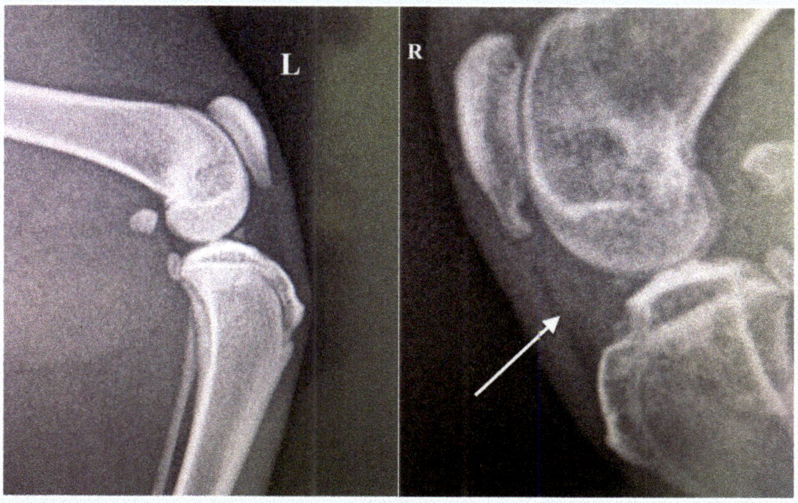

Figure 1. Stifle radiographs. No abnormalities were detected in the left knee. A moderate joint effusion was detected in the right knee (white arrow).

- **Colour:** blood-tinged
- **Volume:** 0.5 ml
- **Viscosity test:** 1–2 cm
- **Estimated cells:** 5% neutrophils; 92% monocytes/macrophages

9. What are the differential diagnoses based on the joint fluid analysis?

A) Immune-mediated polyarthritis.
B) Septic arthritis.
C) Degenerative joint disease (OA).
D) OA or traumatic arthropathy.

Given the fact the lameness was really subtle and the orthopaedic findings were unspecific, a 4-week conservative management was recommended in the form of daily administration of a different NSAID (robenacoxib) and exercise restriction. An orthopaedic recheck was scheduled to evaluate patient response to the conservative treatment.

Four weeks later the patient returned for a recheck. This time, a mild to moderate weight bearing lameness of the right hind limb was observed in the consultation room. According to the owner, no improvement was observed during the four weeks of conservative management. Moderate pain was detected on palpation and manipulation of the right stifle. Joint effusion was more evident compared to four weeks earlier. A CT scan of the stifle was recommended.

10. Why was this advance imaging technique recommended?

A) Because it has superior contrast and resolution compared to MRI.
B) Because it allows better visualisation of structures such as bone and joint surfaces.
C) Because it is more accurate for detection of bone lysis and/or new bone formation.
D) 'B' and 'C' are both correct.

Stifle CT scan images are displaced in Figure 2. Before finishing the CT scan, arthrocentesis of the right stifle was repeated and CT arthrography performed (Figure 3). CT scan images revealed two well defined osteolytic lesions (yellow arrows) at the craniolateral aspect of the right femoral condyle and fibular head. Cytology of the joint fluid was similar to the sample obtained four weeks earlier. Arthrography was unremarkable.

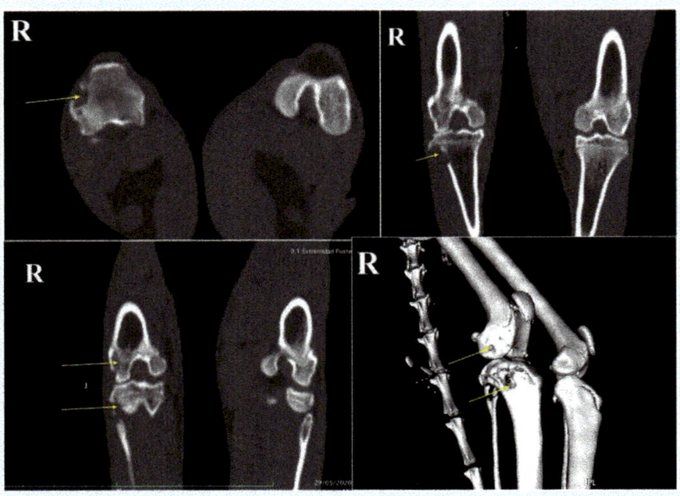

Figure 2. CT of the right stifle revealed well-defined osteolytic lesions (white arrows) at the femoral condyle and fibular head.

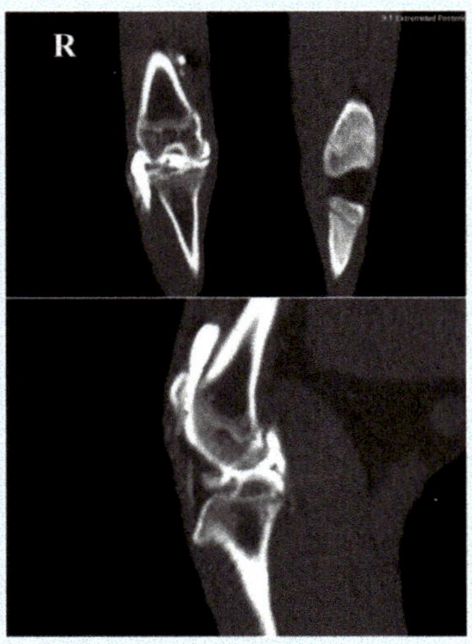

Figure 3. CT arthrography of the right stifle.

11. What are the two main differential diagnoses for these findings?

A) Traumatic lesions on the lateral aspect of the right stifle or degenerative joint disease.
B) Neoplasia or trauma.
C) Infection or trauma.
D) Neoplasia or infection.

Under the same anaesthesia used for the CT scan, ultrasound-guided fine needle aspirates (FNA) of the bone lesions were performed. Samples were submitted for cytology and bacterial culture in a blood culture bottle.

12. Why was a FNA technique chosen instead of a bone biopsy?

A) Because it is less invasive and it can provide a diagnosis in up to 80% of cases.

B) Because it is cheaper than a bone biopsy.
C) Because it carries less risk of post-sampling fracture, it is less invasive and it can provide a diagnosis in up to 80% of cases.
D) Because it is quicker.

13. Why was a blood culture bottle used to submit the sample for bacterial culture?
A) Because it better preserves the microorganisms until the lab can run the test.
B) Because it reduces the number of false negative results.
C) Because it reduces the number of false positive results.
D) Because it is more specific in these types of cases.

Bacterial culture of the samples submitted were negative. Cytology of the bone lesions revealed a population of "abnormal spindle cells" with several criteria of malignancy, including anisokaryosis, anisocytosis and multiple nucleoli.

14. Is it uncommon to find normal joint fluid cytology with this diagnosis?
A) No, it is not. Cell exfoliation does not tend to occur with articular and periarticular tumours. Synovial fluid cytology does not have a diagnostic value for neoplasia.
B) Yes, it is uncommon. It is an abnormal presentation.
C) No, it is not. However, this occurred in this cat because it had a spindle cell tumour.
D) None of the above are correct.

Although cytology did not reveal the origin of the neoplasia and tumour type, the cause of the lameness was identified with the diagnostic tests performed. A pelvic limb amputation was recommended and performed 24 hours after diagnosis. Extensive cartilage defects (yellow arrows) were observed in the specimen after amputation (Figure 4). A soft tissue sarcoma, arising from the periarticular tissue, was diagnosed on histopathology. The cat recovered well after surgery and further follow-ups were performed by oncologists.

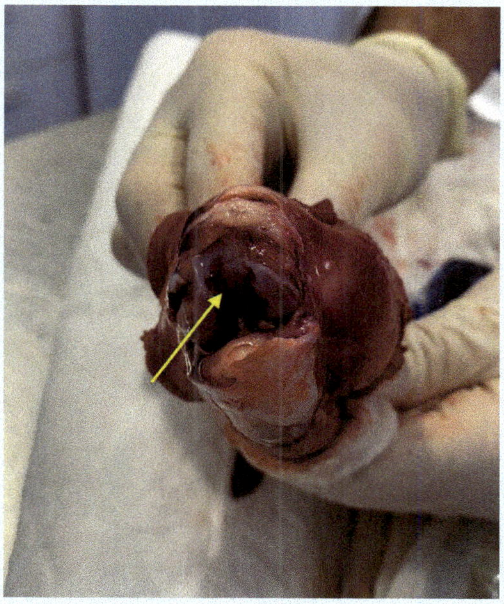

Figure 4. Extensive cartilage defect at the femoral condyle (yellow arrow).

15. In the event that the owner had requested further tests prior to surgery, what would you have recommended?
A) MRI to better assess articular surfaces.
B) Electromyography.
C) Muscle and nerve biopsy.
D) Bone biopsy using a Jamshidi needle.

Answers

1. C	6. D	11. D
2. D	7. D	12. C
3. B	8. D	13. B
4. A	9. D	14. A
5. D	10. D	15. D

Feline anaesthesia

16

Maria Chie Niimura del Barrio, Maria Ángeles Jiménez Lozano

Contents

Introduction

Cats are increasingly popular as pets, with felines representing the most frequently owned pet by the UK adult population (www.cats.org.uk/about-cp/cats-report-2021). Indeed, it is estimated there are about **10.9 million pet cats in the UK**, compared to 10.1 million dogs. However, despite these numbers (pre-pandemic) **cats remain less likely than dogs to receive veterinary care**.

The unique physiology and character of cats makes anaesthesia challenging; they should not be treated as small dogs and **understanding the differences** allows the anaesthetist to prepare a safer anaesthetic. The aim of this chapter on feline anaesthesia is to provide the practitioner with the necessary/basic tools for a safe anaesthetic in the cat.

Anaesthetic risk and mortality rates

The latest and most important study in the UK regarding anaesthetic-related mortality and morbidity (Brodbelt et al., 2008) shows **an overall feline anaesthetic mortality rate of 0.24%** which is higher than dogs. **Healthy cats (ASA I–II) are 10 times more likely to survive anaesthesia** compared to the sick ones (ASA III–V). This highlights the importance of good pre-anaesthetic assessment, consideration of risk factors, and adequate health status classification to plan the anaesthetic and provide the owner with accurate information about the procedure.

Interestingly, **the most dangerous time during the anaesthetic procedure is the post-operative period, with 61% of deaths**, most of them specifically 0–3 hours post-anaesthesia. It is paramount that thorough monitoring continues after extubation. A false sense of safety once the vaporiser has been turned off is to blame for the rapid decrease in monitoring levels and the higher risk of death at this point.

Perioperative risk factors associated with mortality

- **Age**: neonates and geriatric cats are more likely to die under anaesthesia and require special care with anaesthesia or sedation.
- **Weight**: underweight cats are more likely to have comorbidities (e.g. hyperthyroidism, anaemia, kidney disease, hypothermia). Overweight cats are more likely to suffer from cardiovascular disease and hypertension, and a high risk of atelectasis and hypoventilation during anaesthesia.
- **Endotracheal intubation**: it is important to clarify that although endotracheal intubation is not risk-free, it is the safest option as it allows for ventilation and protects the airway. Nevertheless, the CEPSAF (Confidential Enquiry into Perioperative Small Animal Fatalities) study (Brodbelt et al., 2008) reflects that intubated cats were more likely to die. However, in this study the majority of cats intubated were already unwell, and had a higher death risk due to their ASA status rather than the technique per se.
- **Fluid therapy**: cats are more sensitive to intravenous (IV) fluids than dogs and are more prone to suffering fluid overload. The association between fluid therapy and mortality rate could be due to the type of patient which receives intravenous fluid therapy; if only the sickest patients receive fluid therapy they are more likely to die anyway. However, fluid therapy is required under general anaesthesia, especially if the patient has comorbidities (e.g. renal disease).
- **Spay-neuter versus other procedures**: anaesthetic risk in big spay-neuter clinics does not seem to be as high, with anaesthetic related deaths at around 0.05% (Levy et al., 2017) which is lower than in the CEPSAF study. This reflects this type of healthy young population undergoing a routine procedure performed by experienced, skilled clinicians.

Planning the anaesthetic

ASA scale

The American Society of Anaesthesiologists (ASA) created **a physical-status scale to categorise the patients** undergoing general anaesthesia (www.asahq.org/resources/clinical-information/asa-physical-status-classification-system). Patients are assigned a number from 1 to 5: one being a completely healthy patient and five a patient that is moribund. The addition of an E describes an emergency situation. Although it was developed for human patients, the scale is widely used for cats and is useful for identifying patients at risk of developing complications during anaesthesia (Table 1). It has been helpful in several studies (Hosgood and Scholl, 2002; Brodbelt et al., 2008) where its use predicted anaesthetic morbidity and mortality in veterinary patients.

Table 1. ASA physical-status scale for categorisation of patients.

ASA Physical Status Classification System	Examples
ASA Physical Status 1 – A normal healthy patient	OVH/neutering in a healthy cat
ASA Physical Status 2 – A patient with mild systemic disease	Controlled diabetes mellitus, mild cardiac valve insufficiency (no treatment required)
ASA Physical Status 3 – A patient with severe systemic disease	Uncontrolled diabetes, symptomatic heart disease, hepatopathy
ASA Physical Status 4 – A patient with severe systemic disease that is a constant threat to life	Sepsis, organ failure, heart failure
ASA Physical Status 5 – A moribund patient who is not expected to survive without the operation	Shock, multiple organ failure, severe trauma
ASA E – Describes patient as an emergency	Blocked bladder, respiratory distress

It is important to perform **a thorough pre-anaesthetic assessment** in the patient before an ASA is assigned. The decision is based on the current health status of the patient, leaving aside previous anaesthetic experiences or external factors like procedure or the surgeon skill level.

Fasting

In cats, gastro-oesophageal reflux (GOR), occurs in 50% of the cases (Galatos et al., 2001; Sideri et al., 2009; Garcia et al., 2017) and is associated with the potential **complication of aspiration pneumonia**; fasting prior to general anaesthesia is important to decrease this incidence. Moreover, fasting is also important to avoid undesirable effects on the patient such as impairment of ventilation and decrease venous return to the heart. However, there is **no consensus on how fasting should be performed:** withholding time, type and quantity of food offered prior to anaesthesia, and how long water should be withheld. According to Robertson et al. (2018) in the AAFP (American Association of Feline Practitioners) Feline Anaesthesia Guidelines, cats should receive a **wet meal**

three to four hours before anaesthesia and water should be available until the time of pre-medication. However, to the author's knowledge there are no supporting studies in cats; whilst the study by Robertson et al. (2018) does not mention the amount of food offered, however, research performed in healthy dogs (Galatos and Raptopoulous, 1995; Savvas et al., 2009 and Viskjer and Stjostrom, 2017) indicates half of the daily requirements of canned/wet food four to six hours prior to pre-medication is the correct amount. Based on experience, the authors also recommend decreasing the amount of food to 25% of the daily requirements, providing food low in fat and fibre, and avoiding a large amount of water being drunk just prior to pre-medication. **Even if the patient is fasted, chronic oral medications should be administered if appropriate with a small amount of wet food (one to two teaspoons)** or pills coated in an edible paste-like material (Grubb et al., 2020).

Fasting suggestions change in young patients (i.e less than eight weeks) or small sized patients (body weight less than 2 kg). In these cases, the recommendation is to decrease the fasting period to one to two hours (Grubb et al., 2020) and allow free access to water (Adams et al., 2015; Veres-Nyeki, 2016). If the kitten is still sucking, no fasting is required.

Fasting time and the amount of insulin administered prior to anaesthesia to diabetic patients is an ongoing debate and there is no clear consensus. Different authors suggest different protocols, based mainly on personal experiences (Adams et al., 2015; Nelson, 2015; Veres-Nyeki, 2016; Grubb et al., 2020; Adami et al., 2020). The **aim is to cause minimal disruption to the glucose and insulin pattern, and to avoid long fasting periods (>4–6 hours)**. It is vital to know the type and frequency of insulin the patient receives to maintain normoglycaemia and the time of the day the procedure is scheduled for. The day prior to anaesthesia, food and insulin should be given as usual. If the procedure is scheduled in the morning, blood glucose levels should be checked first thing in the morning, prior to insulin administration, and insulin administered according to the patient's blood glucose, aiming for a blood glucose between 8–12 mmol/l. Non-administration of insulin should be avoided (Adami et al., 2020). If the procedure is in the afternoon, breakfast should be provided (half meal of wet food) and insulin administered (normally half dose of insulin, but it should be administered according to blood glucose), and the procedure performed 4–6 hours later. However, this recommendation is not evidence based. Blood glucose levels should be monitored throughout the procedure.

It is worth noting the administration of oral omeprazole (two doses) in cats before general anaesthesia (18–24 and 4 hours before) does not decrease the incidence of GOR (Garcia et al., 2017) despite the increase in gastric and oesophageal pH.

Pre-hospitalisation drugs (trazadone, gabapentin, amitriptyline)

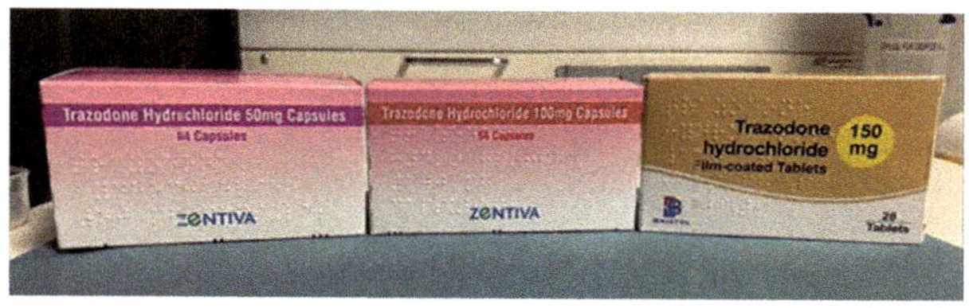

Figure 1. Trazadone.

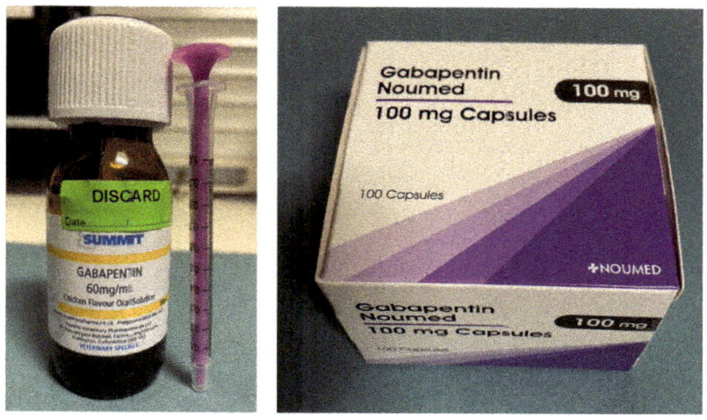

Figure 2. Gabapentin.

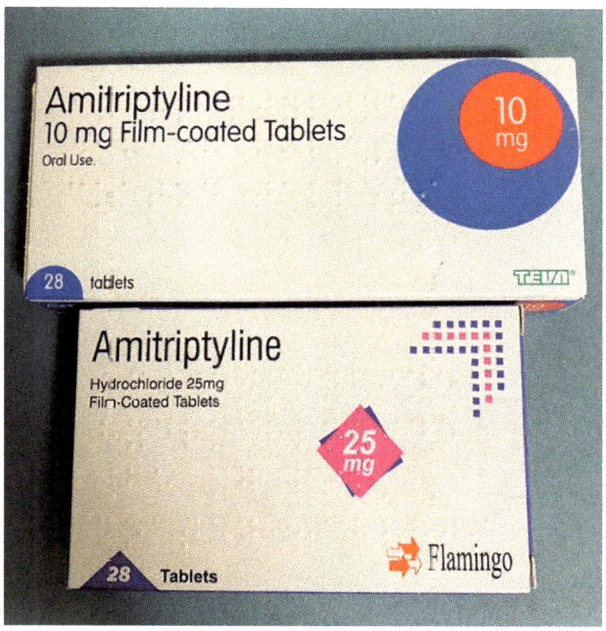

Figure 3. Amitriptyline.

Trazadone

Trazadone is an antagonist of serotonin receptors with anxiolytic, mild sedative, and antidepressant effects. The antidepressant effect is a consequence of the serotonin reuptake inhibition while the sedation effect is due to the alpha-adrenergic blockade and the modest histamine blockade.

It is best used to **control cat anxiety related to travelling**, veterinary visits, fireworks, and other phobias. Trazadone should be administered at least two hours prior to the stressful event. Decreased activity and anxiety without much change in behaviour is to be expected (Stevens et al., 2016).

Although there are few reports, if possible, the concomitant use of acepromazine should be avoided as both drugs act on the same receptors, possibly causing an increase in side effects. Moreover, serotonin syndrome can occur when combined with other serotoninergic drugs.

Trazadone should be used with caution in cats with liver dysfunction as it is predominantly metabolised in the liver.

Oral doses of 50, 75 and 100 mg per cat have been reported to decrease activity with no side effects (Orlando et al., 2016).

Gabapentin

Gabapentin is a structural analogue of the neurotransmitter gamma-aminobutyric acid (GABA) and used as an anticonvulsant drug in humans. The exact mechanism of action is unknown, but it is believed to work through calcium channel blockade on neurons to decrease the release of excitatory neurotransmitters. It has been used in dogs for control of neuropathic pain with the major side effect being sedation. It works well for cats as an oral sedative, especially for fearful, anxious, aggressive cats.

In cats, gabapentin does not undergo liver metabolism but is excreted via the kidneys, therefore it is suitable for cats with normal kidney function. The latest study for cats with chronic kidney disease (Quimby et al., 2022) showed higher gabapentin serum concentration when a dose of 10 mg/kg was used, compared with normal cats administered 20 mg/kg. So, gabapentin may still be **used for cats with kidney disease but at considerably reduced doses**. As it is mainly metabolised in the liver **caution is recommended in cats with liver dysfunction**. Doses of 100 mg per cat or up to 25 mg/kg have been used with success.

Amitriptyline

Amitriptyline is another behaviour-modifying drug like trazodone from the tricyclic antidepressant group (TCA). Its mechanism of action is at central level, blocking the reuptake of neurotransmitters (i.e. serotonin and norepinephrine). It appears to produce sedation in cats and is used as an oral alternative to trazadone or gabapentin. Little is known about its clinical value or even possible side effects. In dogs, depression, and nausea are reported side effects. **The dose per cat is 10 mg PO.**

Pre-medication

Pre-medication is the administration of sedatives and tranquillisers before general anaesthesia. All species, and especially cats due to their cautious nature, benefit from sedation before anaesthesia.

Objectives and indications

- To provide **sedation and anxiolysis**. The patient is calmed down for a minor procedure like an abdominal ultrasound or intravenous catheterisation. The level of stress reduction is important, not only for the cat but also the personnel dealing with the cat.
- To allow **safer handling** of the cat minimising injuries to the handler.
- To provide **analgesia** and preventive analgesia as required.
- To contribute to balanced anaesthetic technique, where the administration of pre-medication will reduce the doses required for induction and maintenance of anaesthesia.
- To provide a smooth stress-free recovery, preventing emergence delirium.
- To counteract side effects of other drugs; one example would be an anticholinergic administered together with an opioid to prevent bradycardia caused by the opioid.

Drugs for sedation and pre-medication

Major tranquilizers: phenothiazines (e.g. acepromazine)

Acepromazine (Figures 4 and 5) exerts its calming, tranquillising effects by blockade of central and peripheral dopaminergic receptors. There is no antagonist/reversal drug, and it has **no analgesic properties.**

- routes of administration: IV, SC, IM and oral
- onset of action: generally slow, it takes at least 20 minutes after IV administration to observe maximum peak effect. It has a long duration of action (4–6 h)
- dosage: 0.005–0.05 mg/kg
- metabolism: hepatic metabolism and renal excretion
- main clinical effects:
  - mild sedation at central level with blockade of dopamine receptors
  - peripheral vasodilation through antagonism of peripheral alpha-1 adrenergic receptors
  - central depression of the thermoregulatory centre
  - weak antihistaminic effect by H1 (histamine) blockade
  - weak antiemetic effect by blocking dopamine receptors in the chemoreceptor trigger zone.

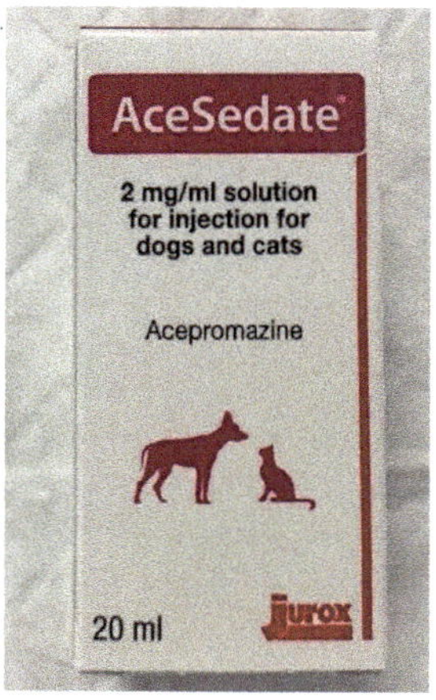

Figure 4. Acepromazine bottle.

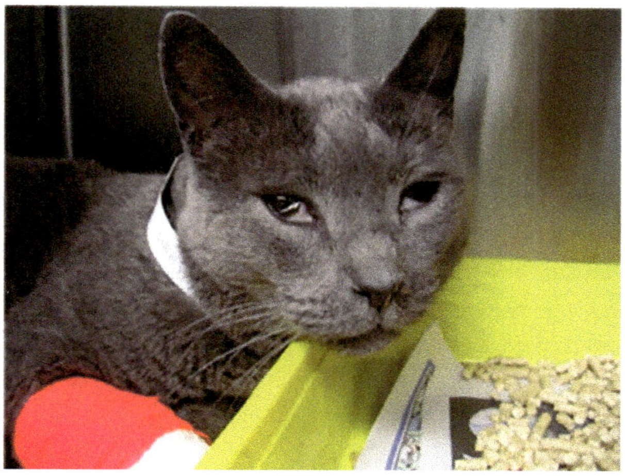

Figure 5. Cat after receiving acepromazine.

- side effects:
  - hypotension due to vasodilation
  - central hypothermia which will worsen due to peripheral vasodilation
  - third eyelid protrusion and priapism.

Clinical use

Acepromazine, combined with an opioid or other sedative drugs, is used as part of the pre-medication or sedation protocol. It is **useful for cats that are more anxious than aggressive**, and it can be administered orally at home in preparation for the veterinary visit. It is often used to counteract possible opioid side effects in cats such as excitation or hyperthermia. It reduces the dose of induction and maintenance inhalant during anaesthesia in cats. Although it can be used on its own it works better as a combo due to its synergistic effects, especially with opioids. It produces only minimal respiratory depression, but its hypotensive effects are dose dependent so **low doses are recommended**. The possibility of hypothermic effect should be considered, as cats tend to become hypothermic under anaesthesia causing prolonged recoveries.

Minor tranquillisers: benzodiazepines (diazepam, midazolam)

Benzodiazepines act centrally through $GABA_A$ receptors. **When used alone they produce a poor sedative effect** and often cause excitation, so they are best used in combination with other drugs. Their **safe cardiovascular and respiratory profile** makes them useful drugs for anaesthesia. They are particularly beneficial for **geriatric or neonate patients** as they produce a good sedation effect when combined with an opioid. They are good muscle relaxants and good antiepileptic drugs. Benzodiazepines are commonly used combined with opioids, ketamine, or as co-induction agents during anaesthesia induction. An antagonist (reversal) drug called flumazenil is available.

Diazepam

Diazepam (Figure 6) is formulated in different preparations and can be administered, orally, rectally, and via IV/IM injection. Commonly, the oral and rectal routes are used for other purposes rather than anaesthesia. In anaesthesia, the only relevant route of administration is intravenously as diazepam is hydrophobic and poorly absorbed if administered intramuscularly. **Diazepam is not suitable for constant rate infusion.**

- routes of administration:
  - IV for anaesthesia
  - oral (appetite stimulant)
  - rectal (seizure treatment)
- onset of action: very fast intravenously and rectally
- dosage: 0.2–0.5 mg/kg
- metabolism: hepatic metabolism via demethylation. Metabolism produces active metabolites
- side effects:
  - slow elimination and accumulation, potential for long term effects
  - **acute hepatic necrosis** reported following repeated oral administration (Center et al., 1996)
  - pain on injection due to the presence of propylene glycol, vein irritation
  - propylene glycol toxicity with cardiac toxicity and cardiovascular depression after repeated injection
  - excitation, aggression.

Midazolam

Midazolam (Figure 7) **is the benzodiazepine of choice in cats.** It is water soluble is appopriate for SC or IM use, besides IV administration, and is, unlikely to cause irritation or liver injury. It prolongs and deepens sedation especially when combined with heavy sedative drugs like alpha-2 agonists or alfaxalone, with synergistic effects allowing dose reduction to get sedative effects and minimise side effects.

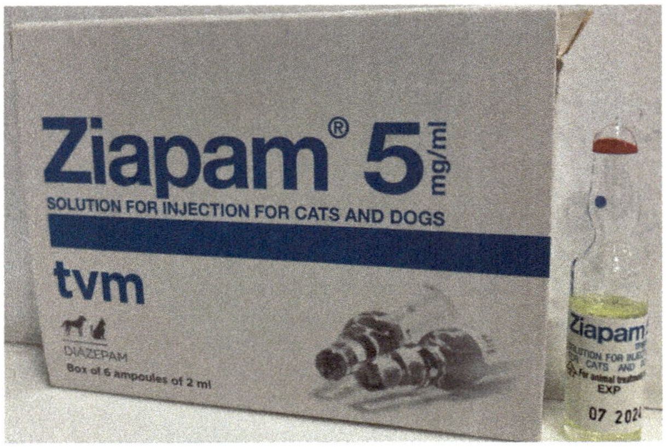

Figure 6. Diazepam.

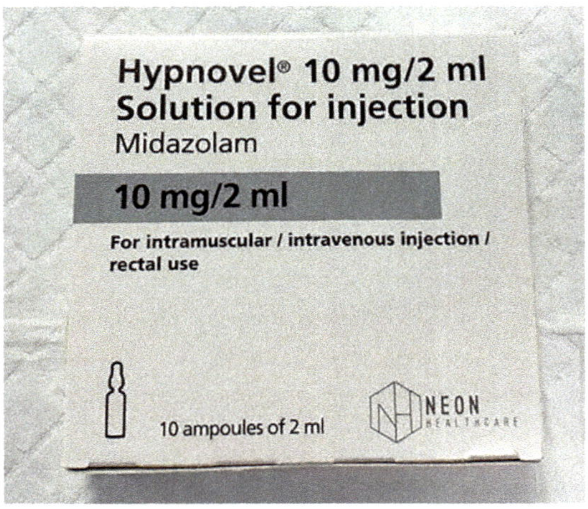

Figure 7. Midazolam.

- routes of administration: IV, SC or IM
- onset of action: very fast either route (fastest IV)
- dosage: 0.2–0.5 mg/kg
- metabolism: hepatic metabolism producing an active metabolite. Limited pharmacokinetic data
- side effects:
  - prolonged recoveries if used as constant rate infusion due to active metabolite accumulation and decreased elimination (glucuronidation)
  - excitation, aggression.

Sedatives: alpha-2 adrenergic receptor agonists (dex-medetomidine)

Alpha-2 agonists (Figure 8) are the best sedatives available for cats. They bind to the alpha-2 adrenergic receptors located centrally to produce **heavy sedation in a dose dependent manner**. As part of the central effect, they increase vagal tone and have major cardiovascular and respiratory effects, which makes them **unsafe for unstable or sick patients**. They have a distinctive peripheral effect where they bind to the alpha-2 adrenoreceptors producing **vasoconstriction and hypertension**. They produce some analgesia, muscle relaxation, hyperglycaemia, and increased urine production. Alpha-2 agonists are useful as part of the anaesthetic protocol as they greatly **reduce the induction agent dose** and have a significant MAC sparing effect too. The sedation level produced allows for a wide range of diagnostic/examination procedures and even minor surgical procedures when combined with good analgesics like opioids. Another important use for these drugs is the ability to treat dysphoria at micro low doses (0.5–1.5 µg/kg) sufficient to **counteract excitement** and avoid self-harm in these extreme situations. Medetomidine and dexmedetomidine are the most widely used alpha-2 agonists in cats.

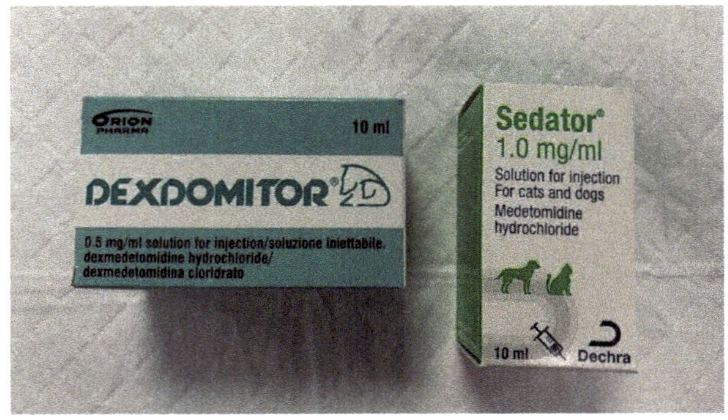

Figure 8. Alpha-2 agonists.

- routes of administration: IV, SC or IM. Oral route in case of dexmedetomidine
- onset of action: very fast IV, only few minutes IM or SC
- dosages:
  - medetomidine 2–40 µg/kg
  - dexmedetomidine 0.5–20 µg/kg
- metabolism: hepatic with renal excretion
- antagonist: atipamezole. Half the volume of medetomidine/dexmedetomidine used should be administered IM (unless an emergency situation)
- clinical effects:
  - heavy sedation
  - muscle relaxation
  - central analgesia inhibiting nociceptive input at spinal cord
  - increased urinary production due to ADH inhibition
  - physiologic stress response suppression
  - decreased intraocular and intracranial pressure
- side effects:
  - central bradycardia and myocardial contractility depression
  - peripheral vasoconstriction, hypertension, and reflex bradycardia
  - vomiting
  - hypothermia
  - hyperglycaemia
  - respiratory depression.

Dexmedetomidine versus medetomidine

Both are highly selective, specific, and potent compared to the oldest xylazine (little used in cats in the UK) but **dexmedetomidine is the purified and active isomer** from the racemic mixture contained in medetomidine. Clinically dexmedetomidine has few advantages over medetomidine but it is a better drug for patients with compromised liver or kidney function as the inactive isomer levomedetomidine is not present, therefore the **metabolic load is lessened**.

Opioids

Opioids are the best analgesics available and play an important role in pre-medication/sedation as part of the neuroleptanalgesia regimes and preventative analgesia. They can be used on their **own for mild sedation or combined with sedatives for a deeper sedative effect**. There are different types which are classified into groups based on their pharmacological properties.

Opioids affect the mood and produce some level of sedation, but this is opioid dependant. Apart from providing analgesia for acute pain, opioids are used as part of sedation, pre-medication, preventive analgesia, and as part of a balanced anaesthetic technique (e.g. opioids have sparing effects of other anaesthetic drugs).

Opioids bind to opioid receptors within the peripheral and central nervous system reducing the release of excitatory neurotransmitters and producing neuronal hyperpolarization. These changes decrease nociceptive input producing analgesia. There are different types of opioids with different effects depending on their receptor affinity, efficacy potency and individual characteristics.

Full mu receptor agonists (e.g. methadone) provide the best analgesia but **their effect on demeanour is variable**, from sedation to dysphoria/euphoria with high doses.

Partial mu-agonists (e.g. buprenorphine) have partial effects so the analgesia provided is not as good as the analgesia provided by full mu-agonists. However, they tend to cause more sedation and sense of calmness and euphoria for cats and less dysphoria compared to full mu-agonists.

Mixed agonists-antagonists (e.g. butorphanol) produce the best sedation due to the agonistic effect on kappa receptors, but as they are mu antagonists they have poor analgesic effects.

The competitive antagonist (e.g. naloxone) is used to reverse opioids effects. It is important to remember that if naloxone is used the analgesia terminates while naloxone remains active.

There are still misconceptions about the use of opioids in cats and some people prefer not to use them due to the morphine mania. This is more of an **urban legend** as the knowledge of opioid pharmacokinetics in cats has improved and this is a problem rarely encountered at clinical doses. Opioids are an important tool for the anaesthetist. However, it is important to select one over another one to maximize their benefits and minimize the side effects.

- clinical effects:
  - analgesia
  - sedation
  - dysphoria
  - euphoria
  - mydriasis (Figure 9)
  - increased vagal tone
  - MAC (minimum alveolar concentration) sparing effects
  - anaesthetic stability as part of balanced technique
- side effects:
  - vagally mediated and dose dependent bradycardia, but no effects on myocardial contractility or systemic vascular resistance
  - nausea, vomiting, hypersalivation
  - decrease in gastric emptying and gastrointestinal motility
  - dose-dependent respiratory depression
  - Increased urethral sphincter tone, inhibiting voiding reflex
  - urinary retention when morphine is used in an epidural injection
  - decreased thermoregulatory mechanisms
  - hyperthermia
  - histamine release risk if morphine and pethidine are administered intravenously.

Methadone

Methadone is a full mu-agonist opioid, widely used in the UK and many other countries in the world. It is

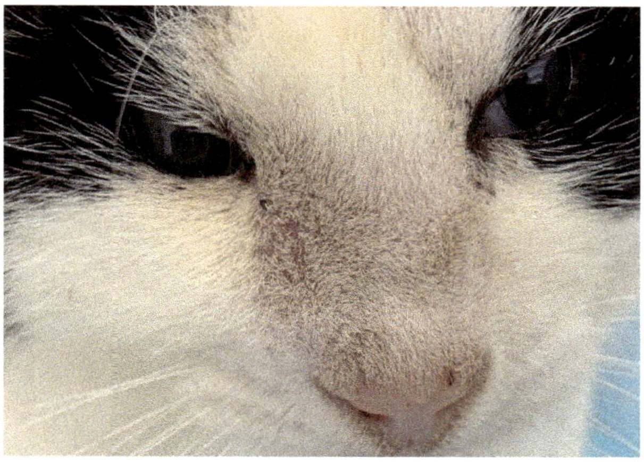

Figure 9. Mydriasis after buprenorphine administration.

licensed for cats and used primarily for its **good analgesic effect**. It does have NMDA receptor antagonist properties, in addition to its overall analgesic effect. It can be used orally but its bioavailability is low, so it is best used injected either SC, IM or IV. The **recommended doses for cats are 0.1–0.3mg/kg**. Although licensed doses are much higher, in the author's experience, cats may become agitated and excited at doses higher than 0.3mg/kg. Its **effects last for 2–4 hours**.

Morphine

Morphine is a full mu-agonist which provides some sedation and great analgesia similar to methadone, but with the disadvantage of not having NMDA antagonist effect. If used **intravenously it must be diluted and administered slowly to avoid histamine release**. It can safely be administered via other routes such as SC or IM. Morphine can cause vomiting, however in dogs this can be avoided by administering acepromazine in advance (Valverde et al., 2004). In the preservative-free form, it can be used epidurally as part of the locoregional anaesthetic techniques with the advantage of providing analgesia for up to 24 hours. Clinically useful **doses are in the range of 0.05–0.2 mg/kg. Its effects last for 4–6 h.**

Pethidine

Pethidine (Figure 10) is a full mu-agonist with a **short duration (1–2 h)**. It provides good sedation and analgesia. It is safe from a cardiovascular point of view as it rarely causes bradycardia (molecular structure resembles an anticholinergic) but it must always be **administered SC or IM**, because IV administration causes histamine release and therefore, never administer pethidine IV. Common clinically used **doses are 2–6 mg/kg**.

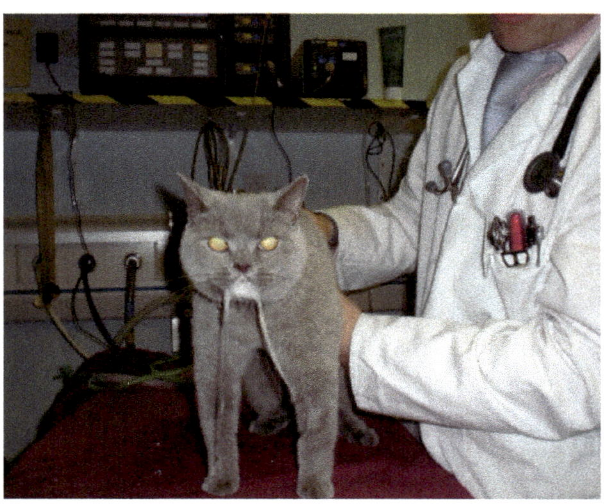

Figure 10. Cat after IM pethidine administration.

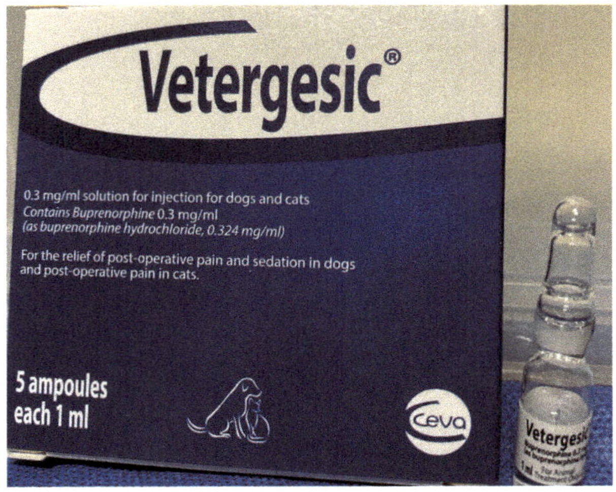

Figure 11. Buprenorphine.

Buprenorphine

Buprenorphine (Figure 11) is a partial mu-agonist opioid. It has all the clinical effects of full mu-agonists, but the efficacy is only partial, therefore the analgesic effect is less than a full mu-agonist opioid. Moreover, **buprenorphine has a ceiling effect** which restricts the possibility of increasing analgesia by administering a higher dose of buprenorphine. Furthermore, if the cat is painful and requires the administration of a full mu-agonist, the analgesic effect is not as effective in the presence of buprenorphine. Buprenorphine binds to the mu receptors more strongly than a full mu-agonist, preventing the full mu-agonist from exerting its complete effect. However, studies that have compared buprenorphine analgesic effect to those of full mu-agonists showed that buprenorphine provides good analgesia in cats despite it being only a partial agonist (Stanway et al., 2002). The advantage of buprenorphine is that it hardly ever causes dysphoria, and all the other side effects are mild. When buprenorphine is administered, cats seem happier (e.g. purring) without excitation. Another advantage **is the oral transmucosal route (OTM) can be used**, plus IV, SC and IM routes. Some studies in cats found similar effects when oral transmucosal route was used compared to IM or SC administration but the analgesic effect was not comparable, providing less analgesia when the OTM route was compared to intravenous buprenorphine (Robertson et al., 2005). Buprenorphine has a slow onset of action and a long duration of action. It may **take up to 45 minutes to achieve peak effect and this will last for 6–8 hours**. Effective **doses of buprenorphine are 0.01–0.02 mg/kg**.

Butorphanol

Butorphanol (Figure 12) is a mixed agonist antagonist. It is an agonist of kappa receptors which produce the best sedation of all opioids and an antagonist of mu

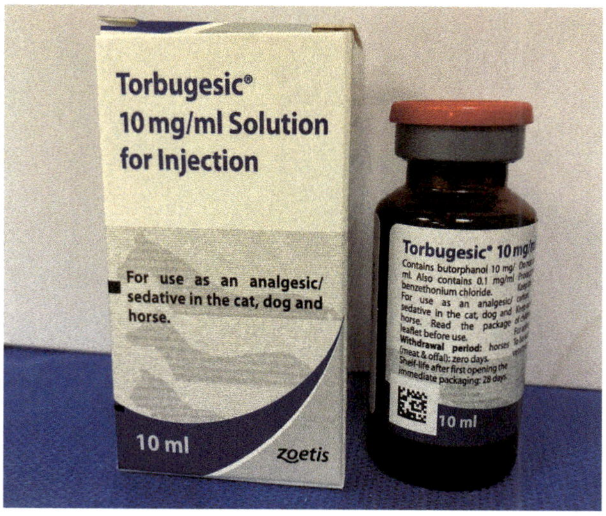

Figure 12. Butorphanol.

receptors which limit its ability to provide analgesia. **Butorphanol is a poor analgesic for cats**, with a fast onset, and the effect lasts **2–4 hours. Clinically useful doses are 0.1–0.4 mg/kg**.

Neuroleptoanalgesia

Neuroleptoanalgesia is the combination of a major/minor tranquilizer or sedative with an analgesic like an opioid. This combination is **synergistic**, therefore, the sedation and the analgesia are more intense compared to when the single agents are administered separately even at higher doses. The advantage is that **a more profound effect is achieved at lower drugs doses** minimizing the appearance of side effects. As opioids are required for any painful procedure the use of a neuroleptoanalgesic combination is widely used in feline medicine.

Anaesthetics used as heavy sedatives (ketamine, alfaxalone, propofol)

(For more information on ketamine, alfaxalone, and propofol see Anaesthesia induction).

Some anaesthetics, such as alfaxalone or ketamine can be used as sedatives at certain doses via IM or SC.

Ketamine

Ketamine is **a dissociative anaesthetic** commonly used in cats. When used in combination with other sedatives it exerts a beneficial effect with a wide safety margin and wide therapeutic index. It is the most effective drug for chemical restraint and therefore it is widely used in wild cats. For the feral domestic cat, it can be used at a dose of 20 mg/kg squirted into the mouth as the cat is hissing to help with handling, however this produces excessive salivation and should only be used as a last resort.

The recommended doses **for IM injection are 3–6 mg/kg**. When used combined with alpha-2 agonists, it should not be antagonised until the effect of ketamine is over.

Alfaxalone

Alfaxalone is aneurosteroid anaesthetic and can be used on its own or in combinations as a sedative via IM route. The doses used are **1–3 mg/kg IM** (up to 5 mg/kg when used alone).

Intravenous alfaxalone and propofol

Either alfaxalone or propofol could be used at very low intravenous doses, to provide heavy sedation if stillness for a brief period is required. However, this may be risky, and the authors do not recommend it due to the lack of scientific evidence, individual variation, and the side effects. Moreover, it is difficult to titrate to a deep sedative state without reaching anaesthesia; the risk of apnoea and unprotected airways with weak/no swallow reflex may end up in catastrophic situations.

Neither propofol nor alfaxalone are licensed for cats to be used intravenously for sedative purposes. When using this technique, supplementary oxygen via mask and full monitoring are mandatory, and a full endotracheal intubation emergency kit should be available before the start of the sedation.

All the drugs discussed above can be combined to provide good sedation. The combination can include two (i.e. double combination) or three (i.e. triple combination) different drugs.

IV/IM/SC sedation with a double combination

Acepromazine + opioid

- great combination for mild diagnostic procedures
- the most common sedative combination is acepromazine and butorphanol
- the combination of both types of drug has a synergistic effect for sedation
- If the patient is in shock, dehydrated or hypovolemic, it is not safe to administer this combination as acepromazine affects the cardiovascular system and it cannot be reversed
- If emesis is contraindicated, the choice of opioid should be carefully considered or acepromazine administered prior to opioid administration.

Benzodiazepine + opioid

- minimal effect on cardiopulmonary system
- very safe combination for critical patients
- reliable sedation effect. Effects depend on individual health status, temperament, and age

- neonates, geriatrics, and critical sick patients sedate well with this combination
- not good combination in healthy wriggly cats as excitation may occur.

(Dex-) Medetomidine + opioid

- potent combination, strong reliable sedation
- suitable for minor surgical procedures (e.g. superficial wound closure), short diagnostic procedures, and invasive examinations
- good muscle relaxation and analgesia.
- suitable for pre-medication for surgical procedures if the correct opioid is chosen (i.e. full mu-agonist)
- careful patient selection, should only be used in healthy animals.

(Dex-) Medetomidine + benzodiazepine

- good for muscle relaxation and positioning the patient for radiographs
- benzodiazepine potentiates sedation caused by medetomidine
- may be insufficient if analgesia is required.

(Dex-) Medetomidine + ketamine

- sedation from medetomidine counteracts excitation caused by ketamine
- the combination produces profound sedation-mild anaesthesia
- adequate for short invasive procedures and minor surgeries (e.g. wound closure, minor wound debridement)
- should only be used in healthy patients as it has cardiovascular effects
- antagonism of the alpha-2 agonist should be at least 45 min from the combination injection, otherwise a rough violent recovery may happen due to the ketamine.

Ketamine + benzodiazepine

- benzodiazepine provides muscle relaxation and counteract agitation and ketamine excitement
- great combination for cats
- safe combination for the cardiovascular system
- induces heavy sedation of short duration (30–45 min)
- disorientation common for a few hours during recovery
- if ketamine is administered at high doses, it provides anaesthesia.

Sedation with a triple combination

A triple combination provides a more profound sedation if the drugs are chosen correctly. Many combinations are possible but should include at least one of the main sedative drugs for optimal sedation effect. A good combination for non-painful procedures is the **combination of medetomidine, ketamine, and butorphanol** which provides a strong sedation and ideal chemical restraint of the fractious cat.

The following chart is a triple combination based on the use of an alpha-2 agonist:

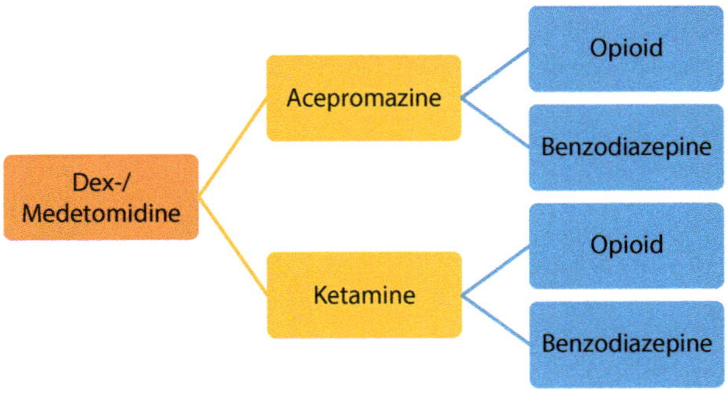

The following chart is for triple combinations based on the use of ketamine:

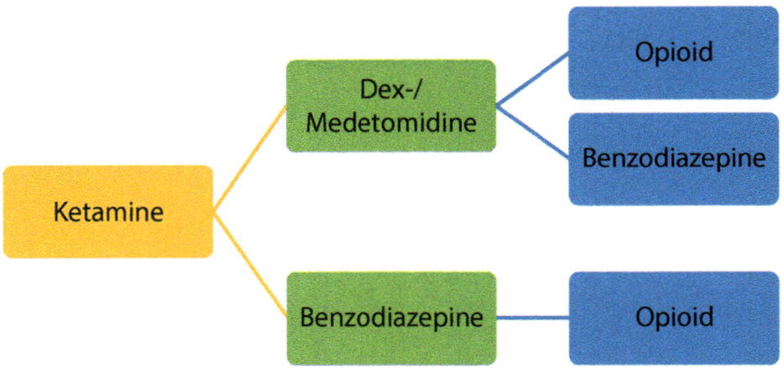

The following chart is good for a relatively safe triple combination, as it spares ketamine and (dex-) medetomidine. It is useful in an IM combination for patients where ketamine and alpha-2 agonists are contraindicated. Depending on the alfaxalone dose it produces heavy sedation without the cardiovascular depression of alpha-2 agonists and without the tachycardia produced by ketamine. Ideal for old cats (e.g. aggressive geriatric hyperthyroid).

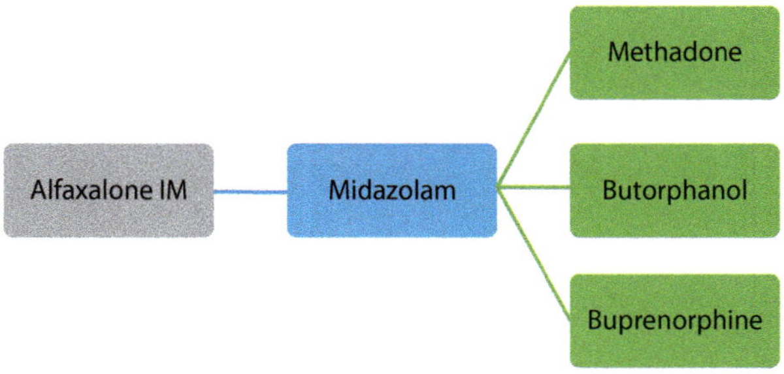

Anaesthesia induction

General considerations

Induction is a critical time in the anaesthesia period. Administration of induction drugs (Figure 13) can

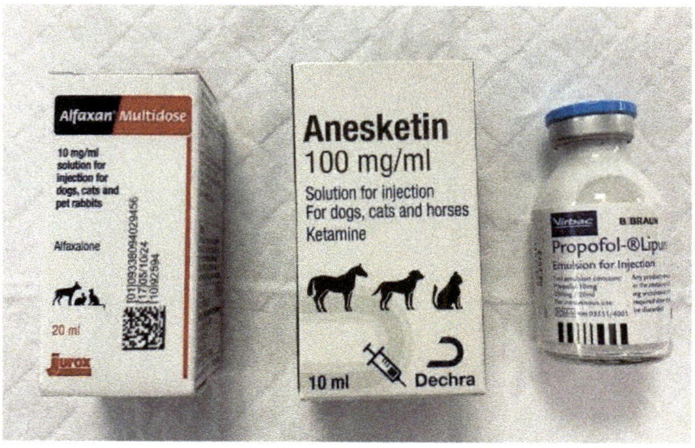

Figure 13. Induction agents.

produce respiratory and cardiovascular depression. **Monitoring appropriately and administration of pre-oxygenation** via face mask or flow-by to minimise oxygen desaturation if apnoea occurs are crucial.

Anaesthesia is often induced with parenteral injectable anaesthetic drugs, whilst some agents (e.g. ketamine, alfaxalone) are injected intramuscularly to induce short periods of anaesthesia which is common practice in spay/neuter clinics. Anaesthesia can potentially be topped up and prolonged by injecting further anaesthetic drugs IM. The disadvantage of this technique is that multiple IM injections may end up causing **drug accumulation and slow recoveries**. However, the advantages include being cost effective and reducing stress in nervous patients (e.g. during intravenous catheter placement). It is important to be aware that parenteral anaesthesia may give a false sense of safety, as some practitioners fail to appreciate the need for intravenous access or/and endotracheal intubation even though the patient is fully anaesthetised. **Intravenous access and endotracheal intubation** for airway protection and assisted ventilation are always required when anaesthesia is induced, regardless of the method chosen, even for short anaesthetics. **Oxygen supplementation** is highly recommended even when an anaesthetic machine is not available. Moreover, an ambu bag suffices to provide assisted ventilation if the patient becomes apnoeic. For long procedures or complicated cases intravenous inductions are recommended, followed by anaesthetic maintenance via total intravenous anaesthesia or an inhalant agent. From the beginning of anaesthesia (even before induction if possible) full monitoring is required; evidence shows **monitoring decreases morbidity and mortality in feline anaesthesia**.

Individual agents

Propofol

Propofol binds to $GABA_A$ receptors within the central nervous system, hyperpolarizing the postsynaptic cell membrane and increasing chloride conductance, which causes inhibition of postsynaptic neurons. It decreases GABA dissociation from receptors, so there is an increase in GABA activity and CNS depression.

Propofol is a lipid emulsion, which is not water-soluble and can **only be administered intravenously**. It contains soybean oil, glycerol and egg lecithin making it easy for bacteria to grow, and therefore once the bottle is opened it should be discarded after eight hours. Current formulation should not be painful on injection, but the author's experience is that occasionally some cats react to propofol injection. Human patients report a cold sensation when propofol is infused but it is unknown if is similar in cats. **Propofol should not be mixed** with any other drug in the same syringe or diluted. In case of accidental perivascular injection current formulations do not cause tissue damage. There is a longer shelf duration propofol marketed called propofol 28 or propofol plus which contains benzyl alcohol as a preservative, which can be used up to 28 days after opening. Although designed to be more cost-effective and to reduce anaesthetic waste, **cats can be sensitive to benzyl alcohol accumulation and toxicity**, so caution is recommended if this product is to be used multiple days or as maintenance agent. Cats seem to be more reactive on injection of this version of propofol. Propofol clear preparation was available for veterinary use, but it is no longer recommended as it caused problems such as pain on injection and phlebitis and even cardiovascular collapse.

Propofol is an intravenous anaesthetic drug for induction and maintenance of anaesthesia. Propofol should be administered slowly, **titrated to effect** to minimise its main side effects, which are reduction in cardiac output and systemic vascular resistance causing hypotension and strong respiratory depression, even apnoea. Propofol does have some use as an antiepileptic drug for treatment of status epilepticus after GABAergic drugs have failed to work (benzodiazepines, barbiturates). It does not have any analgesic properties but is known for producing smooth anaesthesia induction with placid, excitement-free recoveries when used as the sole maintenance agent.

After a single injection propofol reaches the main sites of action in the CNS and body tissues which are highly vascularised. Then it is redistributed in fat and in the rest of body tissues causing a rapid decrease in plasma levels and hence patients recover quickly. **Propofol is considered an ultrashort anaesthetic agent**. It is **metabolised by the liver** into sulphates and glucuronide conjugates and there is a fraction of extrahepatic metabolism with lungs playing a role with high first-pass extraction. Due to cats limited capacity for glucuronide conjugation, **multiple injections or constant rate infusions of propofol in cats may cause prolonged recoveries or anaemia**.

Although the effect of propofol on intraocular pressure is unclear, compared to some anaesthetics (especially inhalants) it decreases cerebral metabolic rate, preserves cerebral blood flow for autoregulatory mechanisms, and preserves the reactivity of cerebral vessels to carbon dioxide. Therefore, propofol has an interesting neuroprotection property and is **the preferred agent for neuroanaesthesia**.

Although it has anticonvulsant properties, propofol occasionally causes opisthotonus, myoclonus, and excitation during very slow inductions. It seems good sedation during pre-medication reduces this risk but if it occurs it should self-resolve as additional propofol is injected and anaesthesia develops.

Propofol is only effective if administered intravenously and its clinical effects last for 3–5 minutes. In general doses of propofol required for cats are higher than those required for dogs. The cardiovascular depression produced by propofol inductions can be profound especially for hypovolemic, sick cats, or those with cardiac disease. A co-induction technique with other agents can be helpful to achieve a smooth induction with less cardiovascular depression. Slow administration to effect is crucial as it minimises cardiovascular depression and apnoea.

Propofol is the agent of choice for head trauma, space occupying lesions, and caesareans but caution is advisable in cases with respiratory or cardiac disease, hypovolemic and geriatric fragile cats.

Cats may sneeze and paw at their ears and face while waking up from propofol. This is normal and hardly ever requires intervention as it is short-lived and self-limiting.

Ketamine

Ketamine (Figure 14) **is a dissociative anaesthetic agent**. It rapidly penetrates the blood-brain barrier, with a slower onset than propofol (e.g. 30–90 seconds). It may take 5–15 minutes for the peak effect when injected via other routes (i.e. intramuscular). Ketamine is fast, reliable, and produces complete immobility and anaesthesia even in the fiercest patient.

Within the CNS it induces a state of dissociation with profound analgesia and amnesia but increased muscle tone. Patients preserve laryngeal, pharyngeal, pineal, and pedal reflexes and keep the eyes wide open with the ability to blink. It is a cataleptic state induced by inhibition of thalamocortical pathways and stimulation of the limbic system.

Ketamine interacts with multiple receptors and binding sites within the CNS, such as the glutamate, nicotinic, muscarinic, cholinergic, monoaminergic, and opioid receptors apart from calcium and sodium voltage channels. But an interesting interaction is the NMDA receptor antagonism accounting for most of the analgesic, amnesic, and psychotomimetic effects.

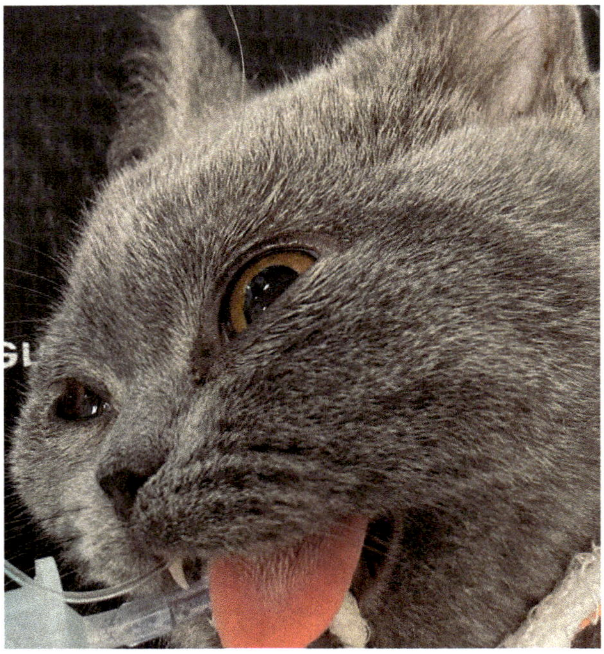

Figure 14. Cat with central eye position due to ketamine.

Although effective as an anaesthetic via intramuscular, the doses required IM are at least double from intravenous and it is painful on injection due to its low pH.

Due to its psychotomimetic effects, hallucinations, and lack of muscle relaxation, **ketamine should not be used alone**. Ketamine should be combined with a heavy sedative drug to counteract those effects and provide muscle relaxation. **Benzodiazepines and alpha-2 agonists** are a great combination, but it is important not to antagonise these drugs unless in an emergency or the ketamine effect has long finished.

After injection, ketamine redistributes, and patients will recover. Ketamine undergoes liver extraction and rapid metabolism with main active metabolite being nor-ketamine. In cats unchanged ketamine is excreted by the kidneys. This is why cats with kidney disease may get drowsier, have slower recoveries, and become more agitated after ketamine.

Ketamine has unique cardiovascular effects. It causes central stimulation of the cardiovascular system by increasing sympathetic tone (e.g. increase in heart rate and blood pressure). This is a notable feature as **ketamine provides a safer induction for patients which are sick, hypovolemic, dehydrated or septic**. On the other hand, the higher oxygen demand and increased myocardial work may be detrimental for specific cardiac diseases like hypertrophic cardiomyopathy (HCM). It is worth mentioning that ketamine has a direct myocardial depression effect, but this is rarely seen as the predominant overall effect is central sympathetic stimulation.

Ketamine has minimal respiratory depression effect but may cause an apneustic breathing pattern after a bolus induction or after a bolus while the patient is anaesthetised.

Recoveries from ketamine anaesthetics can be poor and associated with hyperexcitability especially if ketamine was the only main maintenance anaesthetic agent and sedation during recovery may be required. Therefore, ketamine is not recommended as a main anaesthetic agent in total intravenous protocols.

Ketamine increases salivation and respiratory secretions and may contribute to airway blockage of the small airways. Endotracheal intubation for airway protection and patency is essential but even so endotracheal tubes may become blocked by airway secretion. Thorough continuous monitoring of respiration is necessary.

Ketamine is not good for neuroanaesthesia as it increases cerebral metabolic rate and decreases the threshold for seizures. It is not used for patients with known seizures disorder or known intracranial disease. However, there is evidence to show ketamine may be useful to treat refractory status epilepticus when all GABAergic drugs have failed to work.

Ketamine may increase intraocular pressure and should be avoided for intraocular surgery or ophthalmology cases with bad corneal ulcers or cases where the eye is at risk of rupture.

It is important to recognise ketamine provides a different type of anaesthesia and **the eye remains wide open and central**. This can represent an extra challenge for the inexperienced anaesthetist as to monitor depth of anaesthesia can be sometimes quite challenging. There is also an **increased risk of corneal ulcer formation**, therefore eye lubrication should be used during and after ketamine administration.

Ketofol

The intravenous combination of ketamine and propofol for induction as **per equal doses, 2 mg/kg for each**, minimises side effects and achieves a smoother and safer induction than when used separately as sole agents. However, this combination of two drugs is not licensed for induction.

Propofol provides smooth induction, muscle relaxation and heavy sedation to counteract high muscle tonicity and nightmares from ketamine. On the other hand, ketamine improves the cardiovascular system by increasing the sympathetic tone and overrides the cardiovascular depression produced by propofol. **Propofol (2 mg/kg) should be administered first, followed by ketamine to avoid muscle rigidity and excitation.**

The pharmacokinetics of ketofol CRI (constant rate infusion) has been reported by Zonca et al., 2012.

Alfaxalone

Alfaxalone is a neurosteroid, progesterone derivative. It has similar mechanism of action to propofol or barbiturates; it modulates $GABA_A$ receptors and produces general anaesthesia and good muscle relaxation.

Alfaxalone is not water soluble, so it is included in a cyclodextrin in its current commercial preparation. It is different from the alfaxalone-alphadolone product (Saffan) used for cats many years ago, which caused anaphylactic reactions due to the inclusion of the surfactant agent cremophor EL.

It does not seem to accumulate at clinical doses and can be used as maintenance agent through top ups or constant rate infusion. Nevertheless, in cats dose-dependent disposition occurs and it has slower elimination compared to dogs. Periods of anaesthesia longer than 60 minutes with alfaxalone used for maintenance seem to prolong recoveries in cats (Pypendop et al., 2018).

Alfaxalone induces anaesthesia when injected intravenously but it is also effective via IM route. Alfaxalone produces anaesthesia or heavy sedation depending on the intramuscular dose chosen. It does not cause pain when injected IM as the clear solution has neutral pH. **Subcutaneous injections have been used in hyperthyroid cats for sedation achieving peak effects 45 minutes post-injection** (Tamura et al., 2015).

Alfaxalone is another of the so-called ultrashort anaesthetic agents, **lasting for 5–10 minutes** after an intravenous bolus. Induction quality is smooth but in the authors opinion nowadays there are cats which have become more reactive and jump after intravenous injection. It is possible the recent inclusion of preservatives in the current alfaxalone formulation is more irritant than the previous version. On the contrary, **cats recovering from alfaxalone may become dysphoric, agitated, twitchy and even present with opisthotonus.** This effect can be minimised administering more sedatives in the pre-medication. Cats should be placed in a quiet dark area to recover from alfaxalone anaesthesia, as noise and light may trigger this reaction. Route of administration may influence the recovery quality. Intramuscular routes seem to cause worst recoveries with more excitation than the intravenous route. The anticonvulsant effects of alfaxalone are not as good as propofol but has better neuroprotective activity than ketamine as it decreases cerebral metabolic rate.

Alfaxalone may cause a dose-dependent cardiovascular depression during induction by decreasing systemic vascular resistance and cardiac output. Frequently, pronounced tachycardia is observed during induction.

Alfaxalone produces respiratory depression and even apnoea when administered too fast. For very small cats alfaxalone can be diluted to administer it slowly and minimise side effects.

Is alfaxalone superior to propofol?

Both agents have similar mechanisms of action with similar **dose-dependent cardiovascular depression**, although there are small differences between them. Propofol produces a reset of the baroreceptors, therefore, compensatory tachycardia to the hypotension is not seen. Moreover, instead bradycardia is sometimes observed. During alfaxalone induction, tachycardia is often present however this effect is short lived and resolves quickly in healthy cats. If bradycardia or tachycardia are contraindicated, then caution should be exercised with these two drugs.

Apnoea and respiratory depression are observed with both agents, and both require slow administration to effect to minimise apnoea (Taboada et al., 2010)

Quality of induction is smooth for both agents, achieving quite rapidly good conditions for a smooth intubation. Nevertheless, titration to effect is much easier to achieve with propofol because it is less potent so it requires a bigger injection volume.

Recoveries with propofol tend to be calm and of good quality, occasionally cats want to paw their noses/faces but are otherwise quiet. On the other hand, twitching is fairly common on alfaxalone recoveries, sometimes excitement, paddling and trembling, or muscle rigidity are observed too (Mathis et al., 2012)

Due to its extrahepatic metabolism propofol is the agent of choice in cats with liver disease but continuous infusion or multiple anaesthesia with propofol in cats may end up in prolonged recoveries due to the inability to glucuronidate phenols like propofol. Alfaxalone should be used in cats if total intravenous anaesthesia is required.

Another side effect **from multiple injections of propofol in cats is the oxidative red blood cell injury with Heinz-body formation and anaemia. Propofol should only be administered intravenously**.

Both agents have a similar risk for gastro-oesophageal reflux under anaesthesia as they reduce the cardia sphincter pressure.

Currently alfaxalone is more expensive than propofol. However, the new alfaxalone formulation contains a preservative allowing a longer shelf life once the bottle is broached. This makes alfaxalone much more cost-effective and almost same price especially if sensible doses are used.

Etomidate

Etomidate is an imidazole compound which binds to specific sites at the $GABA_A$ receptors enhancing GABA activity and producing anaesthesia.

Etomidate is an ultrashort anaesthetic agent which produces a smooth anaesthesia with rapid onset. Unfortunately, it can be expensive and there are not many clinical studies in cats, therefore it is not popular in practice. **Its main advantage is the lack of cardiovascular and respiratory adverse effects**. It is the **agent of choice for cats with third-degree AV block** or other complicated severe cardiac conditions. It can be used in critical patients, but it can suppress adrenocortical function in a dose dependant manner, so diminishing the natural physiological stress response. Etomidate has been seen as a contributing cause of death in critical human patients in critical care units due to this effect on adrenal glands. These patients had etomidate infusions for prolonged periods, and it is unclear how clinically relevant this can be for a cat with normal adrenocortical function. However, it is important to **use with caution in patients with abnormal liver or kidney function** due to its possible prolonged elimination and long lasting effects. **Etomidate should be avoided in cats with hypo/hyperadrenocorticism**.

The quality of induction may be poor due to irritation and myoclonus/muscle rigidity, but the addition of a benzodiazepine helps overcome those adverse effects.

Inductions via mask/box with inhalant agents

Induction of anaesthesia with an inhalant agent such as isoflurane or sevoflurane using a cat chamber/box or via tight face mask causes a lot of distress and excitation for the cat and poses an important environment pollution and contaminant hazard for all the personnel involved. Therefore, **authors recommend against its use**.

Maintenance (inhalatory and injectable anaesthesia)

Inhalatory anaesthesia

Inhalants have been around for a long time. The first use of ether was recorded in the UK as early as 1846. Towards late 1950's halothane was discovered as the first modern inhalant, being a safer and improved version than previous inhalants. Nevertheless, newer agents such as **isoflurane, sevoflurane, and desflurane** are currently available and have displaced halothane in most countries. These new inhalants are widely used and trusted due to their wide margin of safety and ease of use. They are the closest version of an ideal inhalant anaesthetic.

The mechanism of action of inhalant agents is still not fully understood. The previous theory of disruption of lipid bilayer of neuron membrane is not necessarily true. Most likely inhalants interact with cell membrane proteins and a range of receptors and ion channels at a central level within the CNS.

In general, inhalant agents impact on different systems:

- **Central nervous system**: inhalant agents cause a reversible dose-dependent depression, increase in cerebral blood flow due to vasodilation, increase in intracranial pressure, and decrease in metabolic rate. They also produce an alteration of thermoregulation and sympathetic/parasympathetic outflow.
- **Respiratory system**: inhalants cause a dose dependent respiratory depression with a decrease in tidal-volume and/or respiratory rate. This causes hypercapnia and cerebral vasodilation and depression.
- **Cardiovascular system**: inhalants depress the heart and the vascular tone. There is a decrease in cardiac output, mean blood pressure and vascular resistance, causing dose-dependent hypotension. Inhalants are also negative inotropes. Some can cause arrhythmias (i.e. halothane). There is also a decrease in regional blood flow.

Minimal alveolar concentration (MAC)

Minimal alveolar concentration (MAC) is defined as the minimal alveolar concentration of an inhalant required to avoid movement in 50% of cats' population when a surgical stimulus is applied. **Hence, MAC is an indication of the potency of the inhalant agent.** MAC can be influenced by many factors as well as by the individual patient, therefore it is important to adjust the MAC to the patient. (Tables 2 and 3).

Individual inhalant agents

Isoflurane

- Fluorinated ether used in veterinary medicine since 1980's, still in use today.
- Shelf-stable product which does not require preservatives.
- Dose dependent cardiovascular depression mainly by reducing systemic vascular resistance with vasodilation

Table 2. Factors affecting MAC.

Increase in MAC	Decrease in MAC
Hyperthermia	Hypothermia
Catecholamines/ sympathomimetics	Hypoxaemia
Hypernatremia	Hypercapnia
Hyperthyroidism	Hypothyroidism
	Drugs causing CNS depression (sedatives, injectable anaesthetics)
	Analgesic agents
	Pregnancy
	Old age
	Hypotension

MAC = minimum alveolar concentration

Table 3. Comparison of isoflurane, sevoflurane and desflurane.

	Isoflurane	Sevoflurane	Desflurane
Blood: gas partition coefficient	Low coefficient	Lower than isoflurane	Lower than isoflurane or sevoflurane
MAC	1.63–2.2%	2.58–3.41%	9.79–10.2%
Liver metabolism	0.2%	2–5%	0.02%
Arrhythmogenicity	No It does not sensitize the heart to catecholamines	No It does not sensitize the heart to catecholamines	No It does not sensitize the heart to catecholamines
Pungent odour Airway irritation	Yes Not recommended for box/mask induction	It has a much more pleasant odour than isoflurane. It is the inhalant of choice for box/mask induction Less irritant than isoflurane	Yes Not recommended for box/mask induction
Price	Cheap	More expensive than isoflurane	Very expensive (special vaporizer)

Blood: gas partition coefficient. This parameter provides information on the speed of onset of anaesthesia and recovery from anaesthesia. The lower the coefficient the faster the onset and recovery.
MAC = minimum alveolar concentration. This parameter provides information about the potency of the agent. The lower the MAC the more potent the agent.

and hypotension. It does not affect cardiac contractility so much. Studies reported minimal cardiovascular depression at 1.3 MAC but hypotension started at 2 MAC (Steffey et al., 2015).
- Respiratory depression in a dose dependent manner is also possible with a reduction of tidal volume and hypercapnia as the dose of isoflurane increases.
- Apnoea has been observed at 2.4 MAC. Isoflurane causes more respiratory depression compared to sevoflurane and desflurane.

Sevoflurane

- Fluorinated ether, used in veterinary medicine since 1990's.
- Dose dependent cardiovascular depression reported at 1.25 MAC. It may produce a reduction in arterial blood pressure, cardiac index, and stroke volume. Some studies reported less hypotension in cats anaesthetised with sevoflurane compared to isoflurane, despite substantial myocardial depression.
- Respiratory depression in a dose dependent manner is also possible but seems to be less severe in cats than other species.
- Not indicated for low flow anaesthesia as sevoflurane may react with carbon dioxide absorbent and produce compound A, which in experimental laboratory conditions was nephrotoxic in rats, however the clinical significance of this is unknown.

Desflurane

- Fluorinated ether, currently used in human medicine but not approved for veterinary species.
- Due to its high vapour pressure (700 mmHg), desflurane is a gas at room temperature, which makes it quite unique as it needs a special double coated glass-plastic bottle where it is kept under high pressure as a liquid. From the bottle passes onto a large special vaporiser which heats desflurane and keeps it as gas that is directly mixed with oxygen in a calibrated and very precise way. Desflurane vaporisers require an electricity source and a warming-up period before use. As it is a more expensive vaporiser and requires an understanding of physics and experience, desflurane use is still limited for veterinary patients.
- Dose dependent cardiovascular depression has been reported in cats at 1.3 MAC and 1.7 MAC (Steffey et al., 2015). It may produce a reduction in mean arterial blood pressure but not much effect on cardiac index. Respiratory depression and hypercapnia in a dose dependent manner has been seen with respiratory rate maintained but tidal volume decreased as desflurane dose increases.
- In humans it has been reported to cause thyroid storms with fast changes in concentration. Nothing has been reported in cats, but caution and monitoring is advisable when using desflurane.

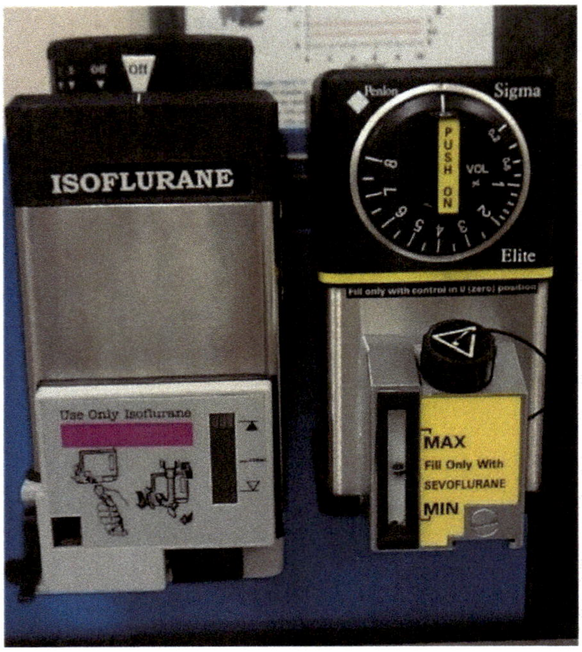

Figure 15. Isoflurane and sevoflurane.

Isoflurane versus sevoflurane

- Both agents are licensed for dogs and cats in the UK.
- Clinically, sevoflurane is similar to isoflurane although isoflurane causes more respiratory depression than sevoflurane. Isoflurane causes respiratory arrest at 2.5 MAC while sevoflurane causes apnoea at 3 MAC.
- Neither sevoflurane nor isoflurane are analgesic.
- Sevoflurane produces more complete recoveries when no other drugs are used. This is potentially of benefit for brachycephalic breeds or any cat which may have complications in recovery due to upper respiratory obstruction or respiratory disease. In these cases, sevoflurane is less respiratory depressant apart from providing a better quality and faster recovery.
- Sevoflurane is the agent of choice if mask or box induction is necessary.

Injectable anaesthesia: total intravenous anaesthesia (TIVA)

TIVA (total intravenous anaesthesia) is a term that includes **any anaesthetic combination with no inhalant, as a constant/variable rate infusion (CRI/VRI) to maintain anaesthesia**. The objective of the TIVA with a constant infusion is to obtain **less variation in plasma concentration with fewer oscillations in cardiovascular, respiratory, and central effects so it is safer for the patient**. Pharmacokinetic models are mathematical descriptions of how a drug disposes in the body and are necessary to design TIVA dosing regimens for a particular species. The latest TIVA advances include **target-controlled infusion (TCI)** techniques, where dosing rates are adjusted to achieve effective drug plasma concentrations, based on the pharmacokinetics of the specific drug. The TCI software used in human anaesthesia includes pharmacokinetic models that are applied to the specific individual: patient data like age and body weight are introduced in the syringe driver. Then the software calculates the specific dose to target the plasma concentration required. A model of TCI has been studied for dogs with propofol, but the clinical application is still far from reality.

The **ideal TIVA drug does not accumulate** so the infusion can be kept constant, but unfortunately there is no ideal injectable anaesthetic drug and over prolonged periods of time distribution occurs. Nevertheless, there are individual and species differences plus surgical stimulation which make constant adjustments to the infusion necessary throughout the procedure. Therefore, the concept of CRI (constant rate infusion) (Figure 16) is becoming obsolete and **VRI** (variable rate infusion) **is gaining popularity**.

The **three main agents used for TIVA are ketamine, propofol, and alfaxalone**. Etomidate is also available and its pharmacodynamics especially in the cardiovascular system make it a safe induction drug. Nevertheless, etomidate use should be restricted to highly critical cardiac patients as a single induction agent. Etomidate is not licensed for veterinary use and it is not indicated as a maintenance agent due to the **depression of the adrenal glands**, which impedes cortisol release and the physiological stress response. This is detrimental for the compromised patient, especially in a critical care setting.

In a surgical setting, ketamine should be administered in conjunction with another analgesic drug since ketamine alone does not provide sufficient analgesia. In addition, **ketamine must never be administered on its own;** it is always necessary the coadministration of a potent sedative or a benzodiazepine to prevent the hallucinatory effects and counteract muscle rigidity. Once the procedure is finished, if ketamine effects are still present it is preferable to recover the animal slowly and not to antagonise the alpha-2 whenever possible.

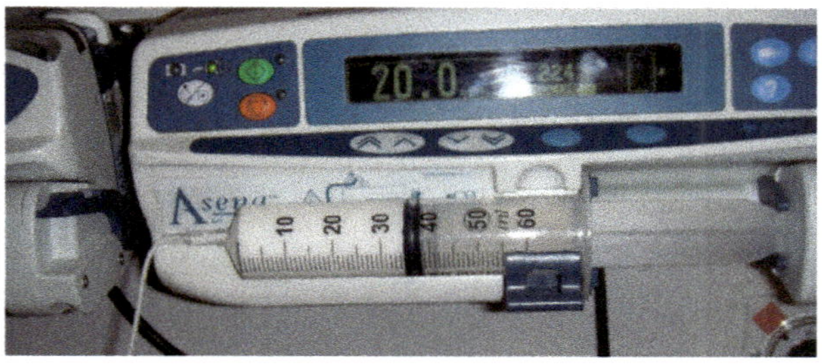

Figure 16. Propofol CRI.

Propofol and alfaxalone have been widely used for dogs and cats as maintenance agents in TIVA protocols. Dose ranges are available for both drugs so they can be infused to effect based on the clinical signs of the individual. Monitoring TIVA can be challenging as the signs to assess anaesthesia depth often differ from the inhalant anaesthetics (e.g. in propofol TIVA, in the author's experience dogs seem to show slight palpebral reflex in a surgical plane for anaesthesia).

Propofol and alfaxalone produce similar dose dependent cardiovascular depression and profound hypoventilation that may require mechanical ventilation.

Propofol TIVA should be avoided in cats as much as possible as they lack the ability to metabolise phenols and the accumulation of propofol could cause toxic changes in RBC's such as Heinz Body formation.

Alfaxalone can be used for TIVA in cats (Schwarz et al., 2014). There are some characteristic face twitches, which appear on recovery, which disappear as the drug redistributes. Some excitement in recovery is possible which is why a quiet and dark environment is recommended when alfaxalone is used as TIVA.

There is little information in veterinary medicine about context sensitive half-life of anaesthetic drugs. But a recent paper published on context-sensitive half-time for alfaxalone in cats showed that after long infusions cats may require more than 50% of plasma level reduction to recover and it may take long time to reach 90% reduction when the cat recovers completely.

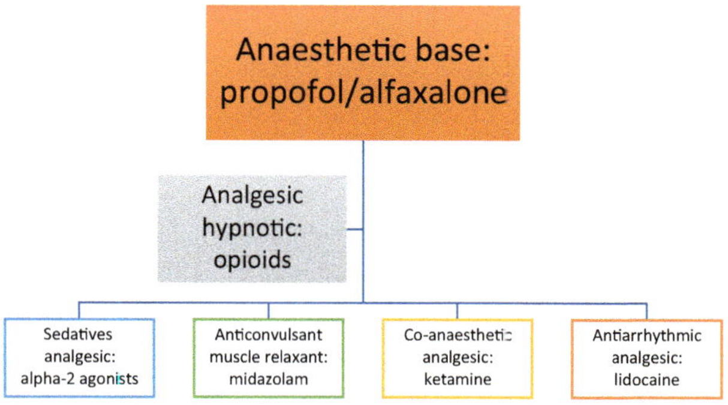

Balanced anaesthesia

Inhalants are still the most used method for anaesthesia maintenance in cats, nonetheless they may produce quite dramatic hypotension and low cardiac output. It is well known that the use of analgesics and/or sedatives decreases MAC. Reduction of the inhalant requirements as much as possible influences positively the cardiovascular stability of the patients. This is the principle of balanced anaesthesia.

By definition, **balanced anaesthesia is the combination of drugs to produce anaesthesia so that the dose of each drug is reduced** so as to decrease the side effects. Balanced anaesthesia is a concept also applied to TIVA, because even TIVA produces a dose dependant cardiorespiratory depression.

Balanced anaesthetic techniques

Opioids

Intravenous

- As predicted in human literature, provides a large reduction of MAC inhalants in a dose-dependent manner.
- Opioids in cats have MAC sparing effects, but less than in other species: large doses of opioids stimulate the sympathetic nervous system, resulting in tachycardia, hypertension, and hyperthermia.
- Different studies with different combinations and different results, but generally high intravenous doses of opioids with inhalant anaesthesia result in good to excellent analgesia blunting autonomic responses to noxious stimuli while increasing blood pressure and heart rate (Pascoe et al., 1997).
- Alfentanil and remifentanil both have shown MAC inhalant reduction in cats (Ilkiw et al.,1997; Ferreira et al., 2009).
- Fentanyl CRIs are commonly used as part of a balanced anaesthetic protocol. When used as a bolus (1–5 µg/kg) followed by CRI 0.1–0.4 µg/kg/min, it produces good analgesia and anaesthetic stability. This is better if decreased/stopped 20–30 min towards the end of the procedure to avoid unwanted effects like dysphoria.
- Bradycardia is not as profound in cats so anticholinergics may not be necessary even during a CRI.

Epidural administration

- Opioids as epidural or subarachnoid injection are great analgesics and reduce overall anaesthetic requirements.
- Morphine (Figure 17) epidural has shown MAC reduction of up to 31%.
- Buprenorphine used epidurally produces adequate analgesia although its effects on MAC are not as good as morphine (Pypendop et al., 2006).
- It appears opioids administered by this route may not be as helpful to improve haemodynamics.

Ketamine

- Ketamine can decrease MAC up to 75% when administered at doses 23–115 µg/kg/min (Pascoe et al., 2007).
- Doses of 10–20 µg/kg/min may help with cardiovascular stability as heart rate and blood pressure increase in cats anaesthetised with inhalants.
- Ketamine combined with remifentanil may improve the MAC sparing effects of remifentanil.
- The full cardiovascular effects of ketamine as CRI's on inhalant anaesthesia in cats have not yet been studied in depth.

Lidocaine

- Lidocaine is a local anaesthetic, which is used for intravenous administration for treatment of arrhythmias and perioperative analgesia. Its benefits have been demonstrated in humans as it reduces requirements of both injectable and inhalant anaesthesia.
- Historically lidocaine was only used as an antiarrhythmic or as part of loco-regional block in cats due to the risk of lidocaine toxicity.
- Evidence shows lidocaine CRI's in cats decreases MAC up to 52% in a dose-dependent manner, but cardiovascular depression was noticed (Pypendop, Ilkiw 2005 and Pypendop et al., 2005).
- Lidocaine CRI is not suitable for cats if the aim is to improve haemodynamics in balanced anaesthesia as it is likely to cause hypotension (Pypendop et al., 2005).
- Lidocaine may be used in balanced anaesthesia in cats if the aim is treatment of ventricular arrhythmias.

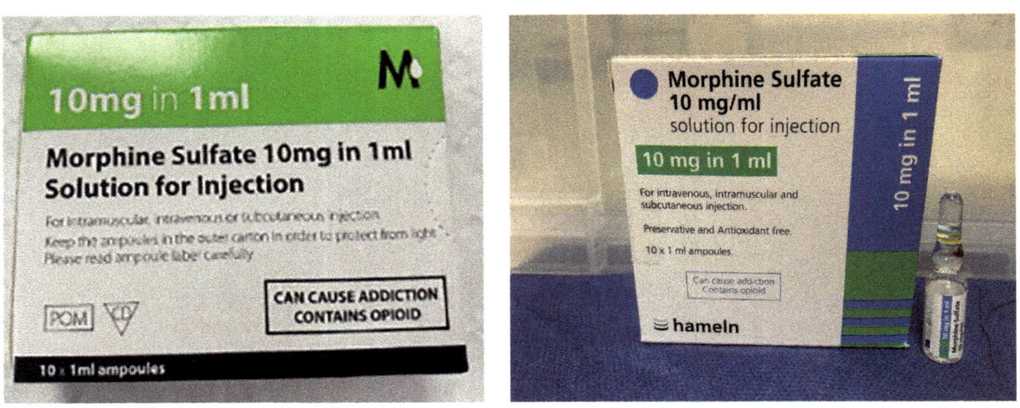

Figure 17. Preservative free morphine.

Dexmedetomidine/medetomidine

- Studies show a decrease in MAC up to 85% in a dose dependant manner with CRI's of dexmedetomidine but decreased cardiac output, oxygen tissue delivery, and increased systemic vascular resistance were observed too (Pypendop et al., 2011).
- Low-rate infusions of dexmedetomidine may be beneficial in some cases when extra analgesia, anaesthesia depth and muscle relaxation is desired, but in general dexmedetomidine / medetomidine infusions should be used with caution and certainly are not indicated for feline balanced anaesthesia if the aim is to improve cardiovascular stability.

Fluid therapy

Administration of a **balanced crystalloid fluid should be part of an anaesthetic plan**. During anaesthesia water balance is affected by the ongoing physiological fluid loss (sensible and insensible loses) and pathological fluid loses related to the procedure (e.g. haemorrhage, evaporation). Moreover, cardiovascular function may be impaired by anaesthetic drugs, as most of these drugs are negative inotropes and decrease the systemic vascular resistance causing hypotension.

Fluid administration is not risk free and it is important to be aware of the possible complications.

Intraoperative fluid administration is associated with a nearly **fourfold increase in the risk of death** compared to those cats that did not receive fluids during anaesthesia (Brodbelt et al., 2007). **Fluid overload has a negative impact on the body.** It produces an increase in body weight and lung water content, decrease in pulmonary function, coagulation deficits, decrease in gut motility, decrease in tissue oxygenation, increase in infection rate, decrease in packed cell volume, total proteins, and temperature. **Cats are more prone to fluid overload than dogs.** This could be due to the different blood volume, and the subclinical cardiac disease (Pascoe, 2018). It is well known that cats have a smaller blood volume compared to dogs. **The blood volume in cats varies from 45 to 60 ml/kg** depending on the study compared to 80–90 ml / kg in dogs. Therefore, for the same amount of fluid administered, cats have a higher percentage increase in blood volume compared to dogs, even though the fluid remaining in the vasculature after redistribution is the same in both species. Special care should be taken **if the patient is obese**, as it is easier to produce fluid overload. Often cats suffer from subclinical cardiac disease which contributes to fluid overload and pulmonary oedema. During the physical exam, **the lack of an audible heart murmur does not rule out cardiomyopathy**. This was demonstrated in one study, where a total 16% of the cats examined had cardiomyopathy and only a third had an audible murmur.

Another important factor when discussing fluid therapy is the **endothelial glycocalyx**. This is a layer of proteoglycans, glycosaminoglycans, glycoproteins, and soluble components lining the vascular endothelium. This layer is important in the maintenance of normal homeostasis (e.g. vascular permeability) (Gaudette et al., 2020). The glycocalyx can be damaged during many diseases (e.g. sepsis or reperfusion injury), however, something as simple as **hypervolaemia can destroy this membrane, increasing the vascular permeability, and allowing passage of fluid from the intravascular system to the interstitium.** Moreover, fast administration of crystalloids can also cause inflammation and damage of the glycocalyx (Smart et al., 2018).

Fluid overload in cats is also aggravated when the intravenous catheter is flushed after pre-medication, induction, and top up drugs with large volumes of saline for a cat (e.g. 2 ml each time). The authors recommend against the use of a 10 ml syringe of saline to flush the intravenous catheter as there is a tendency to administer larger volumes of saline to flush compared to when a smaller syringe is used.

Administration of four times the maintenance rate (i.e. 10 ml/kg/h) was a common practice for patients under general anaesthesia. However, this rate was associated with complications and Davis et al., (2013) suggested a rate of 3 ml/kg/h in healthy adult cats undergoing routine procedures. Moreover, if the patient is stable under general anaesthesia, **a decrease of 25% every hour until maintenance rates are reached is recommended.**

Fluid therapy should always be administered if anaesthesia is longer than 15–30 minutes or in high-risk cases. **Fluid administration should be continued during the postoperative period** until the cat can regulate its intake and output. Usually, in a healthy patient, this is around two to three hours post anaesthesia.

It might be challenging to administer fluids accurately, so it is important to use a fluid pump (Figure 18) or at least a paediatric burette if fluids are administered via gravity.

The most commonly used type of fluid is a balanced crystalloid solution (e.g. Hartmann's). Colloids and blood products are also available, but fluid choice is beyond the scope of this chapter.

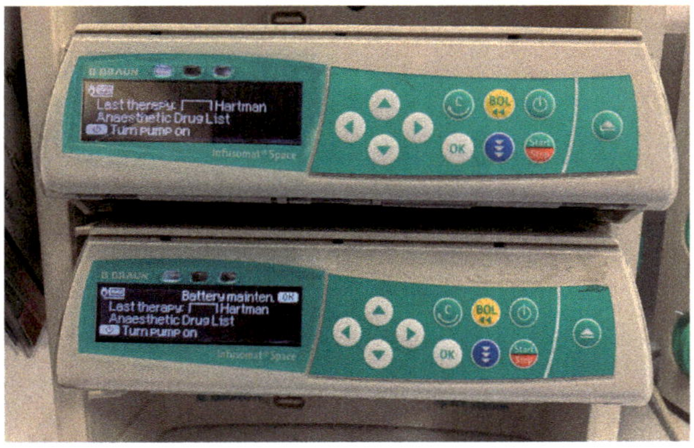

Figure 18. Fluid pump.

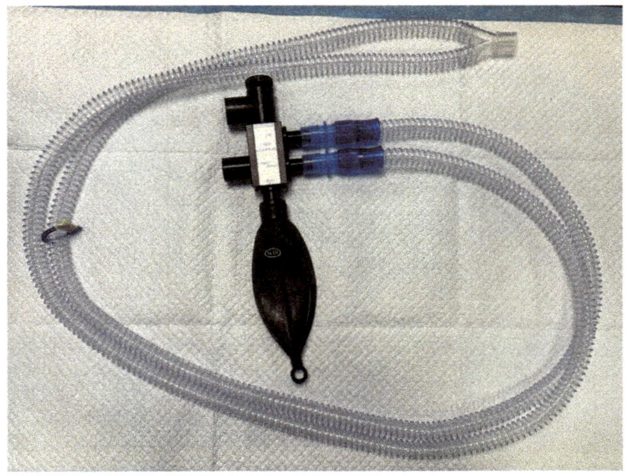

Figure 19. Parallel Mini-Lack breathing system.

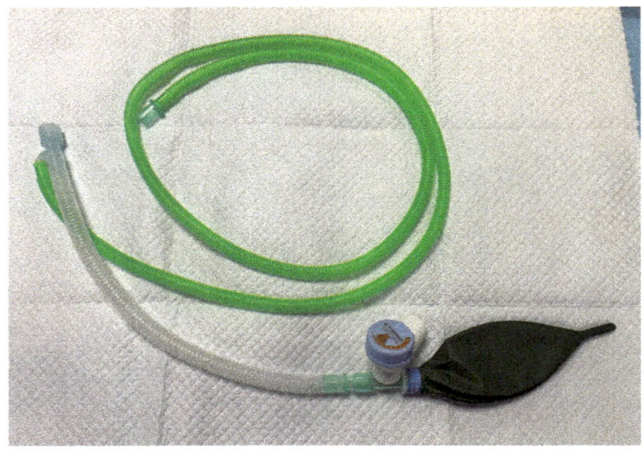

Figure 20. Modified T-Piece breathing system.

Preparation for the procedure

Breathing system

Breathing systems (Table 4) **connect the anaesthetic machine at the common gas outlet to the patient via the endotracheal tube** (**ETT**). Breathing systems are designed to provide oxygen and anaesthetic agent and to remove the carbon dioxide (CO_2) produced by the cellular metabolism of the patient. In cats several breathing systems are suitable: **parallel mini-Lack, modified T-Piece, paediatric circle breathing system, and Humphrey ADE** (Figures 19–21). The size of the reservoir bag should be at least two to three times the tidal volume of the patient. For an average cat a **reservoir bag of 0.5 l** is enough.

It is important to understand the difference between alveolar gas and dead space. **Alveolar gas participates in the gas exchange in the alveoli and hence contains carbon dioxide.** This gas needs to be removed from the breathing system prior to the next breath to avoid rebreathing and hypercapnia. **Dead space gas is the gas that sits in the airway (e.g. trachea) but it does not contribute to the gas exchange**, therefore it does not contain carbon dioxide. This gas is warm and moist so it could be beneficial if it is reinhaled

Table 4. Comparison of breathing systems used in cats. MV = minute ventilation, FGF = fresh gas flow.

Breathing system	Classification	Patient size	FGF	Soda lime	Mechanical ventilation	Reasons for rebreathing
Mini Lack	Mapleson A	2–10 kg	0.8 MV	No	Not efficient	Low FGF
Modified T Piece	Mapleson D	< 8–10 kg	2–3 MV	No	Yes	Low FGF
Humphrey ADE	Mapleson ADE Circle (if soda lime added)	1 kg–10–20 kg	0.7 MV	Could be added	Yes, if used in D position or as a circle breathing system	Low FGF (ADE) If used as circle: – Exhausted soda lime – Malfunction of the one way valves
Paediatric circle	Rebreathing system	>7–10 kg >5 kg cat if a low resistance system is used	Initially 100 ml/kg/min, then 10 ml/kg/min	Yes	Yes	Exhausted soda lime Malfunction of the one way valves

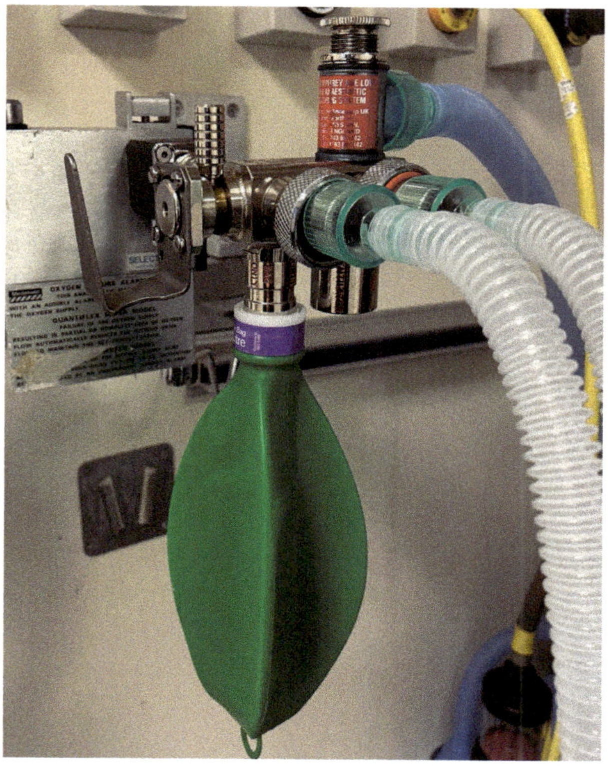

Figure 21. Humphrey ADE breathing system. (Courtesy of Vilhelmiina Huuskonen).

in the next breath. Some breathing systems (e.g. mini Lack) are designed to allow rebreathing of dead space, allowing a reduction in the amount of fresh gas flow (FGF) delivered and hence decrease patient cooling from the inhaled oxygen. Normally, inhaled air is warmed and humidified by the patient's upper respiratory tract, but this function is bypassed in an intubated animal. Therefore, the oxygen delivered is cold and dry and it is the body's job to humidify it and warm it. Both processes, humidification and warming, use body heat.

A **parallel mini-Lack** is classified as a Mapleson A non-rebreathing system. The main advantage of this breathing system is the reinhalation of the dead space during spontaneous ventilation; however, this advantage disappears if mechanical ventilation is required as FGF is increased to remove the carbon dioxide from the breathing system.

The modified T-Piece is classified as a Mapleson D non-rebreathing system. This breathing system offers little resistance to breathing, however, due to the lack of rebreathing of the exhaled dead space, a high FGF is required during spontaneous ventilation (two to three times minute ventilation). The expiratory pause is the time when the carbon dioxide is removed from this breathing system; the longer the expiratory pause the lower the FGF required, hence this breathing system is efficient during mechanical ventilation when the expiratory pause can be controlled.

Many cats may not be big enough to be able to handle a standard small animal circle breathing system but any **cat weighing more than 5 kg may be able to breath spontaneously comfortably through a paediatric circle breathing system which has a series of adaptations in the circle breathing system** like a small reservoir bag (0.5 l), thin limbs and paper-thin very light (non-rubber) one-way valves. Due to these adaptations cats can be connected to circle breathing systems, which are less wasteful and more environmentally friendly, more economical and better preserve temperature while the cat is anaesthetised.

The **Humphrey ADE** is a versatile breathing system which can be used in patients as small as 1 kg body weight. This breathing system offers little resistance to breathing as the inside of the limbs is smooth. During spontaneous ventilation it can be used as a Lack (Mapleson A). During mechanical ventilation it is used as a Modified T-Piece/Bain (Mapleson D). It is easy to change from Mapleson A to D, the lever should be changed from the upright position to the downside position. Moreover, soda lime can be added so it is used as a circle breathing system.

Physical monitoring

Physical monitoring is more important and more reliable than any machine. A trained, dedicated anaesthetist is the best monitor for a patient under general anaesthesia. Using sight, touch, smell, and hearing, anaesthetic depth, heart and respiratory rate and responses to surgical stimulation can be monitored.

Sight

Anaesthetic depth (Figure 22)	Palpebral reflexes, pupil size, eye position, lacrimation, movement, heart and respiratory rate
Respiration	Movement of thorax and abdomen Reservoir bag or ventilator bellows
Equipment leaks	Abnormal capnogram, reservoir bag collapsed, no pressures in ventilator manometer if disconnection
Circulation	Arterial pressure waveform, capillary refill time, surgical site (bleeding, tissue colour) Mucous membranes colour: – Pink: normal – Pale: anaemia, vasoconstriction (Figure 23) – Red: vasodilation, congestion – Blue: cyanosis – Yellow: ictericia, bilirubinaemia – Red-brownish: endotoxaemia

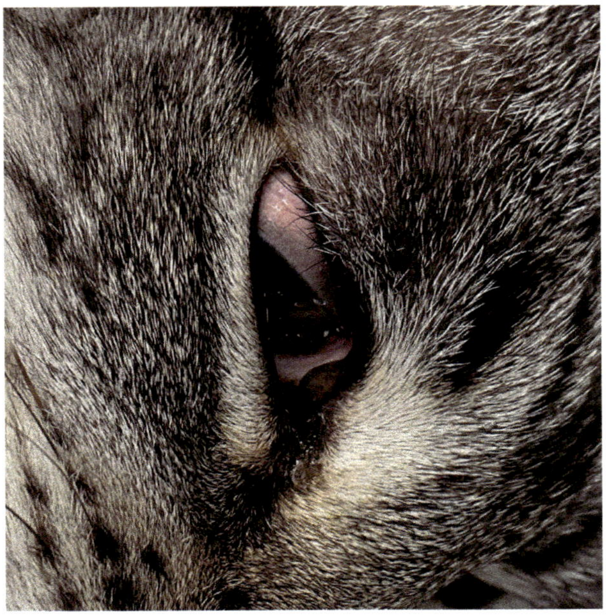
Figure 22. Correct depth of anaesthesia.

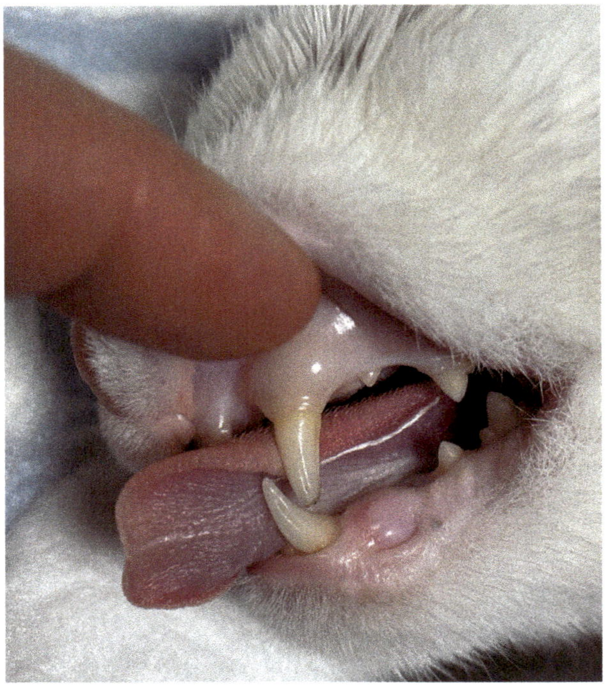
Figure 23. Pale mucous membranes.

Touch

Anaesthetic depth	Muscle tone, pulse rate and strength
Respiration	Manual lung inflation allows lung assessment for compliance and resistance
Equipment leaks	Pressure of the pilot balloon of the endotracheal cuff reflects inflation of the cuff. If cuff is deflated, there is no pressure in the balloon
Circulation	Palpation of peripheral pulses and arterial tone, skin turgor, skin temperature

Temperature	Skin temperature Temperature on the outside of canister for carbon dioxide absorbent • Normal: increase during CO_2 absorption • No temperature: change if absorbent is exhausted • Extreme increase in temperature: absorbent might be dry

Smell

Equipment	Odour from the anaesthetic, leak from the breathing system or the machine

Hearing

Anaesthetic depth	Heart rate (auscultation, Doppler, signal from monitor)
Respiration	Auscultation Pulse oximeter pitch (the higher the pitch the better the oxygen saturation)
Equipment/leaks	Audible leak (e.g. ETT cuff not inflated) Ventilator alarm or abnormal sound in the bellow
Circulation	Cardiac auscultation (Figure 24) Pulse oximeter beep sound, Doppler sound ECG beep sound from monitor

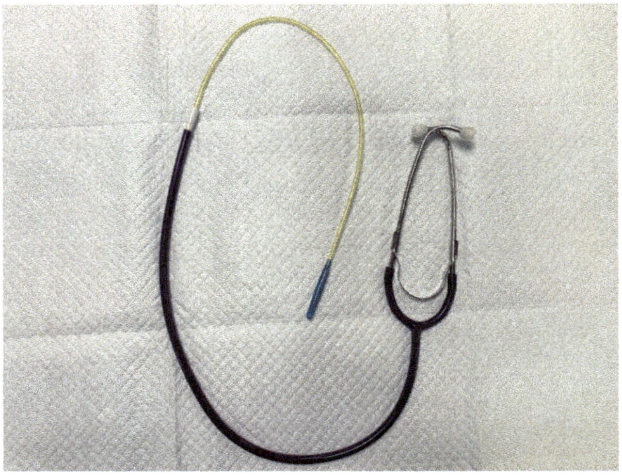
Figure 24. Oesophageal stethoscope.

Capnography

Visualization of the reservoir bag moving, thorax movements, and/or auscultation of a breath via an oesophageal stethoscope indicates the patient is breathing. However, the presence of breathing does not indicate adequate alveolar ventilation, which is the main way of assessing the respiratory system. Direct assessment of ventilation is not easily obtained;

therefore, **capnography is used to measure ventilation indirectly by measuring the partial pressure of carbon dioxide in the exhaled gas**. The relationship between the expired carbon dioxide and ventilation is described by $ETCO_2 = 1/Valv$, where $ETCO_2$ is the partial pressure of exhaled carbon dioxide (CO_2) at the end of expiration and Valv is the alveolar ventilation. As alveolar ventilation increases, expired CO_2 decreases proportionately.

Carbon dioxide is a waste product from metabolism, which enters the blood stream and reaches the pulmonary vessels where it crosses the alveolo-capillary barrier and is then exhaled. Therefore, the exhaled CO_2 ($ETCO_2$) is closely related to the arterial partial pressure of CO_2 ($PaCO_2$). The CO_2 diffuses rapidly from the blood into the alveoli, hence, in normal circumstances the $ETCO_2$ is similar to $PaCO_2$ that is 35–45 mmHg (4.5–6 kPa), with only a difference of 2 mmHg. However, there are times where the difference is higher and carbon dioxide levels do not reflect ventilation accurately. This is related to the presence of alveolar dead space. **Alveolar dead space is defined as an alveolus that is ventilated but it is not perfused.** As a result, gas exchange between the pulmonary blood and the alveolar gas is reduced so that gas in the alveoli at the end of the exhalation is poor in CO_2. The net effect of dead space is to dilute CO_2 from areas of lung participating in gas exchange. The diluted sample has lower $ETCO_2$ (capnography), underestimating the $PaCO_2$.

A capnograph is a non-invasive means of measuring the amount of carbon dioxide present in the exhaled breath of the patient using the absorption of infrared light. The gas sampled is removed from the breathing system, normally at the connection between the ETT and the breathing system. There are **two main capnograph types** based on the sampling technique for measurement: **mainstream and side stream.**

Mainstream capnographs have a plastic sensor located between the endotracheal tube and the breathing system where the measurement is performed. It is a good method for cats due to their small size with small tidal volume and high respiratory rates and provides real time information. However, the sensor is quite heavy and bulky, and can potentially drag on the endotracheal tube. Another disadvantage is the increased apparatus dead space and the tendency of the sensor to get damaged more often due to the action of the water vapour of the sample.

Side stream capnographs measure the carbon dioxide by sampling gas from the breathing system at a rate of 50–200 ml/min. A small plastic connector with an attachment for a small sampling tubing is placed between the endotracheal tube and the breathing system, but the sampling tubing can be attached to the ETT directly or even over the nostrils if the patient is awake or non-intubated. Contrary to the mainstream system, it does not create much drag on the endotracheal tube, but the sampling volume sometimes is too big compared to the small tidal volume so dilution may occur by mixing fresh gas flow and the expired gas from the patient. When everything else is normal but a small cat has an abnormally low expired CO_2, then this sample dilution may be the explanation. This system normally has a water trap between the sampling tubing and the sensor in the machine, preserving the sensor from any malfunction due to the water vapour damage. Another advantage of this system is that the dead space is minimized by choosing a low dead space connector (Figure 25) or even eliminated by attaching the sampling tube directly in the ETT with a needle.

A capnograph (Figure 26) is formed by plotting the patient expired carbon dioxide against time in a graph, where the X-axis represents time, and the Y-axis is carbon dioxide; the result is a rectangular shape wave which represents the respiratory cycle. **The capnogram has different phases.** The first phase is the start with **expiratory upstroke**, followed by the expiratory **pause or plateau** and the **inspiratory downstroke** at the end of the capnograph wave. Always the downstroke or inspiration declines to reach zero provided there is no fault in the equipment and the breathing system is correctly used. The **inspired carbon dioxide should be zero or close to zero meaning there is no rebreathing** (Figure 27).

A capnograph is a valuable piece of equipment as it provides information about three main body systems, 1) **respiratory system (ventilation)**, 2) **metabolic activity (main homeostasis)**, and 3) **cardiovascular system (lung perfusion, circulation, and cardiac output)**.

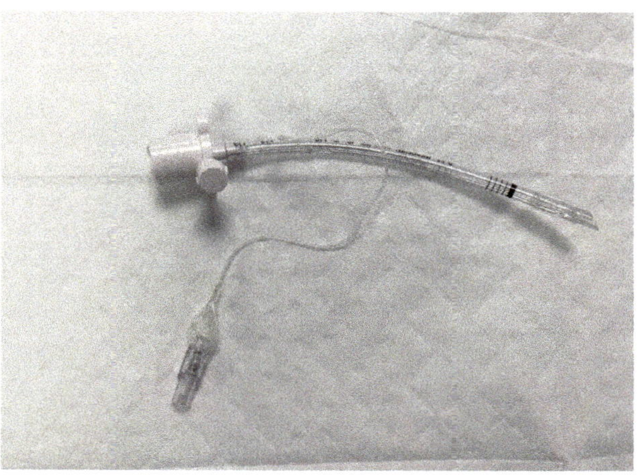

Figure 25. Low dead space connector.

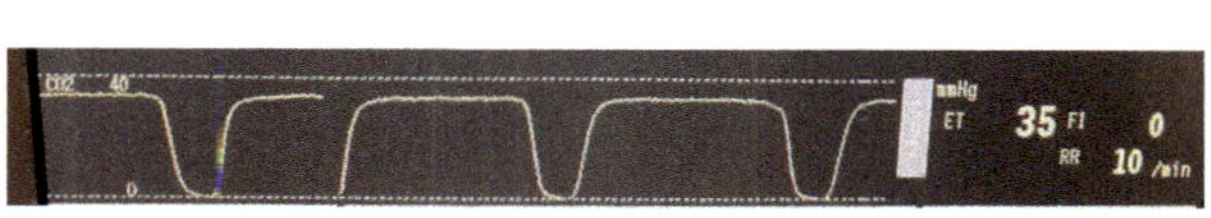

Figure 26. Normal capnogram.

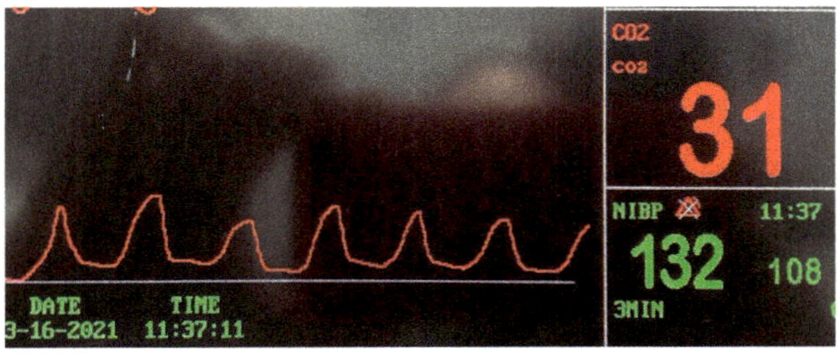

Figure 27. Rebreathing.

End tidal CO_2	Causes
Hypercapnia: increased $ETCO_2$ (>45 mmHg).	• Hypoventilation • Increased cardiac output • Fever, malignant hyperthermia or any condition that increases metabolism • Additional carbon dioxide from laparoscopy • If increased inspired carbon dioxide too, rebreathing due to exhausted carbon dioxide absorbent or insufficient fresh gas flow in a non-rebreathing system
Hypocapnia: decreased $ETCO_2$ (<35 mmHg).	• Hyperventilation • Decreased cardiac output • Pulmonary embolism • Decreased metabolism, hypothermia • Equipment related: leak in the ETT (too small, leak in the cuff), dilution addition of fresh gas flow sampling, rapid respiratory rates and small tidal volume
Absence of exhaled carbon dioxide	• Disconnection • ETT in the oesophagus • Cardiac arrest • Apnoea/respiratory arrest • Obstructed sampling line or kinked tubing
Rebreathing: inspired carbon dioxide above zero	• Insufficient fresh gas flow in a non-rebreathing system • Exhausted carbon dioxide absorbent in a circle breathing system • Increased apparatus dead space • High respiratory rate and small tidal volume when sampling is low

Moreover, capnography also provides information about possible equipment faults. Abnormal capnography caused by equipment fault are quite specific and easy to differentiate but can be confused with a more serious complication. A bronchospasm that looks like a faulty valve in a circle system or the capnograph of a cardiac arrest looks like a simple breathing system-endotracheal tube disconnection. Capnography can also be used during CPR (cardiopulmonary resuscitation). A value of $ETCO_2$ higher than 20 mmHg in cats could be suggestive of an effective cardiac massage and might be associated with better outcomes (Fletcher et al., 2012).

Cardiovascular system

The main goal under general anaesthesia is to **maintain oxygen supply to the tissues**. Understanding oxygen delivery to the tissues, cardiac output, and blood pressure is vital.

Oxygen supply or oxygen delivery to tissues (DO_2) depends on 1) oxygen content (CaO_2) and 2) cardiac output (CO). If there is low oxygen content or if there is low cardiac output the oxygen delivery to tissues can be compromised.

$$\text{Oxygen delivery } (DO_2) = CaO_2 \times CO$$

Oxygen content

The oxygen content is the carriage of oxygen by each unit volume of blood, and it is calculated using the formula shown below.

$$CaO_2 = [1.34 \times Hb \times (SaO_2/100)] + 0.003 \times PaO_2$$

The oxygen content depends on the **oxygen bound to the haemoglobin (i.e. SaO_2)** and the **oxygen dissolved in blood (i.e. partial pressure of oxygen, PaO_2)**. Both parameters are related through the haemoglobin dissociation curve, where saturation of haemoglobin with oxygen depends mainly on the PaO_2. The percentage (%) of haemoglobin saturated with oxygen can be **measured by a pulse oximeter (SpO_2) or using a co-oximeter (SaO_2)**. The partial pressure of oxygen can be measured with arterial blood gas analysis. Each component is important to deliver oxygen to the tissues. Oxygen bound to haemoglobin exerts a bigger effect on the CaO_2, however, the PaO_2 is the driving force for the final release of oxygen to the cells (i.e. mitochondria).

Cardiac output

Cardiac output (CO) measures the volume of blood ejected by the heart per unit of time; this blood flows to the tissues to deliver oxygen and nutrients. Cardiac output depends on stroke volume and heart rate. **Stroke volume (SV) depends on preload, afterload, and contractility.**

$$CO = HR \times SV$$

It is important to maintain cardiac output during general anaesthesia but its measurement although possible is not practical involving expensive equipment and a high level of expertise, hence anaesthetists rely on measurement of parameters which are directly related such as $ETCO_2$ and arterial blood pressure (ABP).

Cardiac output and arterial blood pressure are directly related, as arterial blood pressure is the force exerted by blood flow on the arterial wall and the product of CO and systemic vascular resistance (SVR): ABP = CO × SVR. There must be enough blood ejected from the ventricles in order to perfuse the organs, however, **the main determinant factor for organ and tissue perfusion is blood pressure**. The blood flow to an organ depends on the organ perfusion pressure and the organ vascular resistance (blood flow to an organ = organ perfusion pressure / organ vascular resistance). Therefore, the organ perfusion pressure = mean arterial pressure (MAP) – pressure inside the organ. A classic example is the cerebral perfusion pressure (CPP) = MAP – intracranial pressure (ICP).

There are **three components to ABP: systolic, diastolic, and mean arterial pressure**. Systolic arterial pressure (SAP) is the peak pressure within the arteries after ventricles contract at the end of the cardiac cycle; whilst diastolic arterial pressure (DAP) is determined by the systemic vascular resistance (SVR) and circulating blood volume. Mean arterial pressure is calculated from the other two:

$$MAP = DAP + 1/3(SAP–DAP)$$

MAP is the most important of the three during anaesthesia because it is the main factor to overcome arteriolar resistance and ensure capillary blood flow to the tissue. The most important body systems such as renal, cerebral, and coronary circulation show excellent autoregulation and are able to keep constant organ flow despite perfusion pressures as long as MAP is kept between 50 and 150 mmHg. When MAP falls below 60 the blood flow to main organs can be compromised, hence the importance of monitoring ABP and specifically MAP.

If ABP is very high due to vasoconstriction, oxygen delivery to the tissue may be compromised unless cardiac output is high too; a good ABP does not always guarantee good tissue perfusion. It is important to maximize tissue flow over good ABP values.

Pulse oximetry

The concerning lack of knowledge about pulse oximetry among clinicians, nurses, and students from both veterinary and human medicine has been repeatedly highlighted by several authors (Hofmeister et al., 2005). This occurs even though the use of pulse oximetry and capnography together prevents up to 93% of the preventable anaesthesia-related mishaps in human anaesthesia (Tinker et al., 1989). **Pulse oximeter allows the anaesthetist to assess oxygenation in a non-invasive way**. Moreover, pulse oximeter can detect desaturation much faster than trained eyes can detect cyanosis. This piece of equipment provides **the percentage of oxygen bound to the haemoglobin in the blood**, which is associated to the amount of oxygen dissolved in blood through the oxygen dissociation curve. Pulse oximetry does not inform on the amount of oxygen dissolved in blood (PaO_2). PaO_2 can only be measured by sampling blood from the artery and doing a blood gas analysis. Fortunately, by knowing the SpO_2 and the oxyhaemoglobin dissociation curve, the PaO_2 can be extrapolated to determine if the patient is hypoxaemic. To better understand pulse oximetry the author recommends the following reference: Chan et al., 2013.

The normal value for oxygen saturation is between 98–100%, whether the patient is breathing room air or enriched air with oxygen. The threshold of hypoxaemia is 90%, below which desaturation starts quickly due to the shape of the oxygen dissociation curve and immediate treatment is required. However, the authors recommend troubleshooting when the saturation drops to 95%, especially if the percentage of inspired oxygen is above 21%.

Oxygenation	% Saturation	PaO_2 (mmHg, kPa)
Normoxaemia	98–100%	100 mmHg, 13.3 kPa
Mild hypoxaemia	95%	75 mmHg, 10 kPa
Severe hypoxaemia	<90%	60 mmHg, 8 kPa

When under general anaesthesia, the inspired gas is enriched with oxygen, therefore the inspired fraction of oxygen (FiO_2) increases from 21% to up to 100%. When the FiO_2 increases, the PaO_2 increases, however, the SpO_2 never reads higher than 100%. Provided the PaO_2 is above 100 mmHg, the SpO_2 always reads 100%. It is only when the pulmonary problem is severe when the SpO_2 reading drops; this means **the pulse oximeter only warns the anaesthetist when there is a severe problem**.

% Inspired oxygen	% Oxygen saturation	PaO_2 (mmHg, kPa)
21%	98–100%	100 mmHg, 13.3 kPa
100%	100%	500 mmHg, 65 kPa

The pulse oximeter probe measures oxygen saturation of haemoglobin in arterial blood by passing light waves of a determined wavelength (red and infrared) through a tissue (e.g. tongue) and determining the quantity of light absorbed by oxygenated (oxy-Hb) and deoxygenated blood (deoxy-Hb). Deoxygenated haemoglobin absorbs

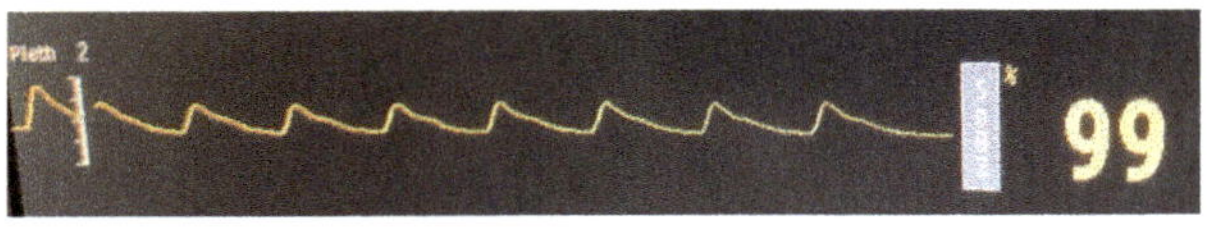

Figure 28. Plethysmograph with good signal.

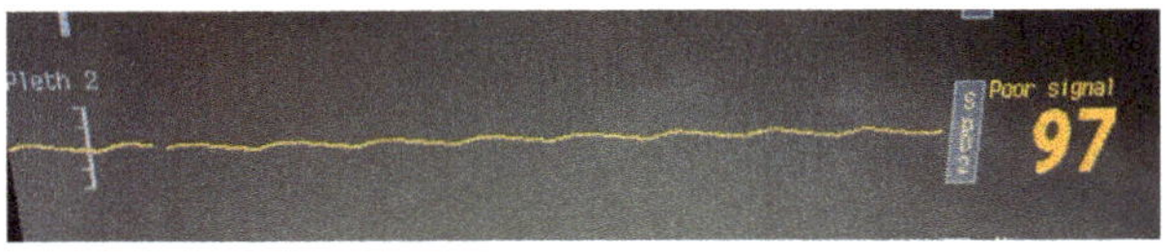

Figure 29. Plethysmograph with poor signal.

red light whereas the oxygenated one absorbs the infrared, so the pulse oximeter calculates a percentage. Red blood cells emit a unique pulsatile signal which is read and interpreted by the pulse oximeter. Signal emitted by non-pulsatile red blood cells is not considered, which is how the saturation of arterial blood is obtained. The screen displays the oxygen saturation (%), the pulse rate (bpm), and the signal quality detected by the probe. Some pulse oximeters also show a **plethysmograph** (Figures 28 and 29), **which is the change in absorbance with time**. This helps confirm if the pulse oximeter is detecting an adequate signal/arterial pulsation. Other pulse oximeters have an indicator panel which shows increased lighting bars as arterial pulsation is detected.

Unfortunately pulse oximetry (Figure 30) does not provide information about ventilation (CO_2), adequacy of oxygen delivery to the tissues, oxygen content in blood, or presence of abnormal haemoglobins (such as carboxy-haemoglobin or methaemoglobin). Contrary to what people think, **anaemia cannot be detected by pulse oximetry**. Moreover, if a patient is anaemic, visual detection of cyanosis is more difficult. Cyanosis can be detected only when the blood's deoxy-Hb content is at least 5 g/dl. Anaemia does not affect SpO_2 unless it is severe (PCV <12% or Hb <4 g/dl). Thus, an anaemic patient can have a normal PaO_2 and haemoglobin saturation even if, due to the low amount of haemoglobin, the total blood oxygen content (CaO_2) is low.

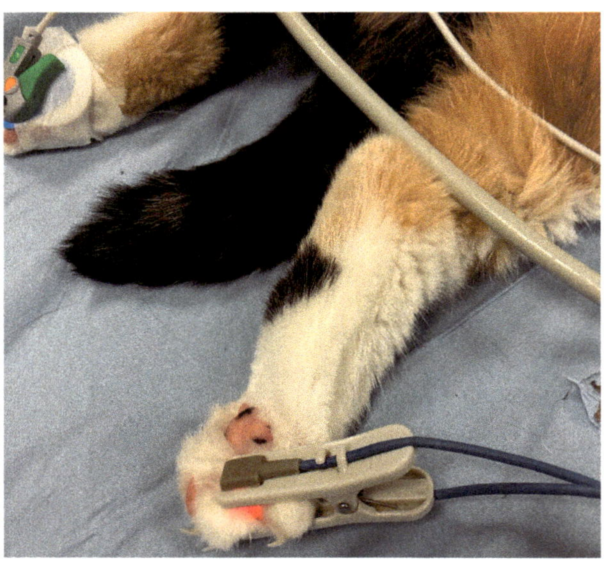

Figure 30. Pulse oximetry on a paw.

There are some other limitations to the use of the pulse oximetry:

- A high concentration of carbon monoxide in blood results in high levels of carboxi-haemoglobin. Pulse oximetry will overestimate the oxyhaemoglobin levels as both carboxihaemoglobin and oxyhaemoglobin absorb light at a similar frequency. **A victim of smoke inhalation may have SpO_2 of 100% but it is not a true reading.**
- **High levels of methaemoglobin result in an underestimated reading**. A patient may not be hypoxaemic but shows an SpO_2 of 80–85%. Methaemoglobin and deoxygenated haemoglobin absorb light at a similar frequency.
- Movement produces artefacts (e.g. shivering in recovery).
- Vasoconstriction and poor tissue perfusion produce poor signal and no readings.
- Ambient light can interfere with the quality of the signal (e.g. fluorescent lighting).
- Abnormal colour of mucosa and pigmented mucosa interfere with readings.
- Venous pulsation.
- Pigmented skin (e.g. Chow Chow).

Troubleshooting a low pulse oximeter reading

Oximeters occasionally give a false reading; however, anaesthetists should use their clinical judgement and suspect the patient may be hypoxaemic. **The ABCDE should be checked** (A: airway clear? B: breathing (ventilating) adequately? C: adequate circulation? D: drugs causing a problem? E: equipment working properly?).

If there is a low SpO_2 displayed the main causes could be poor positioning of the probe, poor perfusion to the area where the pulse oximeter is placed, or true hypoxaemia.

If low SpO_2 is due to poor positioning of the probe, the probe should be replaced as it could be compressing the tissue underneath, or a wet gauze placed on the tongue (Mair et al., 2017), or another location used.

If the low SpO_2 is due to poor tissue perfusion (poor pulse strength seen in the pulse oximeter), this could be due to drugs which have been administered, low blood pressure or hypothermia:

- Drugs that produce peripheral vasoconstriction decrease tissue perfusion especially alpha-2 agonists such as (dex-)medetomidine (also phenylephrine, noradrenaline, adrenaline). This drug produces peripheral vasoconstriction and therefore SpO_2 can provide falsely low readings.

- Blood pressure should be checked. If there is hypotension due to dehydration, hypovolaemia, hypotension, or cardiac problems it should be treated accordingly. The signal will improve when the clinical condition of the patient improves.
- If the patient (or the area where the pulse oximeter is placed) is cold and therefore vasoconstricted, the area should be rubbed gently or a warm-water swab applied; this may restore the perfusion of the area and hence the signal.

If SpO_2 is low due to true hypoxaemia, the most likely causes are:

a) Low FiO_2: equipment should be checked for faults and airway patency should be checked.
b) Hypoventilation while breathing room air (21% FiO_2): supplemental oxygen ±mechanical ventilation should be provided.
c) Anatomical shunt (e.g. PDA) or ventilation/perfusion mismatch (e.g. atelectasis): mechanical ventilation should be applied to maximise lung capacity.
d) Impairment of oxygen diffusion from the alveoli to the arterial blood (e.g. pulmonary oedema, pneumonia) should be treated accordingly (beyond the scope of this chapter).

The no-pulse-detected alarm is commonly caused by the probe coming off the tongue, but also triggered if the **patient is hypotensive, hypovolaemic, or has suffered a cardiac arrest**. The probe site should be checked quickly and then the patient assessed to see if this correlates with the clinical picture.

Blood pressure

Hypotension is the most common complication in veterinary anaesthesia. It is not possible to know if a patient becomes hypotensive under anaesthesia unless blood pressure is adequately measured. Unfortunately, not only sick or old patients become hypotensive, but all patients are at risk. Several survey studies in different veterinary hospitals indicate that up to 33% of all anaesthetized patients (dogs and cats) were hypotensive as systolic arterial pressure was lower than 90 mmHg or mean arterial pressure was lower than 60 mmHg. Research shows even healthy young patients undergoing elective procedures are susceptible to anaesthetic hypotension. Generally, there are few post-anaesthetic complications that can be directly connected to an anaesthetic hypotensive episode but vital organs like kidneys may be injured in the process with no obvious clinical signs: more than 75% of nephrons must be non-functional before changes are shown in BUN and creatinine levels. Consequently, **blood pressure should be routinely measured for all patients** and hypotension addressed adequately should it appear.

Techniques for measurement of blood pressure

The most common techniques used to assess arterial blood pressure are palpation of peripheral pulse, non-invasive techniques (NIBP), and invasive techniques (IBP).

Williamson and Leone (2012) suggest (based on the author's experience) when SAP is greater than 90 mm Hg pedal pulses can be palpated, however when SAP is less than 60 mm Hg neither femoral nor pedal pulses can be palpated. Reineke et al., (2016) show peripheral pulse palpation in conscious cats is another tool to assess abnormalities in arterial blood pressure of the patient as it correlates with SAP and may provide supportive evidence for the presence or absence of hypotension. Metatarsal pulses disappear when there is a decrease in arterial blood pressure and femoral pulses were absent with severe hypotension.

It is important to remember that pulse quality is highly subjective and correct assessment may depend on the level of experience of the clinician. A good pulse pressure is not synonym of good ABP, **pulse pressure only indicates the difference between systolic and diastolic arterial pressures**, and the higher is that difference the stronger the pulse feels. In situations where there is significant vasodilation or low circulating volume the pulse feels strong due to the low diastolic arterial pressure, but ABP may be low too. Fortunately, a well-trained clinician can feel the difference of a healthy patient pulse by depressing the artery and checking if the vessel feels turgid. **If the artery is easy to depress and the pulse disappears with only gentle pressure over the vessel, most likely the ABP is low**. Arterial blood pressure should always be measured whenever possible rather than estimated by palpation.

Another method of measuring NIBP indirectly is by auscultating the Korotkow sounds (Riva Rocci technique). The SAP and DAP is auscultated, and MAP calculated using the following formula:

$$MAP = (SAP - DAP)/3 + DAP$$

However, this method is not accurate in veterinary medicine as the sounds are not heard so distinctly compared to humans.

Non-invasive techniques are used widely, and three main devices are used in veterinary medicine: **Doppler flow meter, oscillometry, and high definition oscillometry**. Invasive blood pressure measurement is mainly used in patients with a higher anaesthetic risk.

NIBP versus IBP

NIBP advantages	IBP advantages
Inexpensive	Gold standard
Easy to use	Continuous reading
Non-invasive	Display of wave form: contractility, SVR
No major complications	
Very available & portable	

NIBP disadvantages	IBP disadvantages
Inaccurate (see specifications of the different NIBP devices): underestimation of SAP, overestimation of MAP in hypotensive patients and hypertensive patients	Expensive
Difficult to measure in very small patients, hypothermic, hypotensive, arrhythmias, movement, vasoconstriction	
Intermittent measurements	Requires experience
Accurate reading depends on cuff location, size	Invasive
	Possible complications (infection, blood loss)

Non-invasive techniques

Appropriate interpretation of arterial blood pressure results from a non-invasive blood pressure device is paramount to provide the correct treatment and this depends on the accuracy and validation of the NIBP monitor. There are no established validation standards in veterinary medicine, except for recommendations from the American College of Veterinary Internal Medicine (ACVIM) Hypertension Consensus Panel and Veterinary Blood Pressure Society Recommendations (AHCP-VBPS Validation). Sadly, according to the ACVIM Hypertension guidelines there are no devices that meet the validation criteria; hence it is recommended **to use current available devices with a degree of caution**.

With a NIBP monitor, accuracy depends on selecting **the appropriate cuff size, cuff location, and cuff attachment** for the patient.

The width of the cuff should be 30–40% of the circumference of the limb. If the cuff is too narrow the arterial blood pressure measurement can be falsely high, conversely if the cuff is too wide the measurement can be falsely low. For most cats, **a cuff width of 2.5 cm** is appropriate.

The cuff should be placed at the level of the right atrium. For cats in sternal recumbency the cuff should be placed at the level of the thoracic inlet; cats in lateral recumbency should have the cuff placed at the level of the sternum. If the cuff is below the right atrium the reading is falsely elevated, if it is placed higher than the right atrium it is falsely low.

The cuff should be placed with the line on the cuff over the artery (part that inflates) and the cuff should be neither too tight nor too loose. The cuff should not be forced around the limb or be taped. If the cuff is too loose, falsely high readings are obtained. If the cuff is too tight, falsely low readings result.

Falsely high readings	Falsely low reading
Cuff too narrow	Cuff too wide
Cuff too loose	Cuff too tight
Cuff placed below the right atrium	Cuff placed over the right atrium

The accuracy and effectiveness of NIBP devices are affected by patient movement and it is often difficult to obtain an audible signal in patients experiencing peripheral vasoconstriction.

Doppler ultrasonic flow detector

This is probably the easiest and most versatile ABP measurement. It **is appropriate for smaller size patients and cats** where other techniques fail or are not practical.

Doppler blood pressure (Figure 31) consists of a cuff attached to a sphygmomanometer (pressure gauge) and a Doppler probe. The Doppler probe consists of two small piezoelectric ultrasound crystals, one is the transmitting crystal and the other one is the receiving

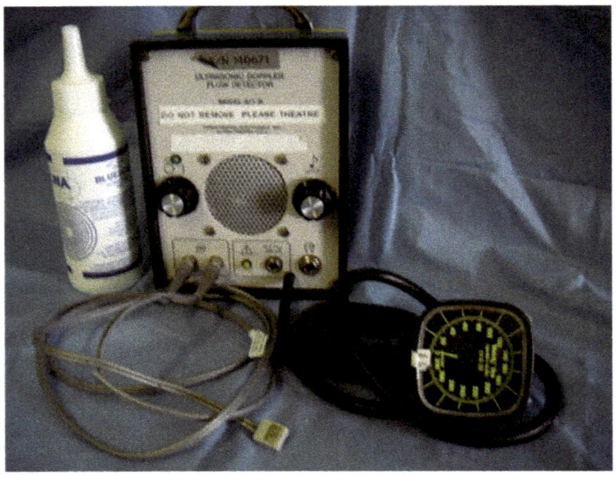

Figure 31. Doppler ABP measurement equipment.

crystal. The emitted ultrasound signal is reflected by the moving red blood cells, causing a change in frequency (Doppler shift or effect) detected by the receiving crystal. This change in frequency is electronically transduced into an audible signal.

A cuff is placed proximally to the Doppler probe and attached to a sphygmomanometer. The Doppler probe with ultrasound gel is placed over an artery (skin area must be previously clipped) and once pulsation is audible the probe is secured in place with tape. The cuff should be inflated until the artery is occluded with the pressure of the cuff and the pulse is no longer audible. Then the cuff is slowly deflated to release the cuff pressure until the first audible sound returns. The pressure at which this first sound was audible corresponds to the highest pressure in the vessel; that is, the SAP value.

Unlike dogs, where Doppler measures SAP, in anaesthetized cats, **Doppler measurement reflects MAP** (Caulkett et al., 1998). The measurement underestimates direct SAP and better predicts direct MAP, obtained from the femoral artery. As a result, it was proposed a calibration factor such that:

Femoral SAP = Doppler SAP + 14 mmHg (Grandy et al., 1992)

It is interesting to note that Doppler measurements as an estimation of SAP values fail to meet the American College of Veterinary Internal Medicine (ACVIM) validation criteria in cats. Therefore, measurements obtained with Doppler should be interpreted with caution. One study found poor correlation between Doppler measurements and IBP. The Doppler reading read the SAP 8.8 mmHg lower than the IBP and 14 mmHg greater than the MAP (da Cunha et al., 2014).

Oscillometry in feline species

Oscillometric ABP monitors (Figure 32) are automated devices which **provide estimates of SAP, MAP and DAP, in addition to heart rate**. A microprocessor controls the sequence of inflation and deflation of the cuff. The cuff is inflated to a pressure above the previous systolic arterial pressure; then it is deflated incrementally. A transducer senses the pressure changes, which are processed by the microprocessor and displayed on the screen of the monitor. This has an accuracy of +/−2%. The mean arterial pressure corresponds to the maximum oscillation at the lowest cuff pressure. The systolic arterial pressure corresponds to the onset of rapidly increasing oscillations. Diastolic arterial pressure corresponds to the onset of rapidly decreasing oscillations. It is calculated from SAP and MAP. The device has a fast rate of inflation and a slow cuff deflation to avoid venous congestion and allow

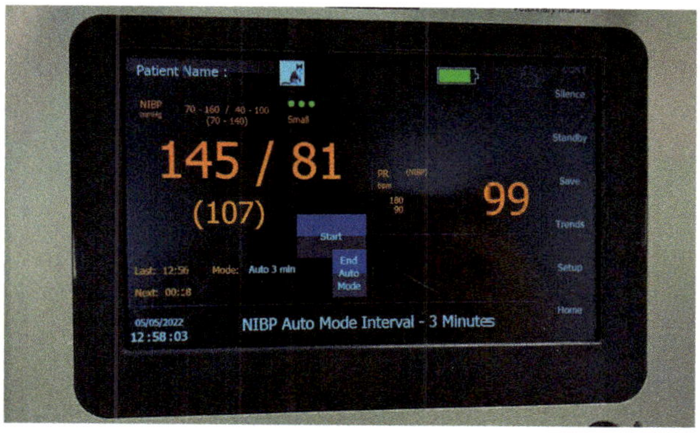

Figure 32. Oscillometric device.

time to detect the artery pulsing. The MAP is considered the most accurate ABP value from oscillometric monitors because it is the measured parameter.

Oscillometric devices may be less accurate in very small patients, patients with very rapid or slow heart rates, arrhythmias, or systemic vasoconstriction, hypotensive animals with low pulse pressure or during patient movement (restlessness, shivering, and seizure activity), or when external pressure is applied on the cuff. Clipping the hair on the limb prior to placement of the oscillometric ABP cuff has no effect on the reading. Normally with alpha-2 agonists drugs the Doppler technique works better than oscillometry.

Many studies showed that oscillometric devices (Dinamap Veterinary Blood Pressure monitor, Cardell and petMAP) are inaccurate in cats (Binns et al., 1995, Caulkett et al., 1998, Acierno et al., 2010, Cerejo et al., 2017). However, Pedersen et al., (2002) found that Cardell used in anaesthetised cats provided a good estimate of MAP and DAP but underestimated SAP, which became worse as ABP increased. When the cuff was placed on the base of the tail it met the AHCP-VBPS validation criteria for MAP evaluation using the Cardell monitor (Zwijnenberg et al., 2011). The petMAP monitor in cats cannot be recommended for clinical use. It has poor estimation of SAP regardless of cuff location (median artery, coccygeal artery) (Acierno et al., 2010, Cerejo et al., 2017).

High definition oscillometric (HDO)

High definition oscillometric (HDO) ABP monitors use a new technology which allows direct measurements of SAP, MAP, and DAP, working with a wide range of pulses (up to 600 beats/min) and pressures (0 to 450 mmHg); this makes this monitor more accurate than traditional oscillometric technology. Despite this, HDO does not meet the AHCP-VBPS validation criteria for NIBP evaluation in cats. **In anaesthetised cats, HDO has poor precision and a tendency to overestimate hypotension**. This is a problem as hypotension might go unidentified if this monitor is used for trending ABP values. (Acierno et al., 2010, Petric et al., 2010).

Invasive blood pressure

This is the **gold standard technique for ABP measurement** but is technically challenging and more expensive than any other technique, which is why its use is not in common practice. Nevertheless, it is without a doubt the best technique for ABP monitoring. First, the artery must be catheterised. A normal intravenous catheter can used but there are **special indwelling arterial catheters** with a stronger sheath made of Teflon to overcome the stronger muscular arterial wall and ease up the introduction of the catheter. Once the catheter is placed and secured, it is connected to a non-complaint plastic tubing filled with heparinized saline. The tubing connects to a pressure transducer, placed at the height of the right atrium, which detects and converts the pulsating signal into an electric signal which is displayed on the screen (Figure 33) as the arterial blood pressure wave trace.

The most common places to catheterise an artery are the **dorso-pedal artery** (Figure 34) **and the coccygeal artery**. However, in cats, catheterization of the dorso-pedal artery can be difficult due to its small size, and it is easier to place a catheter in the coccygeal or femoral artery.

Common reasons for misreading ABP values are small air bubbles within the catheter or connecting tube, blood clots, or small size catheters. All of which cause a considerable damping of the wave form and SAP reading gets underestimated, DAP gets overestimated and only MAP will be close to a true reading.

In addition to a **true real time and continuous reading**, IBP provides extra information about the cardiovascular system: the upstroke of the arterial waveform indicates **the force of ventricular contraction** so the steeper it looks the stronger the contraction is. On the other side the location of the dicrotic notch within the waveform is indicative of vascular tone and the lower it is the more vasodilated the vessel is.

Electrocardiogram

As stated previously, the main goal of anaesthesia is to maintain oxygen delivery to the tissues. Any factor

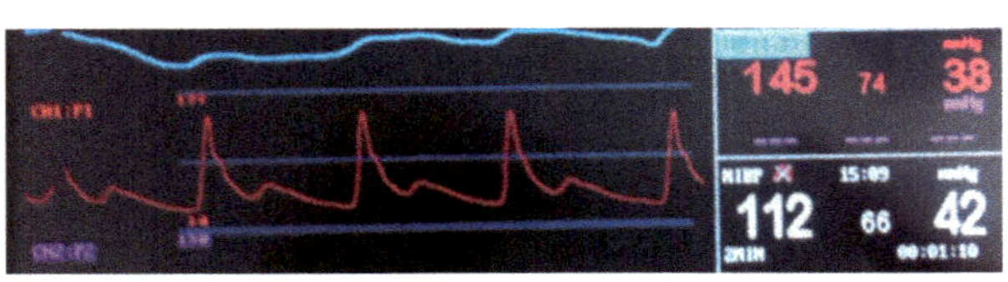

Figure 33. Arterial pressure wave form during invasive blood pressure monitoring.

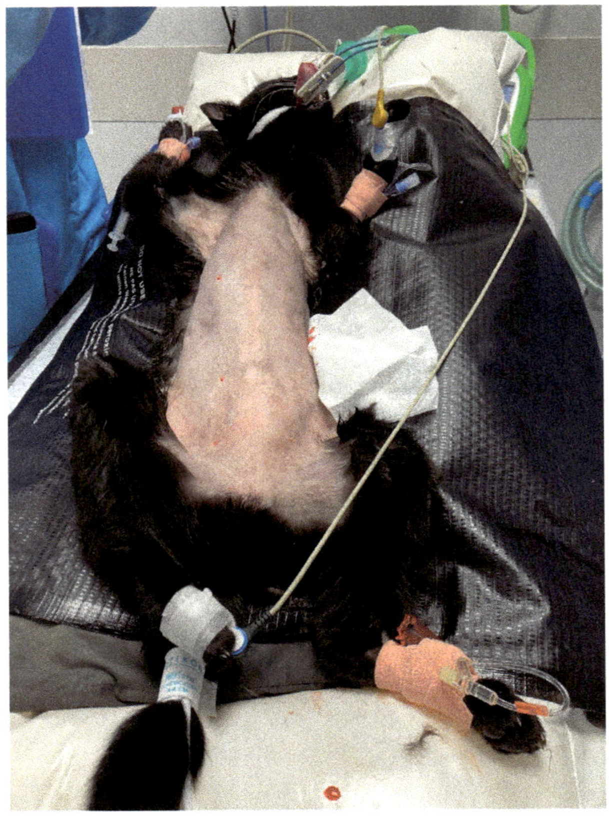

Figure 34. Arterial catheter in dorso-pedal artery.

negatively influencing cardiac output, blood pressure, or oxygen content puts oxygen delivery at risk. **Arrhythmias** (alteration in the normal coordinated sequence of contractility) can have a dramatic effect on the cardiovascular system by affecting stroke volume or heart rate, which could lead to serious consequences under anaesthesia and poor oxygen delivery to the tissues. Moreover, the combination of an arrhythmia with anaesthetic drugs could have a larger negative effect of anaesthetic drugs on the cardiovascular system. In addition, the presence of **hypercapnia and/or hypoxaemia during general anaesthesia, may also exacerbate arrhythmias**. Therefore, monitoring the electrocardiogram (ECG) under general anaesthesia is highly recommended. Arrhythmias can be associated with cardiac disease (e.g. hypertrophic cardiomyopathy) or have a non-cardiac aetiology (e.g. hyperkalaemia).

The electrocardiogram monitors electrical activity of the heart. The normal electrocardiogram has a sequence of waves arising due to electrical activity in the different areas of the heart:

- P-wave marks the depolarization of the atrium.
- P-R interval is the time for the signal to go from atrium to atrio-ventricular node and bundle-of-His.
- QRS complex is the signal conduction and depolarization of the ventricle.
- T-wave is the ventricle re-polarization.

- S-T segment represents the ventricles when completely depolarized.

In veterinary anaesthesia a three-lead system is commonly used, with the heart between two electrodes and the third one acting as the ground electrode. **The best signal is produced when two electrodes are placed on the paws of the front limbs and the third on the paw of a hind limb.** Other positions are possible too, provided the heart falls between two electrodes. When limbs are not available the electrode pads could be placed over the skin along the sternum, neck, and chest area in a base-apex location. Electrodes get a better signal when gel is applied between the skin and the electrode.

In cats, interpretation of the ECG is challenging due to the small size of the heart and the fast heart rate. The small size of the heart makes the amplitude of the ECG trace small and hence the heart rate and the rhythm assessment could be difficult or erroneous. ECG counts QRS complexes to count the heart rate but sometimes the T-waves get counted as QRS.

The ECG has some limitations. **ECG does not assess the cardiovascular system, circulation, cardiac output, or arterial blood pressure.** ECG does not provide information about ventricular contraction; in fact, the ECG still shows electrical activity for a few minutes after the heart has arrested as it displays residual electrical activity that may look like a normal ECG (i.e. pulseless electrical activity).

Bradyarrhythmia, a slow regular or irregular rhythm, can be detected under general anaesthesia and classified as follows:

1) sinus bradycardia
2) sinus arrhythmia
3) sinus block
4) sinus arrest
5) atrioventricular (AV) block (first-degree, second-degree type I, second-degree type II and third-degree)
6) sick sinus syndrome
7) asystole and pulseless electrical activity (cardiac arrest rhythms).

It is beyond the aim of this chapter to discuss each in detail. The most common arrhythmias under general anaesthesia are **sinus bradycardia and second-degree AV block**. Both arrhythmias cause a low heart rate (<110 bpm).

Sinus bradycardia is a regular sinus rhythm. The ECG trace shows that all P-waves are followed by QRS complexes. Sinus bradycardia can be caused by anaesthetic drugs, overdose (e.g. deep plane of anaesthesia), hypothermia, increased vagal tone (e.g. pulmonary disease, shock), hypertension, severe hypoxaemia,

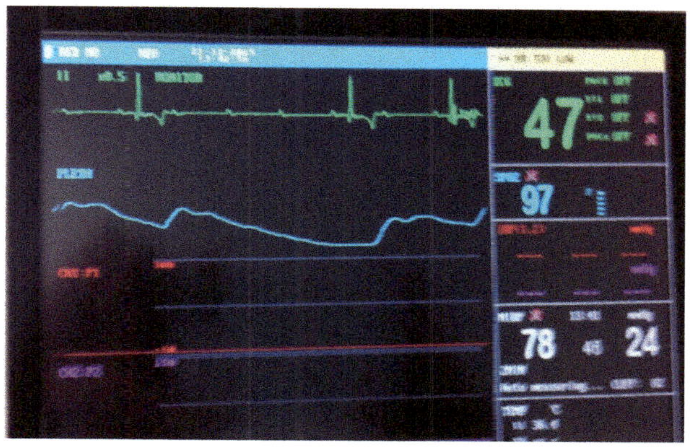

Figure 35. Second-degree AV block.

hypoglycaemia, increased intracranial pressure, severe acidosis, and hyperkalaemia.

Second-degree AV block (Figure 35) produces an irregular rhythm, where some P-waves are not conducted and therefore they are not followed by a QRS complex. These solo P-waves are associated with a pulse deficit. Second-degree AV block is associated mainly to **high vagal tone** and anaesthetic drugs (e.g. opioids and alpha-2 agonists). Usually treatment is not required, however if the arterial blood pressure is low or if the second-degree AV block is a high grade (many P-waves not conducting) this may guarantee treatment. It is important to treat the underlying cause, however administration of an anticholinergic drug (e.g. glycopyrrolate) might be required. Note that low doses of anticholinergics may increase the severity of the bradycardia initially. This problem can be resolved by administering a second dose of the drug. If the patient is hypothermic the anticholinergic may have a poor effect. Anticholinergics should be used with caution if the bradycardia is caused by an alpha-2 agonist because they can increase the myocardial work and oxygen consumption leading to arrhythmias (Short, 1991). In this case the bradycardia should be treated with a low dose of atipamezole intramuscularly, keeping in mind that the patient might become light.

Sinus bradycardia could be associated with spontaneous depolarization of the ventricles without normal AV conduction. This is called synchronous atrioventricular dissociation (Figure 36), a type of

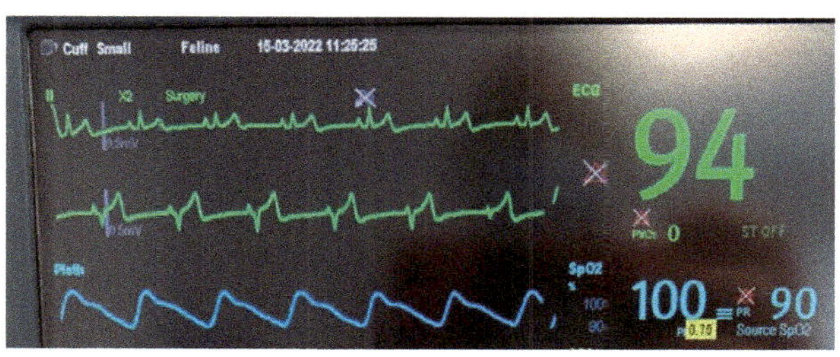

Figure 36. Synchronous atrioventricular (AV) dissociation.

idioventricular rhythm. This arrhythmia generally resolves spontaneously but it may respond to administration of an anticholinergic if treatment is required. The ECG shows sinus complexes and junctional escape beats (largely negative QRS complexes not associated with P-waves).

Tachyarrhythmias, rapid regular or irregular rhythm, can also be detected under general anaesthesia and can be classified as follows:

1) sinus tachycardia
2) atrial fibrillation
3) isolated ventricular premature complexes (VPC)
4) accelerated idioventricular rhythm
5) ventricular tachycardia
6) ventricular fibrillation (cardiac arrest rhythm)
7) bundle branch block.

Sinus tachycardia is a sinus rhythm with a high heart rate (>180 bpm). The ECG shows a P-wave always followed by a normal QRS complex. It can be caused by light plane of anaesthesia, pain/nociception, hypercapnia, moderate hypoxaemia, electrolyte alterations (e.g. hypercalcaemia), hypotension, anaemia, underlying diseases (e.g. hyperthyroidism) and drugs (e.g. atropine). Treatment is focused on the underlying problem.

A VPC (Figure 37) **is a premature contraction of the myocardium with its origin in the ventricle** (i.e. the sinus atrial node is not sending the signal). The VPC is premature (i.e. it occurs sooner than a normal sinus QRS would have occurred for that beat) and its QRS complex is abnormal in appearance; **wide and bizarre** (ventricular depolarization originates and spreads in a different orientation within the ventricles compared to a normal sinus beat) and T-wave with different morphology. Moreover, this complex is **not preceded by a P-wave** and is followed by a compensatory pause to allow the rhythm to return to its previous pattern. The cardiac output is lower or null as it occurs before the heart had time to fill with blood during the diastolic filling. An alternating sequence of one VPC following one sinus beat, repetitively, is referred to as **ventricular bigeminy**, and an alternating sequence of one VPC following two sinus beats or two VPCs following one sinus beat is known as ventricular trigemini. Two VPCs in sequence are termed a couplet, three a triplet and four or more a run of ventricular tachycardia (VT). The differential diagnosis for wide, bizarre QRS complexes on an ECG are:

1) VPC/VT/ accelerated idioventricular rhythm (Figure 38)
2) ventricular escape rhythm
3) sinus rhythm with bundle branch block (right or left)
4) right ventricular enlargement
5) motion artefact.

VPCs occur in 78–90% of healthy cats (Hanas et al., 2009), especially when the heathy cat gets older (>8 years old). VPCs can be associated with structural heart disease, but the underlying cause can also be extracardiac (e.g. hypokalaemia, hypoxaemia, anaemia, hyperthyroidism, pain/nociception).

The presence of sporadic VPCs with no negative impact on the cardiovascular system are usually monitored but not treated. However, if VPCs are polymorphic (different shapes as they are originating from different points of the ventricle), if they are causing hypotension, if they are combined with other arrhythmias, or if there is ventricular tachycardia, treatment is required.

Ventricular tachycardia is the occurrence of four or more VPCs consecutively at a rate of 240 beats/minute or greater. The combination of an elevated heart rate, poor diastolic filling and time leading to low cardiac output and myocardial hypoxia respectively, stimulation of myocardial cells during their refractory period can produce deterioration of VT to ventricular fibrillation (VF).

The **drug of choice to treat VPCs or VT is lidocaine**, however, it is well known that lidocaine has a

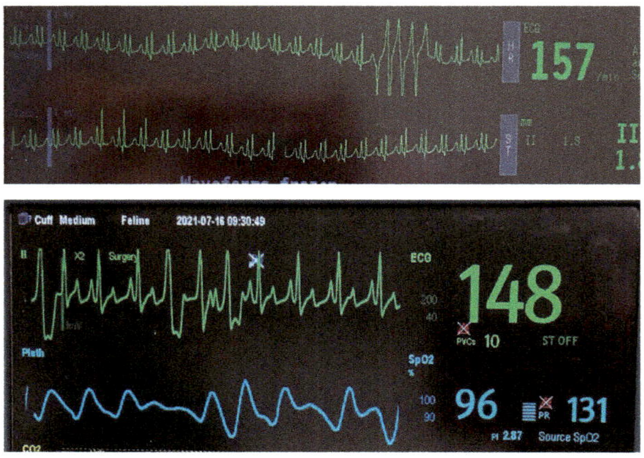

Figure 37. Ventricular premature complexes (VPC).

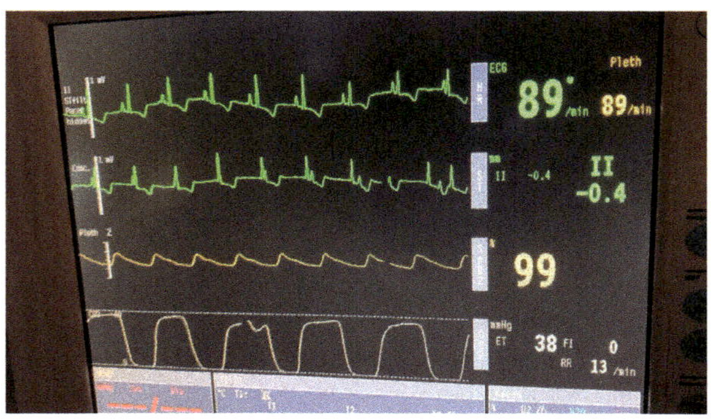

Figure 38. Idioventricular rhythm.

narrow safety margin in cats as they do not metabolize lidocaine well (see metabolism). If the cat develops VT under general anaesthesia and it is associated with an underlying heart condition (e.g. HCM) lidocaine is not recommended as the first-line of treatment as it produces depression of the CV system in anaesthetized cats (Pypendop, Ilkiw 2005). However, a small bolus of lidocaine (0.25–1 mg/kg IV as a bolus) could be administered to a healthy cat with normal systolic function. While lidocaine is being administered close monitoring for signs of toxicity (e.g. bundle branch block, AV block, sinus bradycardia) is mandatory. Ventricular arrhythmias could be the result of stimulation of beta receptors by adrenaline released due to stress or pain, therefore a beta blocker (e.g. esmolol, propranolol) could be an alternative drug to lidocaine in cats. If VT is refractory or there is VF/cardiac arrest, magnesium sulphate can be considered a possible treatment in cats.

It is important to **differentiate a VPC from an escape rhythm**. A ventricular escape rhythm has the same bizarre QRS shape as a VPC, however it occurs at a slower than normal rate (60–120 beats/minute in the cat). This rhythm is saving the patient's life because it prevents asystole. Therefore, even though ventricular escape QRS complexes may be wide and bizarre, **ventricular antiarrhythmic therapy is absolutely contraindicated**.

Temperature

Feline core body temperature should be maintained within normal range (37.8–39.2°C) during general anaesthesia to allow normal homeostasis. Due to their high surface area to body mass ratio, the incidence of hypothermia in cats is high (96.7%) (Redondo et al., 2012). **Hypothermia, defined as a core temperature <37°C**, is associated with undesirable complications intraoperatively and postoperatively. Human literature shows small decreases in temperature (1–2°C) are detrimental for the patient producing increased infection rate, wound healing delay, increased patient discomfort, and even respiratory depression. If there are greater heat losses and temperature decreases ≥5°C more side effects are observed such as bradycardia, arrhythmias, decreased cardiac output, reduced CO_2 production, cardiac fibrillation, and cardiac arrest. During the postoperative period, hypothermia can reduce drug clearance and metabolism, and delay recovery time by affecting the pharmacokinetics of drugs. The solubility of the inhalant agent in blood increases as temperature decreases, slowing its elimination. Moreover, hypothermia depresses the immune system, alters the coagulation, and increases hospital stays (Reynolds et al., 2008, Clark-Price, 2015).

There are key times during the procedure where the anaesthetist can act to improve the postoperative temperature. Redondo et al., (2012) found the patient's body temperature before pre-medication is associated with an increase in the final temperature. On the other hand, Jae Hwa Yoo et al., (2020) found pre-warming human patients for 10 minutes had no additional effect on the prevention of perioperative hypothermia. Although there is no clear evidence to demonstrate the benefits of pre-warming in cats, **the major drop in core body temperature (1–1.5°C) occurs during the first hour of general anaesthesia** due to redistribution of heat from the core to the periphery (Armstrong et al., 2005). The authors recommend the use of methods to keep normothermia before pre-medication (e.g. do not keep cats in cold rooms) or at least soon after induction to follow up during the whole anaesthesia.

The main route of heat loss is via radiation. Radiation contributes approximately 40–50% to the heat loss by transferring heat energy from the body to structures that are not in contact with the cat. Radiant heat loss is increased if the cat is surrounded by cold objects and the room walls have lower temperature than the cat's body temperature. There are three other mechanisms of heat loss from the body, **convection, conduction, and evaporation**.

Convection heat loss occurs when the layer of air in contact with the patient's body surface is heated, becomes less dense and rises. This creates a current that carries heat away from the cat. Here the room air temperature and air currents play a major role. **Conduction** consists of heat transfer when two objects are in contact. The cat may lose heat if in direct contact with stainless steel surgical tables or other hard surfaces with a temperature lower than the patient's body temperature. Heat can also be lost via **evaporation** of water or during respiration. In the case of evaporation of water, the heat lost is due to the loss of latent heat of vaporization of moisture on the skin's surface (when the water on the skin evaporates, it loses latent heat). Surgical scrub and alcohol placed directly on the patient and moisture lost from an open body cavity or respiratory secretions. All these routes of heat loss depend on the total area of skin exposed to the environment. Some of the mechanisms are involved in the same problem that causes heat loss (ventilation causes heat loss by radiation and convection).

General anaesthesia, some sedatives and analgesics may affect temperature by decreasing the thermoregulatory mechanisms. Moreover, there is a decrease in muscle activity and metabolic heat production, vasodilation, and redistribution of central heat towards the periphery.

There are some factors that may accelerate this process, such as the size of the patient, anaesthetic protocol used, length of anaesthesia and type of surgery performed amongst others.

Preventing hypothermia is important as it is easier to prevent than treat once established, so **monitoring of body temperature is paramount**. Temperature probes are available from most multiparameter monitors. Those **temperature probes** can be placed in the oesophagus or on the rectum for continuous monitoring during anaesthesia. Thermometers can be left inserted in the rectum but must be removed and reinserted with each reading. Rectum and oesophagus are easy and accessible under anaesthesia for measuring body temperature. They give the most reliable readings as they are close to core temperature. There are alternatives which have been used in practice like ears or the axillary area which may be useful if cat is awake or sedated. Axillary temperature tends to underestimate body temperature, and there is poor correlation with rectal temperatures. Currently axillary and tympanic temperature measurements are known for being inaccurate and variable.

The list shown below covers the points to prevent/treat heat loss during general anaesthesia.

- **Pre-warming** the patient by placing it on a heat mat under the bed or forced air warming prior to premedication. This is especially important in patients susceptible to suffering from hypothermia (e.g. low body condition score).
- **Passive** surface warming methods by covering patients with bubble wrap and blankets (Figures 39 and 40). Small animals have arteriovenous anastomoses in the limbs, ears and muzzle used to regulate heat loss, therefore bubble wrap can be placed on all four feet, head and ears.
- **Active surface warming** methods (Figure 41) by using heat pads, thermostatically controlled heat mats, and forced air warming devices. Burns and eye ulcers should be prevented by avoiding using >40°C in the heat mats, placing a blanket between the patient and the heat mat, and using eye lubricant if the device delivers warm air.
- **Isolating patients** from cold surfaces by placing a bed or blanket between the table and the patient. Moreover, pre-heat tables/kennels with forced warm air devices can also be applied.
- **Adequate room temperature**.
- Use of a **heat and moist exchanger** (HME). An HME (Figure 42) is a way of providing humidification to the inhaled gas by using a hygroscopic substance. The HME is placed between the endotracheal tube and the breathing system.

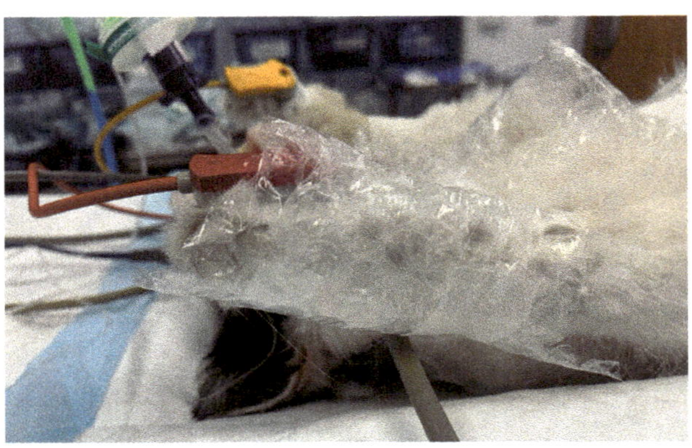

Figure 39. Bubble wrap.

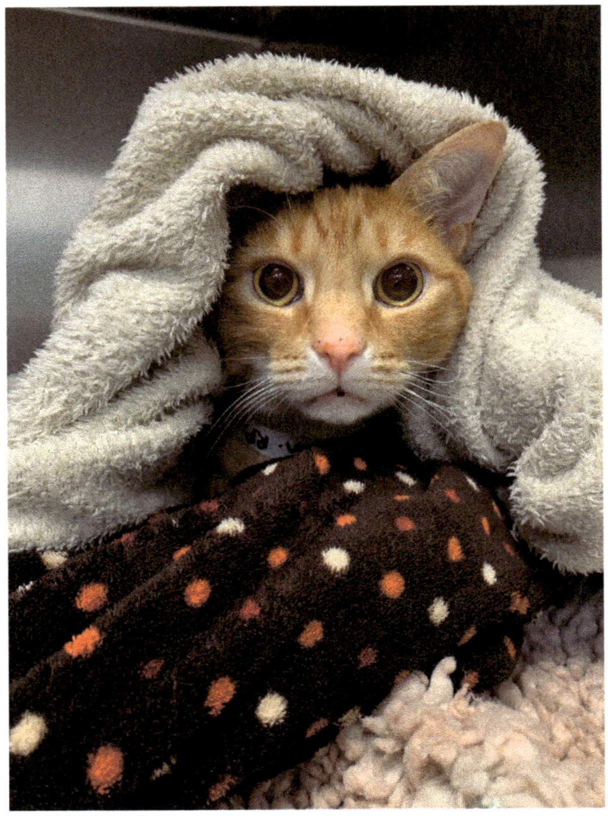

Figure 40. Cat recovering from anaesthesia under some blankets. (Courtesy of Ms. Stace Parker).

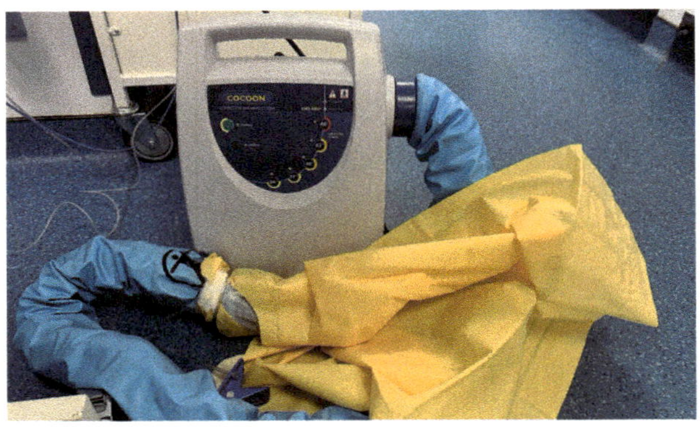

Figure 41. Bair Hugger.

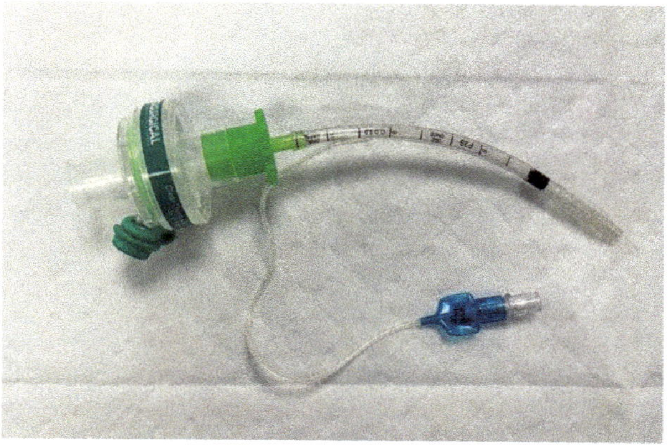

Figure 42. Heat and Moist Exchanger (HME)

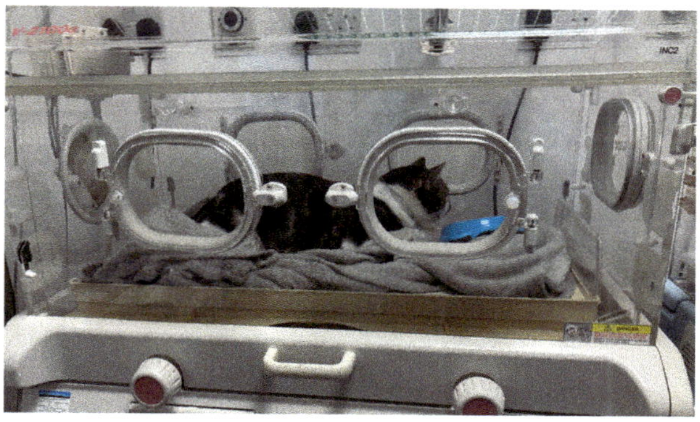

Figure 43. Incubator.

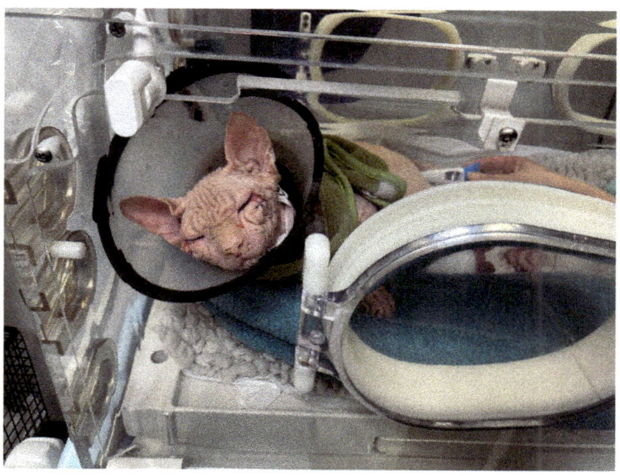

Figure 44. Hypothermic cat with fleece in the incubator.

- Use of the breathing system with the **lowest FGF possible**.
- Placing the patient in an **incubator for recovery** (Figures 43–44).
- Ensuring the **duration of procedures is kept as short as possible**.
- Use of **drugs and doses adjusted to each patient** to avoid high impact on vasomotor tone and prevent long recoveries.
- Use of **peripheral nerve blocks** when possible to reduce the amount of other drugs required and shorten the recovery.

During recovery a hypothermic patient (Figures 40, 43, 44) will start shivering due to muscle activity to increase the temperature. It is vital to **monitor oxygen saturation** and to provide oxygen flow by as this consumes oxygen, and the patient can become hypoxaemic.

Feline-specific complications related to general anaesthesia

Blindness

Postanaesthetic cortical blindness, neurological deficits, and blindness have been reported in cats (Stiles et al., 2012). This has been attributed to its unique anatomy of the blood supply to the brain and location of main blood vessels within the skull.

In cats the maxillary artery plays a major role in the vascularization of the retina, brain, and inner ear. The feline external carotid artery, a branch of the common carotid artery, continues as the maxillary artery at the level of the angle of the jaw. The maxillary artery continues rostro-dorsally forming what is known as the rete mirabile, maxillary rete, maxillary artery, mirabile rete or carotid rete, a network of vessels which connects with the Circle of Willis. This rete has two portions, one extracranial and one intracranial (Kamijyo and Garcia, 1975). The extracranial part is adjacent to the skull and extends from the level of the foramen rotundum over the orbital fissure to the level of the optic foramen. The rete mirabile is surrounded ventrally by the lateral and medial pterygoid muscles and dorsolaterally by the temporal muscle. Arising from this rete, the ophthalmic artery further bifurcates into the long posterior ciliary arteries, which send branches that provide perfusion to the retina (Wong and Macri, 1964). The intracranial portion is formed by the release of several arteries through the orbital fissure into the cavernous sinus to form an intracranial arterial network from which the cerebral arteries (Circle of Willis) arise.

Unlike dogs and humans, perfusion of the feline cerebral cortex depends mostly on the **maxillary artery** (Reneman et al., 1974), therefore **any compromise to this vessel has the potential to cause ischaemia** (Stiles et al., 2012). Usually, the Circle of Willis receives blood from both the internal carotid and the basilar artery. However, in cats, the brain is not supplied by the internal carotid or the basilar artery (as the first one becomes non-patent a few weeks after birth) (Kamijyo and García, 1975; Stiles et al., 2012) and the second one carries blood away from the arterial circle. Thus, mainly the maxillary artery supplies the Circle of Willis. The ascending pharyngeal artery (a branch of the common carotid artery) supplies a small amount of blood to the Circle of

Willis. The pathway of the maxillary artery also plays an important role. The maxillary artery courses around the caudal aspect of the mandible predisposing it to compression and partial or complete occlusion when the cat's mouth is maximally opened. When the mouth is maximally opened, for example when a spring-loaded mouth gag is used, the distance between the angular process of the mandible and the rostro-lateral wall of the tympanic bulla became shorter and alters the morphology of the maxillary artery as it passes between these two bony structures (Scrivani et al., 2014).

Reductions in blood flow through the maxillary arteries can also result in **decreased perfusion to the inner ear**, and this could explain the occurrence of deafness after procedures in which the mouth has been held open (Stevens-Sparks, Strain 2010).

There has been an association between the aggressive / excessive use of mouth gags, more specifically spring-loaded mouth gags (Figure 45), and the development of post-anaesthesia blindness and neurological deficits in cats. Barton-Lamb et al., (2013) showed that the use of spring-loaded mouth gags to open the mouth maximally resulted in alterations in both blood flow and the electroretinogram in some cats. It is common to recommend against the use of spring-loaded mouth gags in cats. If a mouth gag is required for the procedure, it is important to **avoid large or maximal opening of the mouth and to limit the time during which the mouth gag is applied and minimize the time taken for the procedures**. A small mouth gag can be made by cutting a syringe barrel or using a needle cap and placing it on opposing canine teeth to hold the mouth open as minimally as needed (Figure 46).

According to Stiles et al., (2012), blindness is temporary in the majority of cases.

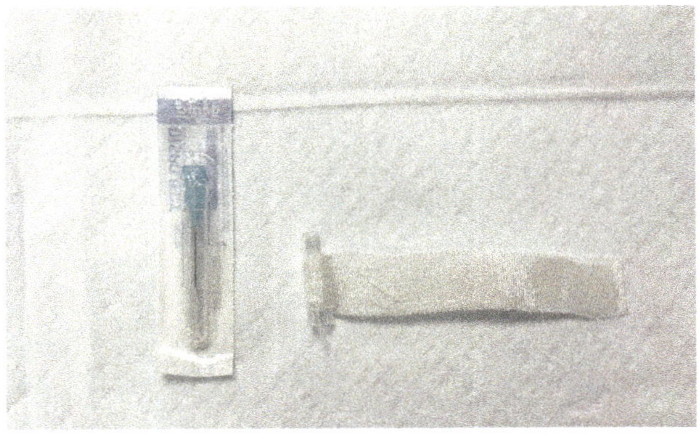

Figure 46. Homemade mouth gag.

Laryngeal spasm

Cats are more susceptible to suffer from laryngeal spasm than dogs. The main reason is their well-developed protective laryngeal reflex and its laryngeal responsiveness to mechanical stimulation. Laryngeal spasm can be produced in experimental decerebrated cats under general anaesthesia by mechanical stimulation of the soft palate, pharynx, larynx, and trachea. Laryngeal spasm can be provoked at **intubation and extubation**. Therefore, desensitization of the larynx with local anaesthetic prior to intubation, proper intubation technique, and early extubation before swallowing and coughing are paramount to avoid laryngeal spasm. Moreover, spasm is more likely to occur if there is a light plane of anaesthesia and an inflamed larynx.

When laryngeal spasm develops **the airway obstruction can be partial or total**. Usually, the laryngeal spasm is self-limiting, and no treatment is required apart from oxygen administration by mask (Figure 47) or by flow-by and administration of more anaesthetic induction agent to deepen the plane of anaesthesia. It is important to avoid stimulating the larynx. Attempts to reintubate the airway, application of more local anaesthetic or mechanical stimulation of the larynx should be avoided. If obstruction is complete or if the spasm does not resolve spontaneously, intravenous administration of a muscle relaxant should be considered (atracurium) followed by intubation and mechanical ventilation.

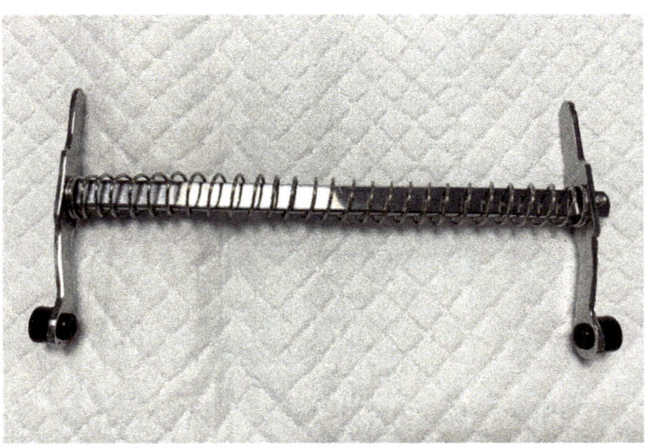

Figure 45. Spring loaded mouth gag.

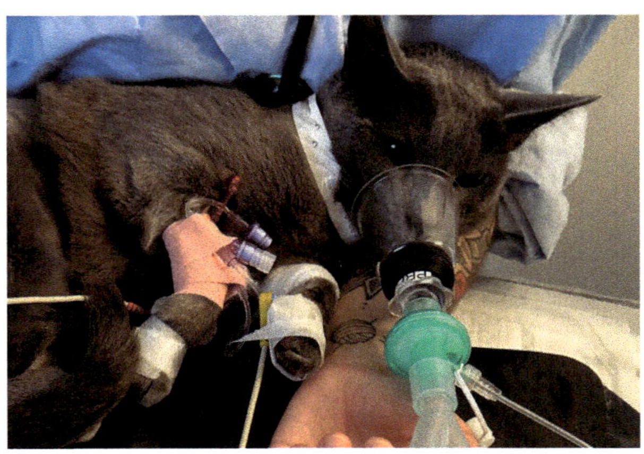

Figure 47. Administration of oxygen via a facemask connected to a breathing system.

The last option is to perform a tracheotomy or to place a large (14G) needle or catheter percutaneously between two tracheal rings.

Difficult airway intubation

Endotracheal intubation is the best approach to manage the patient's airway while under general anaesthesia. However, in cats it has been associated with an increase in anaesthetic-related **deaths** (Brodbelt et al., 2007), **tracheal tears, tracheal avulsion, and bronchial rupture.** Moreover, cats are prone to suffer from laryngeal spasm, producing probably the high incidence of respiratory obstruction leading to deaths within the first three hours of recovery. It is possible that improper intubation technique causes higher number of complications in cats than in dogs.

The reasons behind cat's difficult airway are not clear, however it could be associated to the **small size of the upper airway**, to the increased laryngeal sensitivity to mechanical stimulation, and a delicate dorsal tracheal ligament which ruptures easily with over inflation of the ETT, in combination with multiple position changes during anaesthesia.

Tracheal rupture or tears are associated with subcutaneous emphysema, coughing, gagging, dyspnoea, anorexia, and fever. Management depends on the extension of the lesion and varies from surgery to conservative management. Treatment of injuries that extend to the carina is successful, however if the tracheal tear is present in the intrathoracic region the prognosis is poor.

Selecting the correct size ETT is essential. ETT can be chosen based on the internal diameter (ID), the presence or not of a cuff, and the type of cuff. Briefly, the widest ETT possible should be chosen, as the wider the ID the less resistance the cat encounters during breathing. This is one of the reasons why uncuffed ETTs were traditionally preferred. Cuffed ETTs were bulkier due to the cuff material and a narrower ETT was then used. Nowadays there is better manufacturing processes and materials, and the cuffs are less bulky. Most adult cats require a **3.5–5.0 mm ID ETT but a range from 2.0–5.5 mm should be available.**

Cuffed ETTs (Figure 48) are better at protecting the airway from aspirated, regurgitated material than uncuffed ETTs. However, as stated earlier they have been associated with complications when overinflated (e.g. necrosis of the tracheal mucosa). There are mainly two types of cuffs, **low volume-high pressure (LV-HP) and high volume-low pressure (HV-LP).** LV-HP cuffs are less bulky compared to HV-LP and hence endotracheal intubation is easier (e.g. less trauma during intubation). LV-HP are better at preventing aspiration of any type of content than HV-LP, however LV-HP can exert a high pressure in the tracheal wall.

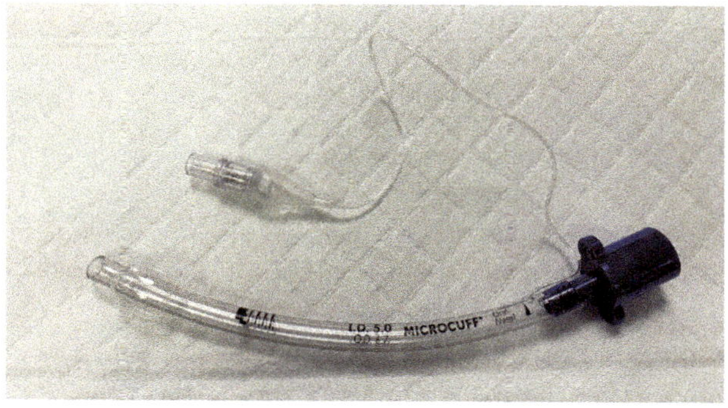

Figure 48. Cuffed ETT.

To avoid complications, it is vital that cuffed ETTs are inflated correctly and disconnected when changing the patient's position. The most common technique to seal the trachea is to listen for air leaks when another person is inflating the lungs up to a maximum peak inspiratory pressure of 15 cm H_2O and to inflate the pitot balloon in 0.5 ml increments until the leak disappears. Another method consists of attaching a manometer to the pitot balloon. Tracheal damage/rupture is also a risk when the patient's position requires changing during anaesthesia since the trachea can move around the tube if the ETT is not disconnected from the breathing system first. Common sites of tracheal damage being at the location of the tube tip and/or cuff.

There is some additional equipment required for feline intubation (**lidocaine spray, stylet and bougie**). Lidocaine spray (Figure 49) without adrenaline is applied topically over the larynx to desensitise the area. After application of the topical lidocaine on the cat's larynx, it is important to wait at least 45 seconds before attempting endotracheal intubation. Stylets and bougies are usually not required however they should be readily available in case they are needed. Stylets are used to stiffen or alter the shape of the ETT. If stylets are used, the tip should be blunt and remain within the lumen of the ETT. The bougie (Figure 50) is used to

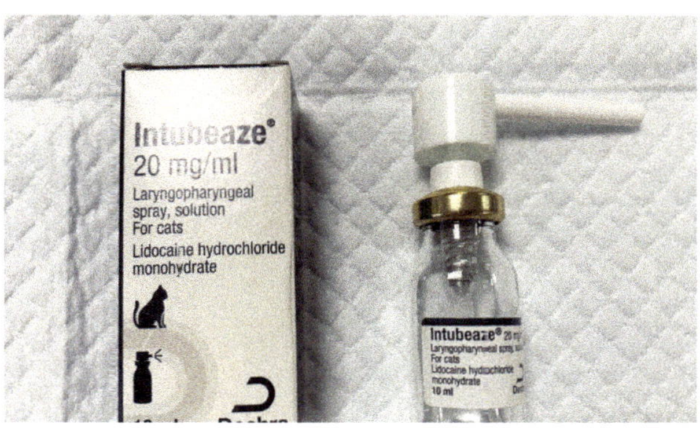

Figure 49. Lidocaine spray.

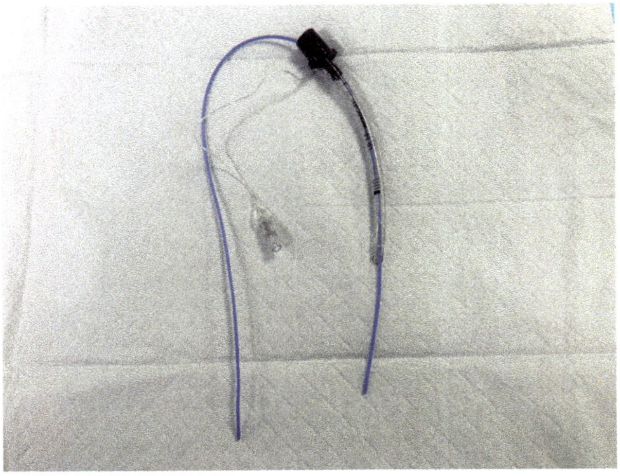

Figure 50. Bougie within an ETT.

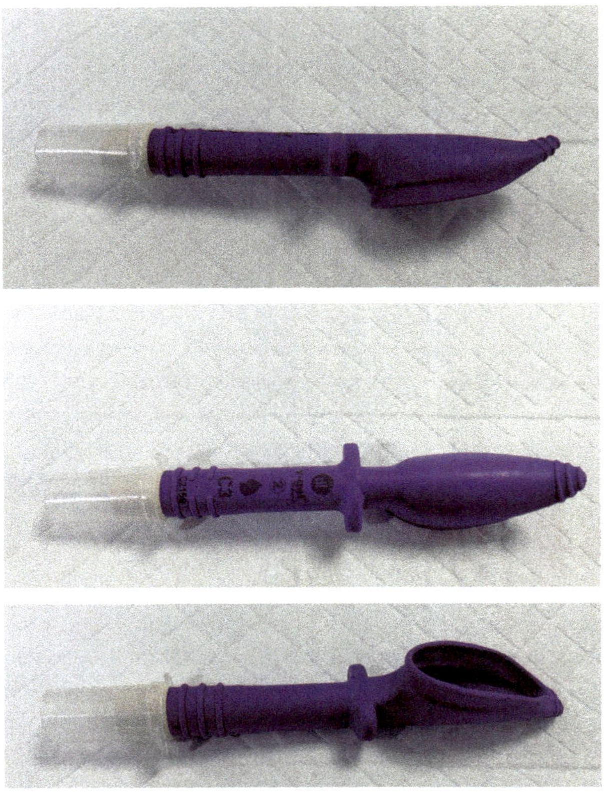

Figure 51. Supraglotic airway devices V-gel®.

guide the ETT. First the bougie is gently placed in the trachea and then the ETT threaded over it.

Feline-specific supraglottic airway devices (SGAD) are an alternative to endotracheal intubation (Figure 51). They were designed to decrease the associated mortality in cats due to intubation. Feline-specific SGAD use soft anatomically-preshaped silicone to form an anatomically precise seal around the airway, whilst at the same time, blocking the proximal oesophagus. This device offers several advantages. They can be placed rapidly and atraumatically, and fewer attempts to intubation and lower propofol is required (i.e. intubated at lighter plane of anaesthesia) (Barletta et al.,

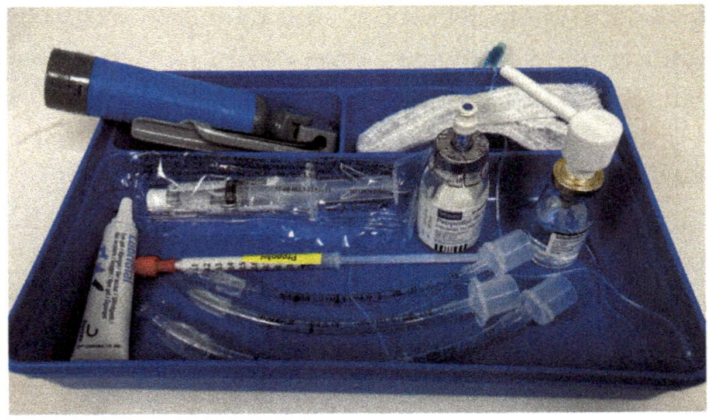

Figure 52. Intubation kit.

2015, Prasse et al., 2016). Moreover, intubation is possible by less experience personnel and they offer much lower resistance to breathing than conventional ETTs because the tubing proximal to the glottis is wider. Postoperatively, less airway discomfort and stridor (van Oostrom et al., 2013) and greater food intake were documented after use of an SGAD compared with an ETT (Barletta et al., 2015). The device is suitable for spontaneous ventilation and for controlled mechanical ventilation up to 16 cm H_2O of peak inspiratory pressure. However, this device has disadvantages. In about 7% of the cases, replacement of the device is required due to **mispositioning or dislocation** (Hecker-Turkovic et al., 2021). Furthermore, complete protection of the airway is not guaranteed especially if there is likely to be a large quantity of refluxed material. Selecting the type of airway management depends on several factors including length of the procedure, patient position, type of anaesthetic and procedure, mechanical ventilation requirement, and the risk of regurgitation.

Drug metabolism

It is well known that cats metabolise certain drugs more slowly than dogs (Court, 2013).

Drug metabolism occurs mainly in the liver, although there are other organs that also metabolize drugs. The main aim of hepatic metabolism is to convert lipid soluble drugs into water soluble compounds which can be eliminated via urine or bile. This conversion takes place in one- or two-phase reactions, depending on the drug.

Phase 1 reactions, also called non-synthetic reactions, include oxidation, reduction or hydrolysis. **The main enzyme system involved in phase 1 reactions is the cytochrome P450 system.** This group of enzymes is divided into families (e.g. CYP 1) and subfamilies (e.g. CYP 1A) and each isoform is in charge of the metabolism of specific drugs. The isoform CYP 2E1 metabolizes fluorinated inhalational agents such as sevoflurane. Cats may have a reduced phase 1 metabolism compared to dogs, due to lower activity of some hepatic cytochrome P450 enzymes. It has recently been reported that the activities of CYP 1A, 2D, 2E, 3A were lower in feline than in canine hepatic microsomes. This may contribute to the differences in drug metabolism observed in cats, compared to dogs. **Phase 2 reactions**, also called synthetic or conjugation reactions, consist of the combination of the result product from phase 1 or an unchanged drug with glucuronide, sulphate, acetate, or glycine radicals. The most important conjugation of **phase 2 is glucuronide conjugation.** This conjugation mainly depends on enzyme systems in the hepatic endoplasmic reticulum. Uridine diphoaphate- glucuronyl transferase (UDP-UGT) is involved in the conjugation of many compounds (e.g. phenolic compounds), however the activity of this enzyme is lower in cats than in dogs. Moreover, cats have a non-functional pseudogene for UGT1A6. Cats also have a deficiency in N-acetyltransferase (NAT) 2, which catalyses N-Acetylation. N-Acetylation is an important route to metabolize some antibiotics and paracetamol.

Cats clear propofol more slowly than dogs, mainly due to the phenolic compound present in the molecule of propofol which requires glucuronide conjugation for its metabolism. This slower metabolism leads to a prolonged recovery when cats receive propofol CRI. Moreover, after three daily doses of propofol red blood cells suffer an oxidative injury and Heinz bodies develop (Andress et al., 1995). After five days of daily dosing, the cat suffered malaise, anorexia and diarrhoea. Benzyl alcohol and benzoic acid compounds are frequently added to drugs as preservatives such as propofol to make the vial last longer once the vial is opened. Benzyl alcohol is metabolized to benzoic acid via oxidation and then conjugated with glucuronide or glycine to produce benzyl glucuronide and hippuric acid. Benzyl alcohol can produce toxicity in cats as they are unable to glucuronidase benzoic acid, however cats can still metabolize some of the benzyl alcohol as glycinate conjugation is not deficient in cats. One study showed that administration of 2% benzyl alcohol with propofol (Figure 53) at normal to high clinical doses did not produce additional adverse effects and toxicity compared to preservative free propofol (Taylor et al., 2012).

Lidocaine (Figure 54) is an amide-linked local anaesthetic that might cause toxicity in cats at lower doses

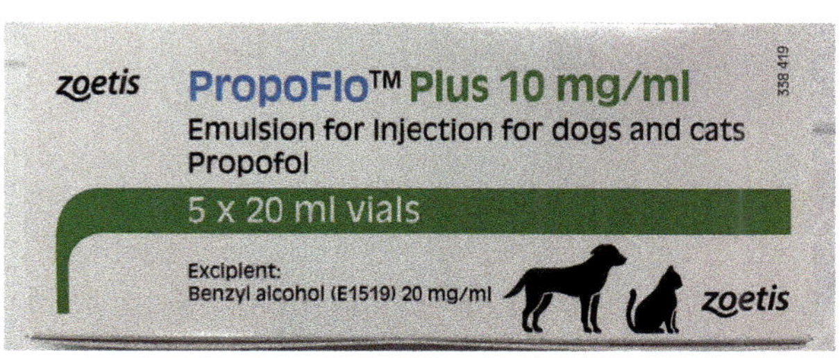

Figure 53. Propofol with benzyl alcohol.

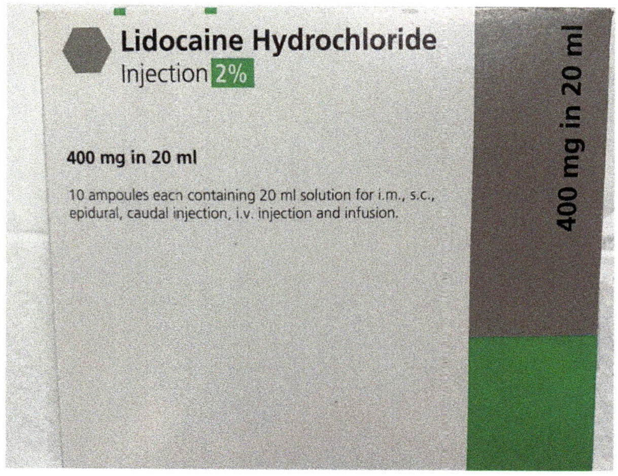

Figure 54. Lidocaine.

than in dogs, especially when under isoflurane anaesthesia (Thomassy et al., 2005). Lidocaine undergoes hepatic hydroxylation (CYP450) and N-methylation and produces two metabolites, glycinexylidide (GX) and monethylglycinexylidide (MEGX) which is an active metabolite with 70% activity of lidocaine. When lidocaine is administered to cats under isoflurane anaesthesia it is important to adjust the dose, dosing interval, or duration of the infusion to avoid depression of the cardiovascular system. It is not recommended to administer a bolus of lidocaine to decrease the MAC of isoflurane (Pypendop and Ilkiw 2005).

Paracetamol (Figure 55) **causes toxicity in the cat** even at low doses due to glucuronidation and NAT2 deficiency. Cats lack UGT1A6 and UGT1A9 which are essential in paracetamol metabolism. Paracetamol undergoes hepatic metabolism, mainly conjugation (glucuronidation and sulphation) and to a lesser extend oxidation. When saturation of the conjugation pathway

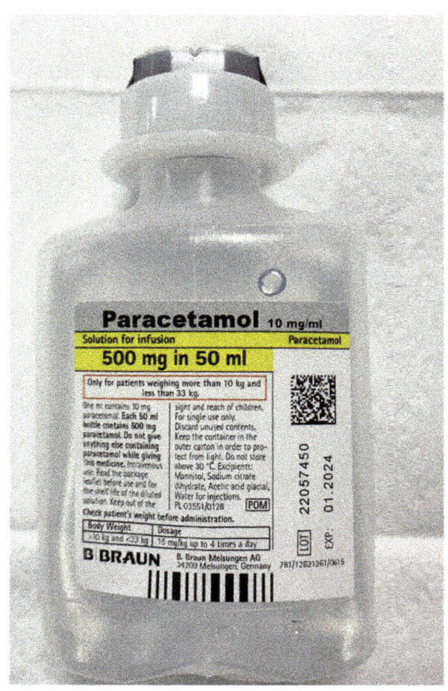

Figure 55. Paracetamol.

occurs, the cytochrome P450 starts metabolizing paracetamol to form a reactive metabolite, N-acetyl-p-quinone-imine (NAPQI). Red cell glutathione conjugates with NAPQI for its elimination, however once this mechanism is saturated, NAPQI causes oxidative cellular damage and methaemoglobinaemic hepatic necrosis occurs. In cats, it is believed erythrocytes have less anti-oxidant capacity and therefore are more sensitive to this oxidative injury. There is another mechanism in cats that contributes to the oxidative injury. Cats produce p-aminophenol by deacetylation of paracetamol. Usually, this compound is reacetytated back to paracetamol by NAT2, however cats have a NAT2 deficiency, therefore, p-aminophenol accumulates in the erythrocytes causing oxidative damage. The half-life of paracetamol is long in cats since the production of the metabolite glucuronide after hepatic glucuronization and its clearance in urine is slow. Toxicity from paracetamol can cause met-hemoglobinaemia and oxidative injury to erythrocytes causing Heinz bodies and anaemia.

Non-steroidal anti-inflammatory drugs (NSAIDs) are well known to cause adverse effects when administered to cats. NSAIDs are mainly metabolized via glucuronidation. Aspirin and carprofen have been shown to have a decrease in clearance due to the reduced glucuronidation. The authors recommend following the guidelines when administering NSAIDs for long-term use (Sparkes et al., 2010).

References

Adami, C. et al. (2020) 'Effect of insulin and fasting regimen on blood glucose of diabetic dogs during phacoemulsification'. *JAAHA*, 56:1–6.

Adams, J.G. et al. (2015) 'Physiology, pathophysiology and anaesthetic management of patients with gastrointestinal and endocrine disease'. Grim KA, Lamont LA, Tranquilli WJ, Greene, S.A., Robertson, S.A. (eds). *Veterinary Anaesthesia and Analgesia*. Lumb and Jones. 5th edition. Iowa: Wiley Blackwell, 641–677.

Acierno, M.J. et al. (2010) 'Agreement between directly measured blood pressure and pressures obtained with three veterinary-specific oscillometric units in cats'. *J Am Vet Med Assoc*, 237:402–06.

American Society of Anesthesiologists (2014) ASA Physical Status System, www.asahq.org/resources/clinical-information/asa-physical-status-classification-system (accessed May 2022) original approval October 2014, last amended December 2020.

Andress, J.L. et al. (1995) 'The effects of consecutive day propofol anaesthesia on feline red blood cells'. *Vet Surg*, 24:277–82.

Armstrong, S.R. et al. (2005) 'Perioperative hypothermia'. *Journal of Veterinary Emergency and Critical Care*, 15:32–37.

Barletta, M. et al. (2015) 'Assessment of v-gel supraglottic airway device placement in cats performed by inexperienced veterinary students'. *Vet Rec*, 177:523–28.

Barton-Lamb, A.L. et al. (2013) 'Evaluation of maxillary arterial blood flow in anesthetized cats with the mouth closed and open'. *Vet J*, 196:325–31.

Binns, S.H. et al. (1995) 'Doppler ultrasonographic, oscillometric, sphygmomanometric and photoplethysmographic techniques for non-invasive blood pressure measurement in anesthetized cats'. *J Vet Int Med*, 9:405–14.

Brodbelt, D.C. et al. (2007) 'Risk factors for anaesthetic-related death in cats: results from confidential enquiry into perioperative small animal fatalities (CEPSAF)'. *British Journal of Anaesthesia*, 99:617–23.

Brodbelt, D.C. et al. (2008) 'The risk of death: The Confidential Enquiry into Perioperative Small Animal Fatalities'. *Veterinary Anaesthesia and Analgesia*, 35:365–373.

Cats protection website: Cats annual report 2021 – www.cats.org.uk/about-cp/cats-report-2021.

Caulkett, N.A. et al. (1998) 'A comparison of indirect blood pressure monitoring techniques in the anesthetized cat'. *Vet Surg*, 27:370–77.

Center, S. et al. (1996) 'Fulminant hepatic failure associated with oral administration of diazepam in 11 cats'. *Journal of the American veterinary medical association*, 209:618–625.

Cerejo, S.A. et al. (2017) 'Comparison of two species-specific oscillometric blood pressure monitors with direct blood pressure measurement in anesthetized cats'. *J Vet Emerg Crit Care*, 27:409–18.

Chan, E.D. et al. (2013) 'Pulse oximetry: understanding its basic principles facilitates appreciation of its limitations'. *Respiratory Medicine*, 107:789–99.

Clark-Price, S. (2015) 'Inadvertent perianaesthetic hypothermia in small animal patients'. *Veterinary Clinics Small Animal*, 45:983–94.

Court, M.H. (2013) 'Feline drug metabolism and disposition'. *Veterinary Clinics Small Animal*, 43:1039–1054.

Davis, H. et al. (2013) 'AAHA/AAFP fluid therapy guidelines for dogs and cats'. *Journal of the American Animal Hospital Association*, 49:149–59.

da Cunha, A.F. et al. (2014) 'Measuring the level of agreement between values obtained by directly measured blood pressure and ultrasonic Doppler flow detector in cats'. *J Vet Emerg Crit Care*, 24:272–78.

Fletcher, D.J. et al. (2012) 'RECOVER evidence and knowledge gap analysis on veterinary CPR'. Part 7: clinical guidelines. *Journal of Veterinary Emergency and Critical Care*, 22:S102–S131.

Ferreira, T.H. *et al.* (2009) 'Effects of remifentanil hydrochloride administered via constant rate infusion on the minimum alveolar concentration of isoflurane in cats'. *American Journal of Veterinary Research*, 70:581–588.

Galatos, A.D. & Raptopoulos, D. (1995) 'Gastro-oesophageal reflux during anaesthesia in the dog: the effect of pre-operative fasting and pre-medication'. *The Veterinary Record*, 4:479–83.

Galatos, A.D. et al. (2001) 'Gastro-Oesophageal Reflux during Thiopentone or Propofol Anaesthesia in the Cat'. *J. Vet.*, A 48:287–94.

Garcia, R.S. et al. (2017) 'Prevalence of Gastroesophageal Reflux in Cats During Anaesthesia and Effect of Omeprazole on Gastric pH'. *J Vet Intern Med*, 31:734–42.

Gaudette, S. et al. (2020) 'The endothelial glycocalyx: structure and function in health and critical illness.' *Journal of Veterinary Emergency and Critical Care*, 30:117–134.

Grubb, T. et al. (2020) 'AAHA Anaesthesia and monitoring Guidelines for dogs and cats'. *JAAHA*. 2020, 56.

Grandy, J.L. et al. (1992) 'Evaluation of the Doppler ultrasonic method of measuring systolic arterial blood pressure in cats'. *Am J Vet Res*, 53:1166–69.

Hanas, S. et al. (2009) 'Twenty-four Holter monitoring of unsedated healthy cats in the home environment'. *Journal of Veterinary Cardiology*, 11:17–22.

Hecker-Turkovic et al. (2021) 'Success of placement and complications during v-gel placement and maintenance of anaesthesia.' *Journal of Feline Medicine and Surgery*, doi: 10.1177/1098612X211050612.

Hofmeister, E.K. et al. (2005) 'Evaluating of veterinarians' and veterinary students' knowledge and clinical use of pulse oximetry'. *Journal of Veterinary Medicine Educations*, 32:272–77.

Hosgood, G., Scholl, D.T. (2002) 'Evaluation of age and American Society of Anaesthesiologists (ASA) physical status as risk factors for perianesthetic morbidity and mortality in the cat'. *Journal of Veterinary Emergency and Critical Care*, 12 (1):9–15.

Ilkiw, J.E. et al. (1997) 'Effect of alfentanil on the minimum alveolar concentration in cats'. *Am J Vet Res*, 58(11):1247–1249.

Jae Hwa Yoo et al. (2020) 'Effects of 10-min of pre-warming on inadvertent perioperative hypothermia in intraoperative warming patients: a randomized controlled trial'. *Anaesthesia & pain medicine*, 15:356–64.

Kamijyo, Y., Garcia, J.H. (1975) Carotid supply of the feline brain. *Stroke*, 6:361–69.

Levy, J.K. et al. (2017) 'Perioperative mortality in cats and dogs undergoing spay and castration at a high-volume clinic'. *Veterinary Journal*, 224:11–15.

Mair, A. et al. (2017) 'Effect of lingual gauze swab placement on pulse oximeter readings in anaesthetised dogs and cats'. *Veterinary Record*, 180:49–54.

Mathis, A. et al. (2012) 'Comparison of quality of recovery from anaesthesia in cats induced with propofol or alfaxolone'. *Veterinary Anaesthesia and Analgesia*, 39:282–289.

Naden, K. (2020) 'Developments in surgical fluid therapy rates in cats and dogs'. *Veterinary Evidence*, 5:2–15.

Nelson, R.W. (2015) 'Canine Diabetes Mellitus'. In: Feldman, E.C., Nelson, R.W., Reush, C.E., Scott-Moncrieff, J.C.R. (eds). *Canine and Feline Endocrinology*, 4th edition. Elsevier. 213–257.

Noel-Morgan, J., Muir, W.W. (2018) 'Anaesthesia-associated relative hypovolemia: mechanisms, monitoring, and treatment considerations'. *Frontiers in Veterinary Science*, 5:article 53.

Orlando, J.M. et al. (2016) 'Use of oral trazadone for sedation in cats: a pilot study'. *Journal offeline medicine and surgery*, 18:476–482.

Pascoe, P.J. et al. (1997) 'Cardiovascular effects of equipotent isoflurane and alfentanil/isoflurane minimum alveolar concentration multiple in cats'. *Am J Vet Res*, 58(11):1267–73.

Pascoe, P.J. et al. (2006) 'The effect of the duration of propofol administration on recovery from anaesthesia in cats'. *Vet Anaesth Analg*, 33:2–7.

Pascoe, P.J. et al. (2007) 'The effects of ketamine on the minimum alveolar concentration of isoflurane in cats'. *Veterinary Anaesthesia and Analgesia*, 34:31–39.

Pascoe, P. (2018) 'Fluid therapy'. In: Steagall P, Robertson S, Taylor P (eds). *Feline Anaesthesia and Pain Management*, 1st edition. New Jersey: Wiley Blackwell, 123–138.

Pedersen, K.M. et al. (2002) 'Evaluation of an oscillometric blood pressure monitor for use in anesthetized cats'. *J Am Vet Med Assoc*, 221:646–50.

Petric, A.D. et al. (2010) 'Comparison of high definition oscillometric and Doppler ultrasonic devices for measuring blood pressure in anaesthetized cats'. *J Feline Med Surg*, 12: 731–37.

Prasse, S.A. et al. (2016) 'Clinical evaluation of the v-gel supraglottic airway device in comparison with a classical laryngeal mask and endotracheal intubation in cats during spontaneous and controlled mechanical ventilation'. *Veterinary Anaesthesia and Analgesia*, 43:55–62.

Pypendop, B.H., Ilkiw, J.E. (2005) 'Assessment of the hemodynamic effects of lidocaine administered IV in isoflurane-anesthetized cats'. *AJVR*, 66:661–68.

Pypendop, B.H. et al. (2005) 'The effects of intravenous lidocaine administration on the minimum alveolar concentration of isoflurane in cats'. *Anaesthesia and Analgesia*, 100:97–101.

Pypendop, B.H. et al. (2006) 'Effects of epidural administration of morphine and buprenorphine on the minimum alveolar concentration of isoflurane in cats'. *American Journal of Veterinary Research*, 67:1471–75.

Pypendop, B.H. et al. (2011) 'Hemodynamic effects of dexmedetomidine in isoflurane-anaesthetised cats'. *Veterinary Anaesthesia and Analgesia*, 38:555–567.

Pypendop, B.H. et al. (2018) 'Pharmacokinetics of alfaxalone infusions, context-sensitive half-time and recovery times in male neutered cats'. *Veterinary Anaesthesia and Analgesia*, 45:630–639.

Quimby, J. et al. (2022) 'Serum concentrations of gabapentin in cats with chronic kidney disease'. *Journal of Feline medicine and surgery*, 1–7.

Redondo, J.I. et al. (2012) 'Retrospective study of the prevalence of postanaesthetic hypothermia in cats'. *Vet Rec*, 170:206–09.

Reineke, E.L. et al. (2016) 'Prediction of systolic blood pressure using peripheral pulse palpation in cats'. *Journal of Veterinary Emergency and Critical Care*, 26:52–57.

Reneman, R.S. et al. (1974) 'Vertebral and carotid blood distribution in the brain of the dog and the cat'. *Cardiovascular Research*, 8:65–72.

Reynolds, L. et al. (2008) 'Perioperative complications of hypothermia'. *Best Practice & Research Clinical Anaesthesiology*, 22:646–57.

Robertson, S.A. et al. (2005) 'PK-PD modelling of buprenorphine in cats: intravenous and oral transmucosal administration.' *J Vet Pharmacol Ther*, 28:453–460.

Robertson, S.A. et al. (2018) 'AAFP Feline Anaesthesia Guidelines'. *Journal of Feline Medicine and Surgery*, 20:602–34.

Smart, L. et al. (2018) 'Large-Volume Crystalloid Fluid Is Associated with Increased Hyaluronan Shedding and Inflammation in a Canine Haemorrhagic Shock Model'. *Inflammation*, 41:1515–23.

Savvas, I. et al. (2009) 'The effect of pre-anaesthetic fasting time and type of food on gastric content volume and acidity in dogs'. *Veterinary Anaesthesia and Analgesia*, 36:539–46.

Schwarz, A. et al. (2014) 'Minimum infusion rate of alfaxalone for total intravenous anaesthesia after sedation with acepromazine or medetomidine in cats undergoing ovariohysterectomy'. *Veterinary Anaesthesia and Analgesia*, 41:480–490.

Scrivani, P.V. et al. (2014) 'Structural and functional changes relevant to maxillary arterial flow observed during computed tomography and nonselective digital subtraction angiography in cats with the mouth closed and opened'. *Vet Radiol Ultrasound*, 55:263–71.

Short, C.E. (1991) 'Effects of anticholinergic treatment on the cardiac and respiratory systems in dogs sedated with medetomidine'. *Vet Rec*, 129:310–13.

Sideri, A. et al. (2009) 'Gastro-oesophageal reflux during anaesthesia in the kitten: comparison between use of a laryngeal mask airway or an endotracheal tube'. *Veterinary Anaesthesia and Analgesia*, 36:547–54.

Sparkes, A.H. et al. (2010) 'ISFM and AAFP consensus guidelines long-term use of NSAIDs in cats'. *Journal of Feline Medicine and Surgery*, 12, 521–38.

Stanway, G.W. et al. (2002) 'A preliminary investigation comparing pre-operative morphine and buprenorphine for postoperative analgesia and sedation in cats'. *Veterinary Anaesthesia and Analgesia*, 29(1):29–35.

Stiles, J. et al. (2012) 'Post-anaesthetic cortical blindness in cats: twenty cases'. *Vet J*, 193:367–73.

Stevens, B.J. et al. (2016) 'Efficacy of a single dose of trazadone hydrochloride given to cats prior to veterinary visits to reduce signs of transport- and examination-related anxiety' *Journal of the American Veterinary Medical Association*, 249:202–207.

Stevens-Sparks, C.K., Strain, G.M. (2010) 'Postanesthesia deafness in dogs and cats following dental and ear cleaning procedures'. *Veterinary Anaesthesia and Analgesia*, 37:347–51.

Steffey, E.P. et al. (2015) 'Inhalation anaesthetics.' In: Grimm, K.A. L.A., Lamont, L.A., Tranquilli, W.J. et al. (eds). *Veterinary Anaesthesia and Analgesia*, V edition. Ames: Wiley Backwell, 297–331.

Taboada, F.M. et al. (2010) 'Induction of anaesthesia with alfaxolone or propofol before isoflurane maintenance in cats.' *Veterinary Record*, 167:85–89.

Tamura, J. et al. (2015) 'Sedative effects of intramuscular alfaxalone administered to cats'. *Journal of Veterinary medical sciences*, 77:897–904.

Taylor, P.M. et al. (2012) 'Evaluation of propofol containing 2% benzyl alcohol preservative in cats'. J Feline Med Surg, 14:516–26.

Tinker, J.H. et al. (1989) 'Monitoring devices in prevention of anaesthetic mishaps: a closed claims analysis'. *Anaesthesiology*, 71:541–46.

Thomasy, S.M. et al. (2005) 'Pharmacokinetics of lidocaine and its active metabolite, mkonoethylglycinexylidide, after intravenous administration of lidocaine to awake and isoflurane-anesthetized cats'. *AJVR*, 66:1162–1166.

Valverde, A. et al. (2004) 'Effects of acepromazine on the incidence of vomiting associated with opioid administration in dogs'. *Veterinary Anaesthesia and Analgesia*, 31:102–108.

van Oostrom, H. et al. (2013) 'A comparison between the v-gel supraglottic airway device and the cuffed endotracheal tube for airway management in spontaneously breathing cats during isoflurane anaesthesia'. *Veterinary Anaesthesia and Analgesia*, 40:265–71.

Veres-Nyeki, K.O. (2016) 'Endocrine diseases.' In: Duke-Novakovski, T., de Vries, M., Seymour, C. (eds). *BSAVA manual of Canine and Feline. Anaesthesia and Analgesia*. 3rd edition. Gloucester: BSAVA, 376–391.

Viskjer, S., Sjostrom, L. (2017) 'Effect of the duration of food withholding prior to anaesthesia on Gastroesophageal reflux and regurgitation in healthy dogs undergoing elective orthopaedic surgery'. *AJVR*, 78:144–50.

Williamson, J.A., Leone, S. (2012) 'Non-invasive arterial blood pressure monitoring'. In: Burkitt Creedon, J.M., Davis, H. (eds). *Advanced Monitoring and Procedures for Small Animal Emergency and Critical Care*. West Sussex: Wiley Blackwell, 134–44.

Wong, V.G., Macri, F.J. (1964) 'Vasculature of the cat eye'. *Arch Ophthalmol*, 72:351–58.

Zonca, A. et al. (2012) 'Pharmacokinetics of ketamine and propofol combination administered as ketofol via continuous infusion in cats'. *Journal of Veterinary Pharmacology and Therapeutics*, 35:580–587.

Zwijnenberg, R.J. et al. (2011) 'Evaluation of oscillometric and vascular access port arterial blood pressure measurement techniques versus implanted telemetry in anesthetized cats'. *Am J Vet Res*, 72:1015–21.

Tests

1. **Calculate the volume in millilitres of 10% ketamine that need to be added to a 20 ml syringe in order to make a 2 mg/ml solution of ketamine.**
   A) 0.4 ml of ketamine in 19.6 ml of saline.
   B) 0.4 ml of ketamine in 20 ml of saline.
   C) 4 ml of ketamine in 16 ml of saline.
   D) 4 ml of ketamine in 20 ml of saline.
2. **A 17-year-old cat is under general anaesthesia for a minor surgical procedure. The fraction of inspired oxygen is 80%, the pulse oximeter reading is 98%, and the respiratory rate is 16 bpm. Is the patient ventilating appropriately?**
   A) Yes, pulse oximeter is within normal limits.
   B) Yes, pulse oximeter and respiratory rate are within normal limits.
   C) No, the inspired fraction of oxygen should be higher.
   D) All above are false.

3. Which of the following statements is correct regarding brain vascularization in cats.
A) Maxillary artery and internal carotid artery play a major role.
B) Maxillary artery and basilar artery play a major role.
C) Basilar artery and common carotid artery.
D) Maxillary artery plays a major role.

4. A cat is pre-medicated intravenously with an opioid and an alpha-2 agonist. Five minutes later anaesthesia is induced with alfaxalone. Soon after induction there is bradycardia and low blood pressure. How should this complication be treated?
A) There is no need for treatment.
B) Administration of an anticholinergic such as atropine or glycopyrrolate.
C) Administration of a full dose of atipamezole intramuscularly.
D) None of the above.

5. Calculate mean arterial pressure (MAP). Systolic arterial pressure (SAP) = 120 mmHg, diastolic arterial pressure (DAP) = 60 mmHg, heart rate = 150 bpm.
A) 60 mmHg.
B) 80 mmHg.
C) 40 mmHg.
D) 120 mmHg.

6. After induction of anaesthesia and tracheal intubation, the capnograph is connected but there is no capnogram. Choose the least likely reason:
A) The endotracheal tube is in the oesophagus.
B) The patient is apnoeic.
C) Capnograph is not functioning.
D) Cardiac arrest.

7. Choose the correct answer regarding buprenorphine:
A) It is a partial mu agonist drug and provides the highest analgesia.
B) It is a partial mu agonist with good transmucosal absorption.
C) It is a mu agonist and provides the maximum analgesia.
D) It is a partial mu agonist with a fast onset of action.

8. Choose the incorrect statement regarding gabapentin:
A) It is a calcium channel blocker.
B) Recommended dose is 25 mg/kg to 100 mg/kg PO.
C) It is excreted via the kidneys.
D) It is an analogue of the neurotransmitter GABA.

9. Choose the correct answer:
A) Diabetic cats should not be fasted prior to general anaesthesia.
B) 61% of deaths occur during the 0–3 hours during general anaesthesia.
C) During anaesthesia fluid rate should be 3 ml/kg/h.
D) Whenever possible uncuffed endotracheal tubes should be used in cats.

10. A 13-year-old aggressive cat with hypertrophic cardiomyopathy requires general anaesthesia for a dental procedure. Which of the following is the best intramuscular (IM) pre-medication:
A) Methadone, ketamine and dexmedetomidine IM.
B) Butorphanol, ketamine and acepromazine IM.
C) Methadone, alfaxalone and dexmedetomidine IM.
D) Methadone, alfaxalone and acepromazine IM.

11. Calculate the inspiratory time if a 5 kg cat is breathing 20 times per minute and the I:E is 1:2. Then calculate the inspiratory flow required to administer a tidal volume of 12 ml/kg in the same cat.
(RR = 60/I:E time, 20 = 60/ I:E, I:E = 60/20 = 3 seconds, if it is 1:2, 1 second inspiration, 2 seconds expiration time. Inspiratory TV = inspiratory time x inspiratory flow 60 ml = 1 x flow)
A) Inspiratory time = 1.2 seconds, inspiratory flow = 60 ml.
B) Inspiratory time = 1 second, inspiratory flow = 60 l.
C) Inspiratory time = 1 second, inspiratory flow = 0.06 l.
D) Inspiratory time = 0.5 seconds, inspiratory flow = 0.06 l.

Clinical Case. Anaesthetic management

Signalment: 18 years old, female, Domestic Short Hair cat, 3.5 kg body weight.
History: chronic kidney disease IRIS 2, losing weight, anorexia, anaemia, poor body condition score.
Reason for anaesthesia: oral exam and possible dental extractions.
Physical exam: BAR, aggressive cat. Not possible to perform a physical exam.
Diagnostic tests: none, aggressive patient.

1. **Choose the correct answer:**
   A) The patient should be fasted for 12 hours.
   B) The owner should administer gabapentin PO prior to the appointment.
   C) Perioperative bloods are not required.
   D) A mouth gag should be used to fully open the mouth.
2. **Which of the following statements is correct regarding anaemia:**
   A) Anaemia causes a low reading for oxygen saturation of haemoglobin.
   B) Anaemia decreases the amount of oxygen dissolved in blood (i.e partial pressure of oxygen).
   C) Anaemia decreases the oxygen delivery to the tissues.
   D) Anaemia affects the pharmacodynamics of anaesthetic drugs.
3. **Which of the following is the most appropriate way of managing the airway of this patient:**
   A) V-gel, it is less traumatic than a normal endotracheal tube.
   B) Uncuffed endotracheal tube. Cuffed endotracheal tubes are not recommended in cats.
   C) Cuffed endotracheal tube to protect the airway.
   D) Face mask, as there is no need for an endotracheal tube.
4. **Which of the following breathing systems would be most appropriate?**
   A) A mini Lack if the patient is breathing spontaneously.
   B) A T-Piece as it is very efficient during spontaneous ventilation.
   C) A mini Lack as it is very efficient during mechanical ventilation.
   D) A circle breathing system if the patient is breathing spontaneously.
5. **Choose the correct answer to prevent/treat hypothermia:**
   A) Lower the fresh gas flow by using a Mini Lack with mechanical ventilation.
   B) Warm the bag of fluids before administration.
   C) Use an HME to decrease the humidity of the inspired gas.
   D) Wrap all 4 limbs with bubble wrap.
6. **Doppler is used to measure blood pressure. Choose the correct answer:**
   A) Doppler provides a reading closer to systolic blood pressure.
   B) A cuff placed too tight provides a falsely low blood pressure reading.
   C) Doppler provides an estimate of the cardiac output.
   D) A cuff placed below the right atrium provides a falsely low blood pressure.
7. **During a dental extraction the screen in the image below can be seen. Choose the correct answer:**

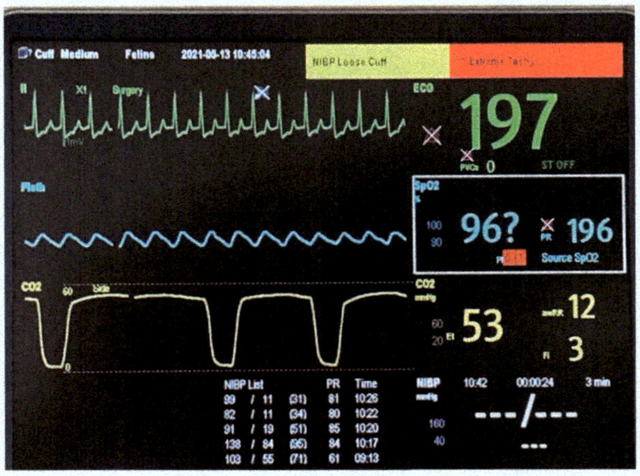

A) Sinus tachycardia, assess depth of anaesthesia.
B) Ventricular premature complexes, no need for treatment.
C) Ventricular tachycardia, start CPR.
D) Tachyarrhythmia. Lidocaine should be administered.

8. Choose the correct answer regarding maintenance of anaesthesia:

A) Isoflurane is not recommended as it is highly metabolised in the kidneys.
B) Sevoflurane is better than isoflurane due to its low blood:gas coefficient.
C) Total intravenous anaesthesia (TIVA) with propofol is better than TIVA with alfaxalone.
D) Sevoflurane is not recommended due to its arrhythmogenicity.

9. During the dental examination the following capnogram is seen. Choose the correct answer:

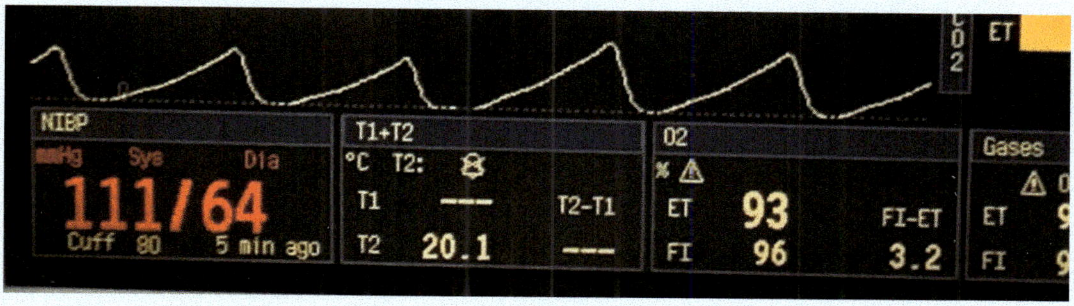

A) The capnograph shows a possible airway obstruction.
B) The capnograph shows a leak in the endotraqueal tube.
C) The capnograph shows rebreathing.
D) The capnograph is normal.

10. See the image below and choose the correct answer:

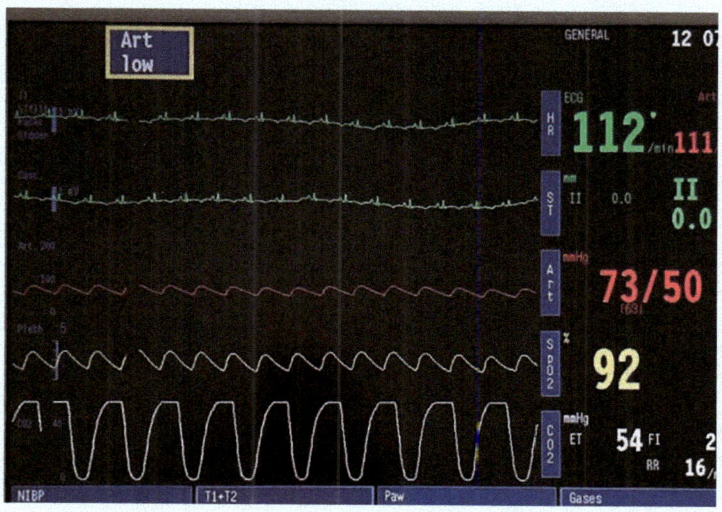

A) Oxygen saturation is low (92%) but this is normal in an anaemic cat.
B) The capnograph shows hypercapnia due to rebreathing.
C) The low heart rate should be treated with an anticholinergic drug.
D) Systolic blood pressure is within normal limits for an anaesthetised cat.

Correct Answers

Test

1. A	6. C	11. C
2. D	7. B	
3. D	8. B	
4. D	9. C	
5. B	10. C	

Clinical Case

1. B	6. B
2. C	7. A
3. C	8. B
4. A	9. A
5. D	10. C

Respiratory system disorders

17

Kerry Rolph

Contents

Cats live in colonies which are predominantly formed of closely related females that come together, often around food sources, to help rear their young. Unlike dogs, cats do not form an interdependent hierarchy but remain solitary hunters without a social survival strategy or a pack mentality, and in their natural environment cats are both a hunter and prey species. **For a cat to show signs of illness would advertise vulnerability to a predator** and places them at increased risk without a pack to protect them.

Therefore, as a solitary hunter and prey species, the cat has an inherent ability to mask the signs of illness. This is especially important to remember when presented with a cat with respiratory compromise.

Initial management of the cat with respiratory compromise

When presented with a dyspnoeic cat, the initial history taking and assessment should be dictated by the cat's condition, rather than the convenience of clinician or client. Patients with dyspnoea, especially severely affected patients, benefit from being **placed in an oxygen enriched environment** whilst the history is taken. It should be remembered that handling a severely dyspnoeic cat (even for something as simple as checking body weight) can result in hysteria, respiratory decompensation, and death. However, in a stable patient a full history and physical examination can be

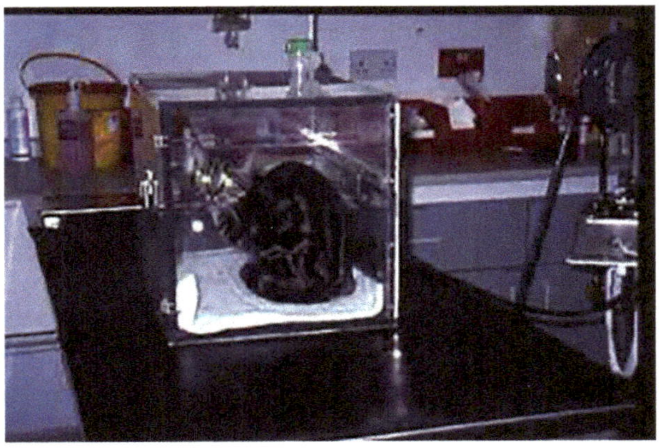

Figure 1. Induction chamber.

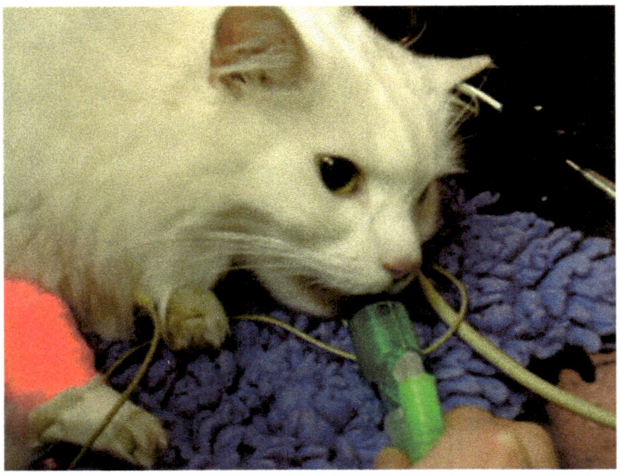

Figure 2. Free flow oxygen.

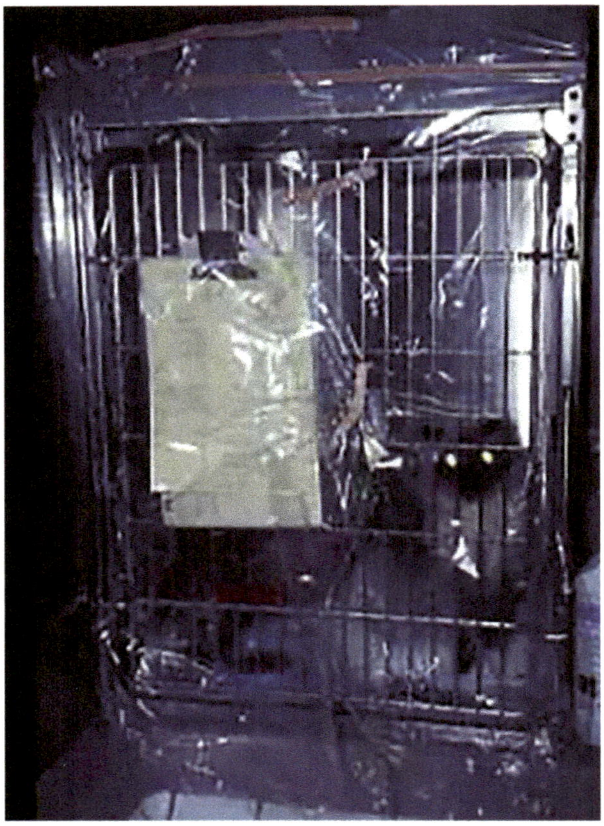

Figure 3. Cellophane cage.

undertaken, whilst taking care not to distress the cat and exacerbate the clinical signs.

Signalment

Whilst waiting for a dyspnoeic patient to arrive or stabilize, **their signalment and the likely differential diagnoses should be considered.**

History

It is helpful to determine the environment the cat lives in, for example access to the **outdoors, travel history, and any previous history of trauma** or disease either affecting this cat or others in the household.

In addition, the veterinarian should ascertain whether or not the cat has been **coughing, sneezing** or if there is any **nasal discharge**; cats with pulmonary oedema rarely cough, whereas it is a common finding in cats with asthma (Simpson, 2013). The presence of

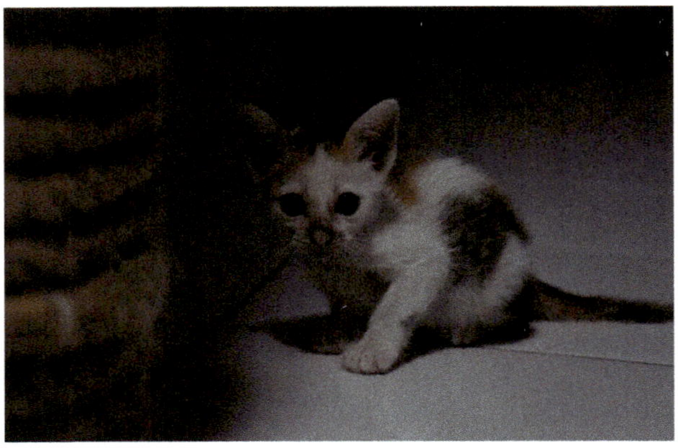

Figure 4. Paediatric or juvenile cats are more likely to contract infectious conditions.

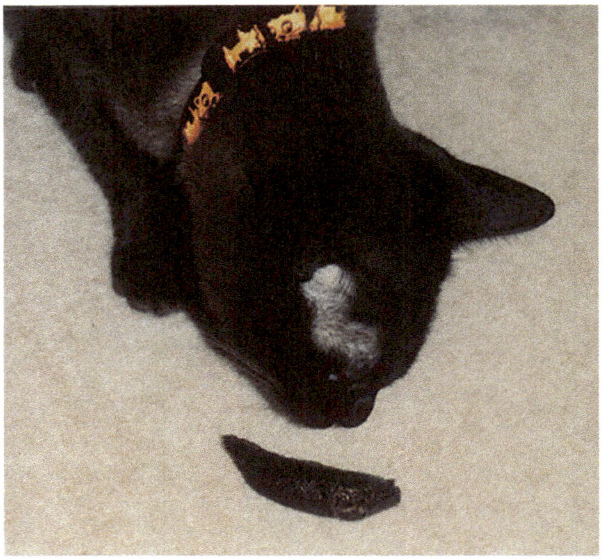

Figure 5. Young male cats which hunt are more likely to present with lung worm infections.

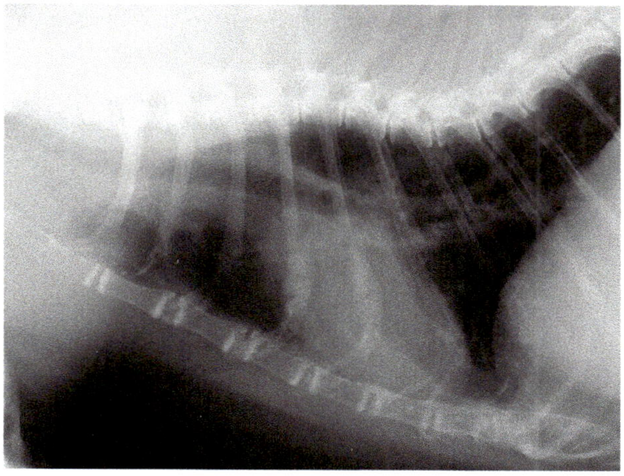

Figure 6. Young to middle-aged cats are more likely to present with asthma (especially middle-aged Siamese or Burmese cats which commonly present with chronic bronchopulmonary disease).

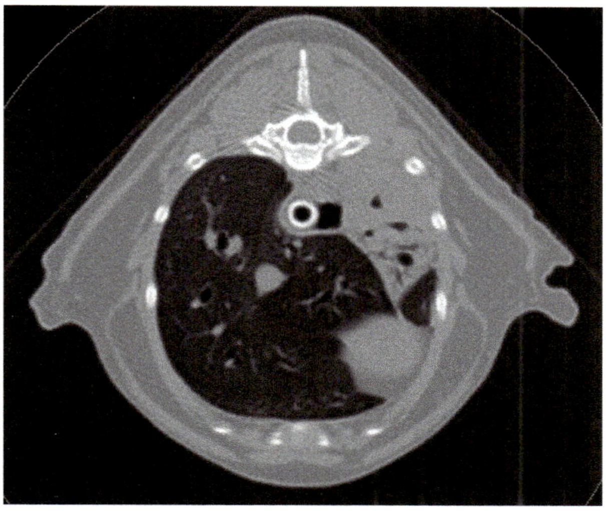

Figure 7. Primary pulmonary parenchymal neoplasms are more common in older cats.

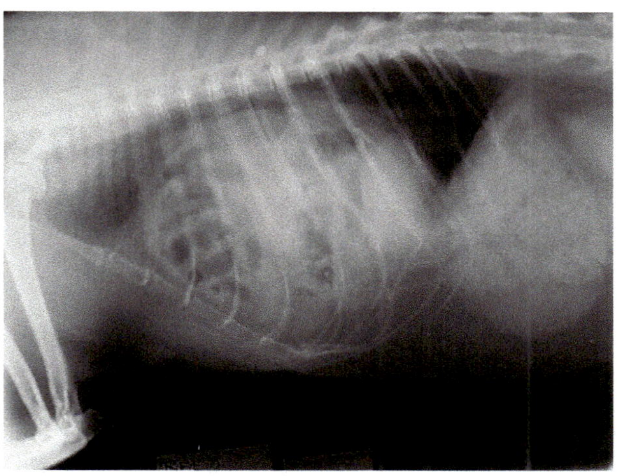

Figure 8. Breed can also be helpful; for example, very young Bengal or Burmese kittens may be seen with 'flat chest' disease, juvenile Siamese cats appear to be predisposed to thymic LSA, young pedigree cats from multi-cat households are at an increased risk of developing FIP, and young Persian or British Shorthaired cats appear predisposed to pericardioperitoneal diaphragmatic herniation.

stridor, voice changes, sneezing, or snoring might indicate upper respiratory tract disease.

Also the duration of signs, rate of progression, severity of clinical signs, history of weight loss, regurgitation, anorexia, exercise intolerance, syncope, vomiting, lameness, trauma, or exposure to possible toxins should be assessed; this can help to determine the cause and significance of any respiratory signs.

Observing the patient

An important part of the initial assessment is **observing the patient to evaluate the respiratory pattern**. This helps the clinician decide if the dyspnoea is most likely due to a non-respiratory cause or originates from the upper respiratory tract (URT), lower respiratory tract (LRT), or results from pleural space disease; and whether the breathing pattern is restrictive or obstructive.

Initially it is important to determine if the dyspnoea is:

- **Inspiratory**: most commonly associated with:
  - URT disease
  - pleural space disease
- **Expiratory**: most commonly associated with:
  - LRT disease
- **Tachypnoeic** (King, 2004) without an increased respiratory effort, is often associated with non-respiratory causes such as:
  - hyperthyroidism
  - metabolic acidosis
  - abdominal enlargement
  - hyperthermia
  - stress, fear, pain

The **respiratory rate and pattern** further helps determine if the dyspnoea is restrictive or obstructive.

- **Restrictive disease**: prevents the lung expanding properly:
  - rapid, short, shallow breaths
  - associated with parenchymal disease and pleural space disease (King 2004).
- **Obstructive disease**: narrowing of the airway or laryngeal paralysis:
  - slower, deeper breathing pattern.
  - associated with feline allergic airway disease, laryngeal disease.

Physical examination

Physical examination findings (even when performed in several short episodes) help narrow the differential diagnoses, to better enable stabilisation of the dyspnoeic patient. When possible, a **complete physical**

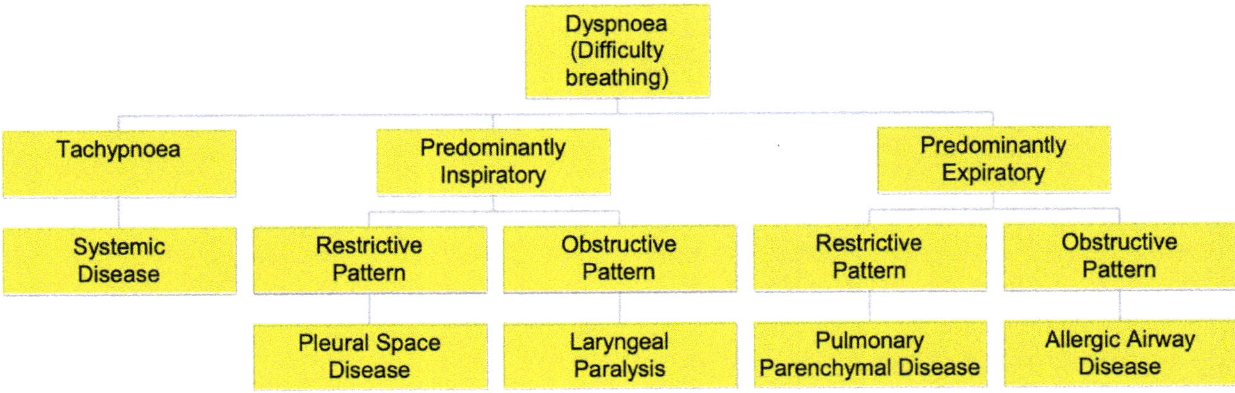

Figure 9. Causes of dyspnoea.

examination should be performed and the cat assessed for **evidence of trauma**. This includes careful palpation of the thoracic cavity and abdomen; and examination of the digits for signs of injury.

Examination of the head and neck

Capillary refill time

For an animal in shock or with reduced cardiac output, the capillary refill time may be prolonged. However, in the majority of animals, the capillary refill time is normal (even in those in heart failure) emphasising that abnormalities are often **only evident in particularly severe diseases.**

Mucous membranes

Mucous membrane colour should be evaluated and any pallor or cyanosis noted. The latter may be due to central or peripheral causes, and it is important to distinguish between the two.

- **Pallor**: associated with fear, anaemia, hypoxia.
- **Cyanosis**: signifies a concentration of deoxygenated haemoglobin > 5 g/dl, indicating severe hypoxia.
  - **Central cyanosis**: generalized cyanosis indicative of arterial hypoxaemia. This can result from:

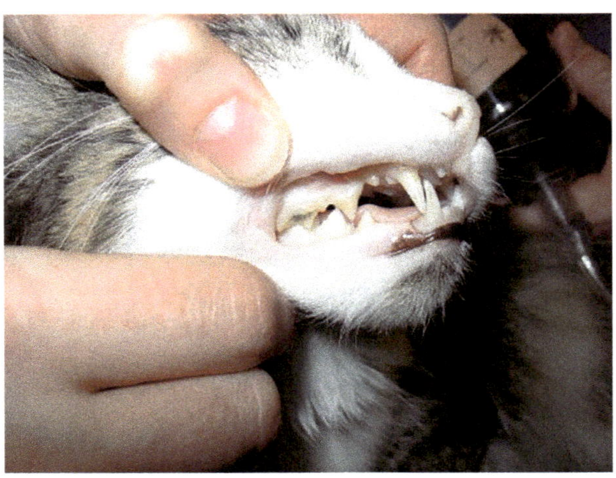

Figure 10. Pale mucus membranes in a severely anaemic cat.

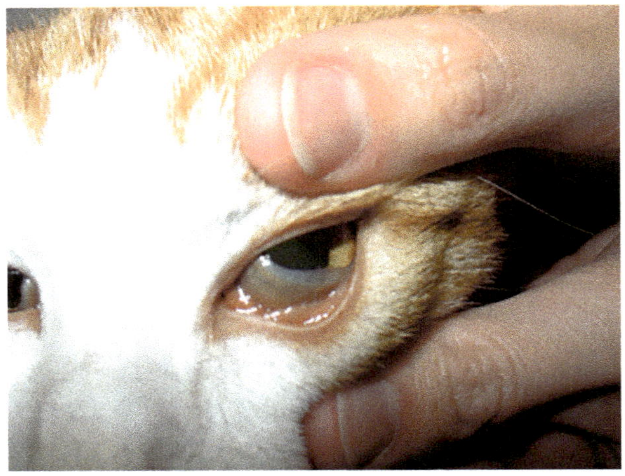

Figure 11. A cat with significant methaemoglobinaemia.

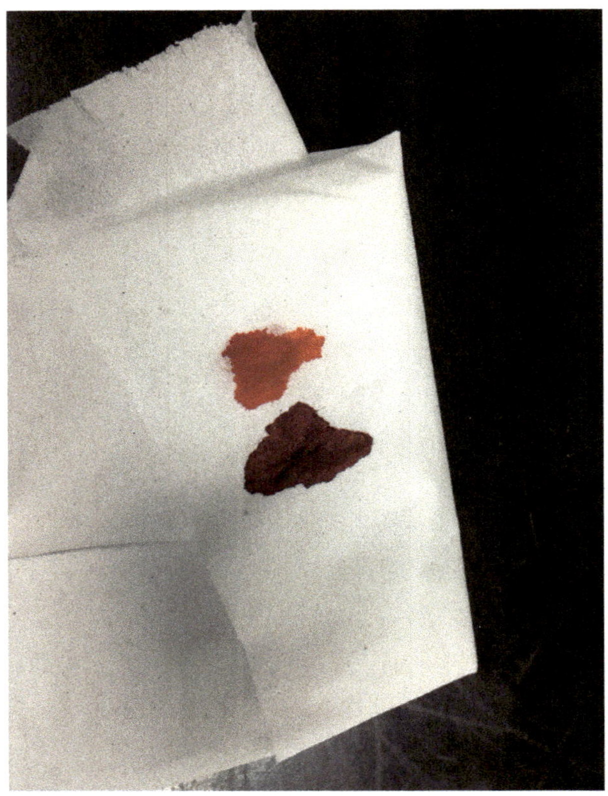

Figure 12. Case with paracetamol toxicity and methaemoglobinaemia; note how dark the blood is compared to a normal blood sample.

    - hypoventilation
    - diffusion impairment
    - ventilation perfusion mismatch
    - inhaled air deficient in oxygen
    - right to left shunting cardiac abnormality.
  - **Peripheral cyanosis**: observed only in the extremities (distal limbs and ear tips). The arterial oxygen content is normal but the capillary or venous blood perfusing the affected area extracts a larger proportion of the oxygen. It occurs due to:
    - decreased arterial blood flow or venous pooling
    - associated with reduced cardiac output, regional vasoconstriction, or vascular obstruction.
- **Brown mucous membranes**: commonly indicate methaemoglobinaemia, associated with paracetamol toxicity (other presenting signs include facial oedema and severe respiratory distress).

Ocular examination

Ocular examination helps determine the presence of exophthalmus (retrobulbar neoplasms or abscesses), anisocoria, Horner's syndrome, hyphaema, or retinal lesions suggestive of hypertension, neoplastic infiltration, fungal or parasitic infections, or taurine deficiency.

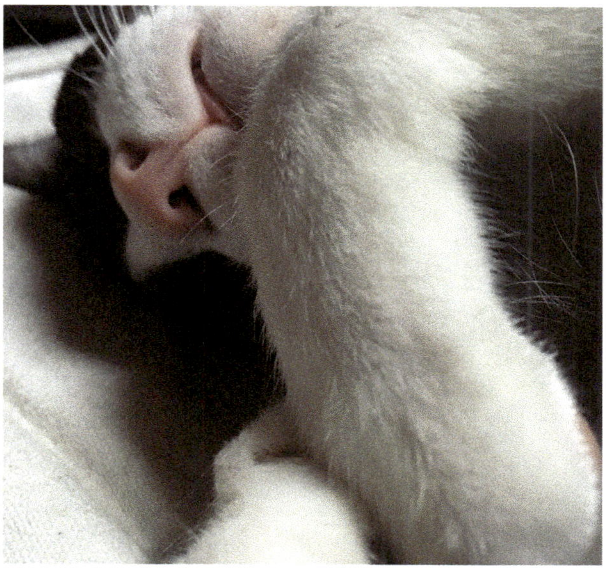

Figure 13. Animals solely suffering from a nasal disorder rarely present with severe respiratory distress. However, since some cats are reluctant to breathe through their mouths, in this species nasal obstruction can present as marked respiratory distress. Palpation over the nasal cavities may reveal pain, asymmetry, or distortion of the nasal cavity. Furthermore, thorough examination of the oral cavity may reveal bony abnormalities, severe dental disease, or palatine abnormalities. Assessment of the patency of the nares helps determine whether there is a unilateral or bilateral disorder. Unilateral nasal obstruction or discharge may be related to a tooth root abscess, oronasal fistular, cyst, haematoma, foreign body or neoplasm, whereas bilateral disease is often related to neoplasia, infection or a disease process occurring caudal to the nasal septum.

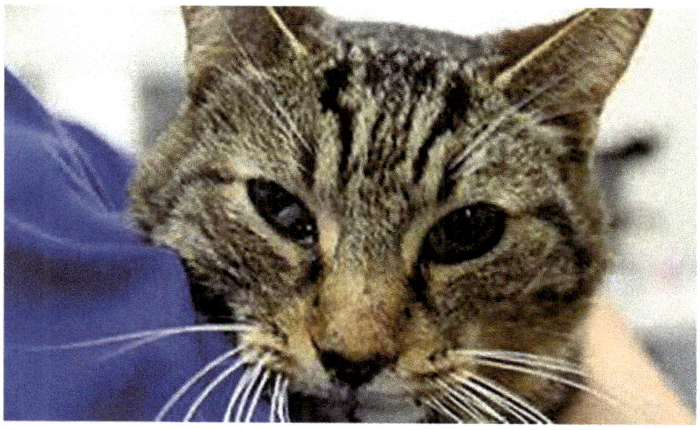

Figure 14. Horner's syndrome in a cat with dyspnoea. The presence of Horner's syndrome suggests interruption of the sympathetic supply to the facial muscles; this can be central or pre/post ganglionic. In this case the cat was dyspnoeic with a restrictive, inspiratory pattern suggesting pleural effusion. The concurrent Horner's syndrome raised a suspicion of involvement of the cranial mediastinum and imaging revealed mediastinal lymphoma.

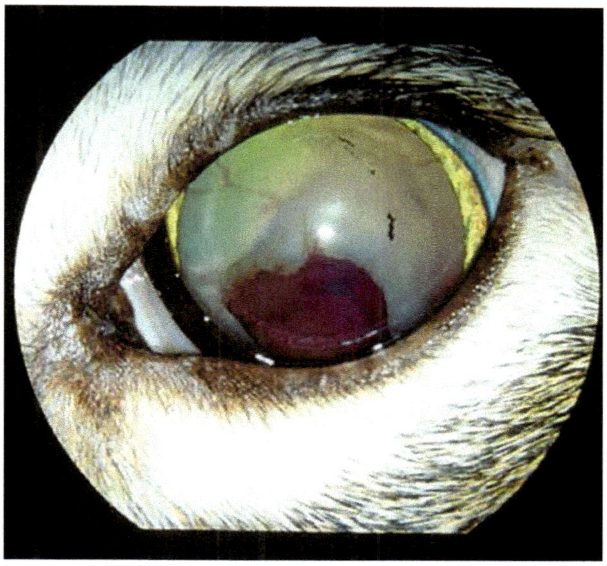

Figure 15. Hyphaema in a 12-year old cat with expiratory (restrictive) dyspnoea. Differentials for hyphaema include uveitis, traumatic injury, ocular neoplasia, retinal detachment or tearing (most often secondary to hypertension), clotting disorders, birth defects, and glaucoma. This cat also had expiratory restrictive dyspnoea, suggesting pulmonary parenchymal disease/pulmonary oedema. She was found to be hypertensive, with retinal detachment and congestive heart failure. (Image courtesy of Prof D Gunn-Moore).

The neck

Careful palpation of the neck, from the pharyngeal area to the thoracic inlet, assessing for pain, asymmetry, swelling or masses helps to localise the disease process e.g. detection of goitre raises a suspicion of hyperthyroidism. In addition, **the lymph nodes should be palpated**, and in cases where cardiac abnormalities are suspected, the extent and nature of **jugular filling** assessed. If upper respiratory tract disease is suspected, gentle palpation of the trachea should be performed.

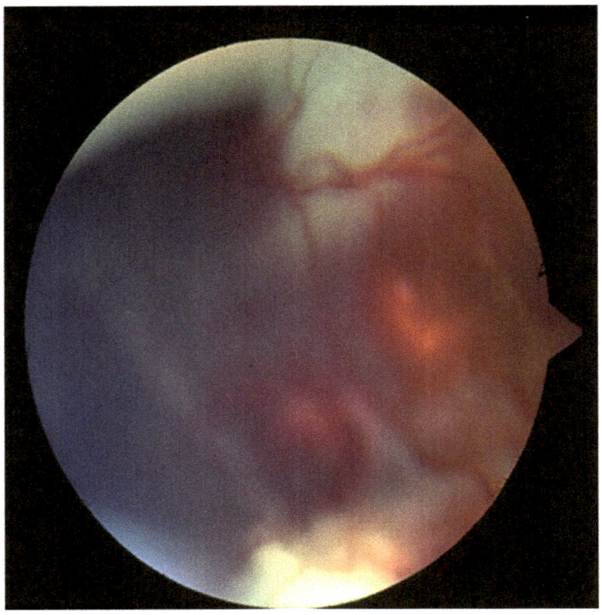

Figure 16. Retinal detachment in the cat described previously. The cat's systolic blood pressure was 310mmHg. She was therefore started on anti-hypertensive medications (amlodipine), alongside frusemide. Blood work was delayed until the hypertension had been sucessfully controlled for seven days (to avoid the risk of a catastrophic event at the time of blood sampling, decreasing BP is advisable to allow the central vasculature time to heal prior to any stressful events). (Image courtesy of Prof D Gunn-Moore).

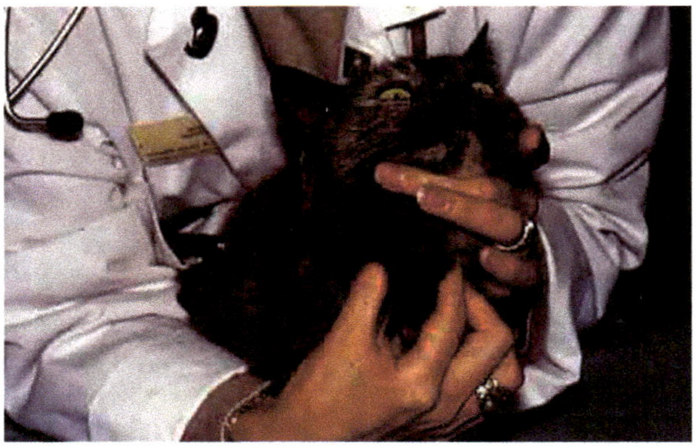

Figure 17. Cervical palpation. (Image courtesy of Prof D Gunn-Moore).

If the trachea is inflamed, a cough is easily elicited. In such instances, auscultation over the trachea often reveals harsh, stridor sounds.

Examination of the thoracic cavity

Thoracic palpation is performed to assess for trauma, congenital defects, to localize the apex beat, and check for the presence of a cardiac thrill. In severely asthmatic cats, the chronic exaggerated expiratory effort can lead to a barrel chested appearance accompanied by a **heave line** (due to the enhanced musculature).

Thoracic compression is useful to assess the residual volume within the thoracic cavity and compliance of the chest wall. This is decreased in cats with an excess of pleural fluid, soft tissue masses within the thoracic space, or air trapping (a feature of chronic obstructive pulmonary disease). Anterior thoracic compression may be decreased in cats with mediastinal masses. However, old cats can demonstrate a decreased compression of the thoracic cavity as a result of ossification of the costrochrondral cartilages.

Percussion assesses the resonance of the thoracic cavity, however, in cases of severe respiratory distress percussion may exacerbate clinical signs and should be performed with caution. Thoracic percussion can help to detect the presence of fluid or soft tissue within the thoracic cavity, resulting in a **decreased resonance** (fluid accumulation may lead to a linear delineation between areas of normal and decreased resonance). Unusual gaseous accumulations result in **increased resonance**, typically dorsally. In addition, thoracic percussion is particularly useful to determine the extent to which the thoracic cavity extends. This is typically increased in cats with chronic obstructive pulmonary disease and air trapping.

Thoracic auscultation identifies the presence of crackles, wheezes, harsh or dull lung sounds. Respiratory noise may be increased in LRT disease, referred from URT disease, or amplified due to air in the pleural space. Harsh lung sounds are pronounced bronchovesicular sounds and signify turbulent flow within the airways.

- **Crackles** are most commonly heard at end inspiration and usually represent air bubbling through fluid, therefore signifying the presence of alveolar fluid.
- **Harsh crackles** can result from the opening and closing of small airways in cats with bronchial disease.
- **Wheezes** are high pitched musical sounds or squeaks which result from the air moving through narrowed airways; these are most commonly heard in cats with bronchoconstriction, as is common in cats with asthma.
- **A decrease in respiratory noise** may indicate air, fluid or tissue within the pleural space.

Examination of the cardiovascular system

Meticulous examination of the cardiovascular system is necessary to differentiate between respiratory and cardiac causes of dyspnoea. However, it should be emphasised that severe cardiac disease can present with no abnormalities on cardiac auscultation; furthermore, primary respiratory disease can be accompanied by cardiac abnormalities.

Heart rate and rhythm should be evaluated. The position of the heart may be shifted if there is collapse of lung lobes, or if there is fluid or soft tissue within the thoracic cavity. It is useful to note whether the heart is in its usual position, or if the apex beat is shifted.

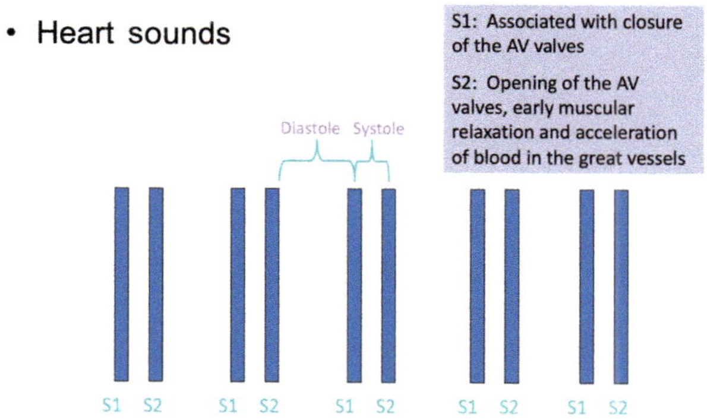

Figure 18. The intensity of the heart sounds should be assessed. In a normal cat, two heart sounds (lub-dub) should be audible. The heart sounds may be diminished in obese animals, but also decreased due to emphysema, pleural or pericardial disease, or when left ventricular contractility and cardiac output are decreased. In contrast the heart sounds are increased in thin or fit animals, or in hyperdynamic states (such as anaemia, pyrexia or hyperthyroidism).

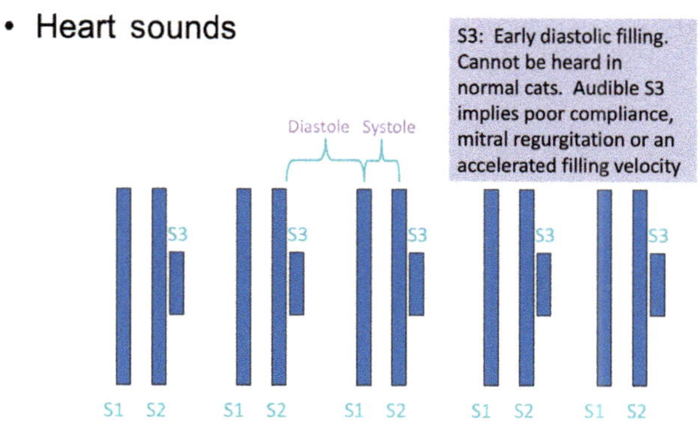

Figure 19. Extra heart sounds may be audible (gallop sounds). These occur due to intensification of either the third or fourth heart sound (or both). Gallop sounds often indicate advanced myocardial disease or heart failure. Rapid ventricular filling generates the third heart sound, the intensity is determined by the speed at which early ventricular filling occurs. An accentuated third heart sound is commonly associated with restrictive myocardial disease, or diastolic ventricular overfilling.

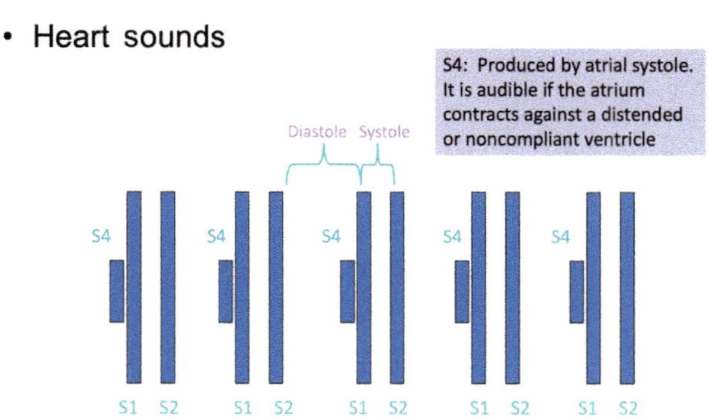

Figure 20. The fourth heart sound is produced by atrial systole and attenuated in conditions in which there is impaired ventricular relaxation, such a hypertension, hypertrophic cardiomyopathy (HCM) or hyperthyroidism.

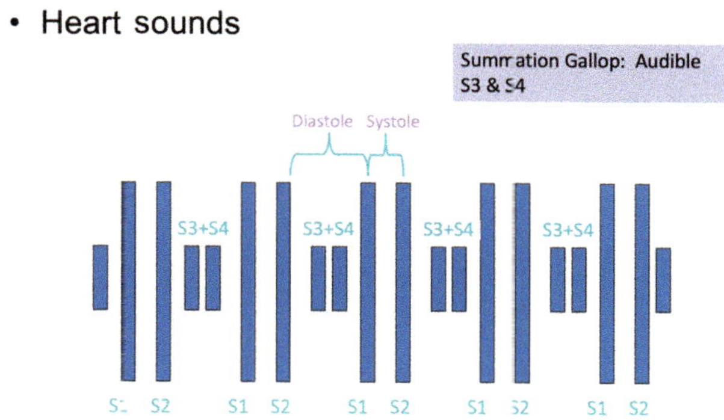

Figure 21. If both the third and fourth heart sounds are audible, a summation gallop may be audible.

Heart murmurs

Note the presence and character of any murmurs. Heart auscultation should include auscultation along the sternum, as murmurs are often heard here. If a murmur is auscultated, the **point of maximum intensity** should be localised, as this helps determine the anatomical structure from where the murmur is arising (while this is useful in the dog, it is of less use in the cats due to the close proximity of the valves in this species). The timing (systolic, diastolic, or both) and intensity of the murmur should be ascertained and a note made whether or not the murmur is dynamic (altering with alterations in heart rate) or static (Simpson, 2013).

- **Diastolic murmurs** are rare in the cat and are most commonly associated with congenital defects (for example, stenosis of the atrioventricular valves).
- **Continuous murmurs** are also rare in cats; again these are typically associated with congenital abnormalities (PDA or multiple congenital abnormalities).
- **Systolic murmurs** however, are frequently identified. Dynamic systolic murmurs are commonly associated

Murmur grade	Description
I	Audible in a localized area, only after prolonged listening with a stethoscope
II	Immediately audible; not as loud as the heart sounds
III	Immediately audible; of equal intensity to the heart sounds
IV	Immediately audible; louder than the heart sounds; no precordial thrill (palpable vibration evident over the heart)
V	Easily audible and associated with a precordial thrill; audible only when the stethoscope is held against the thoracic wall
VI	Easily audible with a precordial thrill; can be auscultated with the stethoscope lifted off the thoracic wall

with ventricular outflow obstruction (which may originate from either the left or right atrium). Unfortunately, the grade of the murmur often varies with heart rate and is therefore not a good representation of the extent of disease (Simpson, 2013).

Heart rhythm

The heart rhythm should be assessed. **Sinus arrhythmia is not a normal finding in the cat** (at least not in the clinical setting). The presence of sinus arrhythmia is suggestive of **increased vagal tone** and is most common with URT obstruction, although it can also be identified with cervical disease or trauma, and is not uncommon in abdominal diseases such as gastritis or pancreatic pathology. In addition, the **character and nature of the peripheral** pulses should be noted. If a cardiac arrhythmia is evident, the presence or absence of any pulse deficits can help to determine the cause of the arrhythmia, for example, there are often multiple pulse deficits in a cat with atrial fibrillation due to the variation in ventricular filling. If the peripheral pulses are weak, it is likely the cat has a reduced stroke volume, increased peripheral resistance, and narrow pulse pressure (the difference between the systolic and diastolic components). Common causes of this type of pulse include left ventricular failure and hypovolaemic shock.

General physical examination

Many intrathoracic diseases have systemic involvement and examination of the other body systems should not be overlooked in the cardiorespiratory patient. Furthermore, since severely dyspnoeic animals have a poor appetite, their **body condition score should always be evaluated**. Severe weight loss is suggestive of an advanced infectious process, neoplasia, systemic disease such as hyperthyroidism, or congestive heart failure.

The **musculoskeletal system** should be examined particularly looking for evidence of trauma or **thromboembolic disease**. Abdominal palpation may reveal a lack of contents in diaphragmatic or pericardiac, peritoneal, diaphragmatic hernias. In some forms of neoplasia abdominal masses or enlargement of the abdominal lymph nodes is apparent. The abdomen should be evaluated for the presence of free fluid, as may occur in FIP, right sided congestive heart failure, hypoproteinaemia, or neoplasia. Generalised or regional lymphadenopathy should be assessed for, as this may be associated with neoplasia or infection. If possible, the cat's temperature should be taken; hypothermia may indicate shock, whereas severe pyrexia may be the cause of tachypnoea, or result from of an infectious or painful process.

Management of the cat with acute upper respiratory tract disease

Acute upper respiratory tract disease in cats is typically infectious in origin, and makes up part of the **feline respiratory disease complex (FRDC).** This refers to the syndrome typified by a combination of rhinosinusitis, conjunctivitis, lacrimation, salivation, and oral ulcerations; a complex frequently referred to as Cat Flu. Due to the infectious origins of this complex, it is frequently seen in unvaccinated cats and kittens, particularly when kept in large groups, either in private homes, or rescue centres. Although viral and/or bacterial pathogens are crucial in the initiation of FRDC, it is complicated by a number of factors related to the environment (such as poor ventilation, high humidity and over-crowding) and host (with disease being more prevalent in kittens and immune suppressed individuals) (Cohn, 2011).

Clinical presentation

The presentation of a cat or kitten with FRDC is similar irrespective of the underlying infection. The severity of clinical signs is variable, with some cats demonstrating mild signs, whereas others are severely affected. Typically, depression, pyrexia and sneezing are the first clinical signs observed, followed by nasal discharge (serous, mucoid or mucopurulent); sneezing; conjunctivitis and ocular discharge; ulcerations of the lips, tongue, gums or nasal planum; salivation; coughing; fever; lethargy; and inappetence. Conjunctivitis can cause the eyelids to become sticky leading to closure, or keratitis and corneal ulceration. The nose may block leading to a total loss of olfaction and mouth breathing. Ulceration of the oral cavity leads to salivation and loss of appetite (Cohn, 2011).

Several **viral and bacterial pathogens** have been identified in cats with FRDC. These frequently occur in combination, with cats testing positive for one pathogen, with a second organism identified in 45.6–48% of cases. Studies demonstrate over 80% of cases are caused by infection with either feline calicivirus (FCV) or feline herpesvirus (FHV-1) (Gaskell et al., 2007, Radford et al., 2007). However, other potential primary pathogens include *Bordetella bronchiseptica* and *Chlamydophila felis* (formerly *Chlamydia psittaci*). In addition, a range of other bacteria and viruses can lead to FRDC, including reovirus, *Pasteurella* and rarely, *Streptococcus equi* subspecies *zooepidemicus* or cetrain influenza viruses (H5N1). Some Mycoplasma species are potentially normal commensal organisms of the upper respiratory tract, although some species may be pathogenic.

Whilst there are no pathognomic clinical signs for specific underlying causes, **the distribution of**

lesions can offer clues as to the aetiological agent. For example, severe oral ulceration is more likely to occur with FCV (although it can be seen in some cases of FHV-1, it tends not to be as severe). In addition, limping can be associated with FCV infection. Keratitis, corneal (dendritic) ulcers are more likely to be associated with FHV-1 infection, as is dermal ulceration. Coughing is seen less commonly and tends to be associated with *B. bronchiseptica*. *Chlamydophila felis* can be involved in respiratory disease, although it is typically regarded as a conjunctival pathogen, resulting in conjunctivitis.

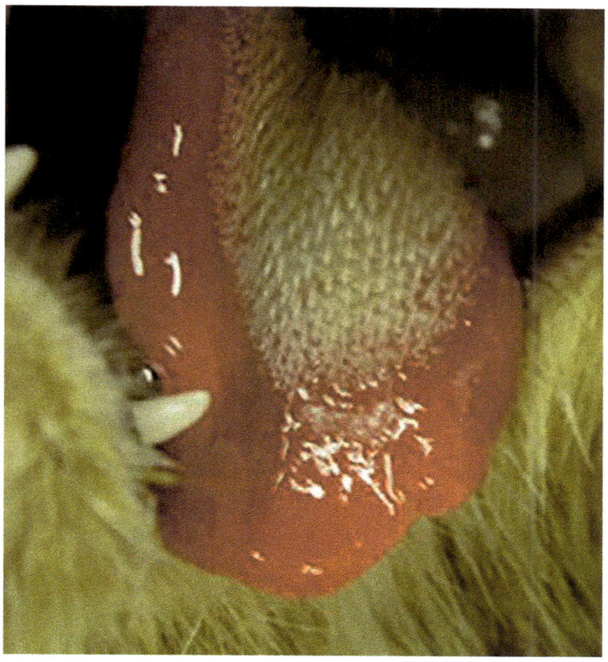

Figure 22. Calicivirus ulcer. Options: FHV-1, FCV, *Chlamydophila felis*.

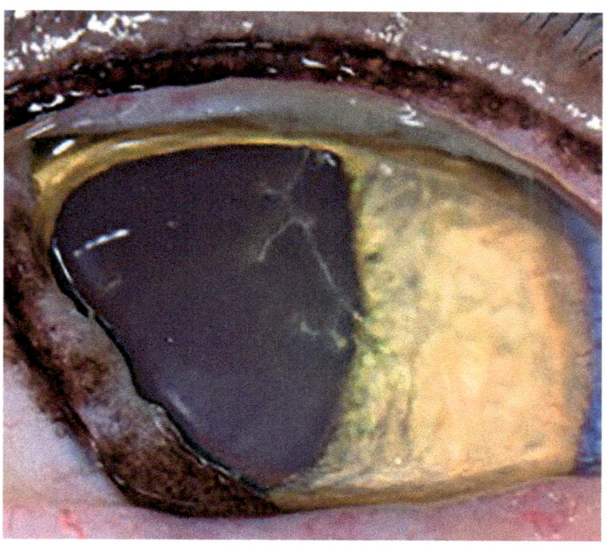

Figure 23. Dendritic ulcer. Options: FHV-1, FCV, *Bordetella bronchiseptica*. (Image courtesy of TAMU Ophthalmology).

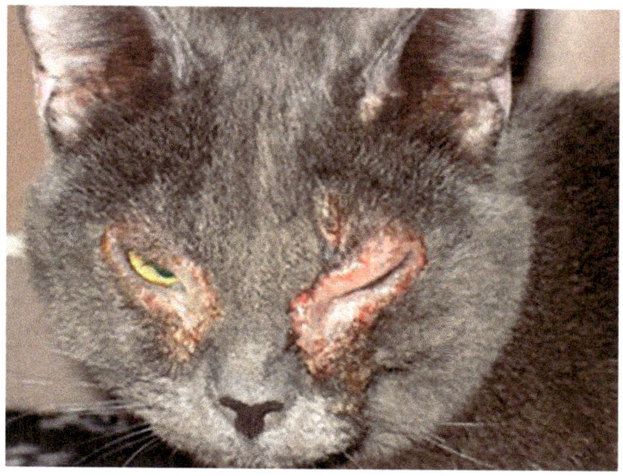

Figure 24. Herpes nose. Options: FHV-1, *Chlamydophila felis, Bordetella bronchiseptica.*

Feline calicivirus

FCV is a widespread, highly infectious pathogen of cats. The virus is a small, un-enveloped, single-stranded RNA virus. Being an RNA virus, FCV demonstrates a wide range of genomic plasticity, leading to a **large number of strains of FCV** which vary slightly in their antigenicity and pathogenicity. Because there are such a large number of strains, the clinical signs of FCV vary greatly; from oral ulceration and ocular-nasal discharge, to pneumonia, febrile limping-syndrome, and viral-systemic disease (see infectious disease) (Radford

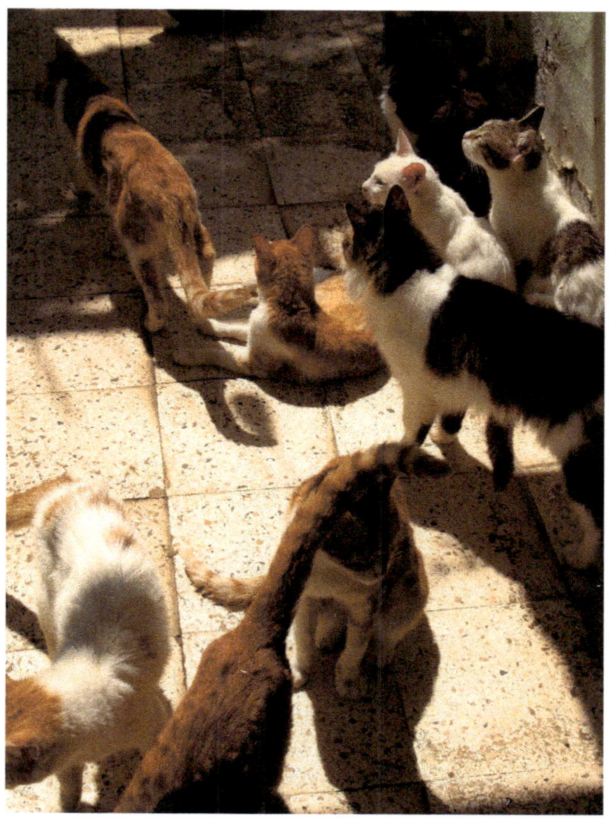

Figure 25. Rescue cats.

et al., 2009). In addition, FCV has been associated with feline oral disease (gingivostomatitis), although this has not been recreated experimentally, and therefore a causative role is debated.

FCV infection is widespread, with the prevalence being related to the number of cats within a household. Pet cats, living in single or small groups typically have a prevalence of around 10%, whereas cats in colonies or shelters often demonstrate a prevalence of 25–40% (although in some reports, up to 90% of cats have demonstrated exposure to the virus) (Radford et al., 2007).

Infection is spread directly by acutely infected cats and carrier cats, but indirect transmission also occurs as the virus persists on dry surfaces at room temperature for days to weeks, and longer in cooler, wet conditions (Radford et al., 2007).

Once exposed (via the oral, nasal or conjunctival mucus membranes), replication typically takes place within the oral and respiratory membranes, presenting as oral ulceration (often along the edges of the tongue), and upper respiratory tract infection. Most cats continue to shed the virus for at least one month after infection. However, some cats shed for significantly longer periods of time (Wardley and Povey, 1977).

Control of FCV is achieved predominantly via vaccination. Vaccination against FCV generally decreases the likelihood of developing significant oral/respiratory disease, however, it does not prevent infection or development of the carrier state (for more discussion on vaccination refer to the Infectious diseases chapter).

There are no specific treatment recommendations for FCV; antiviral treatments that have been trialled include feline interferon therapy (reported to demonstrate some efficacy in *in vitro* trials), but evidence for the efficacy of these treatments is weak, and in all but the most severe cases, treatment is typically cost prohibitive (Radford et al., 2009).

Feline herpesvirus

FHV-1 is a double stranded DNA virus, with a glycoprotein-lipid envelope. It is a relatively fragile virus, which **does not survive well in the external environment** (surviving only 18 hours in damp conditions, less if the environment is dry) (Gaskell et al., 2007). Unlike FCV, FHV-1 demonstrates little strain variation, with all strains belonging to one serotype (although minor differences between isolates do exist). The most important source of this virus is clinical cases, with shedding occurring as early as 24-hours after infection, and persisting for 1–4 weeks (Gaskell et al., 2007). However, most cats that recover from FHV-1 infection become **long-term latent carriers**, and can shed the virus intermittently, typically in response to stress, concurrent disease or following the use of corticosteroids (See figures 22, 23, 24).

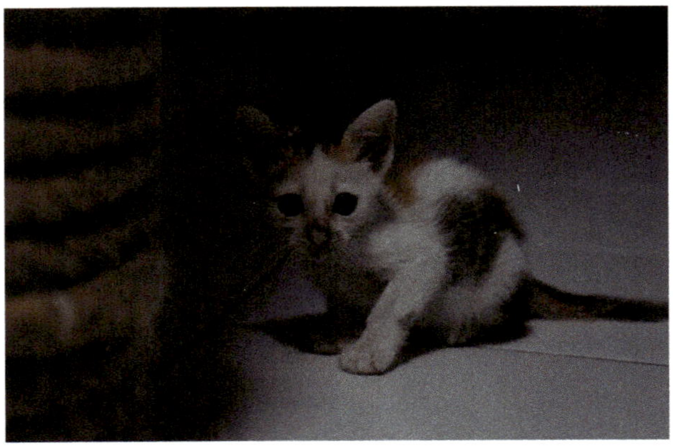

Figure 26. Kitten with herpesvirus.

Typically, cats are infected via the oral, nasal, or conjunctival mucous membranes. Following infection, the virus replicates predominantly within the mucosal surfaces of the nasal turbinates, septum, nasopharanyx, and tonsils; with replication favouring cooler areas such as the respiratory tract, systemic viraemia is rare. As the respiratory epithelium becomes infected, neutrophilic inflammation, multifocal epithelial necrosis and fibrin exudation occurs. Osteolytic changes can also occur within the nasal turbinates.

Clinical signs typically occur 2–6 days after infection; with depression, pyrexia, inappetance, and sneezing seen initially, followed by an ocular-nasal discharge. Ocular signs can be severe and often include conjunctivitis, sometimes with severe hyperaemia, chemosis, and ulcerative keratitis. Discharge gradually becomes mucopurulent and crusting of the external nares and eyelids can occur. In severe cases there is lower respiratory tract involvement, which can result in pneumonia (Thiry et al., 2009).

Although oral ulceration may be present with FHV-1 infection, it is relatively uncommon in comparison to FCV infection. In addition to acute upper respiratory tract disease, **FHV-1 infection can lead chronic ocular lesions** such as stromal keratitis, corneal sequestrae, eosinophilic keratitis, uveitis, and keratoconjuncitivitis sicca (Thiry et al., 2009). FHV-1 is known to cause ulcerative cutaneous lesions, including ulcerative facial and nasal dermatitis (Hargis and Ginn, 1999). A possible role for FHV-1 in chronic gingivostomatitis in cats has been suggested in one study as there was a relatively high viral isolation rate from cases compared to controls.

Vaccination against FHV-1 is generally effective; however, maternally derived antibodies can wane prior to vaccination. In group housed cats, infection can be common and stressors such as pregnancy or lactation can lead to recrudescence and increase shedding.

In many cases treatment of FHV-1 involves non-specific therapy to decrease congestion, maintain hydration and treat secondary infections. The anti-viral agent famciclovir has been shown to be effective in decreasing the morbidity in cats infected with FHV-1. Other treatments, such as L-lysine have been investigated, with variable outcomes (Thomasy and Maggs, 2016).

Chlamydophila felis

C. felis is an obligate intracellular bacterium, and therefore **cannot survive for long periods outside of the cell.** Transmission requires close contact between cats and is spread within ocular secretions (Gruffydd-Jones et al., 2009). For this reason, *C. felis* is most frequently seen in multicat households or at cat shows, and is particularly common in pedigree cats. The majority of cases are under one-year of age, with conjunctivitis being the most persistent clinical feature. In the first 1–2 days post infection, unilateral conjunctivitis may be present but this usually progresses to bilateral disease. Conjunctivitis can be severe, with marked chemosis, erythema of the nictitating membrane, blepharospasm, and ocular discomfort. Ocular discharge is initially serous, but later becomes mucoid, or mucopurulent. In some cases, ocular signs may be accompanied by pyrexia, inappetence, and mild respiratory signs.

Treatment of *C. felis* requires antibiotics, with systemic treatment being more efficacious than topical therapy. The treatment of choice is tetracycline, with **doxycycline preferred**, as it is safer in young kittens and administered once daily (Gruffydd-Jones et al., 2009). However, unless a liquid preparation is used, care should be taken to ensure that tablets are followed by food or water to prevent oesophagitis. There is a minimal risk of tooth discolouration with doxycycline. However, in cases that cannot tolerate this medication, fluoroquinolones can be used; or in very young kittens a four-week course of amoxycillin-clavulanate has been advised.

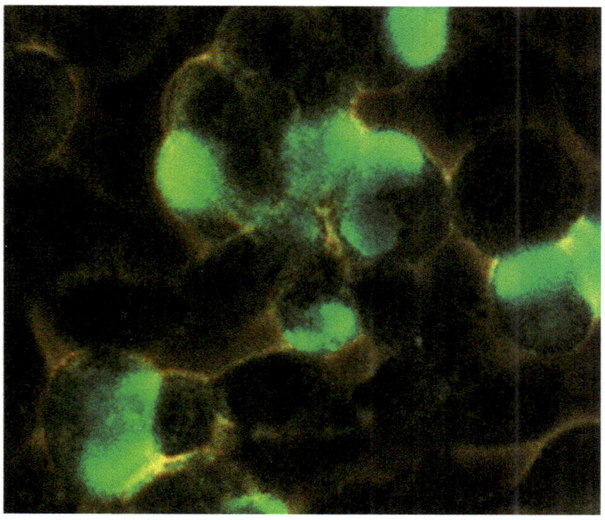

Figure 27. Indirect immunofluorescence in infected cell cultures is used as a serological test to titrate the antibodies against *Chlamydophila felis*. (Image courtesy of The Feline Centre, University of Bristol).

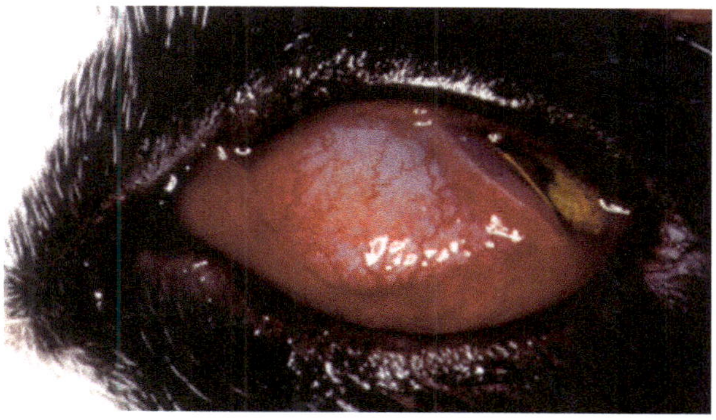

Figure 28. *C. felis* conjunctivitis. (Image courtesy of The Feline Centre, University of Bristol).

C. felis can be isolated from the conjunctiva of cats until approximately two months post infection. However, some cats become persistently infected, with organisms being isolated as long as 215 days post infection. Therefore, in cats at high risk (i.e. in households with known *C. felis* infection) vaccination is advised. The available vaccines have been demonstrated to prevent disease (although not infection itself), and can be administered in addition to the core vaccines. The initial vaccination guidelines are for two vaccines at 8–10 weeks, and then 3–4 weeks later, with annual boosters.

Bordetella bronchiseptica

B. bronchiseptica is a Gram-negative coccobacillus which acts as a respiratory pathogen in a number of species, including rabbits, pigs, dogs (where it is one of the causes of kennel cough), cats and humans (particularly when immuno-compromised). It can cross-infect species and has **potential zoonotic risk** (Egberink et al., 2009).

Infection with *B. bronchiseptica* is associated with over-crowding and poor hygiene. Studies demonstrate the seroprevalence amongst cats in shelter environments is 41–61%. Furthermore, in a study of pathogens associated with respiratory disease in multicat households, *B. bronchiseptica* was detected in 5% of samples, whereas it was only detected in 1.3% of households without respiratory disease (Egberink et al., 2009).

The pathogenesis of *B. bronchiseptica* has not been studied widely in the cat and is extrapolated from other species, particularly the dog. The bacterium can be spread as an aerosol but also survives relatively long periods in the environment, therefore indirect transmission is also likely to occur. After infection, the bacterium colonises the ciliary epithelium of the respiratory tract and is thought to produce toxins which cause ciliostasis and destruction of the cilia (Speakman et al., 1999).

Clinical signs typically last approximately 10 days and consist of pyrexia, cough, sneezing, ocular discharge, and lymphadenopathy. However, in some cases signs may last longer, or involve the lower respiratory tract, leading to pneumonia (Egberink et al., 2009).

Treatment with antibiotics is recommended in infected cats due to the propensity for colonisation of the lower respiratory tract. Ideally, this is based on culture and sensitivity. However, if this is not available, the recommended treatment is doxycycline, as it is suspected that feline isolates are often resistant to amoxycillin clavulanate, and ampicillin (Egberink et al., 2009).

Improved hygiene is recommended in establishments with a high incidence of disease. *B. bronchiseptica* is killed by most common/readily available disinfectants. In many countries a vaccine against *B. bronchiseptica* is available. This is not a core vaccine and is only advised for high risk cases (i.e. those living in environments with known *B. bronchiseptica* infection), or those in high density populations.

Diagnosis

A presumptive diagnosis is based on the presence of typical clinical signs and a history of possible exposure to causal organisms. While different organisms tend to produce characteristic clinical signs in the laboratory setting, in mixed natural infections it is not possible to determine which organisms are involved from clinical signs alone (Cohn, 2011).

Nasal or oropharyngeal swabs can be taken for isolation and culture or PCR. Care is required when interpreting the results since FHV-1 is shed only intermittently, whilst both pathogenic or non-pathogenic field strains of virus cause FCV shedding. PCR may be positive in cases where the infection is present but not the cause of the clinical signs. Bacteriology is generally of little value unless the laboratory is instructed to look for specific agents (e.g. *B. bronchiseptica, Mycoplasma spp.*, or *C. felis*). It is advisable to speak to the laboratory prior to collecting samples, since specific transport media may be required. Some studies have suggested culture of *B. bronchiseptica* is more sensitive than PCR (Egberink et al., 2009, Gruffydd-Jones et al., 2009, Radford et al., 2009, Thiry et al., 2009).

Serology helps determine whether a cat has been exposed to FCV or FHV-1. However, it is of limited value since many cats have been vaccinated. A rising titre against *C. felis* may be detected in unvaccinated cats.

C. felis may be detected as intranuclear inclusion bodies in Giemsa-stained conjunctival smears around seven days post infection. However, the recommended test for *C. felis* is PCR of a conjunctival swab.

Treatment

Antibiotics

Where specific organisms are detected (i.e. *C. felis*), antibiotic selection is based on culture and sensitivity. If not, a safe broad-spectrum antibiotic (e.g amoxycillin-clavulanic acid or a cephalosporin) active against bacteria commonly found in the feline oropharynx should be given for two to three weeks. Since affected cats typically find swallowing painful, syrups or parenteral administration (where available) are preferable to tablets or capsules.

Where *B. bronchiseptica, Mycoplasma spp.* or *C. felis* have been detected, doxycycline should be given at 10 mg/kg/day or oxytetracycline at 20 mg/kg q8h, plus an ophthalmic tetracycline ointment. Oral tetracycline should not be used in kittens, as it discolours the teeth, instead **doxycline** is preferred as it carries a reduced risk of this occurring.

Nutritional, fluid support, and nursing

This often involves **intravenous fluids and placing a feeding tube**. Oesophageal feeding tubes are preferred,

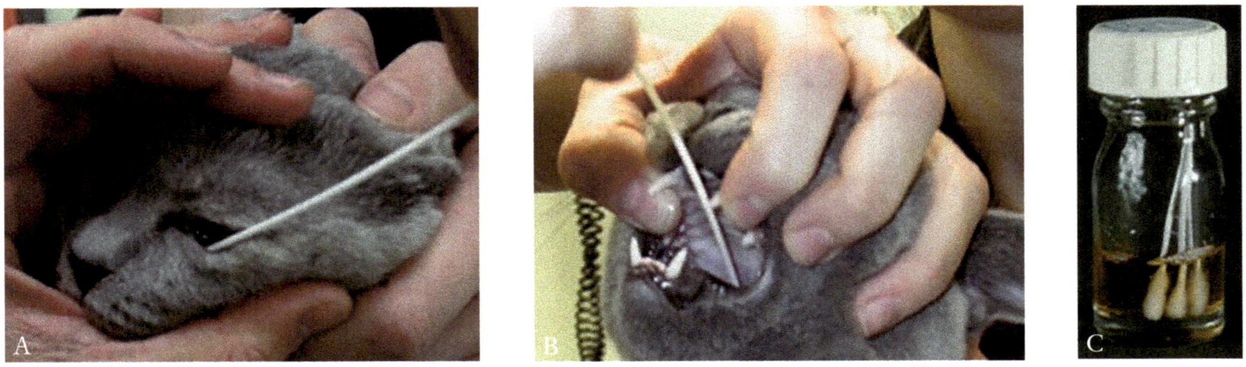

Figure 29. Conjunctive viral swab (A), oral viral swab (B), swab in TM (C). (Images courtesy of Danielle Gunn Moore).

as inflammation of the nasal turbinates makes naso-oesophageal tubes uncomfortable. Cats should be encouraged to eat by offering warmed, tempting foods. Appetite stimulants such as mirtazapine are useful in some cases.

- **Supportive nursing care** – it is important to keep the cat's eyes and nose clean, and coat groomed.
- **Multivitamins** – anorexia can result in a lack of certain vitamins, especially B12, which exacerbates anorexia, therefore, supplementation can be beneficial.
- **Ocular anti-inflammatory drugs** – for use when ocular signs cause significant pain and/or inflammation. However, they can slow the healing of corneal ulcers.
- **Nebulisation** – steam or nebulised water help clear mucus and hydrate the airway (nebulisation of antibiotics/disinfectant solutions is not recommended).

Antivirals

For FHV-1 infection the use of antivirals such as famciclovir can decrease morbidity. In severe cases, oral high dose L-lysine may be added to reduce clinical signs.

Interferon: while many non-specific immune stimulants are currently available, few have proven efficacy and safety.

Corticosteroids are not usually indicated.

Prevention and control

To reduce respiratory disease within a group of cats, it is necessary to address both infectious and non-infectious causes. This involves instigating a suitable vaccination and/or isolation programme, treatment with appropriate antibacterial agents, improved ventilation, and reduced over-crowding.

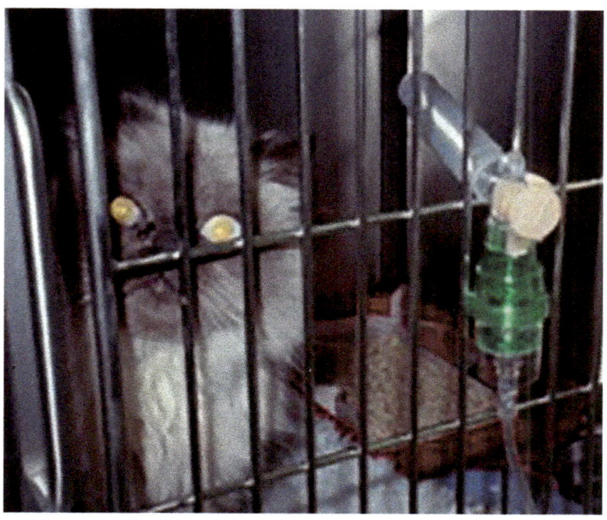

Figure 30. Nebulization in a cat.

Management of the cat with nasal discharge

The nasal cavity provides a portal through which air flows to the lungs. It regulates and filters the air flow, helps determine the heat and water saturation of the inspired air, as well as performing complex motor tasks such as sniffing and smelling.

The nasal cavity is comprised of bony and cartilaginous parts and divided into left and right by the nasal septum. In turn each half of the nasal cavity is divided into four air passages, the dorsal, middle, ventral and common meati. The dorsal, middle and ventral meati are divided by the dorsal nasal concha. Associated with the nasal cavity are the frontal, maxillary, and sphenoidal sinuses.

- **Nasal discharge**: the nature and origin of any nasal discharge is helpful in determining the type and extent of disease (Table 1). Discharge can result from local disease processes or be a sign of extranasal diseases. In addition, the presence of unilateral or bilateral discharge and whether or not the airways are patent, help further differentiate between disease types.
- **Sneezing**: sneezing is a protective reflex which expels foreign particles from the nasal cavity. This manifests as an explosive expiration of airflow from the nasal cavity; any cause of nasal mucosal irritation or nasal discharge can result in sneezing.
- **Reverse sneezing**: Reverse sneezing is a reflex in which powerful contraction of the inspiratory muscles and adduction of the laryngeal cartilages generates a negative tracheal and pleural pressure. A strong tracheal occlusion pressure with a sudden opening of the glottis produces a rapid inspiratory airflow. This rapid inhalation is thought to dislodge irritant particles from the nasal cavity and deposit them in the oropharynx, where they are eliminated by swallowing. It is thought that post inspiratory glottal narrowing and coughing prevent aspiration into the lower airways. The presence of reverse sneezing suggests a problem located within the nasopharynx.

Differential diagnosis: nasal discharge/sneezing

- Infectious
  - viral
    - feline upper respiratory tract infection complex
      - feline herpes virus (FHV-1)
      - feline calicivirus (FCV)
  - bacterial infections

Table 1. Types of discharge.

	Serous	Mucoid	Purulent	Mucopurulent	Sanguineous	Epistaxis
Properties	Clear, acellular discharge	Clear acellular discharge with a high protein content	Opaque, viscous, pale yellow to green. Containing neutrophils and bacteria	A mixture of mucoid and purulent discharges, bacteria are variably seen	Blood mixed with another type of discharge	Predominantly RBC's
Common causes	Increased lacrimation or URT disease	Chronic non-infectious nasal disease	Failure of mucocilliary clearance to oppose bacterial colonisation. May be due to intra- or extranasal causes	Chronic nasal disease with a bacterial component or necrotic focus	Damage to the nasal mucosa	Intranasal disease ie: neoplasia, or extranasal disease, trauma, coagulopathy or hypertension
Location	Uni- or bilateral	Typically bilateral	May be unilateral if due to a foreign body, or bilateral with other causes	Uni- or bilateral	Dependent on the mixed component	Uni- or bilateral

- secondary infection, i.e.: invasion from oropharynx, secondary to anatomical defects, foreign bodies, neoplasia, trauma or immune suppression
- *Bordetella bronchoseptica*
- infection with *Mycoplasmal species*
- mycotic
  - *Cryptococcus neoformans*
- inflammatory
  - post-viral rhinitis / chronic idiopathic rhinitis
  - allergic rhinitis
  - nasopharyngeal or nasonasal polyps
  - nasopharyngeal stenosis
- neoplastic
  - lymphoma
  - adenocarcinoma
  - undifferentiated carcinoma
  - others ie: chondrosarcoma, fibrosarcoma, osteosarcoma
- oral disease
  - palatine defects
  - periapical infections of the upper teeth
  - tooth root abscessation
- trauma
- foreign body
- congenital defects
- epistaxis
  - local disease
    - infectious (especially mycotic infections)
    - neoplasia
    - foreign bodies
    - trauma (including trauma from sneezing)
- systemic disease
  - coagulopathies
  - systemic hypertension
  - vasculitis
  - hyperviscosity syndrome
  - polycythaemia
  - multiple myeloma
  - thrombocytopaenia
  - thrombocytopathia.

Diagnosis

A thorough history and physical examination helps exclude some potential differentials. It is important to rule out systemic causes prior to continuing with a nasal work-up. Where appropriate blood pressure should be assessed (e.g. if hypertensive epistaxis is suspected). Routine haematology (including a manual platelet count), biochemistry, a coagulation profile, and FeLV / FIV status should be assessed where appropriate. In addition, in cases suspected of viral infection (FHV-1 or FCV), swabs taken from the oropharynx should be sent in special transport media for analysis. In cases of suspected bacterial or mycotic infection, swabs should be taken and submitted for culture.

Radiography

Radiographical evaluation is performed under anaesthesia, in order to obtain good quality images. Evaluation includes assessment of the symmetry, bone and turbinate definition, variations in opacity and soft tissue changes. However, interpretation of the radiographic anatomy of the nasal cavity can prove difficult due to superimposition of surrounding structures, the

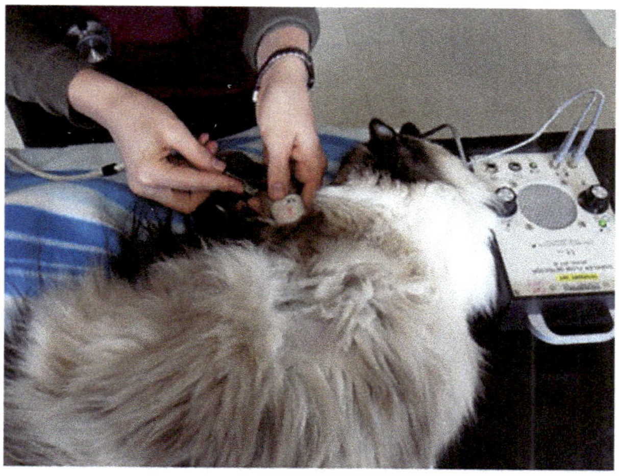

Figure 31. Blood pressure measurement.

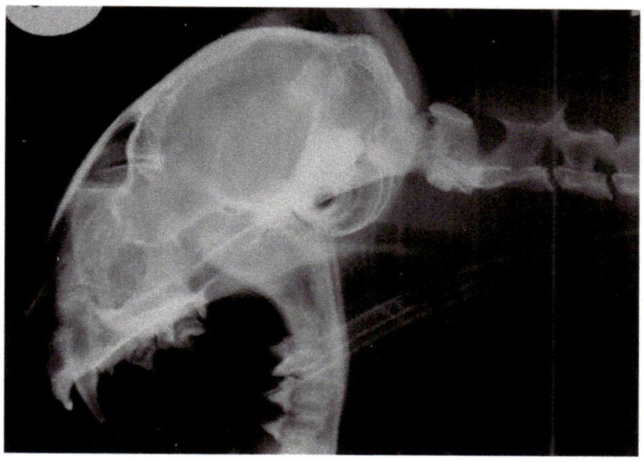

Figure 32. Lateral skull radiography. Superimposition of the teeth and turbinates make lateral radiographs hard to interpret.

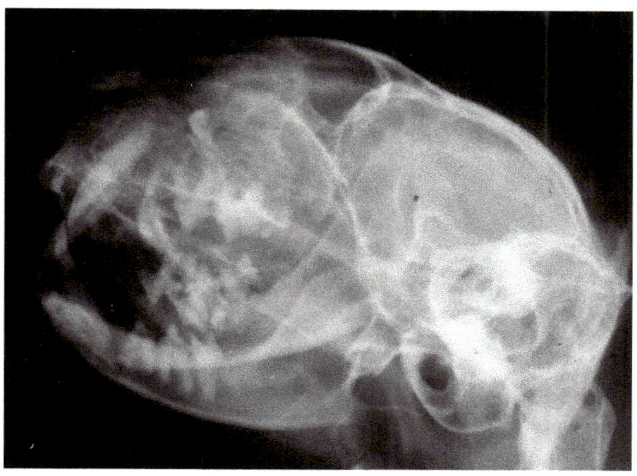

Figure 33. Lateral oblique skull radiography. Taking a lateral oblique radiograph at a 45-degree angle allows better visualisation of the tooth roots and bullae.

intricate nasal anatomy and the wide variation in the normal appearance of the skull.

The intra-oral radiograph is useful for assessment of the nasal turbinates. However, its helpfulness is limited in that it **cannot differentiate soft tissue and fluid.** The image provided demonstrates increased opacity

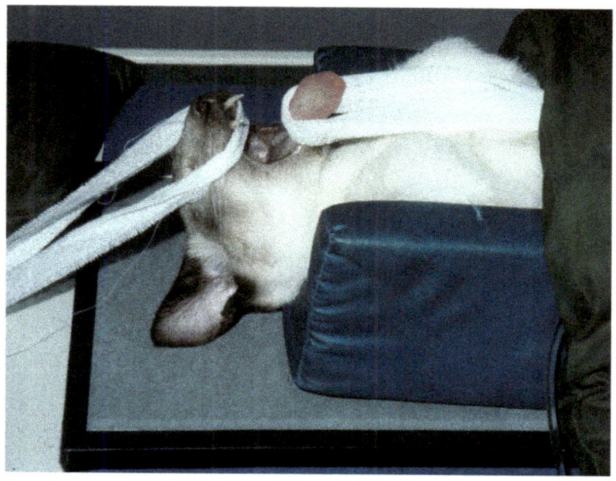

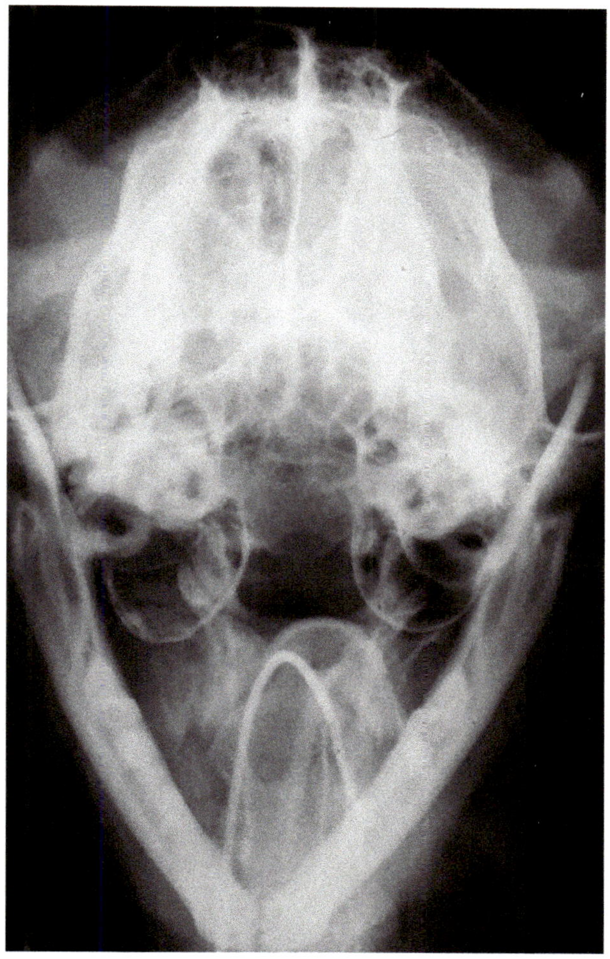

Figure 34. The open mouth view can be used to assess the frontal sinuses and bullae.

and lack of turbinate detail within the left side of the nasal cavity; but this may be due to fluid (i.e. mucus accumulation) or soft tissue inflammation/neoplasia.

Computed tomography

Computed tomography (CT) provides a higher resolution and is more sensitive than radiography. Whilst CT provides better resolution of areas such as the

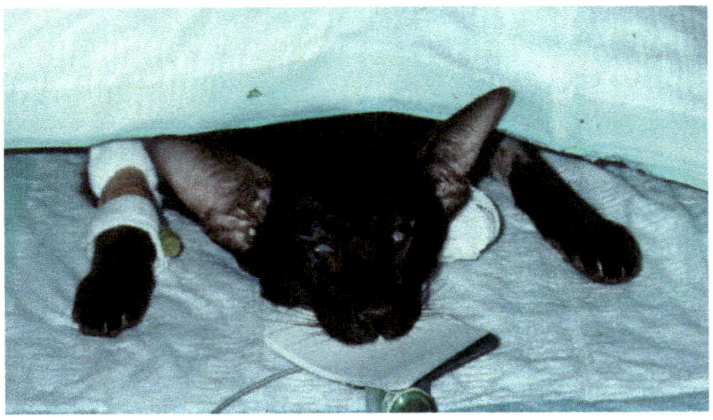

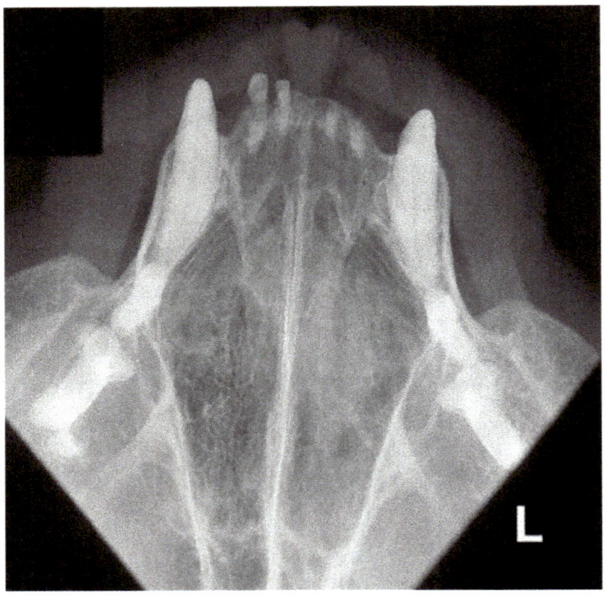

Figure 35. Intraoral and rhinitis radiography. (Images courtesy of Prof D Gunn-Moore).

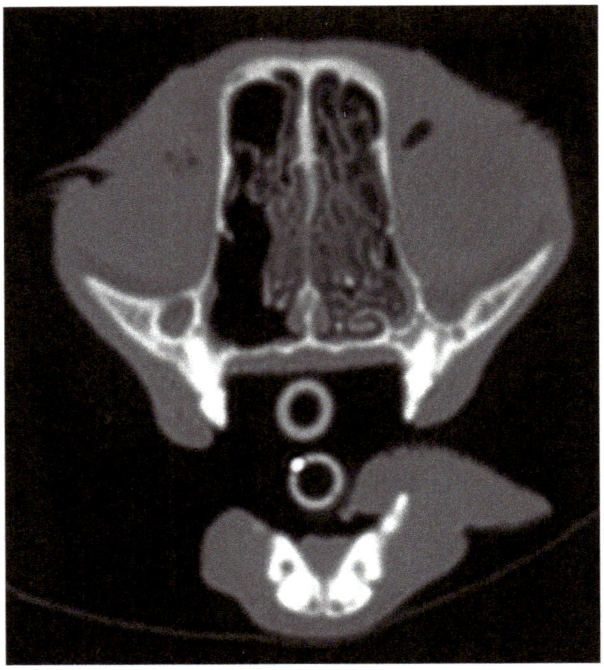

Figure 36. CT is excellent at highlighting areas of turbinate loss (which can occur in infection, rhinitis or neoplasia), identifying nasal masses, and allowing assessment of the paranasal structures (such as the sinuses and bullae). However, in order to obtain a definitive diagnosis biopsy is required.

cribriform plate, which is useful for the early detection of soft tissue masses, however epistaxis, and nasal discharge can be hard to differentiate from soft tissue opacities.

Swabs

If samples have not already been submitted for viral/bacterial infectious disease assessment, oropharyngeal swabs should be taken prior to any possible iatrogenic haemorrhage. Typically, samples are submitted for FHV-1, and FCV virus isolation +/- PCR, culture, and mycoplasma PCR, although other diseases might be considered dependant on the clinical signs. Nasal swabs for culture taken by swabbing the nasal discharge, are of minimal benefit, with most samples demonstrating commensal bacteria of the oropharynx.

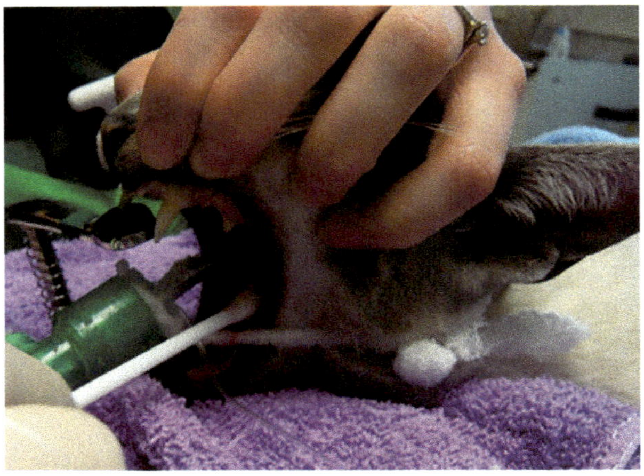

Figure 37. Oropharyngeal swab.

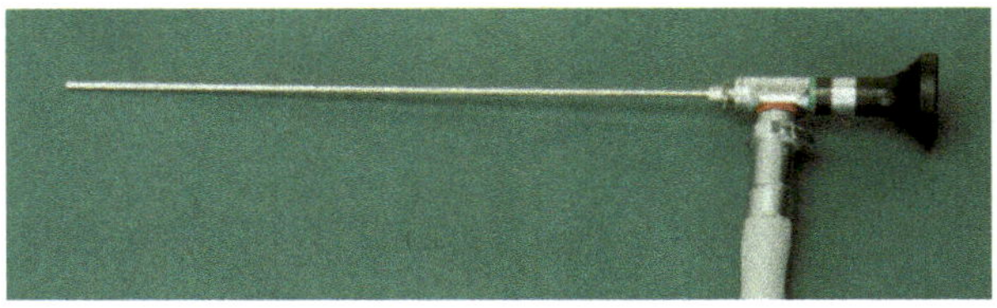

Figure 38. Rhinoscope.

Rhinoscopy

Rhinoscopy and pharyngoscopy are useful techniques which **allow the direct visualization of lesions**, biopsy of samples under guidance, and identification/removal of foreign bodies. If a flexible bronchoscope is available pharyngoscopy should be performed first. The scope is inserted into the pharynx, retroflexed and gently advanced in a rostral direction until the caudal nasopharynx is visualised.

Prior to rostrocaudal evaluation, the pharynx should be packed and a rolled towel placed under the cranial thorax to ensure a downward slope to the nasal cavity. **This encourages blood flow out of the nose, and not into the airway.**

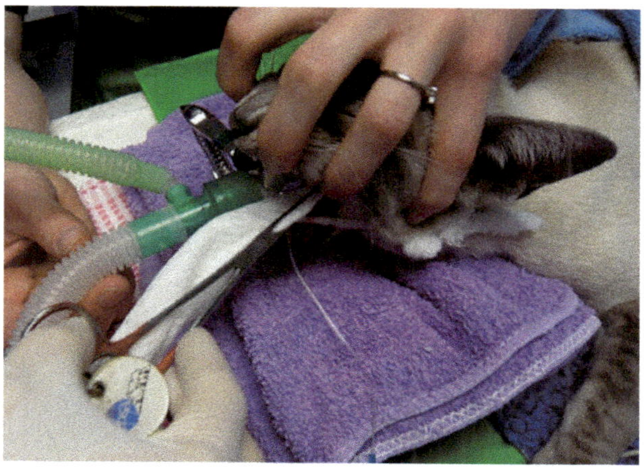

Figure 39. Packing pharynx.

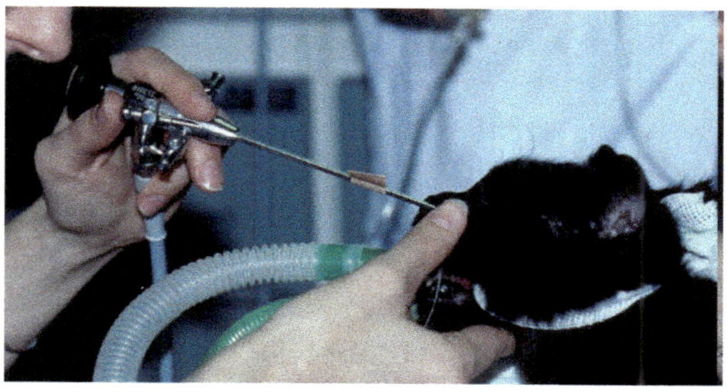

Figure 40. Rhinoscopy. The distance from the medial canthus of the eye to the tip of the nose should be measured against the rhinoscope and marked with a piece of tape. This is the furthest distance that the scope should be advanced to avoid penetrating the cribiform plate. (Image courtesy of Prof D Gunn-Moore).

Rhinoscopic examination requires assessment of both lateral and medial aspects of the nasal cavity, on both the left- and right-hand side. If mucus is present, saline flushed down the scope aids visualisation. Small biopsies of localised lesions can be taken via the scope. However, immediately after the view is obliterated and therefore if there are no localised lesions noted, typically blind biopsies are performed.

If other diagnostic approaches have failed or a foreign body cannot be removed by alternative methods, a **rhinotomy may be required**. However, complications post-rhinotomy include persistent epistaxis and chronic nasal discharge.

Care is required as the cat recovers from anaesthesia. Cats rarely mouth breath and complete **obstruction of the nasal cavity** (due to haemorrhage, soft tissue or inflammation) **can lead to apnoea.** In cases where the nasal mucosa is highly reactive, an anti-inflammatory dose of dexamethasone may be indicated.

Treatment

Treatment of nasal discharge is based on **identifying and treating the underlying condition**. Investigations

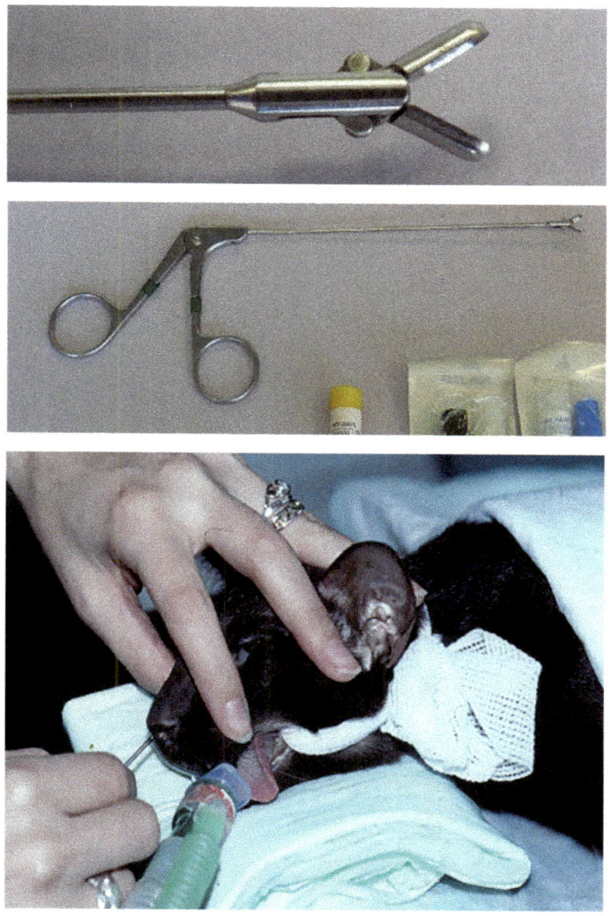

Figure 41. Biopsy tool. Diagnosis of many nasal disorders requires a tissue biopsy. Biopsies can be collected using small biopsy forceps or a rigid tube with suction applied. Again, these techniques require care not to penetrate the cribriform plate: the medial canthus of the eye is generally considered the maximum distance to enter the nasal cavity. Biopsies should be submitted for cytology and culture. Unfortunately, the size of the biopsy is limited, and obtaining deep samples can be problematic. Histopathologic changes should be interpreted alongside imaging and gross findings.

may identify an obvious cause such as a foreign body or nasopharyngeal polyp which can be removed. In other cases, a more chronic disease process is identified.

Clinical presentations

Chronic rhinitis

Feline chronic rhinitis is a condition commonly seen in feline practice. However, it is not well understood and can be frustrating to manage.

In reality, **chronic rhinitis is likely a group of diseases, with various proposed aetiologies**. In some cases, it seems likely the inflammation is related to **post viral infection**, particularly with FHV-1 as turbinate necrosis is a part of the disease pathogenesis. In many cases **bacterial infection** is identified. However, these are frequently commensal bacteria, and therefore, unless there is a pure, profuse growth of a single

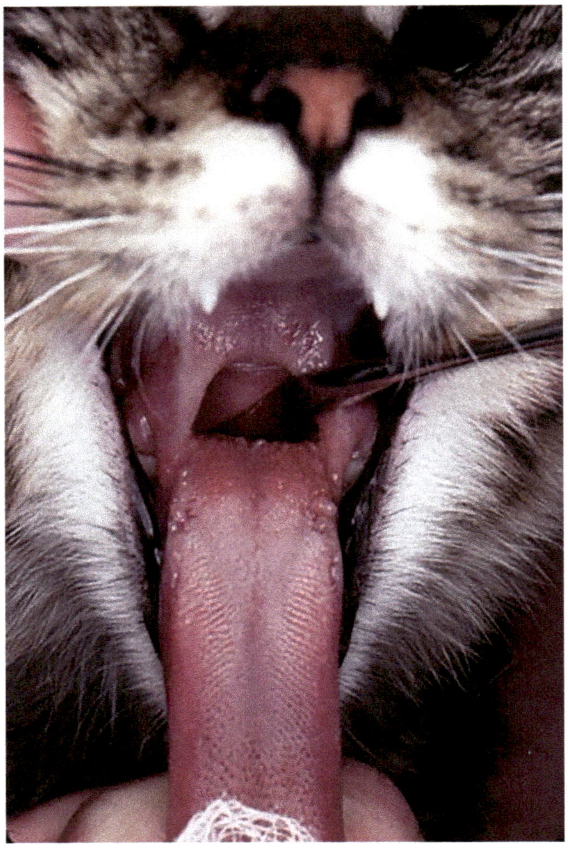

Figure 42. In cases where rhinoscopy is not performed, the clinician should carefully retract the soft palate to ensure there are no foreign bodies, tumours, or polyps within the caudal nasopharynx. A large polyp is observed in the image; this can be removed with gentle retraction. The small stalk is easily dislodged with minimal bleeding.

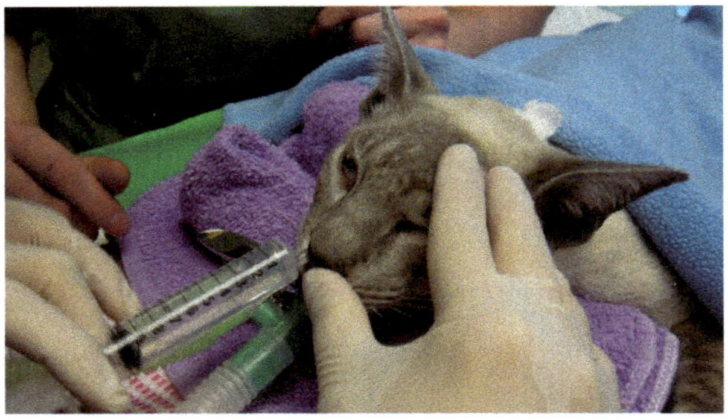

Figure 43. If a large intranasal growth or foreign body is present, a forced flush technique can prove useful. This is performed by placing a collection vessel in the oropharynx and forcibly injecting 5 ml of saline into the nares (this should not be performed if the integrity of the cribriform plate is in question). (Image courtesy of Prof D Gunn-Moore).

organism, in the majority of cases these are secondary or of limited significance. The role of *Mycoplasma* spp. in rhinitis remains unclear. These organisms were considered to be part of the commensal flora in the upper respiratory tract. However, in some studies *Mycoplasma* spp. have been detected in cats affected by chronic rhinitis, but not in control cats, suggesting that they may play a role in this disease complex. Currently, a potential role of *Tritrichomonas foetus* is also being investigated (Reed, 2020).

The role of allergens has not been extensively investigated in cats, despite this being a common cause of rhinitis in people.

Treatment

Many different treatments are suggested for chronic rhinitis, with a highly variable response to treatment.

- **Antibiotics/antivirals**: if an underlying bacterial or viral infection is identified, this should be treated accordingly. In addition, broad spectrum antibiotic cover may be beneficial in cases with secondary bacterial infection.
- **Improving air flow**: often cases demonstrate a significant improvement immediately after nasal work-up, as a part of this process involves nasal flushing. In cases that improve markedly after assessment, periodic nasal flushing may provide clinical relief by removing this mucopurulent material.
- **Nebulization** (Figure 30): theoretically nebulization dilutes viscous secretions and promotes ciliary clearance. Although there are no studies assessing the benefit of nebulisation in cats, the author does advocate its use. If a nebuliser is not available, sitting with the cat in a steam filled room for 20 minutes up to three times daily may be of benefit. Any potential benefit of mucolytics and decongestants has not been assessed in cats.
- **Immune modulation**: glucocorticoids are frequently used in chronic rhinitis, although there are no studies assessing the response to treatment. If viral and bacterial infection have been ruled out, then the anti-inflammatory and immunomodulatory effects of glucocorticoids may be beneficial. Administration can be via the oral route or by inhalation (Reed, 2020). Whilst the author prefers the latter route, it is advisable that any mucus build-up has been cleared first (e.g. by nasal flushing or nebulization) for the drug to contact the nasal mucosa. Then the medication is administered in the same way as it is to an asthmatic cat.
- **Other medications** such as NSAIDs and antihistamines have been proposed by some. NSAIDs should not be given at the same time as glucocorticoids. There is no evidence that NSAIDs are beneficial in the treatment of chronic rhinitis, but anecdotal reports from many practitioners do report improvements with meloxicam administration. In cases where an allergic component is suspected antihistamines may be of benefit, but there is limited information in the literature on the use of these medications. In some cases, with marked eosinophilic

inflammation, the author has trialled a hydrolysed diet, with mixed success.

Chronic rhinitis is rarely cured and management can be frustrating as there are several potential therapies, all with limited evidence of benefit.

Fungal rhinitis

Nasal aspergillosis is rare in the cat, although in the past decade infection has been identified with increased frequency. There are two different forms of disease; sinonasal aspergillosis (SNA) and sinoorbital aspergillosis (SOA), with SOA being the most common form, accounting for 65% of cases (Barrs, 2020).

The major differentials are neoplasia and foreign body, however, both conditions may predispose to secondary fungal infection. Typically cats with fungal rhinitis have involvement of the sinuses and infiltration into the retrobulbar space.

Clinical signs

In cases of SNA, a mucopurulent nasal discharge which may be uni or bilateral (with or without blood); sneezing, nasal pain, inappetence, and lethargy are frequently identified, making it hard to differentiate from chronic rhinitis, neoplasia, or a foreign body. Cases of SOA may also have these signs, but are often presented for clinical signs associated with an invasive retrobulbar fungal granuloma.

Diagnosis

Definitive diagnosis requires identification of fungal hyphae on cytology or histopathology. In addition, culture testing should be performed and where possible the organism typed.

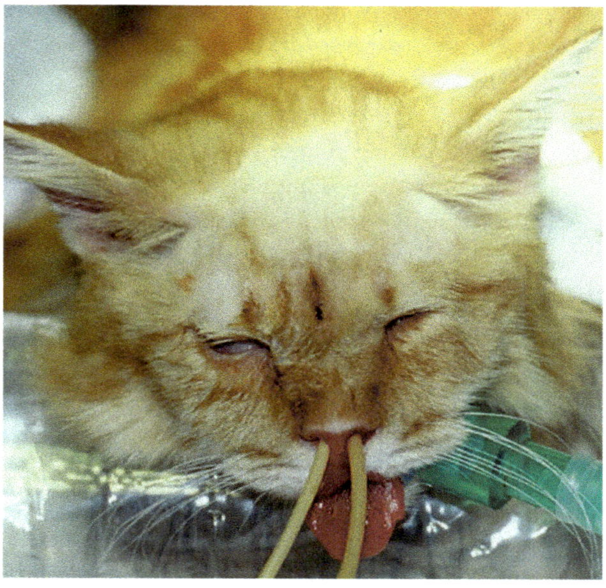

Figure 44. Cat undergoing treatment for aspergillosis. (Image courtesy of Prof D Gunn-Moore).

Treatment

SNA has a better response to therapy, and treatment is similar to aspergillosis treatment in canines. Therefore, prior to therapy, it is advisable to perform CT to rule out SOA, assess the integrity of the cribriform plate, and biopsy to establish if the fungal disease is invasive. Ideally the fungal isolate and its antifungal susceptibility is determined prior to starting therapy. After this, endoscopic debridement of the fungal plaques/lesions from the nasal cavity and frontal sinuses is performed.

For non-invasive infections, an intranasal infusion of 1% clotrimazole in polyethylene glycol is instilled into the nasal cavity for a one hour soak under general anaesthesia. During this time the head is tilted downward to allow drainage. For invasive infections and/or if *Aspergillus felis* is identified, the use of additional systemic antifungal therapy is warranted.

For SOA the prognosis is guarded, with few cases responding to treatment. In addition to the treatment above, systemic antifungals should be administered, the choice dictated by susceptibility testing. Prior to receiving these results, administration of empirical oral posaconazole monotherapy is advisable. This medication is generally well tolerated in cats, but monitoring of the case, and frequent assessment of the liver parameters is advised (Barrs, 2020).

Neoplasia of the nasal cavity

Nasal tumours are predominantly malignant and may extend into the frontal and paranasal sinuses. The most common neoplasm within the feline nasal cavity is nasal lymphoma. However, carcinoma, and sarcoma are not infrequent. (Neoplasia of the respiratory tract is discussed later in this chapter.)

Feline lower respiratory tract disease

Cats with lower respiratory tract disease typically present with **coughing, dyspnoea**, and in severe cases, **central cyanosis** (which is present when there is more than 5 g/dl of deoxygenated haemoglobin present) (Lundsgaard and Van Slyke, 1923).

Cough is a sudden expiratory effort, initially against a closed glottis, producing a forced expulsion of air from the lungs. Coughing results from stimulation of the cough receptors, located in the larynx, trachea and bronchial tree. Therefore, cats with cardiac or pleural space disease rarely cough (although cats with pyothorax may have a concurrent pneumonia which can lead to coughing). In addition, the respiratory pattern should be carefully assessed. Cats with pulmonary parenchymal disease typically show a restrictive expiratory pattern; whereas those with pleural space disease demonstrate an inspiratory restrictive dyspnoea (King, 2004).

Causes of lower respiratory tract disease

- chronic bronchopulmonary disease
  - asthma
  - chronic bronchitis
- pneumonia
  - bacterial
    - *E. Coli*
    - *Pasteurella*
    - *Bordetella bronchoseptica*
    - obligate anaerobes
    - *Streptococcus spp.*
    - *Coagulase + Staphlococcus spp.*
    - *Klebsiella*
    - *Moraxella*
    - *Enterococcus*
    - *Pseudomonas*
    - *Mycobacteria*
    - *Yersinia pestis*
    - others
  - viral
    - avian influenza (rare) H5N1
    - feline calicivirus
    - feline herpes virus
    - feline infectious peritonitis
    - feline pox virus
  - fungal
    - cryptococcosis
    - aspergillosis
    - candidiasis
  - parasitic
    - toxoplasmosis
  - lipid/reactive
- neoplasia
- foreign bodies
- parasites
  - *Aelurostrongylus abstrusus*
  - *Dirofilaria immitis*
  - toxocariasis
- pulmonary contusions
- pulmonary oedema (primarily cardiogenic)
- pulmonary fibrosis.

Feline chronic bronchopulmonary disease

Cats with disease affecting the bronchial tree typically demonstrate **an expiratory, obstructive respiratory pattern.** However, involvement of the surrounding pulmonary parenchyma can lead to an increased respiratory rate, and therefore chronic bronchopulmonary disease is not always easily distinguishable from other lower respiratory diseases (Trzil, 2020). Furthermore, there are several diseases that can affect the bronchopulmonary tissues, and clinically, it is important to differentiate between these diseases and not blanket diagnose all chronic bronchopulmonary disease as feline asthma.

Asthma

Asthma is a common inflammatory disease of the lower airway, reported to affect approximately 1–5% of cats (Trzil, 2020). **It is thought to be allergic in origin**. The hallmarks of asthma are airway inflammation, airway hyperresponsiveness, and airflow limitation. In the long-term, these abnormalities lead to airway remodelling and fixed obstruction.

The pathogenesis is thought to be similar to that in humans, where aero-allergens activate the lymphocytes, which leads to the production of cytokines and prompts an allergic inflammatory response. Importantly, allergen-specific immunoglobulin E (IgE) binds strongly to receptors on mast cells and basophils. With re-exposure to the aero-allergen, the mast cells and basophils degranulate, which promotes a more profound inflammatory response, resulting in bronchoconstriction, inflammation, hyper-responsiveness and, airflow limitation. With this progressive structural changes result from recurrent, chronic exposure to the allergen (Trzil, 2020). **Bronchoconstriction leads to mucus plugging of airways, airway wall remodelling, and oedema; air trapping may also occur as a result.**

Asthma is considered an obstructive lung disease, that **affects young-middle aged cats** (although the median age at presentation is 4–5yrs, many cats have a history of chronic signs at first presentation). Siamese, Oriental, Burmese and Himalayan (colour-point Persian) cats have all been reported as being predisposed to asthma, suggesting a **genetic component** to the disease aetiology. Currently, there are no tests to definitively diagnose asthma. Therefore, it is important to rule out other disorders with similar clinical signs (Garrity, Lee-Fowler and Reinero, 2019).

The clinical signs of feline asthma demonstrate marked overlap with other chronic bronchopulmonary disease and are often complicated by secondary infections. Owners often report bouts of coughing/dyspnoea, where the cat adopts a hunched sternal posture with the elbows adducted and the neck extended.

Clinical signs

- coughing
- wheezing

- increased expiratory effort
- open mouth breathing
- retching/vomiting

Physical examination

- positive tracheal pinch
- end expiratory wheeze
- increased abdominal effort on expiration
- percussion may reveal hyper-resonance of the thorax and air extending to the last rib
- palpation of the thoracic cavity may reveal a barrel chest with eversion of the costochondral junctions and a **heave line** (increased development of the thoracic musculature).

Approximately 20% of cats with feline asthma have concurrent mycoplasma infection within the lower respiratory tract (Reed et al., 2012), which may lead to acute worsening of the clinical signs. It is therefore important to consider secondary infection in these cases; if diagnostics are being undertaken PCR for mycoplasma infection should be considered, and in cases were investigations are not an option, empirical treatment with doxycycline is advised.

Chronic bronchitis

Chronic bronchitis is common is cats and is difficult to differentiate from feline asthma, as both present with similar clinical signs. Chronic **bronchitis is thought to occur as a response to a previous airway insult**, such as infection or irritation. The initiating disease leads to permanent damage to the airways, resulting in clinical signs of chronic bronchopulmonary disease. The conditions can be differentiated by assessing the response to inhaled aeroallergens; with asthmatic cats displaying bronchoconstriction and with this, air-trapping, both of which are not evident in cats with chronic bronchopulmonary disease.

Cats with chronic bronchitis do not have spontaneous bronchoconstriction (Reinero et al., 2019). They can however, demonstrate fixed airflow limitation secondary to cellular infiltrates or remodelling changes. The marked **overlap in presentation** makes differentiating between chronic bronchitis and feline asthma challenging. Radiographic changes may be similar, and although theoretically the **cytology from bronchoalveolar lavage helps to differentiate the diseases; asthmatics present with eosinophilic inflammation, whereas the infiltrate in chronic bronchitis is classically one of non-degenerate neutrophils**. However, the differentiation is not always clear cut, with many asthmatic cats having a neutrophilic component, and cats with chronic bronchitis demonstrating mixed inflammatory infiltrates (Reinero et al., 2019).

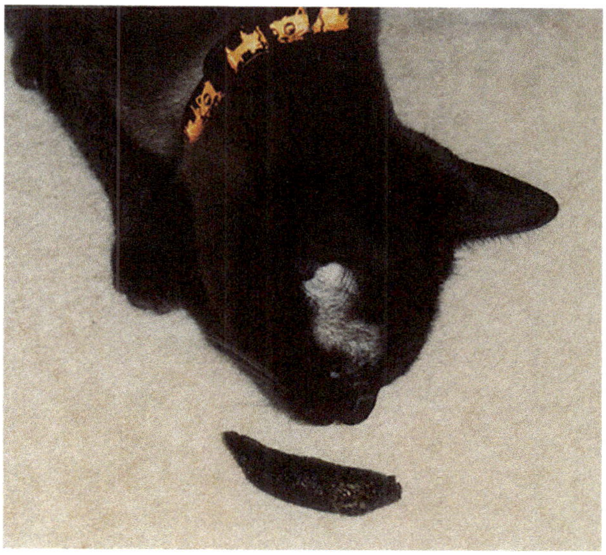

Figure 45. Douglas and the slug.

Aelurostrongylosis

Pulmonary parasitic diseases can mimic feline asthma; amongst these is *Aelurostrongylus abstrusus* infection. ***Aelurostrongylus* is a metastrongyloid nematode that infects cats through ingestion of snails, slugs or paratenic hosts.** Infection has been reported in most areas of the world, including Asia, Australia, Europe, North and South America.

The adult worms are small parasites (males 7 mm, females 10 mm) which reside in the alveoli, alveolar ducts, and terminal bronchioles. Eggs are found in the alveolar ducts and adjacent alveoli, where they form small nodules and hatch to release larvae, which are then coughed up, swallowed, and passed in the faeces (Reinero, 2019a).

Infection with *Aelurostrongylus abstrusus* can cause chronic respiratory disease with clinical signs of chronic bronchopulmonary disease. Histopathological features include multifocal, amber, and subpleural granulomatous nodules up to 1 cm in diameter throughout the lungs. In association with the adult parasites, eggs, and coiled larvae in the bronchioles and alveoli, there can be a catarrhal bronchiolitis, hyperplasia of the submucosal glands and, in advanced cases, granulomatous alveolitis, alveolar fibrosis, and fibromuscular hyperplasia.

Differentiation of *Aelurostongylus* infection from other causes of bronchopulmonary disease is best achieved by **faecal Baermann examination**. However, as parasites are shed intermittently it is advisable to submit three samples. In some cases in which faecal analysis has not been performed appropriately, larvae may be identified on bronchoalveolar lavage (although larvae can become trapped in airway secretions, so negative results do not exclude this differential). **Empirical treatment with an appropriate anti-parasiticide such**

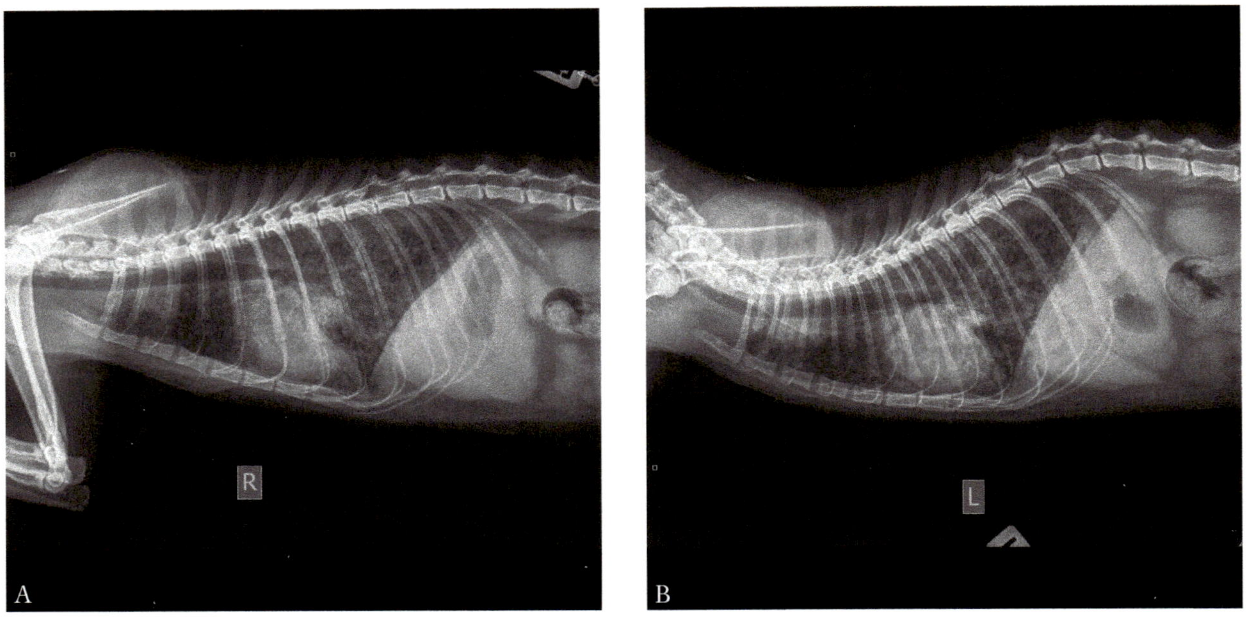

Figure 46. Severe *Aelurostrongylus abstrusus* infection in a cat: right lateral view (A) and left lateral view (B). (Images courtesy of Mette Mortenson).

as fenbendazole is recommended in cats with appropriate history/clinical signs (Pennisi et al., 2015).

Heartworm associated respiratory disease (HARD)

Heartworm (*Dirofilaria immitis*) affected cats may present with clinical signs typical of chronic bronchial disease, or with acute, often fatal, severe dyspnoea associated with pulmonary thromboembolism, particularly when the worms die. However, the natural host for *Dirofilaria immitis* is the dog. Cats are not the preferred target for mosquitoes and are therefore relatively resistant to heartworm infection (HWI) and for the cat to become infected, the mosquito must have fed on an infected dog first. In fact, it has been demonstrated that whilst approximately 12% of cats in the USA have evidence of exposure to *D. immitus*, approximately 80% of these cats clear the infection. One recent study demonstrated HWI in 0.4% of 35,000 cats (Garrity, Lee-Fowler and Reinero, 2019).

Since cats are not the natural host, they often develop amicrofilaraemic infection, with no or few adults and the life cycle is prolonged (7–8 months). However, in the cat, aberrant migration of the parasite is more common and may lead to the development of clinically relevant pulmonary disease even when there are no mature adult worms.

Heartworm associated respiratory disease (HARD) is an inflammatory & proliferative disease of the pulmonary arteries, bronchioles, and pulmonary parenchyma in cats without mature infections.

In HARD the pulmonary intravascular macrophages (PIMs) contribute to the profound inflammatory reaction to immature (S5) and dead worms (adult live worms are not susceptible to PIMs). Therefore, approximately 50% of cats with immature (i.e. S5) infections develop HARD, which produces asthma-like symptoms. As this is a diagnosis of exclusion, it is typically under diagnosed (Garrity, Lee-Fowler and Reinero, 2019).

Reported cases demonstrate a male predisposition, and most affected cats are between 4–6 years old (although they can be any age). Whilst most cases have had some exposure to the outdoors, around 25% of cases are seen in indoor only cats.

Clinical signs vary from none to acute signs often due to dead worm embolization, anaphylaxis-like reaction, or aberrant migration (e.g. into CNS) – dyspnoea, coughing/haemoptysis, shock, ptylism, vomiting/diarrhoea, altered mentation, ataxia, vision loss, seizure,

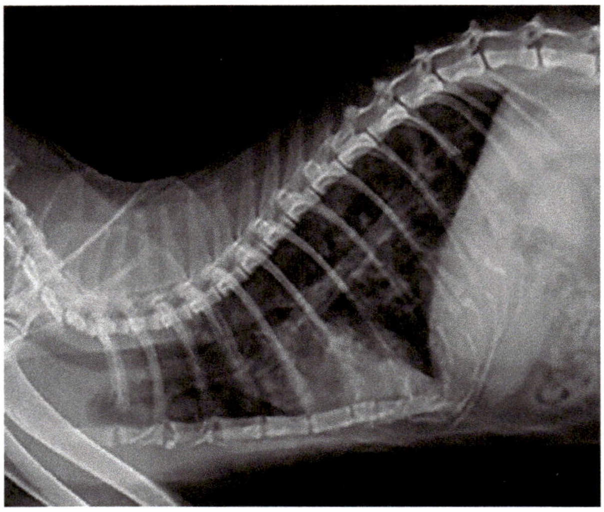

Figure 47. Radiodraphy of a cat with HARD. (Image courtesy of Dr G Norsworthy).

and sudden death may result. With chronic disease coughing, wheezing, dyspnoea, lethargy, hyporexia, weight loss, exercise intolerance, vomiting and/or right sided congestive heart failure have been reported.

Physical exam may be normal, or may include abnormal lung sounds, tachypnoea/dyspnoea, murmur, gallop, weight loss, or ascites.

Wolbachia pipientis **is an intracellular, gram-negative bacteria** which can live in *D. immitis* (and other parasites). *Wolbachia* endotoxins & surface proteins have been implicated in the pathogenesis and adverse reactions associated with HWI and specifically in the bronchial hyperreactivity seen in cats with HARD. Doxycycline is effective at reducing or eliminating *Wolbachia* and reduces & suppresses the larval and adult stages of *D. immitis*. It is therefore, recommended that cats suspected of having HARD are treated with doxycycline (Pennisi et al., 2020).

Diagnosis

Current antigen (Ag) tests detect antigens produced in the reproductive tract of adult female worms, however they are very insensitive for detecting HWI in cats as there are often few/no adults, and therefore, these will be negative if worms are not fully mature or if there are no females (or only 1).

Antibody (Ab)-positive status occurs when larvae develop to stage 4 (L4), so a positive Ab test does not necessarily mean adults are present. If a cat tests Ab positive then an Ag test should be performed (see limitations above). A negative Ab test means there is no HWI or it is too early to detect infection (i.e. <60–90 days post transmission).

Microfilarial testing is not usually performed in cats because they are often amicrofilaraemic (or have very low numbers of microfilaria).

Treatment

Microfilaricidal therapy is not indicated in cats because they are often amicrofilaraemic or have very low numbers of microfilaria. Adulticidal therapy is not recommended in cats as there is a high risk of morbidity and mortality.

Cats with respiratory signs or radiographic evidence of HARD should receive short-term corticosteroid therapy (prednisolone 1–2 mg/kg PO q24–12 h, or parenteral steroid if an emergency). For embolic/anaphylactic emergencies: supplemental oxygen, parenteral corticosteroid (e.g. dexamethasone), and bronchodilator (e.g. terbutaline) may be useful. In addition, it is advised clinicians consider doxycycline (for *Wolbachia*) & clopidogrel (for PTE prevention) (Pennisi et al., 2020).

Prevention

In heartworm endemic areas heartworm preventatives should be used. The macrocyclic lactone drugs are the most common preventatives; however, resistance is developing to this group and alternative drugs are under development.

Toxocariasis

In experimentally infected cats, *Toxocara cati* infection has been shown to induce pulmonary and vascular disease (as pulmonary and transtracheal migration occurs). In addition, experimental infection induced bronchointerstitial lesions on thoracic radiography and is associated with eosinophilic infiltrate on bronchoalveolar lavage, making it an important differential for feline asthma. Notably, cats with T. *cati* infection were asymptomatic, and did not demonstrate airway hyperresponsiveness (a salient feature of feline asthma). Therefore, it is important to rule out Toxocariasis (or treat against these parasites empirically) in cases with suggestive lesions (Garrity, Lee-Fowler and Reinero, 2019).

Pneumonia and pulmonary parenchymal disease

There are various forms of pneumonia described in the cat including bacterial, viral, fungal, and parasitic diseases, as well as a group of poorly described reactive or lipoid pneumonias. In addition, there are several diseases that lead to interstitial lung disease, including pulmonary fibrosis and neoplasia (Reinero, 2019b). Diseases of the alveoli or pulmonary parenchyma typically result in an expiratory, restrictive breathing pattern, however, the same can be said for pulmonary oedema. Therefore, **care should be taken to exclude cardiac involvement** in cases that present with this respiratory pattern.

Bacterial pneumonia

Bacterial pneumonias in cats are not well described in the veterinary literature, with some texts suggesting this is an uncommon disorder. However, with improvements in diagnostic imaging modalities became evident many cats presenting with pyothorax have underlying pulmonary disease (Barrs and Beatty, 2009). The paucity of information makes cats with pneumonia especially difficult to recognise and treat. As many of these cats are critical when they present, bacterial culture is often not performed (as investigations may lead to de-compensation), therefore antibiosis is frequently instigated without knowledge of the underlying pathogen. Common bacterial pathogens that have been isolated in cats include *Mycoplasma spp., Mycobacterial spp., Pasturella spp., Streptococcus spp., Bordetella, E. Coli, Pseudomonas* and the group eugenic fermenter-4 (EF-4a)

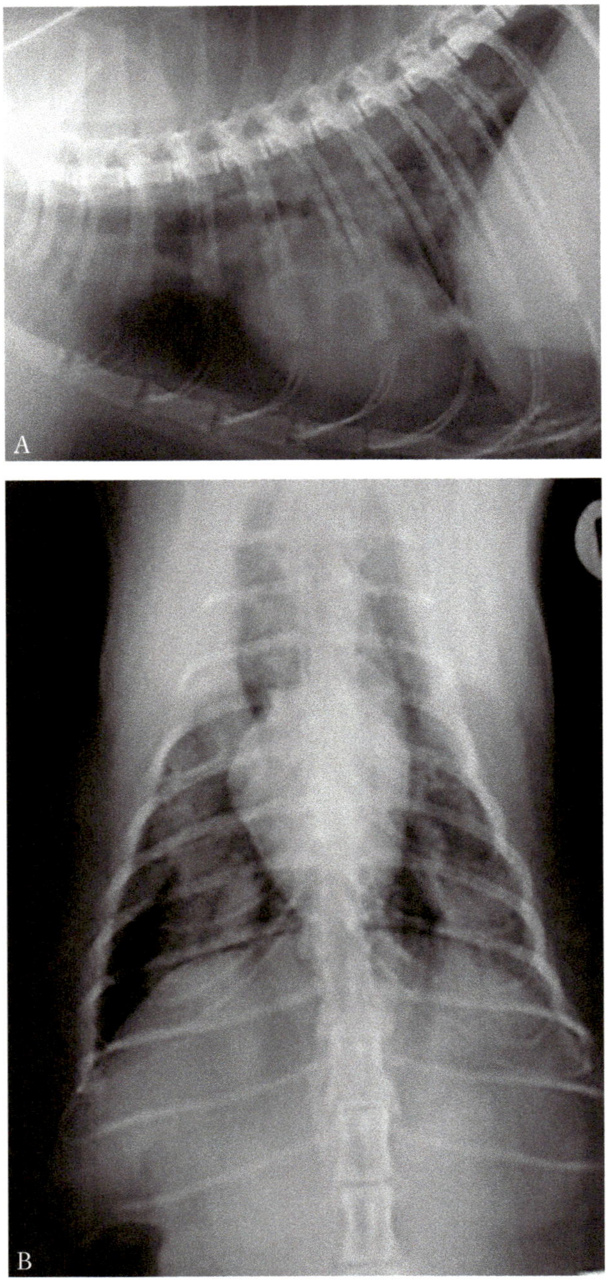

Figure 48. Lateral (A) and DV (B) radiographs of a cat with severe bronchopneumonia demonstrating alveolar infiltrates and bullous lesions.

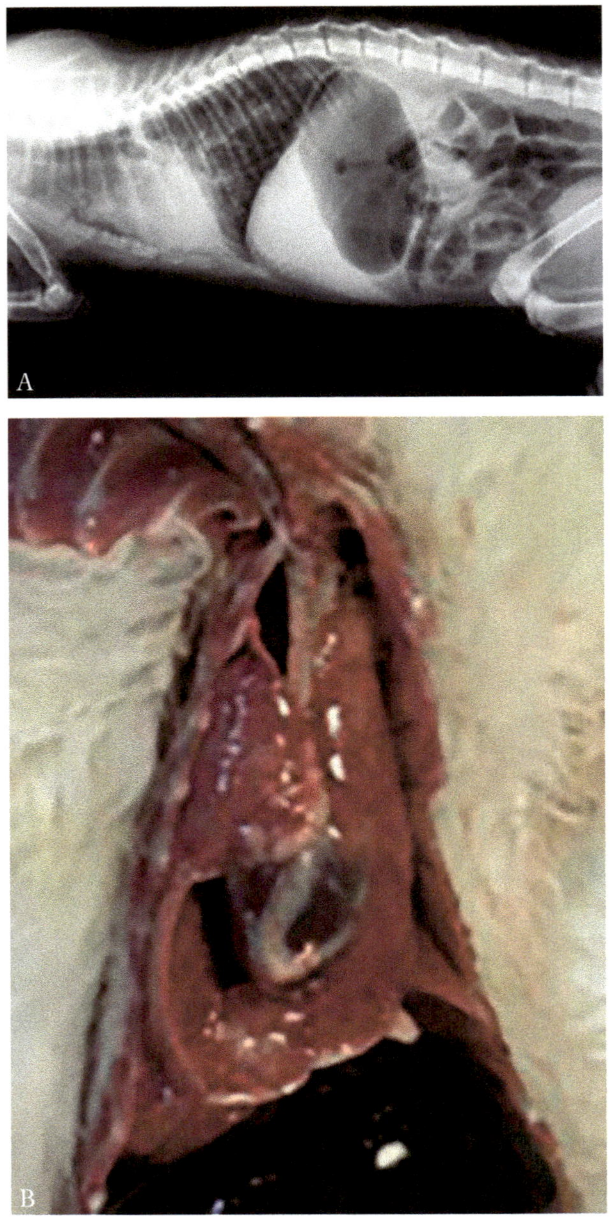

Figure 49. Herpes pneumonia in a young cat, the radiographs demonstrate severe aerophagia, with an interstitial-alveolar lung pattern. On post-mortem the extent of the lesions can be appreciated. (Images courtesy of Prof D Gunn Moore).

bacteria (Dear, 2020). Cats with pneumonia can present with signs of LRT disease with or without concomitant URT signs, but may also have pleural disease, and therefore, a range of respiratory patterns may be evident.

Radiographs are essential for the evaluation of cats with suspected pneumonia, with a variety of radiographic patterns seen. Bronchopneumonia may present as a diffuse bronchointerstitial pattern, with or without localised areas of alveolar consolidation. A multifocal distribution of patchy alveolar infiltrate can occur, which may not be readily distinguishable from metastatic disease. In addition, pleural effusions may be present in severe cases.

Viral pneumonias in cats

Viral pneumonias in cats can be caused by extension of URT viruses (i.e. Calici and Herpes), although the URT signs may no longer be evident, the history of ocular or URT disease helps to narrow the differentials. Cats with FIP typically have systemic lesions or pleural effusion with an elevated albumin:globulin ratio (see pleural effusion section), whereas those with pox virus typically have cutaneous lesions in addition to LRT signs.

Fungal pneumonias in cats

In the UK fungal pneumonias, including aspergillosis, are rare in the cat. Candidiasis is

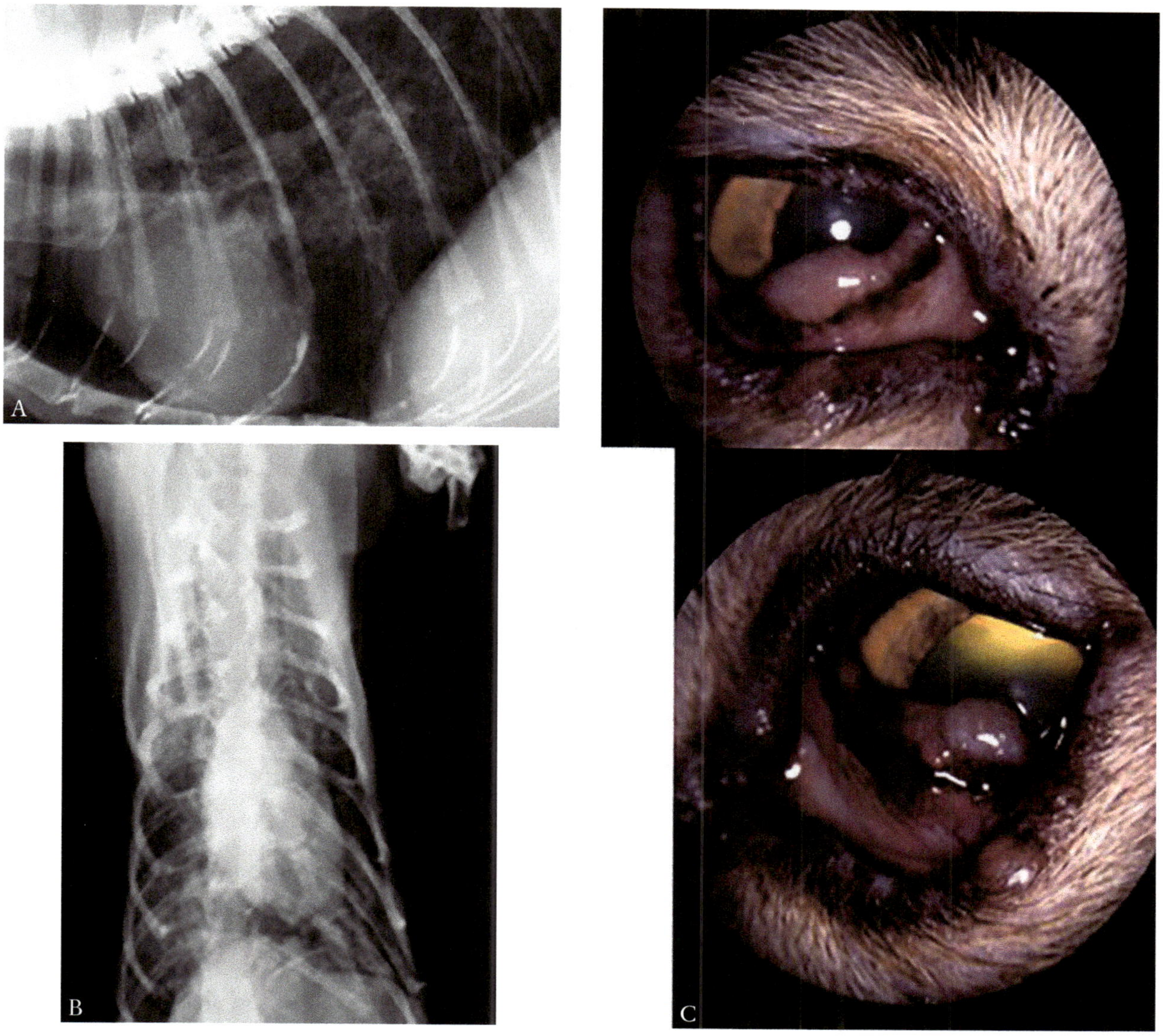

Figure 50. Cryptococcus pneumonia in a cat. Radiographs demonstrating a "reticular" interstitial pattern. Nodules on the eyelids were highly suggestive of cryptococcosis. Scrapings of these lesions and latex-cryptococcal agglutination testing confirmed the diagnosis.

occasionally seen, particularly in immunosuppressed individuals. Systemic crytococcosis can lead to interstitial pneumonia.

Parasitic pneumonias in cats

Systemic toxoplasmosis can result in respiratory involvement. Typically, systemic disease initially affects the interstitium, but later fluid accumulation leads to a mixed alveolar interstitial pneumonia.

Reactive pneumonia

Reactive pneumonia can be seen secondary to systemic diseases, i.e. inhalation of irritant substances such as liquid paraffin inhalation or severe dust/soot.

Pulmonary fibrosis

Idiopathic pulmonary fibrosis (IPF) is a poorly understood disease, which has been identified in cats.

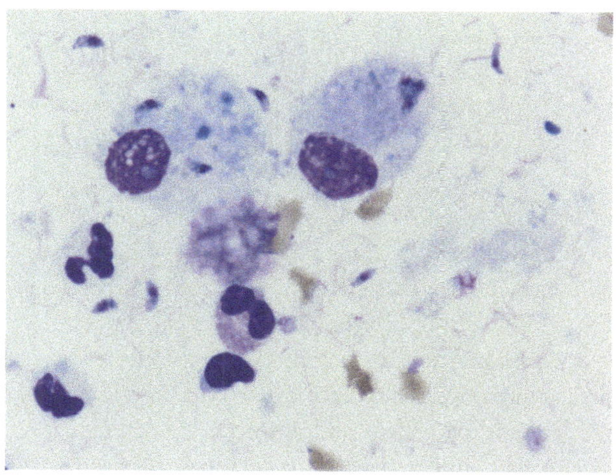

Figure 51. The image demonstrates *Toxoplasma* trophozoites within the BAL of a cat. (Image courtesy of Prof E Milne).

Histopathological lesions have been described and include:

1. **interstitial fibrosis** with fibroblast / myofibroblast proliferation
2. **honeycombing** with alveolar epithelial metaplasia and type II pneumocyte hyperplasia
3. alveolar interstitial smooth-muscle metaplasia. These lesions are heterogeneously distributed (Cohn et al., 2004).

Clinically cats present as severe asthmatics which are refractory to treatment. Typically, cats with pulmonary fibrosis are older (middle to older age) than those presenting with asthma. Cases may have concurrent pulmonary hypertension, and treatment of pulmonary hypertension and inflammation provides temporary stabilisation in some cases. However, 20% of affected cats were found to have pulmonary carcinoma at post mortem (Evola et al., 2014).

Pulmonary neoplasia

Primary pulmonary neoplasia is not common in the cat, but the incidence has increased in the past decade. The tumour which is most commonly diagnosed is carcinoma, but other forms of neoplasia including lymphoma, osteosarcoma, fibrosarcoma, and haemangiosarcoma are occasionally encountered.

Non-cardiogenic pulmonary oedema

In healthy cats, low volumes of fluid and solutes leak through gaps between the capillary endothelial cells to enter the interstitial space. Tight junctions between alveolar epithelial cells prevent the fluid from entering the alveoli. Instead, interstitial fluid moves into the peribronchial space, where it is removed by lymphatics and returned to the circulation. Starling's equation for filtration across a semipermeable membrane describes the factors that determine the amount of vascular leakage.

Noncardiogenic pulmonary oedema occurs when vascular permeability increases as a result of direct or indirect lung injury. This fluid is rich in protein (in contrast to cardiogenic pulmonary oedema) and therefore modifies oncotic pressure gradients, further altering fluid flux.

Accumulation of alveolar fluid, along with decreased lung compliance and airway compression as a result of the oedema, increases pulmonary vascular resistance resulting in hypoxaemia due to ventilation-perfusion mismatch. Removal of alveolar fluid requires active transport of sodium and chloride from the luminal surface through the epithelial cell and across the basolateral membrane. Water movement passively follows sodium-chloride. Injury to the epithelial cells not only leads to oedema formation but impedes the lungs ability to resolve that oedema.

Acute respiratory distress syndrome (ARDS) can occur when there is endothelial and epithelial disturbance of permeability and exit of protein-rich fluid. This can be complicated by coagulation disturbances, perfusion disturbances, and loss of surfactant. ARDS can occur as a complication of primary lung damage such as after inhalation of toxic gas, smoke intoxication, aspiration of gastric content, inhalation of hyperbaric oxygen (pulmonary oxygen toxicity), or pneumonia. ARDS may also occur as a complication of a severe systemic disease such as sepsis, extensive burns, and acute pancreatitis. The prognosis, even with intensive supportive care, is poor.

Investigating lower respiratory tract disease

Introduction

Assessment of serum biochemistry, complete blood count and FIV / FeLV status are useful to generate an overall picture of the cat's health and assess their suitability for general anaesthesia. **Cats with bacterial pneumonia may demonstrate a circulating neutrophilia, whereas those with parasitic infection may demonstrate an eosinophilia.** It has been reported that 17–46% of cats with asthma demonstrate a circulating eosinophilia, but this does not correlate with the degree of airway eosinophilia. In addition, in stable cases, faecal samples should be collected and submitted for Baermann floatation, to detect lungworm (three samples optimises the test sensitivity). However, in practice it is often more convenient to perform a clinical treatment trial.

Imaging

If the cat is stable enough for investigation, thoracic radiographs help to determine the cause of dyspnoea. Radiographs visualize the size and shape of the cardiac silhouette, pulmonary vasculature, local lymph nodes, and patterns within the lungs. In most cases sedation or anaesthesia is required to perform imaging. In cases with suspected bronchopulmonary diseases (and no cardiac concerns) **terbutaline given in the pre-med** may reduce bronchospasm.

Radiography

Thoracic radiographs can provide useful information regarding **the pulmonary parenchyma and allow visualisation of the cardiac shape and size.** A minimum of two well-positioned radiographic views are needed for evaluation (one or ideally both lateral projections, and either a dorsoventral or ventrodorsal projection).

If the lungs are poorly inflated, they appear to have an increased density, and therefore, films should be exposed at peak inspiration.

Interpretation of thoracic radiographs should include assessment of the thoracic wall, the mediastinum, the pleural space, diaphragm, heart and great vessels, and pulmonary parenchyma. Lung patterns can be divided into alveolar, interstitial and bronchial patterns (or often a combination of these).

Alveolar patterns

An alveolar pattern is seen when the **alveoli collapse or fill with fluid**. Radiographs will demonstrate patchy, poorly defined areas of increased density (these have fluffy, indistinct borders which tend to coalesce). In addition, air bronchograms may be seen. There are air filled (i.e. black) tubes highlighted against the white background. Alveolar patterns are seen in cases of pulmonary oedema (in the cat both cardiac and non-cardiogenic oedema can have a generalised distribution); pneumonia and bronchopneumonia, haemorrhage, pulmonary thromboembolism, lung-lobe torsion and atelectasis can all result in an alveolar pattern.

Interstitial patterns

There are different types of interstitial pattern can be seen; nodular densities (with well-defined margins) and a more generalised nonspecific greyness without distinct features and blurring of the vasculature and bronchi. Differentials for the nodular form of interstitial disease include neoplasia, abscessation, and granuloma (i.e. mycobacterial disease); whereas the nonspecific form can be suggestive of pulmonary fibrosis, diffuse neoplasia (i.e. lymphoma), interstitial pneumonia, fungal infection, haemorrhage, or pulmonary oedema.

Bronchial patterns

A bronchial pattern is evident when the walls of the bronchi are more opaque (due to thickening, or when surrounded by fluid or infiltrate). Radiographically this is seen as white/grey circular opacities (doughnuts) or lineal parallel lines (tramlines). A bronchial pattern is seen with bronchopulmonary disease (i.e. asthma, chronic bronchitis, parasitic disease), with bronchopneumonia, or if the bronchi are enlarged and sac like, with bronchiectasis.

Bronchopulmonary diseases typically present with a bronchial or bronchointerstitial pattern. In addition, **collapse of a lung lobe, particularly the right middle lung lobe, is not uncommon** (this is thought to occur due to mucus trapping and atelectasis). Air trapping may also be evident (seen as hyperlucent lung fields and caudal displacement of the diaphragm with flattening of the diaphragmatic silhouette).

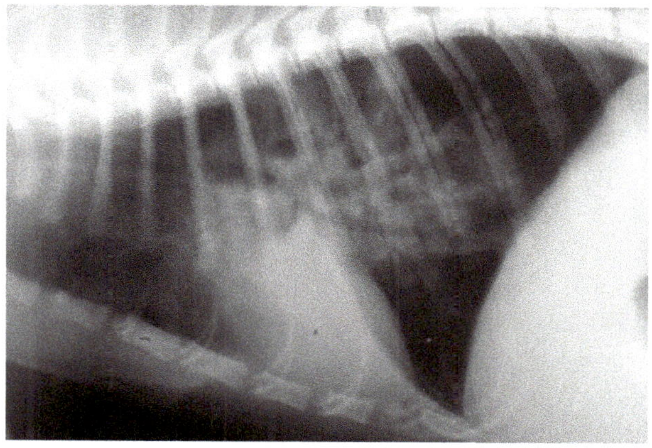

Figure 52. Alveolar pattern in a cat with bacterial pneumonia.

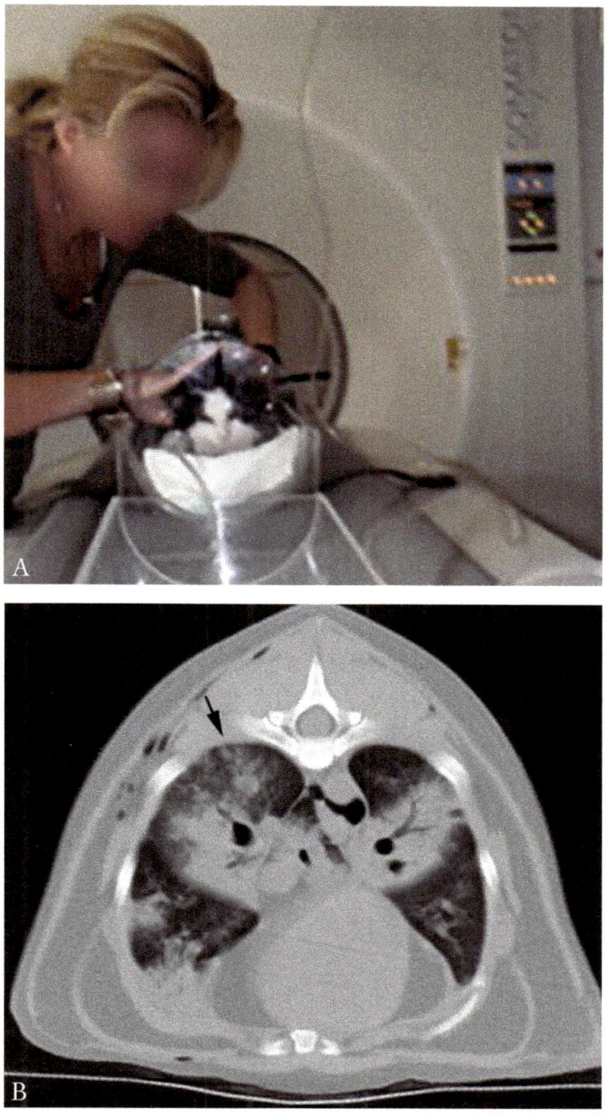

Figure 53. Cat being placed into mousetrap for CT (A). Pulmonary infiltrates on the CT of a cat with aspergillus infection (3).

However, up to 23% of cats with asthma have no radiographic abnormalities and differentiation between different bronchopulmonary diseases is not possible radiographically.

Pneumonia is frequently associated with an alveolar or interstitial alveolar pattern; however, the severity does not always match the severity of the clinical signs.

Computed tomography (CT)

If available, CT provides an alternative to radiography. Thoracic CT allows for a detailed assessment of the pulmonary architecture, allowing identification of bronchial wall thickening, bronchiectasis, alveolar patterns, and assessment of the interstitium. Because CT provides a more detailed examination of the thoracic cavity, it can identify lesions which are not evident on radiography. In addition, in cases that cannot be anaesthetised, a "mouse-trap" CT can be performed (this is a form of plexiglass chamber that can be used to provide an enhanced oxygen environment, whilst restraining the cat during CT).

Whilst radiography and/or CT help locate regional abnormalities and provide information on the type of lung pattern, which narrows down the potential causes but neither provide a definitive diagnosis. **In order to obtain a diagnosis, cytology and culture are required.**

Bronchoscopy and bronchoalveolar lavage (BAL)

Bronchoscopy is useful to **assess the trachea and main stem bronchi**, which are typically inflamed with excessive mucus/mucopurulent secretions present. However, prior to performing bronchoscopy, the status of the cat should be carefully assessed. Bronchoscopy and BAL help reach a diagnosis (by detecting the presence of tracheal inflammation, narrowing, oedema, collapse, foreign bodies, granuloma, neoplasia or helminths), but the risk/benefit ratio must be carefully considered.

For bronchoscopy, the cat's oxygen status should be carefully monitored (in many patients the scope nearly occludes the trachea). In cases where the scope obstructs a large proportion of the trachea, supplementary oxygen given via the bronchoscope port aids maintain saturation.

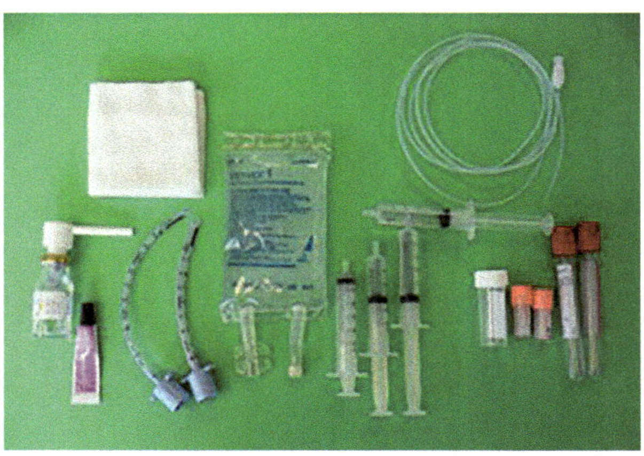

Figure 54. BAL can be performed with the cat in sternal or lateral recumbency, depending on whether the disease is predominantly uni- or bilateral (in unilateral disease, performing a BAL in lateral recumbency with the affected side placed down can help to guide the catheter to the diseased side).

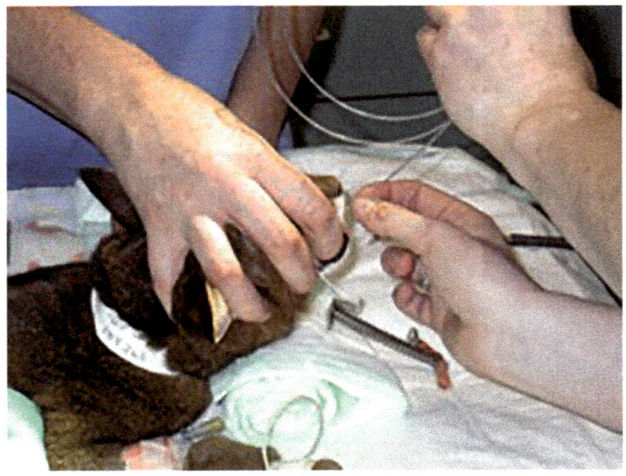

Figure 55. When performing the technique without endoscopic guidance, a sterile catheter should be measured (typically a dog urinary catheter) against the cat's chest and marked approximately two-thirds of the way down. The catheter is then advanced through the sterile endotracheal tube to approximately this level (catheters can sometimes get 'caught' at the tracheal bification, in which case gentle repositioning is required). Once positioned, pre-warmed sterile saline can be flushed down the catheter and then aspirated (approximately 3 ml aliquots are used). Between flushing and aspirating coupàge should be performed on the chest, to release cells into the saline.

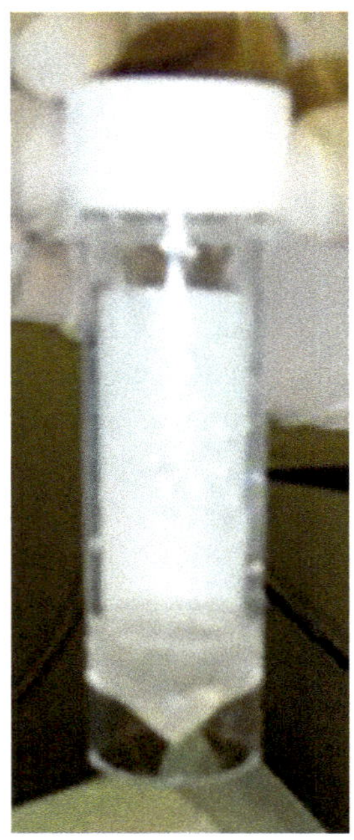

Figure 56. Usually a small volume of fluid is aspirated after the first flush, and therefore three flushes are often necessary. Since the third flush generally has the best cellular harvest, this is ideal for cytological examination. After collection of the BALF (bronchoalveolar lavage fluid), the cat should be provided with increased oxygen for a few minutes, prior to recovery from anaesthesia. Occasionally, performing a BAL stimulates bronchoconstriction. In such cases emergency administration of a bronchodilator such as IV terbutaline, can prove helpful.

It is important to make a note of the orientation of the scope, and bronchial anatomy, in order to note which bronchi are assessed. In cases where a foreign body is suspected, CT examination can be useful in identifying which bronchus/level requires assessment. This allows the investigator to orientate immediately to the affected bronchus and minimize the time taken for extraction.

Bronchoalveolar lavage can be performed with bronchoscopic guidance or by a blind technique. The cat is anaesthetised and pre-medication with terbutaline can be useful, provided there are no contraindications to this drug (i.e. cardiac arrhythmias).

The BALF is submitted for cytology and culture; if anaerobic culture is required, then all air should be evacuated from the container. Most laboratories do not routinely culture for *Bordetella bronchiseptica* or *Mycoplasma species*. Therefore, it is important to request these species are looked for, as we now recognise **up to 20% of cats with chronic bronchopulmonary disease have a *Mycoplasma* spp. infection.** Culture and sensitivity (including anaerobic culture) should be performed (ideally prior to antibiotic administration, although this is not always practical).

Cytological evaluation of tracheal/bronchial fluid should be interpreted with care as there is a massive variation in the population of cells in healthy animals. The presence of leukocytes with intracellular bacteria confirms active infection, whilst the presence of large numbers of neutrophils, especially those with degenerative changes may be highly suggestive. The absence of these cytological changes does not rule out an infectious process. In cats with bronchopulmonary disease cytology is useful to differentiate asthma from chronic bronchitis. Although there is not always a clear-cut distinction on BAL, cats with chronic bronchitis typically demonstrate non-degenerate neutrophilic inflammation, whereas those with asthma should have ≥17% eosinophils.

Further testing

Imaging plus cytology and culture are usually sufficient for definitive diagnosis of pneumonia. However, bronchopulmonary disease is more difficult to differentiate. Therefore, other tests have been suggested to try to differentiate between chronic bronchitis and feline asthma. One such test is allergy testing; to date intradermal skin testing and serum allergen-specific immunoglobulin E have not proved reliable in the diagnosis of asthma. However, with advances in allergen-specific immunotherapy, these techniques may be refined for respiratory cases in the future.

Pulmonary function testing is used in human medicine to assess lung function, and in cats airflow limitation (which can be reversed by the use of bronchodilators) is suggestive of feline asthma. Therefore, there is growing research in the use of barometric whole body plethysmography (BWBP) as a non-invasive test to differentiate chronic bronchitis from feline asthma and in the future this technique may become part of the clinical assessment of chronic lower respiratory tract disease in the cat.

Treatment of feline lower respiratory tract disease

Ideally, the treatment of feline lower respiratory tract disease is based on a diagnosis and in some cases (i.e. foreign body) diagnosis allows for immediate cure.

However, in an emergency it is important to assess the respiratory pattern, perform thoracic percussion to assess for air and fluid, and if possible, a T-FAST to rule out effusion and congestive heart failure. Any severely dyspnoeic cat should be placed in oxygen (ideally humidified as this aids bronchopulmonary clearance in cases of pneumonia, and makes it less irritant to the bronchi in cats with chronic bronchopulmonary disease). In the majority of cases, history and clinical signs are suggestive of either pneumonia or chronic bronchopulmonary disease, but in cases with conflicting findings it may be necessary to treat for both (i.e. treat as for status asthmaticus, but add in nebulisation and antibiotics (See Figure 2).

Status asthmaticus

Acute decompensation of bronchopulmonary disease requires prompt intervention. Stress should be minimised and the cat placed in an oxygen-enriched environment, ideally with humidification, that is free from potential allergens (no cat litter for example). Useful, rapidly acting drugs include:

- Terbutaline 0.01 mg/kg SQ, IM or IV q4hrs (is also absorbed rapidly PO).
- Aminophylline 5 mg/kg IV q8–12 hrs (is also absorbed rapidly PO) but is painful if administered by SQ or IM injection.
- Salbuterol 100 mg metered dose inhaler (MDI), two doses at onset of clinical signs and every 30 mins for up to 2–4 hours (this can be particularly useful in cats where asthma has previously been diagnosed, as it can be administered immediately the owner notices severe signs. However, emergency veterinary attention should be sought if no response is seen within 15 mins). Generally, other inhaled medications are not useful in the emergency situation, as it takes longer for therapeutic concentrations to be reached.

- Methylprednisolone sodium succinate 50–100 mg/cat SQ, IM or IV.
- Dexamethasone 0.2–2.2 mg/kg SQ, IM or IV.

In severe respiratory distress:

- Adrenalin 0.1 ml of a 1:1000 solution SQ, IM, IV or via ET tube.
- Atropine 0.015 mg/kg IV, 0.04 mg/kg SQ-will increase heart rate and can be pro-arrhythmic.

Feline asthma

Long-term treatment of chronic bronchopulmonary disease aims to **control the clinical signs rather than cure**. In mild cases, this may be possible using only environmental control, whereas in more severe asthmatics, therapy aimed at reversing bronchoconstriction and reducing inflammation may be required.

Decrease allergen/irritant exposure

Reducing the exposure to potential allergens can lead to a marked improvement in clinical signs. Common irritants include smoke, cat-litter, aerosols, dust and sudden temperature changes. In addition, drugs that lead to bronchoconstriction (beta-2-blockers, non-specific beta-blockers and aspirin) should be avoided, as should stressful events. Obese cats should be encouraged to lose weight.

It is advisable to discuss the cat's routine with the owner. If the cat has a litter tray, dust-free litter options (such as paper-based litters) are useful. Most owners are happy to avoid using aerosols and perfumes around their cat, and many volunteer to stop smoking (or stop smoking in their house). However, exposure to dust can pose issues. A cat's exposure to dust (and human dander) is often at its highest when it is sleeping on the owners bed. Therefore, the ideal advice is to remove carpets from the house and shut the cat out of the bedroom. However, even in situations where the owners remove the carpets, it is rare the cat is ever shut out of the bedroom. Moderated advice is more likely to be adhered to, such as advising owners to regularly vacuum the mattress and sofa etc with a hepa-filter and limiting dust exposure with the use of mattress and pillow covers made for human asthmatics.

In addition, it is useful to mark the cat's record so that if the cat is admitted to hospital, they have a note to use dust-free litter in their kennel. Typically, in hospitalised patients the litter tray is close to the bed, and this irritant can cause an otherwise stable case to destabilise. Some clinics carry a range of cat litters to allow for individual preference and dust-free options; however, if not, urine collection beads or even shredded paper can provide alternatives in an emergency situation.

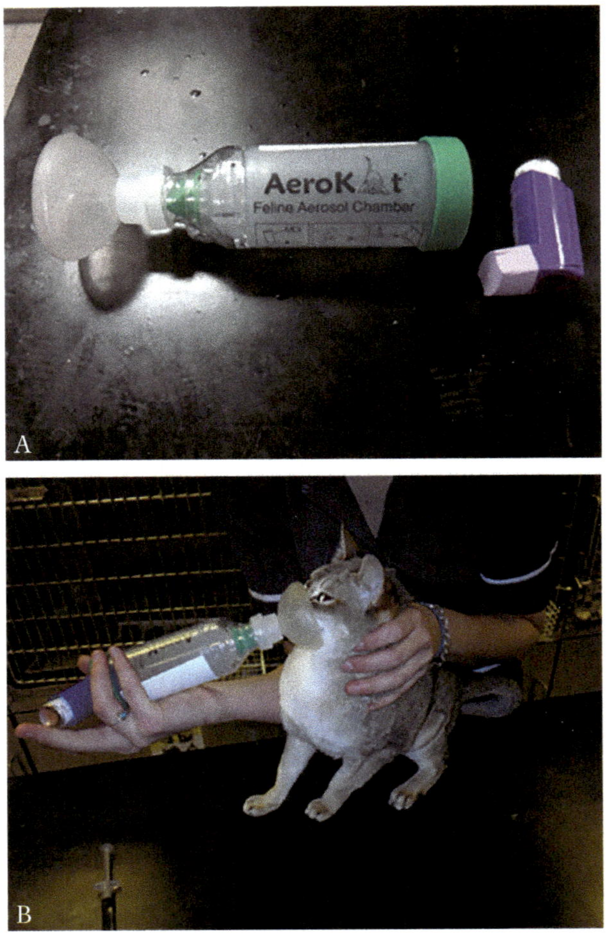

Figure 57. An AeroKat chamber™ and cat being treated with inhaled medications.

Medical therapy

The most consistent and reliable therapy for the long-term management of the chronic bronchopulmonary disease involve **corticosteroid medications**. The aim of therapy is to reduce the underlying inflammation. Inhaled steroids are utilised principally in human asthmatics and can be administered in the cat:

- fluticasone propionate (Flixotide®), 125 MDI, 1–2 doses, twice daily
- beclomethasone bipropionate (Becotide®), 100 or 200 MDI, 1–2 doses twice daily
- budesonide, 125 MDI, 1–2 doses, twice daily

With patience, many cats learn to tolerate inhaled medications. The AeroKat chamber ™ is specially designed for feline use and is the preferred choice. The cat should be introduced to the chamber in the home environment, initially without any drug placed in the chamber, and allowed to get used to the mask being placed over its face. Eventually, once the cat is used to the chamber,

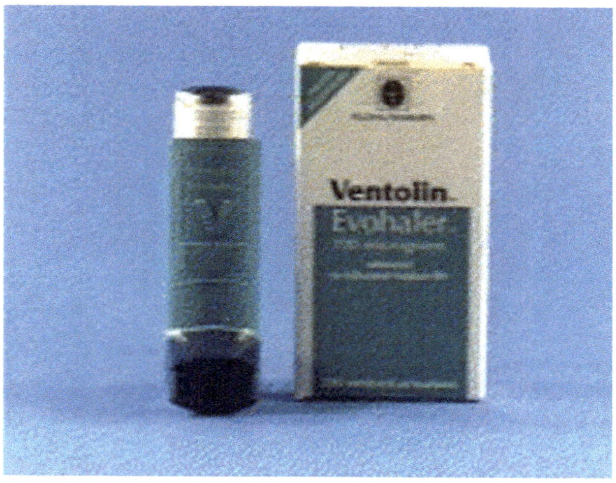

Figure 58. Inhaler device.

the chosen drug should be added. Where more than one dose of the drug is required, one dose should be introduced into the chamber, the mask placed on the cat's face for 5–10 seconds, and then repeated for the second dose.

For cats that do not tolerate inhaled medication or prior to commencing therapy with inhaled medications, oral steroids can be administered:

- Prednisolone 1–2 mg/kg PO, twice daily, for 7–10 days, then tapered to the minimum dose required to control clinical signs.

Bronchodilators are useful during acute exacerbations caused by bronchoconstriction. These drugs can also be used in the chronic management of disease in an attempt to decrease the dose, or side effects associated with chronic corticosteroid therapy. However, there is recent evidence that the chronic use of bronchodilators (salbuterol) may increase airway inflammation. Since the primary goal of therapy is to decrease the underlying airway inflammation, bronchodilator therapy should not be used in place of corticosteriod treatment.

Experimental therapies

There are various treatment options under assessment experimentally. These include allergen-specific immunotherapy (allergy shots), which have been administered by 'rush immunotherapy' in experimental models, offering promising results, as they have been shown to decrease the number of eosinophils in the airways after exposure to allergen (Reinero et al., 2019).

Other experimental therapies include inhaled lignocaine therapy, omega series fatty acid supplementation, tyrosine kinase inhibitors and stem cell therapy.

Cats with chronic bronchopulmonary disease are susceptible to opportunistic infections and therefore, whenever an infection is identified, they should be treated, ideally with antibiotics with proven sensitivity. However, empirical doses of doxycycline (5 mg/kg PO, twice daily), penicillin and fluoroquinolones may be of use in some cases. Where infection is identified, or there is a good response to antibiotic therapy, courses of treatment should be administered.

Monitoring and outcome

Evaluation of clinical response is the usual and most practical method of monitoring response to treatment in the asthmatic cat. If the cat appears not to respond to treatment in the first 2–3 weeks of therapy, it is important to ensure the owner is able to administer the medication properly, review the original diagnosis and ensure that there are no concomitant infectious or neoplastic processes ongoing. In cases refractory to medication, a trial of methylprednisolone acetate can be considered. Whilst the majority of cats respond well to treatment, it should be assumed that life-long medication will be required, as it is rare for spontaneous resolution to occur in the cat.

Chronic bronchitis

Many authors argue that in clinical cases it is not necessary to distinguish chronic bronchitis from asthma. The reasoning for this is that the treatment of these two conditions, currently, is essentially the same. Chronic bronchitis is managed predominantly with steroids, and where necessary additional bronchodilators and treatment of secondary infections. The same medications, and dosages that are used in patients with feline asthma are therefore, used in cases with chronic bronchitis. However, as advances are made in the treatment of feline chronic bronchopulmonary disease, particularly treatment of asthma, there are likely to be some alternative medications which are more effective in one disease compared to the other.

Idiopathic pulmonary fibrosis

Pulmonary fibrosis is rarely diagnosed in clinical cases. However, pathological lesions including interstitial fibrosis, fibroblast proliferation, myofibroblast proliferation, and enlarged airspaces lined by prominent epithelium have been described in affected cats. It is reported that the lungs are heterogeneously affected. Cases can present with severe clinical signs, often presumed to be due to asthma. However, they are typically refractory to treatment. In cats 20% of affected cats have been noted to have pulmonary carcinoma at postmortem. Concurrent pulmonary hypertension may be present (see section later on in chapter); treatment of pulmonary hypertension and inflammation can provide temporary stabilisation in some cases.

Pneumonia

Pneumonia results in various degrees of ventilation/perfusion mismatch (V/Q). Local inflammatory mediators act as vasodilators and over-ride hypoxic vasoconstriction. Oxygen supplementation should be provided if the SpO2 is less than 94% (or if the PaO2 is less than 80 mmHg). Humidification of oxygen is essential to maintain the mucociliary escalator and facilitate coughing of secretions.

Intravenous fluids are often indicated since cats with pneumonia are often inappetent, while panting/pyrexia increases fluid loss. In addition, dehydration changes mucus composition, decreasing mucociliary clearance, and alveolar emptying. Inappetent cats may also benefit from supplemental feeding via parentral nutrition, nasoesophageal tube, or oesophagostomy tube placement.

Atelectasis can exacerbate respiratory insufficiency; therefore, recumbent patients should be turned every 1–2 hours, or ideally supported in sternal recumbency. Nebulisation can help to hydrate the mucocilary system and encourage coughing. It is controversial as to whether or not to coupage as coughing may exasperate the dyspnoea and distress the animal and coupage can increase pulmonary haemorrhage. See figure 30.

People with pneumonia report it to be a painful condition, therefore the use of analgesics, such as buprenorphine should be considered.

Various other treatments have been attempted in refractory cases. These include the use of bronchodilators, mucolytics, and corticosteroids. All of these treatments have potential advantages and disadvantages, with no definitive studies demonstrating proven benefits. Therefore, these drugs should be used with caution, but may be of potential benefit in some cases of bronchopneumonia.

Bacterial pneumonia

In stable cases the choice of antibiotic depends on culture and sensitivity. However, in severe cases antibiotic therapy may be commenced without a definitive diagnosis. Broad-spectrum cover is required and achieved by various combinations of antibiotics. Typically, the first choice of antibiosis for a cat with severe bacterial pneumonia at the authors practice includes a fluoroquinolone and clindamycin (by intravenous injection).

Management of viral pneumonia

If viral pneumonia is suspected, then an appropriate antiviral medication should be administered. In the majority of cases, treatment is non-specific (i.e. feline interferon). However, if FHV is isolated or strongly suspected, then famciclovir should be used.

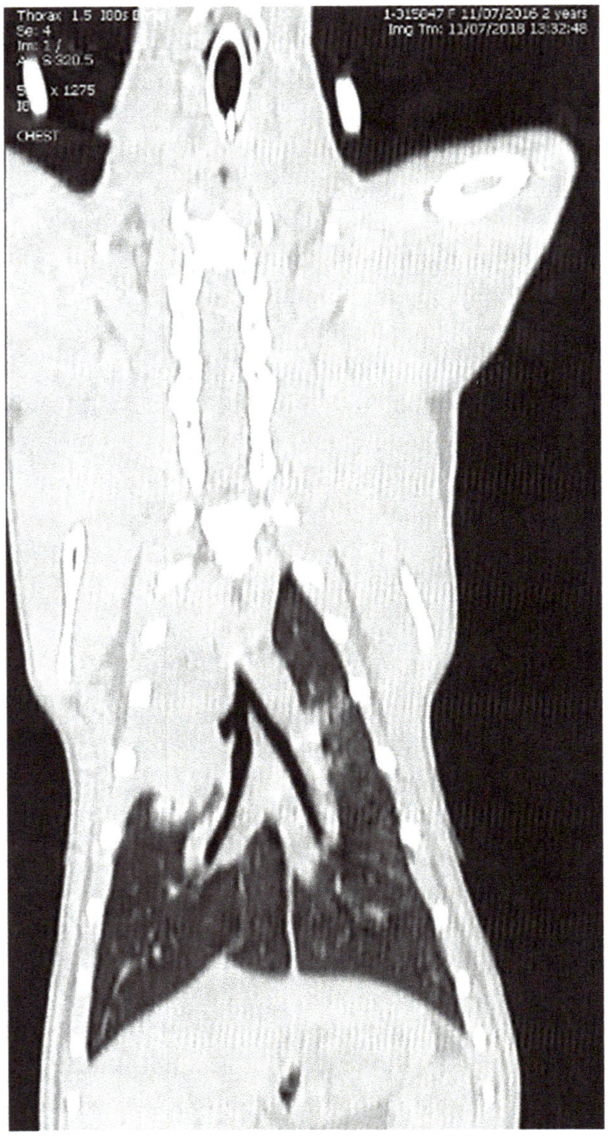

Figure 59. CT of a cat suffering from bacterial pneumonia.

Management of fungal pneumonia

If fungal pneumonia is diagnosed, systemic mycotic infection should be suspected. The most common mycotic infection seen in cats is *Cryptococcus*. There are several different treatment protocols described, which include:

- fluconazole or itraconazole
- amphotericin B can be given SC (0.5–0.8 mg/kg diluted in 0.45% saline containing 2.5% dextrose; 400 ml per cat), 2–3 times per week or amphotericin B lipid complex (1–2 mg/kg per cat) can also be given 3 times/week for 12–15 treatments
- flucytosine can be used alone; however, drug resistance may develop, so combination therapy with amphotericin is recommended.

Of these fluconazole is the least toxic compound, and therefore the treatment favoured by the author.

Parasitic pneumonia

If parasites are identified they should be treated accordingly. In severe *Aelurostrongylus* infestation it is recommended by some authors to initially treat with fenbendazole prior to more efficient treatments as it is hypothesised that if the parasites are killed rapidly then the inflammatory response can overwhelm the cat.

In cats diagnosed with *Dirofilaria immitus*, microfilaricidal therapy is not indicated because they are often amicrofilaraemic or have very low numbers of microfilaria.

Adulticidal therapy is not performed in cats as there is a high risk of morbidity and mortality.

Cats with respiratory signs or radiographic evidence of HARD should receive short-term corticosteroid therapy (prednisolone 1–2 mg/kg PO q24–12h, or parenteral steroid if an emergency). For embolic/anaphylactic emergencies: supplemental oxygen, parenteral corticosteroid (e.g. dexamethasone), bronchodilators (e.g. terbutaline) may be useful. In addition, the use of doxycycline should be considered (vs *Wolbachia*) and clopidogrel (PTE prevention).

Pulmonary hypertension

Pulmonary hypertension (abnormally increased pressure within the pulmonary vasculature) is a well-established syndrome in human medicine and recognised in both canine and feline medicine. However, traditionally there have been difficulties in diagnosing and treating pulmonary hypertension and therefore the veterinary literature has largely avoided this subject. But with advances in our diagnostic capabilities and newly available medications, interest in pulmonary hypertension in veterinary patients has increased and recently, the American College of Veterinary Internal Medicine published a consensus statement of guidelines for the diagnosis, classification, treatment, and monitoring of pulmonary hypertension in the dog (Reinero et al., 2020). To date, no such guidelines exist for feline patients and much of the understanding of this syndrome is extrapolated from either human or canine literature.

Haemodynamic definitions and aetiologies

Accurate assessment of the pulmonary arterial pressure involves catheterisation of the right heart. In humans a mean pulmonary artery pressure of ≥25mmHg at rest, is diagnostic for pulmonary hypertension. However, increased pulmonary arterial pressure is seen in a multitude of different diseases and is not diagnostic for one particular disease process.

Pulmonary hypertension can be further divided based on the absence or presence of pulmonary vascular resistance.

In cases with pulmonary hypertension and increased pulmonary vascular resistance the underlying cause may be pulmonary endothelial dysfunction, pulmonary vascular remodelling, vascular luminal obstruction, increased blood viscosity, arterial wall stiffening or lung parenchymal destruction.

If there is no increase in pulmonary vascular resistance, pulmonary hypertension can occur due to increased pulmonary venous pressure (i.e. left-sided heart disease or compression of a large pulmonary vein), or increased pulmonary blood flow (i.e. left to right shunting cardio/vascular defects).

In cats, invasive measurement of the pressures within the right heart or vasculature is not a routine procedure. Therefore, non-invasive estimates are often substituted for direct measurement. Echocardiography may be used to estimate the pressure within the pulmonary artery. If there is no RV outflow tract obstruction, pulmonary arterial pressure can be estimated from either the peak tricuspid regurgitation velocity (by using the simplified Bernoulli equation to estimate the difference between the right atrial and right ventricular pressure); or by using a pulmonary regurgitant jet to estimate the mean pulmonary artery pressure (again using the simplified Bernoulli equation) (Vezzosi and Schober, 2019). These estimates are subject to user variability and clinicians should interpret the accuracy, variability and precision of such measurements with caution, taking care to assess the history and presentation alongside any such estimates. Therefore, in many cases feline pulmonary hypertension is presumed, based on identification of a known cause, clinical signs, and response to treatment, rather than being accurately diagnosed.

Classification of pulmonary hypertension

The following six groups of pulmonary hypertensive disease are proposed in canine patients (with a similar classification system published for the evaluation of pulmonary hypertension in humans). As many of these diseases are recognised in the cat, a similar classification system appears appropriate.

1. Possible causes of pulmonary arterial hypertension. Possible causes:

- vascular damage leading to medial hypertrophy and intimal proliferation/fibrosis
- idiopathic or heritable
- drug or toxin induced
- congenital systemic-to-pulmonary shunts
- pulmonary vasculitis
- pulmonary vascular amyloid deposition

- pulmonary veno-occlusive disease or pulmonary capillary haemangiomatosis.

In cats, there are no reports of idiopathic or heritable pulmonary hypertension occurring. This may be due to difficulties in diagnosing the condition, and lack of recognition, or the syndrome might not affect felines. However, drug/toxin induced pulmonary hypertension has been reported, predominantly in experimental studies where the right cardiac pressures were assessed in cats receiving infusion of *E Coli* endotoxin (Schützer, Haglund and Falk, 1987). Interestingly, there are also reports of pulmonary vasculitis in cats presenting with *E Coli* septicaemia (Brooks et al., 2013). Congenital left to right cardiac or vascular shunts are well recognised in cats and there are occasional case reports of both pulmonary vascular amyloid deposition, and pulmonary veno-occlusive disease or pulmonary capillary haemangiomatosis (Jaffey et al., 2017; Jenkins and Jennings, 2017; Mawby, Whittemore and Donnell, 2018).

2. Pulmonary hypertension with left heart disease
Elevated left atrial pressure, increases pulmonary venous pressures and results in pulmonary capillary hypertension and ultimately pulmonary artery hypertension.

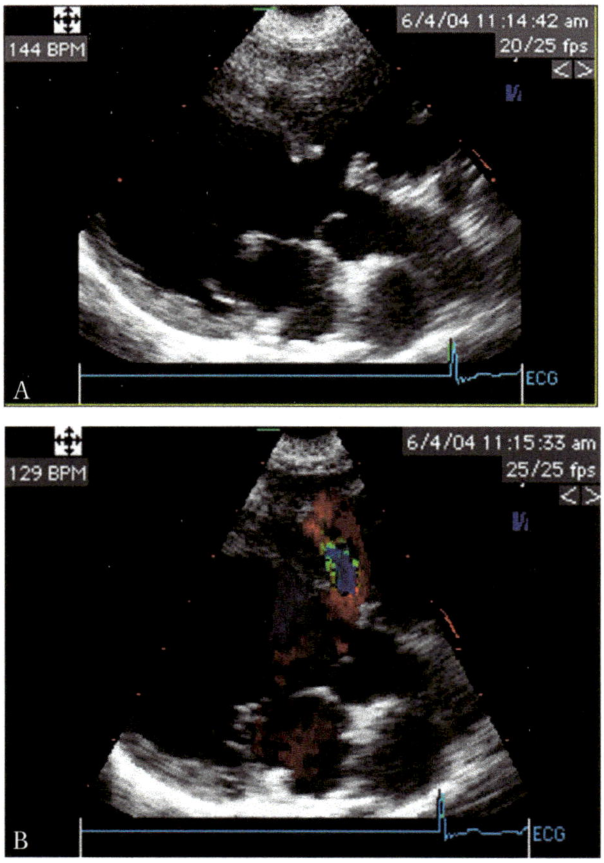

Figure 60. A large VSD in a cat resulting in left-to-right shunting.

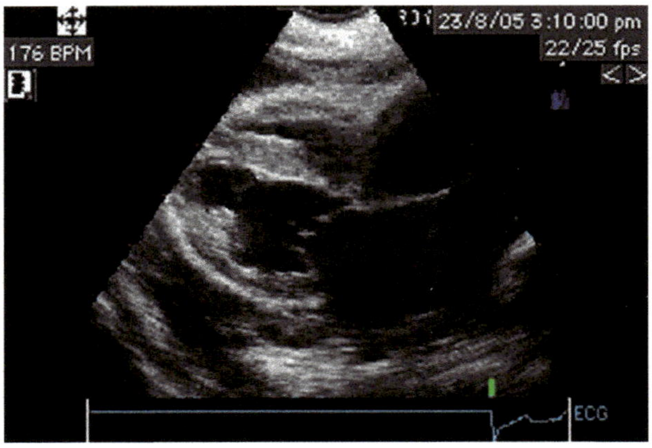

Figure 61. Restrictive cardiomyopathy has been linked to pulmonary hypertension in the cat.

Feline endomyocarditis is rarely reported, and to date there are no reports of pulmonary hypertension occurring in cats with this disease. There is a recent report analysing the prevalence of pulmonary hypertension in cats with left sided heart disease. These authors reported that 17% of cats with left sided heart disease demonstrated echocardiographic evidence of pulmonary hypertension (Vezzosi and Schober, 2019). Further analysis demonstrated this was most common in cats with congenital heart disease (5 of 5 cases), but was present in 3 of 8 cats with restrictive cardiomyopathy (RCM), 2 of 6 with unclassified cardiomyopathy (UCM), 1 of 5 with dilated cardiomyopathy, 3 of 23 with end-stage hypertrophic cardiomyopathy (HCM) and 6 of 80 with HCM, suggesting that pulmonary hypertension may not be uncommon in feline patients with RCM (Vezzosi and Schober, 2019).

3. Pulmonary hypertension with pulmonic disease/ hypoxia
Primary pulmonary diseases result in hypoxia and with this pulmonary artery vasoconstriction. Common causes include:

- chronic obstructive pulmonary disease (COPD)
- interstitial lung disease
- high altitude
- reactive pulmonary artery vasoconstriction
- developmental lung disease
- miscellaneous: bronchiolar disorders, bronchiectasis, emphysema, pneumonectomy.

Despite being recognised as the most common cause of pulmonary hypertension in humans and dogs, there are very few reports of feline pulmonary hypertension secondary to respiratory disease. Cats with pulmonary fibrosis have been recognised as exhibiting pulmonary hypertension (Cohn et al., 2004). However, there are

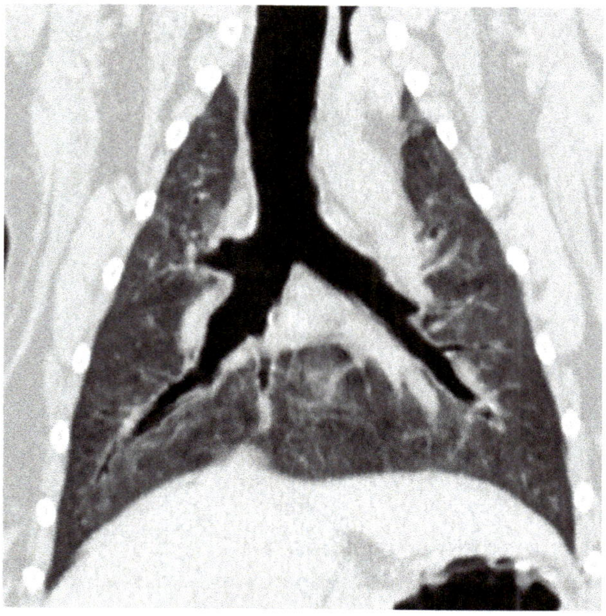

Figure 62. CT of a case with pulmonary fibrosis. The CT demonstrates an interstitial pattern, with the density of the interstitium being increased (up to -500 Housfield units, normal density is approx. -750–850 Housfield units).

no studies assessing the prevalence of feline pulmonary hypertension in common airway diseases such as feline asthma or chronic bronchitis. Experimental studies demonstrate that the feline pulmonary vasculature is highly sensitive to the effects of hypoxia, and therefore it is likely on many occasions pulmonary hypertension exists in feline chronic respiratory disease.

4. Pulmonary hypertension caused by thrombotic or embolic disease

The likely mechanism for pulmonary hypertension in thromboembolic disease is arteriopathy caused by endothelial dysfunction and/or pulmonary arterial vascular remodelling, luminal narrowing, and increased pulmonary vascular resistance.

Despite pulmonary thromboembolism being a relatively rare diagnosis in the cat, there is a report of pulmonary hypertension and cor pulmonale in a cat secondary to thromboembolism (post-surgical debridement of an abscess), and therefore, emboli/thromboembolism is a differential for feline pulmonary hypertension (Sottiaux and Franck, 1999).

5. Parasitic disease

There are several reports of feline pulmonary hypertension secondary to both feline heartworm or lungworms (both *Aelurostrongylus*, and lesser known *Troglostrongylus*, a feline lungworm reported in young cats with increasing prevalence in some Mediterranean and Balkan countries) (Rawlings, 1990; Dirven et al., 2012; Pennisi et al., 2015). (Figure 46).

6. Miscellaneous

Group 6 causes of pulmonary hypertension have not been well described in the cat.

Diagnosis

Diagnosis of pulmonary hypertension relies on evaluation of the signalment, history, clinical signs, and diagnostic tests which support the diagnosis of pulmonary hypertension, along with evaluation of the underlying cause.

Treatment

Recommendations for the treatment of canine pulmonary hypertension include strategies to decrease the risk of progression or complications associated with pulmonary hypertension, treatment of the underlying disease, and specific therapies for pulmonary hypertension (Reinero et al., 2020).

Strategies to decrease the risk of progression or complications from pulmonary hypertension include restricted exercise (which is not usually a consideration in feline medicine), prevention of respiratory infections/parasites, avoidance of high altitude and air travel, and avoidance of nonessential anaesthesia. Thereafter, treatment recommendations depend on the form of pulmonary hypertension.

- **Group 1** disease may improve with withdrawal of drugs, treatment of toxins or closure of left-to-right shunts. If there is right-to-left shunting treatment of hyperviscosity via phlebotomy or the use of hydroxyurea may be beneficial.
- **Group 2** pulmonary hypertension may improve with treatment of the underlying cardiac disease or where indicated (and not detrimental to the underlying cardiac condition) the phosphodiesterase V inhibitor Sildenafil may be beneficial (see later on in chapter).
- **Group 3–6** pulmonary hypertension treatment of an underlying disorder, where possible, is advised. However, in some cases the underlying disease may not be treatable, or the pulmonary hypertension may not resolve; for example residual pulmonary hypertension has been reported after treatment of feline lungworm disease.

The majority of studies assessing specific treatment options for pulmonary hypertension in small animals focus on the phosphodiesterase V inhibitor (Sildenafil) (Reinero et al., 2020). **Sildenafil** increases pulmonary vascular cGMP, thereby increasing the activity of endogenous nitric oxide and decreasing vasoconstriction within the pulmonary vasculature. Studies have suggested the use of sildenafil benefits the patient by decreasing the clinical signs, increasing the quality of life, and in some cases, by decreasing echocardiographically derived estimates of pulmonary arterial pressure. However, the vast majority of these studies were performed on canine patients, with only a few reports of the use of sildenafil in cats with pulmonary hypertension. The author has successfully used sildenafil in several cats with pulmonary hypertension secondary to pulmonary fibrosis and in cases of RCM.

Pleural effusion & mediastinal disease

Diseases of the pleural cavity are not uncommon and **cats frequently present with pleural effusion.** Rapid identification and treatment of this condition can be lifesaving. Dyspnoeic cats can decompensate with excessive handling; therefore, it is useful to place the cat into an oxygen enriched environment, ensure oxygen requirements are minimized (i.e. the environment is cool, quiet and the cat is not stressed) and assess the status in the least invasive manner possible.

Identification of pleural effusion

In general, the following five steps are helpful rule-in or out pleural space disease.

1. **Observation**
   If the pleural space is occupied by gas or fluid, the lungs cannot expand fully. This results in **an inspiratory dyspnoea with a restrictive pattern** (elevated respiratory rate). Recognising this pattern of breathing allows rapid identification of pleural fluid. Deciding whether or not a pattern is inspiratory or expiratory can sometimes be problematic. If **nostril flare** is present this gives an indication as to which phase of respiration is abnormal. In addition, assessing the movement of the tissues overlying the thoracic inlet (i.e. the prescapular area) can also be helpful. It is the author's opinion any cat with such a breathing pattern should be assessed for effusion, which should be drained prior to any other investigation.
2. **Percussion**
   Assessment for pleural effusion includes thoracic percussion. Free fluid within the pleural space decreases resonance. In some cases, the change in resonance forms a line where the fluid accumulation ends or it may be unilateral. If there is free gas within the thorax resonance is increased. It should be remembered that a decrease in resonance is heard with consolidation or infiltration of the pulmonary parenchyma, and an increased resonance is heard with air trapping, as seen with asthma.

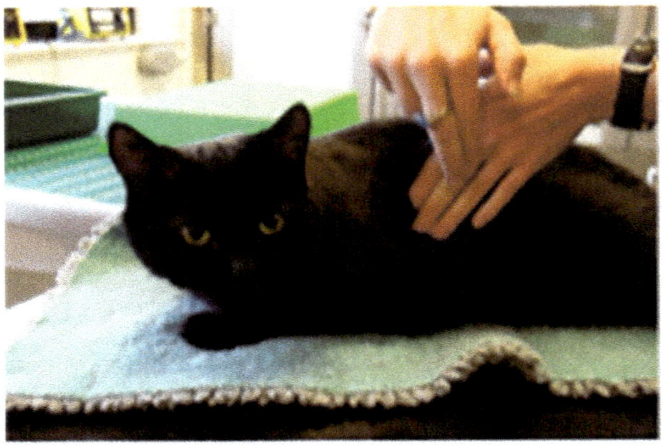

Figure 63. Thoracic percussion.

   However, in these conditions, expiratory dyspnoea is seen.
3. **Compression**
   The thoracic cavity of most normal cats is relatively springy (with the exception of elderly cats, in which the normal compliance in the costrochondral junctions is lost). If there is increased density (be that increased air, fluid, inflammatory cells or neoplasia) within the chest, compressibility is decreased.
4. **Palpation**
   Palpation of the thorax, with identification of the apex beat is particularly useful. In cases of pleural effusion or pneumothorax, traumatic lesions may be noticed or, the apex beat is displaced. The latter is particularly common with effusions secondary to mediastinal masses.
5. **Auscultation**
   Fluid within the thorax often makes auscultation of the lungs and heart hard. Muffled sounds in a dyspnoeic cat increase suspicions that an effusion is present. If possible, careful assessment of the heart sounds and pulses helps identify the cause

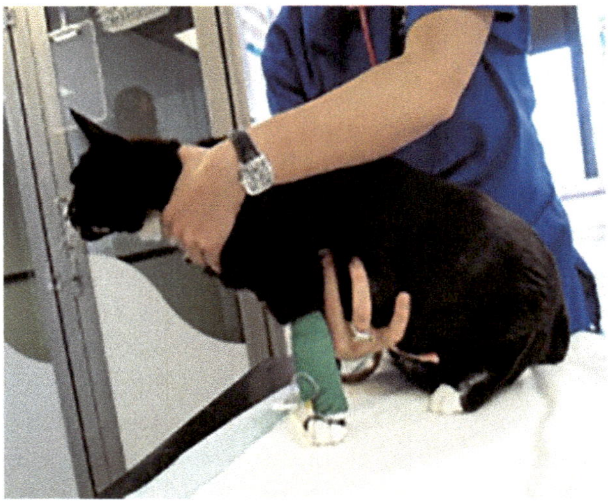

Figure 64. Thoracic compression.

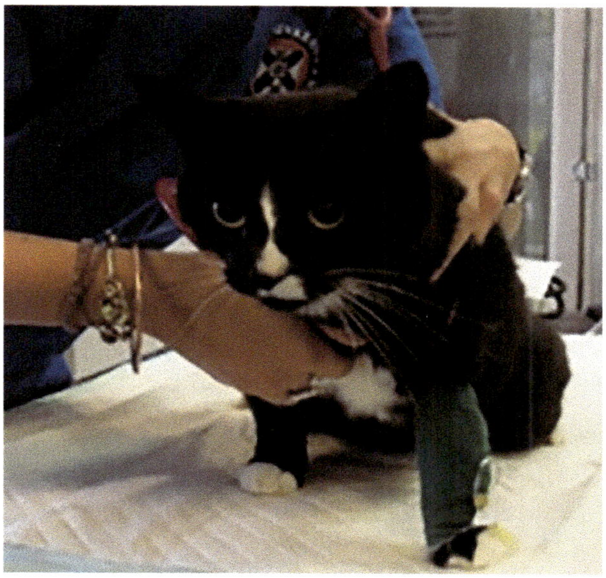

Figure 65. Thoracic auscultation.

of the effusion in cases with congestive heart failure. In addition to the criteria above ultrasound is very useful to confirm the presence and location of pleural fluid. Fluid density (black) with hepatization of the lungs is easily identifiable and can be assessed without removing the cat from the oxygenated environment.

Stabilisation of a cat with pleural effusion

Once the presence of pleural fluid or free gas is confirmed (or highly suspected), the cat should be stabilised prior to any further investigations. This involves draining the fluid or air from the thorax.

If possible an intravenous catheter should be placed at the earliest opportunity. Local anaesthetic cream such as EMLA can be used to decrease the stress involved with placement. In addition, the use of portable quiet clippers (such as those used in hair dressing salons), can reduce stress.

If the dyspnoeic cat is very stressed, **light sedation may be beneficial to reduce anxiety**, as cats in respiratory distress often panic when handled; the increased sympathetic drive increasing their demand for oxygen and leading to worsening of the clinical signs.

Emergency thoracocentesis is often required if the physical examination suggests the presence of an effusion. In such cases thoracocentesis can be life-saving and the risk of causing significant harm is minimal. In addition, obtaining samples of the fluid narrows the list of differentials. If a significant volume of fluid remains within the thoracic cavity further investigations (such as thoracic radiography) will not only be dangerous, but results will be virtually meaningless.

Thoracocentesis

Thoracocentesis is generally well tolerated, often even without sedation or local anaesthetic. Ultrasound-guidance is useful but not essential and can localise pockets of fluid or determine whether the effusion is bilateral or unilateral. However, if ultrasound is not available thoracic percussion may help in this assessment.

A 21- or 23-gauge butterfly needle, extension set and a three-way-tap are attached to a 10 or 20 ml syringe. Ideally the cat is positioned in sternal recumbency and the chest wall clipped and prepared aseptically to provide access to the thoracic cavity from the 7th to 8th intercostal space, at the level of the costrochondral junction. With the bevel facing the chest, the needle is inserted into the skin just caudal to the 8th rib and passed forward at a 45° angle, to enter the thoracic cavity just cranial to the rib (thereby avoiding the intercostal artery). Negative pressure (1–2 ml) should be gently applied to the syringe and the fluid aspirated.

Thoracocentesis is both a diagnostic and therapeutic procedure and samples should be obtained for culture, fluid analysis, and cytology. As much pleural fluid as possible should be removed. As the volume within the thorax decreases, it may be beneficial to angle the needle more ventrally down the thoracic wall. If purulent fluid is present, personnel should wear masks to avoid inhalation of potentially zoonotic material (i.e. *Nocardia* infection).

Thoracic drain placement

Alternatively, there are now thoracic drains available which can be placed in conscious cats. Thoracic drains are particularly useful in cases where repeated drainage, or lavage may be useful (i.e. pyothorax or chylothorax). These drains are introduced via a

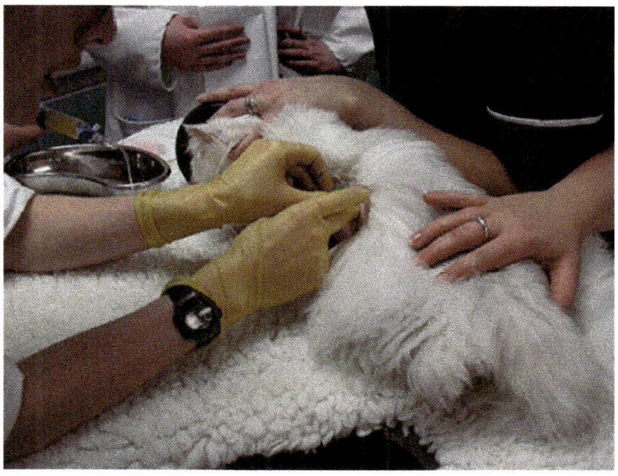

Figure 66. Thoracocentesis being performed in a cat. (Image courtesy of Prof D Gunn Moore).

Seldinger technique (described below) rather than the more traditional trochar drains, which require anaesthesia.

In a conscious patient, local anaesthetic should be injected into the muscle and the subcutis at the point of entry. A small incision should be made with a scalpel blade and the needle introducer introduced in exactly the same way as a needle would ordinarily be introduced into the thorax. A guide-wire should then be inserted into the introducer and fed forward into the thorax until it can no longer be easily advanced (approximately 10 cm in a cat). The needle should be withdrawn and a drain fed along the guide-wire into the thoracic cavity. Lastly, the guide-wire should be removed and a syringe valve placed on the end of the drain. The thorax is then drained, again using gentle pressure. Bilateral chest drains are often required to completely drain the thoracic cavity. As these drains have multiple side ports, very good results can be achieved, and once they have been radiographed to assess their location, they can remain in place and be used to repeatedly drain recurring effusions, or in the case of pyothorax, to lavage the chest.

Types of effusion

The pleural space is lined with mesothelial cells. These cells are supported by a layer of elastic connective tissue which contains arteries, veins, capillaries and lymphatics. The hydrostatic pressure within the parietal (systemic) capillaries is greater than within the visceral (pulmonic) capillaries. Therefore, there is a net movement of fluid out of the parietal capillaries, into the pleural space and then into the visceral pleural capillaries. In addition, the pleural lymphatics remove fluid via stomas between the mesothelial cells of the parietal pleural and endothelial cells of the pleural lymphatics. Pleural lymphatics generate a pressure of approximately 10 cmH20 (i.e. below atmospheric pressure). The rate at which the lymphatics can resorb pleural fluid is highly variable and when necessary, it can increase by approximately 20 times.

Pleural effusion can develop if the lymphatic drainage is impaired by decreased colloid oncotic pressure (i.e. hypoalbuminaemia), if there is increased venous pressure (i.e. congestive heart failure), increased lymphatic permeability (trauma or neoplastic processes), or if there are inflammatory diseases which result in vasculitis (i.e. FIP, pancreatitis, neoplasia), or venous or lymphatic obstruction, as can be seen with a lung lobe torsion or incarceration of a liver lobe through a diaphragmatic hernia. Determining the type of effusion can help to differentiate between potential aetiologies. Therefore, upon drainage samples should be taken for cytology, culture and fluid analysis.

Treatment

The treatment of pleural effusion depends on the underlying cause, for example, in the case of congestive heart failure, drainage and diuretics may be required. In other cases the underlying systemic disease may require specific treatment (i.e. hypoalbuminaemia). However, in certain circumstances pleural space disease requires specific therapy. This is particularly true in cases of chylous effusion and pyothorax.

Chylothorax

The treatment of chylothorax depends on the underlying cause. If a mass or congestive heart failure is identified, then treatment to decrease the pressure on the lymphatics will typically alleviate the effusion. However, often no underlying cause is identified and where idiopathic or traumatic aetiologies are suspected, drainage relieves the cats' distress in the short-term, if the effusion recurs. In such cases placement of a thoracic drain aids subsequent drainage. Typically, the fatty effusion continues to reform, in which case surgical options should be considered (thoracic duct ligation, pericardial strip, shunt placement and/or cisterna chyli ablation). In some cases, conservative management was trialled, involving the administration of the herbal medication Rutin, along with repeated drainage; but the efficacy of this approach has not been compared to that of drainage alone.

Pyothorax

Pyothorax will frequently recur after initial drainage. As the fluid is irritant, potentially leading to fibrosing pleuritis and severe respiratory compromise. Conservative management comprises of oxygen therapy, placement of thoracic drains, appropriate antibiotic cover (or broad-spectrum antibiotic cover until culture is returned), and thoracic lavage with 20 ml/kg warmed sterile saline every 6 hours. If an underlying pneumonia is present, nebulisation may be beneficial. In cases with extensive underlying pulmonary lesions and abscessation, surgical resection of one or more lung lobes may be warranted.

Neoplasia of the respiratory tract

Neoplasia can affect any part of the feline respiratory tract, with lymphoma and carcinoma being relatively common.

Pure transudate	Appearance: clear, colourless fluid
	Protein: Low <25 g/l
	Cellularity: Low <1500 cells/µl
	Specific gravity (SG) <1.015
	Primary cell type: mononuclear-macrophages and mesothelial cells are often present (low numbers) with occasional neutrophils and lymphocytes
		• decreased oncotic pressure
		• hypoalbuminaemia-protein losing nephropathy
		  • protein losing enteropathy
		  • liver failure
		• increased hydrostatic pressure
		• early congestive heart failure
		• pericardial effusion or constrictive pericarditis
		• heartworm infection
		• pulmonary thromboembolism
		• lung lobe torsion
		• caval syndrome
		• translocation of abdominal/retroperitoneal effusion
		• vasculitis (typically modified transudate)

Modified transudate
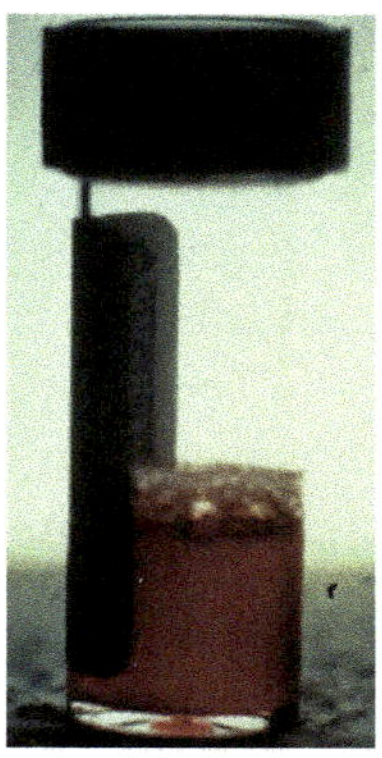
	Appearance: clear to slightly cloudy with a yellow, or pink tint.
	Contains additional protein (20–30 g/l) and/or cells (1500–5000 cells/µl)
	Specific gravity 1.020–1.030
	Caused by either increased hydrostatic pressure or increased vascular or lymphatic permeability
	In addition, to mesothelial cells and macrophages, neutrophils, lymphocytes, mast cells, eosinophils, and neoplastic cells may be seen
		• congestive heart failure
		• neoplasia
		• diaphragmatic hernia
		• systemic inflammation/infection
		  – sepsis
		  – pancreatitis
		  – lung lobe infection
		• immune mediated disease
		• anaphylactic reaction
		• increased hydrostatic pressure (see above)
		• translocation of abdominal/retroperitoneal effusion

Exudate 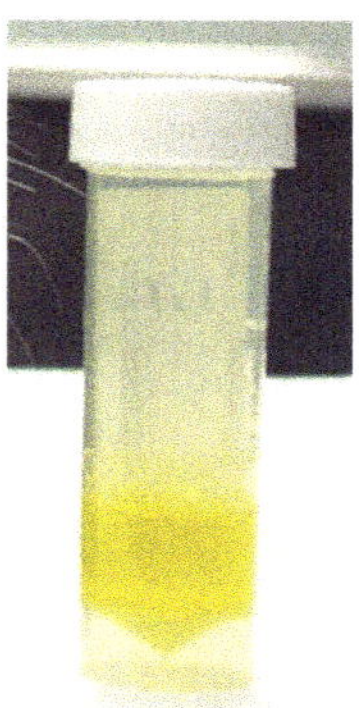	Appearance varies from purulent (pyothorax) to clear viscous fluid High protein content (>30 g/l) and higher nucleated cell counts (>5000 cells/µl) Specific gravity >1.015 Results from increased vascular permeability, decreased lymphatic removal, or both and can be caused by inflammatory or neoplastic processes or by diseases of the lymphatic system In cats if the cause is septic, Glu < 30 mg/dl & pH <6.9 High fibronectin in pleural fluid was 100% sensitive and 57% specific for a malignant effusion in cats Diagnosis of pyothorax is based on fluid analysis: protein count > 30 g/l, SG>1.025, nucleated cell count > 3000 cells/µl with predominant cell type degenerate neutrophils	• FIP • neoplasia • diaphragmatic hernia • lung lobe torsion • pyothorax • Bacterial infection of the pleural space is commonly associated with pyrexia 28–50% and coughing 14–30% – Serofibrinous pleuritis • systemic inflammation/infection • parasitic disease i.e. *Aelurostrongulus*
Blood 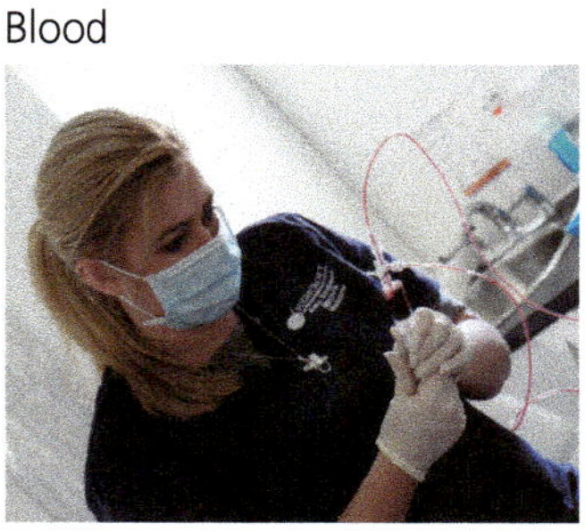	Appearance: resembles blood Assess if the blood is from active haemorrhage (i.e. will clot) or previous haemorrhage. Compare the PCV to circulatory PCV	• trauma • coagulopathy • neoplasia • lung lobe torsion • pulmonary infarction • pulmonary abscessation • heartworm disease • aortic aneurysm • iatrogenic

Chyle 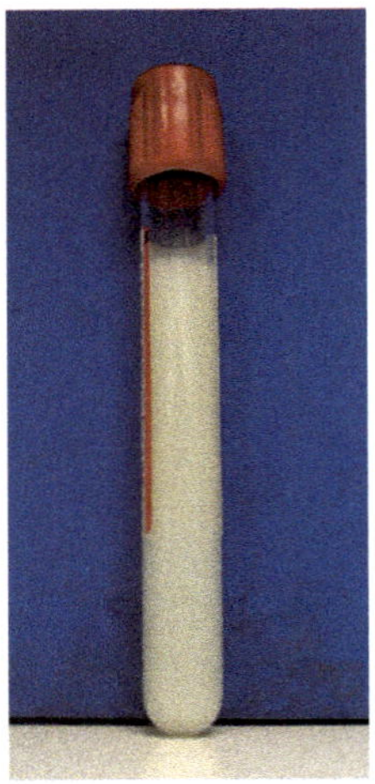	Appearance: pale pink or white Lymphatic fluid, similar to a modified transudate, but with triglyceride levels in the fluid are greater than those in plasma, cholesterol: triglyceride ratio of fluid is less than one; chylomicrons seen microscopically	• lymphangiectasia • congestive heart failure • cranial vena cava obstruction – heartworm – thrombus – fungal granuloma • neoplasia • diaphragmatic hernia • lung lobe torsion • trauma • Pericardial disease • Idiopathic

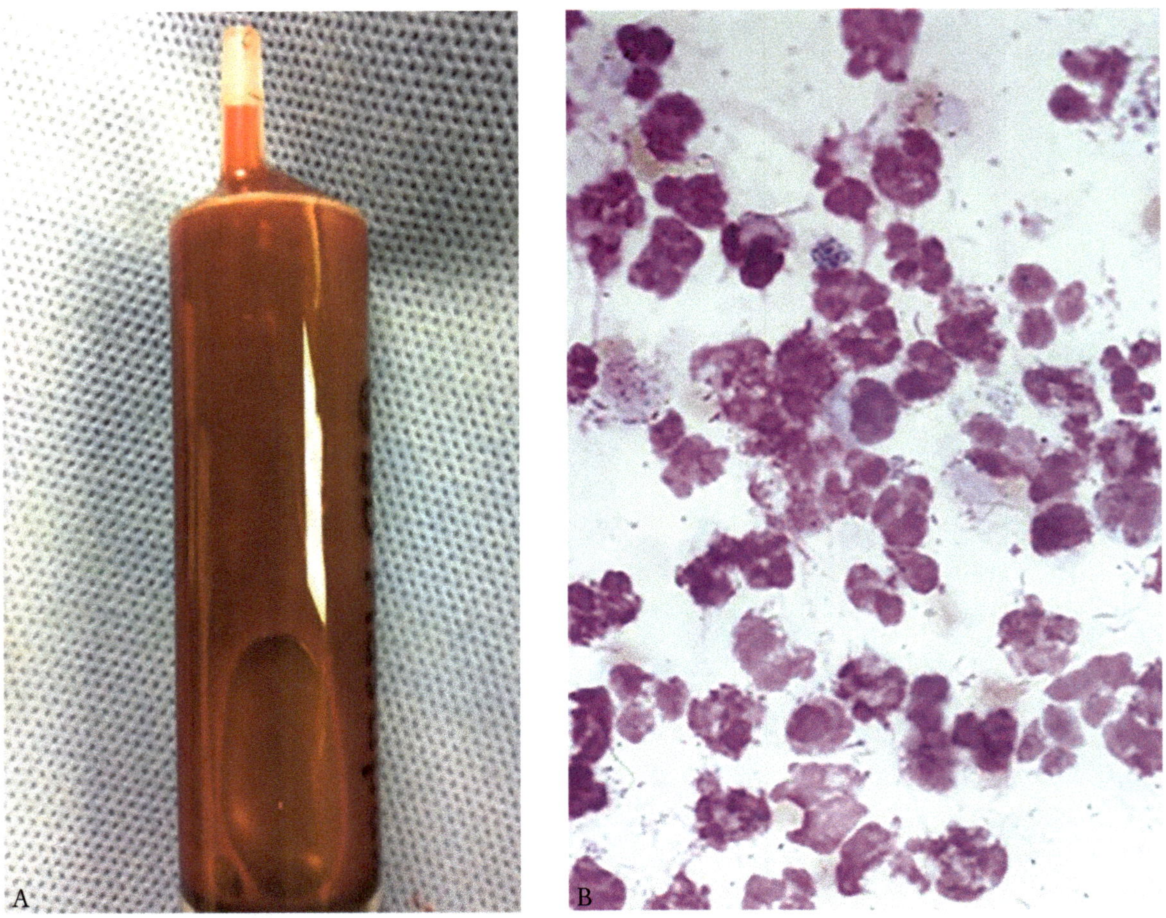

Figure 67. Drained fluid from pyothorax and pyothorax cytology.

Neoplasia by location

Nose and paranasal sinuses

Tumours of the nose and paranasal sinuses account for approximately 1% of all feline tumours. The incidence is higher in males than females, with the mean age at time of diagnosis being 12 years (Taylor et al., 2009; Fujiwara-Igarashi. A. et al., 2014; Santagostino et al., 2015). In the cat, over 90% of nasal tumours are malignant, with lymphoma being the most common, followed by carcinoma. Tumours of the nose and paranasal sinuses are typically very invasive locally but metastasize infrequently and late in the disease process. Common sites of metastasis are the regional lymph

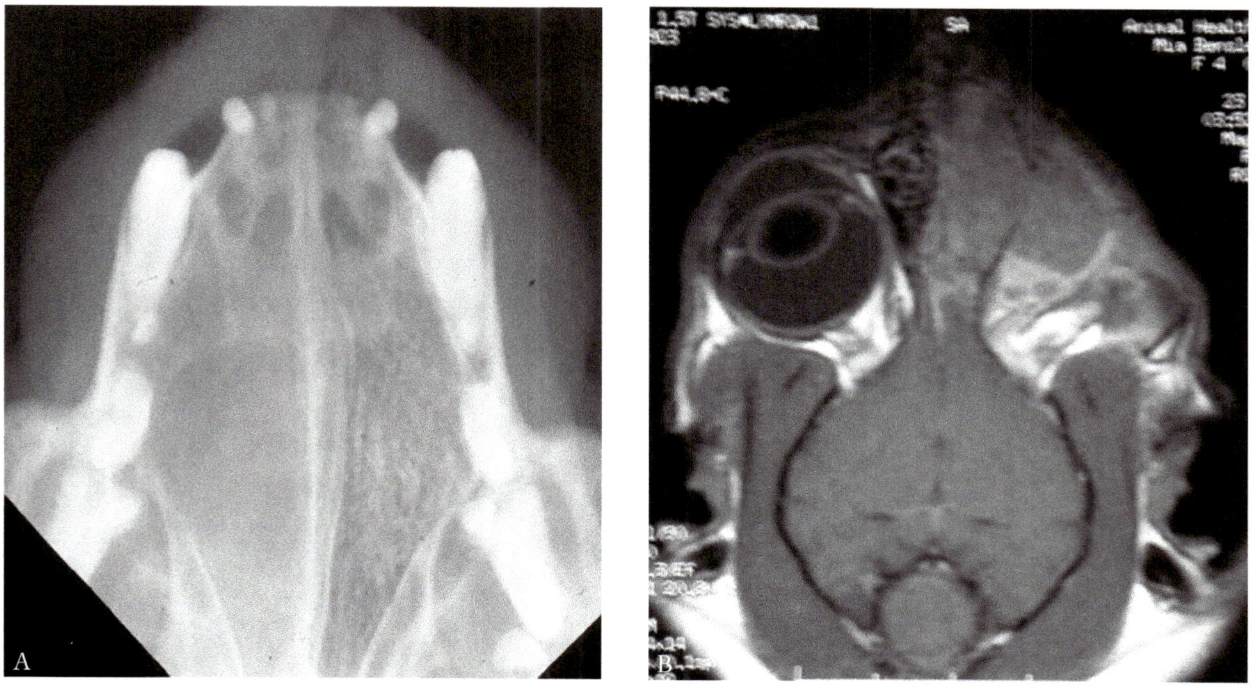

Figure 68. A case of feline nasal lymphoma. On MRI the tumour has penetrated the cribiform plate and entered the brain.

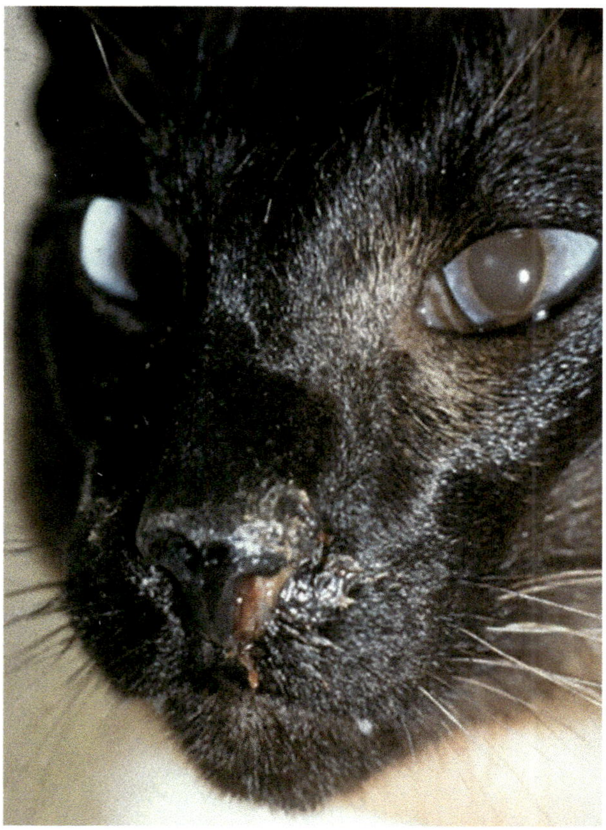

Figure 69. Loss of colour pointing and mucosanguinous discharge in a cat with retrobulbar extension of a nasal mass.

nodes, lungs, and brain. In general, the survival time of untreated animals is 3–5 months after diagnosis.

The most common presenting complaint is chronic nasal discharge of a mucoid, mucopurulent, or serosanguineous nature. Initially, the discharge is unilateral but often becomes bilateral with chronicity. Periodic sneezing, epistaxis, and respiratory stertor can also occur. Facial and oral deformities may develop as a result of destruction of bony or soft tissue sinonasal structures. Retrobulbar extension of these tumours can result in exophthalmos and exposure keratitis, or loss of colour-pointing on the affected side in pointed cats. Secondary epiphora may occur if the nasolacrimal duct is blocked. Late in the disease, neurological signs (e.g disorientation, blindness, seizures, stupor and coma) may develop if the tumour extends into the cranial vault.

Diagnosis is based on history, clinical findings, and elimination of other causes of nasal discharge, sneezing, or facial deformation. Nasal radiographs or CT typically show increased density of the nasal cavity and frontal sinuses as well as evidence of bone destruction. CT is vastly superior to plain radiography in diagnosis of chronic nasal diseases. Definitive diagnosis is based on biopsy of tumour tissue, either with blind biopsy based on CT lesion localization or on rhinoscopic visualization with direct biopsy. Nasal forced flush using a high-pressure saline infusion into the nose often yields diagnostic samples and, if large volumes of tumour tissue break free, nasal obstruction can be relieved immediately.

Treatment largely depends on tumour type and extent of disease. Lymphoma may be amenable to radiation therapy, or chemotherapy. The treatment of choice for nasal adenocarcinoma is radiation therapy. Aggressive surgical excision, chemotherapy, radiation therapy, or combinations for other tumour types

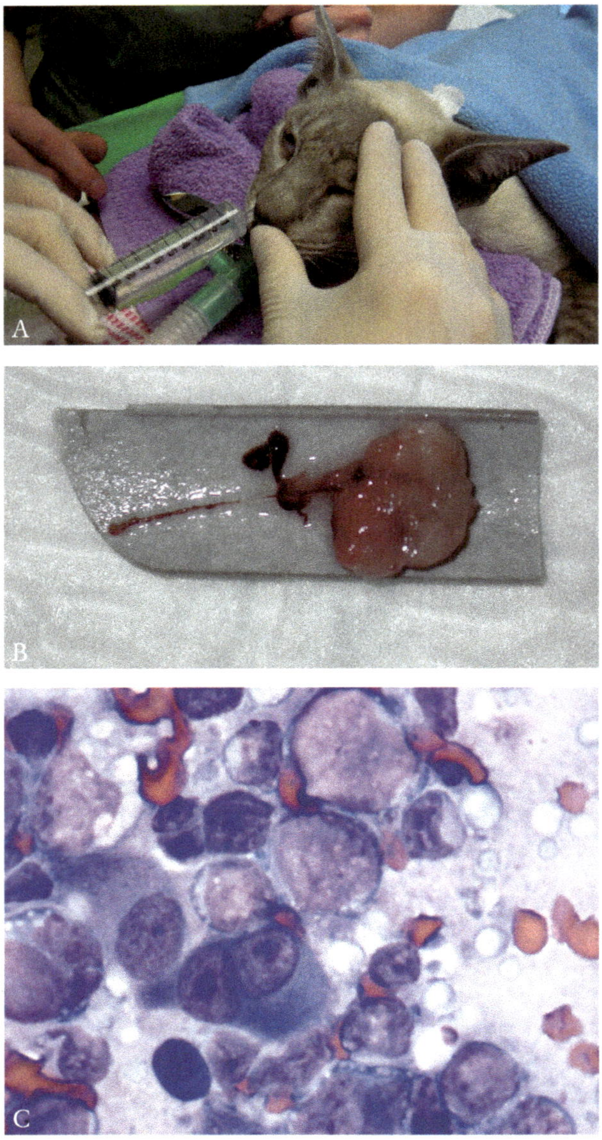

Figure 70. Nasal mass obtained via forced flushing (A, B)). Diagnosed on cytology (C) as nasal lymphoma.

afford a more favourable prognosis when diagnosis is made early.

Unfortunately, in some cases biopsy is non-diagnostic or demonstrates surface epithelial infection/inflammation, whilst CT suggests an aggressive infiltrative disease process. In such cases, carcinoma may be suspected (as lymphoma typically sheds easily), and treatment options discussed prior to further diagnostics (for example if radiation is not an option aggressive biopsy might not be in the cat's best interest).

Larynx and trachea

Tumours of the larynx and trachea are rare in cats. The most frequently encountered tumours of the larynx are squamous cell carcinoma, lymphoma, and adenocarcinoma. Benign inflammatory polyps and cysts of the larynx are also seen. If a cat presents with signs of laryngeal disease, polyp, cyst, or tumour should

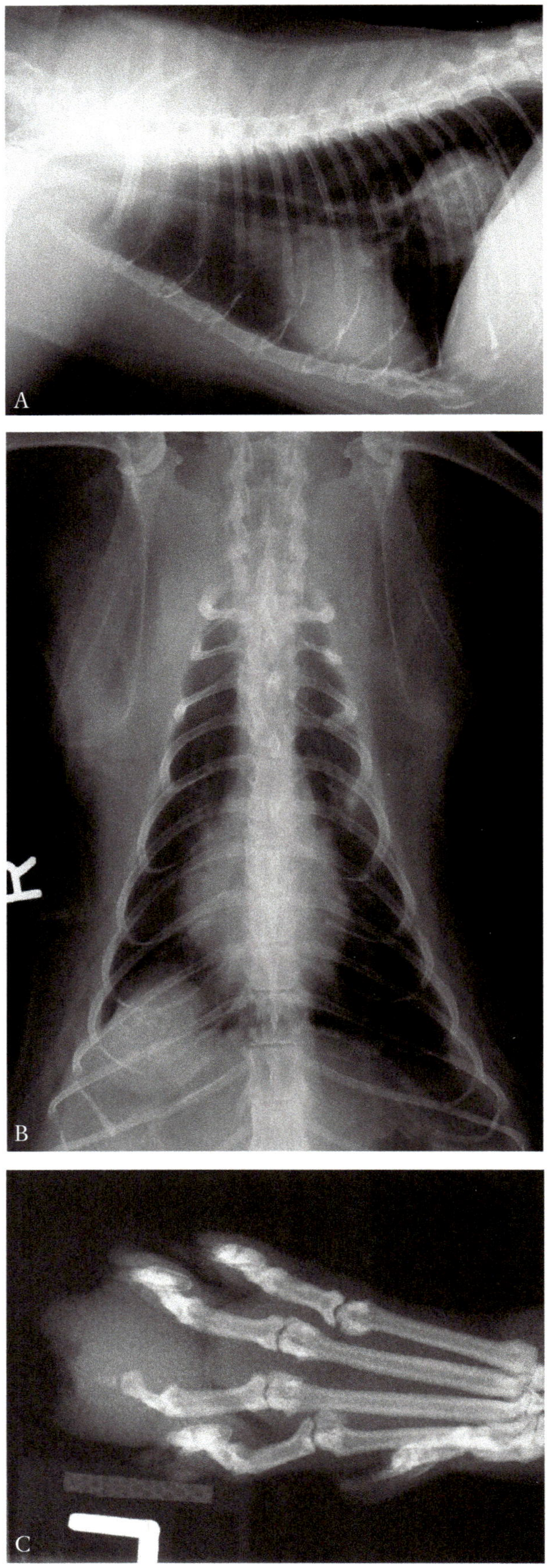

Figure 71. Thoracic and digital radiographs of a cat who presented for lameness and digital swelling. The thoracic mass was found on investigation (there were no clinical signs attributed to this at diagnosis). After digital amputation the cat survived a further five months before developing pleural effusion.

be considered the most likely differentials (unless thyroid surgery has recently been undertaken). Tumours of the trachea are rare.

The most common signs of tumours of the larynx include inspiratory dyspnoea, stridor, voice change, coughing, and exertional dyspnoea, whereas cases with tumours of the trachea typically present with coughing, dyspnoea, stridor, and (rarely) haemoptysis.

Diagnosis is made by eliminating other causes of upper airway obstruction or coughing. The tumour mass may be seen radiographically, on laryngoscopy, or tracheoscopy. Definitive diagnosis is made by cytology (aspirating or brushing the mass with an endoscopically guided cytology brush), or on histopathology, although taking a biopsy of a mass in the trachea is not without risk of haemorrhage and with this potential respiratory failure.

Lymphoma is ideally treated with chemotherapy, whereas other forms of tumour are more amenable to surgical excision (where possible). Radiation therapy may be palliative for radiosensitive tumours such as squamous cell carcinoma, mast cell tumour, and lymphoma.

Primary lung tumours

Primary lung tumours were once considered rare in small animals; however, an increased incidence has been reported within the last 20 years. This is attributed to an increased average life span, better detection and awareness, or possibly increased exposure to environmental carcinogens and better diagnostics. Most primary lung tumours are diagnosed at a mean age of 12 years in cats. There is no consistent breed or sex predilection (Taylor et al., 2009; Nunley et al., 2015; Fowler et al., 2020).

The majority of primary lung tumours in cats are malignant (over 80%), with adenocarcinoma, alveolar carcinoma, and lymphoma being the most common types. Primary lung sarcomas and adenomas are rarely reported. Metastatic spread of primary lung tumours is generally to other areas of the lungs, tracheobronchial lymph nodes, bone, and brain, although metastatic spread to the pleurae, pericardium, heart, and diaphragm may occur and at times extrathoracic sites including the liver, spleen, kidney or digits may be affected (the latter being known as lung-digit syndrome).

Clinical signs

Clinical signs tend to be vague in cats; coughing is uncommon, and presentation is often nonspecific, such as inappetence, weight loss, and occasionally tachypnoea and dyspnoea. This presentation often results in pulmonary neoplasia being diagnosed late in the disease process. Thoracic auscultation may be normal, reflect increased breath sounds compatible with pulmonary airway disease, or be muffled because of pulmonary consolidation or pleural effusion. Percussion can be useful in identifying an area of decreased resonance. If pleural effusion is present an inspiratory restrictive breathing pattern may be seen.

Diagnosis

One-third or more of primary lung tumours are recognized incidentally during radiography for other problems or at necropsy. Thoracic radiographs are essential for a tentative diagnosis in animals exhibiting compatible clinical signs. In cats, single circumscribed mass lesions are not common, whereas a diffuse lung pattern or lobar consolidation is seen more frequently. Pleural fluid accumulation is common and chest wall involvement and hilar lymphadenopathy may be seen. Tentative diagnosis is made by excluding other causes of pulmonary disease with similar radiographic lung patterns. However, definitive diagnosis requires cytology (FNA may be possible in peripherally located lesions) or histopathology (either via Tru-cut in peripherally located lesions, or surgical excision).

Treatment

Pulmonary carcinoma may be amenable to surgery if there is a single nodule. In cats, the median survival time for pulmonary carcinoma is approximately 156 days (Nunley et al., 2015). However, this is highly variable, with survival of cats with lymph node enlargement being 65 days versus 498 days for cats without lymph node enlargement (based on preoperative CT). Furthermore, in the same study, the median survival

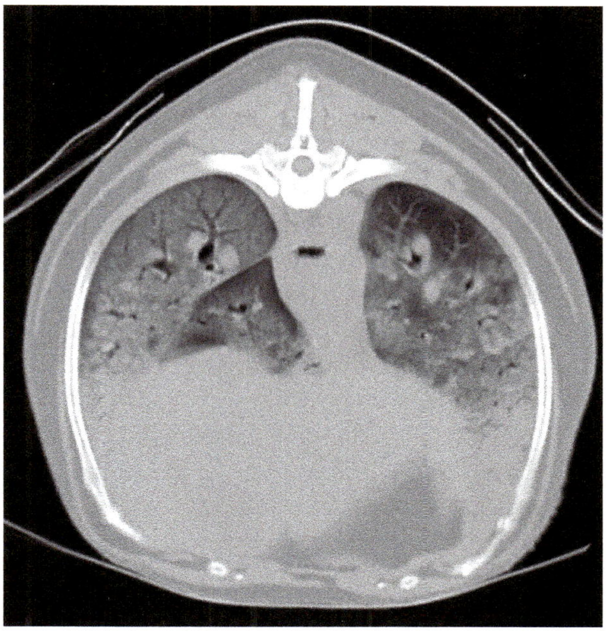

Figure 72. Lymphoma can cause either nodular or diffuse interstitial disease. The latter is often hard to diagnose as the interstitium is difficult to sample.

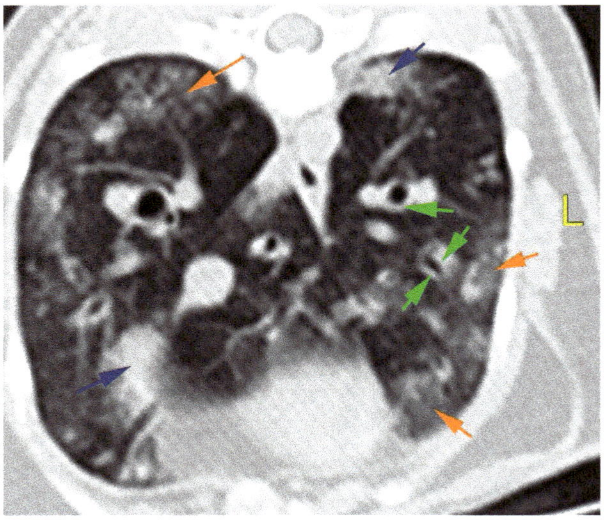

Figure 73. CT of a pulmonary carcinoma.

time for cats with preoperative pleural effusion was 2.5 days versus 467 days for cats without pleural effusion. In addition, cats with low or intermediate grade tumours had a median survival time of 730 days versus 105 days for cats with high grade tumours (Nunley et al., 2015).

Metastatic tumours of the lungs

A localized tumour may extend to the lungs by dissemination through haematogenous or lymphatic routes or by direct extension of tumour cells. Certain primary tumours, such as mammary adenocarcinoma, osteosarcoma, haemangiosarcoma, and oral melanoma commonly metastasize to the lungs. However, in general pulmonary metastasis occurs late in the clinical course of a malignant tumour and the prognosis is poor.

The signs of metastatic pulmonary disease are similar to those of primary lung tumours except coughing is less common. Severity of signs depends on the anatomic location of the tumour and whether the lesions are solitary or multiple.

Establishing a diagnosis is as for primary lung tumours. Because of the limitations of routine radiography, small lesions (≤3 mm in diameter) may not be seen, which are present in over 40% of cases with pulmonary metastasis. Therefore, thoracic CT is the imaging modality of choice.

Radiography or CT of the chest should precede removal of tumours with a known high incidence of metastatic spread to the lungs. The major goal of cancer therapy is prevention of metastasis rather than cancer eradication. Slow-growing or solitary metastatic lesions are best treated by surgical excision. Chemotherapy or radiation therapy may be useful with certain tumour types not amenable to surgical resection. Overall, the prognosis for animals with pulmonary metastasis is poor.

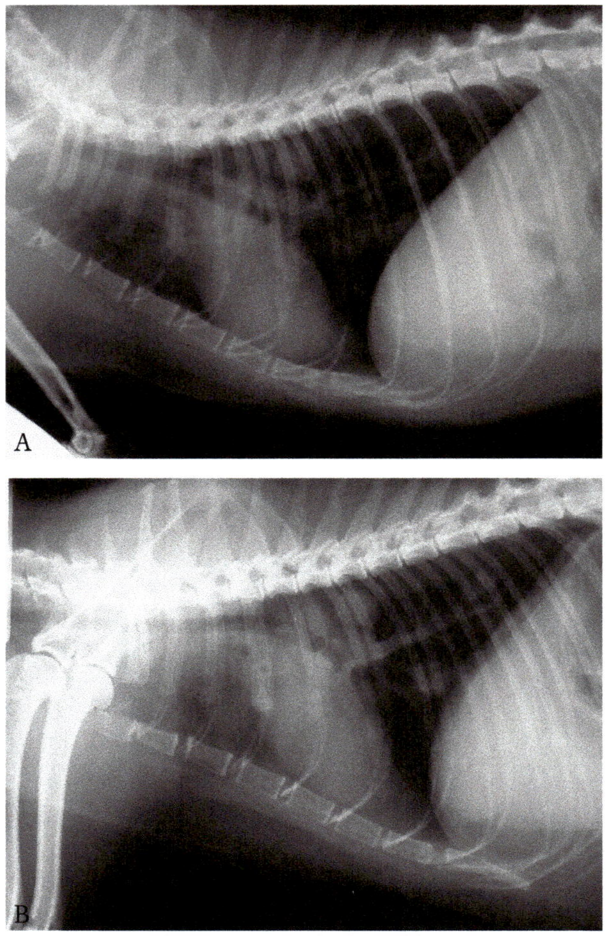

Figure 74. Left (A) and right (B) lateral radiographs of a cat with pulmonary metastases.

Mediastinal disease

Mediastinal disease can occur with trauma (most common), infection/inflammation, neoplasia, or secondary to a foreign body.

Clinical signs

Clinical signs of mediastinal disease are usually associated with pressure on structures within the mediastinum and involve one or more of the following:

- respiratory signs
- laryngeal paralysis
- oesophageal, gastrointestinal signs (regurgitation, dysphagia)
- Horner's syndrome
- vena cava syndrome (head and forelimb oedema)
- right-sided cardiac failure (pericardiodiaphragmatic hernia)
- cardiac dysrhythmia (sinus arrhythmia).

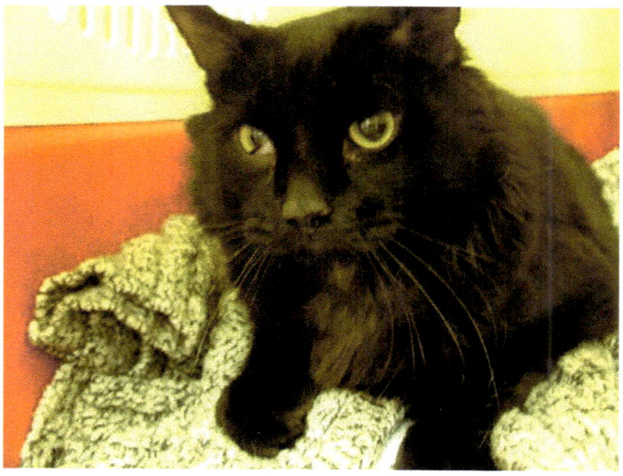

Figure 75. A cat with Horner's syndrome due to a mediastinal lymphoma.

Diagnosis

Imaging of the mediastinum is best performed using CT (although radiography can be used). In addition, fluid or masses may be evident on ultrasonography. The carina should be located at the 6th intercostal space in cats on lateral radiography. Displacement implies the presence of a soft tissue structure within the mediastinum. CT or ultrasound guided aspirates aid in the diagnosis although some cases require surgical biopsy.

In young animals the mediastinum may appear wide, but this may be due to the normal size and shape of the juvenile thymus.

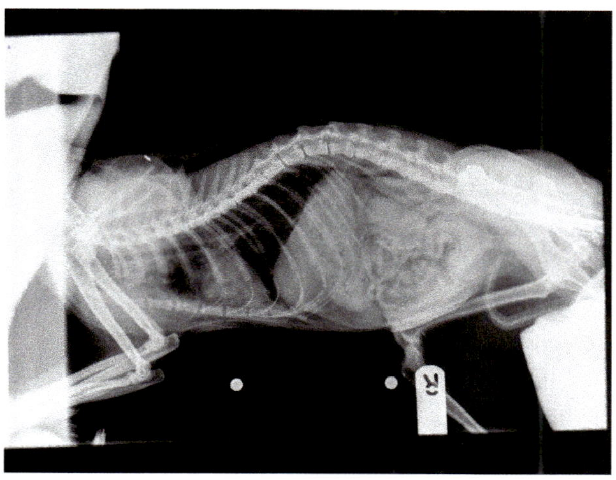

Figure 76. Radiograph of a cat with subcutaneous emphysema and intermittent dyspnoea post trauma (the scapula is also fractured). The cat did not demonstrate respiratory compromise until three weeks after the inciting event, and at the time of radiograph it was mild, with the emphysema seen to be resolving. The tear within the airway (location not identified) was left to heal and the signs resolved over the next few weeks. (Image courtesy of Dr S Radford).

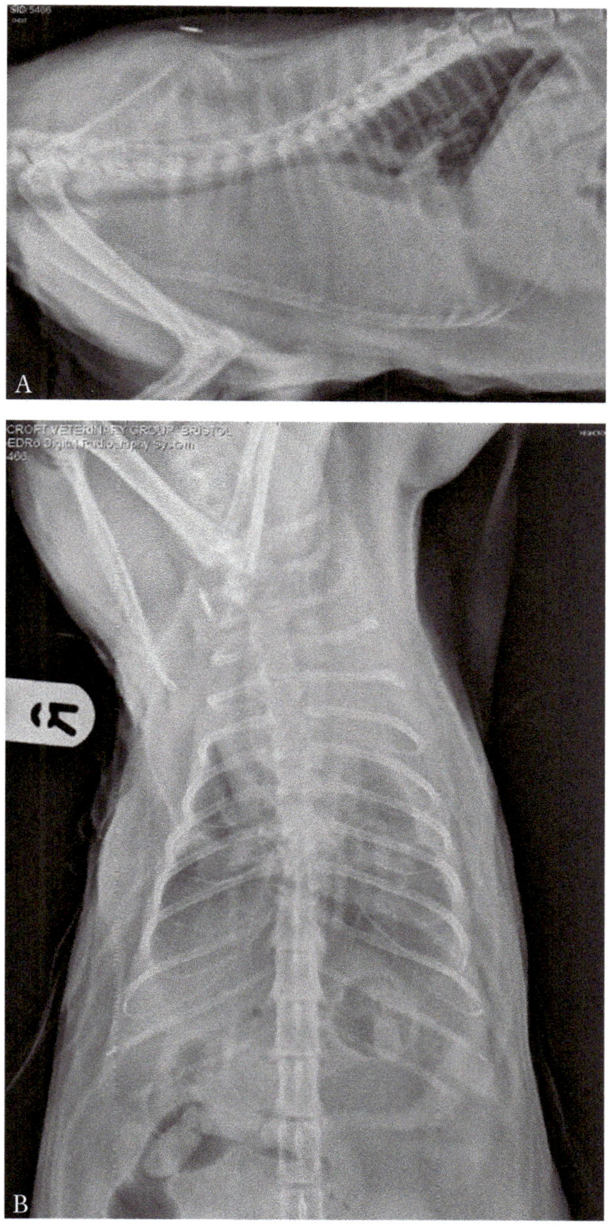

Figure 77. Pleural fluid and a mediastinal mass in a 10 years old cat presented for sudden onset dyspnoea.

Pneumomediastinum

Air enters mediastinal space from the trachea, bronchi, lungs or oesophagus. Affected cases present with **breathing difficulties and subcutaneous emphysema**. This can be a consequence of trauma (most common), neoplastic erosion, or iatrogenic. This results in enhanced visibility of mediastinal structures on radiography; the outer edges of the tracheal wall, azygous vein and major vessels of the mediastinum are often easily visualised. In cats, the most common cause is trauma (a fall or road traffic accident), which results in tearing of the trachea or main stem bronchus. Often the soft tissues stabilise this after the initial insult, and clinical signs may take days/weeks to become apparent. Intubation of these cases can worsen the tear. In some cases, the tear can seal, and the pneumomediastinum resolves, but complete resolution can take up to three weeks. However, in others the breathing is severely compromised and therefore, surgical intervention required.

Mediastinitis

Mediastinitis can occur secondary to oesophageal or tracheal perforation, deep cervical infections extending along fascial planes, extension from the pericardium or from the pleural space. Chronic granulomatous infection with mycoses or bacteria such as *Actinomyces* or *Nocardia* have also been reported. Abscessation may result from chronic disorders or neoplasia.

Cases with mediastinitis can present with signs of mediastinal disease (as above), along with pain and/or pyrexia.

Mediastinal neoplasia

Lesions within the mediastinum are not uncommon. **The most common mediastinal masses in cats are lymphoma and thymoma**, followed by cystic lesions and ectopic thyroid. Mediastinal masses may cause pleural effusion, compression of the oesophagus, increased vagal tone, or occasionally paraneoplastic syndrome (such as myasthenia gravis or exfoliative dermatitis). Therefore, the presentation of cats with mediastinal masses is highly variable.

Common presentations include weight loss, cough and regurgitation, dyspnoea and tachypnoea. Physical examination often detects a sinus arrhythmia, relative bradycardia, decreased thoracic resonance on percussion, decreased compressibility of the thorax, displacement of the cardiac apex beat, and in some cases attributable to pleural effusion.

Thymoma

Thymoma is a tumour of the thymic epithelial cells, typically seen in middle aged or older cats. **Feline thymoma has been associated with paraneoplastic syndromes such as myasthenia gravis or exfoliative dermatitis.** Ultrasound, CT or radiography may demonstrate the presence of a mediastinal mass, which can be solid, cystic, or both. Cytology is often performed to differentiate thymoma from lymphoma (although this can be problematic as small lymphocytes may be present in both diseases). Treatment of choice for feline thymomas is surgery, however, it is advisable to assess the invasiveness of the mass on CT prior to surgery (although typically feline

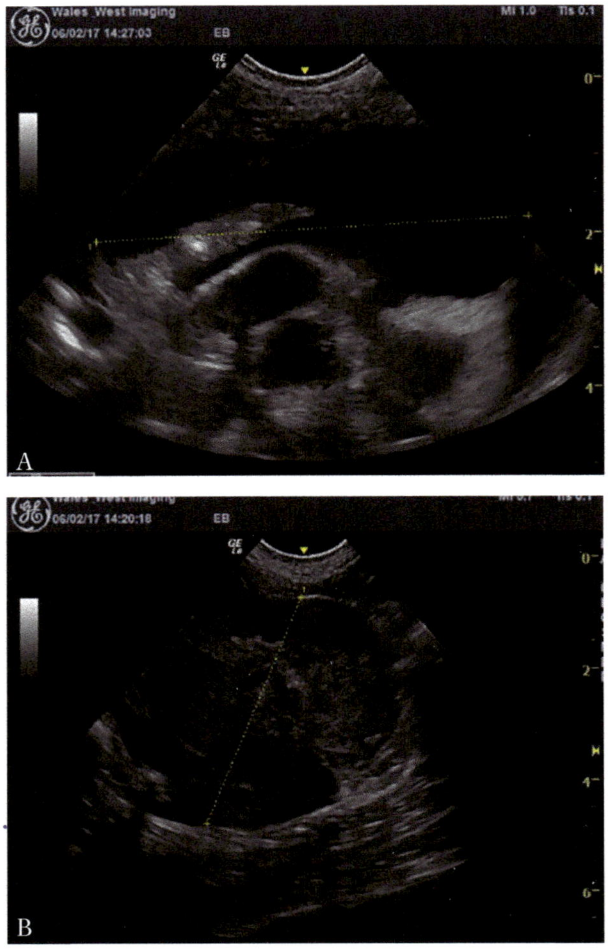

Figure 78. Moderate effusion and mass identified on ultrasound of the 10 years old cat presented for sudden onset dyspnoea (radiographs shown previously). Aspirates of the mass demonstrated this to be a thymoma.

thymoma is more encapsulated than canine thymoma). Thymomas are approached through a median sternotomy or intercostal thoracotomy. In many cases prognosis after surgical resection is excellent (median survival time of 1825 days), however, this may be shorter in cases where there are concurrent paraneoplastic diseases or metastases (Zitz et al., 2008).

Lymphoma

Mediastinal lymphoma in the cat typically affects young cats, and males and Siamese cats are predisposed (Fabrizio et al., 2014). It is no longer associated with FeLV infection. The presentation is similar to that of thymoma, with the two diseases being differentiated on cytology. The treatment of choice is chemotherapy, with the best outcomes achieved with multidrug protocols such as CHOP (vincristine, cyclophosphamide, doxorubicin and prednisolone) or COP (cyclophosphamide, vincristine and prednisolone) (Fabrizio et al., 2014). The prognosis appears highly variable, with some studies reporting response rates of around 90%.

Cats that experience complete remission have been reported to have a median survival time of 262–980 days whereas cats that have a partial response have a reported median survival time of 42 days (Fabrizio et al., 2014).

Bibliography

Barrs, V. R. & Beatty, J. A. 2009. Feline pyothorax – new insights into an old problem: part 1. Aetiopathogenesis and diagnostic investigation. *The Veterinary Journal*, 179, 163–170.

Barrs, V. R. 2020. Fungal Rhinosinusitis and Disseminated Invasive Aspergillosis in Cats. *Veterinary Clinics of North America Small Animal Practice*, 50, 331–357.

Brooks, J. W., Roberts, E. L., Kocher, L., Kariyawasam, S. & Debroy, C. 2013. Fatal pneumonia caused by Extraintestinal Pathogenic Escherichia coli (ExPEC) in a juvenile cat recovered from an animal hoarding incident *Veterinary Microbiology*, 167, 704–707.

Cohn, L. A. 2011. Feline Respiratory Disease Complex. *Veterinary Clinics of North America Small Animal Practice*, 41, 1273–1289.

Cohn, L. A., Norris, C. R., Hawkins, E. C., Dye, J. A., Johnson, C. A. & Williams, K. J. 2004. Identification and characterization of an idiopathic pulmonary fibrosis-like condition in cats. *Journal of Veterinary Internal Medicine*, 18, 632–641.

Dear, J. D. 2020. Bacterial Pneumonia in Dogs and Cats. *Veterinary Clinics of North America Small Animal Practice*, 50, 447–465.

Dirven, M., Szatmári, V., Van Den Ingh, T. & Nijsse, R. 2012. Reversible pulmonary hypertension associated with lungworm infection in a young cat. *Journal of Veterinary Cardiology*, 14, 465–474.

Egberink, H., Addie, D., Belák, S., Boucraut-Baralon, C., Frymus, T., Gruffydd-Jones, T., Hartmann, K., Hosie, M. J., Lloret, A., Lutz, H., Marsilio, F., Pennisi, M. G., Radford, A. D., Thiry, E., Truyen, U. & Horzinek, M. C. 2009. Bordetella bronchiseptica infection in cats. ABCD guidelines on prevention and management. *Journal of Feline Medicine & Surgery*, 11, 610–614. 10.1016/j.jfms.2009.05.010.

Evola, M. G., Edmondson, E. F., Reichle, J. K., Biller, D. S., Mitchell, C. W. & Valdés-Martínez, A. 2014. Radiographic and histopathologic characteristics of pulmonary fibrosis in nine cats. *Veterinary Radiology and Ultrasound*, 55, 133–140.

Fabrizio, F., Calam, A. E., Dobson, J. M., Middleton, S. A., Murphy, S., Taylor, S. S., Schwartz, A. & Stell, A. J. 2014. Feline mediastinal lymphoma: a retrospective study of signalment, retroviral status, response to chemotherapy and prognostic indicators. *Journal of Feline Medicine & Surgery*, 16, 637–644

Fowler, B. L., Johannes, C. M., O'connor, A., Collins, D., Lustgarten, J., Yuan, C., Weishaar, K., Sullivan, K., Hume, K. R., Mahoney, J., Vale, B., Schubert, A., Ball, V., Cooley-Lock, K., Curran, K. M., Nafe, L., Gedney, A., Weatherford, M. & Levine, D. N. 2020. Ecological level analysis of primary lung tumors in dogs and cats and environmental radon activity. *Journal of Veterinary Internal Medicine*, 34, 2660–2670.

Fujiwara-Igarashi. A., Fujimori, T., Oka, M., Nishimura, Y., Hamamoto, Y., Kazato, Y., Sawada, H., Yayoshi, N., Hasegawa, D. & Fujita, M. 2014. Evaluation of outcomes and radiation complications in 65 cats with nasal tumours treated with palliative hypofractionated radiotherapy. *The Veterinary Journal*, 202, 455–461.

Garrity, S., Lee-Fowler, T. & Reinero, C. 2019. Feline Asthma and Heartworm Disease: Clinical Features, Diagnostics and therapeutics. *Journal of Feline Medicine & Surgery*, 21, 825–834.

Gaskell, R., Dawson, S., Radford, A. & Thiry, E. 2007. Feline herpesvirus. *Veterinary Research*, 38, 337–354. 10.1051/vetres:2006063.

Gruffydd-Jones, T., Addie, D., Belák, S., Boucraut-Baralon, C., Egberink, H., Frymus, T., Hartmann, K., Hosie, M. J., Lloret, A., Lutz, H., Marsilio, F., Pennisi, M. G., Radford, A. D., Thiry, E., Truyen, U. & Horzinek, M. C. 2009. Chlamydophila felis infection. ABCD guidelines on prevention and management. *Journal of Feline Medicine & Surgery*, 11 605–609. 10.1016/j.jfms.2009.05.009.

Hargis, A. M. & Ginn, P. E. 1999. Feline herpesvirus 1-associated facial and nasal dermatitis and stomatitis in domestic cats. *Veterinary Clinics of North America Small Animal Practice*, 29, 1281–1290.

Jaffey, J. A., Williams, K. J., Masseau, I., Krueger, M. & Reinero, C. 2017. Vasoproliferative process resembling pulmonary capillary hemangiomatosis in a cat. *BMC Veterinary Research*, 13, 72.

Jennie Mcinerney, J., Papasouliotis, K., Simpson, K., English, K., Cook, S., Milne, E. & Gunn-Moore, D. A. 2016. Pulmonary cowpox in cats: five cases. *Journal of Feline Medicine & Surgery*, 18

Jenkins, T. L. & Jennings, R. N. 2017. Pulmonary capillary hemangiomatosis and hypertrophic cardiomyopathy in a Persian cat. *Journal of Veterinary Diagnostic Investigation*, 29, 900–903.

King, L. G. 2004. *Respiratory Disease in Dogs and Cats*, London, UK, Elsevier Health Sciences.

Lundsgaard, C. & Van Slyke, D. D. 1923. Cyanosis. *Medicine*, 2, 1–76.

Mawby, D. I., Whittemore, J. C. & Donnell, R. L. 2018. Fatal pulmonary hemorrhage associated with vascular amyloid deposition in a cat. *Journal of Feline Medicine and Surgery Open Reports*, 4, 2055116918817993.

Nunley, J., Sutton, J., Culp, W., Wilson, D., Coleman, K., Demianiuk, R., Schechter, A., Moore, G., Donovan, T. & Schwartz, P. 2015. Primary pulmonary neoplasia in cats: assessment of computed tomography findings and survival. *Journal of Small Animal Practice*, 56, 651–656.

Pennisi, M. G., Hartmann, K., Addie, D. D., Boucraut-Baralon, C., Egberink, H., Frymus, T., Gruffydd-Jones, T., Horzinek, M. C., Hosie, M. J., Lloret, A., Lutz, h., Marsilio, F., Radford, A. D., Thiry, e., truyen, U. & Möstl, K. 2015. Lungworm disease in cats: ABCD guidelines on prevention and management. *Journal of Feline Medicine & Surgery*, 17, 626–636. 10.1177/1098612X15588455.

Pennisi, M. G., Tasker, S., Hartmann, K., Belák, S., Addie, D., Boucraut-Baralon, C., Egberink, H., Frymus, T., Hofmann-Lehmann, R., Hosie, M., Lloret, A., Marsilio, F., Thiry, E., Truyen, U. & Möstl, K. 2020. Dirofilarioses in cats: European guidelines from the ABCD on prevention and management. *Journal of Feline Medicine & Surgery*, 22, 442–451. 10.1177/1098612X20917601.

Radford, A. D., Addie, D., Belák, S., Boucraut-Baralon, C.,

Egberink, H., Frymus, T., Gruffydd-Jones, T., Hartmann, K., Hosie, M. J., Lloret, A., Lutz, H., Marsilio, F., Pennisi, M. G., Thiry, E., Truyen, U. & horzinek, M. C. 2009. Feline calicivirus infection. ABCD guidelines on prevention and management. *Journal of Feline Medicine & Surgery*, 11, 556–564. 10.1016/j.jfms.2009.05.004.

Radford, A. D., Coyne, K. P., Dawson, S., Porter, C. J. & Gaskell, R. M. 2007. Feline Calicivirus. *Veterinary Research*, 38, 319–335. 10.1051/vetres:2006056.

Rawlings, C. A. 1990. Pulmonary arteriography and hemodynamics during feline heartworm disease. Effect of aspirin. *Journal of Veterinary Internal Medicine*, 4, 285–291.

Reed, N. 2020. Chronic Rhinitis in the Cat: An Update. *Veterinary Clinics of North America Small Animal Practice*, 50, 311–329.

Reed, N., Simpson, K. E., Ayling, R., Nicholas, R. & Gunn-Moore, D. A. 2012. Mycoplasma species in cats with lower airway disease: improved detection and species identification using a polymerase chain reaction assay. *Journal of Feline Medicine and Surgery*, 14, 833–840.

Reinero, C. 2019a. Interstitial lung diseases in dogs and cats part II: Known cause and other discrete forms. *Veterinary Journal*, 243, 55–64.

Reinero, C. 2019b. Interstitial lung diseases in dogs and cats part I: The idiopathic interstitial pneumonias. *The Veterinary Journal*, 243, 48–54.

Reinero, C. R., Masseau, I., Grobman, M., Vientos-Plotts, A. & Williams, K. 2019. Perspectives in veterinary medicine: Description and classification of bronchiolar disorders in cats. *Journal of Veterinary Internal Medicine*, 33, 1201–1221.

Reinero, C., Visser, L. C., Kellihan, H. B., Masseau, I., Rozanski, E., Clerx, C., Williams, K., Abbott, J., Borgarelli, M. & Scansen, B. A. 2020. ACVIM consensus statement guidelines for the diagnosis, classification, treatment, and monitoring of pulmonary hypertension in dogs. *Journal of Veterinary Internal Medicine*, 34, 549–573.

Santagostino, S. F., Mortellaro, C. M., Boracchi, P., Avallone, G., Caniatti, M., Forlani, A. & Roccabianca, P. 2015. Feline upper respiratory tract lymphoma: site, cyto-histology, phenotype, FeLV expression, and prognosis. *Veterinary Pathology*, 52, 250–259.

Schützer, K. M., Haglund, U. & Falk, A. 1987. The role of prostanoids in the feline intestinal vascular and central haemodynamic responses to i.v. infusion of live E. coli. *Acta Physiology Scandanavian*, 130, 359–366.

Simpson, K. E. 2013. Heart Murmur. *In:* Harvey, A. & Tasker, S. (eds.) *BSAVA Manual of Feline Practice*. BSAVA.

Sottiaux, J. & Franck, M. 1999. Pulmonary embolism and cor pulmonale in a cat. *Journal of Small Animal Practice*, 40, 88–91.

Speakman, A. J., Dawson, S., Binns, S. H., Gaskell, C. J., Hart, C. & Gaskell, R. M. 1999. Bordetella bronchiseptica infection in the cat. *Journal of Small Animal Practice*, 40, 252–256.

Taylor, S. S., Goodfellow, M. R., Browne, W. J., Walding, B., Murphy, S., Tzannes, S., Gerou-Ferriani, M., Schwartz, A. & Dobson, J. M., J Small Anim Pract. 2009 NOV;50(11): 584–92 2009. Feline extranodal lymphoma: response to chemotherapy and survival in 110 cats. *Journal of Small Animal Practice*, 50, 584–592.

Thiry, E., Addie, D., Belák, S., Boucraut-Baralon, C., Egberink, H., Frymus, T., Gruffydd-Jones, T., Hartmann, K., Hosie, M. J., Lloret, A., Lutz, H., Marsilio, F., Pennisi, M. G., Radford, A. D., Truyen, U. & Horzinek, M. C. 2009. Feline herpesvirus infection. ABCD guidelines on prevention and management. *Journal of Feline Medicine & Surgery*, 11, 547–555. 10.1016/j.jfms.2009.05.003.

Thomasy, S. M. & Maggs, D. J. 2016. A review of antiviral drugs and other compounds with activity against feline herpesvirus type 1. *Veterinary Ophthalmology*, 2016, 119–130.

Trzil, J. E. 2020. Feline Asthma: Diagnostic and Treatment Update. *Veterinary Clinics of North America Small Animal Practice*, 50, 375–391.

Vezzosi, T. & Schober, K. E. 2019. Doppler-derived echocardiographic evidence of pulmonary hypertension in cats with left-sided congestive heart failure. *Journal of Veterinary Cardiology*, 23, 58–68.

Wardley R. C. & Povey R. C. 1977. The clinical disease and patterns of excretion associated with three different strains of feline calicivirus. *Research in Veterinary Science*, 23, 7–14.

Zitz, J. C., Birchard, S. J., Couto, G. C., Samii, V. F., Weisbrode, S. E. & Young, G. S. 2008. Results of excision of thymoma in cats and dogs: 20 cases (1984–2005). *Journal of the American Veterinary Medical Association*, 232, 1186–1192.

Case studies

Case 1: "Lucy"

Patient details

2-year old, female neutered, domestic shorthair (DSH)
5-day history of dyspnoea and dysphonia
Indoor/outdoor (hunts, mainly mice)
Fully vaccinated
Not wormed
Housed with 2 cats and one dog (other cat is well. The dog was rehomed from a shelter 10 days ago and so far, appears well)
No overseas travel and no previous medical problems

History

Presented to her vet for difficulty breathing and loss of voice
Temperature 40.2 °C
Amoxycillin clavulanate was given subcutaneously
24-hrs later Lucy was deteriorating so was switched to enrofloxacin (there is a risk of retinopathy in cats with this drug and it is not advised if alternative fluoroquinolones are available)
After 36 hours she continued to deteriorate
Dexamethasone was administered
No other abnormalities noted on physical exam, except for small scab that was removed from her chin

Clinical examination

Stridor, mouth breathing and marked dyspnoea (inspiratory and expiratory)
BCS 3/9
HR 120 bpm
Sinus arrhythmia
RR 28 bpm, crackles and wheezes audible throughout lung fields
No other abnormalities

- **What are the problems identified and their differential diagnoses?**

Lucy has signs of both upper and lower respiratory tract disease. The stridor, dysphonia and obstructive inspiratory (slow rate) pattern suggest larynx/pharynx is affected, and the obstruction/respiratory disease is causing high vagal tone (sinus arrhythmia). The expiratory dyspnoea and crackles suggest lower respiratory tract involvement.

Differential diagnoses for URT disease

FCV
FHV
Bordetella bronchiseptica
Pasteurella
Other bacteria
FCoV (less likely as typically mild, nasal disease)
Neoplasia
Foreign body

Differential diagnoses for LRT disease

FCV
FHV
Bordetella bronchoseptica
Poxvirus
Mycobacterial disease

Other bacteria
Fungal disease i.e. *cryptococcus, aspergillus* or candidiasis
Reactive pneumonia
Neoplasia
Foreign body

- **What tests are appropriate for this patient?**

Investigations

Lucy was severely dyspnoeic (despite the low rate). Therefore, initially investigations weren't pursued. She was placed in an oxygen chamber.

Lucy didn't respond to oxygen therapy or buprenorphine. She looked like she was going to die of respiratory failure and her owner could not afford for her to be placed on a ventilator.

Lucy had received 48-hrs of antibiotics and steroid prior to referral and was still deteriorating.

Therefore, a choice was made to anaesthetize her and further investigate her condition, even though it was uncertain she would recover from the anaesthetic

Complete blood count	Units	Reference range (adult feline)	Result day 1
Red blood cell count	$\times 10^{12}$/l	5.50–10.00	5.80
Packed cell volume	%	0.240–0.450	0.270
Haemoglobin	g/dl	8.00–14.00	9.00
Mean cell volume	fl	39.00–55.00	46.10
Mean cell Hb concentration	%	30.00–36.00	33.40
White blood cell count	$\times 10^{9}$/l	7.00–20.00	13.62
Neutrophil count (segmented)	$\times 10^{9}$/l	2.50–12.80	10.12
Neutrophil count (Band)	$\times 10^{9}$/l	0.00–0.00	0
Lymphocyte count	$\times 10^{9}$/l	1.50–7.00	2.10
Monocyte count	$\times 10^{9}$/l	0.070–0.850	0.800
Eosinophil count	$\times 10^{9}$/l	0.000–1.000	0.560
Basophil count	$\times 10^{9}$/l	0.000–0.200	0.040

- **What abnormalities are identified in the lab report?**

Blood test interpretation

Despite having taken the risk of blood sampling Lucy, the results were unrewarding.

The elevated glucose is appropriate considering how stressed Lucy was.

The CBC was unremarkable, with no neutrophilia or leucocytosis.

Biochemistry	Units	Reference range (adult feline)	Result day 1
Alanine transferase	IU/l	6.00–83.00	6.00
Alkaline phosphatase	IU/l	10.00–100.00	16.00
Calcium	mmol/l	2.10–2.90	2.44
Chloride	mmol/l	117–140	121
Cholesterol	mmol/l	2.00–3.40	2.37
Creatinine	μmol/l	40–177	110
Glucose	mmol/l	3.30–5.00	9.47
Phosphate	mmol/l	1.40–2.50	1.71
Potassium	mmol/l	4.00–5.00	4.50
Total protein	g/l	69–79	69
Albumin	g/l	28–39	29
Globulin	g/l	23–50	40
Sodium	mmol/l	145–156	151
Urea	mmol/l	2.80–9.80	8.30
Bile acids	mmol/l	0.0–7.0	5.0

- **How would you proceed with this case?**

Thoracic imaging:

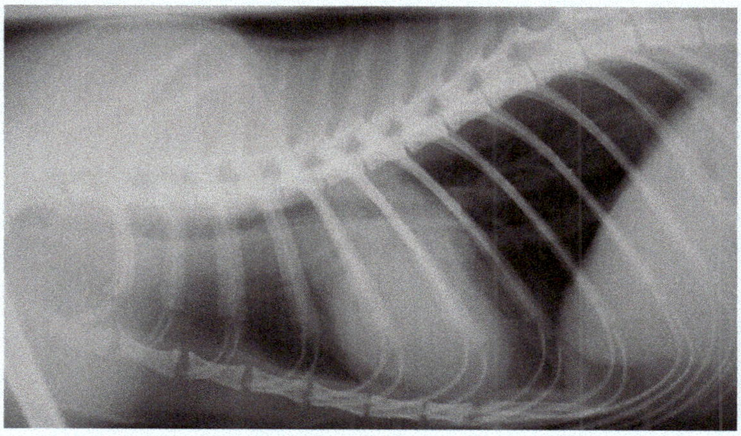

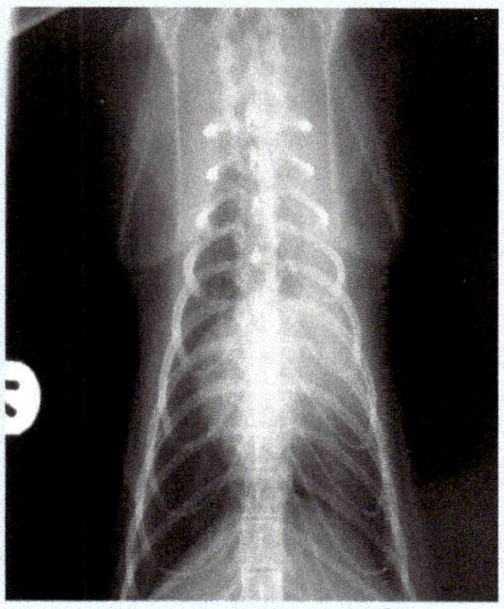

- **Interpret the radiography images**

Radiograph interpretation

There is an area of atelectasis on the left (cranial lung lobe). Lucy had been in left lateral recumbency prior to the radiographs being taken.

The remainder of the thorax was unremarkable despite her having crackles and severe dyspnoea.

On induction of anaesthesia the caudal pharynx/larynx was noted to be very inflammed.

Under anaesthesia Lucy was oxygenating satisfactorally (SpO_2 96–97%).

- **Do the investigation results explain the clinical signs?**

No. She is demonstrating LRT signs, but the radiographs are relatively unremarkable.

We have seen inflammation of the pharynx/larynx but don't know the cause.

- **How would you proceed with this case?**

We need to get samples from the respiratory tract to identify the cause.

- So need to perform BAL (+/– bronchoscopy)
- Take swabs and cytology from pharynx/larynx
- Take blood for FeLV/FIV in case immune suppressed.
- Take blood for Pox serology, Toxoplasma IgG and IgM

Bronchoscopy:

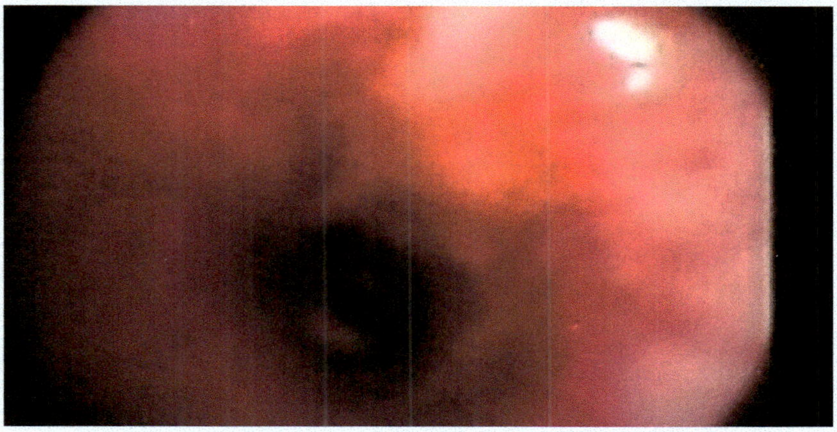

When visualised the trachea demonstrated severe inflammation, erythema with diphtheritic plaques (cream coloured areas). The image is blurred as the scope was not advanced further after seeing how fragile the airway was.

BAL:

BAL final cytology report:

There is a heavy background of mucus sheets and strands and moderate mounts of brightly eosinophilic granular material (lubricant gel) and RBCs. The smears are highly cellular and the nucleated cells comprise approximately 70% non-degenerate neutrophils, 30% macrophages (activated and non-activated) and an occasional multinucleate giant cell.

Diagnosis: Chronic pyogranulomatous bronchitis or bronchopneumonia.

Comments: This appears to be a severe pyogranulomatous bronchitis or bronchopneumonia with mucus hypersecretion. The cause was not identified in the smears but it could be bacterial or viral in origin. No inclusion bodies were seen but cowpox is one possibility. Foreign body is also possible although the diffuse nature of the endoscopic findings seem to make this less likely.

Further bloods:

FeLV	+/–	-ve
FIV	+/–	-ve
Toxoplasma IgG*		<50
Toxoplasma IgM*		<20
Pox Serology*		1/128

BAL culture and sensitivity

Bordetella bronchiseptica	Antibacterial sensitivity in vitro
Tetracycline	S
Amoxycillin/clavulanate	S
Co-trimazole	S
Cephalexin	R
Gentamycin	S
Ciprofloxacin	S
Marbofloxacin	S

Further testing of BAL

Virology testing	Result
BAL	
Pox isolation	**Isolated**
Herpesvirous DNA (PCR)	**High** levels
Oropharangeal swab	
Calici/herpesvirus Isolation	Herpes **isolated**
Feline herpesvirus DNA (PCR)	**High** levels
Scab	
Pox isolation	Positive

Diagnosis

Pox, *Bordetella* and herpes infection

- **What treatment plan would you recommend?**

Oxygen three days 60->25%
Marbofloxacin (2 mg/kg q24) 6 wks
Clindamycin (10 mg/kg q12) 6 wks
Omega interferon (2.5 MU/kg q 48) 8 d
Famciclovir 62.5 mg q12 for 14 d
Intravenous fluid therapy 5 d
Buprenorphine 5 d

Prognosis

Documented to infect cats for over 30 years
Transmitted to cats from voles
Majority of infections occur in hunting cats in the autumn months
Infections are typically cutaneous
Sporadic reports of necrotising pneumonia
Until recently the literature suggested this is a fatal disease, but recent reports suggest 75% of cats treated appropriately can recover (McInerney et al., 2016). Lucy made a complete recovery, she didn't receive Famciclovir as the herpes virus PCR/isolation results returned after she had recovered. She is one of the cases in the paper referenced.

Case 2: "Polo"

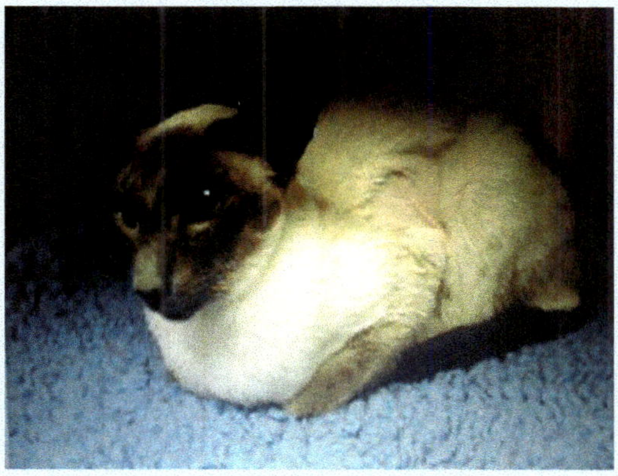

Patient details

2 year old, male neutered Siamese
Fully vaccinated (including FeLV) and regularly dewormed
Lives with 2 other Siamese cats (both well)
Indoor/outdoor
Hunter (rabbits/mice)

History

4 week history of lethargy, inappetance, dyspnoea, tachypnoea, coughing, weight loss and regurgitation
Polo has been hospitalized at the referring veterinarians
They have diagnosed him with pyothorax
He has been having thoracocentesis performed up to three times daily
He is receiving amoxycillin clavulanate, and marbofloxacin

Clinical examination

Body condition score 2/9
Pink mucous membranes
CRT < 2 seconds
Ears, eyes, mouth: No abnormalities detected
Lymph-nodes: mandibular, no abnormalities; prescapular and axial markedly enlarged
Abdomen: no abnormalities detected
Muscle/nerve/retinas: no abnormalities detected
Thoracic auscultation: nothing ventrally, right dorsal breath sounds, RR 60 bpm, increased inspiratory effort
Heart: apex beat-shifted caudally, muffled, no murmurs, but sinus arrhythmia, HR 115 bpm
No pulse deficits
Percussion: dull except right dorsal quadrant
Compression: poor

- **What problems are identified and what are their differential diagnoses?**

Problem: regurgitation

Motility disorders
Megaoesophagus
Congenital
Acquired
Primary (idiopathic)

Secondary

Hiatal hernia
Inflammatory disease
Oesophagitis
Gastroesophageal reflux
Hiatal hernia
Obstructive lesions
Foreign body
Stricture
Vascular ring anomaly
Neoplasia
Miscellaneous
Diverticulum
Bronchoesophageal fistula

Problem: lymphadenopathy

Reactive hyperplasia
Primary or secondary inflammation of the node (lymphadenitis)
Mineral-associated lymphadenopathy
Metastatic neoplasia
Lymph node haemorrhage, infarction, or oedema.
Lymphoma

Problem: coughing

Chronic bronchopulmonary disease
Pneumonia
Viral
Bacterial
Parasitic
Neoplasia
Foreign bodies
Parasites
Pulmonary contusions
Pulmonary oedema
Pulmonary fibrosis

Problems: abnormalities on thoracic examination

Restrictive inspiratory dyspnoea
Pleural space disease
Pneumothorax
Pleural effusion
Decreased resonance
Fluid or soft tissue within the thorax
Decreased compressibility
Sinus arrhythmia and relative bradycardia
Increased vagal tone
Airway obstruction
Mediastinal disease
Cranial abdominal disease
Shifted apex beat
Thoracic mass
Lung consolidation
Muffled heart sounds
Fluid or soft tissue within the pleural space or pericardium
Polo Radiographs supplied from referring vets:

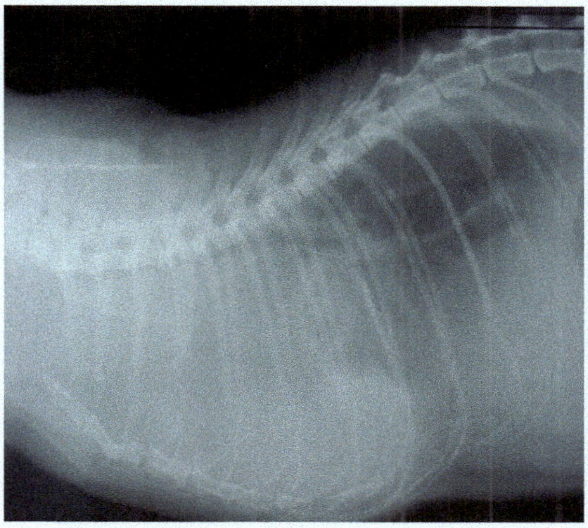

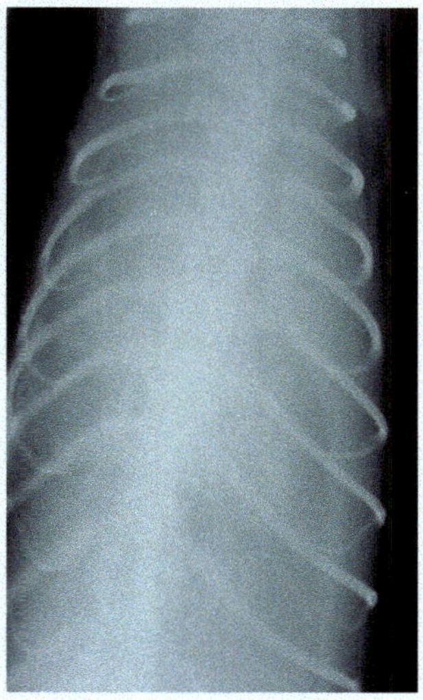

- **What is your interpretation of the radiography images?**

Interpretation: pleural effusion. In addition, the position of the carina is displaced caudally suggesting the presence of a mass within the cranial mediastinum

- **What investigations would you consider for this patient?**

T-FAST
Perform thoracocentesis and submit fluid for culture, fluid analysis, and cytology. Consider thoracic drain placement
FNA LN
Bloods: CBC, Biochemistry, FeLV, Clotting Times

Results

Thoracocentesis
120 ml of fluid removed
Analysis: chylous effusion, culture negative

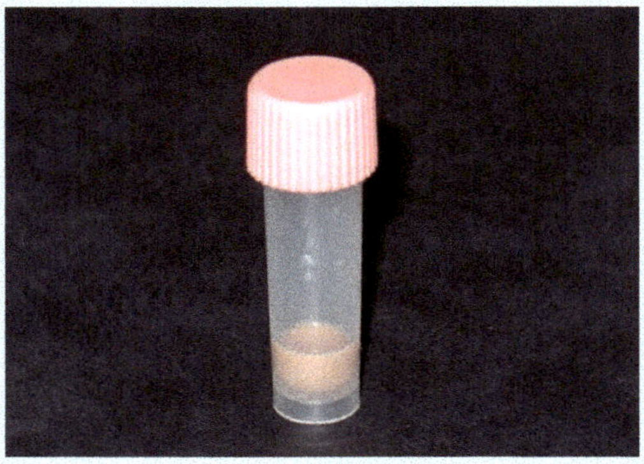

Bloods: FeLV negative
CBC: mild lymphopenia
Biochemistry: no abnormalities
PT and APTT: within normal limits
T-Fast: mass identified within the mediastinum
FNA performed
FNA of prescapular and axial lymph nodes removed

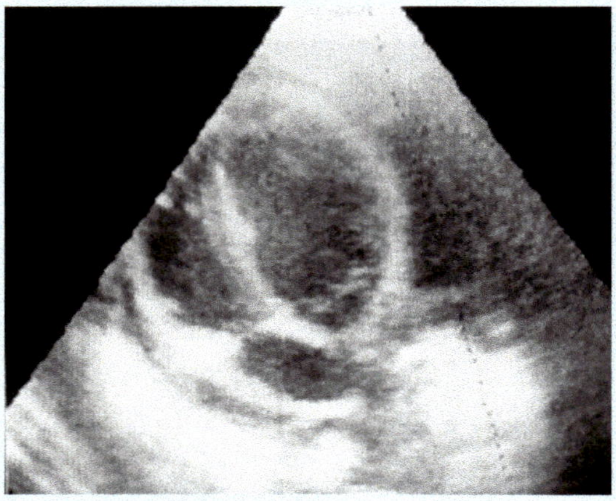

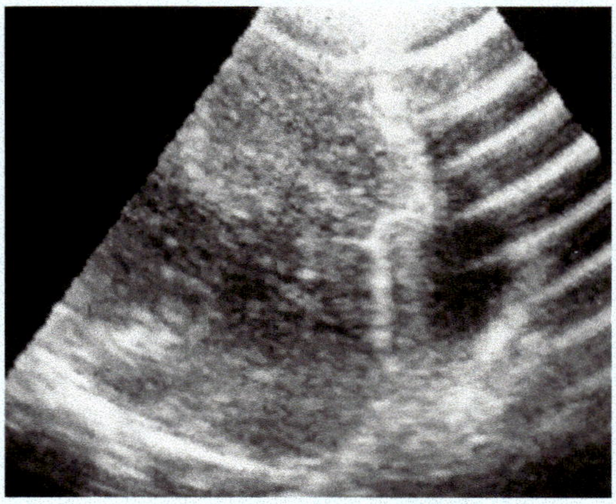

Cytology of effusion
Lymphoma
FNAB cytology
Lymphoma
Cranial mediastinal lymphoma

Diagnosis

Mediastinal lymphoma

- **What treatment plan would you recommend?**

Chemotherapy: CHOP or COP protocol

Follow up

Eating within 24 hours
No regurgitation
Thoracocentesis:
20 ml day 1
7 ml day 2
Culture was negative
Repeat radiographs day 3
Returned home on day 8
Weight gain of 0.4kg
Initial loss of 0.2kg
Weight of tumour
Continued on chemo at referring vets and at home

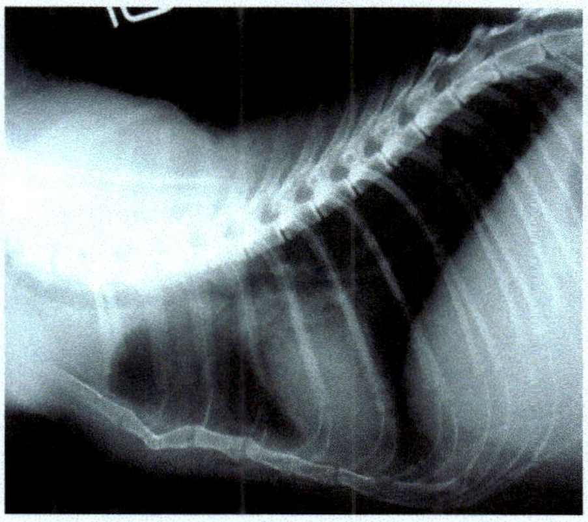

Prognosis

Highly variable; but complete response to chemotherapy is a positive prognostic factor, with a reported mean survival time of 262–980 days. Polo was alive and well 7 years post treatment.

Test

1. **The mean normal pressure within the pulmonary artery is:**
   A) 5 mmHg.
   B) 25 mmHg.
   C) 45 mmHg.
   D) 70 mmHg.
2. **Inspiratory dyspnoea is commonly associated with:**
   A) Pleural space disease.
   B) Chronic bronchopulmonary disease.
   C) Bronchopneumonia.
   D) Lungworm infection.
3. **Cyanosis signifies a concentration of deoxygenated haemoglobin in excess of:**
   A) 2 g/dl.
   B) 0.5 g/dl.
   C) 7 mg/dl.
   D) 5 g/dl.

4. **Which of the following breeds is at an increased risk for developing feline chronic bronchopulmonary disease?**
   A) British short hair.
   B) Persian.
   C) Siamese.
   D) Bengal.
5. **Vaccines can be divided into core vaccines (*) and non-core vaccines. Core vaccines could be considered essential for all cats, whereas the non-core vaccines are given dependent on the individual cat's requirement for them. Vaccines against the following are considered core vaccines:**
   A) Feline herpes virus and *Chlamydophila felis.*
   B) Feline herpes virus and feline calicivirus.
   C) Feline herpes virus, feline calicivirus and feline panleucopenia virus.
   D) Feline herpes virus, feline coronavirus, feline calicivirus and feline panleucopenia virus.
6. **Radiography of cats with chronic bronchopulmonary disease frequently reveals:**
   A) An alveolar pattern.
   B) A prominent bronchial pattern.
   C) An abnormal shaped sternum.
   D) A marked interstitial component.
7. **Approximately 20% of cats with chronic bronchopulmonary disease have been found to have:**
   A) Clay based litter.
   B) Outside access.
   C) *Mycoplasma spp.* infection.
   D) *Bordetella bronchiseptica.*
8. **Methaemoglobinaemia is commonly association with:**
   A) Aspirin toxicity.
   B) Foxglove poisoning.
   C) Paracetamol toxicity.
   D) Raisin poisoning.
9. **Which of the following breeds are recognised as being predisposed to pericardioperitoneal diaphragmatic herniation (PPDH)?**
   A) Bengal and Birman.
   B) Maine Coon and Ragdoll.
   C) Burmese and Siamese.
   D) British Short Hair and Persian.
10. **ABCD guidelines state:**
    A) All cats should be vaccinated every year.
    B) Cats should be vaccinated with core vaccines every 3 years.
    C) Cats should receive a primary course and booster one year later, then never need vaccinated again.
    D) Cats should receive a primary course, and booster one year later, then core vaccines should be given every 3 years.
11. **Type 3 pulmonary hypertension results from:**
    A) Vascular disease.
    B) Left sided heart disease.
    C) Pulmonic disease.
    D) Thrombotic disease.
12. **Oxygen supplementation is advised in cases of bronchopneumonia if the SpO_2 falls below:**
    A) 87%.
    B) 80%.
    C) 97%.
    D) 94%.

13. Cats vaccinated against herpes and caliciviruses:
   A) Will never develop cat flu signs.
   B) Are still at risk, but disease is likely to have a lower morbidity.
   C) Can be cured of pre-existing disease.
   D) Are at risk of herpesvirus but not calicivirus.

14. Expiratory dyspnoea with an obstructive pattern is most commonly associated with:
   A) Pleural space disease.
   B) Asthma.
   C) Bronchopneumonia.
   D) Lungworm infection.

15. Examination of the thorax should include:
   A) Auscultation and palpation.
   B) Auscultation, percussion, compression, and palpation.
   C) Auscultation and percussion.
   D) Auscultation, compression, and palpation.

Answers

1. B
2. A. Pleural space disease, the rest, if they cause dyspnoea are likely to cause expiratory dyspnoea.
3. D
4. C. Siamese, Burmese and Oriental breeds of cat are recognised as being at an increased risk of developing chronic bronchopulmonary disease.
5. C
6. B. Typically radiographs reveal a prominent bronchial pattern, with or without interstitial changes and/or alveolar infiltrates.
7. C. Isolation of *Mycoplasma spp.* has been reported in 20–25% of cats with chronic bronchopulmonary disease.
8. C. Paracetamol poisoning is a cause of methaemoglobinaemia. Aspirin causes renal failure and GI haemorrhage. Foxglove contains digitoxin and therefore can lead to abnormal cardiac rhythms, whereas raisin toxicity has been reported to cause renal failure. Other causes of methaemoglobinaemia include methaemoglobin reductase deficiency, and drug induced toxicity associated with benzocaine and phenazopyridine toxicity.
9. D. The Persian and British Short Hair breeds of cat are predisposed to PPDH.
10. D
11. C
12. D
13. B
14. B
15. B

Notes

Notes

Notes

Notes

Notes

Notes

Notes